Handbook of Sensory Physiology Vol. V/2

Errata

Please, rip off the figure on the right side, moisten it and paste it over Figure 3, page 317.

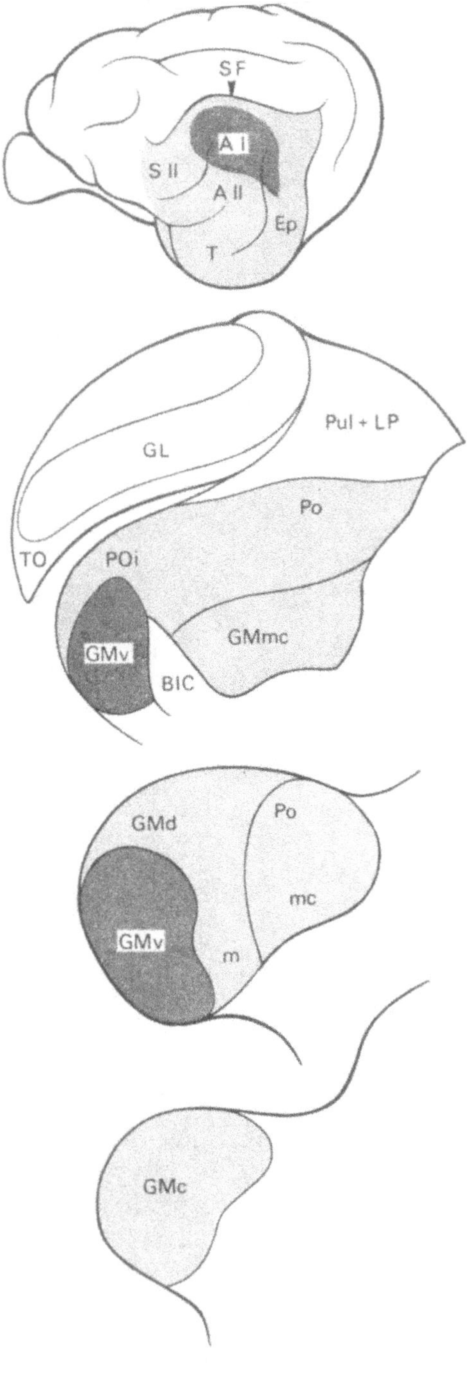

Handbook of Sensory Physiology

Volume V/3

Auditory System

Clinical and Special Topics

By

E. de Boer W. K. Connor H. Davis J. J. Eggermont R. Galambos
C. D. Geisler G. M. Gerken H. E. von Gierke C. S. Hallpike
E. Hawkins Jr. S. A. Hillyard W. D. Keidel D. E. Parker T. W. Picton
W. Rudmose F. B. Simmons G. Stange C. R. Steele J. Tonndorf
M. E. Wigand F. Zöllner

Edited by

Wolf D. Keidel and William D. Neff

With 343 Figures

Springer-Verlag Berlin Heidelberg New York 1976

Wolf D. Keidel

Institut für Physiologie und Biokybernetik (formerly I. Physiologisches Institut) der Universität 8520 Erlangen, Universitätsstraße 17 (Germany)

William D. Neff

Center for Neural Sciences and Department of Psychology, Indiana University, Bloomington, Indiana 47401 (USA)

ISBN-13: 978-3-642-66084-9 e-ISBN-13: 978-3-642-66082-5

DOI: 10.1007/978-3-642-66082-5

Library of Congress Cataloging in Publication Data

Main entry under title: Auditory system. (Handbook of sensory physiology; v. V/3) Bibliography: p. Includes index. 1. Hearing disorders. 2. Hearing. 3. Ear. 4. Electrophysiology. I. Boer, E. de. II. Keidel, Wolf Dieter. III. Neff, William D. IV. Series. QP351.H34 vol. 5/3 [RF290] 591.1'82'08s [617.8'9] 76-44844

Softcover reprint of the hardcover 1st edition 1976

Contents

List of Contributors

de Boer, E., Physical Laboratory, ENT Department, Wilhelmina Hospital, University of Amsterdam, Eerste Helmersstraat 104, Amsterdam - Oud West, The Netherlands

Connor, William, Tracor Inc., 6500 Tracor Lane, Austin, Texas 78721, USA

Davis, Hallowell, Central Institute for the Deaf, 818 South Euclid, St. Louis, Missouri 63110, USA

Eggermont, J. J., Academisch Ziekenhuis, E.N.T.-Department, Rijnsburgerweg 10, Leiden, The Netherlands

Galambos, Robert, Department of Neurosciences, University of California at San Diego, La Jolla, California 92037, USA

Geisler, C. D., Department of Neurophysiology, 283 Medical Science Bldg., University of Wisconsin, Medical School, Madison, Wisconsin 53706, USA

Gerken, G. M., The Callier Center for Communication Disorders, The University of Texas at Dallas, 1966 Inwood Road, Dallas, Texas 75235, USA

von Gierke, Henning, E., 1325 Meadow Lane, Yellow Springs, Ohio 45387, USA (Department of the Air Force, 6570th Aerospace Medical Research Laboratory (AFSC), Wright-Patterson Air Force Base, Ohio 45433, USA)

Hallpike, C. S., Fern Lodge, 44 Ashurst Road, West Moors, Dorset, Ferndown 87, 4418, Great Britain

Hawkins, Joseph E. jr., Kresge Hearing Research Institute, Medical School, The University of Michigan, Ann Arbor, Michigan 48109, USA

Hillyard, Steven A., Department of Neurosciences, University of California at San Diego, La Jolla, California 92037, USA

Keidel, Wolf D., Institut für Physiologie und Biokybernetik der Universität Erlangen, 8520 Erlangen, Germany

Parker, D. E., Department of Psychology, Miami University, Oxford, Ohio 45056, USA

Picton, Terence W., University of Ottawa, Hospital General D'Ottawa, 43 Bruyere, Ottawa, Ontario, Canada, K1N 5C8

Rudmose, Wayne, Tracor Inc., 6500 Tracor Lane, Austin, Texas 78721, USA

Simmons, F. Blair, Division of Otolaryngology, Stanford University, 300 Pasteur Drive, Palo Alto, California 94305, USA

Stange, G., Hals-Nasen-Ohrenklinik der Universität Freiburg, Killianstraße 5, 78 Freiburg, Germany

Steele, C. R., Department of Aeronautics and Astronautics. Stanford University, Stanford, California 94306, USA

Tonndorf, Juergen, College of Physicians and Surgeons, Columbia University, New York, N. Y. 10032, USA

Wigand, M. E., Hals-Nasen-Ohrenklinik der Universität Erlangen, 8520 Erlangen, Waldstraße 1, Germany

Zöllner, F., Hals-Nasen-Ohrenklinik der Universität Freiburg, 7800 Freiburg, Killianstraße 5, Germany

Chapter 1

Sensori-Neural Deafness and Derangements of the Loudness Function: their Nature and Clinical Investigation

C. S. HALLPIKE FRS. FRCP. FRCS., Wimborne (Great Britain)*

With 32 Figures

Contents

Introduction

Sensori-neural deafness — the nerve or perceptive deafness of the earlier text books of Otology — is due, with very few exceptions, to organic disorders which exert their effects, either separately or in combination, upon the sensory cells of CORTI's organ or upon the nerve cells or fibres of the peripheral cochlear neurones.

* Former Director of the Otological Research Unit of the Medical Research Council, National Hospital for Nervous Diseases, Queen Square, London W.C.1.

In accordance with practice in the United States, the use for this group of the descriptive title of Sensori-neural Deafness has in recent years become widely established.

Owing largely to developments in the course of what may be called the "modern" period of audiology, the subject has acquired new perspectives. The period in question can be said to have begun with the observations of POHLMAN and KRANZ (1924) and of FOWLER (1937) on the loudness recruitment phenomenon which soon lead to the recognition that sensori-neural deafness was characterised by a variety of complex derangements of the loudness function.

Many new otoneurological test procedures have since been introduced for their recognition and analysis; these will be described and their principles, practice and clinical value will be discussed in the light of present experience.

It must be stressed, however, that before the tests can be effectively applied the diagnosis of sensori-neural deafness first needs to be accurately established. This diagnosis is largely dependent upon the pure tone audiometric findings. Here, certain difficulties are well known and arise in particular from cross hearing and faulty masking. Consideration of these will not be included in this contribution.

I. Loudness Recruitment: The Nature of the Phenomenon, the Functional Tests Employed for its Investigation, and its Anatomical and Pathophysiological Mechanisms

The diagnosis of sensori-neural deafness, accurately established, has not until the last two decades provided much insight into particular patterns of organic damage to the various anatomical elements of the cochlear apparatus. Since then, however, much progress in this direction has been made. New theoretical concepts have taken shape, and many new test procedures have been devised. As a result, it is now possible to effect a serviceable differentiation between the two main types of sensori-neural deafness: 1. End organ deafness due to organic affections of the hair cells of Corti's organ. 2. Nerve fibre deafness due to organic affections of the nerve fibres and cells of the peripheral cochlear neurones. These diagnostik advances have accrued in large measure from the intensive investigation of certain derangements of the loudness function, in particular, the loudness recruitment phenomenon, found to occur in a substantial proportion of cases of sensori-neural deafness. This will now be considered in some detail.

Early information on the phenomenon of loudness recruitment was provided in 1924 by POHLMAN and KRANZ. This was followed by the well known investigations of FOWLER (1937) carried out upon subjects suffering from "nerve" deafness.

Fowler was responsible for the introduction of the ABLB (Alternate Biaural Loudness Balance) test for loudness recruitment which has continued to hold its place in certain situations, *i.e.*, in subjects with unilateral deafness, as the most valuable of the many that have been prescribed.

The nature of the phenomenon of loudness recruitment is readily appreciated from a brief explanation of its demonstration by means of the ABLB test: The subject wears a pair of telephone receivers each supplied from a pure tone audiometer with arrangements for the independent adjustment of the intensity at the two receivers. The frequency of the stimulus is the same in each receiver and the tester switches alternately between the two. By this means, two series of intensity levels are determined, each point of the left ear series being matched for loudness with a point of the right-ear series. The results are conveniently displayed upon a ladder diagram of the type used by FOWLER. Fig. 1 illustrates the findings in two typical cases of unilateral deafness together with their pure tone audiograms.

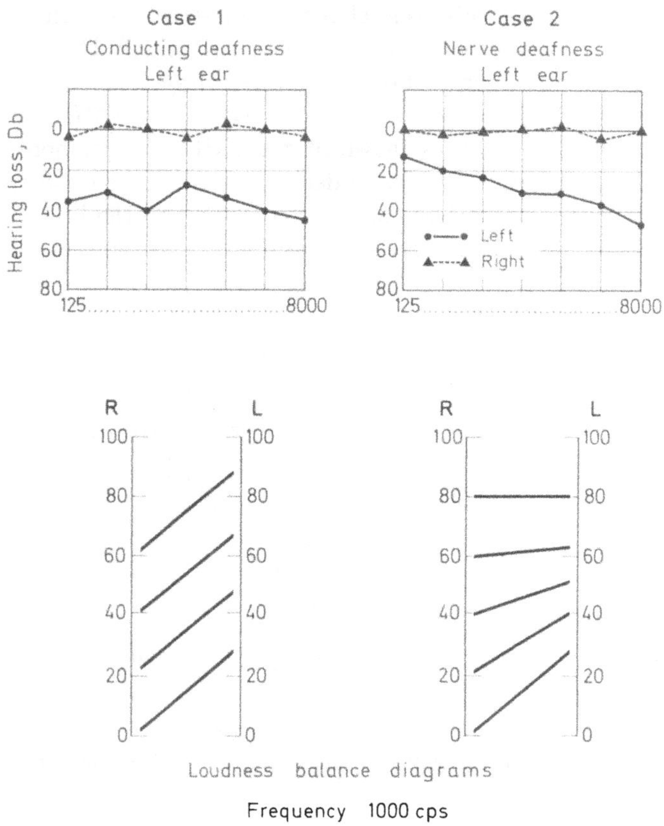

Fig. 1. (Reproduced by permission of Royal Society of Medicine)

In each case, the test frequency is 1000 Hz at which frequency the audiograms show a threshold shift for the affected ear of 30 dB. The test starts with a stimulus of threshold intensity at the right ear; the balancing intensity for the left ear will, of course, be 30 dB higher. Successive stimuli rising in intensity in steps of 20 dB are then applied to the right ear, and, for each level, the equal loudness intensity for the left ear is established by trial, the comparison being made by switching the stimulus backwards and forwards between the two ears. The result obtained in Case 1 indicates that the loss of sensitivity, or deafness, of the affected ear, 30 dB at threshold, remains constant throughout the entire intensity range. This finding is an unvarying one in conductive deafness and is open to the straightforward explanation that the obstruction caused by the middle ear lesion to the passage of sound waves to the inner ear introduces an attenuation factor, in this case 30 dB, which is constant at all intensities.

A different result is obtained in Case 2. The pure tone audiogram is substantially the same as in Case 1 with a threshold shift at 1000 Hz of 30 dB. The balancing points at threshold are identical with those of Case 1 with a 30 dB displacement upwards for the left ear. On ascending the intensity scale, however, it is found that the sensitivity loss or deafness of the left ear becomes progressively less until, at 80 dB, equal intensities at the two ears evoke equal sensations of loudness. In other words, deafness as shown by an elevation of the normal threshold is reduced or disappears at high stimulus intensities. This in its simplest terms constitutes the phenomenon of loudness recruitment.

An alternative form, due to STEINBERG and GARDNER (1937), for the graphic representation of these results is shown in Fig. 2. It is in common use and has many advantages. Sound intensities in decibels above the normal threshold are plotted on the vertical axis for the unaffected ear and on the horizontal axis for the affected ear. Equal loudness levels for the two ears are plotted on this chart as

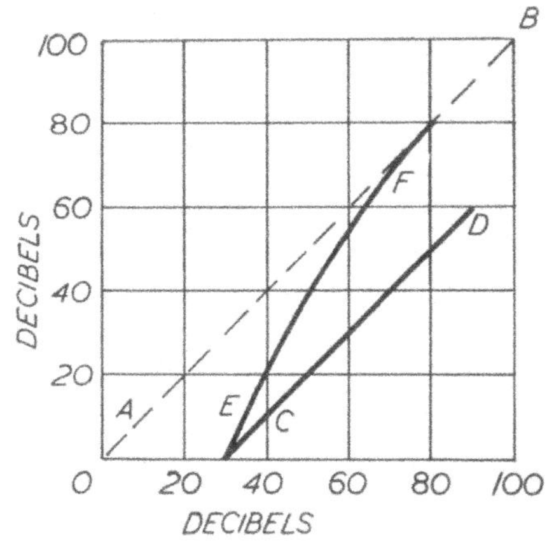

Fig. 2. (Reproduced by permission of Royal Society of Medicine)

a series of points and the line, AB, passing through the origin, connects the points which would be obtained in a normal subject. CD is the corresponding line obtained in Case 1. Here, the sensitivity loss at threshold of the deaf ear is represented by the displacement of the Point C along the base line to the right of the origin. This sensitivity loss remains constant at higher intensities, and the Line CD thus lies parallel to AB. EF is the corresponding line obtained in Case 2. As in Case 1, the same sensitivity loss at threshold is represented by the same displacement of the Point E to the right of the origin. At high intensities, however, the sensitivity loss is progressively reduced and the line EF approaches and finally coincides with the Line AB.

At the time of FOWLER's work, the neurological mechanism of loudness recruitment received much attention. Thus, according to LORENTE DE NÓ (1937) quoted by FOWLER (1939), it was considered to be a physiological consequence of any organic affection which would reduce the number of active neuro-sensory elements, be they nerve fibres or sensory cells. A similar view seems to have been accepted by STEVENS and DAVIS (1938). No closer analysis was attempted of the anatomical basis of loudness recruitment, and the subjects exhibiting it continued to be included with others within the general category of nerve deafness.

In 1946, the subject was examined afresh by DE BRUÏNE-ALTES who confirmed the observational data and stressed the need for further studies in which the results of the clinical tests for loudness recruitment could be correlated with more exact information upon the underlying structural changes in the cochlear sense organs and their associated neural pathways, and, in 1948, a substantial body of information of this kind was presented by DIX, HALLPIKE, and HOOD. This new information was derived from a detailed clinico-pathological study of subjects suffering from two different and clearly defined organic affections of the VIII nerve system, Menières disease of the labyrinth and acoustic neurofibroma.

In the case of MENIÈRES disease, it is known from the work of HALLPIKE and CAIRNS (1938), LINDSAY (1942), ALTMANN and FOWLER (1943) and others that the primary lesion is one of the endolymph system of the inner ear resulting in damage to the sensory cells of Corti's organ. The cochlear nerve fibres and ganglion cells are unaffected, at any rate, until the disease is of long standing.

In the case of acoustic neurofibroma, the observations of HARDY and CROWE (1936) upon the very early stages in the development of this tumour indicate its

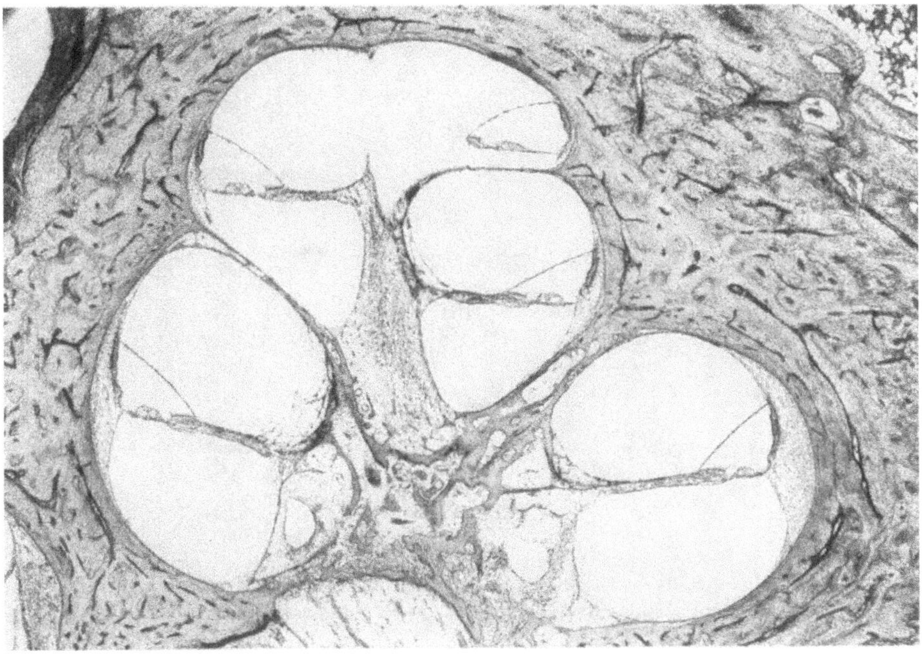

Fig. 3. Cochlea of a human subject showing degeneration of the spiral ganglion cells and cochlear nerve fibres resulting from tumor pressure upon the VIII nerve. The peripheral sensory apparatus, including the hair cells of Corti's organ, is well preserved. (Reproduced by permission of Royal Society of Medicine)

origin to be from the vestibular portion of the VIII nerve in the region of SCARPA's ganglion. With growth of the tumour, pressure is exerted upon the fibres of the VIII nerve. It should be noted that, in the case of the cochlear nerve, this pressure point is central to the spiral ganglion cells, and the implications of the laws of Wallerian degeneration would accordingly lead to no expectation of lasting changes in these cells. However, for reasons that are still not fully understood, the cochlear nerve exhibits a special vulnerability, and, as a result, a constant feature of acoustic neurofibroma is the degeneration and disappearance of the spiral ganglion cells and their associated nerve fibres. A typical example of this disorder is shown in Fig. 3.

DIX, HALLPIKE, and HOOD examined 30 typical cases of Menières disease. In all of these cases, they found loudness recruitment to be present and complete. A few exhibited the phenomenon of over-recruitment. That is to say, with high stimulus intensities, the affected ear was found to be the more sensitive of the two. The audiograms and loudness recruitment diagrams, in three cases characteristic of the group, are shown in Fig. 4.

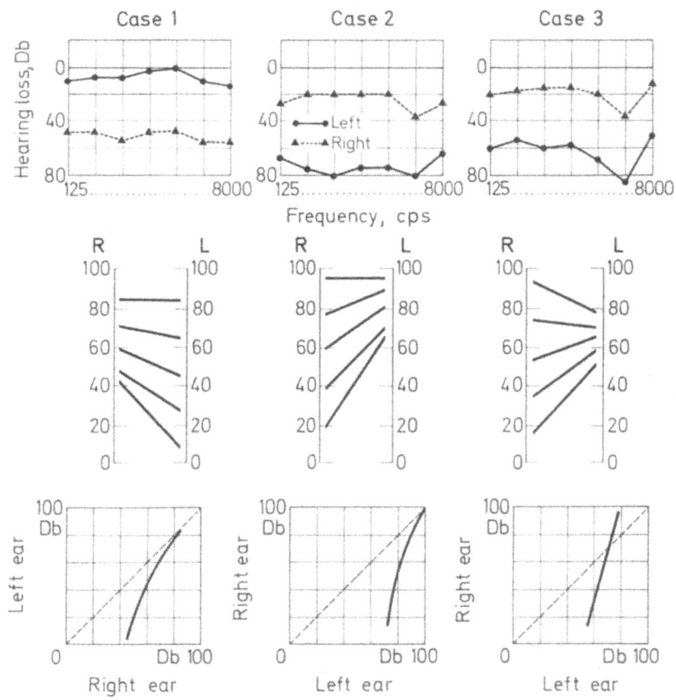

Fig. 4. Loudness balance diagrams in three cases of Menière's disease. Frequency: 1000 Hz. Showing full recruitment of loudness. (Reproduced by permission of Royal Society of Medicine)

Another group of subjects described by DIX, HALLPIKE, and HOOD consisted of 11 cases of acoustic neurofibroma and 9 of other varieties of tumour of the cerebello-pontine angle, all with involvement of the VIII nerve. In all 20 cases, the diagnosis was confirmed at operation or post-mortem. In 14 of the cases, loudness recruitment was completely absent. In the remaining 6, it was present but incomplete. The audiograms and loudness recruitment diagrams in 3 representative cases are shown in Fig. 5.

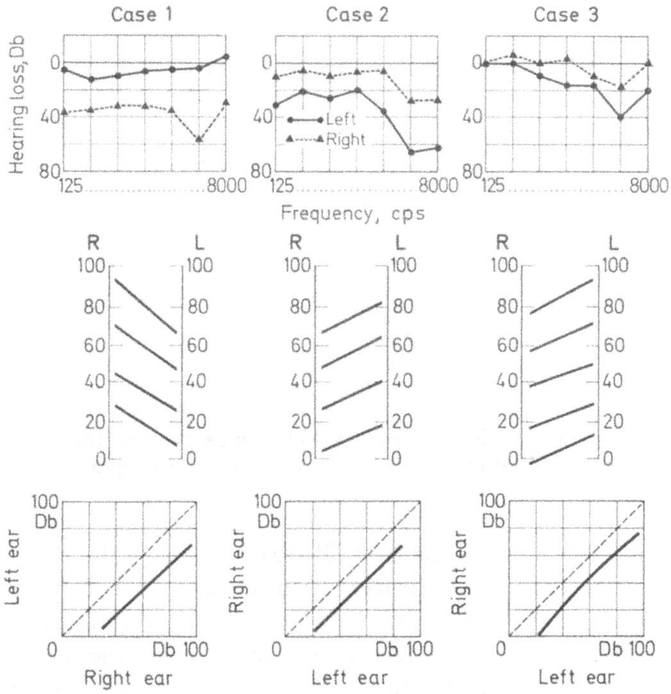

Fig. 5. Loudness balance diagrams in three cases of degeneration of the cochlear nerve due to VIII nerve neurofibroma. Frequency: 1000 Hz. Showing absence of loudness recruitment. (Reproduced by permission of Royal Society of Medicine)

Dix, Hallpike, and Hood endeavoured to provide a theoretical basis for their findings. This part of their work will be considered under two headings: 1. The occurrence of loudness recruitment in association with affections of the cochlear end organs. 2. Absence of loudness recruitment in association with affections of the cochlear nerve fibres.

A. The Occurrence of Loudness Recruitment in Association with Affections of the Cochlear End Organs

Dix, Hallpike, and Hood argued that the damage to the hair cell complex, known to occur in Menières disease, must derange its microphonic function, and, because of this, loudness recruitment would occur. In a later paper (Hallpike and Hood, 1959) the matter was considered more closely. The clinical material for this 1959 study consisted of 200 subjects with unilateral deafness due to Menières disease; loudness recruitment, as revealed by means of the ABLB test, was present in all, and the results were recorded for analysis upon the conventional STEINBERG-GARDNER chart. The principles of the analysis are indicated in Fig. 6, which shows the findings in two subjects with unilateral deafness. In each of

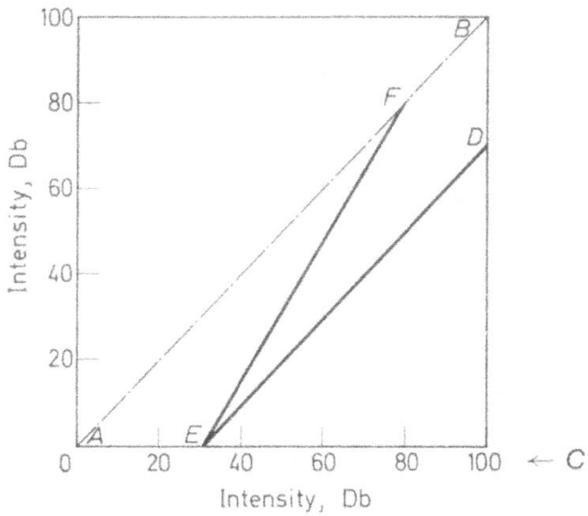

Fig. 6. Recruitment diagram: loudness recruitment is present when the recruitment angle FEC exceeds 45°. (Reproduced by permission of Acta Otolaryngologica [Stockholm])

these cases, the threshold elevation is 30 dB. *ED* is the curve obtained in Subject 1 whose deafness was due to a conductive lesion. Its form is that of a straight line and it makes an angle of 45°, *DEC*, with the base line. Loudness recruitment being absent, this is defined as the no-recruitment angle. *EF* is the curve obtained in Subject 2 whose deafness was due to Menières disease. It, too, takes the form of a straight line which meets the normal line at *F* and makes an angle, *FEC*, with the base line. This angle was described by HOOD as the recruitment angle and provides a useful quantitative index of recruitment. HOOD found further that, in subjects with Menières disease, the straight-line form of the recruitment curve was a constant feature, and, furthermore, that the value of the recruitment angle showed a linear relationship to the amount of the deafness. HOOD's results are summarised in Fig. 7 in which are shown the recruitment angles which correspond to hearing losses of 0, 20, 40, and 60 dB with the shaded areas indicating the 2σ limits of variation. The wide distribution along the base line of the lower ends of the curves and their convergence at their upper ends upon a point very close to the normal was thought by HALLPIKE and HOOD to convey a clear impression of a loudness function subserved by two mechanisms. Of these, that for the low intensities showed varying degrees of derangement. That for high intensities was little affected.

This situation was explained by HALLPIKE and HOOD in terms of the dual excitation mechanism proposed by HALLOWELL DAVIS (1957, 1958). It had been shown by DAVIS and his collaborators that, in addition to the cochlear microphonics (CM), there existed also another variety of cochlear electrical responses, the summating potential (SP). The SP, like the CM, originated apparently in the hair cell complex. It consisted of a negative D.C. potential and made its appearance only at high levels of sound intensity. Davis postulated that the CM played an essential part in the transduction mechanism but operated only at sound intensity levels up to 60—80 dB above the normal threshold. At higher intensities, another mechanism was thought to come into play, a mechanism associated with the SP and the *inner* hair cells.

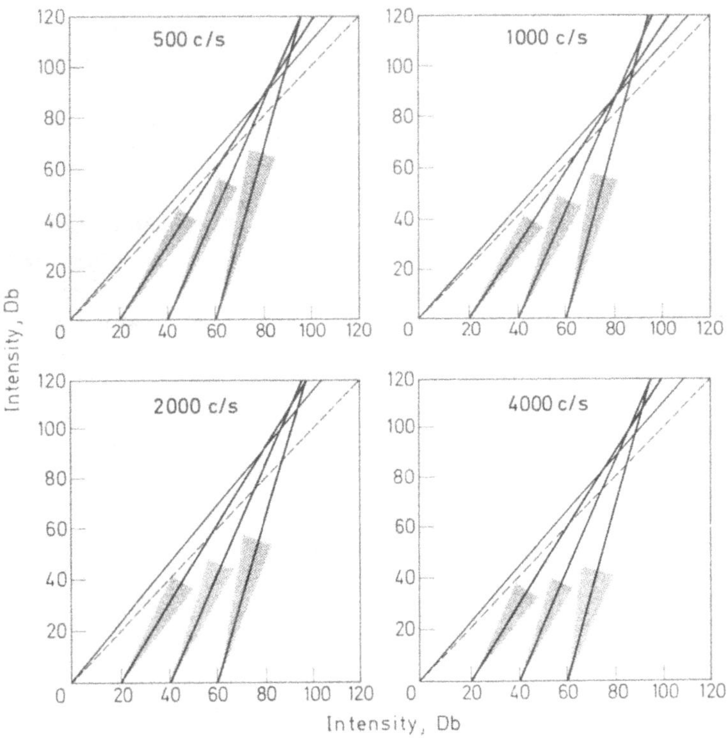

Fig. 7. The loudness recruitment/amount of hearing loss relationship. Showing 2σ limits of variation. (Reproduced by permission of Acta Otolaryngologica [Stockholm])

An explanation of the loudness recruitment phenomenon in terms of the theory proposed by Davis would clearly be favoured by histological data indicative of a particular pattern of distribution of the end organ damage found to occur in Menières disease, *i.e.* with selective sparing of the inner hair cells. Some evidence of this kind was accordingly examined by Hallpike and Hood (1959) and found by them to be suggestive but inconclusive.

However, the subject is one of great difficulty, much beset by fixation and other kinds of artefact, and Hallpike (1965), reviewing the situation in the light of additional histological and other evidence including, in particular, the finding by Engstrom (referred to by Hallpike, 1965) and recently confirmed by Spoendlin (1972) of a particularly rich innervation of the inner hair cells, concluded, that as part of the derangement of the hair-cell complex found to occur in Menières disease, a selective sparing of the inner hair cells must be accepted as highly probable.

B. The Absence of Loudness Recruitment Occurring in Association with Degeneration of the Cochlear Nerve Fibres

In explanation of this finding, Dix, Hallpike, and Hood (1948) developed a working hypothesis based upon the assumption that the degenerative condition consisted of a progressive reduction, *evenly distributed throughout the nerve* in the number of its nerve fibres. This was coupled with certain implications of the Weber-Fechner relationship which predicts that equidistant levels on a scale of loudness will show a straight line relationship to the values, plotted upon a logarithmic scale, of the sound intensities to which they correspond. It was argued too that the same straight line relationship would also exist between these loudness levels and the numbers, also plotted upon a logarithmic scale, of activated nerve fibres.

In Fig. 8 is shown the application of the Dix, Hallpike, and Hood hypothesis to the derangement of the loudness function occurring in a subject with a unilateral reduction (90%) in the number of normal cochlear nerve fibres. Each point on the graph represents a sensation magnitude subserved by a particular number of nerve fibres and corresponding to a particular value of sound intensity.

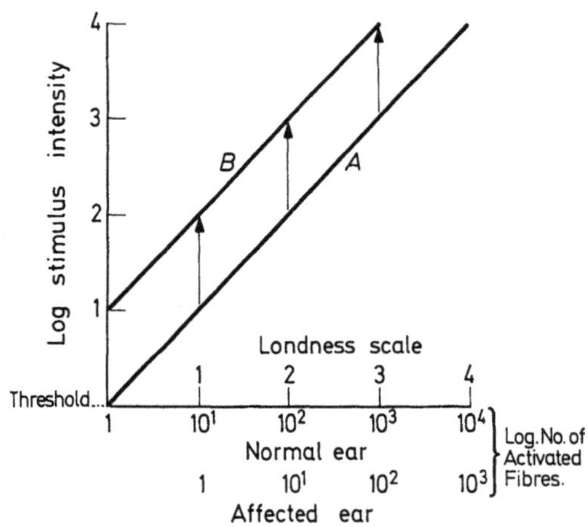

Fig. 8. The absence of loudness recruitment in diffuse degeneration of the cochlear nerve. Diagram showing a suggested explanation of the stimulus intensity/loudness relationship

The line, A, is obtained with the subject's normal ear. At the log 1 level on the stimulus intensity scale the number of activated nerve fibres will be 10. For the affected ear however, (line B) the corresponding number will be 1. The full complement of 10 is regained, as indicated by the arrow, at the log 2 level of the stimulus intensity scale. This situation is repeated at at all levels of the scale. The line B is thus the result obtained from the affected ear and is representative of the absence of loudness recruitment observed to occur in cochlear nerve degeneration. The hypothesis could clearly be extended to cover situations in which the nerve fibre degeneration is not evenly distributed throughout the nerve. For example, should there be a selective involvement of the fibres associated with the outer hair cells, then, as in Ménieres disease, loudness recruitment would be expected to occur, as indeed it does, in a minority of cases of angle tumor.

In a later paper (1958), DIX and HALLPIKE reported their findings in 95 additional cases of sensori-neural deafness due to tumour pressure on the VIII nerve. In 70, the tumours were acoustic neurofibromata, arising in the nerve itself. In a second group of 25 cases, the nerve was secondarily affected by tumours arising in or invading the cerebello-pontine angle. The results of the ABLB tests for loudness recruitment are shown in Figs. 9 and 10. In all but some 10 of the 95 cases, full loudness recruitment was absent.

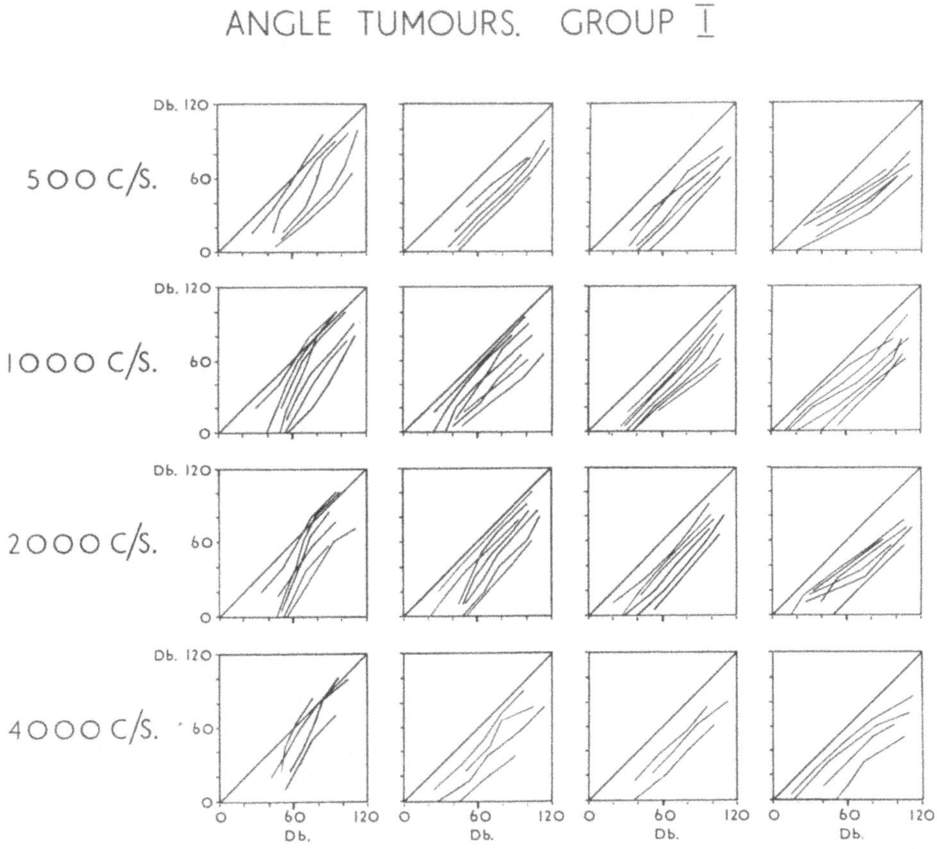

Fig. 9. Loudness recruitment diagrams: angle tumours. Group I. (See text.) (Reproduced by permission of Royal Society of Medicine)

The possibility presented by these findings of using the tests for loudness recruitment for the differential diagnosis of two kinds of sensori-neural deafness has attracted much attention. On the whole, the findings have been widely substantiated (LÜSCHER, 1950; EBY and WILLIAMS, 1951; LUNDBORG, 1952; KRISTENSEN and JEPSEN, 1952; SCHUKNECHT and WOELLNER, 1955; STENGER, 1956). Certainly, the contention that loudness recruitment is strongly indicative of an organic disorder of the cochlear end organs now seems to be accepted (VON BÉKÉSY, 1965).

Nevertheless, certain difficulties persist and are concerned almost entirely with the absence of loudness recruitment claimed by DIX, HALLPIKE, and HOOD to be a characteristic feature of the nerve fibre type of sensori-neural deafness resulting from tumour pressure on the cochlear nerve. Noteworthy in this connection is the work of JERGER (1961), DENNY (1955) and others who have claimed that the test is of doubtful value for the diagnosis of VIII nerve tumours. Several reasons can be cited for this lack of agreement. First, is the mixed effects of the tumours,

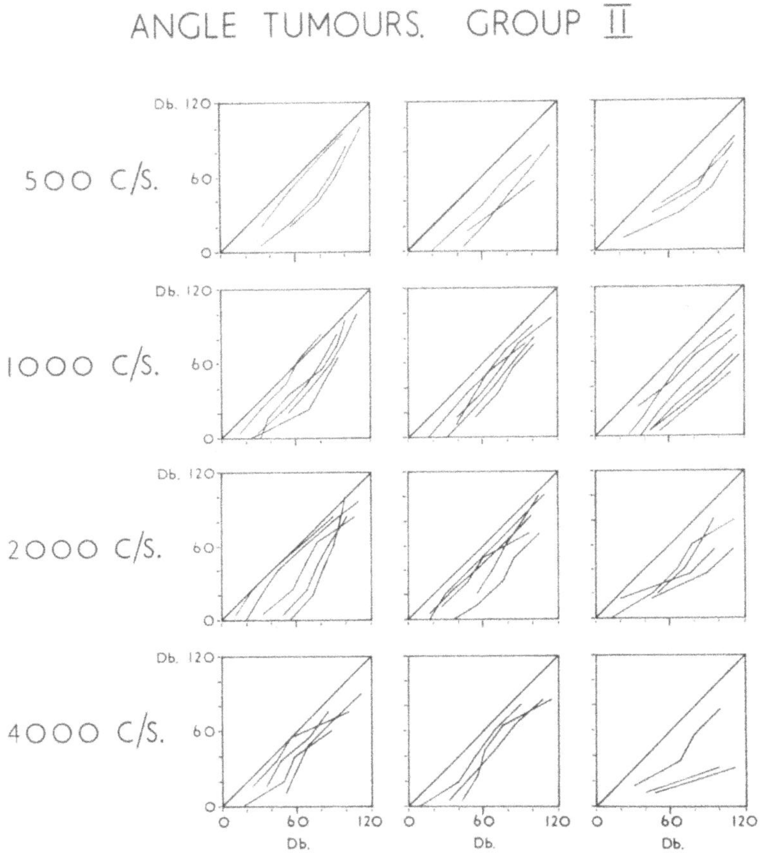

Fig. 10. Loudness recruitment diagrams: angle tumours. Group II. (See text.) (Reproduced by permission of Royal Society of Medicine)

whereby a direct pressure action upon the nerve fibres may be combined with a loss of blood supply to the cochlear end organs. The latter factor may predominate and loudness recruitment will then result. Evidence in support of this occurrence has been presented by DIX and HOOD (1953) and by SIMONTON (1956) who have described several cases of early VIII nerve tumour with good preservation of hearing in whom loudness recruitment was present. Following removal of the tumours, cochlear function was retained, but loudness recruitment was found to be abolished. DIX has also reported (1965) the results of tests for loudness recruitment in a number of cases of unilateral deafness due to multiple sclerosis affecting the peripheral cochlear neurones in the neuroglial part of their course within the brain stem. In these cases, there would appear to be no possibility of any interference with the vascular supply of the cochlear end organs. Loudness recruitment however was found to be absent.

An additional factor which seems to have caused much misunderstanding is a lack of uniformity in the graphic recording of the ABLB tests for loudness recruitment. A ladder type of diagram was originally employed by FOWLER and is still in common use. As stressed by HOOD (1969), the Steinberg-Gardner type of graph has many advantages, in respect especially of the more penetrating analysis which it permits of loudness function derangement. This applies in particular to situations where loudness recruitment is present but incomplete, partial loudness recruitment, as it is usually called. It must be admitted that, even when the STEINBERG-GARDNER chart is used to depict partial loudness recruitment, ambiguities of interpretation are common, and it appears that loudness recruitment is said by some to be present only if complete; by others, to be absent if only incomplete. In this situation, little purpose can be recognised in seeking to attach much statistical significance to the numerous published reports on the results of clinical tests. Progress requires a rational and agreed system of quantification of loudness recruitment.

One other factor, which has led to much confusion, is the fact that sensorineural deafness, in addition to loudness recruitment, frequently exhibits a number of other derangements of the loudness function. One or more of these derangements sometimes occur with loudness recruitment, sometimes without it. One of them, an alteration of the time constants of adaptation to sustained stimulation is of particular importance; HOOD's studies (1950) of its physiological basis have provided much information of value and will be briefly outlined.

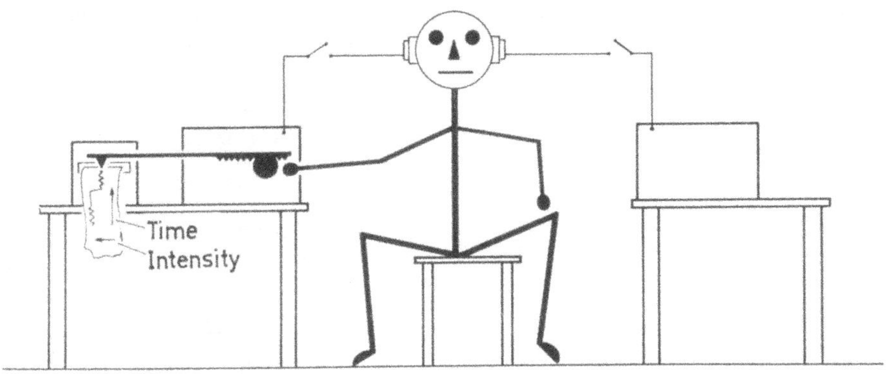

Fig. 11. (Reproduced by permission of Acta Otolaryngologica (Stockholm)

The experimental procedure used by HOOD is shown in Fig. 11. A normal subject wears a pair of receivers, each supplied by a pure tone audiometer with the frequencies set at 1000 Hz. The intensity at the left, or test ear, is maintained at 80 dB; that at the right, or control ear, is varied by the subject, in the manner shown, about a level which gives a loudness sensation equal to that derived from the left ear. The result is shown in Fig. 12. At the start, loudness equality is obtained with equal intensities, 80 dB at the two ears. Once the loudness balance has been established, the right ear is rested. Stimulation of the left ear is continued.

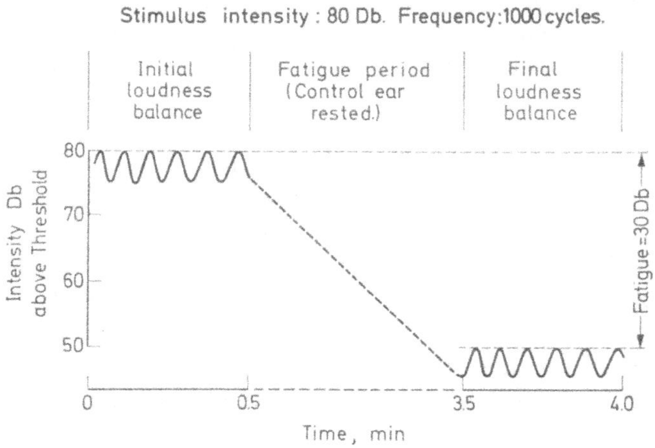

Fig. 12. (Reproduced by permission of Acta Otolaryngologica (Stockholm)

After a period which may be determined at will, the variable tone is reapplied to the control ear, and it is then found that a loudness balance is attained with an intensity which is less than 80 dB by an amount which may be considerable and depends, within certain limits, upon the intensity and duration of the constant stimulus applied to the test ear. The amount in question (in this case, 30 dB) is a measure of the sensitivity loss caused by the stimulus. In Fig. 13 is shown

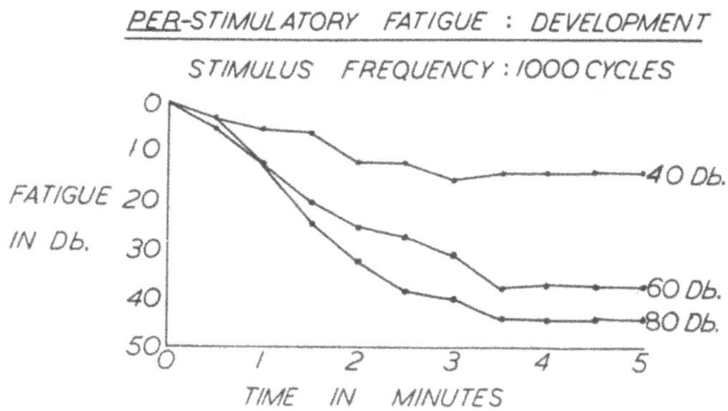

Fig. 13. (Reproduced by permission of Acta Otolaryngologica (Stockholm)

how this sensitivity loss, per-stimulatory fatigue as HOOD has called it, varies with the intensity and duration of the fatiguing stimulus. It will be noted that, with all intensities, the fatigue reaches its maximum after about $3^1/_2$ min.

Hood also studied the time course of the recovery process. Following the induction of perstimulatory fatigue in the manner illustrated in Fig. 12, the left ear was rested for periods which were increased in successive experiments from 10—60 sec. At the end of each rest period, the stimulus was reapplied to the left ear, and the balancing procedure was renewed. The result is shown in Fig. 14. Recovery is most rapid in the first 10 sec. Thereafter, it slows progressively and is complete at 60 sec. It will be noted that, under the conditions of the test, the sustained tone used to induce the hearing loss was continued during the application of the simultaneous balancing procedure used to demonstrate it. If, following the induction of the fatigue as shown in Fig. 12, the loudness loss is investigated instead by means of short duration stimuli applied to the two ears in alternation, viz the alternate binaural balancing procedure, it is found that no sensitivity difference can be detected.

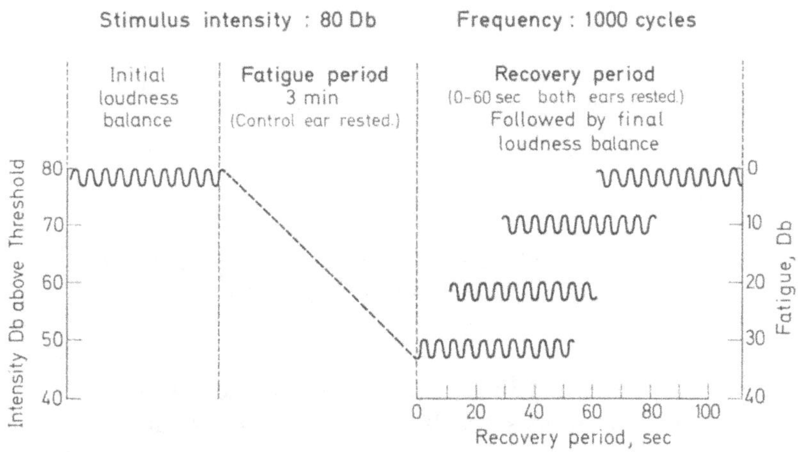

Fig. 14. (Reproduced by permission of Acta Otolaryngologica (Stockholm)

Hood explained the result, illustrated in Fig. 12, in terms of certain time constants derived from Matthews (1931) studies of adaptation in single end organs of muscle.

Matthews results are summarised in Fig. 15. If a constant tension is suddenly applied to a stretch receptor, then the action potential response in the associated nerve fibre will consist of an initial high frequency discharge known as the on-effect. Its duration is brief, being of the order of 0.2 sec, and is followed by a slow decline of its frequency to a new level at which it is maintained; this constitutes the adaptation process and is completed in some $3^1/_2$ min. If, following full adaptation, the stimulus be removed and then reapplied after a rest period greater than about 1 sec, the "on effect" is present and indeed undiminished. This is the phenomenon of on-effect normality. But continued stimulation then results in a rapid relapse of the response, *i.e.* an accelerated adaptation to the previous low level; this is the phenomenon of relapse. If the rest period is less than 0.2 sec, the on effect is absent; if between 0.2 and 1 sec, it is present but diminished.

An impressive similarity is thus revealed between the time characteristics of the adaptation processes of stretch receptors and of the cochlear end organs.

The phenomena of on-effect normality and relapse are of particular importance inasmuch as they appear to be represented in the behaviour of cochlear end organs affected by disease or injury, *e.g.*, Menières disease or acoustic trauma. In the case, for instance, of a cochlear end-organ rendered insensitive by Menières disease, on-effect normality is retained as an essential constituent of the loudness

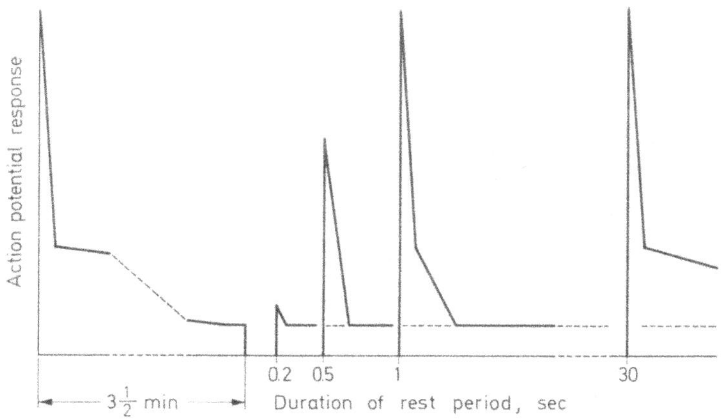

Fig. 15. Adaptation and recovery in muscle stretch receptors (Matthews). (Reproduced by permission of Journal of Physiology)

recruitment phenomenon and finds expression in the normal loudness response revealed by means of Fowler's ABLB test for loudness recruitment. It must be emphasised that the result in question will only be obtained if the test is carried out with due regard to the time constants of the physiological processes which are involved. Attention must be given to the durations of the stimuli and of the intervals between them; for the former, Hood recommends 0.3 sec; for the latter, 1.5 sec. If the stimuli are prolonged with rest periods which are too short, the findings will be distorted by the supervention of "Relapse" and quite different results will then be obtained. Instead of loudness recruitment, there will now be seen the phenomenon known as loudness reversal. Corollaries of recruitment and reversal are of course the compression and expansion of the loudness scale. The matter is illustrated in Fig. 16 (Dix and Hood, 1953) which shows the responses obtained in a subject with unilateral Menières disease with a hearing loss at threshold of 30 dB. Graph A shows the results given by the ABLB test, using stimuli and rest periods of the correct duration. Over-recruitment is present, the recruitment Curve *DC* having an angle, *DCE*, exceeding 45°. Compression of the loudness scale is also shown. Thus, the loudness scale, covered in the normal ear by the intensity range 0—100 dB, is covered in the affected ear by an intensity range of 30—80 dB. Similarly, the fraction of the loudness scale, covered in the normal ear by the intensity range 20—40 dB, will, in the affected ear, be contained within the intensity range 40—50 dB. The results are in sharp contrast to those shown in Graph B and obtained in the same case by means of a loudness balance procedure involving the simultaneous application of sustained tones to the two ears. The angle of the recruitment curve, *DCE*, is now much less than 45°. Recruitment is therefore absent. In addition, the loudness range, covered in the normal ear by the intensity range 20—40 dB, is no longer compressed but is expanded in the affected ear to 60—90 dB.

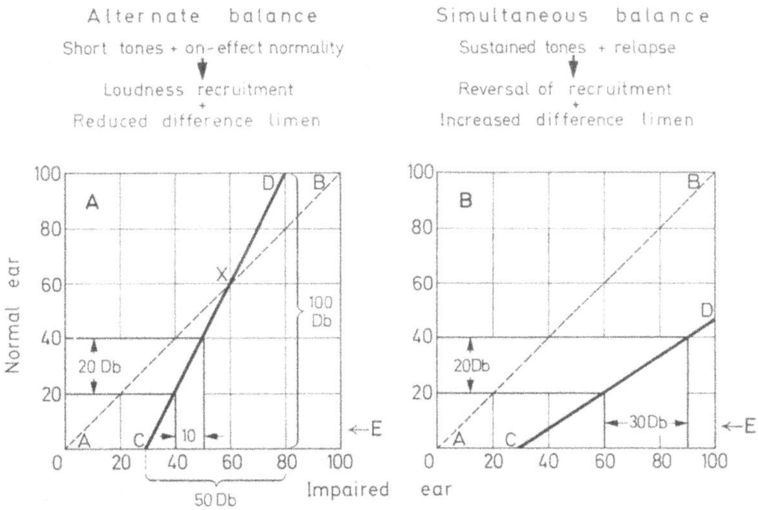

Fig. 16. (Reproduced by permission of Journal of Laryngology & Otology)

II. Other Tests Employed for the Investigation of the Loudness Function in Sensori-Neural Deafness

It is clear, from the nature of the ABLB test, that it can only be used in subjects with unilateral deafness. In many instances, however, the deafness is bilateral. For these cases, monaural testing methods are essential. Five well known monaural tests of this kind are the following:

A. Determination of the intensity difference limen (Lüscher and Zwislocki).

B. Békésy audiometry.

C. The SISI (Short Increment Sensitivity Index) test of Jerger.

D. Determination of the loudness discomfort level (Hood and Poole).

E. Middle ear impedance measurements (Metz) for the determination of the reflex contraction threshold of the middle ear muscles.

A. Determination of the Intensity Difference Limen

For their investigations, Lüscher and Zwislocki (1948) used pure tones modulated in the manner shown in Fig. 17. The modulation frequency was 3/sec with rise and fall times described as abrupt (Lüscher, 1950). Intensity levels were specified in dynes/cm^2, and the smallest perceptible intensity difference was taken as the difference limen and expressed as a percentage. The findings for a normal subject at four different levels above threshold are shown in Fig. 18.

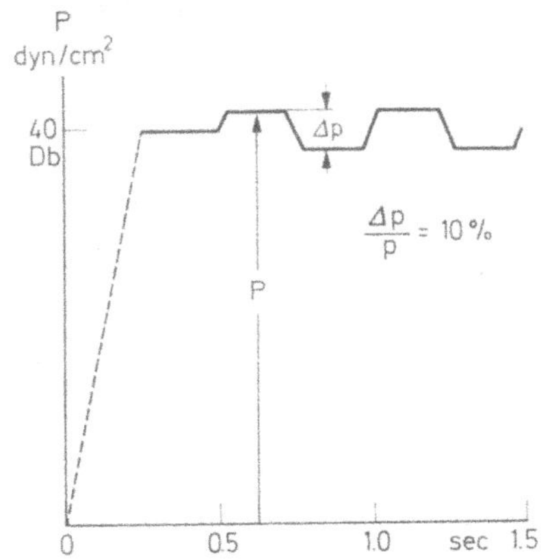

Fig. 17. Difference limens of sound pressure; absolute: ΔP, and relative: $\frac{\Delta P}{P}$ (LÜSCHER). (Reproduced by permission of Royal Society of Medicine)

In accordance with the well known findings of KNUDSEN (1923) and of RIESZ (1928), the magnitude of the DL depends, among other things, upon the intensity level of the stimulus. For instance, with stimulus intensities of 20 and 80 dB above threshold the DL has values as shown in Fig. 18 of 12—18% and 3—4%,

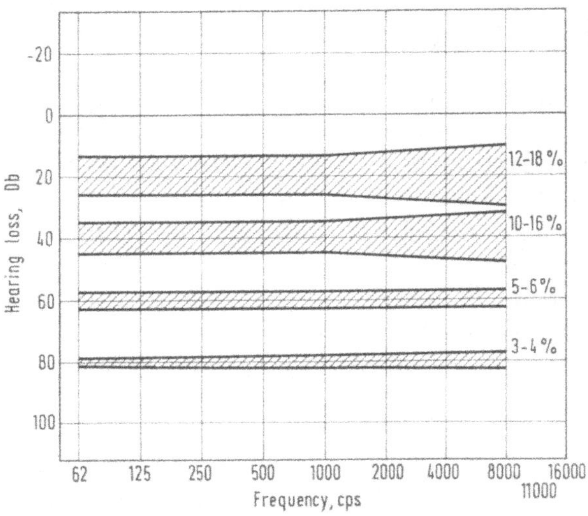

Fig. 18. Relative difference limens, expressed as percentages in normal subjects showing relationship to frequency and intensity (LÜSCHER and ZWISLOCKI). (Reproduced by permission of Royal Society of Medicine)

respectively. In subjects with end organ disorder, LÜSCHER (1950) found the DL to be decreased (Fig. 19). In subjects with deafness due to tumour pressure upon the cochlear nerve, it was found (Fig. 20) that the DL was within normal limits.

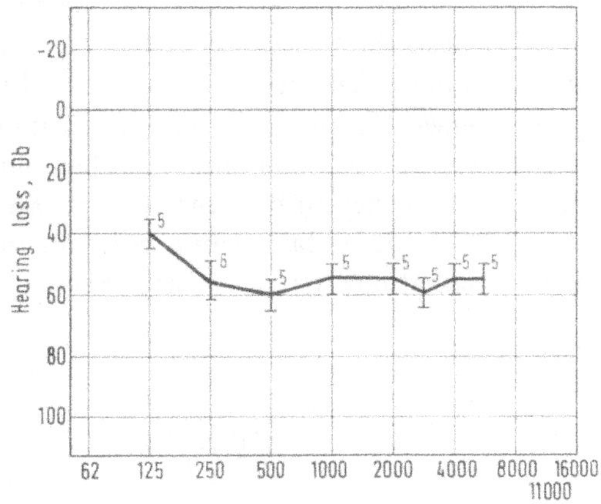

Fig. 19. Relative difference limens (percentages) in 6 subjects with Menières disease. The values are low (LÜSCHER and ERMANNI). (Reproduced by permission of Royal Society of Medicine)

Determination of the DL can be carried out at any level of stimulus intensity relative to the subject's threshold. In routine clinical work, the number of determinations needs to be limited. LÜSCHER and ZWISLOCKI (1948) recommend that the test be applied at the 40 dB level above threshold. DENES and NAUNTON (1949) recommend levels of 2—16 dB and 40 dB.

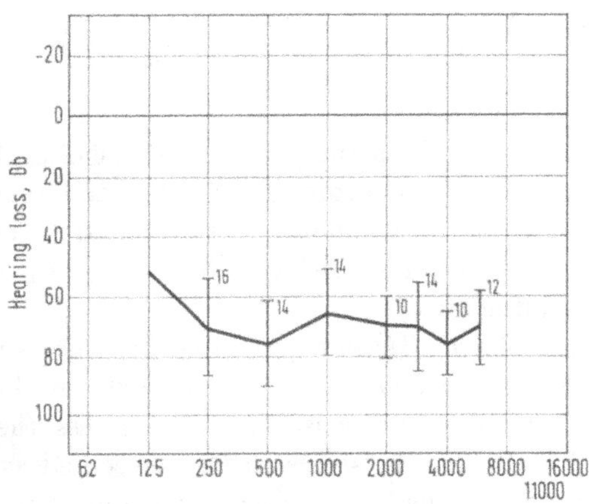

Fig. 20. Relative difference limens (percentages) in a subject with a cerebello-pontine angle tumour. The values are high (LÜSCHER and ERMANNI). (Reproduced by permission of Royal Society of Medicine)

B. Békésy Audiometry

The essential feature of the BÉKÉSY audiometer (1947) is a motor operated attenuator, whereby, the intensity of a pure tone stimulus is caused to rise or fall at a steady rate (2.5 dB/sec is usual). The direction of the intensity change is controlled by the subject by means of a reversing switch. The intensity is increased from a sub-threshold level. When the "just heard" point is attained, the switch is reversed and so maintained until the "just not heard" level is reached. At this point, the switch is again reversed. The intensity variations are recorded by a pen writing upon a moving chart. At the same time, another motor operated mechanism causes the stimulus frequency to be continuously varied over the whole audible frequency range. The results obtained in a normal subject are shown in Fig. 21. The peaks of the oscillations, or to be more precise, their mid-points,

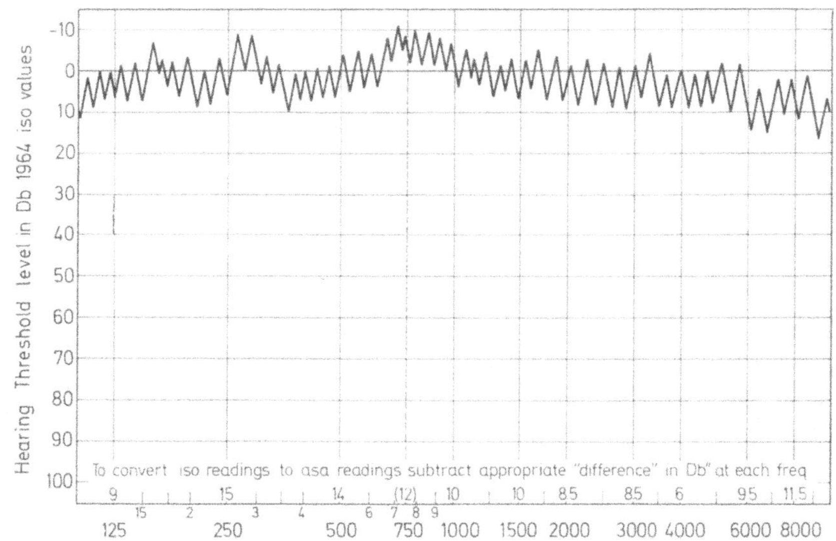

Fig. 21. BÉKÉSY audiogram. Normal subject

represent a continuous recording of the pure tone thresholds. This level and the amplitude of the tracing is also important and is found to be significantly related to certain derangements of the loudness function found to be associated with sensori-neural deafness, in particular with the phenomena of pathological adaptation and loudness recruitment.

In his original paper (1947), BÉKÉSY noted that in subjects who exhibited the loudness recruitment phenomenon and were assumed, on this account, to be suffering from the end organ type of sensori-neural deafness, the amplitude of the oscillations were reduced. This, he seems to have accepted as a natural consequence of the compression of the loudness scale which must result from loudness recruitment. Later (1952), LUNDBORG reported the results obtained with the Békésy audiometer in a large series of subjects of whom 50 were normal. His series also included 25 cases of acoustic trauma, 26 of Menières disease, and 21 with a variety of retrocochlear lesions including tumours of the VIII nerve. In agreement with BÉKÉSY he found that in Menières disease and acoustic trauma there occurred a marked reduction in the amplitude of the oscillations. With retrocochlear lesions, however, this feature was characteristically absent.

An important development in the technique of Békésy audiometry has been the use of interrupted as well as the normal continuous stimulus or, to be more precise, the continuously varying stimulus. This would seem to be a logical requirement arising from the work of DIX and HOOD (1953) on pathological adaptation in organic disorders of the cochlear end organs. If, in such cases, continuous stimulation is used, on-effect normality, which is the essence of loudness recruitment, is interfered with. The phenomenon itself is thus masked and may, in fact, be replaced by loudness reversal. If, as seems reasonable, loudness recruitment has as its corollaries, a compression of the loudness scale and a narrowing of the Békésy tracing, then, these too will be masked but will be restored if the continuous stimulus is replaced by a series of short interrupted stimuli. The situation is illustrated in Fig. 22.

Performance figures for the widely used Grason-Stadler, Model E 800, type of BÉKÉSY audiometer are as follows:

Rate of change of stimulus intensity: 2.5 dB/sec. Rate of change of frequency: 1 octave/min. Frequency of stimulus interruption: 2.5/sec. JERGER has described

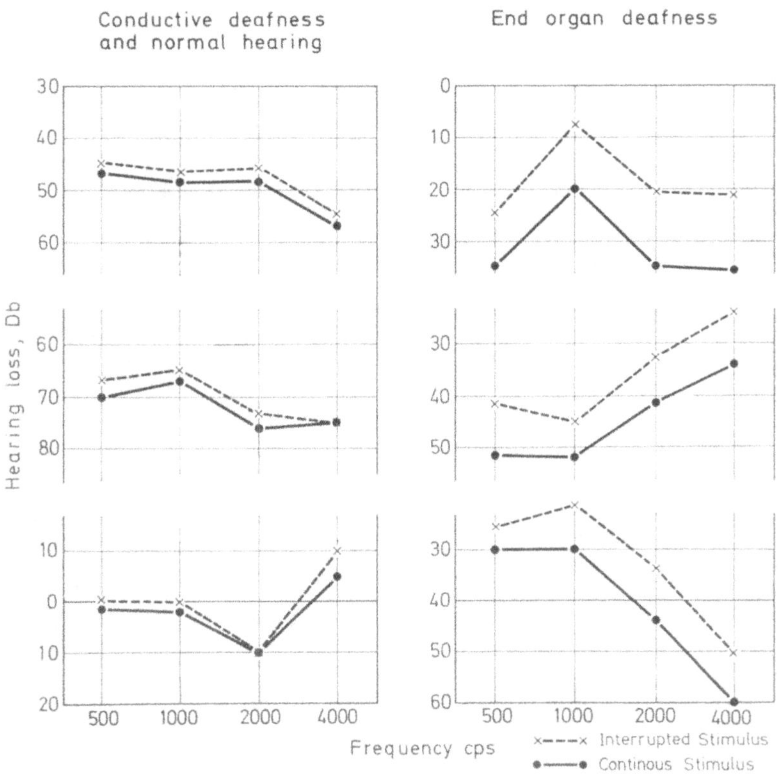

Fig. 22. (Reproduced by permission of Journal of Laryngology & Otology)

four basic types of Békésy audiogram. These are shown in the following figures, reproduced from his paper (1960a). In each, two tracings are shown: One (C) is obtained with the usual continuous (continuously varying) stimulus; with the other (I), the stimulus is interrupted. Types I and II are shown in Fig. 23. Type I is found in normal subjects or in cases of conductive deafness.

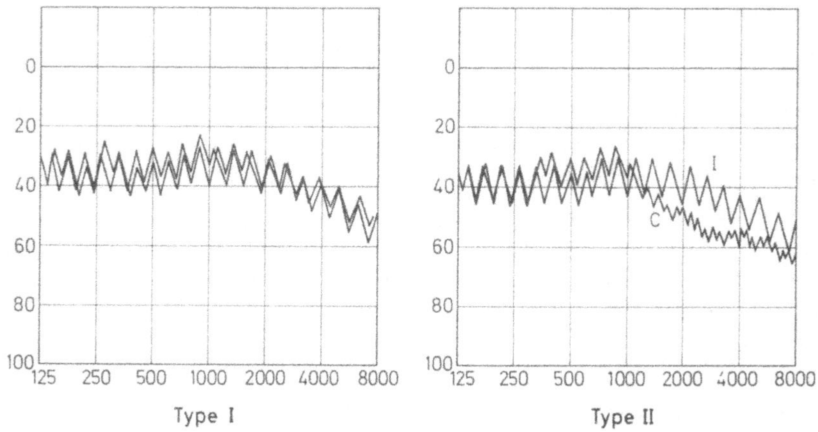

Fig. 23. Békésy audiograms. Types I and II (JERGER). (Reproduced by permission of Journal of Speech and Hearing Research)

Type II presents two notable features:

1. Relative to the I tracing, the C tracing is depressed over the higher frequency range.

2. Combined with this depression of the C tracing, its width is reduced. Type II tracings were found by JERGER in 26 of 32 cases of Menières disease and in 15 of 22 cases of acoustic trauma. A Type II Békésy audiogram would, therefore, appear to be diagnostic of the end-organ type of sensori-neural deafness. It would seem likely that the threshold elevation connoted by the depression of the C tracing is attributable to some degree of pathological adaptation to the continuous stimulation. The reduction in width of the C tracing is more difficult to explain. It may reflect a decrease of the intensity difference limen secondary to some further compression of the loudness scale, resulting, in turn, from the pathological adaptation. The fact that these two features of the C tracing are not present in the I tracing would seem to be attributable to the elimination of pathological adaptation.

Types III and IV tracings, according to JERGER, are shown in Fig. 24.

Type III is remarkable in that the C tracing begins to fall at low frequencies, often fails to stabilise at all, and may disappear from the chart in the manner shown. Its width is usually normal; meanwhile the I tracing runs horizontally throughout.

In Type IV, the C tracing falls below the I tracing at frequencies well below 500 Hz. Thereafter, this level difference is maintained throughout the full frequency range. The width of the C tracing remains within normal limits.

Békésy audiograms of Types III and IV are particularly common in sensori-neural deafness resulting from tumours of the VIII nerve. Thus, in 10 such cases, JERGER found Type III audiograms in 6. In the remaining four cases, the audiograms were of Type IV.

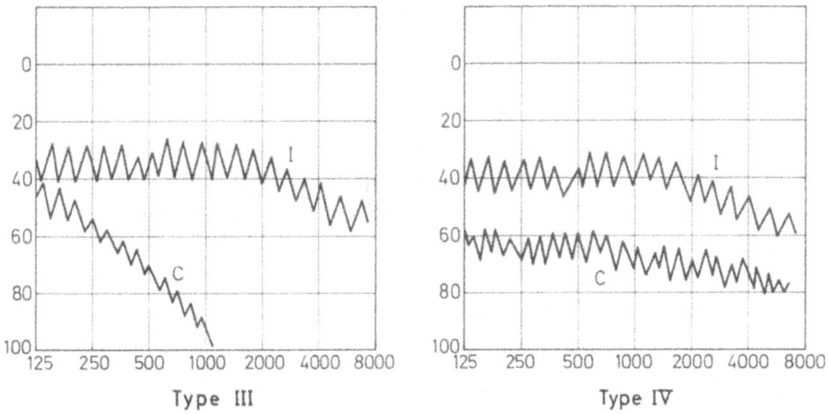

Fig. 24. Békésy audiograms. Types III and IV (JERGER). (Reproduced by permission of Journal of Speech and Hearing Research)

It should be noted that no case of acoustic neurofibroma showed a Type II audiogram. Furthermore, of 32 cases of Menières disease, none showed a Type III and only one, a Type IV.

C. The SISI (Short Increment Sensitivity Index) of Jerger (Jerger, Shedd, and Harford, 1959)

The procedure for the SISI test is as follows: A steady tone is applied to the subject's ear at an intensity level of 20 dB above threshold. At intervals of 5 sec the stimulus intensity is increased by 1 dB for 0.2 sec. Twenty such increments are presented in succession, and the subject's score is presented as a percentage of the 20 that are perceived. In subjects with normal hearing or in others with deafness due to lesions of the conductive apparatus or of the cochlear nerve, scores within the range of 0–20% are the rule. When the deafness is due to Menières disease or acoustic trauma, the SISI scores are much higher and usually lie within the range of 60–100% for frequencies above 1000 Hz. For lower frequencies, the SISI scores are lower. The test is easy to perform and much used for the diagnosis of sensori-neural deafness of the end-organ type. The physiological basis of the SISI test would appear to rest upon the principles involved in the ABLB test for loudness recruitment and in Lüschers test for reduction of the intensity difference limen. It is right, however, to stress that JERGER himself (1962) rejects this interpretation and insists, instead, that the SISI test is not an indirect test of loudness recruitment or of anything else. He prefers the view, empirical and pragmatic, that the interest and value of the test should be allowed to reside in its established usefulness in the diagnosis of organic disorders of the cochlear end organ.

D. Determination of the Loudness Discomfort Level (Hood and Poole)

In 1959, HALLPIKE and HOOD reported the results of a statistical survey of loudness recruitment in 200 cases of unilateral Menières disease. As shown in Fig. 7, reproduced from their paper, the loudness recruitment curves, as presented on Steinberg-Gardiner charts, all converge upon a point which is approximately 90 dB above the normal threshold. It follows that, if in a case of unilateral sensori-neural deafness, the ABLB test of FOWLER shows a loudness balance at 90 dB, or thereabouts, then, on this evidence alone, the chances are high that the deafness is due to an end organ affection, probably Menières disease. Clearly, this short cut to diagnosis would be possible only in subjects in whom the binaural ABLB test can be applied. However, when the deafness is bilateral, so requiring a monaural test, a similar short cut can sometimes be achieved by means of the loudness discomfort level test of HOOD and POOLE.

Working with normal subjects, HOOD and POOLE (1966, 1971) found that, at an intensity level of about 90 dB, the onset of pure tone stimuli caused a sharp feeling of discomfort. This did not occur in subjects with conductive deafness and, for this and other reasons, the basis for the discomfort was considered to have its origin within the cochlea. Since the critical loudness discomfort level (LDL) was found to correspond so closely to the full recruitment level established by means of the ABLB test for cases of unilateral Menières disease, HOOD and POOLE concluded that it could as well be used for the recognition of full recruitment of loudness with the added and conspicuous advantage that, as a monaural test, it could be used in cases of bilateral deafness. The test has certain limitations. Thus, if the deafness is due to a conductive lesion, the LDL is increased by an amount equal to that of the threshold elevation. If this is 30 dB, then the LDL will be 120 dB. Since this is the normal maximum intensity provided by an audiometer, it follows that the LDL determinations are impracticable in cases of conductive deafness in which the threshold elevation exceeds 30 dB. This limitation applies with equal force to cases of sensori-neural deafness in which loudness recruitment is absent or partial. The situation is explained in Fig. 25. *AB* is the recruitment curve for a subject with Menières disease: threshold elevation, 30 dB; loudness recruitment, full; LDL, at 90 dB. If the recruitment were incomplete, its amount could still be represented on the line *X—X'* provided that the LDL point lay between *B* and *C* but not beyond *C*. *C* is the recruitment curve for a subject with the nerve fibre type of sensori-neural deafness: threshold elevation, 30 dB; recruitment angle 45°; loudness recruitment, absent. LDL can be recorded at 120db and this indicates absence of loudness recruitment. *AD* and *AE* are loudness recruitment curves in other subjects with the same kind of deafness. Threshold elevations are 30 dB; recruitment angles are less than 45°; and loudness reversal is, therefore, present. In both cases, the LDL points lie to the right of Point C on the line $X-X$ and cannot be recorded. Although this fact alone is clear evidence of loudness reversal, its extent cannot be specified.

Within the limitations that have been noted, it would seem right to conclude that its ease of application, the fact that it is a monaural test requiring no equipment other than a conventional type of pure tone audiometer, confer upon the LDL procedure some very special advantages in the field of practical audiology. Evidence relating to its diagnostic value is available from a number of sources (Bosatra, 1969; Stephens and Anderson, 1971).

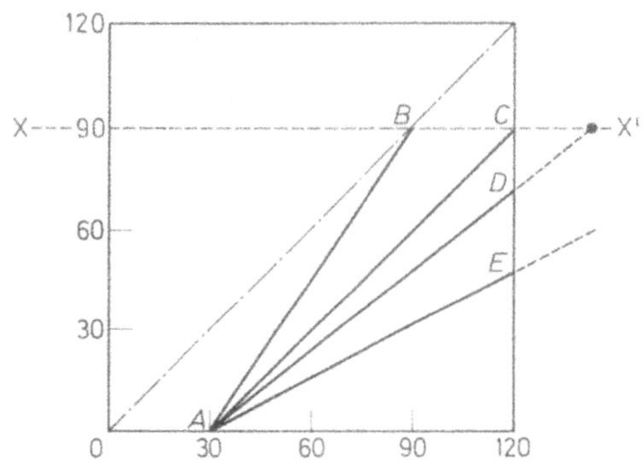

Fig. 25. Quantitative estimation of loudness recruitment by means of the loudness discomfort level test (Hood and Poole): showing the range and limitations of the test

E. Middle Ear Impedance Measurements (Metz) and their Use for the Determination of the Reflex Contraction Threshold of the Middle Ear Muscles

For a concise statement of the essential data relating to the mechanism and effects of sound induced contractions of the middle ear muscles in the mammal, reference may be made to the publications of Hallpike and Rawdon-Smith (1934) and of Hallpike (1935). Using cats under light anaesthesia and pure tone stimuli within the frequency range 200—2000 Hz, Hallpike and Rawdon-Smith observed brisk contractions at intensity levels of 80 dB above the human threshold. As judged from recordings of the cochlear microphonics, the effect of the contractions was a reduction of the energy level of the sound transmitted to the cochlea. This protective action of the muscles was found to have a latency, varying inversely with stimulus intensity, of approximately 30 msec.

In 1936, Lindsay, Kobrak, and Perlman confirmed the earlier findings in human subjects of Lüscher (1929) of contractions of the stapedius tendon induced by sound stimuli, crossed or uncrossed, and observed through post-otitic perforations of the tympanic membrane. The contractions occurred at stimulus intensity levels of 65—85 dB above the hearing threshold.

Following the introduction by Metz (1946), of the electro-acoustic impedance bridge, this and similar instruments have been widely used for the indirect determination of the reflex contraction threshold of the middle ear muscles. The apparatus and its working are diagrammatically represented in Fig. 26. The sound stimulus is generated at A and is applied to the subject's right ear; the equipment for the detection of the crossed muscle contraction threshold is applied to his left ear. A pure tone of 250 Hz is generated at B and delivered to the ear at an intensity of 60 dB above the threshold of hearing. At this level, it is well below that of the reflex contraction threshold. The sound reaching the meatus is

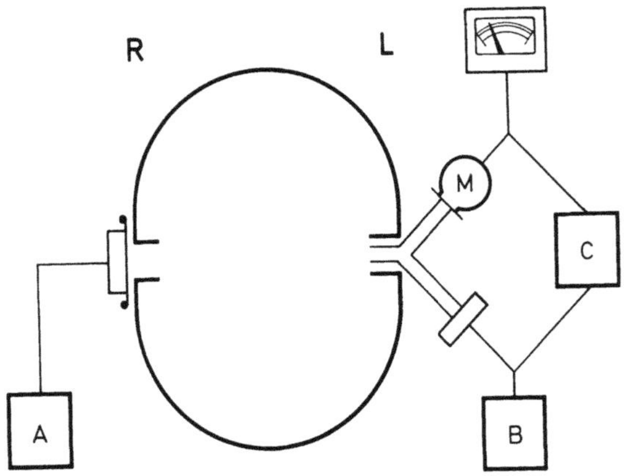

Fig. 26. Impedance bridge (METZ) showing electro-acoustic arrangements

reflected from the tympanic membrane and passes to the microphone, M. The voltage output of B is also passed to a network, C, where it can be adjusted for phase and amplitude. The voltage outputs of C and of the microphone are mixed and applied to a sensitive voltmeter. The controls at C are then used to bring into balance the two voltages reaching the voltmeter in order to obtain a null reading. The sound stimulus, a pure tone, usually within the frequency range 500—2000 Hz, is now applied at increasing intensities to the subject's ear. When the reflex contraction threshold is reached, the left middle ear muscles will contract, altering the elastic constants of the tympanic membrane and consequently the phase of the reflected sound. The voltages reaching the voltmeter will no longer be in balance and a reading will result.

The results for a normal subject appear in audiogram form in Fig. 27, reproduced from JEPSEN (1963). The upper curve shows the hearing thresholds of the right ear, the lower curve the thresholds of reflex contraction of the left middle ear muscles. With both curves, the sound stimuli are applied to the right ear. The difference in levels (70 dB) between the two curves provides a measure of the average normal stimulus intensity at the threshold of the reflex. If deafness is present, the threshold level will be depressed by an amount which depends upon the cause of the deafness. If it is due to a conductive lesion or is sensori-neural and of the nerve fibre type, the muscle reflex thresholds will be depressed by an amount equal to that of the deafness, *e.g.*, with deafness of 50 dB, the level of the muscle reflex threshold will lie at 120 dB, the intensity limit of the audiometer. If, however, the deafness is sensori-neural and of the end organ type, then loudness recruitment will occur and the depression of the muscle reflex threshold will be less than 50 dB. Within these limits, therefore, the test is capable of providing diagnostic information of considerable value. Essentially, the test is a binaural one, involving the sensory function of one ear and the motor function of the other. Usually, the latter is assumed to be normal and test results are interpreted in terms of the former. To this extent, the test has a certain theoretical insecurity.

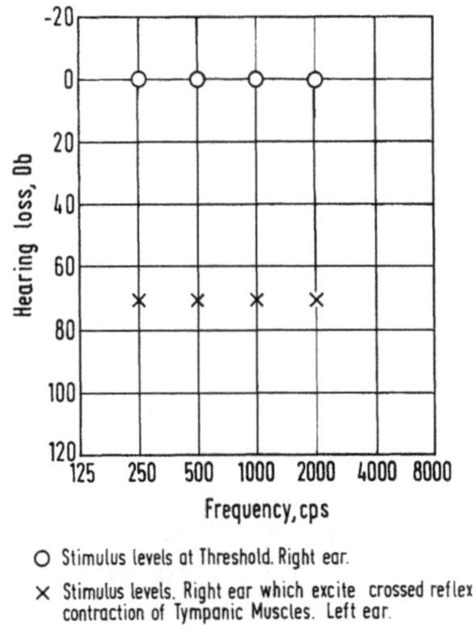

Fig. 27. See text

The value of measuring the response of the middle ear muscles (often referred to as acoustic reflex) lies in the objective character and diagnostic significance of the information which it is capable of providing. It has, too, a considerable usefulness in the investigation of non-organic hearing loss.

III. Speech Audiometry: Its Use for the Investigation of Derangement of Speech Intelligibility Found to Occur in Association with Sensori-Neural Deafness

Although the hearing of speech had long been accepted as the most important function of the human ear, the clinical methods in use for its investigation continued to be of notable inefficiency until the publication in 1929 of HARVEY FLETCHER's book, "Speech and Hearing". This was a compendium of information derived from the investigations of communications engineers and others, many working at the Bell Telephone Laboratories, and all directed towards improving the efficiency of the telephone transmission of speech. The area of knowledge, so covered, included the audiometric determination of the thresholds of hearing for pure tones in normal and deaf subjects, with the establishment in this context of the decibel notation, with the phenomena of masking, with loudness scales and the intensity difference limens for pure tones. In addition, much information was provided relating to the selection and use of phonetic material (words, syllables and sentences) required for the direct measurement of speech transmission efficiency.

In the course of the Second World War, the test methods that had been developed were widely used for the improvement of communications equipment required by the combatant forces for use in armoured fighting vehicles and other situations in which speech intelligibility was debased by high levels of ambient noise. In many ways, the problems encountered and the solutions devised were paralleled by those of deafness due to ear disease, and towards the end of the war, the health authorities in the United Kingdom and the U.S. lost little time in seeking to apply the substantial body of new knowledge made available in the fields of electro- and psycho-acoustics to systematic studies designed to improve the scientific bases for the design and application of audiometers and hearing aids used for the investigation and alleviation of deafness in the civil population. The British findings were embodied in a report (1947) to the Medical Research Council.

The section of the report relevant to the diagnosis of sensori-neural deafness is that concerned with speech audiometry — the theoretical basis and practical application of tests of hearing for speech, with the graphic recording and interpretation of the results.

The test methods recommended by the Medical Research Council's Committee, were, with certain differences, in close accord with those presented in earlier reports from U.S. sources (1942 and 1944). The latter also contained much valuable test material, in the form of phonetically balanced lists of words and sentences, of which the Committee were able to make use. The understanding of meaningful sentences and phrases (sentence intelligibility) was considered by the Committee to be the function of the hearing mechanism most directly related to a subject's social needs, and account was taken of this in the graphic recording of the test results embodied in the speech audiogram form which the Committee proposed. This form is shown in Fig. 28.

Test Procedure. The test were carried out in a sound-proofed, well damped room with the subject's ear located at a fixed distance from a loud speaker by means of which the test sentences and words were reproduced at controllable

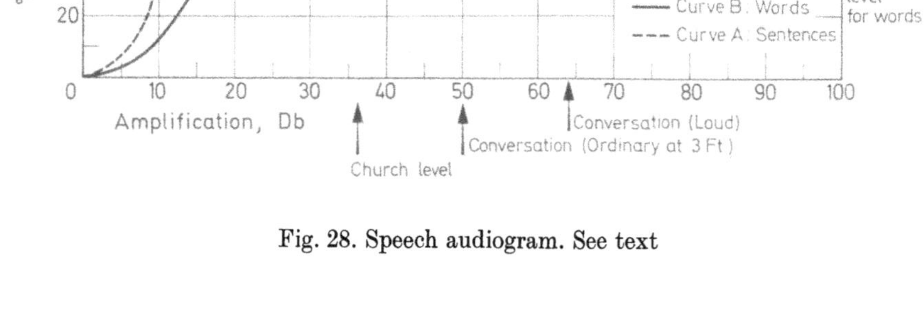

Fig. 28. Speech audiogram. See text

intensities. Curves *A* and *B* show the results obtained in normal subjects. The words used for the word lists were monosyllables and have a consonant-vowel-consonant structure. Words of this kind vary in their "intrinsic intelligibility". That is to say, some are understood only at an amplifier setting which may be considerably higher than is needed for others. If the word lists used are homogeneous in respect of "intrinsic intelligibility", Curve *B* will be steep in form and will approximate to that obtained with spondaic words. In practice, a flatter form, as shown in Fig. 28, is preferred and the word lists are prepared to provide this. The form and siting of Curves *B* and *A* denote a relationship between word articulation and sentence intelligibility scores which approximates to the earlier finding by investigators in the Bell Telephone Laboratories and by others. This relationship makes it easy to express any word articulation score on Curve *B* in terms of sentence intelligibility on Curve *A*. This indirect evaluation of the latter from word articulation scores is important since word articulation tests, being less time consuming, are almost exclusively used for clinical work.

The amplifier settings are given in db. on the horizontal axis of the graph in Fig. 28, the reference point of the scale being taken as the level at which 50% of the words are detected. Three special levels are indicated:

1. Church level (36 dB).
2. Ordinary conversation at 3 feet (50 dB).
3. Loud conversation at 3 feet (64 dB).

It was considered that the articulation scores obtained at these levels by deaf subjects would be of help in assigning them to one or other of the three categories of social disability due to deafness suggested by Beasley (1940). The 40% level of word articulation calls for particular attention. Thus, the articulation Curve *B* for a normal subject, cuts this level at an amplification setting of about 15 dB, at which the sentence intelligibility curve reaches the crest of a plateau with a score of 90%. Above this point, the intelligibility score gains little; below it, there is a steep fall. It follows that the attainment, at any given amplification, of an articulation score of 40% provides a serviceable assurance of social adequacy. The matter is illustrated by the articulation Curves, *C*, *D*, and *E*, which are shown in Fig. 29 and which were obtained in subjects with increasing degrees of

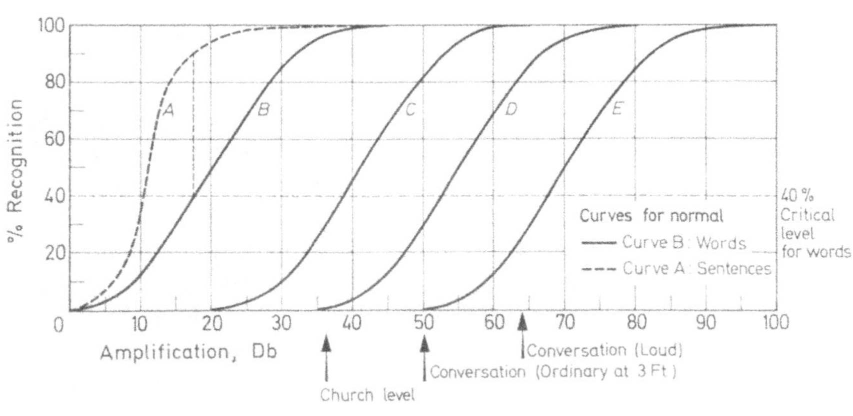

Fig. 29. Speech audiogram. See text

conductive deafness. In each, the amount of the speech deafness is given by the amount of the curves displacement to the right of the normal curve as measured in db along the 40% articulation level. For Curve *C*, the displacement is 22 dB; for Curve *D*, 35 dB; and for Curve *E*, 50 dB. For Subject *C*, the articulation score is well above 40% at the ordinary conversation level but below it at Church level. The Beasley Grading will therefore be No. 1. Subjects *D* and *E* will similarly fall into Grades II and III, respectively.

Speech Audiometry in Sensori-Neural Deafness

Striking abnormalities are frequently exhibited by the articulation curves obtained in subjects with sensori-neural deafness. For this clinical group, therefore, speech audiometry has a special diagnostic value. The subject has recently been reviewed by HOOD and POOLE (1971) in a series of 43 cases of Menières disease, cases that exhibited the end-organ type of sensori-neural deafness.

In Fig. 30 is shown a collection of articulation curves derived from a group of subjects with sensori-neural deafness due to Menières disease. The amount of their hearing loss for pure tones was calculated in terms of the average loss for

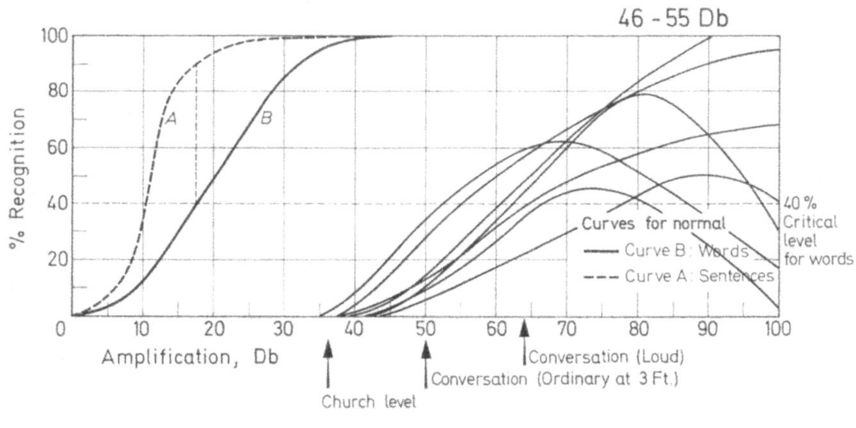

Fig. 30. Speech audiogram in subjects with sensori-neural deafness showing typical discrimination loss. (Reproduced by permission of "Sound")

the speech frequencies, 500, 1000, and 2000 Hz, and lay within the range 46—55 dB. Compared with the findings in conductive deafness shown in Fig. 29, the curves all show a flattening towards the higher levels of amplification. Many, after reaching a peak, fall off with further amplification. Few reach the full 100% level of recognition for words or sentences. The term "discrimination loss" is used to describe this defect which is measured in terms of the amount by which a curve's maximum falls below the 100% level. This discrimination loss provides, of course, an obvious explanation of the well known fact that sensori-neural deafness of the end-organ type is so characteristically insusceptible to correction by means of hearing aids. As shown in Fig. 31, reproduced from HOOD and POOLE's paper (1971), discrimination loss is a function of the pure-tone hearing loss. The articulation curves shown were obtained in five groups of subjects with increasing degrees of deafness for pure tones due to Menières disease. In each case, the limits of the values are enclosed by the shaded area. The average of the values is given by the dark line. With a pure tone hearing loss within the range of 26—35 dB, there is no discrimination loss, and the form of the articulation curve approximates closely to that of a case of conductive deafness. With higher degrees of deafness, however, discrimination loss makes its appearance and increases progressively. In all of the cases concerned, full loudness recruitment was present, a fact which it is reasonable to apply to the explanation of the discrimination loss which is so

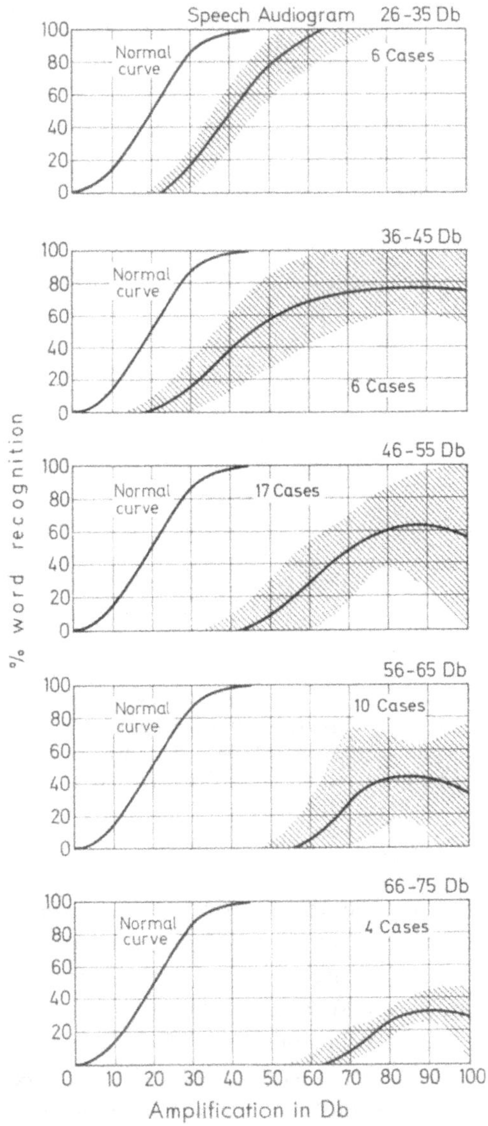

Fig. 31. Speech audiograms in subjects with sensori-neural deafness: showing relationship between discrimination loss and hearing loss. (Reproduced by permission of "Sound")

characteristic a feature of this end-organ type of sensori-neural deafness. As to how loudness recruitment is able to exert this effect, it is impossible to speak with any certainty. However, there is one possibility which must obviously invite attention. For instance, loudness recruitment must of necessity be associated with a compression of the loudness scale over which speech sound enters the periphery of the nervous system. Further, the degree of this compression must vary with the degree of the hearing loss from pure tones. It follows that discrimination loss, if it is due to loudness compression will increase "pari passu" with hearing loss. According to the findings of HOOD and POOLE, this appears to be the case.

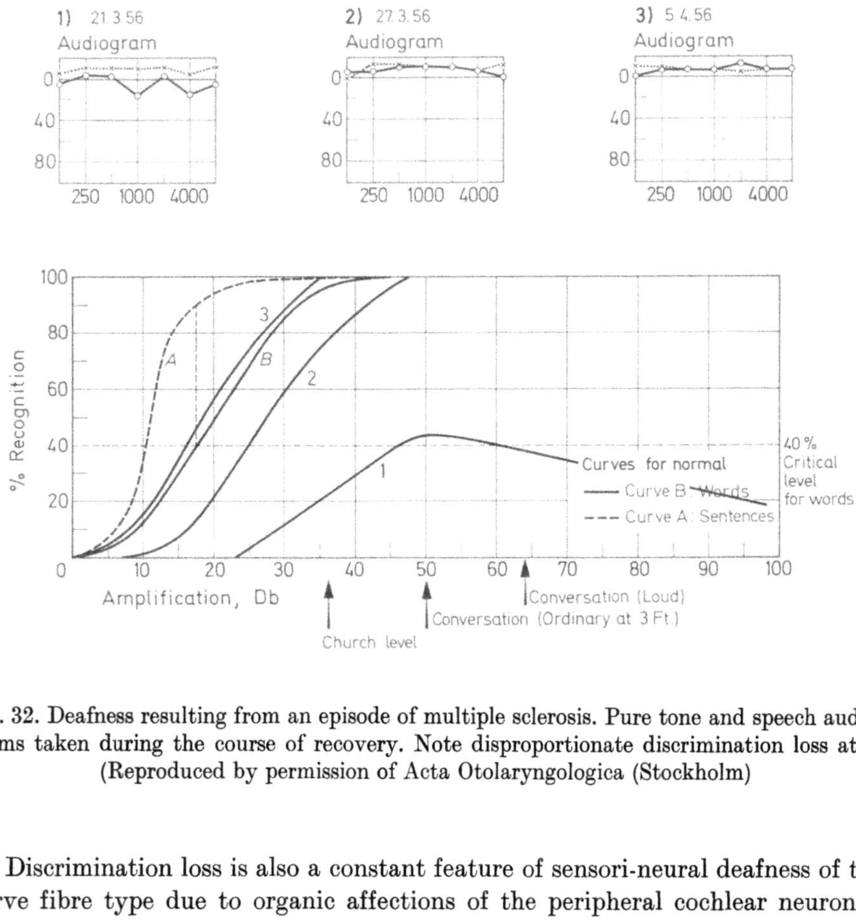

Fig. 32. Deafness resulting from an episode of multiple sclerosis. Pure tone and speech audiograms taken during the course of recovery. Note disproportionate discrimination loss at 1. (Reproduced by permission of Acta Otolaryngologica (Stockholm)

Discrimination loss is also a constant feature of sensori-neural deafness of the nerve fibre type due to organic affections of the peripheral cochlear neurones. The amount of the discrimination loss is again related to the amount of the hearing loss though less constantly than in the case of the end-organ type of sensori-neural deafness. It would seem, on the whole, that, within this clinical category, discrimination loss, although constant in its occurrence, is unpredictable in respect of its amount and often surprisingly large. This estimate would seem to agree with those of SCHUKNECHT and WOELLNER (1955) and of JERGER (1960b) in their consideration of the deafness of subjects with tumours of the VIII nerve.

The surprising character of the speech audiometric findings in subjects with deafness due to organic affections of the peripheral cochlear neurones is exemplified by the findings of Citron and others (1963) in a subject whose hearing was closely studied in the course of an episode of multiple sclerosis affecting the left cochlear nerve fibres in the neuroglial part of its course. Deafness, at first severe, was recovering at the time of the 1st audiogram on 7 March 1956. This is marked 1 on the pure tone audiogram shown in Fig. 32. Also included are the findings recorded on the 9th, 15th, and 21st of March.

Pure tone and speech audiograms recorded on the 21st and 27th of March and on the 5th of April appear in Fig. 32 and show the final stages of hearing recovery. Pure tone audiogram (1) corresponds to the articulation curve marked 1 on the speech audiogram. Although the pure tone audiogram shows that hearing at threshold of pure tones is virtually normal, the speech audiogram reveals a surprising and wholly disproportionate degree of discrimination loss.

References

Altmann, F., Fowler, E. P.: Histological findings in Ménière's symptom complex. Ann. Otol. (St. Louis) **52**, 52—80 (1943).

Beasley, W. C.: The general problem of deafness in the population. Laryngoscope (St. Louis) **50**, 856—905 (1940).

von Békésy, G.: A new audiometer. Acta oto-laryng. (Stockh.) **35**, 411—422 (1947).

von Békésy, G.: Loudness recruitment. Trans. Amer. otol. Soc. **53**, 85—93 (1965).

Bosatra, A.: On the semeiological value of the loudness discomfort level. Int. Audiol. **8**, 164—171 (1969).

de Bruïne-Altes, J. C.: The symptom of regression in different kinds of deafness. Doctoral Thesis Groningen. Groningen: Wolters 1946.

Citron, L., Dix, M. R., Hallpike, C. S., Hood, J. D.: A recent clinico-pathological study of cochlear nerve degeneration resulting from tumor pressure and disseminated sclerosis, with particular reference to the finding of normal threshold sensitivity for pure tones. Acta oto-laryng. (Stockh.) **56**, 330—337 (1963).

Davis, H.: Biophysics and physiology of the inner ear. Physiol. Rev. **37**, 1—49 (1957).

Davis, H.: A mechano-electrical theory of cochlear action. Ann. Otol. (St. Louis) **67**, 789—801 (1958).

Denes, P., Naunton, R. F.: Methods of audiometry in a modern deafness clinic. J. Laryng. **63**, 251—275 (1949).

Denny, W. R.: Diagnosis of acoustic neuroma. J. Laryng. **69**, 608—616 (1955).

Dix, M. R.: Observations upon the nerve fibre deafness of multiple sclerosis, with particular reference to the phenomenon of loudness recruitment. J. Laryng. **79**, 695—706 (1965).

Dix, M. R., Hallpike, C. S.: The otoneurological diagnosis of tumours of the VIII nerve. Proc. roy. Soc. Med. **51**, 889—897 (1958).

Dix, M. R., Hallpike, C. S., Hood, J. D.: Observations upon the loudness recruitment phenomenon, with especial reference to the differential diagnosis of disorders of the internal ear and VIII nerve. Proc. roy. Soc. Med. **41**, 516—526 (1948).

Dix, M. R., Hood, J. D.: Modern developments in pure tone audiometry and their application to the clinical diagnosis of end-organ deafness. J. Laryng. **67**, 343—357 (1953).

Eby, L. G., Williams, H. L.: Recruitment of loudness in the differential diagnosis of end-organ and nerve fibre deafness. Laryngoscope (St. Louis) **61**, 400—414 (1951).

Fowler, E. P.: The diagnosis of diseases of the neural mechanism of hearing by the aid of sounds well above threshold. Laryngoscope (St. Louis) **47**, 289—300 (1937).

Fowler, E. P. (Ed.): Medicine of the ear. New York: Nelson 1939.

Hallpike, C. S.: On the function of the tympanic muscles. J. Laryng. **50**, 362—369 (1935).

Hallpike, C. S.: Clinical otoneurology and its contributions to theory and practice. Proc. roy. Soc. Med. **58**, 185—196 (1965).

Hallpike, C. S., Cairns, H.: Observations on the pathology of Ménière's syndrome. J. Laryng. **53**, 625—655 (1938).

HALLPIKE, C. S., HOOD, J. D.: Observations upon the neurological mechanism of the loudness recruitment phenomenon. Acta oto-laryng. (Stockh.) **50**, 472—486 (1959).

HALLPIKE, C. S., RAWDON-SMITH, A. F.: The function of the tensor tympani muscle. J. Physiol. (Lond.) **81**, 25P—27P (1934).

HARDY, M., CROWE, S. J.: Early asymptomatic acoustic tumor. Arch. Surg. **32**, 292—301 (1936).

HOOD, J. D.: Studies in auditory fatigue and adaptation. Acta oto-laryng. (Stockh.), Suppl. 92 (1950).

HOOD, J. D.: Basic audiological requirements in neuro-otology. J. Laryng. **83**, 695—711 (1969).

HOOD, J. D., POOLE, J. P.: Tolerable limit of loudness: its clinical and physiological significance. J. acoust. Soc. Amer. **40**, 47—53 (1966).

HOOD, J. D., POOLE, J. P.: Speech audiometry in conductive and sensorineural hearing loss. Sound **5**, 30—38 (1971).

JEPSEN, O.: In: JERGER, J. (Ed.): Modern developments in audiology, p. 194. New York: Academic Press 1963.

JERGER, J.: Békésy audiometry in analysis of auditory disorders. J. Speech Res. **3**, 275—287 (1960a).

JERGER, J.: Audiological manifestations of lesions in the auditory nervous system. Laryngoscope (St. Louis) **70**, 417—425 (1960b).

JERGER, J.: Recruitment and allied phenomena in differential diagnosis. J. Res. **2**, And. 145—151 (1961).

JERGER, J.: Hearing tests in otologic diagnosis. ASHA **4**, 139—145 (1962).

JERGER, J., SHEDD, J. L., HARFORD, E.: On the detection of extremely small changes in sound intensity. Arch. Otolaryng. **69**, 200—211 (1959).

KNUDSEN, V. O.: The sensibility of the ear to small differences in intensity and frequency. Phys. Rev. **21**, 84 (1923).

KRISTENSEN, H. K., JEPSEN, O.: Recruitment in otoneurological diagnostics. Acta oto-laryng. (Stockh.) **42**, 553—560 (1952).

LINDSAY, J. R.: Labyrinthine dropsy and Ménière's disease. Arch. Otolaryng. **35**, 853—867 (1942).

LINDSAY, J. R., KOBRAK, H., PERLMAN, H. B.: Relation of the stapedius reflex to hearing sensation in man. Arch. Otolaryng. **23**, 671—678 (1936).

LORENTE DE NÓ, R.: Discussion of paper by FOWLER. Trans. Amer. otol. Soc. **27**, 219—220 (1937).

LÜSCHER, E.: Die Funktion des *Musculus Stapedius* beim Menschen. Z. Hals-, Nas.- u. Ohrenheilk. **23**, 105—132 (1929).

LÜSCHER, E.: The difference limen of intensity variations of pure tones and its diagnostic significance. Proc. roy. Soc. Med. **43**, 1116—1128 (1950).

LÜSCHER, E., ZWISLOCKI, J.: A simple method for indirect monaural determination of the recruitment phenomenon. Acta oto-laryng. (Stockh.), Supplement 78, 156—172 (1948).

LUNDBORG, T.: Diagnostic problems concerning acoustic tumors. Acta oto-laryng. (Stockh.), Supplement 99, (1952).

MATTHEWS, B. H. C.: The response of a single end organ. J. Physiol. (Lond.) **71**, 64—110 (1931).

Medical Research Council: Committee on electro-acoustics: Hearing aids and audiometers. Spec. Rep. Ser. Med. Res. Coun. (Lond.), No. 261 (1947).

METZ, O.: The acoustic impedance measured on normal and pathological ears. Acta oto-laryng. (Stockh.), Supplement 63, (1946).

POHLMAN, A. G., KRANZ, F. W.: Binaural minimum audition in a subject with ranges of deficient acuity. Proc. Soc. exp. Biol. (N.Y.) **21**, 335—337 (1924).

Reports on Articulation Testing Methods. I (1942): National Research Council (USA), Committee on Sound Control. II (1944): Office of Scientific Research and Development, Psycho-Acoustic Laboratory, Harvard, No. 3, 802. Cited in: Spec. Rep. Ser. Med. Res. Coun. (Lond.), No. 261 (1947).

RIESZ, R. R.: Differential intensity sensitivity of the ear for pure tones. Phys. Rev. **31**, 867 (1928).

SCHUKNECHT, H. F., WOELLNER, R. C.: An experimental and clinical study of deafness from lesions of the cochlear nerve. J. Laryng. **69**, 75—97 (1955).

SIMONTON, K. M.: End-organ deafness. Diagnosis and significance. Arch. Otolaryng. **63**, 262—269 (1956).

SPOENDLIN, H.: Innervation densities of the cochlea. Acta oto-laryng. (Stockh.) **73**, 235 (1972).

STEINBERG, J. C., GARDNER, M. B.: The dependence of hearing impairment on sound intensity. J. acoust. Soc. Amer. **9**, 11 (1937).

STENGER, H. H.: Otologische Befunde bei Kleinhirnbrückenwinkeltumoren. Arch. Ohr.-, Nas.-, u. Kehlk.-Heilk. **169**, 285—287 (1956).

STEPHENS, S. D. G., ANDERSON, C. M. B.: Experimental studies on the uncomfortable loudness level. J. Speech Res. **14**, 262—270 (1971).

STEVENS, S. S., DAVIS, H.: Hearing: its psychology and physiology. New York: Wiley 1938.

Chapter 2

Bone Conduction

J. TONNDORF, New York N. Y. (USA)

With 28 Figures

Contents

I. Introduction

Bone conduction testing, that is, the application of audio-frequency vibrations to the head, their conduction to the structures of the ear, and eventual perception as "sound", is an important audiometric tool of considerable clinical significance. It helps to differentiate conductive from sensorineural lesions.

Knowledge of the fact that audio frequencies might be transmitted to the ear in the form of structural vibrations is quite old. GIROLAMO CARDANO (1501–1576), better known as the inventor of the universal joint, is usually credited with having first described this phenomenon. Its first introduction as a clinical tool was due to HIERONYMUS CAPIVACCI (died 1589) who employed it for diagnosing "disorders of the tympanic membrane", *i. e.*, conductive lesions. However, the phenomenon found its first real and rather wide-spread use for a different purpose: as a primitive hearing aid for helping people with conductive lesions to enjoy music. A rod was held between the teeth at one end, while the other was put in contact with the instrument being played. Beethoven, at the time when he first became deaf, is said to have tried this method but found it sadly wanting for his needs. (The concensus of opinion today is that Beethoven suffered from a sensorineural disorder.)

Capivacci's application of bone conduction testing for diagnostic purposes was apparently forgotten until it was "rediscovered" in the early part of the 19th century. WHEATSTONE (1827), when experimenting with the occlusion effect, which much later became known as the test of BING (1891), noticed the phenomenon of lateralization, but also the relative improvement of hearing for low-frequency sounds, for example in the perception of one's own voice. TORTUAL, also in 1827, is said to have been the first to have recognized the diagnostic implications of such observations. WEBER (1834) reported observations of his own, once more on the occlusion effect and largely similar to those of WHEATSTONE. His contribution is still commemorated in the test of Weber that was named for him. RINNE (1855) and SCHWABACH (1885) directly described the tests that still carry their names and assessed their clinical significances. [Note — Much of the above information was taken from FELDMANN: A History of Audiology (1960)]; see also: The Development of Bone Conduction Testing, Trans. Beltone Inst. Hear. Res. 28, (1974).

Reception of air-borne sound by bone conduction — There is another kind of bone conduction that ought to be mentioned, although it has not found any important clinical application. As demonstrated by BÉKÉSY (1948), aerial sound is capable of setting the entire skull into vibration, and, when high enough in intensity, energy thus received and transmitted will exceed threshold and is then added to that entering the ear via ear canal and tympanic membrane. This contribution of bone conduction becomes first noticeable at about 60 dB SL, a value which thus sets a limit to which transmission of aerial sounds might be attenuated by experimental blocking of the ear canal, canal atresias, or ossicular discontinuities. It is in this respect that the phenomenon has some, although indirect, clinical significance.

Bone conduction and industrial hearing loss — WITTMAACK (1917), who had been interested in the problem of noise-induced cochlear lesions for some years, made the suggestion, on the basis of animal experiments with histological follow-up controls, that vibrations of the floor produced by noise-generating machinery might contribute to cochlear damage. Such vibratory energy was thought to reach the ears by transmission via the feet and the entire body. SIEBENMANN (1917) was unable to duplicate WITTMAACK's findings. Over the years, more experiments were performed by both men and their respective students, and, after heated and often bitter debates, SIEBENMANN's opinion finally prevailed, *i. e.*, a contribution to cochlear lesions due to vibrations of the floor transmitted via bone conduction could not be demonstrated. For one thing, it was hard to see how appreciable amounts of energy could reach the ears in this manner, considering the attenuation that is bound to occur across each of the many joints along the pathway involved.

In some older audiological surveys conducted in industry (*e. g.*, TEMKIN, 1933), groups of workmen were found who displayed signs of apical-turn lesions, *i. e.*, low-tone hearing losses for air *and* for bone. Such lesions could not be expected to results from exposure to air-borne sounds because of the low-frequency attenuation of the middle ear. Although WITTMAACK's explanation, which was frequently invoked in such reports, does no longer appear tenable, such apical-turn lesions could conceivably be caused by bone conduction components of high-intensity noise in the sense of BÉKÉSY (1948). — As far as I am aware of, no newer studies have been conducted in this problem area, and the older experiments and/or surveys were done at times before signal parameters could be precisely controlled or measured.

A detailed, critical review of the older studies on the potential contribution of bone-conducted energy to industrial hearing loss and its underlying pathology may be found in Werner (1940) who, incidently, favored SIEBENMANN's point of view.

Osseous and osseo-tympanic modes of bone conduction — Some of the earliest writers on bone conduction formed opinions on the theory of this phenomenon. Despite of continuing efforts, a consensus of opinion was not reached. By the second half of the 19th century, two schools of thought had emerged which were held to be mutually exclusive by the majority of writers. One school maintained that energy was transmitted to the receptors exclusively via the bones of the skull; this mode became known as the *osseous route* of bone conduction. The other school held that vibrations of the skull set up relative displacements of the auditory ossicles, which would then be conducted via the air conduction pathway. This mode was referred to as the *osseo-tympanic route* of bone conduction. There was some evidence in favor of each theory, *i. e.*, there are some phenomena that can best be explained in terms of one theory, and other phenomena that are better accounted for by the opposing theory. A few writers (*e. g.*, POLITZER, 1869) pointed out that such a strict dichotomy could not really be maintained, but the separate concepts have survived in some form or another. In present-day terminology, the osseous mode represents the *compressional* response of the inner ear; the osseo-tympanic mode, the *inertial* response of the middle ear.

The reason for the dichotomy of opinion appears to lie in the fact that many writers have tried to explain *all* bone-conduction phenomena on the basis of one *single*, unifying concept. If recognizing the existence of the other mode at all, they usually downgraded its importance. The present chapter will provide evidence indicating that such attempts, laudable as they may be from a general scientific standpoint, were doomed to failure. Bone conduction, in my opinion, is quite a complicated phenomenon, in a way more complex than air conduction which can be presented by a relatively simple series-network (MØLLER, 1961; ZWISLOCKI, 1962).

The question as to how vibratory energy is being transmitted to the temporal bone from inputs anywhere about the head is an important part of the whole problem. However, its discussion will be postponed in favor of a description of the mechanism operating in the ear itself.

Reception of bone-conducted signals — From the early years of bone-conduction theory well into the 20th century, the notion was frequently expressed that bone conducted energy might bypass the inner ear and stimulate the cochlear nerve directly, the assumption being that the bone of the internal meatus might vibrate around the stationary nerve. This idea was apparently first formulated by WEBER (1834). To dispel such notions once and for all (which are not really tenable on a variety of theoretical grounds), BÉKÉSY (1932) performed a simple, ingenious experiment. He masked one ear by noise, as bone conduction affects both ears to essentially equal degrees. Then, he led identical sine-wave signals to the other ear, simultaneously by air and by bone. By suitable adjustment of signal phase and amplitude in one of the channels, his subjects were able to achieve a clear auditory null, *i. e.*, they were able to cancel both signals. LOWY (1943) repeated this experiment in guinea pigs using the cochlear microphonic response as indicator. He found that, once cancellation had been achieved for one given electrode position, the electrode could be moved to any other place around the cochlea, but the response never re-appeared. These experiments clearly indicate that both modes of signal transmissions utilize, at least in part, identical routes in the mechanical domain; particularly, both must enter, and thus be processed by, the cochlea.

II. Components of Bone Conduction Responses

Several years ago, the present author, in collaboration with a number of co-workers, conducted a series of experimental studies on the problem of bone conduction in experimental animals, mainly in cats (TONNDORF and TABOR, 1962; TONNDORF, 1962; 1964; TONNDORF *et al.*, 1966; TONNDORF, 1968). These studies confirmed some of the classical notions, while refuting others. They gave evidence, both qualitatively and quantitatively, for the fact that the ultimate reception of bone-conductions signals results from a number of contributing *factors* that may be conveniently identified with the outer, the middle, and the inner ear. That is to say, each of these structures is capable of reacting in some specific manner to vibratory stimulation. After it received additional energy from the two other sites, the cochlea forms a consolidated response which then leads to stimulation of its hair cells.

On the strength of the findings by BÉKÉSY (1932) and LOWY (1943) just mentioned, *i. e.*, that bone conducted energy is ultimately received by the cochlea, cochlear microphonic responses were employed as indicator and measured under a variety of experimental conditions. Since some of the experiments involved occlusion of the cochlear windows, differential electrodes in the basal turn were used in most experiments. To avoid creating new cochlear windows, the electrodes were sealed in by means of silicone and dental cement (Fig. 1).

To maintain uniform inputs, the experimental situation was rigidly standardized with respect to the support of the animal's head (foam rubber cushion), application of the vibrator (cemented to the mastoid region), and monitoring its input, both with respect to its phase and its amplitude of acceleration (in Ref. to 1 g). Likewise, both phase and amplitude of the responses were measured.

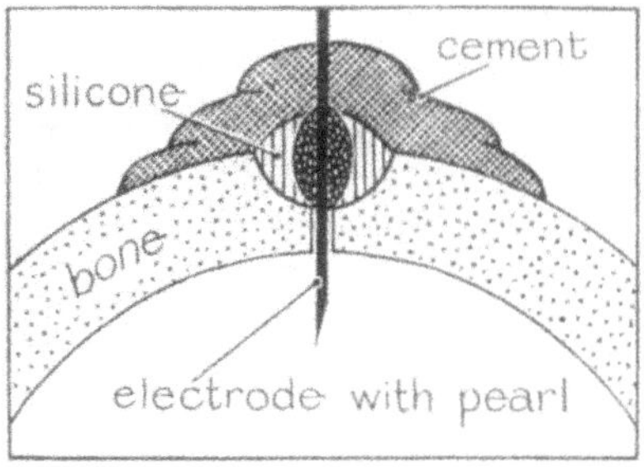

Fig. 1. Intra-cochlear, sealed-in electrode, designed to prevent leakage through the perforation; for experimental details reference is made to the original publication. (From TONNDORF and TABOR, 1962)

A. Inner Ear Component

The inner ear is capable of receiving bone-conducted signals on its own as demonstrated by the common clinical experience that a person's hearing by bone conduction is only slightly impaired following radical mastoidectomy. For reasons that will become obvious in the present discussion, bone-conduction hearing levels may even improve to some extent with time after surgery, a fact that may have contributed to the widely-held notion that hearing levels for bone conduction are not affected when the middle ear is missing. However, in our own experience that notion is not correct, as will be shown presently.

A mechanism of direct cochlear reception of vibratory energy was first suggested by REJTÖ (1914). HERZOG and KRAINZ (1926)[1] later formulated its concept in greater detail. It was called the *compressional mode* of bone conduction.

The speed of propagation of vibratory energy in bone was thought to be so high as to prevent the development of phase differences over the space occupied by the cochlea. Furthermore, the cochlear fluids had to be considered incompressible within the range of audio-frequency vibrations. Thus, the entire cochlear capsule was assumed to contract ("to be compressed") and expand in an alternating manner, in synchrony with an applied steady-state signal. Figure 2 shows a hypothetical case: Suppose that both cochlear windows had the same compliance and that the cochlear capsule were symmetrically built. In that case, changes in cochlear volume due to the contraction of its capsule, being in phase in both perilymphatic scalae, would have to be compensated for by equal displacements of both cochlear windows, but could not produce volume and/or pressure differentials across the partition (Fig. 2a). In reality, however, (1) the cochlear windows are not of equal compliance, the oval-window membrane being stiffer than the round-window membrane, and (2) the perilymphatic scale are not of equal volume,

[1] The 1926 proceedings of the German ENT Society contains two separate papers: HERZOG presenting the theory and KRAINZ the experimental results. Nevertheless, it is customary to list both of their names together when reference is made to the concept they developed.

scala vestibuli being larger than *scala tympani*, especially when the perilymphatic space of the vestibular system is taken into account. Figure 2b and c show the consequences of these two conditions: (1) The lesser displacement of the oval window is compensated for by an appropriate displacement of the cochlear partition; and (2) the larger volume of fluid displaced from *scala vestibuli* is likewise compensated for by an appropriate displacement of the partition. Note that both mechanisms shown in Fig. 2b and c operate *in phase* with each other. — While Fig. 2 illustrates the situation upon capsular contraction, capsular expansion ought to produce displacements of opposite sign.

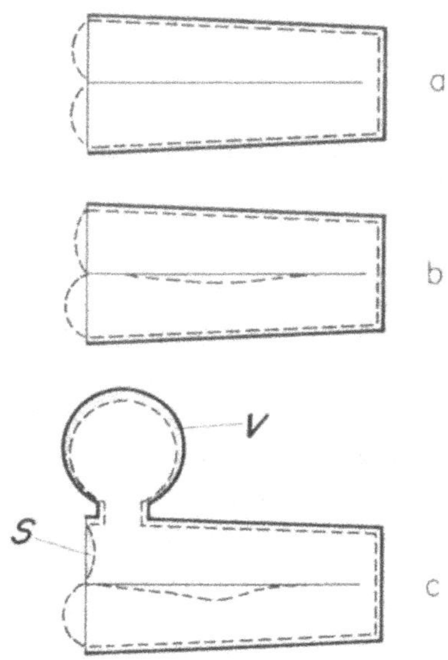

Fig. 2. Compressional mode of bone conduction, according to HERZOG and KRAINZ; for explanation see text. (From BÉKÉSY, 1932)

In order to respond properly to bone-conduction signals, then, the cochlea, according to HERZOG and KRAINZ, requires its perilymphatic scalae to be of unequal volume and its windows of unequal compliance, although, obviously, only the round window needs to be mobile.

First doubts about the correctness of the HERZOG-KRAINZ hypothesis were raised on account of the following observation: HOUSE (1959), while following a number of clinical patients with otosclerosis of long standing, noted that in some of the cases losses, both for air and for bone conduction, gradually accumulated with time and eventually became quite severe. Reasoning that severe reductions of bone conduction responses is precisely what ought to happen according to HERZOG and KRAINZ, when both windows are becoming occluded, HOUSE opened some of these ears surgically. He was able to confirm his diagnosis, but failed to restore hearing, either for air or for bone, by remobilizing the two windows. Most likely, these ears had been functionally dead for some time, and it appeared that the bone conduction losses observed could not be explained in terms of the HERZOG and KRAINZ concept.

1. Experimental Occlusion of the Cochlear Windows

The question remained as to the effects of simultaneous occlusion of both cochlear windows on bone-conduction responses. Before this question could be studied in experimental animals (cats), it was first necessary to find a reliable way of sealing the cochlear windows by experimental means (TONNDORF and TABOR, 1962; TONNDORF *et al.*, 1966a). The need for such preliminary exploration had become evident from the widely divergent results obtained by a number of previous authors on the effects of experimental occlusion of the *round* window. According to a list compiled by GISSELSON and RICHTER (1955), 12 out of 25 writers reported cochlear responses to diminish, 9 others found improvements, and the remaining 12 saw no changes. Obviously, the quality of the seals achieved must have varied widely between experimenters and, perhaps with some of them, even from one experiment to the next one.

Experimental method — In our own study, the problem of sealing the cochlear windows was eventually solved in the following manner — so that results became consistent from animal to animal (Fig. 3): First, the round window niche was filled with high-viscosity silicone, its advantages being that it is chemically inert,

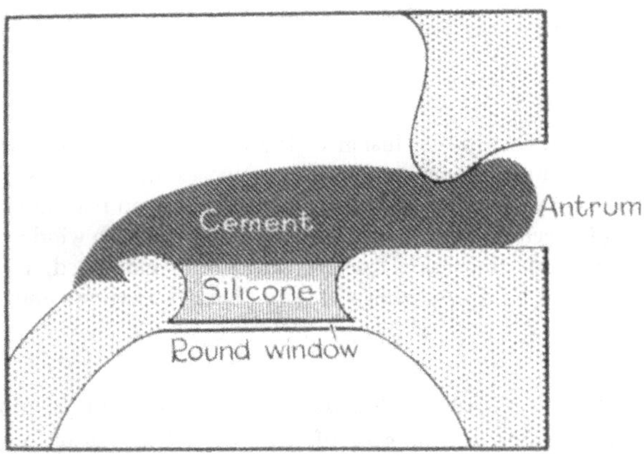

Fig. 3. Experimental method for occlusion of the round window in cats; for details reference is made to the original paper. (From TONNDORF and TABOR, 1962)

and that it permits visualization of air bubbles, which must be eliminated if a proper seal is to be achieved. Then, several undercuts were made into the promontory so as to provide a firm hold for the layer of dental cement by which the niche was eventually capped over. In the case of the round window, such seals could be applied and subsequently removed again, several times in succession, each time restoring full mobility of the membrane, as judged by the return to pre-occlusion responses. The oval window was occluded in a similar manner, the only difference being that its seal could not be removed again without interruption of the ossicular chain and fracture of the stapes footplate.

Bone conduction losses due to window occlusion — Figure 4 shows losses in bone conduction responses, in terms of changes in cochlear microphonics, induced by experimental occlusion of the round window alone, the oval window alone, or both windows simultaneously.

The round window curve possessed a negative slope with frequency. — It ought to be mentioned also that good-quality seals invariably produced losses, not only for bone, but also for air (not shown in Fig. 4). However, when air bubbles, even small ones, were deliberately left in the round-window niche, air-conduction responses showed small *gains*, up to a maximum of 6 dB, but limited to a narrow portion of the audio-frequency range; this was obviously due to resonances of the entrapped air bubbles and had been predicted by WEVER and LAWRENCE (1954).

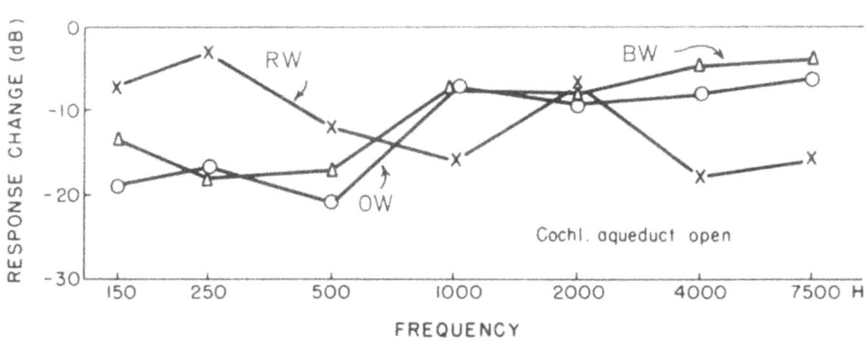

Fig. 4. Effects of the experimental occlusion of the round window, oval window, and both windows simultaneously upon bone conduction responses in cats: Cochlear microphonic response shifts *vs* frequency; cochlear aqueduct open. There is no real difference between the two curves pertaining to occlusion of the oval window alone and both windows simultaneously. In these early experiments, zinc-oxide cement, which was employed, produced relatively severe response changes (cf. Curve *B* of Fig. 12). (From TONNDORF and TABOR, 1962)

The loss curves for the other conditions showed positive slopes. However, none of the losses obtained under any of the three conditions were very severe. Most importantly from the standpoint of the present problem, the losses upon the simultaneous occlusion of both windows never exceded those produced by occluding the oval window alone (Fig. 4).

A finding by GROEN and HOOGLAND (1958) provided the needed next clue. These authors had seen a patient with an otosclerotic occlusion of the round window. The audiogram had revealed a small loss and the curve displayed a negative slope with frequency, very much like the round-window curve of Fig. 4. GROEN and HOOGLAND reasoned that in such cases the cochlear aqueduct, whose opening in *scala tympani* is close to the round window, might act as a bypass. The aqueduct is a narrow tube, and frictional resistance in such tubes varies with flow velocity — or with frequency in the case of ac signals, hence the negative slope of the audiometric curve.

Cochlear aqueduct effect — Figure 5 shows the results of the same three occlusion experiments as those of Fig. 4, but this time carried out after the cochlear aqueduct had been experimentally sealed beforehand. The slope of the *round-window curve* had changed, mainly because of increased losses at low frequencies which, obviously could no longer benefit from the bypass. Thus, the original hypothesis of Groen and Hoogland was confirmed. The findings also support a notion of Ranke (1953) who held that the various communications between the cochlea and the endocranial space (both aqueducts and the sum total of all perineural and perivascular spaces) might affect bone conduction — something to which he applied the term "*third-window*" *effect*.

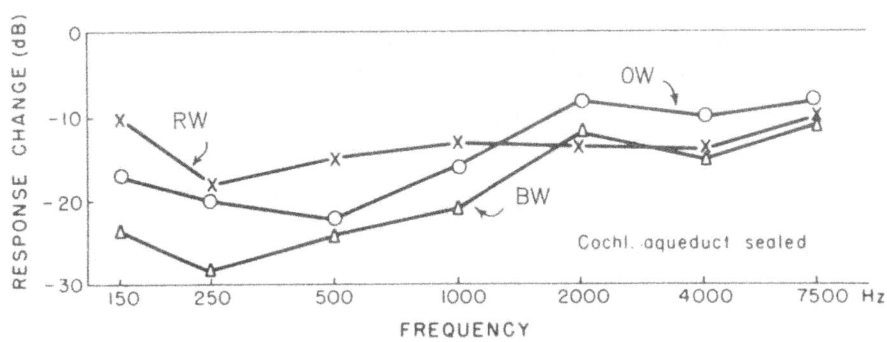

Fig. 5. Same experiments as Fig. 4, but after sealing off the cochlear aqueduct. In comparison to Fig. 4, note the change in slope of the round-window curve and also the clear separation between the curves pertaining to the occlusion of oval window alone and both windows simultaneously. (From Tonndorf and Tabor, 1962)

Since this point will become important later on (*cf.* Section II A 2b), it must be noted that there was never a change in the response for *air conduction* when the cochlear aqueduct was sealed and the round window occluded (not shown in Figs. 4 and 5).

When compared to the results of Fig. 4, the *oval-window curve* had not changed. However, when both windows were occluded simultaneously, bone-conduction losses now exceeded consistently those produced by occlusion of the oval window alone. In the earlier experiments (Fig. 4), the bypass throught the cochlear aqueduct had evidently obscured this effect. Nevertheless, its small magnitude is clearly at variance with the Herzog and Krainz concept. One might argue at this point that sealing off the vestibular aqueduct (which might technically be feasible) and all perineural and perivascular channels leading into the cochlea (which is hardly feasible), in other words the occlusion of the entire "third window" of Ranke, should render more pronounced losses to bring them in line with the concept of Herzog and Krainz. Be that as it may, such a procedure would not be compatible with the survival of the organ of Corti, and there would be no microphonic responses left to be measured.

2. Model Experiments: Distortional Vibrations

It was for the reasons given above that the next experiments were conducted using a mechanical cochlear model that was made so as to have no openings whatsoever (Tonndorf, 1962). When its shell was being driven by sinusoidal vibratory signals, the partition of this model displayed typical traveling-wave patterns, although of rather low amplitudes. These traveling waves appeared but under one condition: only if the two perilymphatic scalae were not equal to each other in crossectional area, *i. e.*, in volume.

Since there were no windows, a different mechanism had to exist providing the necessary yield for the incompressible cochlear fluids. To study this mechanism, drops of liquid immiscible with water were placed at points proximal to the elastic partition, *i. e.*, at places where the yield of the partition would not complicate matters unnecessarily. Initially, mercury was used for this purpose. Since it was feared that this material might be subject to inertial forces, it was later replaced by a special, light-weight oil. The latter oil, although not mixing with water, has almost the same specific gravity as water so that, for all intents and purposes, the oil drops floated in the perilymphatic fluids, thus minimizing inertial effects.

Figure 6 illustrates the reaction of the oil drops to vibrations of the cochlear shell. While, by definition, preserving their volume, they changed their *shape* in synchrony with the applied signal, a mode known as *distortional vibrations*.

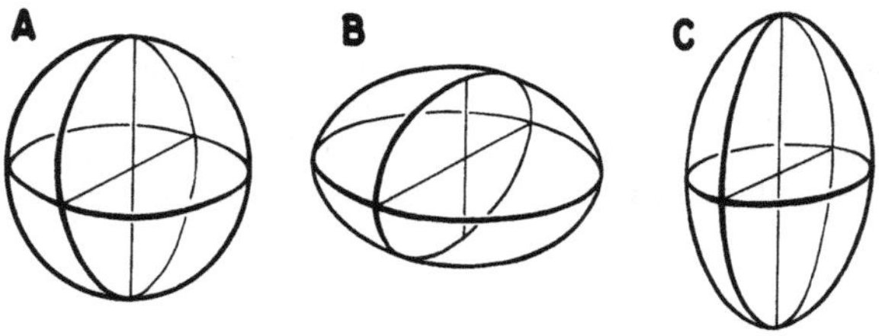

Fig. 6. Distortional vibrations of a spherical body. The vibratory sequence is A-B-A-C-A, etc. (From TONNDORF, 1962)

Although this type of vibration is by no means limited to fluid-filled shells, their internal plasticity aids its occurrence. Depending upon the particular shape of a given body or shell, distortional vibrations may become quite complicated. Hence, the simple-mode vibrations of Fig. 6, executed by the fluid drops within an unrolled cochlear model, should only be taken as indicating the *type* of vibrations the shell of a real cochlea might be undergoing. They do not demonstrate the exact mode which, in all likelihood, is much more complicated. Nevertheless, further considerations of Fig. 6 will indicate why displacements of the partition occured only when the perilymphatic scalae were unequal in volume. Suppose the vibrating sphere of Fig. 6 were divided into two *symmetrical* compartments by a partition placed exactly at its equator; in that case, the volume ratio of the two compartments would remain unaltered during an entire vibratory cycle, and the partition would stay at rest, quite similar to the situation of Fig. 2a.

If, however, the partition would be placed so as to divide the sphere into two *asymmetrical* compartments, which thus have unequal volumes, their volume ratio should change in a push-pull manner during a vibratory cycle as is schematically shown in Fig. 7. Moreover, if the shell is allowed to stretch slightly at the points corresponding to Figs. 7b and c, as theory permits, the total volume enclosed by the shell may be preserved at all times during the entire cycle, even though the shell possesses no openings whatsoever. Such an arrangement would then lead to appropriate displacements of the partition as was indeed observed in the model experiments.

The suggestion that a real cochlea might undergo the same kind of distortional vibrations as found in the model experiments is supported by several observations.

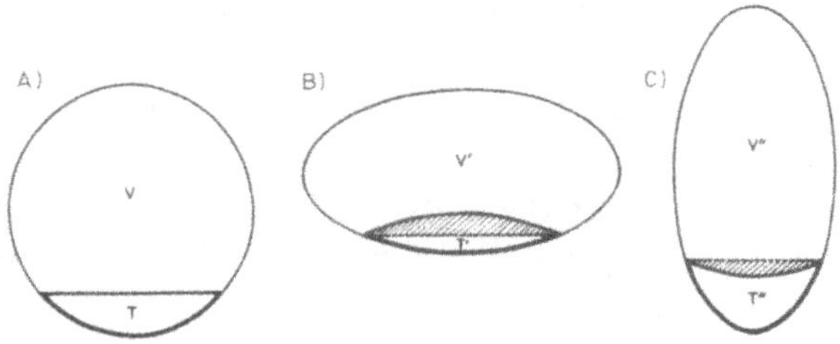

Fig. 7. Displacement of the cochlear partition, when placed in an asymmetrical position, in response to distortional vibrations of the cochlear shell (cross-section). The difference in cross-sectional area between the two perilymphatic scalae has been overstated for the sake of illustration. Vibratory sequence as in Fig. 6. Note that the upward displacement of the partition in graph (b) is larger than the downward displacement in graph (c). (From Tonndorf, 1962)

(a) *Second-harmonic distortion* — As may be noted from Fig. 7, the displacements of the cochlear partition toward the larger compartment (Fig. 7b) were higher in amplitude than those in the opposite direction (Fig. 7c). Such asymmetrical displacement is a direct corollary of the structural asymmetry, as simple considerations will indicate. It was actually observed in the model experiments, once its mechanism was properly understood. It represents an even-harmonic distortion.

Recently, Khanna and the present author (Khanna *et al.*, 1972) had occasion to perform air-bone cancellation experiments in the manner of Békésy (1932). As soon as cancellation was achieved, and provided that sensation levels due to either signal when presented individually exceeded 50 dB, the subject reported hearing the second harmonic very clearly. At such a level, neither tranducer showed any distortion in its output, nor could aural overload have occurred. This observation suggests that it was the asymmetrical displacement of the partition, in the sense of Fig. 7b and c, that caused the appearance of the second harmonic, and, by the same token, the explanation of the occurrence of distortional vibrations in the cochlea is supported.

(b) *Patency of the cochlear aqueduct* — As was already mentioned in connection with Fig. 5, the cochlear aqueduct acted as a round-window bypass only for bone conducted signals, but not for air-conducted signals. This finding indicates that, when the ear is receiving air-conducted signals, the cochlear capsule, which is penetrated by the aqueduct, remains rigid, and consequently, the aqueduct is not patent for ac signals. When, however, bone-conducted signals are applied to the skull, the aqueduct is periodically opened: this can only be brought about when its capsule undergoes distortional vibrations.

(c) *Distortional vibrations in temporal-bone specimens* — In an attempt to assess bone-conduction responses of isolated middle ears in temporal-bone specimens of cat (TONNDORF *et al.*, 1966d), displacements of the stapes footplate were measured by means of a capacitive probe applied via the widely opened internal auditory canal. [BÉKÉSY (1941) had first used this technique with air-conducted signals.] In spite of all efforts, it turned out to be impossible to fasten the probe to the specimen so that it recorded nothing but the relative displacement of the footplate. In fact, while tolerably small at low frequencies, displacements of the probe tip relative to the lateral vestibular walls surrounding the footplate increased with frequency at the rate of 12 dB/octave so that, at 5000 Hz, they became as large as the vibratory displacement of the specimen as a whole. Although this failure made it impossible to use the probe for the intended purpose, these findings indicated once more the occurrence of distortional vibrations within the temporal-bone specimen.

The model experiment, supported by the observations just described, strongly suggest that the cochlear capsule undergoes distortional vibrations in response to vibratory stimulation. (A fourth piece of supporting evidence will be mentioned later in Section IV 1.) In order that displacements of the partition be brought about, it is only required that it divides the perilymphatic space into two asymmetrical compartments, *i. e.*, that the volume of *scala vestibuli* is not equal to that of *scala tympani*. This, as recalled, was one of the two conditions postulated by HERZOG and KRAINZ (1926). Mobile windows, the other condition they had specified, are not a mandatory requirement. To describe this mode of direct cochlear response the term *distortional bone conduction* has been suggested (TONNDORF, 1968).

3. The Influence of the Cochlear Windows

The foregoing statement does not imply that the cochlear windows have no effect upon bone-conduction responses. Such a notion is clearly refuted by the results given in Figs. 4 and 5.

In order to illustrate the effects of mobile windows upon bone-conduction responses, Fig. 8 is presented. In this figure, the line of reference represents the situation in which both windows are occluded simultaneously. To avoid a round window bypass, the cochlear aqueduct was sealed beforehand. With the round window uncovered, as it were, there is a sizable improvement, especially of low-frequency responses. This latter gain is only being exceeded, at least at the two lowest frequencies, upon the additional removal of the stapes. When both windows are uncovered, but the stapes footplate is left intact, the gain is only moderate, but still bigger that than upon mobilizing the oval window alone.

These results indicate the following: (1) A mobile *round* window *aids* the distortional bone-conduction responses of the inner ear. Significantly, both factors were found to be *in-phase* with each other. (2) A mobile *oval* window with the footplate present acts as a *shunt* with respect to inner-ear bone-conduction responses, more so at low frequencies than at high ones for reasons explained in connection with Figs. 4 and 5. This latter view is supported (a) by the finding (Fig. 8) that, when only the round window was uncovered, the gain in bone-conduction responses was larger than when both of them were mobilized; (b) by the additional observation that the two factors, representing releases through the oval and round windows respectively, were in or near *phase opposition* with each other at most frequencies. (3) After stapedectomy, the cochlear fluids are only restrained by the round-window membrane, which is much more compliant than that of the oval window. [According to KIRIKAE (1960), the ratio in compliance between the two windows membranes is 1:20.] Apparently, such mobilization of the cochlear fluids produces quite a strong effect, completely overriding the shunt effect of the oval window.

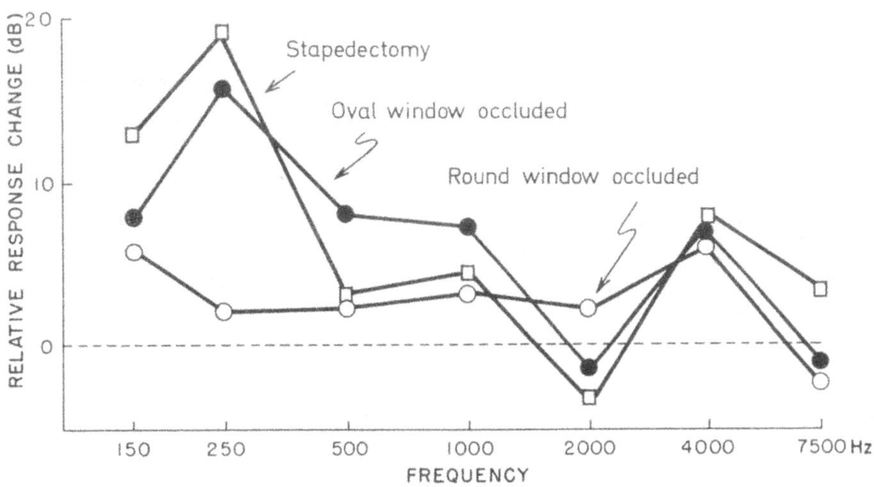

Fig. 8. Results of occlusion experiments as in Fig. 5, but presented in reference to the situation: both windows occluded simultaneously. The curves then depict response shifts *vs* frequency, when the round window, the oval window, or both windows simultaneously are re-opened, as it were, and no middle ear structures are present. (From TONNDORF *et al.*, 1966a)

Figure 8, thus, gives tangible evidence for the existence, at least at low frequencies, of an *inertial response* of the inner-ear fluids, an effect postulated earlier by WEVER and LAWRENCE (1954) and by KIRIKAE (1959). — Mobilizing the oval window alone was seen to result in a small improvement (Fig. 8). This finding is taken to indicate that the oval window might be the functional opposite of some openings on the other side of the partition belonging to the "third" window, an arrangement that will facilitate a small inertial response of the cochlear fluids.

The bone conduction responses of the inner ear are thus seen to be given primarily by the *distortional vibrations of the cochlear capsule* and, to a lesser extent, by the *moment of inertia of the cochlear fluids*. These basic responses are being modified by the yielding of the cochlear windows, *i. e.*, the oval, the round, and also the "third" window.

4. Bone Conduction and Cochlear Wave Travel

The question may be raised as to why there are traveling waves along the cochlear partition in response to distortional vibrations of its capsule. If these vibrations occur over the entire capsule, as indeed they do, it is not easy to see why the traveling waves must progress from base to apex — or why there should be any wave travel at all.

The answer to this question lies in cochlear mechanics. BÉKÉSY (1941, 1955) had originally shown in experiments on cochlear models that, no matter where one puts the cochlear openings wave travel occurs invariably from the stiffer, basal end of the partition, where the impedance is high, toward its more compliant, apical end, where the impedance is lower. The above question can thus be answered as follows: [This answer was first given by ZWISLOCKI (1953) in mathematical terms and, later, by TONNDORF (1962) in the present from.] The cochlea consists of a series of spatially distributed, low-pass filters. Their cut-off points decrease systematically from base to apex, a direct corollary of the stiffness gradient. Suppose a high-frequency signal is applied to the capsule in the region of the cochlear apex. Since its frequency is outside the pass-band of that section of the partition, it cannot directly procedure a displacement there. The signal must first find a filter section that includes its frequency, and that section must necessarily be located farther basally. Now, the part of the partition lying basalward from this point, the fluids on either side, and the two windows can undergo their characteristic displacements that are in phase opposition in the two perilymphatic scalae. The potential energy aquired by the cochlear partition by virtue of its displacement is then released in the form of wave travel toward places of lesser impedance, *i. e.*, toward the apex. Therefore, bone-conduction vibrations whose input is widely distributed over the cochlear capsule may lead to exactly the same kind of wave travel as a signal brought in by air conduction via the oval window. Otherwise, BÉKÉSY's cancellation experiments (1932) would not have succeeded.

B. Middle Ear Component

That the middle ear contributes to the bone-conduction responses of the entire ear was already mentioned. In an effort to elucidate its action, E. BÁRÁNY (1938) performed a series of experiments in human subjects, employing BÉKÉSY's (1932) bone/air cancellation technique. The responses he observed were elicited mainly by the *moment of inertia* of the ossicular system; this was, therefore, dubbed the *inertial mode or middle-ear bone conduction.*

1. Ossicular Inertia

Using the air-conduction signals of each bone/air pair as reference, BÁRÁNY mapped the bone-conduction responses in terms of relative amplitudes and phases of the applied signal for various locations about the head. In order to keep the situation as simple as possible, he employed but one low frequency (435 Hz) at which the skull is known to vibrate in its lowest mode, *i. e.*, to move simply to and fro in relation to the point of input (*cf.* Section IV). By means of this technique, BÁRÁNY found bone-conduction responses to be minimal for inputs along the sagital midline ("line of indifference") and to be maximal for inputs from either side of the head; in the latter two cases, bone-conduction signals received by one and the same ear, but applied to either side of the head, were found to be approximately in phase opposition to each other.

These and other, additional, findings permitted formulation of the following concept (Fig. 9): The major middle-ear ossicles, malleus and incus, may be considered to constitute a pendulum whose support is being vibrated. Such a pendulum would be unable to respond when its moment of inertia were zero, *i. e.*, as long as its mass center would lie directly on the axis of rotation (Fig. 9d). Neither could it respond to vibrations applied in its own plane (Fig. 9c) or that parallel to the axis of rotation, *i. e.*, along the "line of indifference". The pendulum responds maximally to inputs perpendicular to its axis of rotation. It matters little whether it is in its labile configuration (Fig. 9a) or in its stabile one (Fig. 9b), as long as there exists some moment of inertia.

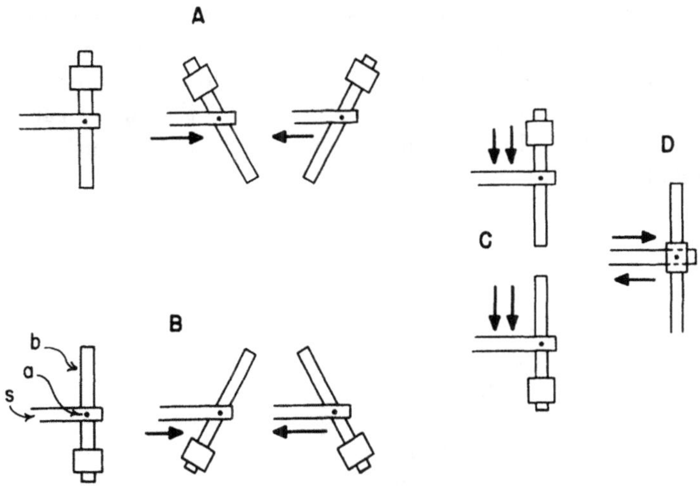

Fig. 9. The concept of ossicular, inertial, bone conduction. (From BÁRÁNY, 1938)

The pendulum concept presupposed that the major ossicles, malleus and incus, rotate around a common axis, running in an anteroposterior direction, specifically from the anterior mallar ligament to the incudal ligament, and, in doing so, move in phase with each other; that is to say, the incudo-mallar joint must essentially be immobile. In BÁRÁNY's opinion, the mass center of the ossicular chain lies below the axis of rotation, but only by a small amount so that its moment of inertia is relatively small. There were slight, but systematic deviations of BÁRÁNY's experimental findings from what should ideally be expected: *i. e.*, responses were not zero for inputs along the "line of indifference", nor were they exactly 180° out of phase with each for inputs to either side of the head. These deviations may be accounted for by the fact that the results had been "contamined" by inner-ear responses which, after all, cannot be eliminated experimentally.

(a) *Loading of the tympanic membrane* — BÁRÁNY's concept is further supported by the finding, first demonstrated by his own father, R. BÁRÁNY (1910), and later confirmed by a number of others (*e. g.*, KIRAKAE, 1959; ALLEN and FERNANDEZ, 1960; a. o.), *i. e.*, that bone-conduction responses can be modified by loading the tympanic membrane. Small weights (drops of mercury) placed at the umbo improve bone-conduction responses to low frequencies, while decreasing those to high frequencies. In an effort to study this phenomenon further, loading experiments were conducted in four different animal species: cat, dog, guinea pig, and rat (TONNDORF *et al.*, 1966b). Once again, cochlear microphonics were employed as indicator of the induced response changes. Figure 10 gives an example of the results, indicating that in all four species changes are similar to one another and also to those subjectively measured in man. By the time these experiments were conducted, a number of factors contributing to the bone-conduction responses of the feline ear had been identified and qualitatively assessed (*cf.* Figs. 21—23, below), making it possible to account for the loading phenomenon in some detail.

The following considerations are based upon BÁRÁNY's original concept: A load placed upon the umbo should increase the moment of inertia of the affected system, and, at the same time, shift its resonance point towards lower frequencies. In this manner, responses to frequencies around and below the newly acquired resonance point would be improved, but those to higher frequencies lessened. At very high frequencies, at which the contribution of the middle ear component becomes insignificant (*cf.* Fig. 21), the loading effect should vanish as was borne out by the findings of Fig. 10.

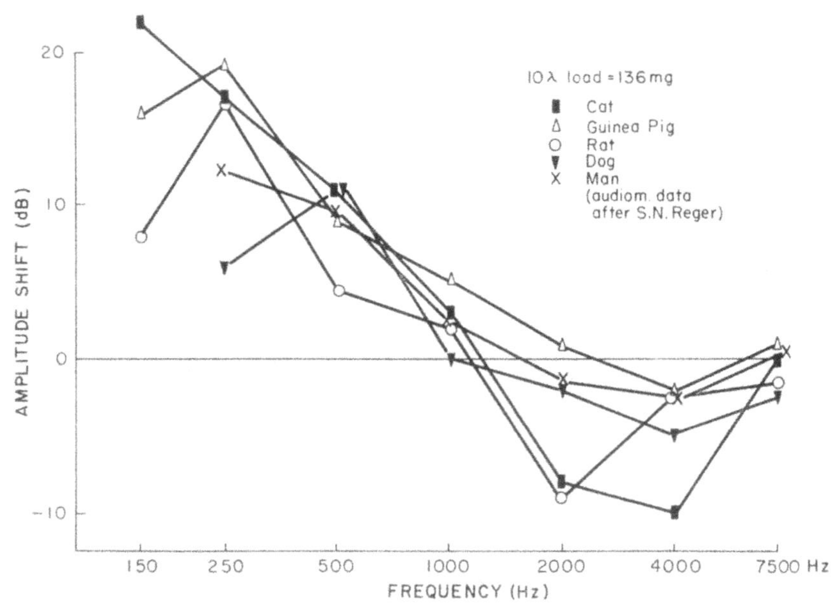

Fig. 10. Loading of the tympanic membrane; response shifts *vs* frequency at a load of 136 mg (10λ of mercury) in the four different animal species listed. The results of audiometric measurements obtained by Reger (unpublished data) for the same load condition are included for the sake of comparison. (From TONNDORF *et al.*, 1966b)

The system affected by placing a load on the umbo was identified as being composed of two inertial components, that of the ossicular chain and that of the inner ear fluids, and to include also the compliance of the air enclosed in the middle ear, the latter being part of its elastic restraint. That is to say, it was only for this combined system that the results fitted the above criteria. For the sake of clarity, Fig. 11 shows only the two extreme conditions of loading used in the actual experiments.

Inspection of Fig. 11 indicates the relationships between load and frequency shifts on the one hand and load and low-frequency gain on the other to be nonlinear. That is not surprising in view of the following facts: (a) The affected system is a composite of three separate factors, only one of which, ossicular inertia, is directly altered by the load; (b) the moment of inertia of the ossicular chain does not grow linearly with loads placed at the umbo, since the distance of the mass center from the axis of rotation approaches a fixed value as soon as it reaches the position of the umbo; and (c), for larger displacements, the restraint of the middle ear becomes nonlinear as the tympanic membrane is excessively stretched. In view of the above findings, it might be more appropriate to refer to the phenomenon as *loading of the ossicular chain*, instead of the tympanic membrane.

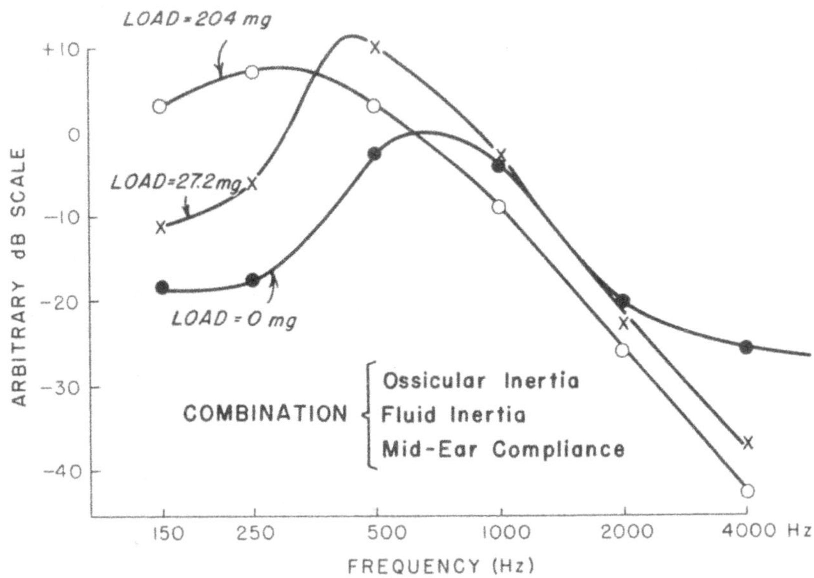

Fig. 11. Loading of the tympanic membrane. Bone conduction responses in dB (arbitrary reference) *vs* frequency calculated for a responding system consisting of the following bone-conduction components (cf. Figs. 21 and 22): (1) ossicular inertia; (2) inner-ear fluid inertia; and (3) middle-ear compliance. For the sake of clearer illustration only the zero-load condition as well as the smallest (27.2 mg) and the largest (204 mg) of a total of four loads actually used in the present experiments are shown. (From Tonndorf *et al.*, 1966b)

(b) *Location of the center of gravity of the major ossicles* — As was just mentioned, Bárány placed the mass center of the ossicles slightly *below* the axis of rotation. Kirikae (1960), however, using stroboscopic observations in human cadaver specimen, found this axis to run somewhat lower than usually thought. The conclusion of his findings was that the ossicular mass center lies slightly *above* that axis. On first sight, the loading experiments seem to support Bárány's viewpoint, since the low-frequency gain was found to rise as a monotonic function of the load. The smallest load that was usually employed in such experiments, including our own, was 27.2 mg (equal to 10 λ of mercury). However, such a load may be too large and thus might have missed proving KIRIKAE's contention. This notion is supported by an accidental finding that must be related here.

The bone-conduction losses following experimental occlusions of the cochlear windows, presented in Figs. 4 and 5, had only been attained after a lengthy period of trial and error. Figure 12 shows how the degree of loss had changed as the quality of the oval-window seal was being improved in several steps (TONNDORF and TABOR, 1962; TONNDORF *et al.*, 1966a). First attempts had led to relatively large losses (Curve *A* of Fig. 12). However, on subsequent inspection, there had hardly been a seal at all; only a lump of cement had been found to be deposited on the stapes superstructure. When the quality of the seal was gradually improved, the degree of loss actually decreased (Curves *B* and *C* of Fig. 12). It ought to be noted, however, that a really firm seal (Curve *C* of Fig. 12) produced about the same degree of loss as that achieved by a much simpler technique: SMITH (1943) had also carried out bone conducted experiments in cats. He "immobilized" the stapes by slinging a thin thread through the obturator foramen and around one crus, and then pulling the stapes firmly against the promontory. His results are also included in Fig. 12.

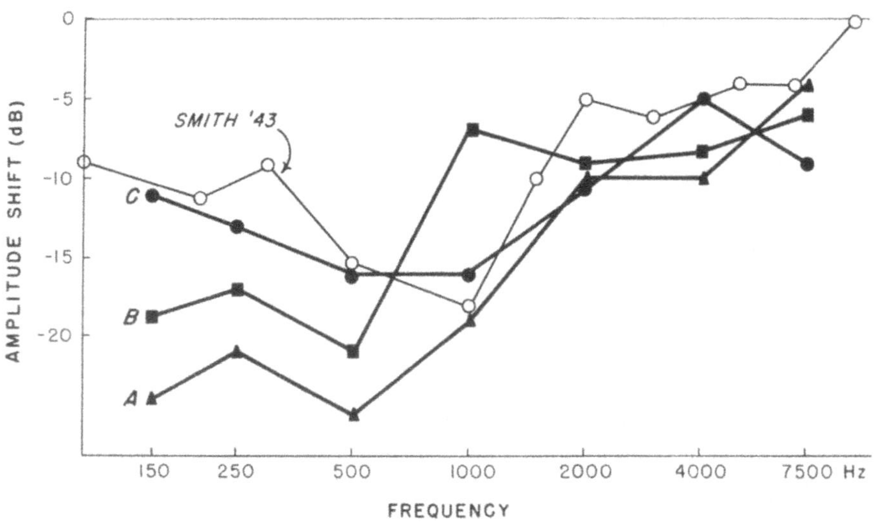

Fig. 12. Experimental occlusion of the oval window in cats: bone conduction response shifts *vs* frequency. The sequence of the three heavy Curves, *A* to *C*, demonstrates the lessening of such losses as the degree of occlusion was improved. Curve *A*: poor adhesion of cement (zinc oxide) to surrounding bone; large lump of cement deposited on the stapes superstructure; Curve *B*: improved adhesion, owing to complete removal of muco-periosteum from stapes and window area, and thorough drying of bone before cement application (zinc oxide); Curve *C*: best adhesion (acrylic cement); application as under *B*. For the sake of comparison, the results of an experiment by SMITH (1943) are included. In his experiment, the stapes was "immobilized" by passing a thin string through the obturator foramen and around one crus and then pulling the stapes firmly against the promontory. (From TONNDORF, 1964)

It was thus seen that a good-quality seal of the oval window, or a "massless immobilization" of the stapes, produced lesser bone conduction losses than a small load placed on the stapes that was not really immobilized. Moreover, this small load of approximately 2—3 mg was acting upon the shorter arm of the ossicular lever, making its effect even less than those of the larger loads that were used in the loading experiments (27.2 mg up to 204 mg), and that were acting upon the umbo, *i. e.*, on the longer arm of the ossicular lever. The fact that such very small loads produced bone-conduction *losses*, whereas larger ones produce *gains*, is in favor of KIRIKAE's notion. That is to say, small loads apparently pull the mass center of the ossicles down towards the rotational axis, thus reducing the moment of ossicular inertia, and minimizing the contribution of the middle-ear component to the total bone-conduction responses. [Significantly, the effect was limited to the frequency range in which the middle-ear component is dominant (*cf.* Fig. 21 later)]. However, when the mass center is shifted farther to points below the rotational axis by application of larger loads, the moment of ossicular inertia increases once more in some proportion to the degree of loading, and so must the contribution of the middle-ear component to the total bone-conduction response.

2. Compliance of the Air Enclosed in the Middle Ear

Listed above among the factors affected by ossicular loading was the compliance of the air enclosed in the middle ear. That this factor plays a role in bone-conduction responses was first recognized by GROEN (1962) who calculated its effect for the case of the human ear and differentiated its action upon the tympanic membrane from that upon the round-window membrane. GROENS's concept was confirmed in our own bone conduction experiments (TONNDORF *et al.*, 1966a) which demonstrated that the bone-conduction responses are concistently more sensitive when the bulla is open than when it is closed. [Incidently, it was known for some time that air-conduction responses are affected in the same manner (BÉKÉSY, 1941).] By repeating the bulla open/bulla closed experiments with the round window occluded, it became possible to separate the (stronger) effect upon the tympanic membrane from the (lesser) one upon the round-window membrane. As GROEN had already stated, the effect upon the tympanic membrane is the stronger of the two because its area is larger than that of the round-window membrane.

It is quite conceivable, although I have no clinical data to back up this statement, that bone-conduction responses in the presence of tympanic membrane perforations show a slight relative improvement. The "lost-baffle effect" so prominent in air-conduction responses (MCARDLE and TONNDORF, 1968) does not apply here, since, in the case of bone conduction, the tympanic membrane does not act as the receptor of energy.

3. Carhart's Notch

In man, stapedial fixation produces bone-conduction losses of about 15 dB maximally, centered around 2000 Hz, the well-known Carhart's notch. In our cat experiments (*cf.* Figs. 4 and 5), bone-conduction losses following experimental fixation of the stapes were somewhat more severe, about 22 dB maximally, and centered around 600 Hz. This discrepancy prompted us to study the changes in bone-conduction responses due to the experimental fixation of the tympanic membrane as well as to the amputation of the middle ear in the same four species already used in the loading experiments: cat, dog, guinea pig, and rat (TONNDORF, *et al.*, 1966c). Fixation of the tympanic membrane was carried out in lieu of stapedial fixation as the latter procedure could not be executed with consistent reliability in guinea pigs and rats. Figure 13 presents the findings after middle-ear amputation. The resultant losses were most severe in the guinea pig and least in the dog, the difference amounting to about 20 dB at the frequency of maximal loss, which happens to be identical for the two species in question. The frequency value varied also with the species, being lowest in the cat (600 Hz) and highest in the rat (2000 Hz). Fixation of the tympanic membrane produced similar variations among the four species, exept that the notch of the loss curve was much broader, and that, quantitatively, the losses were slightly less than those after middle-ear amputation.

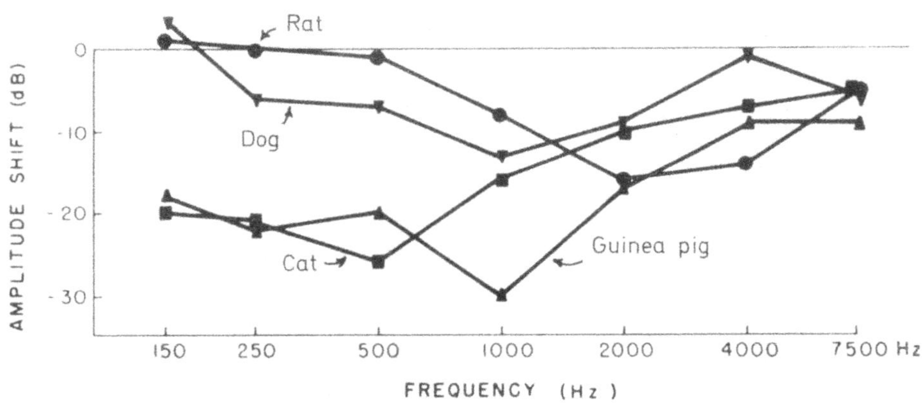

Fig. 13. Amputation of the middle ear in cat, dog, guinea pig, and rat: bone conduction response shifts *vs* frequency. (From TONNDORF *et al.*, 1966c)

For reasons that will be given later (Section III), one cannot directly equate the losses shown in Fig. 13 with the middle ear component of bone conduction. Nevertheless, the losses reflect that component sufficiently well to permit a gross comparison between species.

It is clear, then, that the contribution of the middle ear to the total bone conduction response varies to a considerable degree among animals. Recognition of this fact allows us now to explain the mechanism underlying the phenomemon of Carhart's notch. At the time CARHART first observed it in patients with stapedical fixation (1950), it seemed difficult to associate the relatively high frequency at which the loss happened to be maximal (2000 Hz) with the elimination of the middle-ear component of bone conduction. The term "inertial" bone conduction had apparently misled most people into believing that the effectiveness of the middle-ear component should be highest at very low frequencies and decrease as frequency goes higher, a notion KIRIKAE (1959) once expressed graphically (*l. c.* Fig. 72). However, as Fig. 11 had already indicated, the middle ear is a tuned system and as such has a resonant point. (This will be more definitely shown in Fig. 21.) There is no reason why this resonant point could not be as high as 2000 Hz, as implied by the configuration of Carhart's notch in man. In fact, in one of the animals tested in our study, the rat, it was equally high in frequency, although lower in others.

Carhart's notch, as observed in stapedial fixation is thus seen to be due to the elimination of the middle-ear component of bone conduction. The remaining response represents that of the inner ear with the oval window occluded.

Clinicians have repeatedly made the statement that, in man, there is no loss of bone conduction following amputation of the middle ear. This is contrary to our observations in experimental animals (*cf.* Fig. 13). The negative clinicals results may have several causes. In some cases, measurements were said to have been carried out directly on the operating table, which is not a very reliable method considering the patient's general condition. In other cases, the audiometric tests might have been done too late after surgery, *i. e.*, after scars in the oval-window niche had partially immobilized the stapes footplate, thus minimizing oval-window leakage. At any rate, a number of bone-conduction tests were performed at my request in this institution by Mr. A. Wolfe. The tests were done at the time when the surgical packs were first removed from the ear — on the sixth post-operative day in our cases. Bone-conduction losses showed the same configuration as found in Carhart's notch, except they were slightly more severe. Clearly, the elimination of the middle-ear component of bone conduction was aggravated by the oval-window leakage, as was already mentioned.

Fixation of malleus or tympanic membrane — It has been stated, in connection with Fig. 13, that fixation of the tympanic membrane produces bone-conduction losses that are slightly less than those following amputation of the middle ear, but that the notch of the resulting curves is much broader under this condition. According to Goodhill (personal communication, 1968), tympano-sclerosis with mallar fixation, a comparable condition, produces essentially similar audiograms in human patients, that is to say, the audiometric curves stay flat and fail to rise at 4000 Hz.

In the guinea pig, the difference in bone-conduction losses between the two conditions, middle-ear amputation and tympanicmembrane fixation, was rather small compared to the three other species. The guinea pig does not possess an incudo-mallar joint. These two facts may provide a clue for the explanation of the loss following tympanic-membrane fixation. It stands to reason that in the animals possessing an incudo-mallar joint, man probably included, some slippage may occur in this joint, permitting an inertial response of the incus. In other words, tympanic-membrane fixation may then lead only to a partial elimination of the middle-ear response.

4. The Resonance Point of the Middle Ear

The question may be raised as to why the resonant point of the feline middle ear, as seen by bone conduction, is as low as 600 Hz. It is a well-established fact that, when seen by air conduction, it is about one octave higher, *i. e.*, 1000 —1200 Hz. As shown in detail elsewhere (Tonndorf *et al.*, 1966c), the mechanical circuit of the middle ear looks different for air and bone inputs. In the first case, the tympanic membrane serves as the coupler, *i. e.*, the receptor of the incoming energy; in the second case, this task is taken over by the ossicular chain, the tympanic membrane then merely acting as a back spring. It is quite conceivable, therefore, that bone-conducted sounds see mainly the resonant point of the ossicular chain, 600 Hz in the cat, whereas air-conduction sounds see that of the tympanic membrane, 1000—1200 Hz in the cat. In man, the differences are less pronounced; presumably, the two resonant points are closer to each other.

5. Middle-Ear Bone Conduction Component

In has been shown in this section that the bone-conduction response of the middle ear is primarily given by the moment of inertia of the major ossicles, malleus and incus, as originally suggested by E. BÁRÁNY. This response is being modified by the compliance of the air enclosed in the middle ear. The responses remaining after elimination of the middle ear are determined by the state of the inner ear, *i. e.*, not only by the precense or absence of sensorineural hearing losses, but also by the mobility of its windows.

C. External-Ear Component

The notion that the external ear canal might contribute to the total bone-conduction responses in a manner similar to those of middle and inner ears was first expressed by TONNDORF (1964) and by TONNDORF *et al.* (1966e). However, the phenomenon, whose analysis had led to this suggestion, the *occlusion of effect of the external ear canal*, had been known for a much longer period of time. Clinically, it is referred to as the test of BING (1891), although it was first described by WHEATSTONE (1827) in some detail and also observed by WEBER (1834)[2].

1. Occlusion Effect

Suppose a normal-hearing subject is listening to a bone-conducted signal, preferably at a frequency below 1000 Hz. He will report perceiving a single image located in the middle of his head, regardless of whether the point of input is on the forehead or on one of his mastoids. If one ear canal is now occluded by insertion of a finger, firm pressure on the tragus, or by covering it over by an earphone, the subject will report the image to be *lateralized* to the side of the occluded ear. This phenomenon has formed the basis of a great number of theoretical considerations on bone conduction.

Canal resonances (Rinne/Huizing) — RINNE (1855) expressed the opinion that the lateralization might be due to increased loudness in the occluded ear, and that this in turn could be caused by altered canal resonances. As is well known, the resonance point of an air column within a given tube is different when it is open and when it is closed. RINNE's notion was recently revived by HUIZING (1960).

[2] In German-speaking countries, the term: BING test, is rarely, if ever, used. More often and correctly so, it is simply called the "physiological WEBER test" to distinguish it from its pathological counterpart which is of course utilized for the differentiation of conductive impairments from sensorineural ones.

Cochlear "outflow" (Mach) — The explanation that was most widely accepted for the longest period of time was due to MACH (1863), his so called "Outflow theory". He reasoned as follows: If the middle ear serves as an impendance-matching device between the air of the ear canal and the fluids of the inner ear, it must do so equally well for an energy flow going in the opposite direction — an application of the Reciprocity Theorem of HELMHOLTZ. When, under such conditions, vibratory energy is brought into the cochlea by the osseous route, some of it must escape, *i. e.*, "flow out", via the middle ear, unless it is prevented from doing so by blockage of this pathway. In the latter case, more energy will be retained in the cochlea, making the signal sound louder on that side and the image lateralized accordingly.

Masking (Dean, Hallpike, a. o.) — Another idea that must have been in the air for some time was concerned with the notion that, with the ear canal occluded, bone-conduction signals might be masked by air-borne sounds entering the cochlea via ear canal and middle ear. If one canal would then be occluded, masking should be minimized in that ear, the outcome being that bone-conducted signals would once more appear relatively louder in that ear, with subsequent lateralization to the same side. This notion was expressed independently, but practically simultaneously, by DEAN, HALLPIKE, and POHLMANN in 1930, and some time later by GUILD (1936).

Lower-jaw mechanism (Békésy) — BEKÉSY (1933) was the first to demonstrate that occlusion of an ear canal does indeed increase the loudness of a bone-conducted signal on that side, more so for low than for high frequencies (Fig. 14). The demonstrated variation with frequency, which, in this respect, grossly parallels the occlusion effect, argued convincingly for the fact that the lateralization is due to a difference in loudness between the two ears.

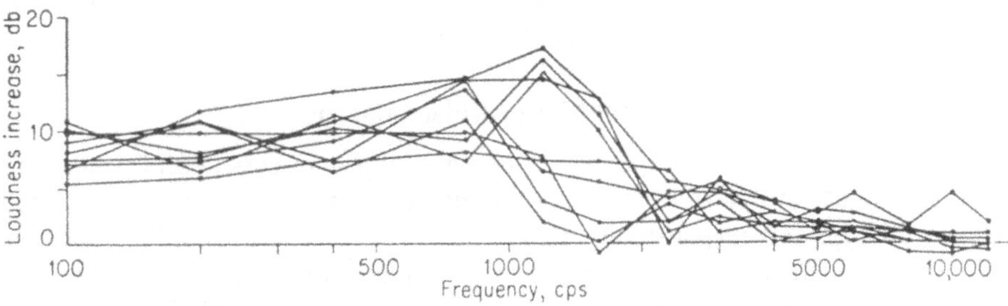

Fig. 14. The increase in loudness of bone-conducted signals following occlusion of one ear canal. (After BÉKÉSY, 1939)

BÉKÉSY (1941) then proceeded to present his own explanation of the phenomenon itself. Upon setting the skull into vibrations, he saw the lower jaw undergo the same vibrations, but, as its coupling to the skull is rather loose, at amplitudes and phases of its own. In this manner, a relative motion is being set up between the head of the mandible and the adjacent wall of the cartilagenous portion of the ear canal, the latter being forced to alter its shape in synchrony with the applied signal. Upon occlusion of the ear canal, the alternating changes in shape ought to create appropriate changes in volume, and hence, in pressure, of the enclosed air.

These pressure changes should in turn be transmitted to the cochlea via the middle ear in the manner of air-conducted signals. This concept is in line with the clinical experience that the occlusion effect cannot be elicited when middle-ear function is impaired. Moreover, when occluding the ear canal in its osseous portion, *i. e.*, beyond its compressible outer section, BÉKÉSY could no longer detect an occlusion effect, a finding that also appeared to support his concept.

The out-of-phase movement of skull and lower jaw was experimentally confirmed by FRANKE *et al.* (1952). Nevertheless, the overall validity of BÉKÉSY's concept was questioned by ALLEN and FERNANDEZ (1960) on the basis of the following observations: They saw two patients in whom the lower jaw had been surgically resected on one side. Yet, in both of these patients, the occlusion effect could be elicited at approximately equal magnitudes in either ear. Another such patient was observed by REGER (personal communication, 1962).

Phase-shift hypothesis (Groen) — LEGOUIX and TARAB (1959) had observed that the cochlear-microphonic responses to bone-conducted signals change their phases upon experimental impairment of middle-ear function. In line with these findings, GROEN (1962) argued that some forms of middle-ear pathology, if occurring unilaterally, ought to set up phase differences between the two ears, resulting in lateralization upon performance of the WEBER test. (As is well known, lateralization of an auditory image in a binaural situation may occur either on the basis of differences in *time or intensity* between the two ears.) In particular, GROEN employed this concept to account for the changes in direction of lateralization that he found to occur rather rapidly from one side to the other and back again as frequency was gradually raised beyond 1000 Hz, a range in which the Weber test is obviously of little, if any, clinical value.

In the following, we will first evaluate the older concepts and then proceed to offer a new explanation that has to do with the fact that, in its unoccluded state, the ear canal constitutes a *high-pass filter*.

2. Evaluation of Older Concepts

Masking — In our own experiments on this subject in cats (TONNDORF *et al.*, 1966d), we first established the fact that, upon occlusion of the ear canal, the cochlear-microphonic responses are affected in the same manner as the subjective response of human subjects (Fig. 15). This finding indicates that the phenomenon cannot depend upon masking as Dean, Hallpike, a. o. had suggested, since microphonic responses are not subject to masking.

Lower jaw mechanism — In cat, the animal used in our experinemts, the lower jaw and the cartilagenous ear canal are not in the same close proximity as they are in man. Moreover, resection of the mandibular capitulum and the entire ascending ramus did not affect the magnitude of the occlusion phenomenon. These findings were in agreement with the observations of ALLEN and FERNANDEZ (1960), indicating that the relative movements of the lower jaw described by BÉKÉSY (1941), although they constitute a real effect, cannot be wholly responsible for the occlusion phenomenon.

Cochlear "outflow" — The validity of Mach's "Outflow theory" had been questioned earlier on a variety of valid grounds (*e. g.*, by BÁRÁNY, 1938). We

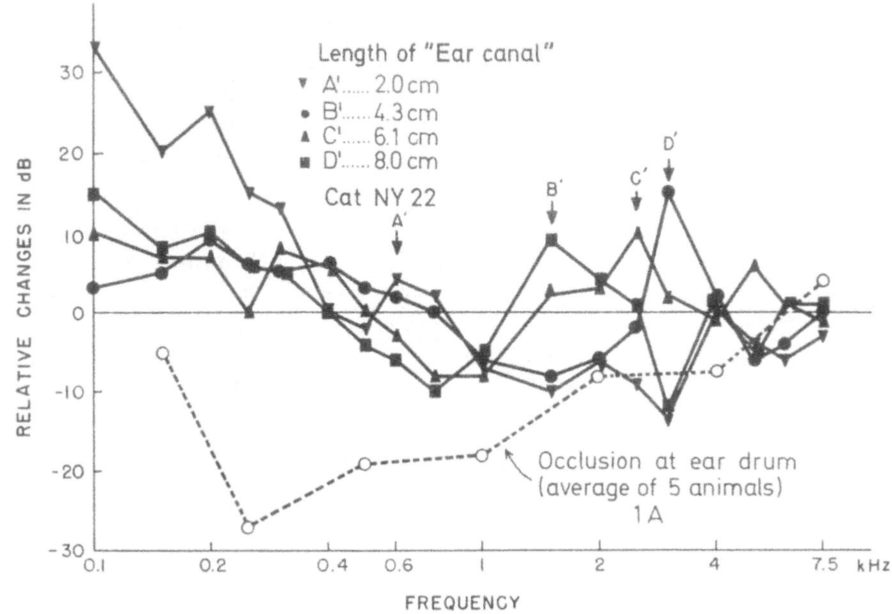

Fig. 15. Occlusion effects for ear canals of various lengths in a single animal: response shifts *vs* frequency. Ear canals of various lengths were fashioned from polyethylene tubing. Note that the occlusion effect was strongest for the shortest canal length. Note also the resonance points at various mid-frequencies for the different canal lengths. (Presenting averaged results from several animals would have smoothed out these resonance peaks). The dotted curve on the bottom gives the response shift observed when the occlusion was affected directly in front of the tympanic membrane, without allowing for any air space between the membrane and the occluding material. (From Tonndorf *et al.*, 1964)

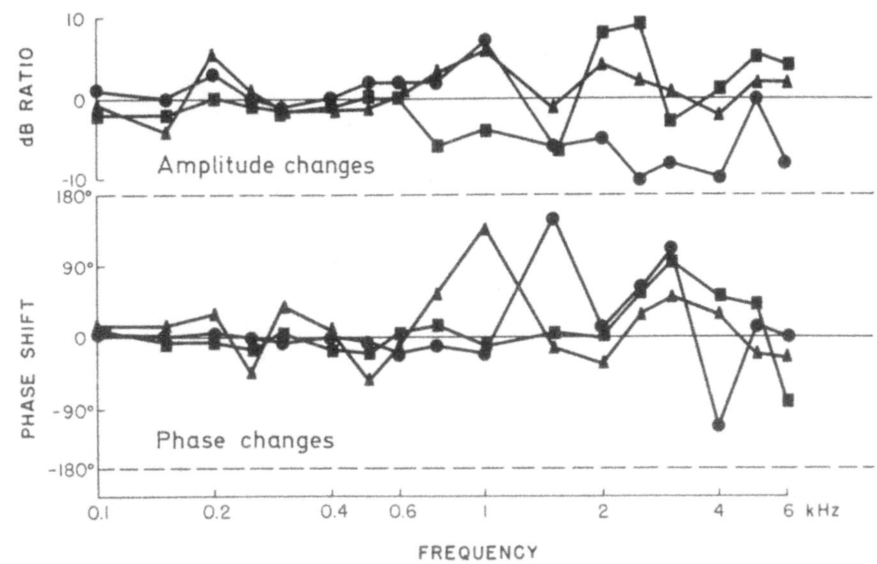

Fig. 16. Removal of the tympanic membrane: effect upon the sound pressure registered by a probe microphone in the external ear canal during bone conduction stimulation; changes in amplitude and in phase *vs* frequency. (From Tonndorf *et al.*, 1966e)

conducted an experiment designed to prove or disprove it directly. A probe microphone was placed into the ear canal to register the sound pressure produced there when bone-conducted signals were applied to the head. If this microphone would really receive an "outflow" from the inner ear, as many early experimenters had reasoned who had performed similar experiments, removal of the tympanic membrane, the tranducer involved in this process, should profoundly affect the microphone readings. In the range of interest, that is, for frequencies below 1 kHz, there were absolutely no changes after resection of the tympanic membrane (Fig. 16), *i. e.*, there was no evidence for any "outflow". Small changes observed at higher frequencies resulted from the fact that, for such frequencies, the size of the space the probe microphone is looking into becomes significant. Removal of the tympanic membrane had made this space considerably larger. The result of this experiment then disproves Mach's outflow theory.

Canal resonances — Figure 15 shows the occlusion effect for ear canals of four different lengths. When these lenghts were normalized for each signal frequency, in terms of its wavelength in air, the ensuing curves were found to form a maximum at $^1/_4\ \lambda$ and a minimum of $^1/_2\ \lambda$, with the canals unoccluded (Fig. 17a).

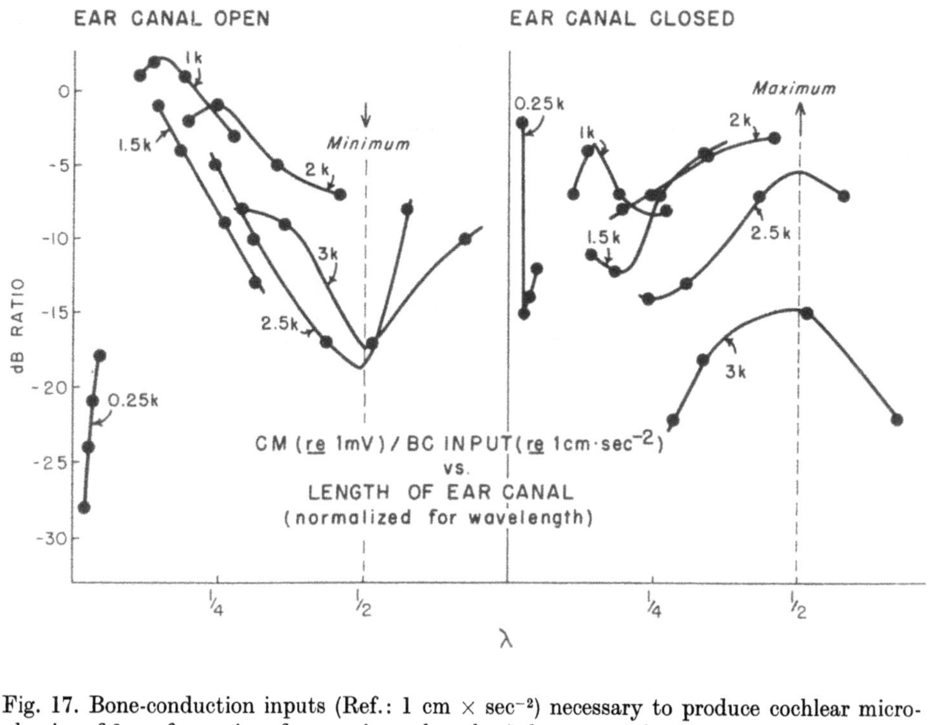

Fig. 17. Bone-conduction inputs (Ref.: 1 cm $\times$ sec^{-2}) necessary to produce cochlear microphonics of 1 μv for various frequencies *vs* length of the ear canal; results are normalized for wavelength in air. Left: ear canal open; right: ear canal occluded. For mid-frequency signals (given in kHz), the minima and maxima formed under two conditions reflect the resonances of tubes open on both ends (canal open) or closed on one end (canal occluded); that is to say, on account of the impedance matching of the middle ear, the tympanic membrane was transparent to the signal, as if the canal were open at its end. Note that, with the ear canal occluded, the low frequencies, for which only one example (250 kHz) is given, do not conform to the above rule. (From TONNDORF *et al.*, 1966e)

Upon their occlusion, maxima and minima changed places, the minima shifting to $^1/_4\,\lambda$ and the maxima to $^1/_2\,\lambda$ (Fig. 17b), exactly as theory predicts. However, these changes were limited to the mid-frequency range. The curves pertaining to low-frequency signals, *i. e.*, in the range of the actual occlusion effect, did not participate in the formation of the maxima and minima, especially with the canal occluded (Fig. 17b). The alteration of canal resonances upon occlusion of the ear canal, thus demonstrated, accounts only for the sharp peaks and dips that, as shown in Fig. 15, were occurring at different frequencies for each canal length. This may be considered a partial confirmation of the contention of RINNE (1855) and HUIZING (1960), although it does not account for the occlusion effect proper, the improvement of *low-frequency* responses.

3. High-Pass Filter Concept

First, some additional experimental findings must be reported. Their order of presentation was chosen so as to make a number of points in sequence.

Transmission of energy from the external canal into the cochlea — Provided the frequency response of the middle ear for bone conduction was taken into account, the cochlear microphonic voltages in response to bone-conduction signals, and at frequencies up to approximately 1500 Hz, were found to vary in the same manner as the sound pressure registered in the outer-ear canal (Fig. 18a). In particular,

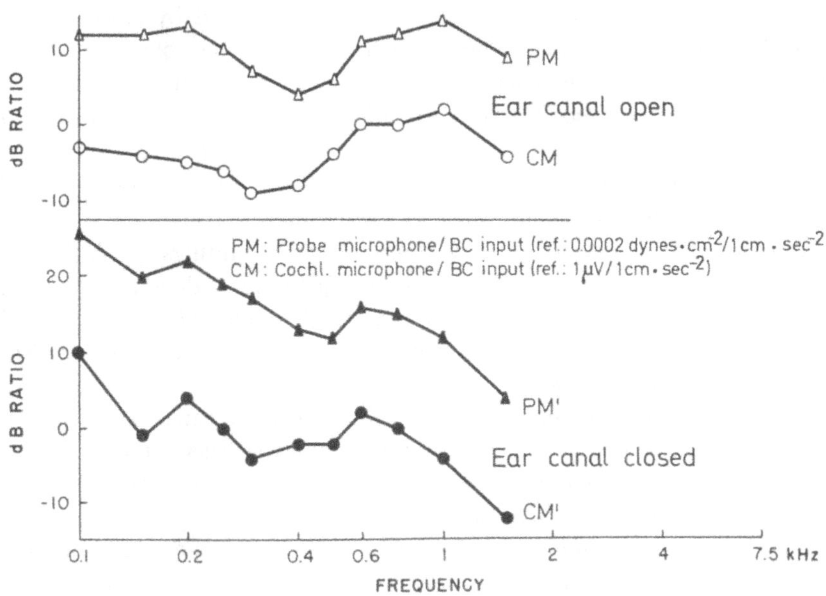

Fig. 18. Comparison between sound pressure registered in the external ear canal and cochlear-microphonic voltages in response to bone-conducted signals. Probe-microphone readings (in Ref. to 0.0002 dynes/cm^2) in the external ear canal and cochlear-microphonic voltages (in Ref. to 1 μv), both normalized for bone-conduction inputs of 1 cm $\times$ sec^{-2}. Furthermore, the cochlear-microphonic responses have been corrected for the bone-conduction response curve of the middle ear (cf. Fig. 23) which does, of course, not affect the microphone readings. Top: ear canal open; bottom: ear canal occluded. (From TONNDORF *et al.*, 1966e)

microphonic responses and sound pressures shifted upward in the same proportion upon occlusion of the ear canal, but only at low frequencies (Fig. 18b). However, when middle-ear transmission was impaired, there was no such dependence of the microphonic responses upon the sound pressure in the ear canal, and there was no occlusion effect. A good example was provided by one particular animal preparation, in which anesthesia was not satisfactory so that the muscles were never really relaxed; the occlusion effect could not be demonstrated until the *tensor tympani* muscle had been severed. Moreover, when the occlusion was affected directly in front of the tympanic membrane, not allowing for any air space between seal and membrane, there was a substantial loss of bone-conduction responses (dotted curve of Fig. 15). In this case, there was not only blockage of transmission through the middle ear, but, in addition, the middle-ear component of bone conduction itself was eliminated by fixation of the tympanic membrane. All of these experiments point out that a functioning middle ear is essential for the registration of the occlusion effect by the cochlea, or, expressed differently, that *acoustic energy is transmitted from the external canal into the cochlea.*

Radiation of energy into the canal lumen — The question may be raised as to where the energy in the canal may come from. It stands to reason, especially on the basis of the evidence presented in Figs. 16 and 18, that the sound pressure that is registered in the external canal is due to energy *radiated into its lumen* by its own walls which are participating in the vibratory responses of the skull as a whole. This viewpoint is supported by a number of additional observations. (a) When the tympanic membrane was widely exteriorized by resection of the canal walls, there was a small bone conduction loss at the low frequency end, although it was not as extreme as that found upon canal occlusion at the level of the tympanic membrane (see Fig. 15). Apparently, *when there was no canal lumen to contain this energy, it could not be transmitted to the cochlea.* (b) When, in the experiments providing the data for Fig. 15, the ear canals were extended in lateral length, there were small gains in low-frequency responses, even before such canals were occluded, results that confirmed earlier findings by W. TONNDORF (1924) in human subjects. (The mode of presentation of Fig. 15 does not demonstrate these gains.) Evidently, *more energy was radiated into and subsequently contained in such extended canals.* (c) On the basis of experiments on human subjects, FELDMAN (1971) reported that the sound pressure in the ear canal was increased, and the occlusion effect became stronger, when the entire canal was sealed over by a circumaural earphone. Since the lenght of the canal was not varied in Feldman's experiments, the *sound pressure under the seal must depend upon the size of the surface area radiating sound into the enclosed cavity.*

Leakage of energy through and around the occluding material — In spite of the fact just mentioned, *i. e.*, that there were small gains in low-frequency responses upon extending the length of the external canal, Fig. 15 shows that the degree of the occlusion effect became larger, the shorter the canal lenght. In fact, the effect was optimal, when the occluding plug was closest to the outer opening of the *osseous* ear canal, *i. e.*, when there was *the least leak around the seal.* Although this was not ascertained systematically, but only by casual observations, the higher the impedance of the occluding material, the stronger was the occlusion effect. Otherwise, sound would be lost by leakage *through* the seal.

High-pass filter effect — We are now in a position to explain the occlusion effect. [It is only fair to mention that ONCHI (1954) may have expressed a similar view. However, the English translation of his paper was such that one cannot be sure of understanding his explanation.] Figure 19 will serve to illustrate the points to be made. Consider first the canal in its unoccluded state (Fig. 19a). When the skull is subjected to audio-frequency vibrations, the osseous and cartilaginous walls of the external canal participate in such vibrations and radiate sound into its lumen. Some of this energy is picked up by the tympanic membrane, mainly in the range around and below the canal's resonant point (1000 Hz in the case of cat), and is transmitted into the cochlea via the middle ear. However, on account of its outer opening, the canal acts as a *high-pass filter* as illustrated

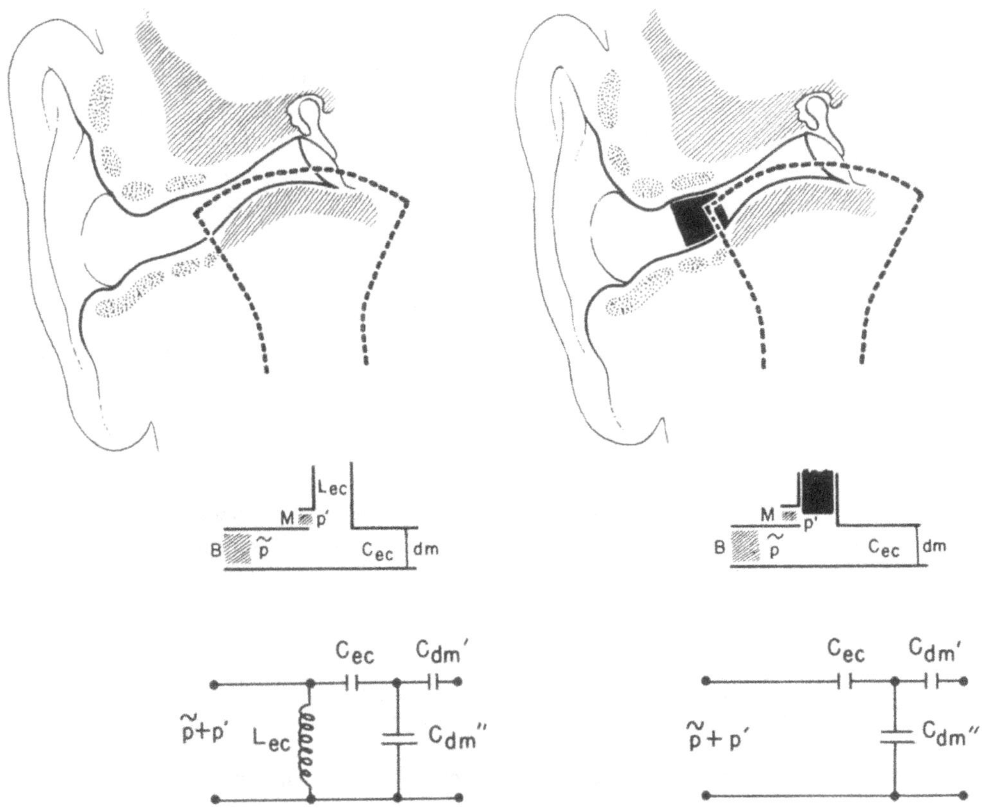

Fig. 19. Occlusion effect: When sound energy is radiated into its lumen from its own vibrating walls, the open ear canal (left) represents a high-pass filter with respect to further transmission of this sound into the cochlea. This filter effect is eliminated by occlusion of the ear canal (right). On top, the anatomical situation is schematically shown and, below, the equivalent mechanical and electrical circuits, illustrating both situations. In the mechanical circuit, a piston B (bone) produces an ac pressure *(p)* within a tube, which has a mass (L_{ec}) in shunt — the outer opening, its enclosed air having the property of a spring (C_{ec}); it is terminated by the drum membrane (*dm*). The mandible *(M)* acts as an ancillary pressure source *(p')*. In the electrical circuits, the outer opening is given by inductance L_{ec}, the air in the ear canal by capacitance C_{ec}, and the drum membrane by capacitances C'_{dm} and C''_{dm}. (From TONNDORF *et al.*, 1966e)

by the accompanying mechanical and electrical equivalent circuits. In other words, most of the low-frequency energy is dissipated by the external opening into the environment, and its transmission into the inner ear is attenuated accordingly. When the canal is occluded (Fig. 19b), the canal resonance is shifted in frequency, but, more importantly, the high-pass filter effect is minimized. Once more, accompanying mechanical and electrical circuits serve to illustrate this point. The low-frequency sound pressure in the external canal increases in some proportion to the surface area that lies medial to the point of occlusion and participates in radiating sound into the canal lumen. It is adversely affected by leakage around or through the occluding material. Obviously, results would be optimal when the occluding material and the walls of the ear canal could be made to form an integral whole. The more low-frequency energy is retained in the ear canal, the more of it can be transmitted into the cochlea via the middle ear. As shown by the low-frequency loss upon exteriorization of the tympanic membrane, and also by the gains upon lateral extensions of the ear canal, the ear canal itself preserves some low-frequency energy, on account of its narrowness and associated resistance, thus providing some small degree of an "occlusion" effect of its own. It is quite conceivable that the relative displacements of the mandible observed by BÉKÉSY (1941) play a minor role in this process. The alternations of canal resonances following its occlusion, as originally suggested by RINNE (1855) and by HUIZING (1960), affect the mid-frequency range.

When the occluding seal is moved deep into the ear canal (as BÉKÉSY has done in his experiments of 1941, in which he found the occlusion effect eliminated) the air space between the seal and the tympanic membrane becomes very small and may ultimately be eliminated altogether. This has three consequences: (a) The surface area of the canal radiating sound into its own lumen is reduced; thus less energy is transmitted into the ear canal. (b) The resonance of the air column enclosed in the canal is shifted to higher frequencies; thus, the low frequencies which are ordinarily favored by the elimination of the high-pass filter effect are attenuated. (c) And ultimately, the tympanic membrane is immobilized, an event that impairs transmission through the middle ear as well as its own bone-conduction responses. Hence, BÉKÉSY's observations are quite compatible with the present concept.

Occlusion of the external canal affects bone conduction quite prominently, at least in the low-frequency region. The reason for this lies in the fact that the contribution of the external canal to the total bone-conduction responses constitutes a major bone-conduction component as will be shown in the following section (Section III).

The bone conduction threshold with the ear canal occluded is often referred to as the "absolute bone conduction threshold". On the basis of the explanation given in the preceding paragraphs, I can no longer see any need for making such a distinction.

4. The Tests of Bing, Runge, Weber, and Gellé

We are now in a position to discuss the results of a number of different clinical bone conduction tests, those of BING, RUNGE, WEBER, and GELLÉ. All of these tests are utilized for the diagnosis of middle-ear impairment, especially otosclerosis. They lead to lateralization of low-frequency signals, but their underlying mechanisms are not identical. Figure 20 presents a tabulation including schematic audiometric curves.

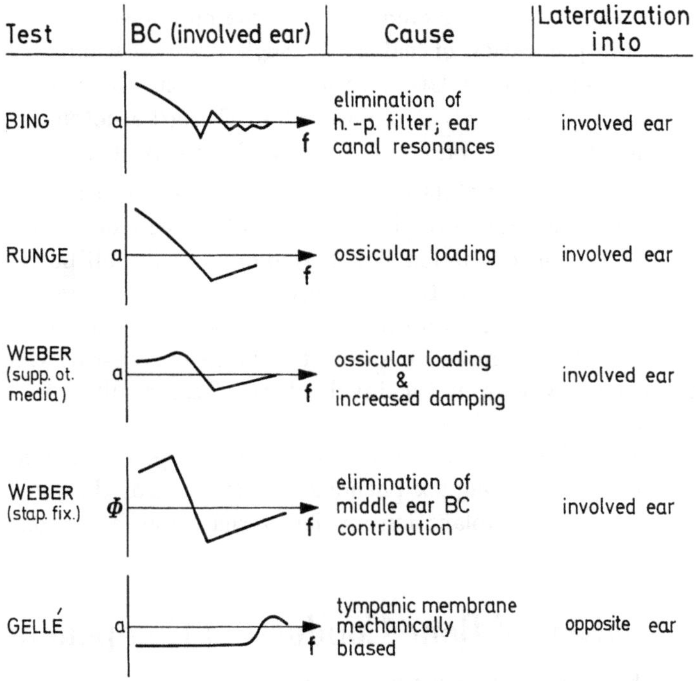

Fig. 20. Lateralization of low-frequency signals, as occurring in a number of clinical bone-conduction tests, and explanations of the lateralization. The second column shows, in a schematic manner, the response shifts with frequency in the occluded ear. Note that in the fourth row, labeled "Weber (stapedial fixation)", *phase* shifts are presented instead of the amplitude shifts given in all other situations

Bing test — The test of Bing (1890), *i. e.*, the occlusion of the external canal results in improved low-frequency responses for bone-conduction signals in the involved ear and some lesser, but sharply delineated, changes in the mid-frequencies. As was just described, these changes are caused by the elimination of the high-pass filter effect, produced by the unoccluded external canal, and alterations in canal resonances. Lateralization occurs towards the involved ear.

Runge test — In the test of Runge (1923), bone-conduction responses are first measured with the ear canal open and then after its having been filled with water. In the latter case, bone conduction is found improved for low frequencies, but decreased for higher ones. [It is interesting to note that this phenomenon was described by Wheatstone in 1827]. The effect is caused by ossicular loading and lateralization occurs once more towards the involved ear. Test results are negative when the middle-ear transmission is impaired.

Weber test — In the test of Weber, two situations must be distinguished. With *suppurative otitis media*, there is a combination of ossicular loading, due to the edema of the tissues covering the ossicles, and increased damping, due to the presence of free fluid in the middle ear, giving the audiometric curve its peculiar shape that, shown in Fig. 20, was first described by LIERLE and REGER (1946). Lateralization occurs into the involved ear. Upon *fixation of the stapes,* there are considerable phase advances at low frequencies, and some phase lags occur at higher ones. The cause lies in the elimination of the middle-ear bone-conduction component and the prevention of leakage through the oval window. The phase advance leads, of course, to a lateralization towards the involved ear and is capable of overcoming the loss that, being due to Carhart's notch, is still small at low frequencies. Lateralization occurs towards the involved ear.

Gellé test — In the test of GELLÉ (1885), the air pressure in the external ear canal is slightly modified, for example, by means of a Siegle otoscope, while the subject listens to a bone-conduction signal. Audiometrically, all but the highest frequencies are slightly impaired. In this case, the tympanic membrane it mechanically biased by being displaced inward (increased pressure) or outward (decreased pressure) with respect to its resting position. This is the only test in which lateralization takes place away from the involved ear. Test results are once more negative on middle-ear involvement.

The tabulation of Fig. 20 may serve to illustrate the point made above, *i. e.*, that bone conduction is a complex phenomenon. In each of the five situations shown, there is a separate explanation for the laterilazation that is common to all of them.

III. Analysis of Bone Conduction Components

Changes in bone-conduction responses following specific interventions, such as resection of the middle ear, occlusion of the cochlear windows, etc., point to a number of components which, each in its own way, have been shown to contribute to the response of the entire ear. After having identified these components *qualitatively*, as described in the foregoing sections, we wish, of course, to asses them *quantitatively*. In some instances, this assessment is quite a simple matter. For example, responses obtained after resection of the middle ear represent, by definition, the bone conduction contribution of the inner ear for a given input.

In other cases, such direct assessments are not feasible. For instance, comparison of responses before and after occlusion of the round window — especially with the cochlear aqueduct sealed off beforehand — revealed a separate factor, the release through the round window. However, this component could not be determined by simply forming the difference between responses obtained before and after window occlusion. In a system possessing resistive as well as reactive elements, response changes upon given interventions invariably involve *both magnitude and phase*. Therefore, *vectorial substraction* had to be employed. Differences were computed, frequency by frequency, between two *vectors*, each of them combining phase and magnitude data (the latter, of course, in *linear* terms) obtained under each condition. For each frequency, the remainder, which is once more a vector, gives the desired result, which can be separately presented in terms of phase and magnitude.

In still other cases, for example, the fluid-inertia component of the inner ear, several vectorial subtractions had to be carried out sequentially in order to determine a given component. For the exact definition of components employed in the computations underling Figs. 21—23 below, reference must be made to Tonndorf *et al.*, 1966a and f. The definitions are too lengthy to be repeated here. Admittedly, some of these definitions are somewhat arbitary, reflecting limitations in carrying out the necessary analyses. For example, the "third-window" effect is represented by only one of its sub-factors, the cochlear-aqueduct effect, the only one that was experimentally accessible. The fluid-inertia component of the inner ear was somewhat arbitrarily separated from the releases through the oval and round window. Clearly, the releases through the two windows must be affected by the distortional vibrations of the cochlear capsule as well as the fluid inertia, and one may argue where and how to draw the dividing line. Nevertheless, it should be noted that the analysis is consistent in itself in that the sum of all components yields the response curve of the intact ear.

Actually, these are quite elementary facts concerning the analysis of any network containing non-resistive elements. They would hardly be worth mentioning, were it not for the fact that they are *being continually disregarded by some writers in the field of bone conduction*. Needless to say, conclusions based upon such simplistic considerations are, more often than not, quite fallacious.

A. Individual Bone Conduction Components

Frequency responses curves of the eight bone-conduction components we were able to identify as separate entities, plus two sub-components of one of them, are shown in Figs. 21—23. They had to be distributed over three graphs merely for the sake of presentation. Each graph contains the bone-conduction response curve of the intact, healthy, feline ear as a reference.

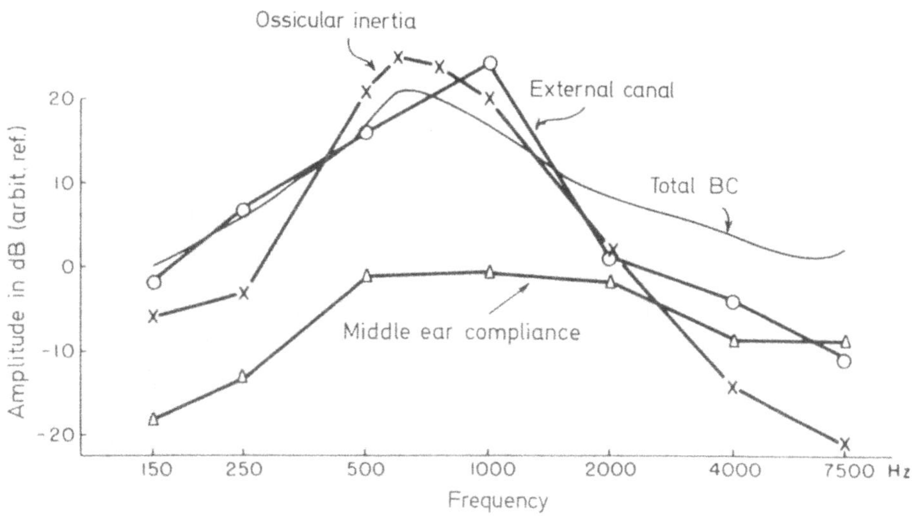

Fig. 21. Bone-conduction components in cat: Response curves calculated from experimental results for (a) external canal; (b) ossicular inertia; (c) middle-ear compliance. The bone-conduction response curve of the healthy, intact, feline ear is included as a reference. (From Tonndorf *et al.*, 1966d)

The following three components are illustrated in Fig. 21: (1) external ear canal; (2) ossicular inertia; (3) middle-ear compliance — the latter component is once more given in Fig. 23, together with its two sub-components acting upon the tympanic membrane and round window, respectively. Figure 22 contains four more components, all belonging to the inner ear: (4) capsular distortion; (5) fluid inertia; (6) round-window release; (7) oval-window release. The eighth component, the cochlear-aqueduct effect (in lieu of the "third window" release), is shown in Fig. 23, together with the aforementioned sub-components of the middle-ear compliance.

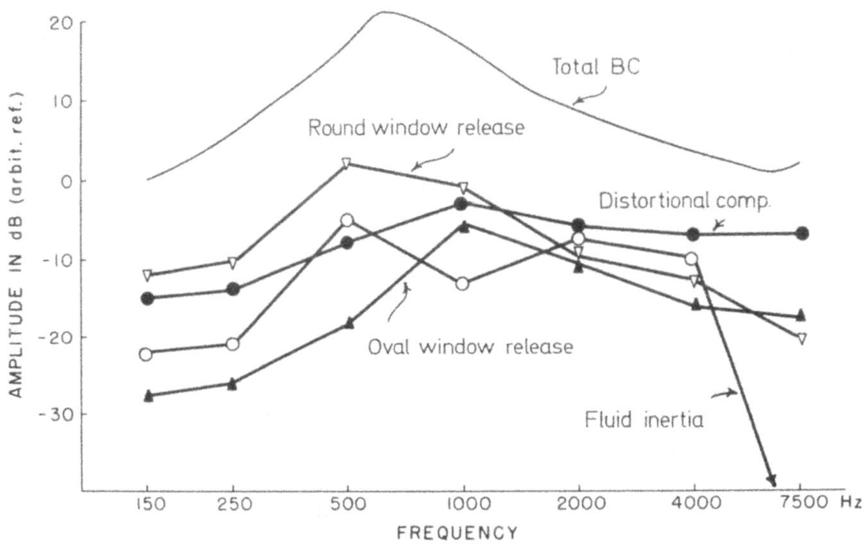

Fig. 22. Bone-conduction components in cat: Response curves calculated from experimental results for (a) capsular distortion, (b) fluid inertia, (c) round-window release, (d) oval-window release. Once more, the bone-conduction response of a normal ear is included as a reference. (From TONNDORF *et al.*, 1966d)

It is seen in all figures that the response curve of the intact ear is far from being flat, its point of maximal sensitivity being located at 600 Hz. Responses around this point are completely dominated by the components respresenting the outer ear canal and the ossicular inertia (Fig. 21). The resonance point of the feline ear canal lies at 1000 Hz and that of the ossicular chain at 600 Hz. The component labeled middle ear compliance is of minor importance. However, as seen in Fig. 23 its two subcomponents possess resonances both at 500 Hz and 2000 Hz. As might be expected on account of their push-pull action upon the middle ear system, responses of these two subcomponents were found to be in phase opposition at these two points, smoothing out the response curve of the total component. The fact that the response acting upon the (smaller) round window runs consistently below that acting upon the (larger) tympanic membrane confirms the correctness of GROEN's earlier considerations (1962).

Taken as a group, none of the inner-ear components of Fig. 22 are very prominent. In particular, they do not contribute to the overall response curve in the region of maximal sensitivity. The curve depicting the distortional component rises gradually with frequency to form a shallow maximum at 1000 Hz. The fluid-inertia component shows two peaks, one at 500 Hz and the other at 2000 Hz. The fluid-inertia component is of minor importance, but, as was just mentioned, its definition, for the sake of the present analysis, was somewhat arbitrary. The release through the round window is relatively prominent at low frequencies, whereas, because of the lesser compliance of the oval window, the release through that window plays a lesser role throughout.

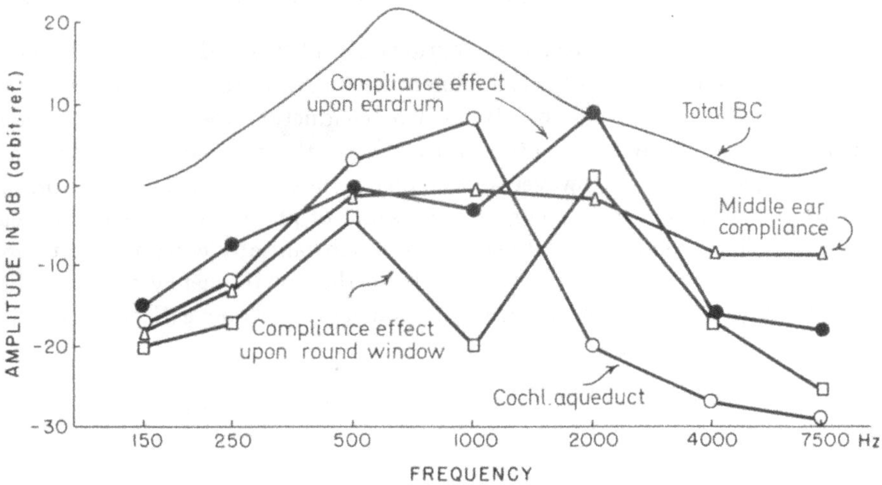

Fig. 23. Bone-conduction components in cat: Response curves calculated from experimental results for (a) middle-ear compliance (same curve as shown in Fig. 21) and its two sub-components, those acting (b) upon the tympanic membrane, and (c) upon the round window, (d) cochlear aqueduct. Once more, the bone-conduction response of a normal ear is included. (From Tonndorf *et al.*, 1966d)

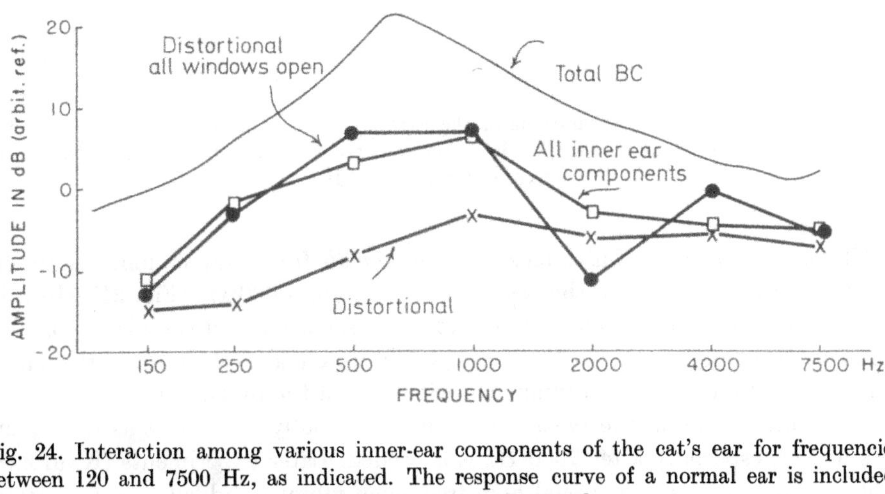

Fig. 24. Interaction among various inner-ear components of the cat's ear for frequencies between 120 and 7500 Hz, as indicated. The response curve of a normal ear is included. (From Tonndorf *et al.*, 1966d)

The curve representing the release through the cochlear aqueduct (Fig. 23), although running relatively high at low frequencies, decreases sharply with frequency beyond 1000 Hz.

Figure 24 illustrates the interaction between the various inner-ear components, showing that the response due to the distortional component alone are substantially improved when both windows are unoccluded, whereas, the addition of the fluid-inertia component has only minor effects, mainly in smoothing out an anti-resonance at around 2000 Hz.

B. Lumped Contributions of Outer, Middle, and Inner Ear

Figure 25 gives the lumped contributions of outer, middle, and inner ears. It so happens that each of them is dominant in a certain frequency region.

The *outer* ear contributes mainly to bone-conduction responses in the *low*-frequency region. The only exception to this rule is the resonant point of the ear canal at around 1000 Hz. However, this resonance has no marked effect upon the shape of the overall response curve as it is out-of-phase with the middle ear component. Thus, the above statement is still substantially correct. The reason why the outer ear canal contributes mainly to the low-frequency responses lies in the "occlusion" effect of the unoccluded canal, described above (Section II, C, 3).

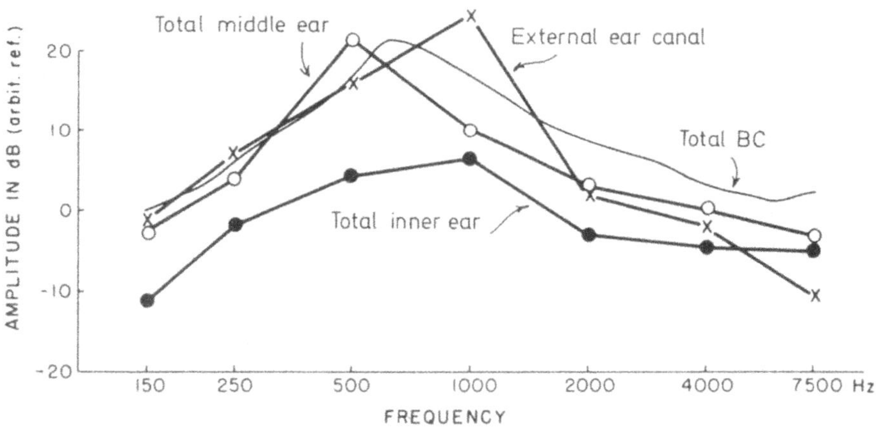

Fig. 25. Bone-conduction contributions of the external, middle, and inner ears of cats for frequencies between 150 and 7500 Hz. The response curve of a normal ear is included. (From TONNDORF *et al.*, 1966d)

The *middle* ear contributes mostly in the *middle*-frequency region, mainly on account of the resonance of the ossicular chain around 600 Hz (Fig. 21). (In this respect, Fig. 25 has not been corrected after determination of the exact point of the ossicular chain resonance. If this correction were made, the peak of the curve would have also coincided in frequency with that of the overall response.)

The contribution of the *inner* ear becomes gradually prominent as frequency goes higher, especially after 7500 Hz is exceeded. Later experiments (KAUFMAN *et al.*, 1968), employing a special high-frequency vibrator, added two more data points at 14000 and 20000 Hz, respectively; these points are not shown in Fig. 25. At 14000 and 20000 Hz bone-conduction responses were found to be completely independent of the conditions of outer and middle ears.

Figures 24 and 25 should also dispel the notion that is occasionally expressed, *i. e.*, that there are no inner-ear responses at low frequencies. It is seen that both the distortional component (Fig. 24) and the contribution of the total inner ear (Fig. 25) have relatively flat frequency-responses curve, extending without a precipitous drop toward relatively low frequencies. (This point will be taken up once more in the following section, Section IV.) The only reason for the lesser importance of the inner ear contribution at low to middle frequencies lies in the relative dominance of the outer and middle ear contributions, as was already mentioned.

The reader may wonder how the individual bone-conduction components of Figs. 21–23 with their response curves, most of which are for from being smooth, finally combine to a relatively smooth overall response curve of the entire ear. The reason, as I see it, lies in the fact that several components actually work in a push-pull manner with respect to one another. Two examples of this kind have just been cited: the interaction between the two subcomponents of the middle-ear compliance, smoothing out their common response curve (Fig. 23), and the interaction between the outer and middle ear contribution in the region of the response peak of 600 Hz (Figs. 21 and 25). Such interactions, of course, occur at the expense of sensitivity. Note in Fig. 25 that, in the region around 600 Hz, the level of the overall response curve is less than the levels due to outer and middle ear contributions separately.

IV. Skull Vibrations

The foregoing description was concerned with the transmission of bone-conducted energy within the ear and its eventual reception by the cochlea. We must now discuss in some detail how such energy may be transmitted from any point of input about head to the temporal bone and the ear.

A. Vibrations in Solids

Vibrations in elastic solids and in response to steady-state signals may occur in several forms or *modes*, depending primarily upon the relationship between the size of such bodies to the wavelength and, to some lesser degree, also on the absorption of energy with distance, which is small in most solids. It is only when such bodies are large, at least in one spatial dimension, *i. e.*, when the effects of *boundaries* can be neglected, that *pressure* waves may travel through the bulk of their material, When structures are relatively small, their displacements are merely *translational*. When structures are larger in one or two dimensions (thin rods or plates), displacements become transversal, usually, combined with compressional-wave travel along the long axes of these structures. When restricted in some manner, *e.g.*, by being clamped at one end, such rods or plates display *flexural* displacements.

Finally, when they become thicker so that the remaining dimensions are no longer small, but not too large either, *distortional* vibrations will occur; that is, displacements take place simultaneously, and in a complex manner, along two or three spatial dimensions, resulting in *shearing* displacements *within* such bodies. Needless to say that, in response to impulse-type signals, there is wave travel in all three dimensions. The steady-state responses shown in Fig. 26 are the result of interferences between the incoming energy and reflections from the boundaries. As mentioned earlier in relation to cochlear displacements, distortional vibrations occur prominently in inhomogeneous bodies, such as fluid-filled shells, but their occurrence is by no means limited to such bodies.

Looking at the problem differently, one may state that a given body undergoes translational vibrations (in its first or fundamental mode) when the wavelength is large, but it will display increasingly higher modes of distortional vibrations as the wavelength is being decreased. This is simply the three-dimensional equivalent of flexural displacements of thin plates which, starting out from a simple basic mode at low frequencies, become increasingly complex in their higher modes when frequency goes higher. For further details on this rather brief account, reference must be made to standard texts such as LOVE (1927) or CREMER and HECKL (1967).

B. Modes of Skull Vibrations

BÉKÉSY (1932) examined the mode of skull vibrations in response to steady-state vibratory inputs, the type of signal employed in clinical testing. He found responses as shown in Fig. 26, that is, in essence, those of a fluid-filled sphere. There is a *translational* mode at low frequencies, and the first higher, *distortional*, mode makes its appearance at 800 Hz, to be followed by the next higher one at 1600 Hz, the first having two *nodal* planes; the second, four. Note the phase opposition between adjacent segments at higher modes which is typical for such modes of vibration and implies that the flat skull bones, when considered on their own, display *flexural* vibrations.

KIRIKAE (1959) enlarged upon BÉKÉSY's findings by demonstrating other, higher modes and also transitional patterns at frequencies between resonant modes. He further showed individual differences among skulls. KIRIKAE conducted additional experiments employing skull models made of Araldite. This plastic allows stress lines that are brought about by a one-time deformation of the model to be fixated for later visualization on appropriate sections. Although he himself did not explicitly state so, KIRIKAE's findings (*cf.* Figs. 47 and 50a, l. c.) show that the thick bones at the base of the skull and, to a lesser degree, even the flat bones of the cranial vault undergo displacements of the *distortional* type, with the attending shear between their various layers. It stands to reason that the cochlear space, which, from this standpoint, represents nothing but a discontinuity of the bones at the base of the skull, participates in these distortional vibrations, a fact for which other evidence has been presented in Section II 2. At the base of the skull, distortional vibrations may actually come about at lower frequencies than were demonstrated by BÉKÉSY for the upper vault of the skull. This statement is based upon the finding shown in Fig. 22 that, even in cats with their relatively small skulls, the distortional component has a frequency response that is nearly flat down to the lowest frequency tested, *i. e.*, 150 Hz, and shows no sign of a precipitous drop in the low frequency region.

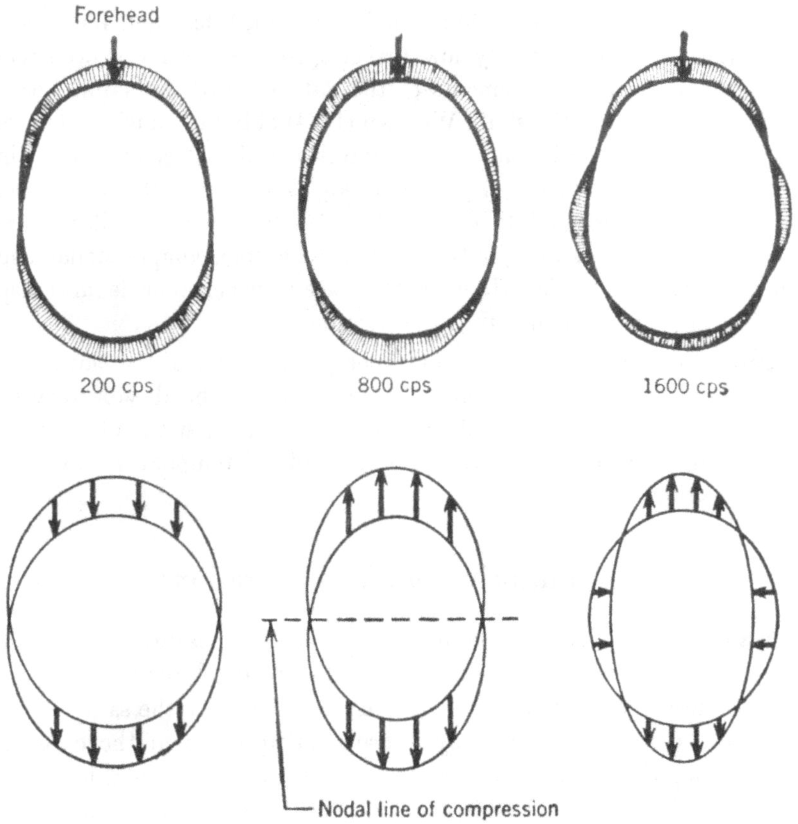

Fig. 26. Response patterns in the horizontal plane of the skull for various frequencies. (From Békésy, 1932.) Since, at least at higher frequencies, these responses occur in all three dimensions, they are in reality even more complicated (cf. Fig. 8, Kirikae, 1959)

Attenuation with distance — In most solid materials, the absorption of vibratory energy with distance is rather small. Furthermore, in bodies of limited size responding to steady-state signals, reflections from the boundaries produce a fairly even distribution of energy, except, of course, at true nodes (*cf.* Fig. 26). It is probably for both of these reasons that, from inputs anywhere about the head, vibratory energy reaches both ears with about the same intensity, pointing to the need of *masking* for the non-treated ear in bone-conduction audiometry. I am not aware of any study which has attempted to clarify which of the two factors mentioned might be the more important from the present standpoint.

Speed of propagation — The speed of propagation of vibratory energy varies with the density and the impedance of a given solid material. However, this rule applies mainly to travel *through* the bulk of a given body, *i. e.*, to the compressional mode. Whenever boundary phenomena are involved, as in flexural or distortional waves, travel speeds are much lower, by almost a whole order of magnitude.

Along the flat bones of the skull, the speed of vibratory transmisson, measured for impulse signals, has variously been given as 570 m/sec (BÉKÉSY, 1948); 100—300 m/sec (FRANKE, 1956); 260 m/sec (ZWISLOCKI, 1962); and 400—800 m/sec (WIGAND, 1964). These relatively low travel speeds confirm the occurrence of predominantly flexural displacements of the flat bones of the skull. For transmission along the base of the skull, WIGAND (1964) obtained much higher values, *i. e.*, up to 2600 m/sec, indicating that compressional displacements occur in this region. There is no contradiction between this and the earlier statement concerning the occurrence of distortional displacements of the base of the skull. Such modes may co-exist. As already stated, in thin rods, for example, compressional displacements may travel along its length, while there are transversal or flexural displacements going on perpendicularly to that direction.

The rate of propagation of vibratory energy, even that of the slower flexural mode, is so high that, from any point of input about the head, vibratory energy arrives at both ears practically at the same time, *i. e.*, with intra-aural time differences that are below or barely at the limit of the temporal resolving power of dichotic hearing.

C. Monitoring of Skull Vibrations

When a vibrator is placed in contact with the head, a measure of the *admittance* of the applied energy may be obtained by monitoring displacement, acceleration, force, or pressure at the vibrator. Such measures then serve the same purpose as sound-pressure readings obtained by a probe microphone in the external ear canal, monitoring the input of air-borne sound to the ear. This point is of practical importance for the calibration of bone-conduction vibrators on so called *artifical mastoids* or *head bones*, electro-mechanical devices that are designed to duplicate the mechanical impedance of the head for the purpose of presenting a proper load to the vibrator being calibrated.

Of the entities mentioned, the easiest to monitor is acceleration, but, apparently, it is not the best as was revealed in recent experiments of KHANNA *et al.* (1972). According to BÉKÉSY (1939; personal communication, 1971), it is the ac pressure that agrees best with the perceived loudness of a bone-conducted signal, up to frequencies of approximately 2500 Hz, *i. e.*, apparently, until skull vibrations become too complex. What is also important is that results are then nearly independent of the effects of soft tissues, interposed between vibrator and bone. BÉKÉSY's findings have apparently received little attention, for acceleration is still the most widely-used measure. However, as pressure-monitoring devices have recently become commercially available, there is no longer a reason why BÉKÉSY's recommendation should not be generally adopted.

Earlier experiments (BÁRÁNY, 1938; BÉKÉSY, 1939) confirmed the general notion that transmission is improved as the dc force of application is increased, a saturation value being reached around a force of 1 kg. Unless ac pressure is monitored (BÉKÉSY, 1939), as was just mentioned, the situation is complicated by interposition of skin and soft tissues between bone and vibrator. In this respect, skin has visco-elastic properties; its mass can be neglected (BÉKÉSY, 1939). According to FRANKE (1952), the mechanical resistance of the skin varies with the dc force of application of the vibrator and also with the area of contact; its compliance depends only on the dc force and is independent of the area of contact. There are considerable individual differences, mainly with respect to compliance. Magnitude of the mechanical skin resistance was found to be approximately proportional to the thickness of the soft-tissue layer.

KÖNIG (1957), on the basis of the foregoing evidence and the results of some experiments of his own, recommended that the vibrator be applied to the head with a constant force, near its saturation value; 0.8 to 1 kg appeared to be a suitable choice.

In our own animal experiments (TONNDORF *et al.*, 1966), we encountered another problem, and at the time of this writing, I am not sure whether or not pressure-monitoring after BÉKÉSY will alleviate it. As already mentioned, signals were monitored by an accelerometer that was directly incorporated into the vibrator tip, and the latter was cemented to the bone, in order to avoid problems of skin interference. Despite these precautions, results of our early experiments varied widely between trials. The source of variations turned out to be the support of the animal's head. In this particular case, the problem was solved in a pragmatic manner, *i. e.*, by rigidly standardizing the experimental situation with respect to the manner of head support, application of the vibrator, as was outlined above (*cf.* Section II). KIRIKAE (1959), apparently, experienced similar difficulties in his experiments on skulls and skull models. He found a solution essentially similar to our own. This problem is, of course, peculiar to laboratory experiments. It will not be encountered in human bone-conduction tests, when the head is free of additional support.

D. Osseous Discontinuities

In adult man, the various bones forming the skull are so intricately dovetailed or even fused with one another that the skull may be treated, in good approximation, as if it were a solid shell of bone. However, in addition to human neonates, there are some other, adult, animals in which the situation is different. Either the cochlea is not fused with the temporal bone (whales) or the temporal bone is not an integral part of the skull (bats, rats). The thought has been expressed (whales: REYSENBACH de HAAN, 1957; bats: HENSON, 1961) that this feature might serve to "protect" the ear against the transmission of audio-frequency vibrations, something that BÁRÁNY (1938) had already postulated.

The effect of discontinuities between the temporal bone and other parts of the skull was tested in experiments on laboratory rats (TONNDORF *et al.*, 1966f). In this animal species, the temporal bone, after its surgical exposure, can be moved to quite some extent with little effort in relation to its neighbors, the parietal and occipital bones. Cochlear microphonic responses were first recorded with the temporal bone exposed, but in its normal, mobile state; the vibrator was applied to the parietal bone, firm union being affected by dental cement. Recordings were repeated after the temporal bone had been securely cemented to the parietal and occipital bones. Separate experiments were conducted (a) with the ear intact and (b) with the middle ear removed.

Figure 27 shows the changes in bone-conduction responses occurring upon fixation of the temporal bone. The presence of the middle ear affected responses by 2—5 dB, but only in the low-frequency range. At higher frequencies, however, it made no difference whether the middle ear was present or absent. There was a relatively large gain of approximately 14 dB at 2000 Hz, followed by a loss of about 4 dB at 4000 Hz, and again a small gain of 3—4 dB at 7500 Hz.

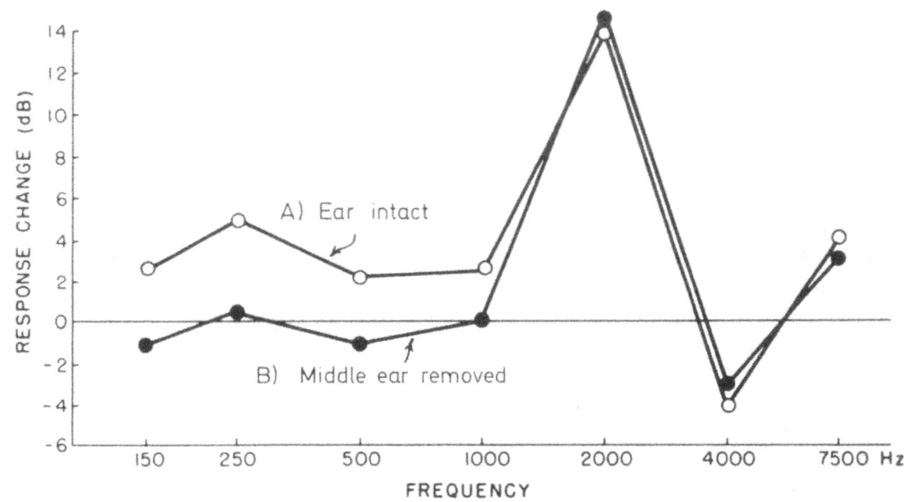

Fig. 27. Experimental fixation of the temporal bone to the surrounding bones in rats: changes in cochlear-microphonic responses *vs* frequency. Vibrator is on the parietal bone. Changes are given (a) for the intact ear and (b) after removal of the middle ear. (From TONNDORF *et al.*, 1966g)

The results of Fig. 27 do not support the notion that the ear is being "protected" by osseous discontinuities against the transmission of vibratory energy. They rather point to the possibility that conduction along the skull bones may not constitute the sole mode of transmission of vibratory energy across the skull. The assumption of multiple pathways of comparable conductivity could easily account for the findings at 2000 Hz and 4000 Hz of Fig. 27. When one of the pathways, for example that along the skull bones, is eliminated owing to osseous discontinuities, interferences between their respective outputs at the level of the temporal bone would be altered accordingly.

In this respect, RANKE's (1953) "third-window" concept must come to mind. RANKE, as will be recalled, proposed that communications exist between the cochlea and the interior of the skull via the aqueducts, and the perineural and perivascular channels. Present Figs. 4 and 5 provided experimental evidence in favor of this concept, although limited to the cochlear aqueduct. SCHNEIDER (1959), on the basis of experiments of his own, thought he had disproved RANKE's notion. However, SCHNEIDER limited himself to one test signal, 6000 Hz; Fig. 23, above, has shown that, at such high frequencies, the degree of transmission through a narrow channel, like the cochlear aqueduct, is quite low. Therefore, SCHNEIDER's argument is not really valid.

It is proposed, therefore, that, in addition to the skull bones, vibratory energy is also transmitted through the interior of the skull, which, in this respect, may have the properties of a viscous fluid. The efficiency of these two pathways appears to be approximately equal. Energy arriving by this second route may enter via RANKE's "third window" or affect the temporal bone as a whole; otherwise the inertial change in the response of the middle ear in Fig. 27 might have been higher than actually observed.

Surface waves along the skin and soft tissue layers that originate from the point of contact and were observed stroboscopically by BÉKÉSY (1959) ought to play a minor role. In our own experiments on rats (*cf.* Fig. 27), their effects were excluded, since the skull bones, that is, the temporal and parts of the parietal and the occipital bones, had been completely exposed. Moreover, with surface waves, in which displacement decreases with depth, there can be very little transmission of energy to the underlying solid material, bone in the present case.

V. Summary

All that remains now is to present the findings reported in this chapter in some integrated form. Figure 28 shows a block diagram, in the manner of an equivalent electric network, that should serve such a purpose. It is recalled (MøLLER, 1961; ZWISLOCKI, 1962) that, with respect to air conduction, the middle ear can be represented as a simple, serial system. With respect to bone conduction however, the situation is considerably more complicated. In this respect, the ear constitutes a *multiple-input* system.

From the vibrator, energy may travel along three different pathways: along the skin, through the bone, and through the skull interior. Energy transmitted by these three pathways is brought together once more at the level of the temporal bone, although the contribution from the skin pathway plays, most likely, a very minor role in this respect. From here on, there is a *signal line* that goes to three separate points of input: (1) the walls of the external canal, (2) the middle ear ossicles, and (3) the cochlear capsule and its contained fluids. In addition, the cochlea has an independent input from the skull interior via the "third window". At each of these points, which represent separate inputs to the outer, middle, and inner ears, respectively, the responses are altered by a number of *modifying factors*.

The walls of the external canal *radiate* sound into its lumen (air), the modifying factor being the external opening, acting as a high-pass filter. The middle ear ossicles respond owing to their *moment of inertia*, this response being modified by the tympanic membrane and the air enclosed in the middle ear, both acting like backsprings. The cochlear capsula undergoes *distortional* vibrations. (The phase inverter signifies the fact that the two perilymphatic scalae are out of phase with each other in this respect.) The mass of the contained *fluid*, being unequally distributed, responds once more in an inertial manner. This cochlear response is modified by the oval and round windows which have not only different compliance values of their own, but face different impedances in the middle ear: the oval window, the ossicular chain; the round window, the air enclosed in the middle ear.

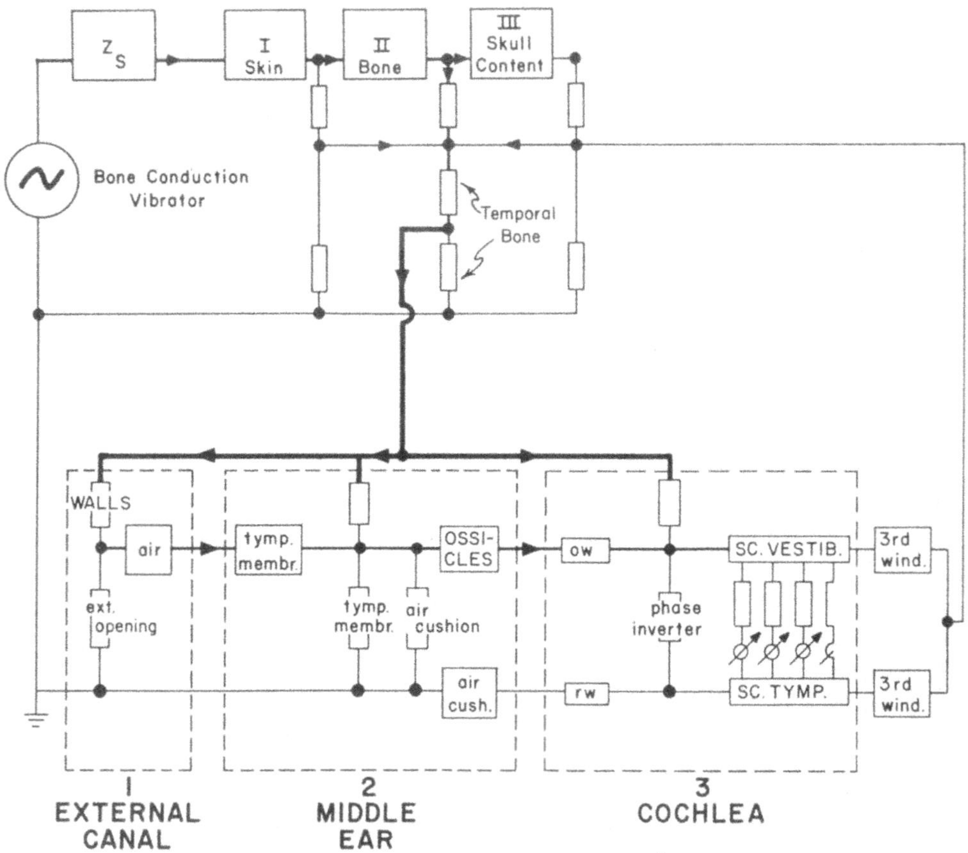

Fig. 28. Block diagram of the mechanism of bone conduction. (From TONNDORF, 1968)

Finally, along what might be called the *response line*, *i. e.*, the air in the external canal — the tympanic membrane — the ossicular chain — the oval window — and the cochlea, all of these various responses are collected and integrated with one another, according to their phase relations, and the integrated response, finally, leads to hair cell stimulation.

Since it makes direct connection with the original input, the "third window" plays a special role. It is a moot question in this *multiple-input system* whether one should consider it a modifying factor, in the sense of being an outlet, or a point of input.

The rigorous analysis of such multiple-input systems is not an easy task and depends not only upon the circuit in general, but also, quite critically, upon the quantitative aspects of its constituents.

References

Allen, G. W., Fernandez, C.: The mechanism of bone conduction. Ann. Otol. (St. Louis) **69**, 5—28 (1960).

Bárány, E.: A contribution to the physiology of bone conduction. Acta oto-laryng. (Stockh.) Suppl. **26** (1938).

Bárány, R.: As cited in Bárány, E. (1910).

Békésy, G. von: Zur Theorie des Hörens bei der Schallaufnahne durch Knochenleitung. Ann. Phys. **13**, 111—136 (1932).

Békésy, G. von: Über die piezoelektrische Messung der absoluten Hörschwelle bei Knochenleitung. Akust. Z. **4**, 113—125 (1939).

Békésy, G. von: Über die Schallausbreitung bei Knochenleitung. Hals-, Nasen- u. Ohrenheilk. **47**, 430—442 (1941).

Békésy, G. von: Über die Messung der Schwingungsamplitude der Gehörknöchelchen mittels einer kapazitiven Sonde. Akust. Z. **6**, 1—6 (1941).

Békésy, G. von: Vibrations of the head in a sound field and its role in hearing by bone conduction. J. acoust. Soc. Amer. **20**, 749—760 (1948).

Békésy, G. von: Paradoxical direction of wave travel along the cochlear partition. J. acoust. Soc. Amer. **27**, 155—161 (1955).

Békésy, G. von: Similarities between hearing and skin sensations. Psychol. Rev. **66**, 1—22 (1959).

Bing, A.: Ein neuer Stimmgabelversuch. Wien. med. Blätter **14** (1891).

Carhart, R.: Clinical application of bone conduction audiometry. Arch. Otolaryng. **51**, 798—808 (1950).

Cremer, L., Heckl, M.: Körperschall. Berlin-Heidelberg-New York: Springer 1967.

Dean, C.: Audition by bone conduction. J. acoust. Soc. Amer. **2**, 281—296 (1930).

Feldman, A.: Studies of the occlusion effect. Dept. of Otorhinolaryng. State Univ. of New York, Upstate Med. Center, Syracuse, N.Y. Techn. rep. Nr. 8, 1—33, Nov. 1971.

Feldmann, H.: Die geschichtliche Entwicklung der Hörprüfungsmethoden. Stuttgart: Thieme 1960. (Translated into English and edited by the Beltone Inst. f. Hear. Res. **22**, 1970).

Franke, E. K.: The impedance of the human mastoid. J. acoust. Soc. Amer. **24**, 410—411 (1952).

Franke, E. K.: Response of the human skull to mechanical vibrations. J. acoust. Soc. Amer. **28**, 1277—1284 (1956).

Franke, E. K., Gierke, H. E. von, Grossman, F. M., Wittern, W. W. von: The jaw motions relative to the skull and their influence on hearing by bone conduction. J. acoust. Soc. Amer. **24**, 142—146 (1952).

Gellé, M.: Épreuve de pression. Trans. Int. Congr. Med., 7th session **3**, 370 (1881).

Gisselson, I., Richter, O.: Ein Beitrag zur Frage des Hörvermögens bei Verschluß des runden Fensters. Arch. Ohrenheilk. **166**, 410 (1955).

Groen, J. J.: The value of the Weber test. In: Schuknecht, H. (Ed.): Intern. Symp. on otosclerosis. Boston: Little, Brown 1962.

GROEN, J. J., HOOGLAND, G. A.: Bone conduction and otosclerosis of the round window. Acta oto-laryng. (Stockh.) **49**, 206—212 (1958).

GUILD, S. R.: Hearing by bone conduction. Ann. Otol. (St. Louis) **45**, 736—754 (1936).

HALLPIKE, C. S.: Some observations on bone conduction. J. Laryng. **45**, 1—24 (1930).

HENSON, O. W., Jr.: Some morphological and functional aspects of certain structures of the middle ear in bats and insectivores. Kans. Univ. Sci. Bull. **42**, 151—255 (1961).

HERZOG, H.: Das Knochenleitungsproblem. Theoretische Erwägungen. Z. Hals-, Nasen- u. Ohrenheilk. **15**, 300—306 (1926).

HOUSE, W. F.: Oval window and round window surgery in extensive otosclerosis. Laryngoscope **69**, 693—701 (1959).

HUIZING, E. H.: Bone conduction. Acta oto-laryng. (Stockh.) Suppl. **155**, (1960).

KAUFMAN, R. S., MCARDLE, F. L., TONNDORF, J.: Experimental round window surgery. Ann. Otol. (St. Louis) **77**, 243—254 (1968).

KHANNA, S. M., TONNDORF, J., COE, R.: Bone conduction testing by a specially designed magnetostrictive vibrator. J. acoust. Soc. Amer. **51**, 124 (1972).

KIRIKAE, I.: An experimental study of the fundamental mechanism of bone conduction. Acta oto-laryng. (Stockh.) Suppl. **145**, 1—111 (1959).

KIRIKAE, I.: The structure and function of the middle ear. Tokyo: Univ. of Tokyo Press 1960.

KÖNIG, E.: Variations in bone conduction as related to the force of pressure on the vibrator. Transl. Beltone Inst. Hear. Res. **6** (1957).

KRAINZ, W.: Das Knochenleitungsproblem. Experimentelle Ergebnisse. Z. Hals-, Nas.- u. Ohrenheilk. **15**, 306—313 (1926).

LEGOUIX, J. P., TARAB, S.: Experimental study of bone conduction in ears with mechanical impairment of the ossicles. J. acoust. Soc. Amer. **31**, 1453—1457 (1959).

LIERLE, D. M., REGER, S. N.: Correlations between bone and air conduction acuity measurements over wide frequency ranges in different types of hearing impairment. Laryngoscope **56**, 187—224 (1946).

LOVE, A. E. H.: A treatise on the mathematical theory of elasticity (4th ed.). London-New York: Cambridge Univ. Press 1927.

LOWY, K.: Cancellation of the electrical response with air- and bone-conducted sound. J. acoust. Soc. Amer. **14**, 156—158 (1943).

MACH, E.: Zur Theorie des Gehörorgans. S.-B. Akad. Wiss. Wien, math.-nat. Kl., Abh. II **48**, 283—300 (1863).

MCARDLE, F L., TONNDORF, J.: Perforations of the tympanic membrane and their effects upon middle-ear transmission. Arch. Klin. exp. Ohren-, Nasen- u. Kehlkopfheilk. **192**, 145—162 (1968).

MØLLER, A. R.: Network model of the middle ear. J. acoust. Soc. Amer. **33**, 168—176 (1961).

ONCHI, Y.: The blocked bone conduction test for differential diagnosis. Ann. Otol. (St. Louis) **63**, 81—96 (1954).

POHLMANN, A. G.: Correlations between the acuity for hearing and bone-transmitted sounds in RINNE-negative and RINNE-positive cases. Ann. Otol. (St. Louis) **39**, 927—960 (1930).

POLITZER, A.: Untersuchungen über Schallfortpflanzung und Schalleitung in Gehörorganen im gesunden und kranken Zustand. II. Über die Schalleitung im Kopfknochen. Arch. Ohrenheilk. **1**, 318 (1869).

RANKE, O.: Physiologie des Gehörs. Gehör, Stimme und Sprache (RANKE-LULLIES). Berlin-Heidelberg-New York: Springer 1953.

RETJÖ, A.: Beiträge zur Physiologie der Knochenleitung. Verh. dtsch. Otol. Ges. **23**, 268—285 (1914).

REYSENBACH de HAAN, F. W.: Hearing in whales. Acta oto-laryng. (Stockh.) Suppl. **134** (1957).

RINNE, A.: Beiträge zur Physiologie des Ohres. Vjschr. Prakt. Heilk. Prog. **46**, No. 1, 71—123, **47**, 45—72 (1855).

RUNGE, H. G.: Über die Lehre der Knochenleitung und über einen neuen Versuch zu ihrem weiteren Ausbau. Z. Hals-, Nas.- u. Ohrenheilk. **5**, 306 (1923).

SIEBENMANN, F.: Entgegnung auf die bevorstehende Abhandlung von WITTMAAK: Über experimentelle Schallschädigung, etc. Passow-Schaefers Beitr. **9**, 38—53 (1917).

SCHNEIDER, W.: Gegenbeweis gegen Knochenleitung mittels Druckwellen über den Kanal des nervus acusticus. Z. Laryng. Rhinol. **38**, 723—734 (1959).

SCHWABACH, D.: Über den Wert des Rinneschen Versuches für die Diagnostik der Gehörkrankheiten. Z. Ohrenheilk. **14**, 1—147 (1885).

TEMKIN, J.: Die Schädigung des Ohres durch Lärm und Erschütterung. Mschr. Ohrenheilk. **67**, 257—299; 450—479; 527—553; 705—736; 823—834 (1933). Engl. Transl. Beltone Inst. Hear. Res. **27**, 1973.

TONNDORF, J.: Compressional bone conduction in cochlear models. J. acoust. Soc. Amer. **34**, 1127—1131 (1962).

TONNDORF, J., TABOR, J. R.: Closure of the cochlear windows. Ann. Otol. (St. Louis) **71**, 5—29 (1962).

TONNDORF, J.: Animal experiments in bone conduction. Ann. Otol. (St. Louis) **73**, 659—678 (1964).

TONNDORF, J., CAMPELL, R. A., BERNSTEIN, L., RENEAU, J. P.: Quantitative evalution of bone conduction components in cats. Acta oto-laryng. (Stockh.) Suppl. **213**, 10—38 (1966a).

TONNDORF, J., DUVALL, A. L.: Loading of the tympanic membrane: its effect upon bone conduction in experimental animals. Acta oto-laryng. (Stockh.) Suppl. **213**, 39—54 (1966b).

TONNDORF, J., DUVALL, A. J., VOOTS, R. J.: Comparative studies on bone conduction in cats, dogs, guinea pigs, and rats. Acta oto-laryng. (Stockh.) Suppl. **213**, 55—71 (1966c).

TONNDORF, J., GREENFIELD, E. C., KAUFMAN, R. S.: Bone conduction experiments in isolated middle ear specimens of cats. Acta oto-laryng. (Stockh.) Suppl. **213**, 72—79 (1966d).

TONNDORF, J., GREENFIELD, E. C., KAUFMAN, R. S.: The occlusion of the external ear canal. Its effect upon bone conductions in cats. Acta oto-laryng (Stockh.) Suppl. **213**, 80—104 (1966e).

TONNDORF, J., GREENFIELD, E. C., KAUFMAN, R. S.: The relative efficiency of air and bone conduction in cats. Acta oto-laryng. (Stockh.) Suppl. **213**, 105—123 (1966f).

TONNDORF, J., OLESEN, M., KING, A. F., COTTLE, R. D., BAKER, D. C. III: The effect of osseous discontinuities upon transmission of vibratory energy across the skull of rats. Acta oto-laryng. (Stockh.) Suppl. **213**, 124—132 (1966g).

TONNDORF, J.: A new concept of bone conduction. Arch. oto-laryng **87**, 595—600 (1968).

TONNDORF, W.: Zur Schallabflußtheorie von MACH. Z. Hals-, Nas.- u. Ohrenheilk. **9**, 548 (1924).

TORTUAL: Cited after BÁRÁNY (1938).

WEBER, E. H.: De pulsu, resorptione, auditu et tactu. Leipzig: C. F. Koehler 1834.

WERNER, CL. F.: Das Labyrinth. Leipzig: Thieme 1940

WEVER, E. G., LAWRENCE, M.: Physiological acoustics. Princeton: Princeton Univ. Press 1954.

WHEATSTONE, C.: Experiments on audition. Quart. J. Sci. Lit. and Art **24**, 67—72 (1827).

WIGAND, M. E., BORUCK, H.-J., SCHMITT, H. G.: Zum Knochenleitungshören von Impulsen. Acta oto-laryng (Stockh.) **58**, 95—104 (1964).

WITTMAAK, K.: Über experimentelle Schallschädigung mit besonderer Berücksichtigung der Körper-Knochenleitungsschädigung. Passow-Schaefers Beitr. **9**, 1—37, 225—227 (1917).

ZWISLOCKI, J.: Wave motion in the cochlea caused by bone conduction. J. acoust. Soc. Amer. **25**, 986—989 (1953).

ZWISLOCKI, J.: On the propagation velocity of sound in the human skull. J. acoust. Soc. Amer. **30**, 186—187 (1958).

ZWISLOCKI, J.: Analysis of the middle-ear function. Part I. J. acoust Soc. Amer. **34**, 1514—1523 (1962).

Chapter 3

Electric Response Audiometry, with Special Reference to the Vertex Potentials*

HALLOWELL DAVIS, St. Louis, Missouri (USA)

With 1 Figure

Contents

I. Scope

This chapter is organized to give a systematic account of the various auditory evoked responses (AER) which may be recorded from the human head and which may, in principle, be used clinically to evaluate the sensitivity or other properties of the auditory system. It includes an outline of the conditions and procedures recommended by the author for electric response audiometry (ERA), together with his reasons for choosing the conditions and the particular values of important parameters. On the other hand, it does not attempt to describe animal experiments or to give detailed physiological interpretations. Neither does it consider several late electric responses which are of great psychological and physiological interest but which do not seem to be serviceable for clinical determination of auditory thresholds. These items, and also the important question of the location

* The preparation of this manuscript was supported by Public Health Service Grant No. NS-03856 from the National Institute of Neurological Diseases and Stroke.

of the generators of the various auditory potentials and the similar electric responses in other systems, are covered in a companion chapter written by Prof. Dr. W. KEIDEL.

II. Physiological Audiometry

The need for some form of physiological audiometry, sometimes called "objective" audiometry, is almost as old as clinical audiometry itself. Voluntary or "subjective" audiometry, in which the subject responds, according to verbal instructions, with an arbitrary response whenever he hears the test signal, is quick and simple, and it is the method of choice whenever we can trust the understanding, the attention span and the motivation of the subject. Physiological audiometry, however, does not require the voluntary cooperation of the subject, and it enables us to deal more or less successfully with infants, with older children who are hyperactive, mentally retarded, autistic or otherwise uncooperative, and with adults who are suspected of feigning or of suffering from psychogenic hearing loss.

Physiological audiometry can be based on any one of a great variety of reflex responses to sound. These include the startle reflex, blinking, awakening from sleep, grimacing, changes in heart rate or the rhythm of respiration, orienting to the source of sound and changes in electrical resistance of the skin. Many of these methods are very useful indeed in the clinic for rough assessment of hearing in infants. More elaborate methods include some form of "conditioning" of a response by associating the auditory signal with some other simple reflex, as in the usual form of electrodermal audiometry, or with operant behavior that yields a reward, as in the so-called "peep-show" and in conventional "play audiometry". When such conditioning is possible, the sensitivity and the precision of physiological (behavioral) audiometry are both greatly increased. We shall not, however, consider any of these forms of physiological audiometry further; we shall confine our attention to electrical responses of the auditory system which do not require any form of motor response by the subject. Voluntary cooperation is required only to the extent of keeping general motor activity within reasonable limits—and, if necessary, this requirement can be implemented by testing during sleep or under sedation.

III. Historical Development of ERA

The earliest form of electric response audiometry, excluding electrodermal reactions, was based on alterations in the pattern of the on-going electroencephalogram. The alterations included "blocking" of the alpha rhythm, alterations associated with changes in the depth of sleep, or the appearance of the "K-complex" (MARCUS *et al.*, 1949; PERL *et al.*, 1953; YAMAMOTO *et al.*, 1953; WITHROW and GOLDSTEIN, 1958; ORTIZ-ESTRADA *et al.*, 1963). The K-complex is a nonspecific response to almost any sudden sensory stimulus given during a particular stage of sleep. Some of these reactions are very clear when they do occur, but they do not always occur. The method is very tedious, as long intervals between stimuli are needed, and classical electroencephalic audiometry has now been almost completely replaced by methods based on instrumental averaging of small responses to many stimuli.

Specific localized cortical responses to sensory stimuli have long been observed in animal experiments but, until quite recently, only with intracranial electrodes. The first identification of evoked auditory (and other) responses in the human extracranial electroencephalogram in the waking state was by P. A. DAVIS in 1939. In exceptional subjects, responses were detected to auditory, visual or electrical stimuli. The vertex, with a reference electrode at or near the ear, was the position where the responses were strongest, and this led later to the designation of these evoked potentials as "vertex potentials" (DAVIS, P. A., 1939; BANCAUD *et al.*, 1953; GASTAUT, 1953; DAVIS *et al.*, 1966). The responses were small, however, and the signal-to-noise ratio usually so unfavorable that they were practically neglected until after the introduction of the method of signal averaging. DAWSON reported his method of summating small evoked potentials in 1954, and with the advent of modern computers, both large and small, progress was rapid thereafter (see WHIPPLE, 1964).

Computer technique also made available, as possible tools for audiometry, the peripheral responses of the cochlea, eighth nerve and (probably) the brain stem, the small early cortical potentials, and late cortical responses averaged during sleep. In this historical survey, the early recordings of cochlear microphonics from the round window (in man) by FROMM *et al.* (1935), ANDREEV *et al.* (1938, 1939), PERLMAN and CASE (1941), and by LEMPERT *et al.* (1947, 1950), without averaging, deserve special mention.

IV. Classification of Auditory Evoked Responses (AER) by Latency

Evoked potentials are usefully classified on the basis of their latency from the onset of the stimulus to the peak or trough of each characteristic wave. These latencies must be stable for a given condition because the method of recording requires the averaging of time-locked responses. Any variability of latency during the collection of responses reduces the amplitude and broadens the contour of the waves.

There are three major ranges of latency which fortunately seem to correspond broadly to major differences in origin and physiological significance of the responses. We shall call them the *fast* (or early), the *slow* and the *late* AERs, respectively.

The fast responses have latencies up to 50 msec. The voltages are usually less than a microvolt, and hundreds of responses must be summed to obtain measurable patterns. There are many generators of such fast responses, and for each there is a preferred placement of electrodes. They represent the responses of various neural structures along the auditory pathway, including the cortex, and also a new class of audiogenic muscle reflex. To the extent that the fast responses can be related to particular anatomical sources, they have great potential value for ERA as an adjunct to otoneurology. The classes that have been so identified will be described separately below.

The slow responses have peak latencies from 50 to about 300 msec. Rather similar patterns are evoked by auditory, visual and somatosensory stimuli. These are the "vertex potentials"; they are usually from 1–50 μv in amplitude. Vertex (C_z) to a reference anywhere at the base of the skull (*i.e.* mastoid, ear lobe, nose, chin, *etc.*) is a good electrode combination for all three modalities, although, as shown in another chapter, the generator seems to be the primary cortical projection area of each sensory system. These AEPs have been the basis of most clinical ERA to date.

The late responses are those that reach their peak or plateau at or after 300 msec. There are several classes of late response, but only one of them, the AERs of sleep, will be considered in detail in this chapter. The AERs in sleep are included because they are the basis of most ERA in infants and uncooperative children and are, therefore, of great clinical importance. Other late responses, treated in Chapter 41, are the positive "expectancy wave" (P_{300}), the "contingent negative variation" (a DC shift after a warning signal but prior to a conditional motor response), and the positive DC shift that develops during continued auditory stimulation (KEIDEL, 1971). All of these have been suggested for use in ERA. It is possible to elicit P_{300} and CNV with "meaningful" stimuli — for example familiar words as opposed to nonsense syllables, and thus carry out a novel form of speech audiometry. It is not the sensitivity of hearing that is measured but the ability to attach meaning to spoken word. This interesting possibility has been demonstrated, but as a method of audiometry it is still in the experimental stage and full reports of the pilot studies are not yet available. The use of the DC shift faces formidable technical difficulties.

V. Fast (Early) Evoked Potentials

The fast evoked potentials may be recorded from many electrode placements on the head. Most, if not all, of the neurogenic responses that we shall describe can be recorded from vertex re ear lobe or mastoid if enough responses are averaged, particularly if special precautions are taken to reduce muscle potentials by relaxation of the subject (GEISLER *et al.*, 1958; GOLDSTEIN and RODMAN, 1967; MENDEL and GOLDSTEIN, 1969; JEWETT *et al.*, 1970). For study of the action potential of the cochlear nerve, however, a placement in or very near the external auditory canal is more efficient (SOHMER and FEINMESSER, 1967; YOSHIE, 1968; COATS and DICKEY, 1970; SALOMON and EBERLING, 1971) or within the middle ear on the promontory (RUBEN *et al.*, 1961, 1962; ARAN *et al.*, 1969). The practical complications of passing an electrode through the tympanic membrane are offset by the larger signal that is obtained. Placement on the hard palate is recommended by KEIDEL (1972).

The early myogenic responses of the "sonomotor" reflex will be described first, partly for historical reasons. These responses are not likely to be as useful for audiometric purposes as the neurogenic potentials, but, in principle, they might be used to test the integrity of certain reflex arcs low in the brain stem.

They may, however, confound or mask neurogenic responses, and, historically, they distracted attention from the early neurogenic potentials.

The myogenic responses are best recorded when one electrode is over or very near the responding muscle. Such positions are inion (*m. rectus capitis*) (BICKFORD *et al.*, 1964b), high on the mastoid process (*m. postauricularis*) (CODY and BICKFORD, 1969), temporal region (*m. temporalis*) (MAST, 1965), or over many muscles of the limbs (BICKFORD *et al.*, 1964b). A necessary condition for a myogenic response is on-going tonic activity of the muscle in question. When loud clicks are presented to the subject, some of the muscle units no longer discharge at random but become more or less time-locked to the clicks. BICKFORD calls this the "sonomotor reflex". The averaged response from inion is rhythmic, with peaks as follows: inion-positive 9, neg. 14, pos. 24, neg. 31 msec. (CODY and BICKFORD, 1969). The threshold for a clear sonomotor response is high, about 90 dB SPL, and the non-auditory labyrinth can be the channel of sensory input (BICKFORD *et al.*, 1964a). Other investigators believe that small sonomotor responses can be evoked also by the cochlear route and by clicks of medium intensity (MAST, 1965).

In some individuals, the postauricular muscle is an excellent reflex source (CODY and BICKFORD, 1969). This response habituates rather rapidly within a test session and across sessions. It presumably is part of a vestigial orienting reflex ("pricking up the ears"), and is of some physiological interest because the latency of its first peak (*ca.* 10 msec) is very short for a muscle reflex.

The sequence of early neurogenic responses begins with the action potential of the auditory nerve. The still earlier "cochlear microphonic", generated by the hair cells, can be recorded in man as noted above (*cf.* also RUBEN *et al.*, 1959), but, in so-called "electrocochleography" (ARAN and others), this response usually is deliberately cancelled out by presenting alternate condensation and rarefaction clicks.

The basis of cancellation of the cochlear microphonic is that the microphonic response reproduces the waveform of the acoustic signal and consequently reverses its polarity with the sound waves and, therefore, cancels out. The action potentials, however, do not reverse polarity but simply shift their latency by half a cycle of the sound wave. If the acoustic wave front of a click is abrupt, with a high-frequency acoustic spectrum, the shift of latency is negligible. This is true also for tone bursts of high frequency (4000 Hz and higher) with brief rise times (DAVIS, 1961), but, at lower frequencies, the shift results in two neural responses, separated by half a cycle, which may blur the total pattern and hinder measurements.

As the frequency of a tone burst is made still lower (1000 Hz or lower), the auditory nerve responds to each sound wave separately. This is the "volley principle" of WEVER (1949). (See DAVIS, 1961, and other chapters of this volume for relevant animal experiments.) The result is that it is easy, with sharp-fronted clicks or high-frequency tone bursts, to obtain a large well-synchronized first volley of nerve impulses. This is not possible with medium or low-frequency signals. The use, in audiometry, of the action potentials of the auditory nerve will always suffer from this inescapable limitation. The result is that the basal turn of the cochlea is open to study by electrocochleography, but, practically speaking, the higher turns are not. The electrocochleogram may nevertheless provide types of information other than a threshold audiogram, derived from the waveform of the neural response to standardized clicks or from the input-output relation of amplitude of the neural wave to sound intensity. Analysis of the waveform by the technique described by TEAS *et al.* (1962) of masking a broad-band click with successive narrow bands of noise offers considerable promise. Both of these avenues of approach are being studied vigorously at the present time, and rapid advances are being made in the use of the electrocochleogram for the study of abnormal ears, both in children and in adults (ARAN *et al.*, 1969; PORTMANN and ARAN, 1971; ARAN, 1971; YOSHIE, 1968).

Fast neurogenic responses of the auditory nerve and (probably) mid-brain auditory centers have been recorded from vertex (RUHM *et al.*, 1967; JEWETT, 1970) and from the hard palate (KEIDEL, 1972). The first neural volley can be identified with some confidence by its latency of about 1 msec. The identification of a larger response at about 5 msec and of a series of later vertex-negative waves at 7.6, 27, and 54 msec (MENDEL and GOLDSTEIN, 1969; KEIDEL, 1972) is still in doubt. Data from depth electrodes in animals and in human patients and from cortical electrodes during surgery (CELESIA *et al.*, 1968; CELESIA and PULETTI, 1971) will be needed to settle this complicated problem. At present, it is not clear that any of the responses between 1 msec (auditory nerve) and 16 msec (upper brain stem or auditory cortex or both) will be of much use in ERA. Fundamental difficulties are the very small voltages available and the practical problems encountered in applying electrodes in the more favorable positions. Consequently, large numbers of responses must be summed. Masking by muscle "noise" or by sonomotor responses is difficult to avoid.

The very early responses require precise synchronization of the nerve impulses in each volley, as explained above. The wavelength of the responses of longer latency is longer, however, (perhaps due to physiological variability in conduction times through the lower synaptic areas), and a greater spread of the initial neural response over two or more successive sound waves is permissible. In thalamic and cortical areas, tone bursts at 500 Hz or even 250 Hz, with rise times up to 6 msec, may give adequate synchronization for reliable detection of the "fast" responses generated there.

Two important general properties of the fast responses (earlier than 50 msec) are: (1) that they may be evoked at interstimulus intervals as short as 200 msec or even 100 msec without loss of average amplitude or undue interference by late components of previous responses, and (2) that they are not significantly depressed by sleep or sedation (MENDEL and GOLDSTEIN, 1969; PULETTI and CELESIA, 1970), although surgical anesthesia does modify the early cortical responses considerably (CELESIA and PULETTI, 1971). With repetition rates of 10 per second, it is feasible to sum as many as 1000 responses for each endpoint and still obtain a reasonable number of tests in a single sitting or surgical operation. The great stability of the response patterns in sleep and anesthesia gives an advantage, in principle at least, to the fast responses for the audiometric testing of uncooperative children for whom sedation is required. As we shall see, the slow V potentials are greatly modified by sleep or sedation.

VI. Slow Auditory Evoked Potentials the "Vertex Potentials"

The fast AERs described above resemble closely the AERs studied in detail in animals and employed in mapping the various sensory systems. Their interpretation involves no new difficulties beyond those of identification of the source or sources of each characteristic wave. The slow AERs, however, present some novel properties, and their interpretation in terms of neuronal activity or physiological significance is very obscure. They do bear a general resemblance to the familiar on-going spontaneous semi-rhythmic electrical activity of the cortex, but we do not really understand the alpha, the beta, the delta, the theta or the lambda rhythms of the cortex. They and the vertex potentials share a slow time-course, certain anatomical distributions and a dependence on the "state of the subject", whether awake or asleep. A major purpose of this chapter is to present a summary of properties of this set of slow potentials that are evoked in the cerebral cortex by auditory stimuli. The AERs are not unique, however. A very similar pattern of response occurs in the visual and somatosensory (and perhaps other) systems as well (ALLISON, 1962; GASTAUT *et al.*, 1967). Most of our information about slow cortical responses is derived from extracranial recordings in man. It is uncertain to what extent similar EPs occur in animals.

The time-course of the vertex potential (VP) is slow. The characteristic pattern of auditory VP is a vertex-negative wave (N_1) at 90 msec, positive (P_2) at 170 msec and negative at 250 (N_2) msec. An earlier positive wave (P_1) at 50 msec is often present but is more prominent in somatosensory responses.

The distribution of the slow AER on the scalp is widespread, but, with reference at ear, mastoid, nose, or chin, the optimum position is vertex (C_z). For somatosensory stimulation of a limb, the best position is over the contralateral primary projection area; for visual, it is at the occiput (O_z) with a strong secondary maximum near the vertex (VAUGHAN, 1969; VAUGHAN and RITTER, 1970). These distributions are compatible with the hypothesis that each set of evoked potentials is generated in the corresponding contralateral cortical projection area(s), with strong secondary responses from the corresponding homolateral area(s). The hypothesis is strongly supported by evidence from cases with known cortical lesions (STOHR and GOLDRING, 1969; JERGER *et al.*, 1969), as discussed by ELDREDGE and MILLER (1971). The potentials spread widely by volume conduction, but they do not represent a diffuse non-specific cortical response, as originally suggested (*cf.* WALTER, 1964). Some of the "late" responses, including those in sleep, are much more diffuse than the "slow" set under consideration here. (All of this is discussed more fully in Prof. KEIDEL's chapter.)

The VP is an on-effect and also a weaker off-effect (ROSE and MALONE, 1965; DAVIS and ZERLIN, 1966; SPYCHALA *et al.*, 1970). Prolongation of a stimulus of moderate strength beyond about 30 msec does not significantly modify the amplitude or latency of VP (ONISHI and DAVIS, 1968), but the temporal integration time near threshold is not yet known. Similar on-effects are produced by small changes, positive or negative, in either the frequency or the intensity of a steady tone (SPOOR *et al.*, 1969; MCCANDLESS and ROSE, 1970; NICHOLS and

TANENHOLTZ, 1970). During continued stimulation (seconds) a positive DC potential appears (KEIDEL, 1971), but this is a late response and is discussed in Chapter 4.

The latency of the auditory VP is stable above 20 dB sensation level but it may increase from 90 to nearly 200 msec (N_1) as the stimulus approaches threshold (BEAGLEY and KNIGHT, 1967). The differences across individuals are relatively small, except that latencies are somewhat longer in infants (ENGEL and YOUNG, 1969).

Under favorable conditions the practical threshold for detection of VP is close to the subject's behavioral (voluntary) threshold. Precise definition of this relation is difficult for reasons explained in the next section.

The voltage, usually measured peak-to-peak, N_1—P_2 or P_2—N_2, is of the order of 10 μv for moderate stimuli. There is a considerable range of variation across individuals.

The voltage of VP is sensitive to the interstimulus interval (ISI). An ISI of at least 10 sec is needed for maximal voltage. At an ISI of 1 sec, the amplitude is about 30% of maximal. From 500 msec to 10 sec, the amplitude is roughly proportional to log ISI (DAVIS *et al.*, 1966; NELSON and LASSMAN, 1968; GJERDINGEN and TOMSIC, 1970). Below an ISI of 500 msec, the VP is very small, and the slow components are difficult to separate from late components of the previous responses. With regular ISI, there is a gradual decline over the first several responses to a final steady-state voltage (RITTER *et al.*, 1968; FRUHSTORFER *et al.*, 1970). For a given average ISI, the responses are slightly larger with an irregular sequence of ISIs than with a constant ISI (ROTHMAN *et al.*, 1970). The variability of amplitude in ISI experiments across trials, across individuals and from one response to the next (ZERLIN and DAVIS, 1967) is large.

As the intensity of stimulus is increased from threshold to about 20 dB SL, the voltage of VP increases rather rapidly and its latency diminishes. (The increase in amplitude may be due in part indirectly to a reduction in the variability of the latency.) Above 20 dB SL, the amplitude increases slowly to about double the 20 dB voltage at 80 dB (see Fig. 1). At higher intensities, the responses may be considerably larger but with great individual differences. There is no clear simple relation such as the "power law" to the intensity of the stimulus, as discussed in Chapter 4.

If a masking noise is present, the auditory VP becomes detectable slightly above the masked behavioral threshold and increases rapidly until, at about 25 dB above masked threshold, the amplitude is as large as it would be with no noise background (DAVIS *et al.*, 1968). This effect resembles recruitment of loudness.

For frequencies from 500 Hz upward, the VPs evoked by tone bursts of different rise times, from 5—30 msec, are indistinguishable. At lower frequencies, short rise times result in an audible click, which must be avoided. As a function of frequency, the responses are slightly larger and clearer in the middle range (500–2000 Hz) than at higher or lower frequencies at the same loudness level (DAVIS *et al.*, 1968; ANTINORO *et al.*, 1969).

The V potential is strongly affected by the state of the subject. Most favorable is a state of high attention or vigilance (HAIDER *et al.*, 1964) such as may be induced by forcing the subject to make a rather difficult discrimination or decision concerning the stimulus (Davis, 1964). It is not clear to what extent attention must be specific to the modality of the stimulus (Näätänen, 1967). The general level of arousal is certainly important. Simple counting of stimuli is no more effective than casual reading or looking at pictures. Restlessness and boredom reduce the responses, and drowsiness is still worse. Other emotional states, such as anxiety, apprehension, and physical discomfort, probably affect the V potentials in ways that are still undefined. Simple closing of the eyes has no effect in itself, but it may invite drowsiness, and the increased alpha activity may make detection of small responses more difficult. Much has been written about "habituation" of the V potentials, but it is probable that the general state of arousal of the subject is more important than specific habituation to a particular stimulus (Fruhstorfer and Bergstrom, 1969; Fruhstorfer, 1971). The slight advantage of irregular ISI is usually attributed to a higher arousal or attention level.

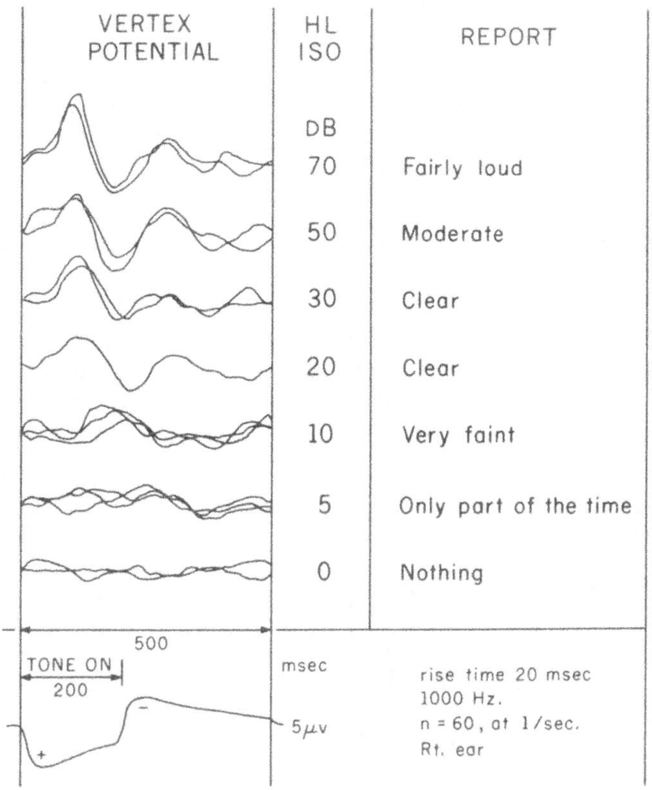

Fig. 1. The form, amplitude, and latency of the vertex (V) potential in response to 1000 Hz tone bursts at various hearing levels are shown in the tracings in the left column. The corresponding reports of the subject are given on the right. Two or three trials were made at most of the hearing levels. Note the very slight reduction in amplitude of the V potential, its constant latency from 70—20 dB, and the rapid fall in amplitude and prolongation of latency from 20—5 dB. (From Hearing and Deafness, third edition, edited by Hallowell Davis and S. Richard Silverman. Copyright 1947, (c) 1960, 1970 by Holt, Rinehart, and Winston, Inc. Reprinted by permission of Holt, Rinehart, and Winston, Inc.)

Light sleep depresses the V potential, particularly N_1 ; P_2 and N_2 may persist. In medium sleep, a larger P_2 and a large delayed N_2 appear. Their latencies are slightly longer than in the waking state, with the peak of N_2 at 320 msec or later. This "sleeping P_{200}–N_{320}" complex increases in amplitude and may be prolonged as a negative plateau (or a second wave) that terminates, often quite abruptly, at about 400–500 msec. In deep sleep, the voltages of these and still later waves may be considerable, but the late waves are erratic and are immersed in high-voltage delta waves. Reliable identification of AER in sleep is more difficult than in the waking state, with many misses in light sleep and more false positives than in the waking state. The best criterion is the P_{200}–N_{320} wave, for which the threshold may be as low as 10 dB (sensation level) in deep sleep. In light sleep, the threshold of the electric response may be 30 or 40 dB SL (DAVIS and ONISHI, 1969; OSTERHAMMEL *et al.*, 1972).

The late evoked potentials in sleep, and perhaps P_{200}–N_{320} also, are probably diffuse in origin and closely related to the spontaneous delta waves and to the K complexes that are sometimes evoked by more widely spaced stimuli.

More study is needed to define the possible specific effects of various classes of drugs such as the barbiturates and other sedatives, and also the maturation of AER in early infancy. Clear sensory evoked responses are seen in neonates (BARNET and GOODWIN, 1965; ENGEL and YOUNG, 1969), and an excellent summary, including clinical applications, is given by GRAZIANI and WEITZMAN (1971). The latencies of AER are somewhat longer in neonates than in older infants, but it is not always clear in these reports whether the depth of sleep or the degree of (waking) arousal were comparable.

A final feature of V potentials is the depressive interaction that may occur when a secondary stimulus, different from the primary stimulus, is interpolated shortly before each primary stimulus. The secondary stimulus may be in the same or a different modality from the primary (DAVIS *et al.*, 1968b). The depression that it produces is least for different modalities and it increases as the two stimuli are made more and more alike (BUTLER, 1968). Relative intensities and also the length of the ISIs are important parameters. Details concerning these various intramodal and cross-modal interactions for both the slow potentials and the DC shifts are given in Chapter 4.

VII. Identification of AER in ERA

ERA depends on recognizing time-locked AERs. Several factors combine to make this a difficult task when the responses are small, such as (1) the poor signal-to-noise ratio between the AER and spontaneous EEG waves of similar wavelength, (2) the intrusion of major electrical artifacts associated with movements of eyes, head or arms, (3) variability of AER across subjects, (4) variation of AER with the degree of arousal of the subject, if awake, or the depth of his sleep, (5) the change in latency near (voluntary) threshold, and perhaps (6) cross-modality interference from visual or tactile stimuli. In epileptic subjects, there may be spontaneous seizure waves in the EEG. On the other hand, it is fortunate for ERA that the threshold for identification of AER under favorable waking circumstances is not more than 5 dB above the subject's voluntary behavioral threshold.

Movement artifacts, the state of the subject, and cross-modality interference are to some extent under the control of the tester. Variability of response patterns across subjects is handled by obtained a clear response at a high stimulus level, which is usually possible unless the threshold is near the limit of the audiometer. In the latter case, a response to tactile (vibratory) stimulation gives a useful although less perfect guide. The superposition of tracings taken at lower intensities on one (or more) "guide patterns" improves immensely the probability of correctly recognizing small reponses, perhaps with increased latency, that are partly but not completely deformed by the EEG "noise" mixed with it. Visual comparison by superposition makes use of all features of the response — not merely the latencies and amplitudes of the peaks.

The signal-to-noise ratio is a fundamental problem. "Noise" outside the frequency band of the response can be greatly reduced by well-chosen electrical filtering, usually retaining only the band from 1—15 Hz. Within the passband, the signal-to-noise ratio can in principle be improved to any desired extent by increasing the number of responses that are summed, but the improvement is proportional to $\sqrt{n}$, not to n itself. The number to be summed will be a practical compromise between the signal-to-noise ratio that is achieved and the number of minutes budgeted for each collection. The duration of each collection and the total length of time that a subject will stay in a favorable state determine how many thresholds can be estimated in a single clinical session. (Recommended numbers will be given in the next section.) Here, we use the term "estimate" advisedly because the value finally written on the audiogram blank is often an interpolation between the intensity of a clearly positive trial and that of a clearly negative trial, and the range of the operator's uncertainty will usually be at least ± 10 dB.

The most difficult question is the definition of what constitutes a "positive" response. When the range of uncertainty has been narrowed so that the estimate turns on a single "doubtful" response, it is usually worth a minute or two of time to repeat that particular trial. When the two tracings are superimposed, this effectively doubles the number of responses summed, but indefinite repetitions are not permissible. Ultimately, each operator must establish for himself his own criterion of what is an acceptable positive response. He knows that he will miss some actual responses that are obscured by EEG "noise", and he knows that he will make some "false positive" judgments. By experience, he learns to minimize the sum of the two errors, or he may deliberately make his criterion more rigid or more lax, depending on whether a miss or a false positive would lead to the more serious error in the overall clinical evaluation of the case. He may also be influenced in doubtful decisions by the overall plausibility of the audiogram he obtains, knowing that statistically there are strong correlations between the thresholds at neighboring frequencies and, in many situations such as congenital hearing loss, between the thresholds for the two ears.

The establishment of a criterion for a positive response is more difficult for sleep than for the waking state. The depth of sleep varies and is not under the operator's control. With it, the amplitude of the response and of the noise in which it is embedded (delta waves) increases. The responses seem to be less reliable than in the waking state, and both misses and false positives are more frequent. Apparently also, as noted above, the threshold of detectability of responses in light sleep is well above the waking voluntary behavioral threshold (OSTERHAMMEL *et al.*, 1972). It is unfortunate that the uncertainty of identification of responses is greatest in exactly the situation in which ERA should be of greatest clinical value, namely, for threshold audiometry in young children under sedation. However, further study of the electric responses in sleep and of the effects of drugs, including optimal dosages, and appropriate allowances for the stage of sleep, as estimated from the amount of delta activity seen in a simultaneous monitor EEG record, should improve the reliability of the method considerably.

VIII. Recommended Procedure for Electric Response Audiometry based on the V Potential

The following summary of practical procedures is based on the experimental findings presented above and on clinical experience of approximately seven years, chiefly with children under 12 years of age (*cf.* DAVIS *et al.*, 1967; DAVIS and NIEMOELLER, 1968). The routine is designed to obtain a 3- or 4-frequency audiogram for each ear in a single session of one hour, including the time for application of electrodes. With the help of an attendant who is skilled in the handling of children and adept at keeping them amused with appropriate books, pictures and toys, this goal can usually be attained with children over three years of age. The child's mother assists in waking tests of those under four or five years, holding the child in her lap, but the importance of the skilled attendant cannot be overemphasized.

The routine is based on an instrument which delivers the audiometric signals automatically and produces an on-line write-out of the averaged evoked potentials on a semitransparent paper (Princeton Applied Research Corp. Evoked Response Audiometer System, Model 140). The successive tracings of summed responses are cut from the tape, labeled, and compared with one another (preferably by superposition) on a viewing surface illuminated from beneath. This maneuver allows on-line judgments to be made rapidly, with only a few seconds delay between successive trials.

The audiometric signals are delivered through earphones mounted in a standard headband, if the child will tolerate them. A sponge-rubber pad on the top of the child's head makes the headband more comfortable, and most children accept the earphones as well as the electrodes if their confidence is gained and they are not hurried. Pictures of children wearing earphones and a mirror held to allow the child to see himself are very helpful. A loudspeaker, properly calibrated, may be used if necessary, but for sound pressure levels above 90 dB and for testing the ears individually earphones are necessary. 110 dB hearing level (ISO) should be available from 500–6000 Hz.

Standard audiometric tone bursts of 200 msec duration and rise and fall times of 5 msec are satisfactory. Bursts as short as 30 msec can be used, but the 200 msec duration brings the test signals within the limits set by the American National Standard for Audiometers (1969). This standard is also followed with respect to the audiometric reference zero (ISO, 1964), the accuracy of calibration of intensity and frequency, and the provision of masking noise for the contralateral ear.

The number of responses averaged in a trial and the interval between stimuli are at the discretion of the operator. With intervals of 1 sec, the voltage accumulated in one minute (60 presentations) is maximum. At intervals of 2 sec, the individual responses are larger but the total in one minute (30 presentations) is slightly less than with the faster rate. Collections of one minute give a good compromise of adequate voltage per collection and the number of collections that can be made within the practical limit of testing time. At intervals of one second or of two seconds, sufficient voltage with an adequate signal-to-noise ratio is accumulated in one minute. The writer prefers regular 1 sec intervals if the child is awake. The slight possible advantage from a carefully planned irregular sequence does not justify the additional complexity of instrumentation in the clinical situation.

Electroencephalographic electrodes are applied at the vertex (C_z), to one earlobe or mastoid area (A_1 or M_1), and a ground electrode elsewhere on the head, either on the forehead or opposite ear. The writer prefers miniature non-polarizable electrodes mounted in plastic cases which can be attached to the skin by double-surfaced adhesive wafers (BECKMAN). The miniature electrode at the vertex requires cutting the hair (with curved scissors) in an area 15 or 20 mm in diameter. The skin is also cleaned with dilute alcohol, rubbing vigorously enough to reduce the interelectrode DC resistance below 20000 Ω. Gold or silver cup electrodes may be used if preferred, but their attachment is usually less secure or may require an odorous adhesive (such as collodion) or adhesive-remover. Such odors, suggestive of a hospital, are quite disturbing to some children and are out of place in a hearing clinic. Of course, an electrode jelly appropriate to the preferred type of electrode is employed.

The EEG is best recorded with limited band-width, usually 1–15 Hz, with conventional EEG roll-offs (6 dB per octave). A 60 Hz "notch" filter to reduce AC interference may also be necessary. With it and a well-designed EEG amplifier, there may be no need for special electrical screening or shielding. Amplification is adjusted arbitrarily to produce V potential records of convenient size. The "window" of the averager should be 500 msec if 1 sec intervals are used. The moment of stimulation must be signalled on the recording tape so that latencies can be measured and separated records can be accurately superimposed. A slowly moving tape allows adequate but economical monitoring for gross EEG artifacts from movement, etc. Useful information is added, even with a slow tape, if the contents of the memory are written out after each stimulus, thus showing whether the growth of the response pattern is regular or erratic. An adjustable peak-limiter to prevent EEG artifacts from contributing unduly to the accumulation in the memory is desirable but not essential.

For "control" responses, a vibrator, to be applied to the palmar surface of the child's fingers, and a photostimulator, such as is used to "activate" the EEG, are very useful. They are operated by the same trigger circuit as the audio generator. (These different forms of stimulation are best administered about midway during the test session, just before a five-minute recess during which the child is allowed to move arms, legs and head more freely than during the collection of evoked potentials.) The purpose of these control responses is to demonstrate the responsivity of the child's brain if no clear auditory responses appear. The form of the tactile responses helps in identifying small auditory responses. The degree of resemblance between two successive vibratory or flash responses gives a strong clue to the amount of "noise" or electrical background from the EEG that accumulates in addition to the responses.

It is not feasible to obtain, in a single session, audiograms of more than four or perhaps three frequencies for each ear. A restless child may effectively terminate the test at almost any moment. In dealing with children with moderate to very severe hearing losses, the writer employs the following sequence: 1000 Hz (two or three collections from each ear), 250 Hz (one or two from each ear), 3000 Hz (one or two from each ear), then control responses (two vibratory and two flash trials). Note that the single frequency 3000 Hz is substituted for 2000 and 4000 Hz. In the second half of the session, after a brief recess, 500 Hz is added, one or two trials with each ear, and additional trials are made near the apparent threshold at the other frequencies.

A. Modification for Tests during Sleep

The chief modification for sleep tests is to employ a "window" of 1 sec instead of 500 msec in order to see possible late components of the V potential of sleep. The longer window requires a longer interstimulus interval, for which 2 sec is satisfactory. The higher voltage of both the background (delta waves) and responses requires also a reduction of the amplification employed. The tester should assess the depth of sleep, on the basis chiefly of the average width of the EEG tracing on the slow tape, and should note it under the final fast write-out of each collection. The criteria for recognizing a positive response vary with the depth of sleep, and in light sleep the threshold of detection of responses no longer coincides with the expected behavioral (voluntary) threshold.

B. Strategy of ERA

We shall not discuss in detail the strategy of efficient electric response audiometry based on the V potentials, but the writer offers the following guiding principles that he has found useful in testing young children.

1) Train an attendant to keep children alert and interested in something, but not too active.

2) Test young children awake if possible but sedated if necessary.

3) Plan a sequence of trials in advance. Alternate trials between the two ears. Three frequencies are sufficient in the initial sequence.

4) 70 dB hearing level (ISO) at 1000 Hz is a good starting point. Change the intensity by large steps, usually 20 dB. The strategy is like the game of "twenty questions".

5) Waste no time between trials. An assistant should label the final write-outs ready for comparison by superposition when cut from the tape.

6) Obtain early in the sequence, if possible, three or four clear positive responses to serve as "guide patterns" for identification of smaller responses.

7) After each ear has been tested at three frequencies, obtain control responses to vibration and flash unless audio responses are very clear. Pause a few minutes while planning exactly the sequence of eight or ten final trials.

8) Defer tests with masking or by bone conduction to a later session. Twenty-five to thirty collections at one minute each usually reach the limit of the period of a child's good behavior.

9) In judging records, reproducibility is the key to correct identification of responses, but background EEG will often obscure or distort true responses and, on the other hand, will sometimes mimic the guide pattern perfectly. P_{180} is the most stable single feature, awake or asleep; N_{250} is next, and N_{100} is the least stable.

10) Responses are usually quite clear in the waking state at 20 dB above behavioral threshold. The response is small and latency prolonged at 10 dB SL. On the basis of a set of two or three well-spaced trials at a given frequency, it is legitimate to interpolate or even extrapolate the final estimate of the threshold.

11) If the child is asleep, it may be necessary to use the loudspeaker, but very frequently an earphone, removed from the headband, can be held against the child's ear to great advantage. In a young child, a reliable estimate of threshold at 1000 Hz in each ear is often sufficient clinically, but this may require many trials. Obtain an endpoint on one ear before moving the child's head. Arousal by sound to a lighter stage of sleep can be very useful evidence of hearing, regardless of evoked potentials.

IX. Summary

Electric potentials evoked by auditory stimuli may be recorded from the human head by the technique of summing or averaging the time-locked responses. This method allows the study of certain properties of the auditory central nervous system and it also can be used for electric response audiometry.

The early responses have latencies (to peak) of 50 msec or less and voltages less than 1 μV. For the very earliest wave, generated by the auditory nerve, electrode placements in or near the ear are best. The identification of the sources of waves later than 1 or 2 msec is still tentative. The "electrocochleogram" has promise for audiometry but it yields very poor responses to the lower audio frequencies.

A vertex recording (C_z- ear or C_z-mastoid) yields fast responses from midbrain or auditory cortex or both. The voltage is small (about 1 μV), but the fast responses are not much affected by the state of the subject. Like the electrocochleogram, the fast vertex responses offer certain advantages for audiometry, notably the stability of the response.

The slow vertex potentials, probably generated in the primary auditory cortex, are 1 to about 25 μV. They show several unique physiological properties, such as a long recovery period (up to 10 sec), appearance only in response to on or off of a tone or to a *change* in intensity or frequency, variability from trial to trial, slight relation of voltage to acoustic intensity, and major modifications in sleep. They can be used effectively for audiometry, even in young or uncooperative children. With appropriate procedures and strategy, clinical useful estimates of auditory sensitivity at all audible frequencies can be obtained.

Late cortical evoked potentials, after 300 msec, and DC shifts of the base-line show interesting relations to psychological factors such as expectancy, and novel forms of audiometry may be based on them in the future, but they lie outside the scope of this chapter.

References

ALLISON, T.: Recovery functions of somatosensory evoked responses in man. Electroenceph. clin. Neurophysiol. **14**, 331—343 (1962).

American National Standards Institute: Specifications for Audiometers. ANSI S3.6-1969. New York: American National Standards Institute, Inc. 1969.

ANDREEV, A. M., ARAPOVA, A. A., GERSUNI, G. V.: On the cochlear potentials in man. Bull. Biol. Méd. Expér. **6**, 495—496 (1938).

ANDREEV, A. M., ARAPOVA, A. A., GERSUNI, G. V.: On the electrical potentials of the human cochlea. J. Physiol. U.S.S.R. **26**, 205—212 (1939).

ANTINORO, F., SKINNER, P. H., JONES, J. J.: Relation between sound intensity and amplitude of the AER at different stimulus frequencies. J. Acoust. Soc. Amer. **46**, 1433—1436 (1969).

ARAN, J.-M.: L'électro-cochléogramme: I. Principe et technique. Cahiers de la C. F. A. **12**, 3—45 (1971).

ARAN, J.-M., PORTMANN, CL., DELAUNAY, J., PELERIN, J., LENOIR, J.: L'électro-cochléogramme: Methodes et premiers résultats chez l'enfant. Rev. Laryng. (Bordeaux) **90**, 615—634 (1969).

BANCAUD, J., BLOCH, V., PAILLARD, J.: Contribution EEG à l'étude des potentiels évoques chez l'homme au niveau du vertex. Rev. Neurol. **89**, 399—418 (1953).

BARNET, A. B., GOODWIN, R. S.: Averaged evoked electroencephalographic responses to clicks in the human newborn. Electroenceph. clin. Neurophysiol. **18**, 441—450 (1965).

BEAGLEY, H. A., KNIGHT, J. J.: Changes in auditory evoked response with intensity. J. Laryngol. **81**, 861—873 (1967).

BICKFORD, R. G., JACOBSON, J. L., CODY, D. T.: Nature of average evoked potentials to sound and other stimuli in man. Ann. N.Y. Acad. Sci. **112**, 204—223 (1964a).

BICKFORD, R. G., JACOBSON, J. L., CODY, D. T., LAMBERT, E. H.: Fast motor system in man: Physiopathology of the sonomotor response. Trans. Amer. Neurol. Ass. **89**, 56—58 (1964b).

BUTLER, R. A.: Effect of changes in stimulus frequency and intensity on habituation of the human vertex potential. J. Acoust. Soc. Amer. **44**, 945—950 (1968).

CELESIA, G. G., BROUGHTON, R. J., RASMUSSEN, T., BRANCH, C.: Auditory evoked responses from the exposed human cortex. Electroenceph. clin. Neurophysiol. **24**, 458—466 (1968).

CELESIA, G. G., PULETTI, F.: Auditory input to the human cortex during states of drowsiness and surgical anesthesia. Electroenceph. clin. Neurophysiol. **31**, 603—609 (1971).

COATS, A. C., DICKEY, J. R.: Nonsurgical recording of human auditory nerve action potentials and cochlear microphonics. Ann. Otol. Rhinol. Laryngol. **79**, 844—852 (1970).

CODY, D. T., BICKFORD, R. G.: Averaged evoked myogenic responses in normal man. Laryngoscope **79**, 400—416 (1969).

DAVIS, H.: Peripheral coding of auditory information. In: ROSENBLITH, W. (Ed.): Sensory communication, Chapter 7. Cambridge: M.I.T. Press 1961.

DAVIS, H.: Enhancement of evoked cortical potentials in humans related to a task requiring a decision. Science **145**, 182—183 (1964).

DAVIS, H., BOWERS, C., HIRSH, S. K.: Relations of the human vertex potential to acoustic input: loudness and masking. J. Acoust. Soc. Amer. **43**, 431—438 (1968a).

DAVIS, H., HIRSH, S. K., SHELNUTT, J., BOWERS, C.: Further validation of evoked response audiometry (ERA). J. Speech Hear. Res. **10**, 717—732 (1967).

DAVIS, H., MAST, T., YOSHIE, N., ZERLIN, S.: The slow response of the human cortex to auditory stimuli: recovery process. Electroenceph. clin. Neurophysiol. **21**, 105—113 (1966).

DAVIS, H., NIEMOELLER, A. F.: A system for clinical evoked response audiometry. J. Speech Hearing Dis. **33**, 33—37 (1968).

DAVIS, H., ONISHI, S.: Maturation of auditory evoked potentials. Int. Audiol. 8, 24—33 (1969).

DAVIS, H., ZERLIN, S., BOWERS, C., SPOOR, A.: Some interactions of the vertex potentials. Electroenceph. clin. Neurophysiol. **24**, 285 (1968b).

DAVIS, H., ZERLIN, S.: Acoustic relations of the human vertex potential. J. Acoust. Soc. Amer. **39**, 109—116 (1966).

DAVIS, P. A.: Effects of acoustic stimuli on the waking human brain. J. Neurophysiol. **2**, 494—499 (1939).

DAWSON, G. D.: A summation technique for the detection of small evoked potentials. Electroenceph. clin. Neurophysiol. **6**, 65—84 (1954).

ELDREDGE, D. H., MILLER, J. D.: Physiology of hearing. Ann. Rev. Physiol. **33**, 281—310 (1971).

ENGEL, R., YOUNG, N. B.: Calibrated pure tone audiograms in normal neonates based on evoked electroencephalographic responses. Neuropädiatrie **1**, 149—160 (1969).

FROMM, B., NYLÉN, C. O., ZOTTERMAN, Y.: Studies in the mechanism of the Wever and Bray effect. Acta Oto-Laryngol. **22**, 477—486 (1935).

FRUHSTORFER, H.: Habituation and dishabituation of the human vertex response. Electroenceph. clin. Neurophysiol. **30**, 306—312 (1971).

FRUHSTORFER, H., BERGSTROM, R. M.: Human vigilance and auditory evoked responses. Electroenceph. clin. Neurophysiol. **27**, 346—355 (1969).

FRUHSTORFER, H., SOVERI, P., JÄRVILEHTO, T.: Short-term habituation of the auditory evoked response in man. Electroenceph. clin. Neurophysiol. **28**, 153—161 (1970).

GASTAUT, Y.: Les pointes négatives évoquées sur le vertex. Leur signification psychophysiologique et pathologique. Rev. Neurol. **89**, 382—399 (1953).

GASTAUT, H., RÉGIS, H., LYAGOUBI, S., MANO, T., SIMON, L.: Comparison of the potentials recorded from the occipital, temporal and central regions of the human scalp, evoked by visual, auditory and somato-sensory stimuli. In: COBB, W., MOROCUTTI, C. (Eds.): The evoked potentials, pp. 19—28. Amsterdam: Elsevier 1967.

GEISLER, C. D., FRISHKOPF, L. S., ROSENBLITH, W. A.: Extracranial responses to acoustic clicks in man. Science **128**, 1210—1211 (1958).

GJERDINGEN, D. B., TOMSIC, R.: Recovery functions of human cortical potentials evoked by tones, shocks, vibration, and flashes. Psychon. Sci. **19 (4)**, 228—229 (1970).

GOLDSTEIN, R., KENDALL, D. C., ARICK, B. E.: Electroencephalic audiometry in young children. J. Speech Hearing Dis. **28**, 331—354 (1963).

GOLDSTEIN, R., RODMAN, L. B.: Early components of averaged evoked responses to rapidly repeated auditory stimuli. J. Speech Hear. Res. **10**, 697—705 (1967).

GRAZIANI, L. J., WEITZMAN, E. D.: Sensory evoked responses in the neonatal period and their clinical application. In: RÉMOND, E. (Ed.): Internat. Handbook EEG and Clin. Neurophys. Amsterdam: Elsevier 1971.

GROSS, M. M., BEGLETTER, H., TOBIN, M., KISSIN, B.: Auditory evoked response comparison during counting clicks and reading. Electroenceph. clin. Neurophysiol. **18**, 451—454 (1965).

HAIDER, M., SPONG, P., LINDSLEY, D. B.: Attention, vigilance, and cortical evoked-potentials in humans. Science **145**, 180—182 (1964).

HILLYARD, S. A., SQUIRES, K. C., BAUER, J. W., LINDSAY, P. H.: Evoked potential correlates of auditory signal detection. Science **172**, 1357—1360 (1971).

JERGER, J., WEIKERS, N. J., SHARBROUGH, F. W., JERGER, S.: Bilateral lesions of the temporal lobe. A case study. Acta Oto-Laryngol. Suppl. **258**, 1—51 (1969).

JEWETT, D. L., ROMANO, M. N., WILLISTON, J. S.: Human auditory evoked potentials: possible brain stem components detected on the scalp. Science **167**, 1517—1518 (1970).

KEATING, L. W., RUHM, H. B.: Some observations on the effects of attention to stimuli on the amplitude of the acoustically evoked response. Audiology **10**, 177—184 (1971a).

KEATING, L. W., RUHM, H. B.: Within average variability of the acoustically evoked response. J. Speech Hear. Res. **14**, 179—188 (1971b).

KEIDEL, W. D.: D.C.-potentials in the auditory evoked response in man. Acta Oto-Laryngol. **71**, 242—248 (1971).

Keidel, W. D.: The use of fast correlators in electrocochleography in man. Proceedings of the First Conference of the British Society of Audiology. London. In press, 1972.

Lempert, J., Wever, E. G., Lawrence, M.: The cochleogram and its clinical application. Arch. Otolaryngol. **45**, 61—67 (1947).

Lempert, J., Meltzer, P. E., Wever, E. G., Lawrence, M.: The cochleogram and its clinical application. Arch. Otolaryng. **51**, 307—311 (1950).

Marcus, R. E., Gibbs, E. L., Gibbs, F. A.: Electroencephalography in the diagnosis of hearing loss in the very young child. Dis. Nerv. Syst. **10**, 170—173 (1949).

Mast, T. E.: Short-latency human evoked responses to clicks. J. Appl. Physiol. **20**, 725—730 (1965).

Mast, T. E., Watson, C. S.: Attention and auditory evoked responses to low-detectability signals. Percept. & Psychophys. **4**, 237—240 (1968).

McCandless, G. A., Rose, D. E.: Evoked cortical responses to stimulus change. J. Speech Hear. Res. **13**, 624—634 (1970).

Mendel, M. I., Goldstein, R.: The effect of test conditions on the early components of the averaged electroencephalic response. J. Speech Hear. Res. **12**, 344—350 (1969a).

Mendel, M. I., Goldstein, R.: Stability of the early components of the averaged electroencephalic response. J. Speech Hear. Res. **12**, 351—361 (1969b).

Näätänen, R.: Selective attention and evoked potentials. Ann. Acad. Sci. Fenn B **151**, 1—226 (1967).

Nelson, D. A., Lassman, F. M.: Effects of intersignal interval on the human auditory evoked response. J. Acoust. Soc. Amer. **44**, 1529—1532 (1968).

Nichols, T. L., Tanenholtz, S. D.: Effect of increments in a sinusoidal pedestal on the vertex potential. J. Acoust. Soc. Amer. **47**, 97 (A) (1970).

Onishi, S., Davis, H.: Effects of duration and rise time of tone bursts on evoked V potentials. J. Acoust. Soc. Amer. **44**, 582—591 (1968).

Ortiz-Estrada, P., Deutsch, E., Hernandez-Orozco, F.: An electroencephalographic method for evaluation of hearing in children. Ann. Otol. Rhinol. Laryngol. **72**, 135—147 (1963).

Osterhammel, P. A., Davis, H., Wier, C. C., Hirsh, S. K.: Adult auditory evoked vertex potentials in sleep. Audiology (in press) (1972).

Perl, E. R., Galambos, R., Glorig, A.: The estimation of hearing threshold by electroencephalography. Electroenceph. clin. Neurophysiol. **5**, 501—512 (1953).

Perlman, H. B., Case, T. J.: Electrical phenomena of the cochlea in man. Arch. Otolaryngol. **34**, 710—718 (1941).

Portmann, M., Aran, M.-M.: Electrocochleographie sur le nourrison et le jeune enfant. Acta Oto-Laryngol. **71**, 253—261 (1971).

Puletti, F., Celesia, G. G.: Functional properties of the primary cortical auditory area in man. J. Neurosurg. **32**, 244—247 (1970).

Ritter, W., Vaughan, H. G., Jr., Costa, L. D.: Orienting and habituation to auditory stimuli: a study of short term changes in average evoked responses. Electroenceph. clin. Neurophysiol. **25**, 550—556 (1968).

Rose, D. E., Malone, J. C.: Some aspects of the acoustically evoked response to the cessation of stimulus. J. Auditory Res. **5**, 27—40 (1965).

Roth, W. T., Kopell, B. S.: The auditory evoked response to repeated stimuli during a vigilance task. Psychophysiology **6**, 301—309 (1969).

Rothman, H. H., Davis, H., Hay, I. S.: Slow evoked cortical potentials and temporal features of stimulation. Electroenceph. clin. Neurophysiol. **29**, 225—232 (1970).

Ruben, R. J., Knickerbocker, G. G., Sekula, J., Nager, G. T., Bordley, J. E.: Cochlear microphonics in man. Laryngoscope **69**, 665—671 (1959).

Ruben, R. J., Bordley, J. E., Lieberman, A. T.: Cochlear potentials in man. Laryngoscope **71**, 1141—1164 (1961).

Ruben, R. J., Lieberman, A. T., Bordley, J. E.: Some observations on cochlear potentials and nerve action potentials in children. Laryngoscope **72**, 545—554 (1962).

Ruhm, H., Walker, E., Jr., Flanigin, H.: Acoustically-evoked potentials in man: mediation of early components. Laryngoscope **77**, 806—822 (1967).

SATTERFIELD, J. H.: Evoked cortical response enhancement and attention in man. A study of responses to auditory and shock stimuli. Electroenceph. clin. Neurophysiol. **19**, 470–475 (1965).

SALOMON, G., ELBERLING, C.: Cochlear nerve potentials recorded from the external ear in man. Acta Oto-Laryngol. **71**, 319—325 (1971).

SOHMER, H., FEINMESSER, M.: Cochlear action potentials recorded from the external ear in man. Ann. Otol. Rhinol. Laryngol. **76**, 427—435 (1967).

SPOOR, A., TIMMER, F., ODENTHAL, D. W.: The evoked auditory response (ear) to intensity modulated and frequency modulated tones and tone bursts. Int. Audiol. **8**, 410—415 (1969).

SPYCHALA, P., ROSE, D. E., GRIER, J. B.: Comparison of the "on" and "off" characteristics of the acoustically evoked response. Int. Audiol. **8**, 416—423 (1969).

STOHR, P. E., GOLDRING, S.: Origin of somatosensory evoked scalp responses in man. J. Neurosurg. **31**, 117—127 (1969).

TEAS, D. C., ELDREDGE, D. H., DAVIS, H.: Cochlear responses to acoustic transients: an interpretation of whole-nerve action potentials. J. Acoust. Soc. Amer. **34**, 1438—1459 (1962).

VAUGHAN, H. G., Jr.: The relationship of brain activity to scalp recordings of event-related potentials. In: DONCHIN, E., LINDSLEY, D. B. (Eds.): Average evoked potentials: Methods, results and evaluations. NASA (Natl. Aeronautics and Space Admin.) SP-191, Washington Chapter **2**, 45—94 (1969).

VAUGHAN, H. G., Jr., RITTER, W.: The sources of auditory evoked responses recorded from the human scalp. Electroenceph. clin. Neurophysiol. **28**, 360—367 (1970).

WALTER, W. G.: The convergence and interaction of visual, auditory, and tactile responses in human nonspecific cortex. Ann. N.Y. Acad. Sci. **112**, 320—361 (1964).

WEVER, E. G.: Theory of Hearing, p. 484. New York: John Wiley & Sons 1949.

WHIPPLE, H. E. (Ed.): Sensory evoked response in man. Ann. N.Y. Acad. Sci. **112**, 1—546 (1964).

WITHROW, F. B., Jr., GOLDSTEIN, R.: An electrophysiologic procedure for determination of auditory threshold in children. Laryngoscope **68**, 1674—1699 (1958).

YAMAMOTO, K., NISHIKAWA, H., NAGATA, M., ITAKURA, S.: Objective hearing test in young children and deafness. Nagoya J. med. Sci. **16**, 79—84 (1953).

YOSHIE, N.: Auditory nerve action potential responses to clicks in man. Laryngoscope **78**, 198—215 (1968).

ZERLIN, S., DAVIS, H.: The variability of single evoked vertex potentials in man. Electroenceph. clin. Neurophysiol. **23**, 468—472 (1967).

A more recent review, with emphasis on brainstem responses and the electrocochleogram is:

DAVIS, H.: Principles of Electric Response Audiometry. Ann. Otol. Rhinol. Laryngol. Supplement 28. Vol. 85, May-June, 1976, No. 3, Part 3.

Chapter 4

The Physiological Background of the Electric Response Audiometry

Wolf D. Keidel, Erlangen

With 76 Figures

Contents

I. Introductory Remarks

In the chapter written by Professor HALLOWELL DAVIS the clinical use of ERA (Electric Response Audiometry) in audiology is described in full detail including the early response (BERA) and the perstimulatory DC-shift. Hence, this most important subtopic of the auditory evoked responses can be omitted here. We therefore feel that our contribution in this handbook should deal with all those questions and solutions – as far as they have been elaborated – which are related to explanations from a neurophysiological background. Thus, it should be obvious that a response as complex as the auditory evoked potential must be looked at under a great variety of aspects. Even then our present knowledge does not allow us to get more than a feeling about possible avenues of the basic physiological principles involved.

After some preceding works about auditory evoked potentials (KORNMÜLLER, 1933; BREMER and DOW, 1939; BREMER, 1943, 1952; LILLY and CHERRY, 1954) it was in the middle to the late fifties, especially in the Communications Biophysics Research Laboratory Group of the Massachusetts Institute of Technology – headed by WALTER A. ROSENBLITH – that a very productive ensemble of researchers including N. Y.-S. KIANG, TOM SANDEL, MOISE GOLDSTEIN, LARRY FRISHKOPFF, BILL PEAKE, DAN GEISSLER and others tried to attain a new stage of technology with (i) *electronic averaging* and (ii) *auto-* and *cross-correlation* both of which were most favored ideas of NORBERT WIENER, and further developed by BARLOW.

Although in those years the concept of correlation functions looked more promising, in the long run it turned out that computerized *averaging* would prove more and more useful as *the* technique for ERA, as labelled by HALLOWELL DAVIS one or two decades later. At that time, undoubtedly the explosive power of this new tool in neurophysiology – introduced and applied ingeniously almost solely by WALTER ROSENBLITH and his group – became a decisive step forward toward the old dream of neurophysiology in general, namely, the objective measurement of complex brain functions which could be correlated to psycho-physical data and to conscious experiences. This was actually the first realization of WUNDT'S speculations and his idea of a meaningful neurophysiology of mentality, a concept which then – again after decennia – became emphatically favored in many countries.

It was as early as 1939 that the late PAULINE A. DAVIS (the first wife of HALLOWELL DAVIS), in her classical paper entitled "Effects of acoustic stimuli on the waking brain", reported the later so-called "K-complex", a relatively large response to acoustical stimulation in human subjects. It could be detected as a single response in the EEG trace, quite similar to an evoked response in the visual system, without the need for improvement of the signal to noise ratio by a computer. Similarly, in light sleep even larger responses could be detected in man with scalp electrodes by HALLOWELL DAVIS, P. A. DAVIS, A. L. LOOMIS, E. N. HARVEY, and G. HOBART in 1939. In 1957, DAN GEISLER and LARRY FRISHKOPFF performed experiments which clearly showed the development of the K-complex during sleep. This is shown in the first Figure.

With the improvement of computer technology and its application to these studies, DAN GEISLER at WALTER ROSENBLITH' laboratory was first able to record not only from the animal's projection areas AI and AII, but also from the intact human (and monkey's) scalp. The ongoing electrical activity of the brain was treated as "noise" – certainly some sort of an oversimplification.

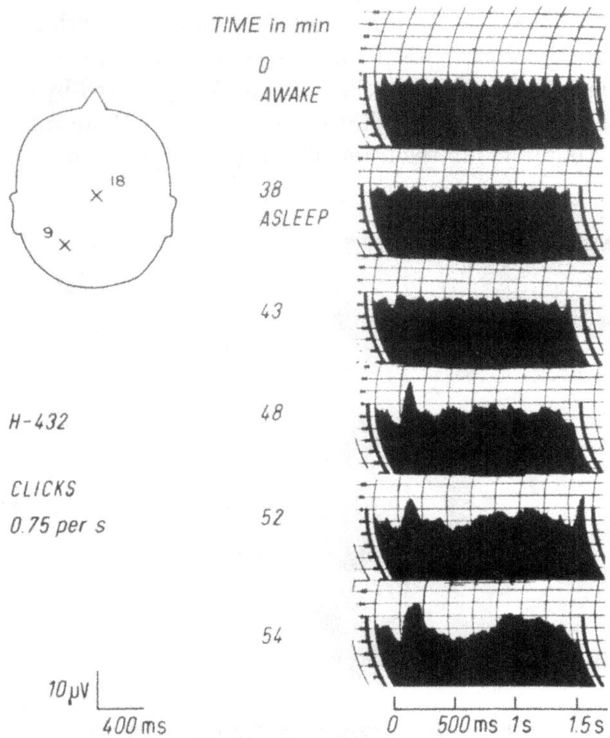

Fig. 1. Development of the K-complex in sleep. Stimulus a medium-intensity click delivered binaurally. Crosses in insert: location of electrodes. In the two lower graphs, the amplitude is reduced by a factor of approximately 3. (According to D. GEISLER and L. FRISHKOPFF, 1957)

II. Animal Research

A. Early Slow Responses in the Anesthetized Cat

1. Classical Cortical Response to Clicks ("On-Effect")

Let us go back to the cat's responses to auditory stimuli. After the first trials of LILLY and CHERRY (1954); BREMER and DOW (1939); BREMER (1943, 1952); KORNMÜLLER (1933), in the middle fifties, again at WALTER ROSENBLITH's laboratory, great effort was made to explore the evoked responses embedded in the *anesthetized* cat's electrocorticogram. Although later on it was possible to demonstrate that to record under anesthesia means a serious restriction of the early responses and a clear neglect of the late and even of the middle latencies responses, it is still of great value to first describe and analyse those responses.

As the next figure (2) shows, in acoustical stimulation by clicks, four peaks can be clearly separated when recording from AII bipolary with a sufficient amplification: Figure 2a shows the location of the electrode and one response, Fig. 2b represents a superimposed photograph of 10 sweeps (bipolar electrode). A first negative deflection N_1 with a latency of 11 to 12 ms with moderate intensities is the first event. This peak is small, highly uniform in size within a long train of clicks. Next is a large positive wave P_1, about 4 times as large as N_1, latency ranging around 15 ms again uniform in size. This peak is followed by a similarly large negative response, the size of which decreases visibly with an increasing number of consecutive stimuli within the train. The latency of N_2 is on the order of 25 ms

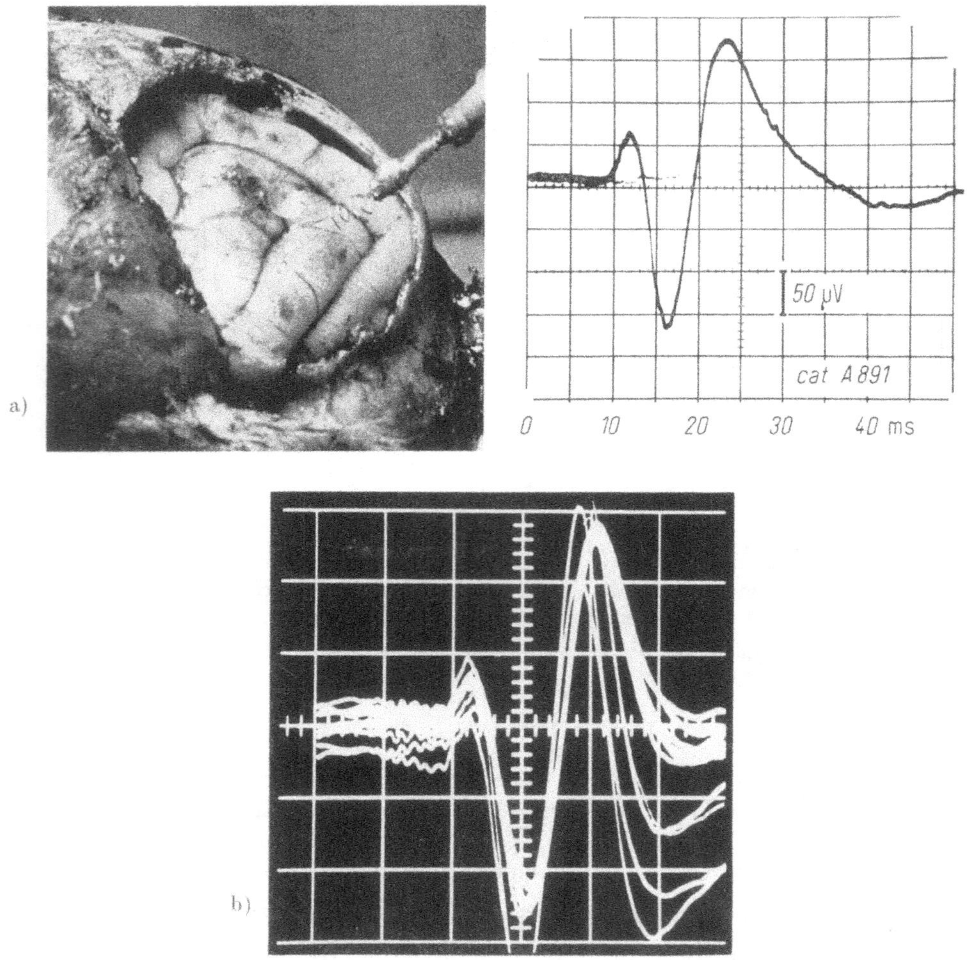

Fig. 2. (a) Location of monopolar electrode and one single sweep. AII. (b) Same as (a), but 10 superimposed responses to a train of clicks, bipolar electrode, AII. One horizontal division 5 ms, one vertical division 50 microvolts. KEIDEL, KEIDEL, and WIGAND (1958). Dial anesthesia

with moderate intensities. The last recordable event is a middle sized second positive deflection, P_2, which starts with an amplitude as great as P_1. This response, as can be seen in Fig. 2b, flattens out completely after the fifth or sixth stimulus within the train.

Recordings from AI produced clearly shorter latencies than recordings from AII. This is shown in Fig. 3. Here, the first peak with positive polarity, P_1, appears as early as 10 to 11 ms after the click with an onset of P_1 at 7 ms, while the negative deflection follows the P_1 with an absolute latency of 19 ms at moderate intensities. This holds only for the animal anesthetized under Nembutal or Dial whereby all later responses are suppressed by the anesthesia.

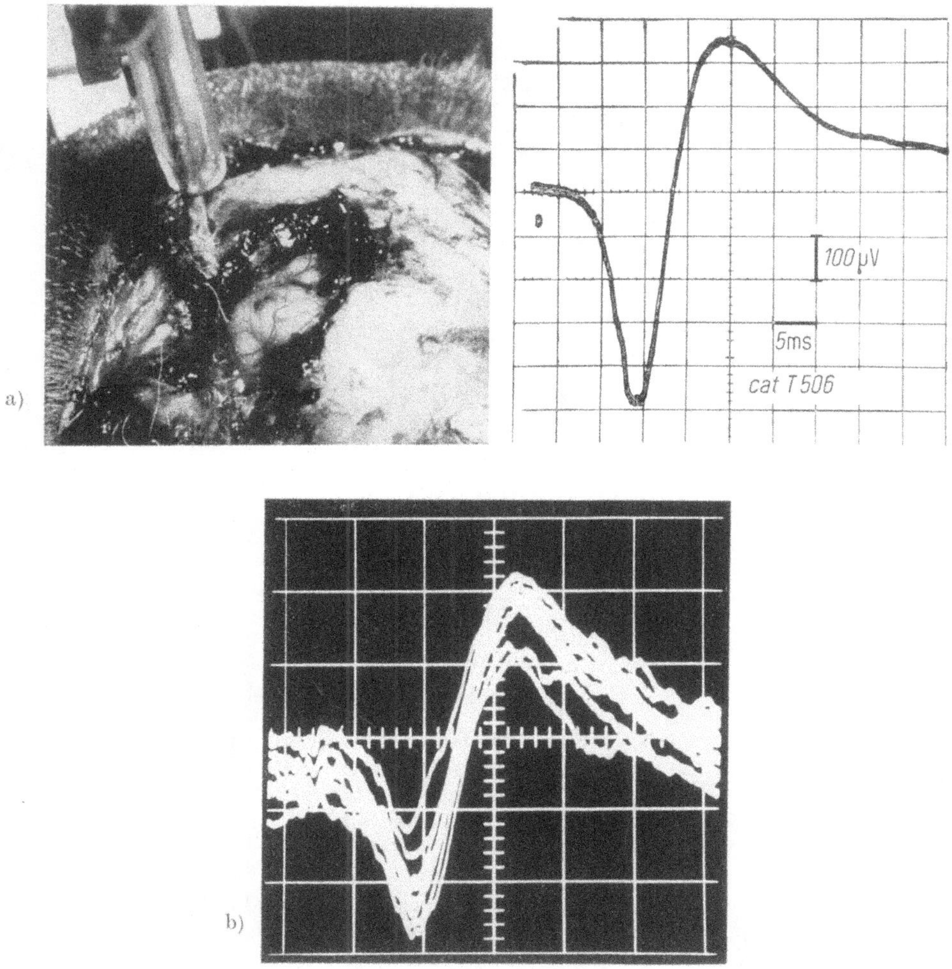

Fig. 3. (a) Location of monopolar electrode and one single sweep. AI. (b) Same as (a), but 10 superimposed sweeps of responses to a train of clicks, bipolar electrode, AI. One horizontal division 5 ms, one vertical division 100 microvolts. Dial anesthesia. KEIDEL, KEIDEL, and WIGAND (1958)

Notice that the size of the responses at AI at identical intensities is about twice those at AII; at AI there is only a very moderate adaptation or habituation within a train of clicks compared to that at AII.

It might be tempting to compare the responses to auditory stimulation with somesthetic cortical responses to vibratory stimuli delivered to the cat's vibrissae. After delivering vibratory stimuli to the cat's vibrissae and recording from SI, the first onset to a positive deflection, P_1, begins for this modality as early as 4 ms after the tactile "click", with a maximum positive deflection at 6.5 ms (Fig. 4). A large negative response N_1, revealing a maximum deflection at 10 ms follows at SI. In contrast to that observation, records from SII show a first small negative deflection at 6 ms, followed by the positive P_1 response at about 9 ms. The last event is a flat negative N_2 with a maximum deflection at approximately 14 ms.

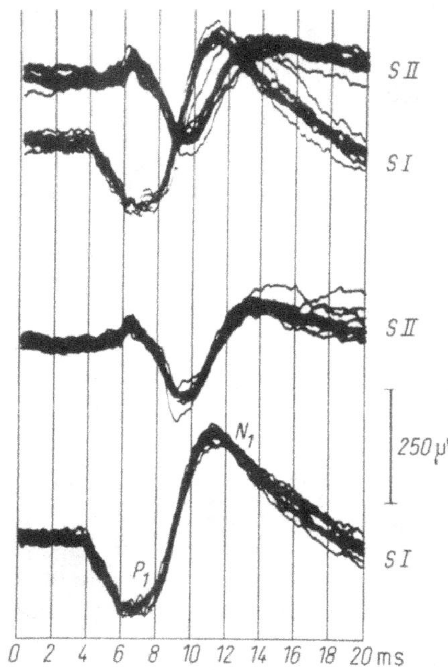

Fig. 4. Bipolar records from SI and SII of the Dial anesthetized cat. All latencies are shorter for this modality. Again the size of the responses at the primary projection area is about twice that at the secondary. Notice that the amplification is about half that of the auditory responses. (Unpublished data by KEIDEL, KEIDEL, and KIANG, 1957)

Hence, a clearly different temporal pattern can be observed in the anesthetized cat when comparing responses to stimuli of different modalities, such as auditory and vibrotactile. The intermodal specific responses of the somesthetic system have clearly shorter latencies (4 ms versus 7 ms) in regard to the first arrival of sensory information at the cortical level. On the other hand the transfer of information from the primary to the secondary cortical projection area needs additional time, on the order of some milliseconds. The shape of the response trace is also profoundly influenced. Finally, late responses in the deeply anesthetized cat are completely suppressed. Under anesthesia, however, the animal cannot hear, just as in sleep or in any other kind of unconscious state. Therefore, what does "intermodal specifity" mean under these conditions? One of the best ways to explore and possibly to answer this question is to try mapping the results along the cortical surface. This indeed is what has been done (Fig. 5).

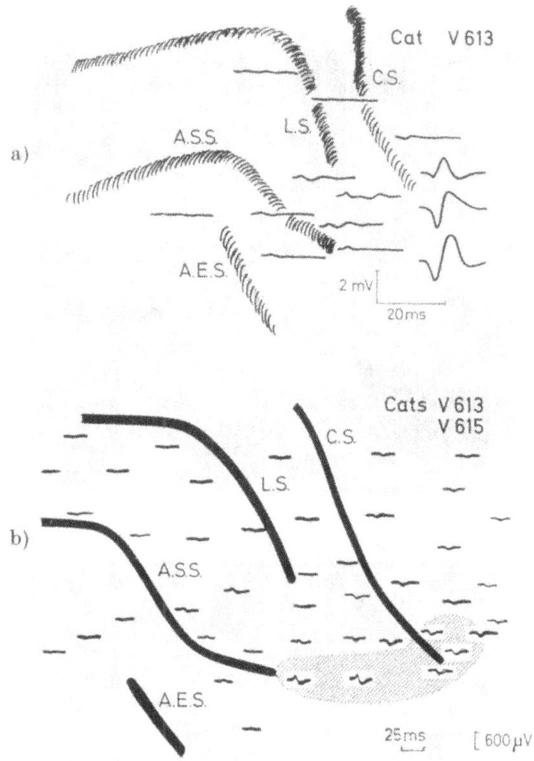

Fig. 5. (a) Nembutal anesthetized cat. Strychninization by means of small pieces of paper 4 mm² in size situated where each trace begins. Vibratory stimuli to the cat's vibrissae. Intermodal specific restriction of the projection area to SI (and SII). No response at AI and AII. (Unpublished data by KEIDEL, KEIDEL, and KIANG, 1957). (b) Same as (a), but without strychninization

The results prove that vibratory stimuli excite the somesthetic projection areas, SI and SII, at the cortical level. Numerous experiments have been performed to elaborate the analogous results for auditory stimuli at AI and AII and the corresponding visually evoked responses at VI and VII. In addition, there are convergent informations conveyed to the association area for all modalities and even to the cerebellar cortex. The consecutive excitation of the precentral cortex is a secondary phenomenon which has to do with the preparation of the motor reactions for sensory stimuli. This also is the place where GREY WALTER's "nonspecific cortex" is located and where the link to the contingent negative variation from the neurophysiological aspect has its counter-part in the structural domain.

There is, however, another observation which ought to be mentioned: The different size of ipsilateral versus contralateral responses is highly significant for those early responses in contrast to the late slow evoked responses, which will be discussed later in this chapter. The difference in size for the early P_1 is as large as a factor of two, in other words, it is on the order of 6 dB, while that for the late responses (as BUTLER, KEIDEL, and SPRENG, showed in 1969) is at best not greater than 1 dB.

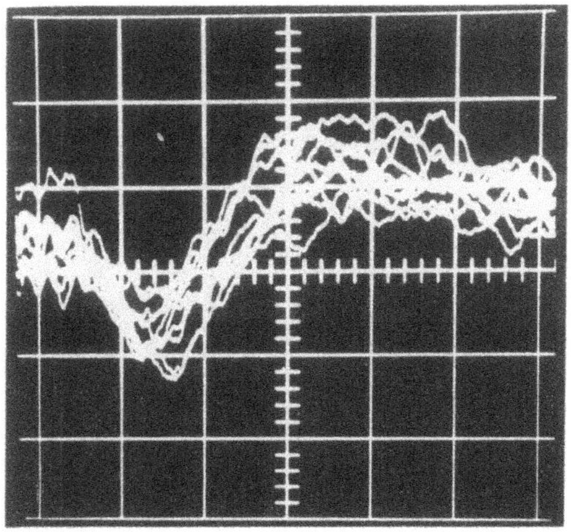
a)

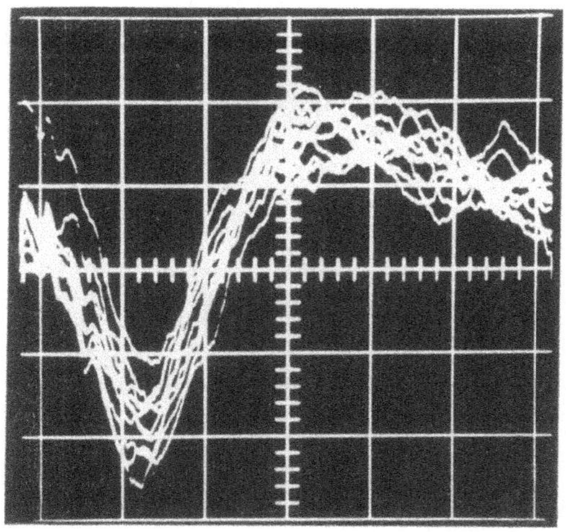
b)

Fig. 6a and b. Comparison of the ipsi- (a) and contralateral (b) responses to the same stimulus of moderate intensity. (Unpublished data by KEIDEL, KEIDEL, and WIGAND, 1958.) Each horizontal division equals 5 ms

The absolute latency – which also differs slightly for the two hemispheres – fits fairly well into the classical concept of approximately one millisecond per synapse. With respect to SHERRINGTON's relay-hypothesis and to MAGOUN and MORUZZI's idea of nonspecific information transfer via the reticular formation, for the transfer of information along the specific pathway of each modality this would mean 5 synaptic relay nuclei for the auditory and fewer for the somesthetic system.

A very thorough study of the effect of anesthesia upon the pattern of responses was performed by TEAS and KIANG in 1964. The loss of the late responses under the influence of Nembutal is shown in Fig. 7 of their work.

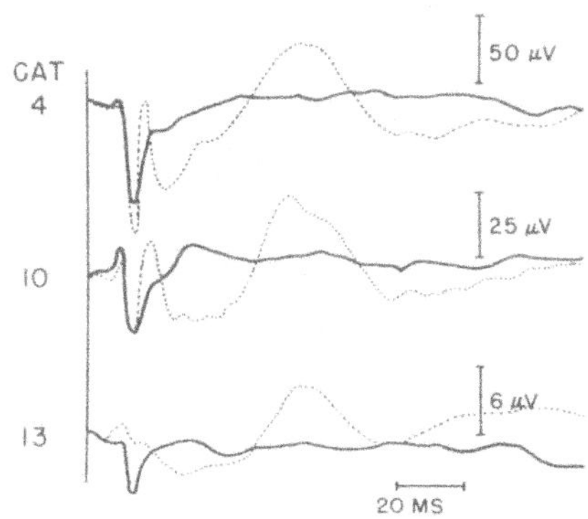

Fig. 7. Effect of intraperitoneal injections of Nembutal on the Electrocorticogram in three cats. Records approximately one hour after the first injection. Dotted traces show the ECC in the awake animals; solid traces, the wave form of average responses after anesthesia was administered. (According to TEAS and KIANG, 1964)

In each case, the dotted line is recorded from the unanesthetized animal's cortex. Under these "physiological" conditions the early peaks are followed by the late slow responses with relatively long latencies. An additional positive peak and, later on, a large negative slow wave become visible. The latency of the peak ranges around 66 ms. The trace then crosses the zeroline to another flatter positive deflection with a mean latency around 100 ms. Although these latencies are shorter than those obtained from the human scalp in ERA, one could compare these three late peaks with the ERA's P1, N1 and P2. After approximately one hour after Nembutal has been injected in dosages of 17.5 mg/kg (Cat number 4), 6.6. mg/kg (Cat number 10) and 11.2 mg/kg (Cat number 13), these three late deflections disappear. This can be seen in the solid traces as the most striking effect of anesthesia.

In another paper, KIANG and GOLDSTEIN (1957) detected an additional positive notch in the first early positive deflection, P_1, of the cat's response to clicks. This P_{1b} disappears as a result of the intravenous injection of Nembutal (concentric electrodes sitting in the primary auditory cortical projection area). Notice this effect in the middle and right columns of Fig. 8a. All records are single traces. In the left column of Fig. 8a, the notch, P_{1b}, can clearly be seen in the unanesthetized cat.

After averaging the responses (Fig. 8b), P_{1b} shows up very clearly in the awake animal and disappears just as markedly after injection of intravenous Nembutal. Note the marked late negativity in the unanesthetized animal, as described above. Finally, in Fig. 8c a typical single sweep response pattern to a click recorded from the unanesthetized cat's AI shows the animal's early P_1 and N_1 and late P1, N1 and P2, as these deflections were later labelled in ERA.

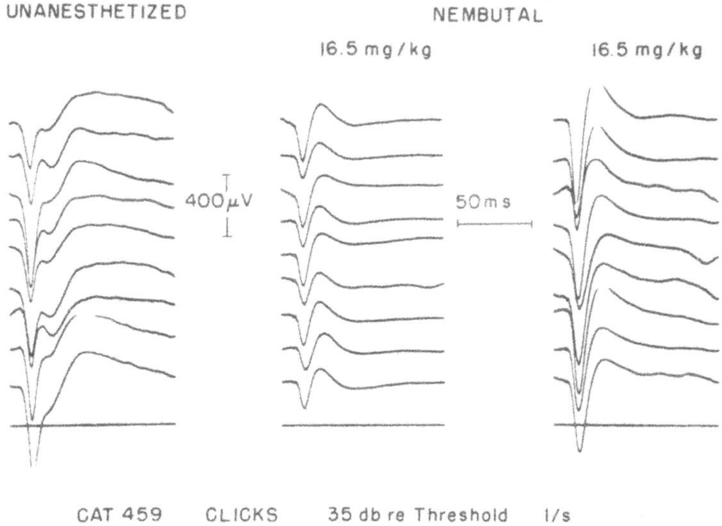

Fig. 8.(a) Effects of intravenous Nembutal on the configuration of the evoked cortical responses. Concentric electrodes were situated in the primary auditory area AI. Upward deflection represents surface negativity as in all other figures in accordance with the conventional custom displaying surface positive deflections downward. (According to KIANG and GOLDSTEIN, 1957)

b)

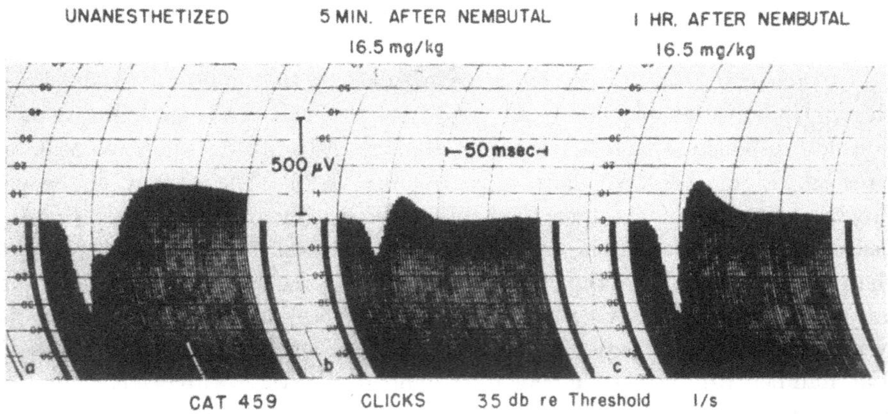

c)

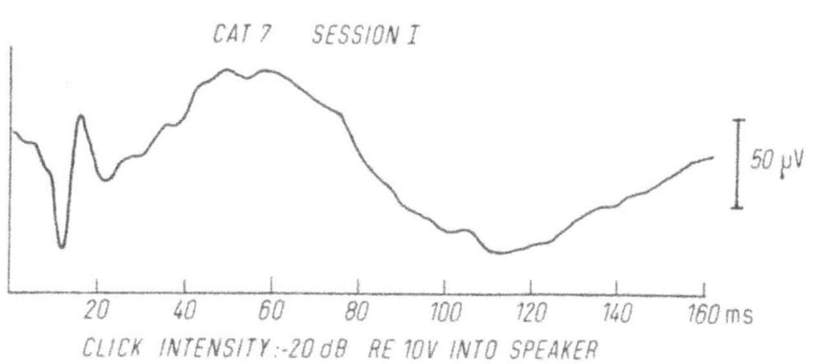

Fig. 8. (b) Effects of intravenous Nembutal on the configuration of the *averaged* evoked cortical responses. Each curve represents the average of 300 responses to successive clicks. Notice the notch, P_{1b}, in the unanesthetized animal. (According to KIANG and GOLDSTEIN, 1957). (c) Average responses to acoustic clicks. Responses were recorded from an electrode at AI. Note the "late" P1, N1, and P2. (According to TEAS and KIANG, 1964)

One more general consideration might now be discussed concerning the *early* responses in the cat: At first sight, one could consider evoked responses as an event elicited by the stimulus alone. There is, however, clear evidence that usually a *change* of the conditions of the surroundings in which the animal (and man) lives excites the brain to a response, as well as just some sort of a single stimulus triggered event. Even changes of the state of the brain itself can play an important role. More precisely, responses can be elicited by any variation in intensity, frequency, complexity of the stimulus or state of the animal (or subject) such as alertness, vigilance, attention, habituation, adaptation, etc. It is in fact the *comparison* between the stored information and the particular *actual* ongoing activation by a given stimulus that is performed by the brain and that is responsible for the type, pattern, size, and latency of the response. Hence, this implies one of the old concepts of philosophy, namely the concept of "tabula rasa": Each animal starts its life with highly selected and specialiest information (inborn behaviour) and with no information (experience) about its surroundings. This state therefore characterizes the new born animal and the new born child. With increasing life time, by means of the increased experience, the animal (and the human subject) stores more and more (auditory) information, and, hence, the response to one and the same auditory stimulus will be changed drastically until it reaches the stage of the adult animal (and man), where it even varies intraindividually at any given age. This is the place where "memory" comes in as an important factor. This is also one of the reasons why an analog transfer from results obtained from ERA responses of adult subjects quite often disappoints the clinician when applying ERA, BERA and cochleography techniques and data to young hearing-impaired children and newborns. It is not the technique, it is this neurophysiological variance

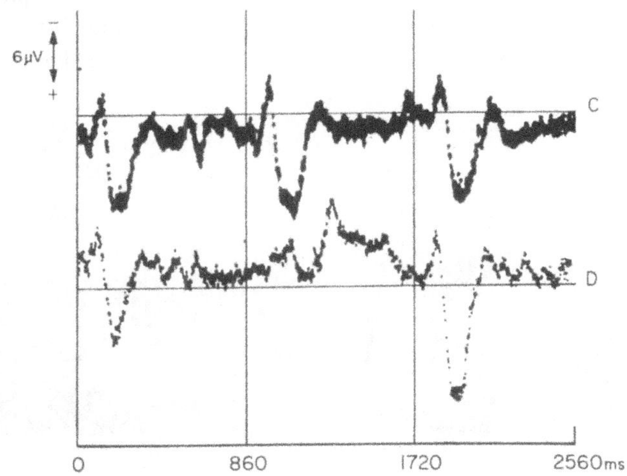

Fig. 9. Upper trace: evoked responses to trains of vibratory stimuli grouped in triplets, one hundred repetitions. Lower trace: same, but each second stimulus missing. Note the responses at a time when the second stimulus within the triplet group has been conditioned and, therefore, has been "expected". The pattern of this stimulus response differs from the normal one in size and latency. Note that also the third response looks different. (According to KLINKE, FRUHSTORFER, and FINKENZELLER, 1968)

which has caused some disappointment during the history of ERA, BERA, and electrocochleography.

Based upon the above reasoning, in adult human subjects, even the *omission* of a conditioned stimulus within a repetitive train of stimuli – obviously also a change of condition in a negative direction – can be responded to as an "evoked" response. Actually, however, it is the retrieval of earlier stored information: In a first set of experiments, groups of three stimuli of equal time intervals were repeated 100 times, and three averaged responses could be recorded from the cat's projection area under these conditions. Thus, the animal was conditioned to expect the second stimulus between the first and the third. The second set of experiments contained only the first and the third stimulus within each group of the series. Every second one was not present. Since the response to the third stimulus was greater than normal in the averaged trace and since there was indeed a response to the nonexistent second stimulus, although smaller in size and with a changed latency, a simple model can be imagined, namely, that the normal response is the difference between the actual and the stored information in the modal specific part of the cat's brain. It turns out that this model is too simple. It leads one, however, in the right direction. The above experiments were performed at our laboratory in 1968 by KLINKE, FRUHSTORFER, and FINKENZELLER.

2. "Off-Effect"

Similarly, the end of a longer stimulus also means a marked change of the stimulus conditions, and hence, is followed by a response, the "off-response". It was first described by KIANG and SANDEL in 1957 at MIT. Those authors could clearly demonstrate off-responses to bursts of noise in *un*anesthetized cats. In the anesthetized animal this type of response is absent. One example is shown in Fig. 10. These records were obtained from the cat's AII using BREMER's technique of "éncephale isolée". A typical off-response can be seen in the left trace. When

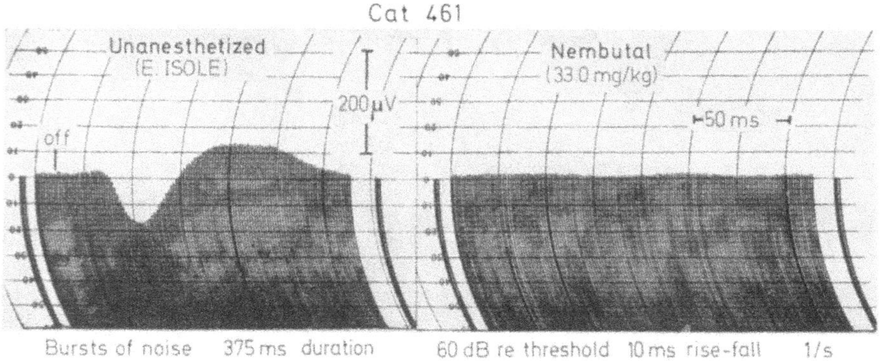

Fig. 10. Off-responses to bursts of noise in the unanesthetized cat (left trace) and effects of intravenous Nembutal on the off-response. Each curve is the computed average of 300 responses to successive bursts. Each pen line represents a 1.25-ms time interval separation. Latency of the onset of the average off-response is approximately 20 ms from the instant at which the fall of the noise burst begins. Recordings with concentric bipolar electrodes in area AII of the auditory cortex. Deflection above the zero-line represents surface negativity as usual. (According to KIANG and SANDEL, 1957)

Nembutal anesthesia is administered this response is clearly cancelled as demonstrated in the right trace. This again strongly stresses the idea that it is the cortex, the awake cortex, which detects this change rather than deeper layers of the auditory pathway. We shall discuss this topic once more when we deal with the human auditory electric response in audiometry.

Latencies, and less so amplitudes of the off-responses, depend upon the rise and fall time of the auditory stimulus, in this particular case of the burst of noise and in general upon the shape, pattern, and intensity of the preceding auditory event (see for example FRUHSTORFER, 1966; SPRENG, 1975; and others).

B. Link between Early and Late Slow Responses in the Unanesthetized Cat

Our next problem concerns the neurophysiological link between the early and late slow evoked responses in the unanesthetized cat as described before. In this context, one could think of many plausible hypotheses, only a few of which can be touched upon in this rather review-like article:

(i) Within the same ensemble of cortical cells a slow change of the membrane potential may possibly be responsible for the relatively long of about 100 ms between the early and the late components. One argument in favor of this hypothesis is based upon the fact that anesthesia (and ablation) of the cortical layer abolishes the late responses completely, as shown in Fig. 7 of this chapter. Another even more striking argument has been suggested very recently by GOLDSTEIN and ABELES (1975). Those authors recorded intracellularly in single units of the cat's cortical auditory projection areas by means of the micropipette technique. They discovered two different types of neurons which they labeled "grouper"-type and "locker"-type with respect to the two different types of the related perstimulus-time-histograms. Although the histograms differ considerably in shape, they have one feature of the two neuronal ensembles in common: when single clicks are delivered to the periphery, the intracellular membrane potential hyperpolarizes for about 100 ms in an almost identical time pattern for both groups of neurons. Finally in the locker group even a depolarization follows simultaneously with the occurrence of the late slow evoked potentials. In both cases a steady state is established between 100 and 150 ms. An example is shown in Fig. 11.

(ii) We know from many experiments that the thalamic nuclei, as well the medial geniculate (KEIDEL, 1969, 1970, 1971a, 1974a, b, 1975a; DAVID, FINKENZELLER, KALLERT, and KEIDEL, 1969a); (KEIDEL, ENGELEN, and RIX, 1971) as the lateral (BURKE and SEFTON, 1966a,b,c) and other nuclei (ANDERSEN, 1966; ANDERSEN *et al.*, 1964a, b) produce periodic changes in excitability and in the degree of spontaneous activity in groups of cells. Those neurons therefore can be considered as "clocks" for all types of timing procedures going on in the brain (KEIDEL, 1969). Although the absolute timing of these clocks, which act as relaxation oscillators, varies between a few cycles per second and approximately 70 per second as an upper frequency limit, the average lies around 10 Hz.

This is also true for the visual system whose relation between the geniculate's clocks and the Alpha-rhythm is well known. These clocks also play an important role in the decoding processes for the pitch perception of tonal stimuli within the specific branch of the auditory pathway (KALLERT *et al.*, 1970; DAVID *et al.*, 1969a). Hence, it might be possible that the latencies around 90 to 120 ms are intimately related to the neuronal network which is the source of the 10 Hz oscillations in the normal EEG. Furthermore, 100 to 180 ms is the time domain of the so-called

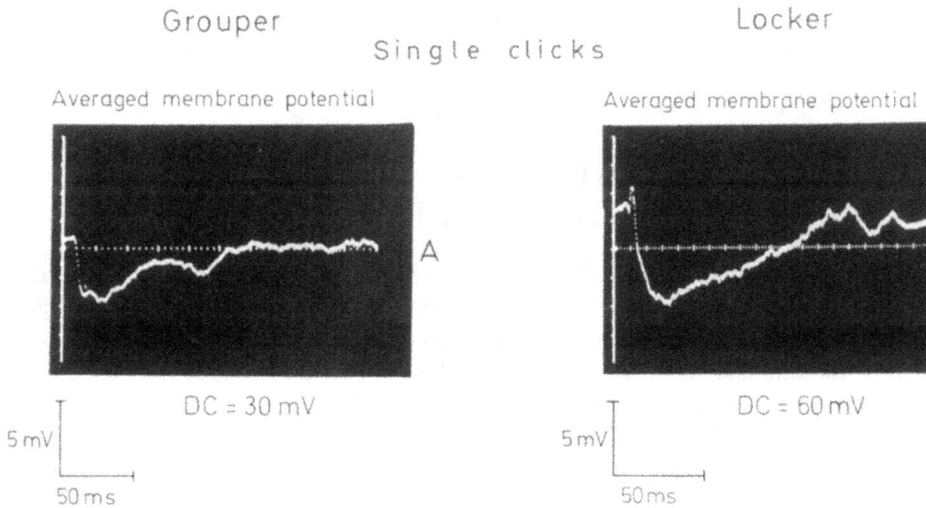

Fig. 11. Change of membrane potential of single cortical neurons at AI and AII. After a period of hyperpolarization of about 100 ms a steady state is reached without (left) or with (right) depolarization between 100 and 150 ms. (According to GOLDSTEIN RIBAUPIERRE, YENI-KOMSHIAN: Cortical coding of periodicity pitch. In: SACHS, M. B. (Ed.): The physiology of the Auditory System, Baltimore: National Educational Consultants 1971.

"physiological moment" (v. BAER, 1864; v. UEXKÜLL, 1949). In the two-click experiment performed by ROSENZWEIG and ROSENBLITH in 1953, this is the time order within which the brain's excitability climbs again to its original steady state value after the first click and following the abrupt drop.

Periodic changes of the brain's excitability during trains of clicks have been observed in the same range of 100 ms by MOLNAR and WEISS, 1960. They are known as "repetitives", examples of which are shown in Figure 12a. Figure 12b demonstrates the resulting long time variations of the anesthetized cat's projection areas as described by KEIDEL (1958).

(iii) Finally a third hypothesis was formulated by GREY WALTER in 1964 stating that the late responses should be due to the delay originated by the flow of information through the complex nonspecific network of the brain and ending up in the precentrally located "nonspecific cortex". Experiments in man with implanted electrodes furthered this idea. In the cat, however, contradictory data were obtained using the technique of implanting 32 supradural electrodes and recording from the completely awake and *un*anesthetized cat! Electrodes were situated on the projection areas and vicinity in this case (DAVID *et al.*, 1966). The result is shown in Fig. 13.

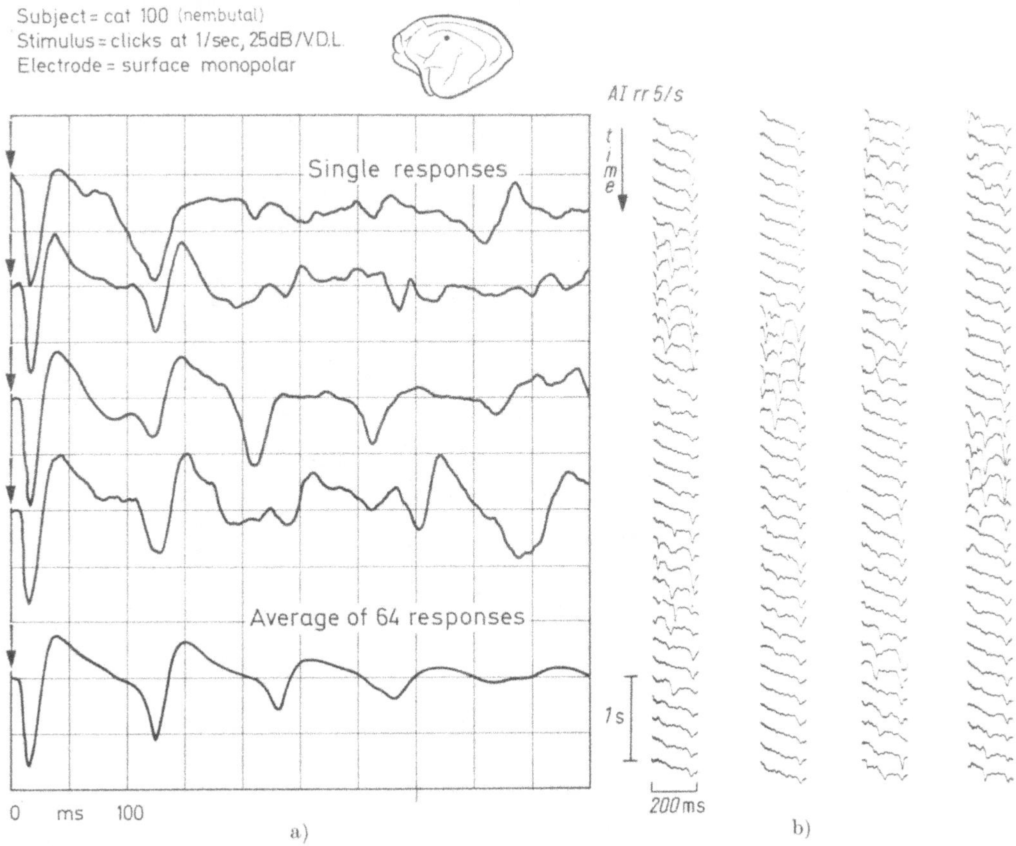

Fig. 12. (a) Stability of averaged repetitive responses to acoustic clicks as a function of time in the experiment. Location of monopolar electrode can be seen in the inset. Nembutal anesthesia. According to Molnar and Weiss (1960). (b) Trains of clicks elicit not only repetitives in the order of 10 Hz, but also longlasting periodicities ranging around 3 s. Read records up to down and left to right. (According to Keidel, 1958)

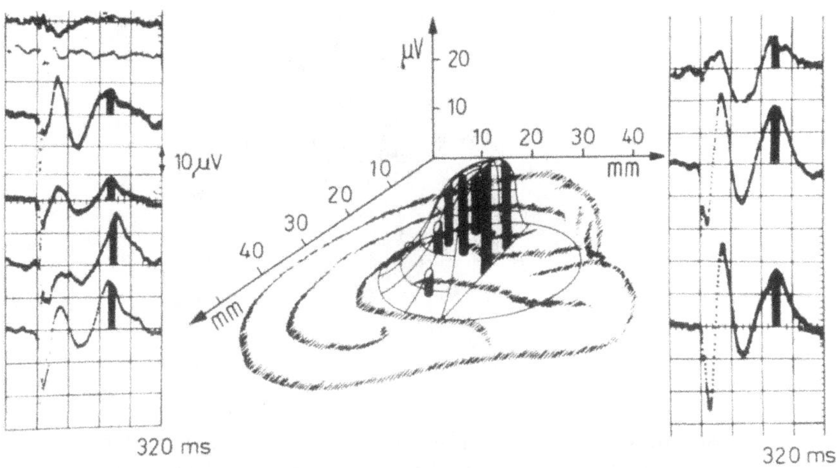

Fig. 13. Threedimensional plot of the amplitude of the late responses to auditory clicks in the awake cat by means of implanted electrodes. Original averaged responses on both sides. Each horizontal spacing equals 64 ms. (According to David *et al.*, 1966.) Nine electrodes

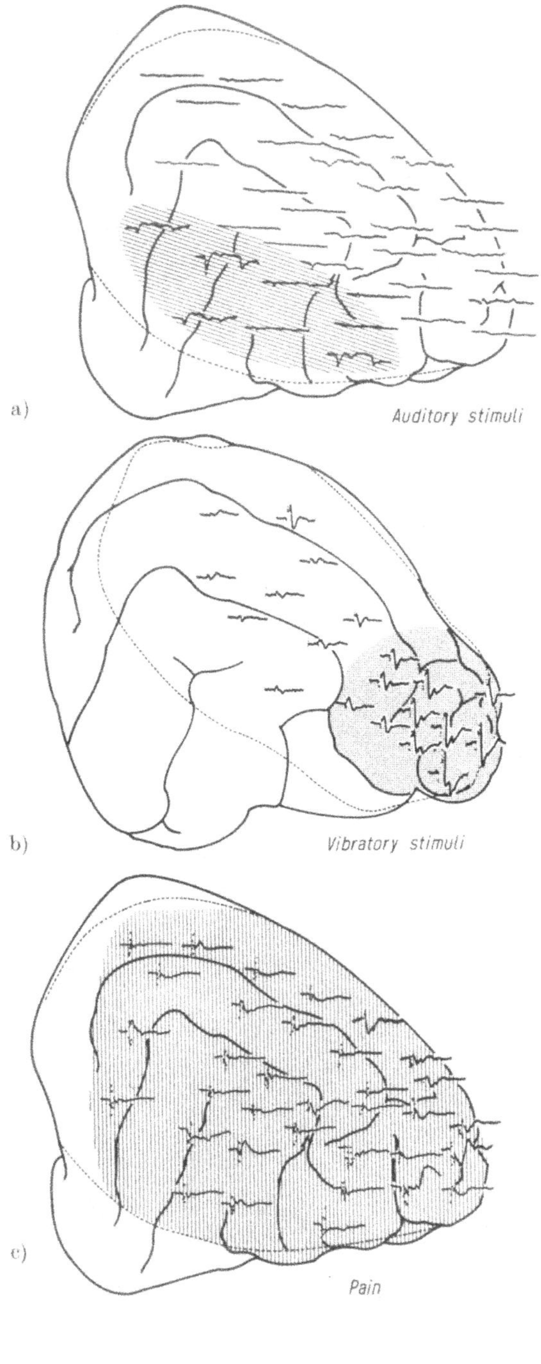

Fig. 14. (a) Awake cat. 32 supradural implanted electrodes. Tone-bursts, 320 ms. Length of records 500 ms. Responses are clearly restricted to AI and AII. (b) Same as (a), but vibratory stimuli which are projected to SI and SII. (c) Pain elicited by electric shocks is projected primarily to SI and SII but spread over the entire surface of the cortex. Discussion, see text. (According to Wilsman, 1969; and v. Kietzell, 1971. Dissertations Erlangen.)

In continuation of DAVID's experiments, WILSMAN in 1969 performed highly interesting *mapping* studies together with v. KIETZELL in 1971. Their results are demonstrated for three different modalities, namely, auditory, vibratory, and painful stimuli in Fig. 14a, b, c. All data converge into the clear conclusion that the origins of the late slow evoked responses in the unanesthetized cat are located in the specific primary projection areas, in AI and AII for auditory, and in SI and SII for vibratory stimulation. Only pain is an exception, that in addition to the spatial location in the somesthetic system, a general excitation all over the cortex could be observed. This is in good agreement with the theory for pain perception. As old as the concept of HEAD, that protopathic and epicritic pain exist, ZOTTERMAN could also prove that the information transfer for pain is performed in two different fiber systems: namely the $A_{\delta 2}$ for fast conducting fibers and in C-fibers for slow conducting fibers. For the auditory system, the source of the late (and the early) slow evoked cortical responses is clearly in the intermodal specific auditory projection areas AI and AII and not at all at the precentral cortex before the beginning of motor and behavioral reactions, which will be described later. Hence, these responses are the neurophysiological representation of entirely sensory and perceptual character. They last over a period of time which is normally the quantum of time perception for man and animal, namely the "physiological moment" of 180 ms.

C. Perstimulatory DC-Potential in the Unanesthetized Cat

In the late 19th century DC-currents from sensory stimulation were recorded from the exposed cortical surface even in man, although the technological equipment at that time was very simple (galvanometer, multiplicator etc.). Moreover, the researches performed by v. MARXOW (1890) and by BECK (1890) are of considerable historical value. With the improvement of the available electronic devices, the collection of data was expanded considerably especially by the KÖHLER-group in 1952 and later. In 1959, CASPERS and SCHULZE, BROOKHART *et al.* (1958), GUMNIT (1960, 1961), GUMNIT *et al.* (1961) succeeded both in mapping different modalities and in discovering the possible origin of those sensory DC-shifts caused by different intermodal stimulation. They were clearly able to prove that auditory stimuli elicit DC-potentials almost all in AI and AII, visual stimuli in the cuneus and related areas, and tactile stimulation above the gyri postcentrales. This was in excellent agreement with the motor reactions obtainable by stimulation of the gyrus precentralis (FRITZSCH and HITZIG, 1871; FLECHSIG, 1876). As to the origin of these potentials, evidence was brought together that they represent dendritic potentials with a fairly wide but rather restricted spread along the cortical surface. This finding corresponded also with the observation that the size and pattern changed in a typical manner with the depth of the recording electrodes within the first few millimeters of the cortical layer (JASPER, 1954). This was very similar to the behavior of peripheral nerves after application of positive and negative artificial electric direct current; in other words, from catelectrotonus and anelectrotonus, changes in size and even polarity of evoked potentials resulted. Other possible sources of these potentials might be chemical alterations across the blood-liquid barrier or/and metabolically involved changes in the glia – neuronal membrane potential.

From all the above data strong support could be gathered for the well-known general problem in sensory physiology, namely, the organisation of the so-called "optimizing function" of the sensory part of the brain's function: Based upon measurements of POLLAK, MILLER (*e.g.* 1956), and others, the information flow per second of conscious experience in man is estimated to be aproximately 60 to 100 bits per second. STEINBUCH (1971), KEIDEL (1963a) and others calculated the maximal possible input via all sensory channels as some 10^9 bits per second. Other estimates (TOMAN, 1973) prefer smaller numbers, on the order of 10^7 bits per second. The output has been suggested as 10^7 bits per second consisting of inborn and conditioned (learned) programs. This is shown in the sketch in Fig. 15.

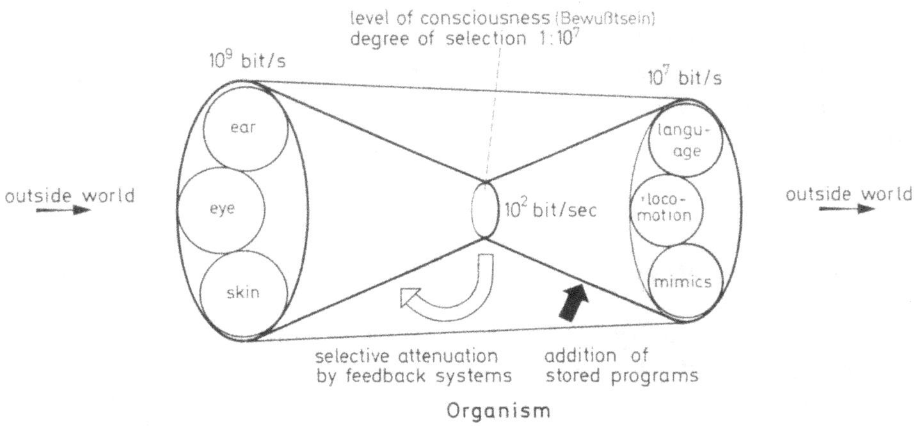

Fig. 15. Information flow to and from a human-being. A strong optimizing selection from input of sensory organs to conscious experience takes place in man on the order of 10^{-7} bits per second. (According to KEIDEL, 1963a)

Bearing in mind that the continuous flow of conscious experience in man is as small as 100 bits per second (short term memory 10 bits per second, long term memory 1 bit per second), one realizes that a remarkable "optimizing selection" of information entering the human subject via the sensory organs must be performed by the brain (KEIDEL, 1962, 1963). Up to now, we did not know exactly how these very important selective processes for decision making were organized neurophysiologically. One of the consequences of the DC-measurements discussed earlier was the preference model suggested by KEIDEL in 1971b, 1972a, b. This model contains the specific and the nonspecific pathways of each sensory channel. It proposes that the selective process is based upon electrotonic DC-changes controlled by either the association area and/or the reticular formation in connection with thalamic and diencephalic structures, thus selecting, that sensory channel to which attention is given. In the case of a catelectrotonus of the specific projection area, this would mean a facilitation, a long-lasting surface negativity. In the case of an anelectrotonus a surface-positivity as a DC-shift would result in an inhibition of that particular sensory channel. The model is in agreement with all known experimental data and hence the DC-potential is the objective correlate to the "optimizing selective process" which switches the attention from one to the other sensory channel. In this sense the DC-potential, the perstimulatory DC-potential, seems to be strictly intermodal specific. The model is shown in Fig. 16.

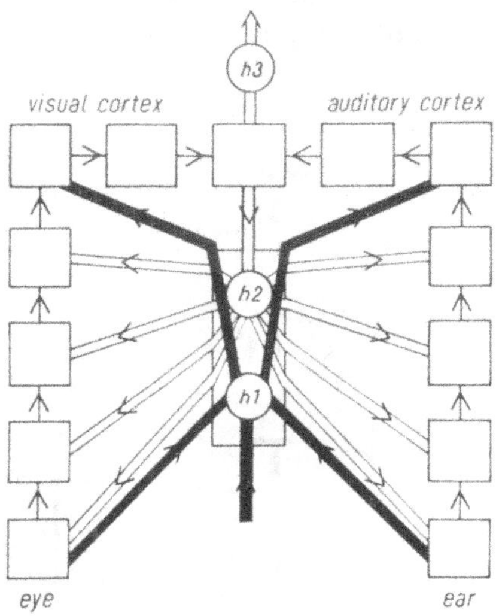

Fig. 16. Model for the optimizing selection of sensory information proposed by KEIDEL (1963). Black: nonspecific system, white: specific system. *h*1 nonspecific thalamic integration, *h*2 descending thalamic system which "selects" the specific system intermodaly, *h*3 decision making structure between association area (white box) and the precentral motor cortex

According to the considerations mentioned above, one would expect to find the perstimulatory DC-shift in unanesthetized awake animals only. With respect to anesthesia, this is true when recording from AI and/or AII. In sleep, the results are contradictory and not clearly consistent. Here more research about the potentials recorded from the *association* areas is necessary. A few data have been collected from the association areas: GOLDRING *et al.* (1967) claim that the dipole which generates the response during sleep was different in the unanesthetized cat with implanted electrode from the one which gave rise to the response when the animal was attentive. They wrote: "These observations suggest that sensory input to association areas is plastic and in contrast to primary sensory areas the pattern of activation is largely determined by unknown factors that might include experience and environment" (GOLDSTEIN *et al.*, 1967). But this is exactly what we label optimizing selection. POLIAKOVA in 1972 presented a review of her experiences with the association area. Although she used somesthetic stimuli her results may also be of interest for auditory information processing. She found practically the same early and late components as those described here for the auditory system. In experiments in which the cortex was separated from the subcortical structures, the early components disappeared. She, therefore, concludes that the early responses are generated locally in the association area (as in AI and AII), and, hence, she believes that these early components of the association area are not due to diffusion of thalamic activities. This means an intracortical connection exists between primary and secondary projection areas and the association areas as AMASSIAN discussed in 1954. In addition, however, POLIAKOVA introduced possible convergence from the nonspecific pathway by saying that those early responses could be provoked by impulses of specific origin relaying in the ventral posterior nucleus of the thalamus. In other words, they are produced by messages having a specific

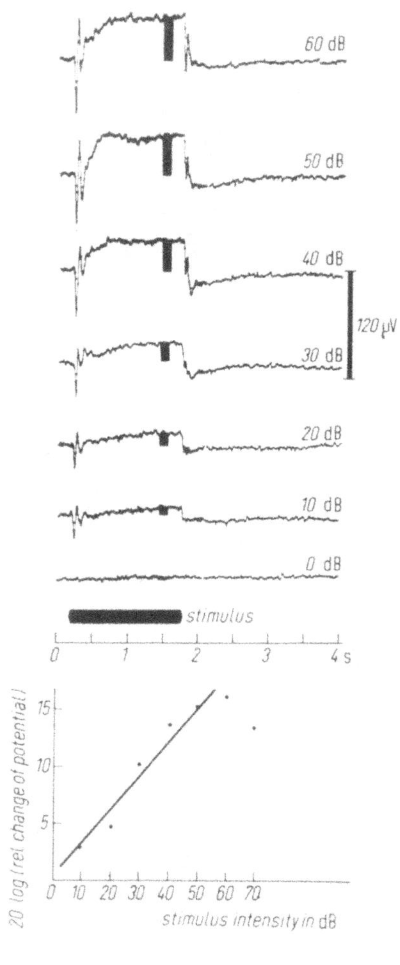

Fig. 17. DC-potential recorded with implanted electrodes from the awake cat's auditory projection areas. Latency is on the order of 200 ms. Pattern depends upon intensity (bottom drawing). Preceeding the on-effect, following the off-effect. (According to DAVID, FINKENZELLER, KALLERT, and KEIDEL, 1969b)

character. But the late responses, in her opinion, are generally supposed to be due to messages passing through nonspecific thalamic nuclei in the sense of ALBE-FESSARD and FESSARD in 1963 (see also BUSER, 1966; BIGNALL, 1967; NARIKASHVILI, 1969). Although this does not involve the problem of DC-generation, all of her results and conclusions fit the model described above, especially with respect to the convergence of nonspecific and specific pathways of the different sensory modalities between the thalamic and the cortical level (probably with descending feedback fibers between cortex and thalamus). Here, we see the link between the sensory and the motor part of the brain: the specific messages all converge at the association area to enable multimodal "Gestalt" detection, storage and retrieval including the decision-making processes. From there, then the clasical transfer of information toward the precentral motor cortex may have its structural origin. Unfortunately, no data concerning DC-changes at the association area and at the precentral motor cortex under sensory stimulation are available at present. It is to be expected, however, that their temporal pattern ought to be of a very high degree of complexity, representing the highest level of cortical activities for the entire spectrum of events ranging from perception to behavioral responses. In the light of these considerations, the importance of the highly consistent specific DC-potentials obtainable at the primary and secondary projection areas of the different modalities is clearly stressed for basic research in audiometry. This is one of the reasons why at our laboratory we put so much emphasis upon the auditory perstimulatory DC-responses from AI and AII.

At the auditory projection areas, AI and AII, perstimulatory DC-potentials of longlasting tonal and filtered and unfiltered noise can be recorded. The records, as Fig. 17 shows, begin with a marked P1, N1, and P2 (the on-effect, P2-latency ranging around 120 ms). About 200 ms after the onset of the click free, tone-burst, a surface-negative DC-potential develops relatively slowly, reaches a steady state value not earlier than approximately 300 to 500 ms, and stays constant then (at high intensities) until the stimulation is finished. The last event when recording with supradural implanted electrodes from the awake cat's cortex is the already described off-effect with its different components. The steady state value of the DC-potential, over a range of more than 50 dB, as indicated by black rectangles, fairly well follows a power function in S. S. STEVENS' sense ($n = 0.29$) and, for higher intensities, flattens out or even drops in amplitude. For the lower intensities, the steady state value will not be reached even for stimuli lasting as long as 1.6 s. A double-logarithmic plot of the intensity function is drawn at the bottom of the Figure. Experiments have been performed by DAVID, FINKENZELLER, KALLERT, and KEIDEL, 1969b, c, d. A survey of this potential and its features was given by KEIDEL in 1971b, and 1972a.

Figure 18 demonstrates the intermodal specific character of the perstimulatory DC-potential. Fully DC-amplified and averaged potentials of the awake cat are recorded here with 32 implanted electrodes from the entire cortex. Two typical average traces are shown as insets. Stimulus duration in each case was 300 ms (tone bursts). Source of each trace was on the underlying cortical surface. In Fig. 18b, the best responding area is cross-hatched. Experiments were performed by FINKENZELLER (1969) and WILSMAN (1969) respectively.

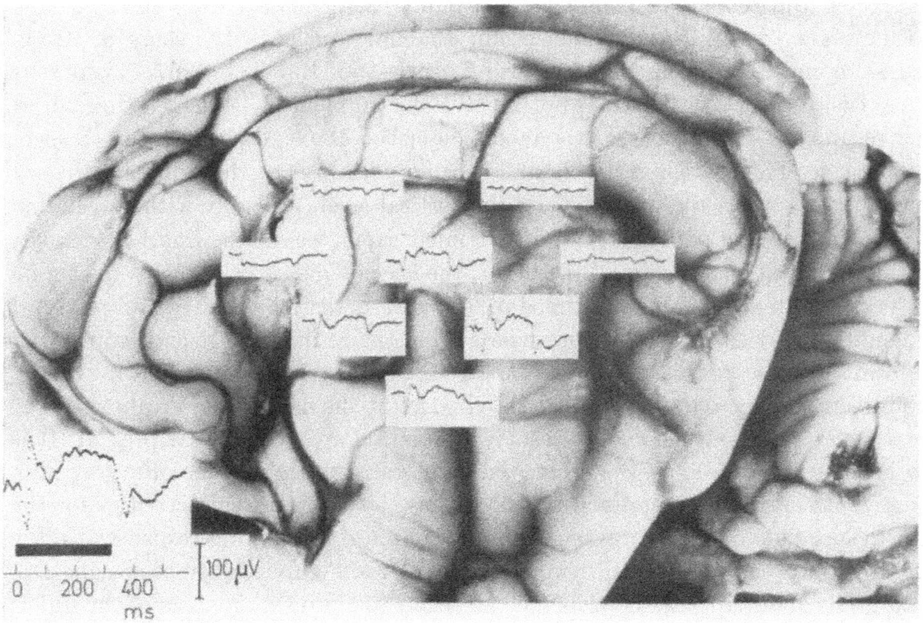
0 200 400
ms
100 µV

a)

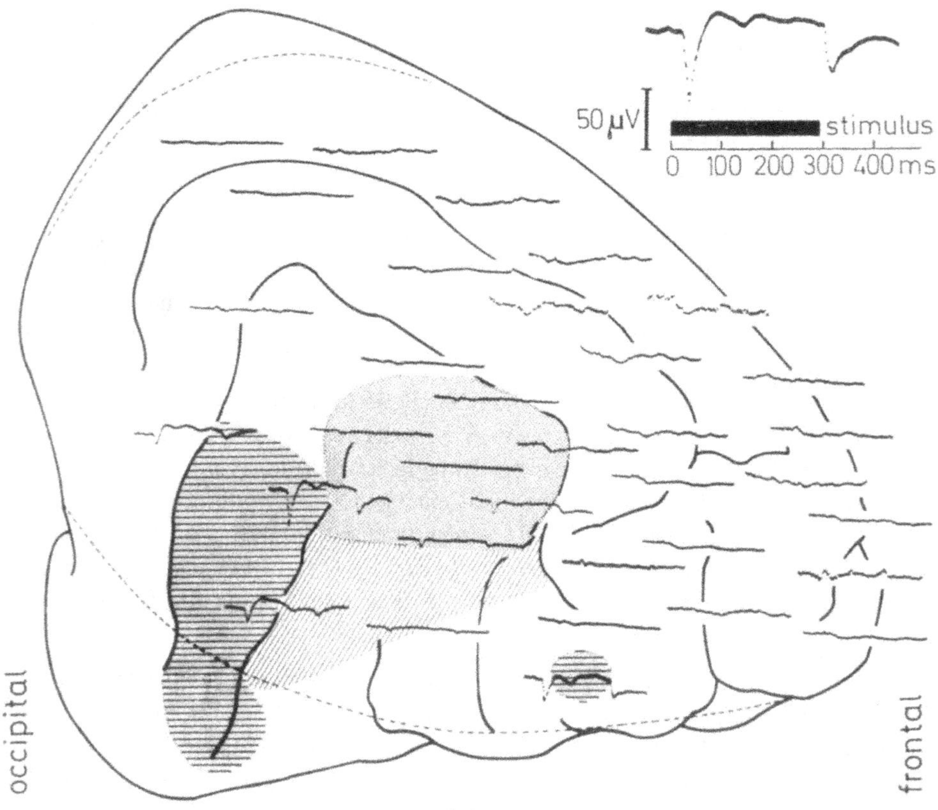
50 µV
stimulus
0 100 200 300 400 ms
occipital
frontal

b)

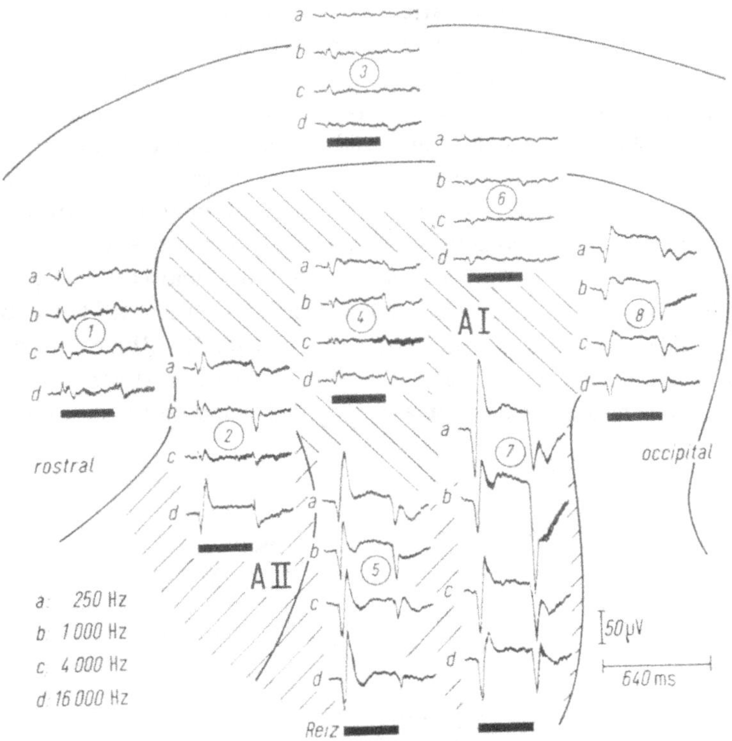

c)

Fig. 18. (a) Mapping of the DC-potential recorded from the awake cat's cortex. Full DC-amplification and averaging. The trace begins where the annealed electrode was located. Inset shows the typical time pattern. According to FINKENZELLER *et al.* (1969). (b) Records same as in (a), but simultaneous use of 32 implanted electrodes. The cross-hatched areas represent AI and AII. According to WILSMAN (1969). Responses (DC upward surface negative) are restricted to the specific projection areas. (c) Frequency dependence. (According to FINKENZELLER, Thesis Erlangen, 1969)

In addition a clear dependence of the DC-potential upon the frequency of the tonal stimuli can be demonstrated, with largest amplitudes between 500 and 2000 Hz. This is shown for middle intensities in Fig. 19.

The problem of the intramodal specificity of the perstimulatory DC-potential was discussed by KEIDEL in detail in 1972b. He compared single unit activity at geniculate level with the pattern of the complex cortical response in the cat (and in man). It is well known (AITKIN, 1973; AITKIN and WEBSTER, 1971; DUNLOP *et al.*, 1969; KALLERT, 1972, 1974) that the PST-histogram at midbrain and geniculate level reveals many different patterns, according to which the neuronal groups of single cells can easily be classified. One of them, for example, is the primary type, another the chopper type and so on. There is, however, one prevailing shape, namely, first a marked on-response with a very high firing probability, followed by a silent period. Then, after a few hundred milliseconds following a long-lasting stimulus, a long-lasting activity is observable. Interestingly enough, it is this third period within the PST-histogram which obviously contains the intramodal specific auditory information. This can be concluded from the fact that different types of stimuli — noise versus sinusoidal tones — can be clearly separated there. For noise, the envelope of this activity appears random. If tonal stimuli are delivered, the same envelope is clearly periodic. This is not the place to discuss the topic of demultiplication, which is involved in tonal stimuli as an effect of the transfer of information through the subsynaptic membranes. It might, however, be mentioned in passing that as a result of this general synaptic feature within the decoding processes, those periodicities have relatively low frequencies but are time-locked and demultiplicated by a factor up to a few hundred. This problem is described elsewhere in detail (Keidel, 1956, 1962, 1969, 1972b, 1974a; v. Békésy, 1960). Figure 20 shows one example obtained by Keidel (1972b), comparing PST-histograms to tonal as well as to noise stimuli with the cat's AI corticogram (after DC-amplification) and the extracranially recorded response to the same type of stimuli in man.

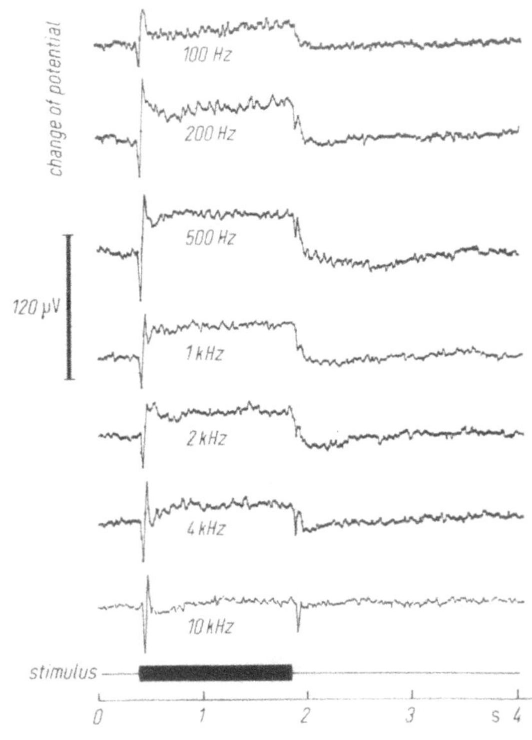

Fig. 19. Frequency dependence of the perstimulatory DC-potential recorded from the awake cat's specific projection area with implanted electrodes. Largest responses between 500 Hz and 2 kHz. (According to David et al., 1969b)

The above comparison clearly shows that the DC-potential in the cat at the cortical level (and in man) is synchronized in time fairly well with that part of the activity in single units at geniculate level, which contains the auditory intramodal specific information. Hence, it is this part of the response where the histogram is random for noise and periodic for tones. If we consider the work of GOLDSTEIN and ABELES (1975) (see p. 117f.), it makes sense to compare the silent period of the histogram to the time needed for the change of the membrane potential from hyperpolarization to normal values, on the order of 100 ms at the cortical level.

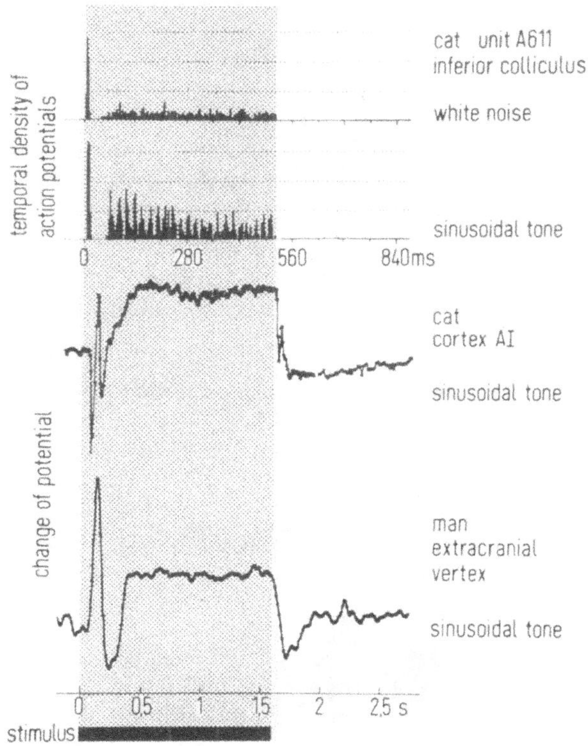

Fig. 20. Comparison of PST-histograms to noise (top trace), to tonal stimuli (next trace), single unit activity from the cat's midbrain, with the corticogram of the AI area of the cat (next trace) and the extracranially recorded response from man's vertex. The perstimulatory DC-potential is synchronized with that part of the PST-histogram which contains the intramodal specific auditory information, whether noise or sinusoidal tones have been used as stimuli. (According to KEIDEL, 1972b)

This was demonstrated in Fig. 11. It also fits experiments performed by CREUTZFELDT, ROSINA, ITO, and PROBST for cortical single unit activity (1969). They proved that facilitatory and inhibitory processes overlap in the integrative process. Particularly, the inhibitory neurons may be responsible for the silent period following the first marked on-effect which tells the brain "there was something". Much later, the brain decodes what sensory channel it was and – during the perstimulatory DC-potential – what intramodal specific auditory stimuli (noise or tones) was delivered. Although CREUTZFELDT *et al.* (1969) did not record the DC-potential (they used some filtering in the amplifiers), this point is still of great interest. Their results are shown in Fig. 21.

Experiments demonstrating the effect of subthalamic brain lesions and section of parts of the auditory channel have been described by quite a few laboratories. Lindsley, Zaroodny, and Morton in 1967 based their experimental work on the following considerations: Following up the concept of an ascending reticular

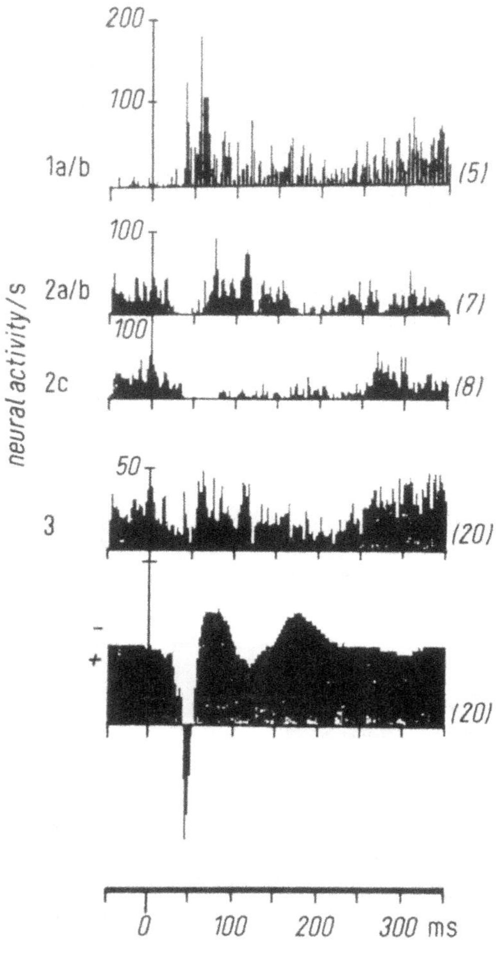

Fig. 21. Single cell activity from the animal's cortex. The top trace shows histograms of facilitatory neurons, 2a/b and c are activities from short term and long term inhibitory cells responsible for the silent period in our histogram (Fig. 20). 3 is the sum of 1 and 2. The bottom trace represents the classical evoked response pattern (without the perstimulatory DC-component which could not be recorded with their device). (According to Creutzfeldt *et al.*, 1969)

system involved in sleep, wakefulness and arousal advanced by Moruzzi and Magoun (1949), attention was directed to descending influences on the reticular formation (Adey, Buchwald, and Lindsley, 1960; Adey, Dunlop, and Sunderland, 1958; Adey, Segundo, and Livingstone, 1957; French, Hernandez-Peon, and Livingstone, 1955). Adey and Lindsley (1959, 1961) showed that tonic subthalamic facilitatory influences are necessary to maintain the responsiveness of the RF to sensory input. Likewise, HUGELIN, and BONVALLETT (1957) demonstrated subthalamic facilitatory and ventral thalamic inhibitory influences on a monosynaptic trigeminal motor reflex. Also, an EEG-synchronizing influence was shown to originate from the lower brain-stem (BATINI, MORUZZI, PALESTINI, ROSSI, and ZANCHETTI, 1959) and a bulbarascending, deactivating influence which functions concurrently with midbrain reticular activation was described by BONVALLET and BLOCH in 1961. Thus, it appears that there are multiple excitatory and inhibitory influences converging on the brainstem RF from the subthalamus, as well as the ventral thalamus and lower brain-stem. In addition to, and probably related to its role in modulation of reticular input, the subthalamus was shown to be importantly involved in EEG arousal and attentive behavior. ADEY and LINDSLEY (1959) observed that cats and monkeys with chronic subthalamic lesions were unresponsive to sensory and emotional stimuli. ADEY, WALTER, and LINDSLEY in 1962 demonstrated that cats with chronic bilateral subthalamic lesions were impaired during brightness discrimination and delayed-response tasks, and concurrent hippocampal Thetaactivity was severely reduced or abolished, perhaps, because of sensory "inattention". FELDMAN and WALLER in 1962 showed that posterior hypothalamic and subthalamic lesions led to behavioral somnolence even during periods of EEG arousal induced by midbrain RF tetanization. NAQUET *et al.* (1966 and 1965) found that cooling of the subthalamus was most effective in inducing sleep and EEG synchronization, even more so than cooling of the midbrain RF. Therefore it seems clear that the subthalamus is involved in the production and maintenance of attention, but its precise role still remains to be demonstrated. It is evident from the work of JASPER (1960) on the thalamic RF, and particularly the lateral midbrain lesions experiments of SPRAGUE *et al.* (1961, 1963), that other areas are also involved in attentive behavior.

In their study of 1967, LINDSLEY, ZAROODNY, and MORTON aimed to examine the cortical and brainstem distribution of these subthalamic facilitatory influences and to determine whether they acted on reticular input in general, as implied by the findings of sensory "inattention" following subthalamic lesions. They summarized their results as follows:

"Knowledge that descending subthalamic influences act to determine responsivness of the RF to various sensory inputs has been confirmed and extended. Subthalamic lesions not only led to reduction of sciatic evoked potentials in the RF but also decreased *click* and flash evoked potentials. Because RF conducted evoked potentials were reduced following subthalamic lesions, it appears that subthalamic facilitatory influences are effective by virtue of their action on the basic excitability of RF neurons themselves and not as a result of alterations of strictly sensory input mechanisms. The distribution of these facilitatory influences to the RF is widespread; evoked potentials in the anterior and posterior midbrain RF were severely affected and those in the medullary RF were also reduced, though not as consistently as in the midbrain. It also appears that subthalamic lesions are capable of altering the later components of the primary sensory, cortical response to sciatic stimulation. Amphetamine was not capable of restoring the depressed reticular evoked potentials. Sequential lesions of the subthalamus revealed that the facilitatory influences are diffusely organized and not limited to any specific region of the subthalamus. Subsequent ventral thalamic lesions demonstrated the existence of inhibitory influences passing through areas dorsal to the subthalamus."

MAJKOWSKY and MORGADES in 1969 studied the influence of sectioning the brachium of the inferior colliculus upon primary auditory evoked potentials. They started from the following considerations:

"there is rather general agreement that the first positive component of the cortical positive-negative primary sensory evoked potentials depends on the lemniscal system; the negative component depends on the multisynaptic unspecific system. In their previous studies, the disappearance of primary auditory evoked potentials in the auditory cortex was considered as an indicator of completeness of the section of the brachia of the inferior colliculus (BIC) (MAJKOWSKI, 1964). GALAMBOS *et al.* (1961) confirmed this finding in experiments in which Nembutal anesthesia was used. However, with chloralose or in the absence of anesthetics, the auditory evoked potentials in auditory cortex persisted unchanged after sectioning of BIC. Recently, ADRIAN *et al.* (1966) using chloralose came to the conclusion that the sectioning when confined to the lateral quadrant of the midbrain may abolish the evoked potential from auditory areas, but they also stated that the short-latency, positive-negative potentials may be recorded from the auditory cortex after complete sectioning of BIC. The same conclusion was reached by GOLDBERG and NEFF (1961). On the other hand, there is agreement that the secondary evoked potentials with long latency, duration and lability which can be recorded outside of primary auditory areas, *e.g.*, in middle suprasylvian, anterior lateral gyri and in somato-motor cortex (LOMBROSO and MERLIS, 1957; BUSER and BORENSTEIN, 1959; BUSER *et al.*, 1959; THOMPSON and SINDBERG, 1960), are not influenced, in a recordable way, by sectioning of BIC. The question of the mediation of auditory impulses by the specific or unspecific systems is very important from the point of view of neurophysiological mechanisms of auditory discriminative learning in cats with sectioning of BIC (KRYTER and ADES, 1943; RAAB and ADES, 1946; GOLDBERG and NEFF, 1961; MAJKOWSKI, 1964). It seems that the phylogenetically newer lemniscal pathways, with their fast conduction fibers, play an important role in carrying meaningful information. It was found that after sectioning of BIC, learning to respond to clicks took 2–3 times longer than in intact cats (MAJKOWSKI, 1964). However, when the sectioning was not complete, even on one side, and some fibers (about 10%) were not cut, the learning was not changed. Thus, the extent of the lesion seems to be very critical for behavioral and electrophysiological results. In 1969, the primary auditory evoked potentials were studied in acute and chronic experiments before and after sectioning of the BIC under Nembutal and alpha-chloralose anesthesia, without anesthesia, and during electrical stimulation of inferior colliculi. The sectioning of BIC resulted in disappearance of evoked responses recorded from auditory cortex AI, regardless of the type of anesthesia and in cats without anesthesia, during auditory and electrical stimulation of inferior colliculus. This effect lasted for several months."

CHOW, RANDALL, and MORRELL in 1966 studied the effect of brain lesions on conditioned cortical electropotentials based upon the following considerations:

"Considerable speculation exists concerning the role of various central nervous system structures in the mediation of the various types of such responses. With tone and flashing light constituting the paired stimuli, three different types of conditioned responses were described: general cortical activation, the repetitive response, and local cortical activation (MORRELL and JASPER, 1956; MORRELL *et al.*, 1957). Tentative assignments of the mesencephalic reticular formation as the substrate for conditioned generalized activation (GASTAUT, 1958) and the thalamic reticular system as the structure important in conditioned localized activation were made (GASTAUT, 1958; MORRELL, 1958). A number of hypotheses have been advanced with regard to the anatomical basis of the conditioned repetitive response: MORRELL (1957) proposed that this response depends upon a state of hyperexcitability and hypersynchrony in the visual cortex; MORRELL and others (1960) raised the question of the relation of hippocampal Theta rhythms to the conditioned repetitive response. GASTAUT (1958) proposed that hypersynchronous discharges induced by the conditioned stimulus are due to inhibition of the diffusely projecting thalamic system. The present study attempts to evaluate the effects of destroying or isolating various midbrain and forebrain regions on those conditioned electrocortical responses in cats with the following results: Conditioned repetitive responses were abolished in cats with neocortical lesions in auditory cortex or between auditory and visual cortex. Knife-cuts separating visual and auditory cortex also abolished conditioned repetitive responses. All other conditioned electropotentials were seen in cats with these cortical lesions. Conditioned local activation was abolished in cats with lesions of the rostral thalamus. All other conditioned electropotentials were seen in these cats with lesions in the rostral thalamus. All conditioned cortical electropotentials developed normally in cats with lesions in the septal region, midline dorsal thalamus, midbrain reticular formation, and frontal neocortex. The importance of cortico-cortical connections for the appearance of conditioned repetitive responses and the importance of the rostral thalamus for the appearance of conditioned local activation were emphasized by that study."

All these many details have been cited so thoroughly because they are of the greatest importance for understanding the neurophysiological difference between the inter- and intramodal specific DC-potential described above and the intermodal (at least partly if not almost) nonspecific contingent negative variation first described by GREY WALTER (1964). He demonstrated beautifully that after conditioning of an animal (and of course of man) to a given type of stimulus such as a brief click, drawing of attention to a behavioral response even of a different modality, was preceded by an inclining DC-shift and the motor response was followed by an immediate drop of the DC-shift to the original baseline. The CNV has latencies on the order of 240 ms to the click and outlasts the stimulus by more than a second. One example of that response which possibly may play an important role in practical audiometry in the future is shown in Fig. 22.

Similarly KORNHUBER and DEECKE in 1965 first demonstrated that corresponding to each motor-reaction, a DC-potential can be observed, which he labelled "Bereitschaftspotential". This is independent of any sensory stimulus given before and can also be recorded in cases with no sensory stimulation

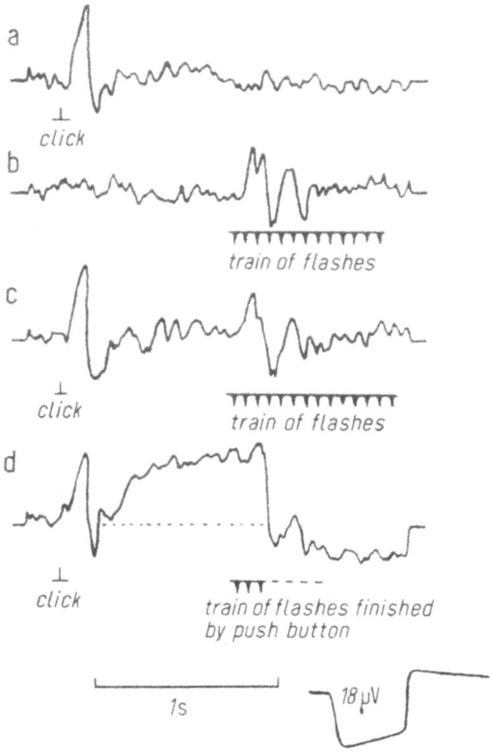

Fig. 22. (a) Click only. (b) Train of flashes only. (c) Click followed by a train of flashes, subject's attention not drawn to flashes and behaviour passive. (d) Click plus train of flashes as in (c), but subject's attention drawn to task of pushing a button when the train of flashes appears and by that means abolishing or finishing the flashes. A clear inclining "expectancy-potential" only in this case can be observed. (According to GREY WALTER, 1964)

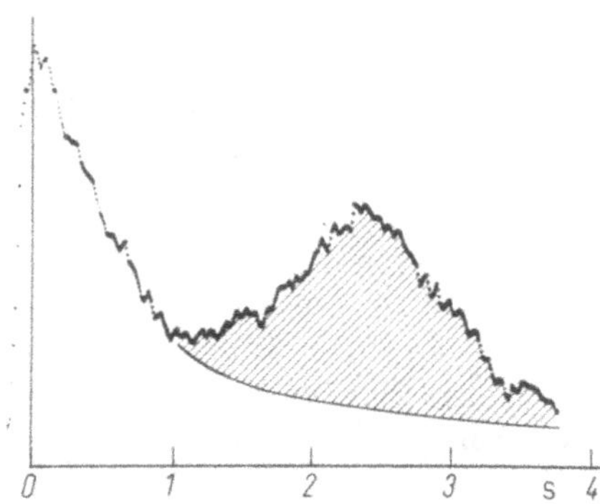

Fig. 23a. Autocorrelated responses from the human skull to voluntary "intentions" of movements of the big toe. Size of electrode above the superior frontal cortex. Full time range 4 seconds. Voluntary period time for intentions, 2 seconds. A clear potential shaded can be observed. It might precede that motor potential described by KORNHUBER, but differs from the motor reaction potential itself which must be triggered by a sensory stimulus. This trigger is absent in this experiment. KEIDEL (1976)

at all. This can be proved by the following experiment (KEIDEL, unpublished data): If a subject sits in an anechoic room and just imagines moving say a big toe at his forehead a DC-potential can be obtained which is not followed by a motor reaction potential at that place of the skull. Since no trigger stimulus of a sensory type is necessary for this experiment, autocorrelation technique is preferable to simple averaging. What is difficult for the subject is only the task of concentrating when thinking of the toe's movement in regular intervals, of say 2 seconds. Surprisingly, this task can be performed easily after some training. Care has to be given to avoid intervals which would be multiples of the heart beat frequency, to avoid EKG artifacts. One example of these experiments is shown in Fig. 23.

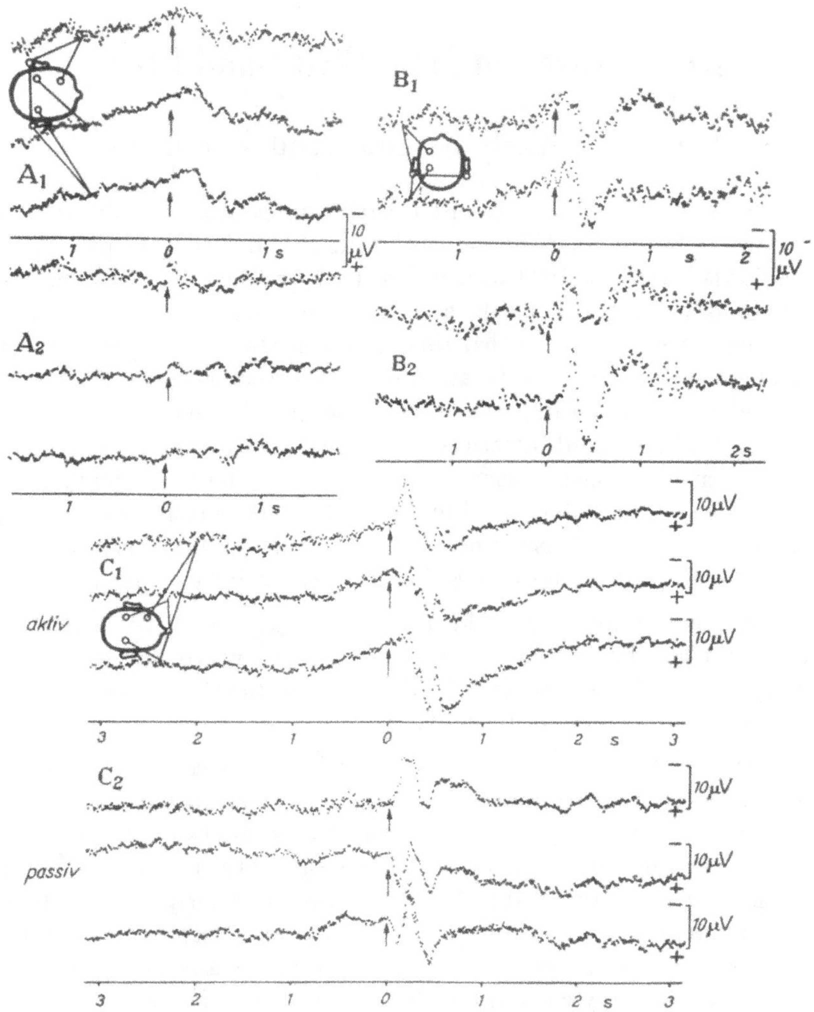

Fig. 23b. "Bereitschafts"-potentials according to KORNHUBER and DEECKE, 1965. A_1, B_1, and C_1 ascending DC-shift before the stimulus (arrow). A_2, B_2, and C_2 absence of this potential in case of "passive" motor response. For details see the original paper

We have now discussed the three types of DC-potentials that play a role in audiometry: (i) the perstimulatory DC-potential during ongoing stimulation (KEIDEL), (ii) the contingent negative variation, or expectancy potential, following a brief stimulus like a click, preceding a behavioral task of a second stimulus (GREY WALTER) and (iii) the DC-potential preceding a motor reaction (KORNHUBER). A clear separation of these different DC-shifts within the complex response to an auditory stimulus is possible only in man. Since we here tried to describe the features of the evoked responses in the cat, we prefer to conclude this part of the chapter and to continue the discussion of those DC-responses in the chapter entitled "auditory responses (ERA, ECG, and BERA) in human subjects."

III. Research in Man. BERA and ERA

A. Classical Early Response and V-response

The very first attempts to record electrical responses to auditory stimuli from the intact human skull in the awake human subject were performed by PAULINE DAVIS as early as 1939, as mentioned earlier. The response of the normal EEG-trace was visible in the awake state and even more clearly in the sleeping state. No computer was used at that time; nevertheless, it was a great discovery The "great era" in ERA, and the break-through to real clinical use could not occur, however, before a marked improvement of the signal-to-noise ratio had been methodologically introduced by means of *electronic computers*. The reason is, that contrary to visually evoked responses, K-complexes of auditory stimuli recorded from the intact human skull occured in rare cases. Normal responses to moderate stimulus intensities, and intensities near behavioral threshold responses to auditory stimuli are usually hidden in the on-going electrical activity of the human EEG.

Therefore, the introduction of the *averaging technique* to ERA in 1957 was a milestone in the history of electrical recording of central nervous system responses to auditory stimuli. Again it was the MIT Communication Biophysics Group that obtained the first computed averaged data.

After trials on the cat – which have already been discussed – DAN GEISLER first studied the distribution of responses from monkey's exposed pia in 1959. He performed mapping studies for the early responses and discussed the problem of a hidden auditory projection area, "hidden" in the case of the primates, particularly monkey and man. As early as July 15, 1957 in the "Quarterly Progress Report" with FRISHKOPF and BROWN, he reported "early" responses to clicks in awake human subjects. As Fig. 24 shows, however, his averaged responses – even vertex versus mastoid – actually contain the classical late N1 response with its latency of 90 ms, although he concentrated his attention on the early response with latencies of 20 to 30 ms and did not mention the late response in his first report.

In their paper, the authors dealt with the topic of intensity function and the influence of repetition rate upon the response. A more detailed account about the early response only was reported in 1960 by DAN GEISLER. He found then the largest responses not at the vertex but at the inion location of the electrode. This is shown clearly in Fig. 25.

Randomized trains of clicks were used as stimuli. The first peak with a latency of 30 ms at the inion is negative in polarity. This is, however, in accordance with our present knowledge of those responses, if one considers the inversion of polarity

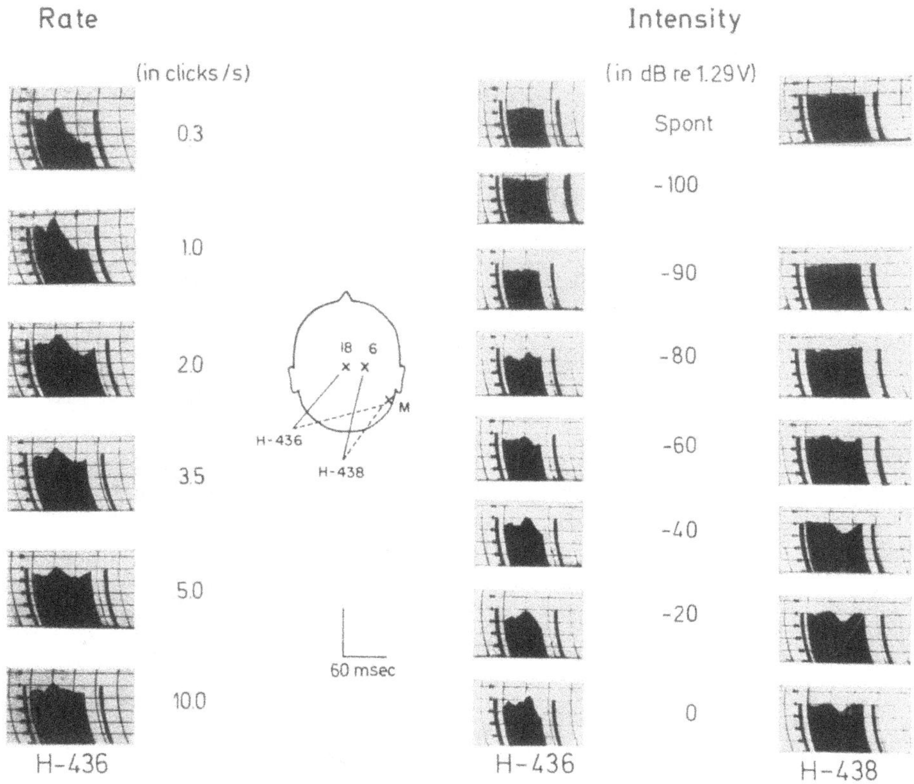

Fig. 24. "Early" responses to clicks. For the rate function, the click intensity is —20 dB re 1.29 volts across the earphones; sample size is 250 times the click rate. For the intensity functions, the rate presentation is 1 per second; sample size, 250. The indicated amplitude calibration is 10 microvolts for H-436 and 20 microvolts for H-438. The zero-potential line is at —6 for H-436, and at zero for H-438. Note that upward deflection represents positivity at electrode 18 for H-436, and at electrode 6 for H-438. (According to GEISLER, FRISHKOPF, and BROWN, 1957.) The late N1 can be seen best in the two left top records

as a function of location of electrodes. This was studied carefully in later mapping experiments (see the monograph of REGAN, 1972). Interestingly enough, GEISLER's own conclusions about his experiments read as follows:

"In summary, then, bilateral responses to clicks have been obtained from the scalp of many human subjects. The responses have amplitudes of a few microvolts, and the largest responses are recorded from the occipital regions. The behavior of

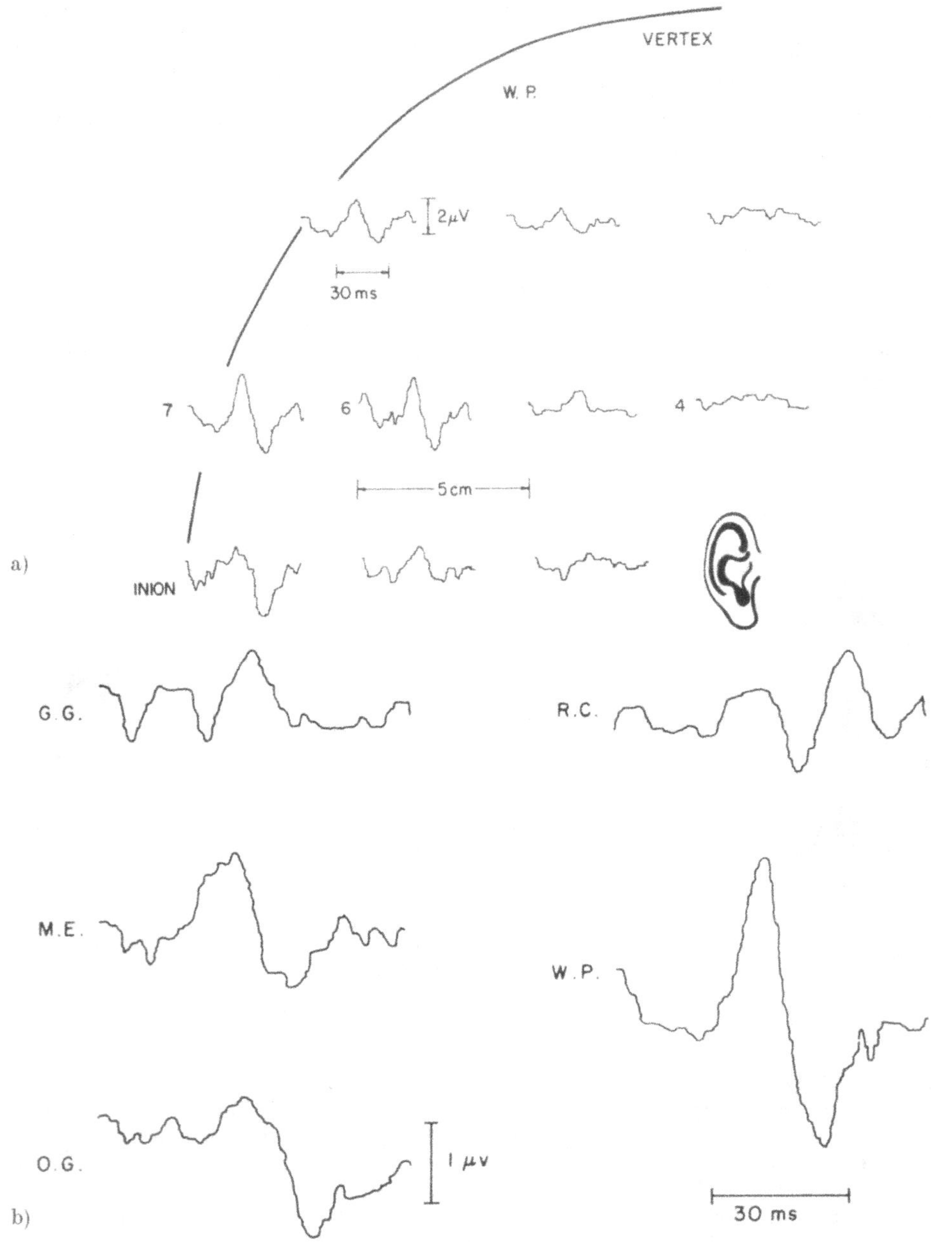

Fig. 25. (a) Distribution of responses on the scalp. Recording electrodes were approximately 5 cm apart. Each trace is the average of 2000 responses. In this and the following figures, negativity with respect to the reference electrode is plotted upwards. Reference electrode was placed on the nose. Clicks were presented periodically at the rate of 14/s; the intensity was —30 dB re 2.2. volts delivered to the earphones. (b) Average responses from 5 different subjects. Clicks were delivered at 14/s or 15/s at an intensity of —45 dB; 4000 responses were averaged from subject M.E., and 8000 from the others. Potentials were recorded between electrode No. 6 (see Fig. 25a) and reference electrode which was either electrode No. 4 or an electrode on the nose (M.E., G.G.). (According to GEISLER, 1960)

the response as the rate and intensity of the click stimuli are varied is quite repeatable and is similar to cortical response data obtained from cats. The latency and spatial distribution, however, argue against a site of origin in the auditory projection areas of the cortex. This is not a dismaying fact, for in addition to the responses obtained from classical auditory areas, "secondary" responses have been recorded from many parts of cat and monkey cortex (BUSER and BORENSTEIN, 1957; STARZL and WHITLOCK, 1952). It is concluded that these responses recorded from human scalp are most probably cortical in nature, but are generated elsewhere than in the Sylvian fissure". (See also GEISLER, FRISHKOPF, and ROSENBLITH, 1958.)

What followed was the so-called "*postauricular electric response*" recorded by N. Y.-S. KIANG *et al.* (1963). Electrodes were placed just behind the ear a bit above the mastoid. The reference electrode was the opposite ear lobe. Again, the first response to clicks was a negative peak, followed by a positive one. The latencies, which were shorter than DAN GEISLER's, ranged between 10 and 15 ms. Amplitude was dependent upon intensity as shown in the lower part of Fig. 26. A log-log plot has been added to the original semi-log plot by the reviewer for comparison. Obviously, over an intensity range of some 50 dB this log-log plot (broken) is nearly linear. Its exponent, n, to the underlying power function is of the order of 0.35 and 0.92 respectively. The negative peak was measured versus the baseline.

Since the tension of the neck muscles influenced the amplitude of the postauricular response drastically (Fig. 26c), the authors concluded their paper with the following remarks:

"The postauricular responses are obtainable with other transient stimuli, such as bursts of tone or bursts of noise. All subjects were healthy. No responses could be detected in records obtained from two subjects with severe hearing losses. The lability of the response... resembles the behavior of certain responses recorded from the brains of unanesthetized cats (TEAS and KIANG, 1961)" and "It is possible that the response arises from activity of either ear or neck muscles. The sensitivity of the response to changes in electrode location and the effects of head position support such a view. The response is unlikely to be the result of stapedius muscle activity in the middle ear, since a clear response was obtained in a subject who had undergone stapes surgery with resultant severing of the muscle".

During the following years the muscular origin (myogenic) was emphasized, if not overemphasized from the standpoint of our present knowledge, by BICKFORD and others in 1964. DAVIS *et al.* write, for instance, in 1964: "We identify both varieties (DAN GEISLER's response and the postauricular response) as muscle responses. They can be separated by the fact, that postauricular response 'habituates' rapidly, while GEISLER's 'early' response from inion is well sustained and reproducible". (BICKFORD *et al.*, 1964; BICKFORD, 1963; BICKFORD *et al.*, 1963; DAVIS *et al.*, 1964). One example of BICKFORD's experiments is shown in Fig. 27.

BICKFORD could also demonstrate that comparable responses could be recorded even from the forearm and from the leg with correspondingly longer latencies up to as much as 60 ms. Along the same line, COBB and MOROCUTTI stressed the

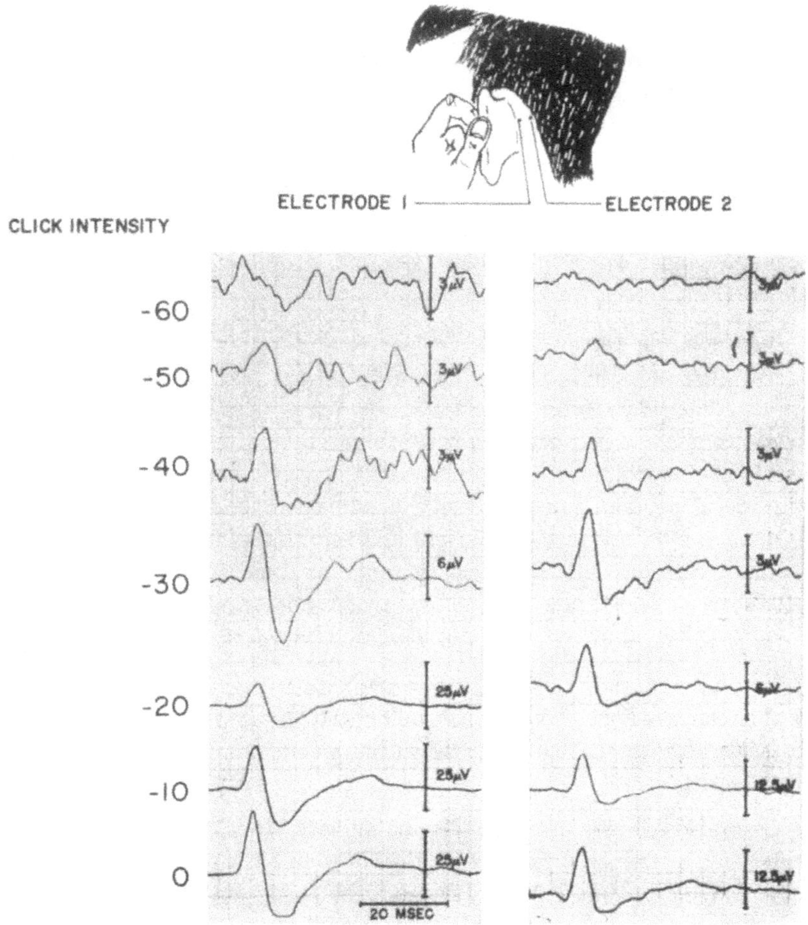

Fig. 26. (a)

Fig. 26. (a) Averaged responses to clicks for two electrode locations behind the left ear. The electrodes were stainless steel needles. The reference electrode was clipped to a saline-moistened cotton pad on the right earlobe. Negative polarity for the active electrodes is plotted upward. Responses are shown for 7 stimulus intensities. Clicks were produced by applying a 10 micro-second rectangular pulse to the terminals of an Altec 1-755A loud speaker located 4 feet in front of the subject who was seated in a sound-proof room. Clicks were presented at a 10/s rate; reference level (0 dB) = 13 volts into the speaker. With this stimulus arrangement, the psycho-physical threshold was approximately —65 dB for this subject. (The beginning of each trace in this and subsequent figures marks the instant at which a monitoring microphone placed near the ear detects the arrival of the click). Number of responses averaged for each trace, N = 1000. (b) Latencies and amplitudes of the negative peaks in the traces of Fig. 26a as functions of click intensity. Latencies are measured from the beginning of each trace; amplitudes are measured from baseline to peak. (Dashed log-log plot of intensity function reviewer.) (c) Post-auricular responses influenced by head position. The head was first oriented in an upright position. Then the head was allowed to fall back until it rested comfortably on a support. Finally, the head was brought forward in a bending position. Changes in head position often had dramatic effects on the responses, but at other times did not. Checks of the recording arrangement were always made to ensure that no electric connections were disturbed as a result of head movements. (All according to KIANG, CRIST, FRENCH, and EDWARDS, 1963)

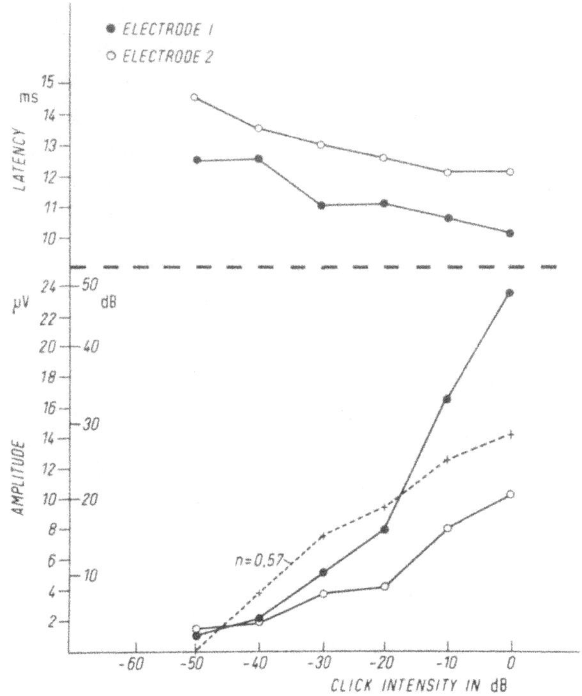

Fig. 26. (b)

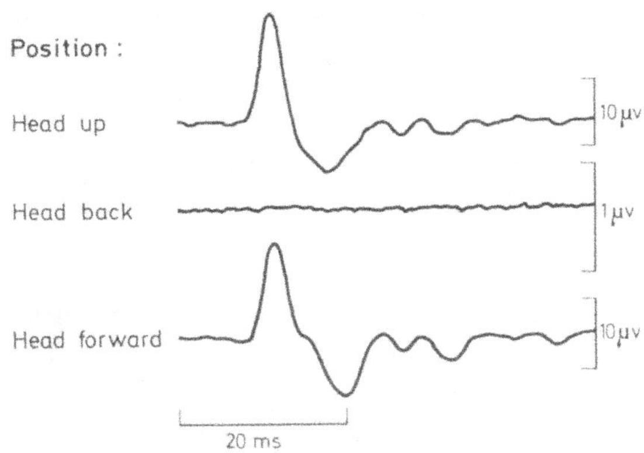

Fig. 26. (c)

possible involvement of the eye blinking muscles and the eye blinking reflex in the late responses (1967). BICKFORD, in addition, used curarization to *nearly* completely abolish the responses to auditory stimulation. This is recorded in Fig. 28.

So the myogenic origin of the inion response has almost been confirmed. However, although a purely myogenic response to a sound may still be used as an auditometric indicator, the small section of sensory (auditory) origin (STANGE, 1973) begins to play an increasingly important role in modern audiometry.

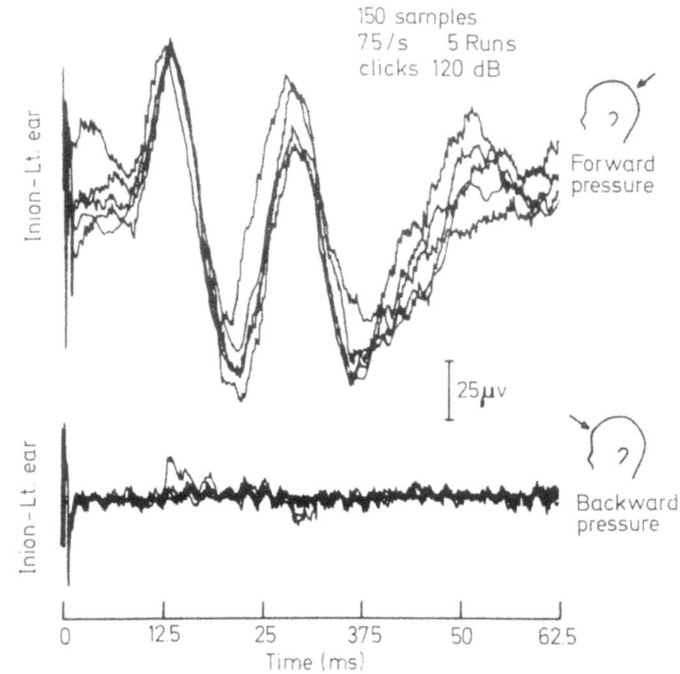

Fig. 27. Inion-response. Effect of muscle tension on response. Modal display of five averages. Above pressure is applied to back of head increasing tension in neck muscles. Below pressure on forehead reflexes relaxes neck muscles and abolishes response. (According to BICKFORD *et al.*, 1964)

In the same paper, BICKFORD, JACOBSON, and CODY (1964) were also able to record *intracerebrally* in the brain of an epileptic patient. This is one of the first records of the late slow potentials to auditory stimulation in man. Therefore one record is shown in Fig. 29.

Similarily CHATRIAN, PETERSEN, and LAZARTE in 1960 were successful in recording intracerebrally from the primary auditory cortex in man. Again, BICKFORD discussed whether their response was primary or secondary in origin: "Experience with depth recording indicates that potentials arising from the primary auditory areas are difficult to record, although occasional successful results have been reported. When averaging techniques are used, intracerebral components to sound stimulation can be recorded at considerable distances from known receiving areas and presumably represent secondary responses."

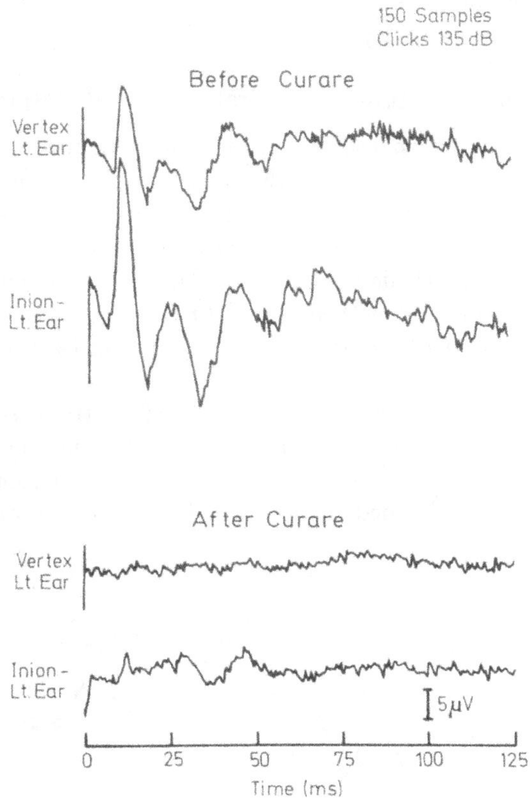

Fig. 28. Effect of partial curarization upon the inion-response. Responses recorded simultaneously from the vertex and inion in human subject. After curarization (sufficient to necessitate assisted respiration) suppression of response was complete at the vertex and almost complete at the inion. Subject was supine with pillow support. No anesthesia. (BICKFORD *et al.*, 1964)

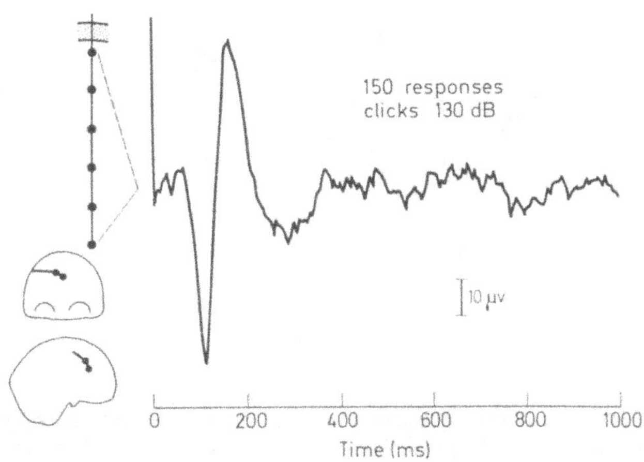

Fig. 29. Intracerebral response to sound in a patient with focal epilepsy. Recordings from upper and lower electrodes to a depth lead in position, shown in roentgenogram, in the frontal lobe. There is a 1 cm separation between depth-electrode contacts. (BICKFORD *et al.*, 1964)

B. Late Averaged Slow Potentials in Man as Audiometric Indicators (ERA)

1. General Features; Temporal Pattern of Responses

The recording of brain responses to auditory stimuli in man was strongly related in its efficiency to the type of technique that was used. Hence, all older assessments were not completely successful because the technique which was applied was too simple. This is not only true for the K-complex, but also for DAWSON's technique of superimposition on a cathode ray display or on a photographic film (1950). The first authors who used this method for audimetric purpose were SUZUKI and ASAWA in 1957, based upon studies performed by ABE in 1954, who had also used the superimposition technique.

The crucial step forward was the introduction of electronic superimposition of trains of stimuli with synchronization of all traces following the onset of stimulus sequence, in other words the use of averaging by means of computers. The first records which could be obtained by a self-made small electronic computer with

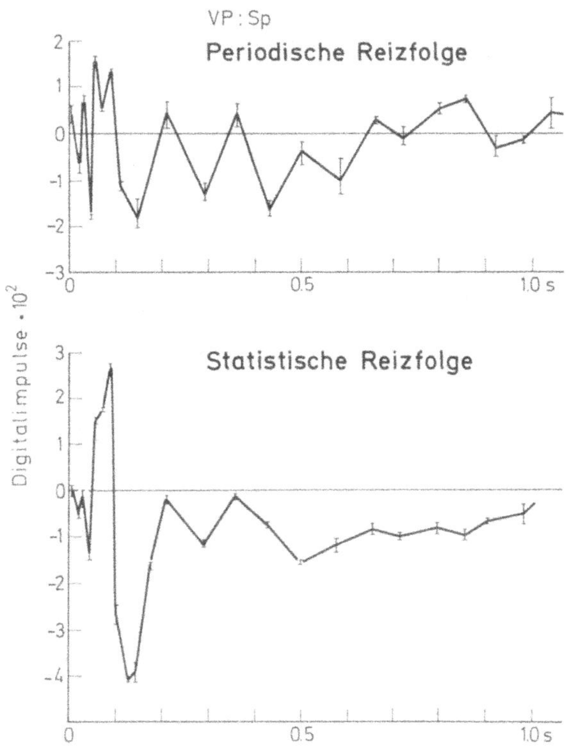

Fig. 30. First electronically averaged late slow responses in man to trains of periodic (top) and randomized (bottom) clicks. Original figure. "Periodische Reizfolge" means periodic trains, "statistische Reizfolge" means randomized train of clicks. Besides the early responses, the late P1, N1 and P2 shows up clearly in the bottom trace. The corresponding latencies are on the order of 60, 90 and 140 ms. (According to KEIDEL, 1962a, b; and KEIDEL and SPRENG, 1963)

tubes (KEIDEL, 1958) were reported by KEIDEL in 1962 at the CORLAS meeting in Athens (published with SPRENG in 1963 in Acta Oto-laryngologica) with the declared intention of using the late slow responses (P1, N1, and P2) for "objective" audiometry. In Fig. 30, the original Figure of this paper is shown. It clearly contains the early and the late slow responses which are most emphasized. Since periodic and random stimulation are compared, the enhancement of Alpha-rhythms in the case of periodic stimuli proved that the late P1, N1, and P2 in the record for random stimulation were not originated by eye-blinking artifacts.

Simultaneously in St. Louis the group of Professor HALLOWELL DAVIS was working on the late slow responses for audiometry and gave a paper about it in Würzburg in 1964 at the CORLAS group where KEIDEL also gave a paper about the same topic. At that time, HAL DAVIS introduced recording from the vertex instead of parietal location of the "hot" electrode in accordance with the electrode location used by P. DAVIS, D. GEISLER, ABE, and SUZUKI. One typical example of the slides hc showed at Würzburg is shown in Fig. 31.

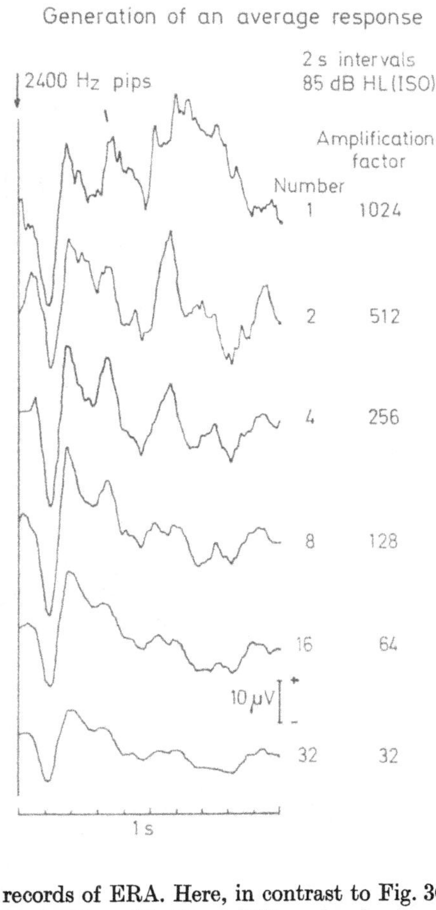

Fig. 31. First St. Louis records of ERA. Here, in contrast to Fig. 30, upward means positive deflection for vertex electrode. Thus, P1, N1, and P2 can be clearly seen for late slow responses. Recorded by HALLOWELL DAVIS (1964). Earlier trials at that laboratory (using only superimposing, but not computerized technique) were done by ATZE SPOOR in 1957 (cited by DAVIS *et al.*, 1966). Clicks

Careful studies about the influence of electrode location upon the pattern of the Auditory Evoked Response in man were performed by FINKENZELLER (Thesis Erlangen, 1969). He recorded with tone bursts of 300 ms duration from the ipsi- and contralateral temporal bone, from the vertex and from the glabella versus the chin. Repetition rate was 0.33 per second. He simultaneously computed the standard deviation, which was the thickness of the traces. In addition, at the bottom of each record, a dark profile three times the standard deviation as a function of time is computed and displayed. His records gave a good standard for adult awake subjects since all intra- and interindividual variations including those due to changes in vigilance are excluded. His standard traces with P60, N90, P160, and N300 are shown in Fig. 32.

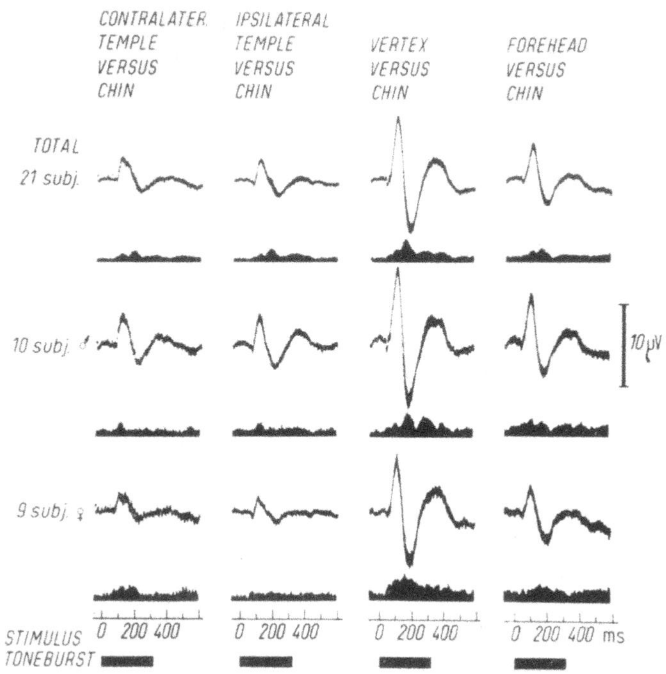

Fig. 32. Standards for ERA responses recorded from the intact human scalp. Mean of 21 subjects. The standard deviation can be seen as the dark profile. In each figure the bottom trace is three times the standard deviation. Stimuli: bursts of tones. (According to FINKENZELLER, Thesis Erlangen, 1969)

Based upon records during the years 1958 to 1961, KEIDEL and SPRENG first tackled the two main problems of frequency and intensity dependence of the late slow responses (ERA) in man. The first results along this line were published at the Würzburg meeting of the CORLAS in 1964. Thus, Fig. 33 shows a continuous series of records of different intensities ranging from threshold to +80 dB SPL. After recording from the temporal bone versus the neck, measuring N1 (150 ms) versus zero base line and plotting that three dimensionally (Fig. 34), the first "objective" audiometric threshold curve could be obtained by extrapolation in the log-log plots of all intensity functions for the different audio frequencies. Those results were also presented by KEIDEL in 1962 at Munich, in 1964a, b, c, d, e at Bremen, Copenhagen, Paris and Tübingen and at the meeting of the German Audiological Society at Erlangen 1965.

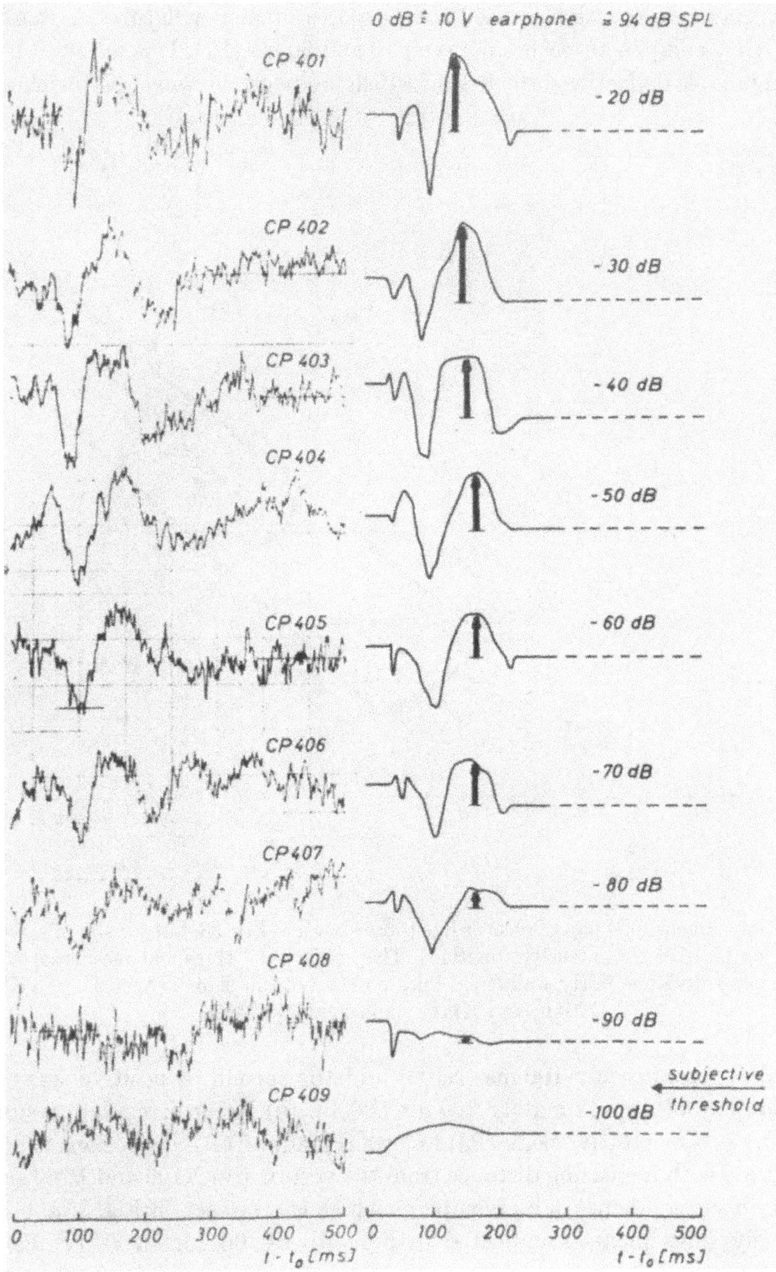

Fig. 33. Original records in adult human subjects to tone bursts. The size of N1 (150) was drawn versus zero base line in the right column (arrows). The intensity ranged from subjective threshold to +80 dB. (According to KEIDEL, 1964b; and KEIDEL and SPRENG, 1965)

At the same time quite a few fundamental papers have been published and/or presented at meetings by HALLOWELL DAVIS and his group (1964ff).

Very thorough mapping was done by VAUGHAN and RITTER in 1970. The authors elaborated the results of their numerous experiments: (i) Auditory evoked responses in adult human subjects are maximal at or near the vertex, so that their wave form at that location is used for purposes of nomenclature. A small and variable early component occurs between 16 and 60 ms (P1). It is followed by two large and reliable deflections, the first of which is a negative wave (N1) with a peak

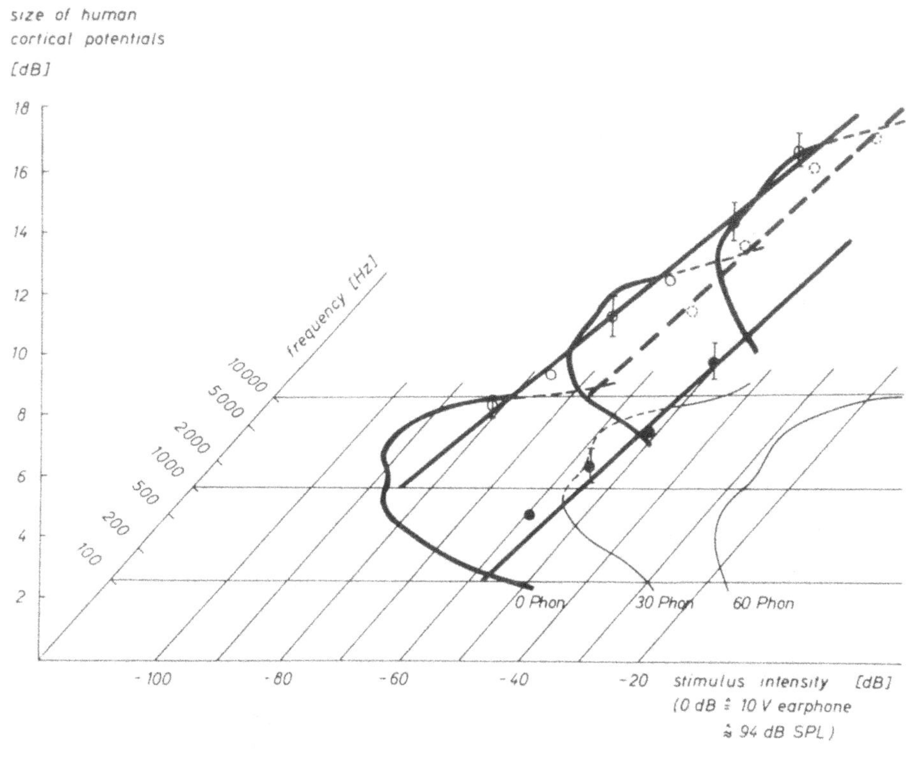

Fig. 34. Three dimensional plot of records like those shown in Fig. 33, but for all audio frequencies. Log-log plots of the intensity functions. The "objective" threshold measured this way fitted the subjective one fairly well (solid lines on the bottom plane). (According to KEIDEL, 1964b; and KEIDEL and SPRENG, 1965)

latency of approximately 100 ms (N100) and the second, a positive wave (P2), with a latency of approximately 200 ms (P200). (ii) When irregular stimuli are delivered, another positive peak (P3) follows (P300). (iii) All deflections decreased in amplitude with increasing distance from the vertex. (iv) N100 and P200 showed a polarity inversion beneath a given plane which can be seen in Fig. 35a, b and c, respectively. This plane is indicated in Fig. 35b by 00 for P200. (v) P300, in contrast, does not change polarity but shows nearly a continuous decrease in amplitude as demonstrated in Fig. 35c. Numbers are percentages of the amplitudes recorded from the vertex equalling 100%. The authors therefore concluded: "The observed distribution, when compared with that predicted from a multi-shell volume conductor model, was most consistent with dipol layer sources within the *primary auditory projection cortex* in the supratemporal plane. AERs to monaural stimuli were larger over the contralateral hemisphere, also supporting their

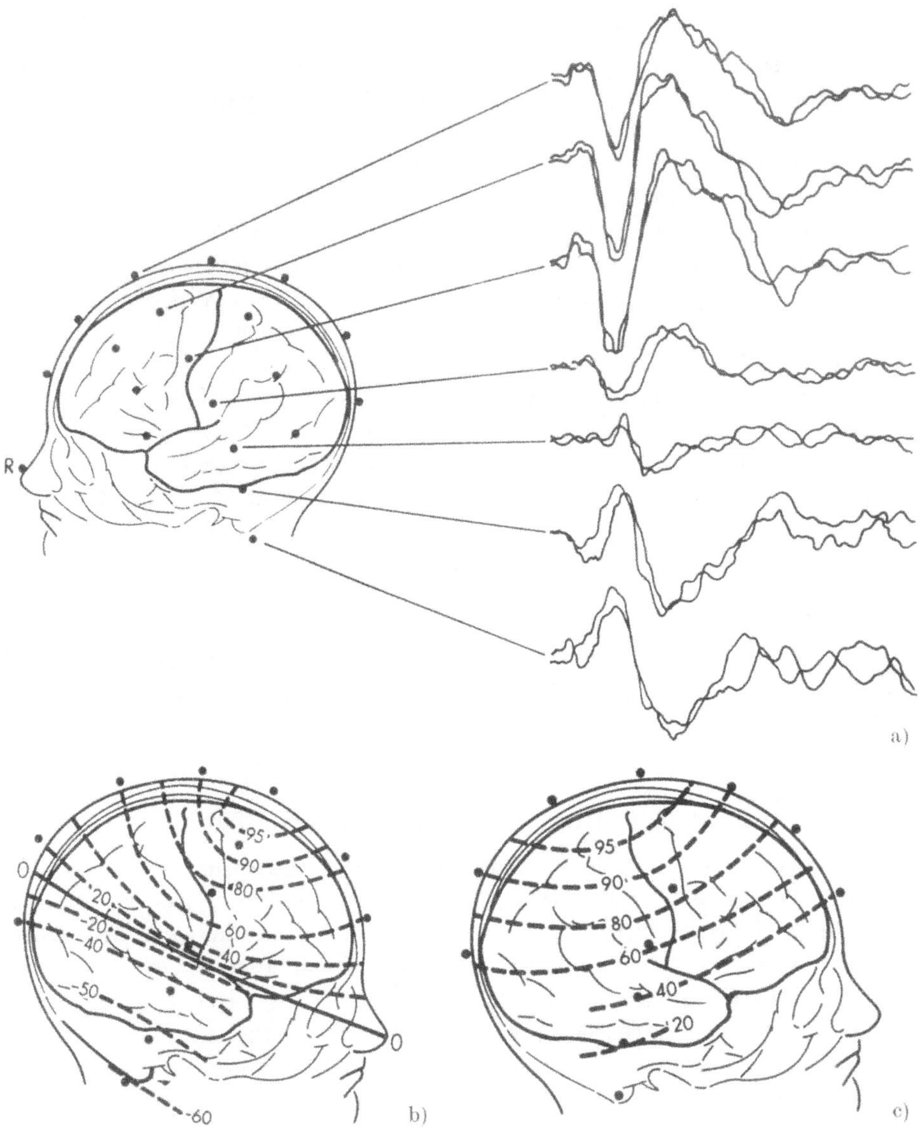

Fig. 35. (a) Records of AERs from the indicated locations on the skull of adult awake human subjects. (b) Distribution of the AERs for peak N200. The numbers indicate percentage of amplitude, with vertex potentials equalling 100%. This peak shows polarity inversion across a plane indicated by the 00 line. (c) Distribution of peak N300 differs from N200 in that no polarity inversion occurs, the maximum peak deflection is more occipital from vertex and amplitude decreases continuously with increasing distance from location of maximum amplitude. Numbers have the same meaning as in b. Surface positive deflections upward. (According to VAUGHAN and RITTER, 1970)

specific origin. In contrast, the longer latency (300 ms) component appearing in AERs elicited by infrequent aperiodic stimuli possessed a different distribution consistent with its origin in parietotemporal association cortex. It was possible to differentiate the myogenic postauricular response which possessed a quite circumscribed distribution, from the early AER components."

The results of the authors related to the early responses were quite striking. Two types of early responses were found. The first type showed one or two positive peaks between 40 and 60 ms, sometimes preceded by a negative deflection at 16 to 20 ms. This complex showed a reversal in polarity below the Sylvian fissure, thus having a distribution similar to N100 and P200. A second type of early response occurred near the inion and the mastoid. This component was markedly enhanced by tension of the muscles near the recording sites and reduced by relaxation. The first type of early response recorded from suprasylvian electrodes was presumed to be of intracranial origin. The myogenic sonomotor responses were generated by contraction of the postauricular muscle (BICKFORD *et al.*, 1964 – establishment of origin by nerve blockade). Those responses could be seen with greater regularity by utilizing loud clicks (greater than 90 dB SL). When the electrode was placed directly over the muscle at the posterior superior margin of the pinna, this response was quite large even during the relaxed state. Its largest components were a sharp negative deflection with a latency of 10–15 ms with peak at 16–20 ms, followed by a somewhat broader positive wave with a peak at approximately 30 ms. Small negative and positive deflections followed at 50–60 and 70–80 ms. This myogenic activity was concurrent with the other type of early activity (intracranial of origin). The authors concluded from those observations that only AERs from electrodes in close proximity to the cranial muscles may contain myogenic components during the initial 60–80 ms, since their location is restricted to a circular area of 2 cm radius.

2. Mapping from the Human Cortical Surface

By means of chronically implanted electrodes (for therapeutic reasons) SEM-JACOBSEN *et al.* in 1956 and CHATRIAN *et al.* in 1960 were the only ones to record directly from the cortical surface of the human brain. The number of their electrodes necessarily had to be restricted because of the technique applied. Therefore, it was a considerable advancement, when, in 1968, CELESIA, BROUGHTHON, RASMUSSEN, and BRANCH succeeded in recording from nearly the entire neocortex in man in seven neurosurgical cases where the surface of the human brain had been exposed. They also compared their results with those obtained by recording from the intact scalp. In Fig. 36a, the sites are shown from which they were able to record, and, in Fig. 36b, the shaded area within the brain's surface indicates the area from which averaged responses to clicks were obtained.

The authors examined 96 cortical points, exploring a maximum of 28 cortical points in each single patient. They found that the early positive wave was limited to a small area of the lateral surface of the cortex including the posterior two-thirds of the first temporal gyrus, the parietal and frontal operculum, as shown in Fig. 36b. In four patients, following temporal lobectomy, the exposed insula was explored but no evoked responses were obtained. They state, that it certainly appeared possible to record responses to auditory stimulation from the human cortex and, moreover, only from a limited area around the lips of the posterior two-thirds of the Sylvian fissure, possibly originating in the Heschl gyri. Since the peak latencies of the first positive events were rather long, these responses might also represent an area analogous to the cat's auditory areas AII and Ep (WOOLSEY and WALZL, 1942; ADES, 1943; DOWNMAN *et al.*, 1960; WOOLSEY, 1960). Their finding, that pre-central responses had longer latencies than responses in the first temporal gyrus and persisted after removal of the temporal lobe including HESCHL's gyri, further suggests, in the opinion of the authors, that these potentials either originated locally or were transmitted by volume conduction from adjacent regions other than the primary auditory area (upper bank of Sylvian fissure ?). This again, they

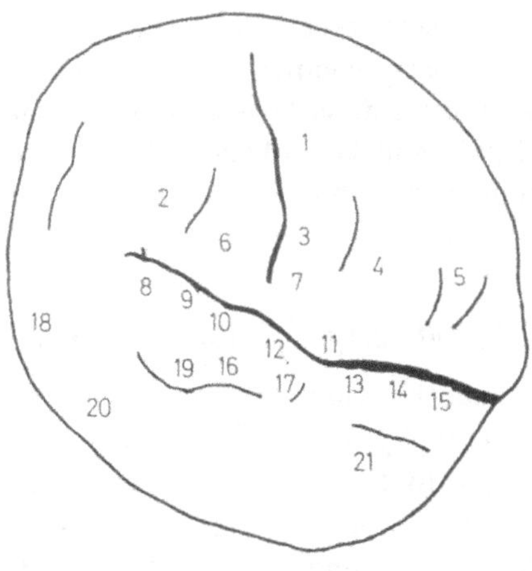

a)

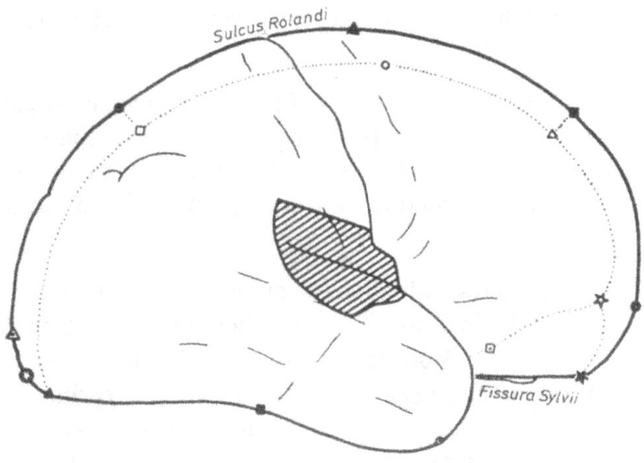

b)

Fig. 36. (a) Electrode-sites from which direct records from the exposed human brain were performed in seven neurosurgical patients by CELESIA, BROUGHTHON, RASMUSSEN, and BRANCH (1968). (b) Cortex of man showing shaded areas from which averaged responses to clicks were obtained conclude, may be a region analogous to the auditory areas AII and Ep or to SII. In contrast to the data of CHATRIAN *et al.*, they were unable to observe evoked potentials in single sweeps and could not find auditory responses from the insula. In accordance with CHATRIAN'S as well as CELESIA'S patterns, responses were closely comparable to those reported in monkeys by PRIBRAM *et al.* (1954). The CELESIA group, which compared direct obtainable surface potentials to responses recorded from the intact scalp, found that they were in agreement with the responses described by several authors including WILLIAMS *et al.* (1962), DAVIS and YOSHIE (1963), MORRELL and MORRELL (1966), CODY and BICKFORD (1965), DAVIS and ZERLIN (1966). The same is true for those responses obtained by KEIDEL (1962), KEIDEL and SPRENG (1963 and 1965). However, several deflections existing in the scalp response were not recorded from the human cortex. Therefore, CELESIA *et al.* concluded, in agreement with BICKFORD *et al.* (1964), that the early scalp deflections in an awake subject were myogenic potentials, whereas, the slow responses recorded from the scalp seemed to represent a mixture of myogenic and neurogenic potentials. The early components of the evoked activity which they recorded from the human cortical surface were one or two positive waves 10 to 25 microvolts in amplitude and 20–40 ms in latency. Direct evidence for the origin of the late deflections in man is still lacking.

3. Intensity Functions of AERs

The problem of the quantification for input-output relations in ERA is as old as psychophysics and neurophysiology. This problem is discussed in detail in Volume I of this handbook by Professor S. S. STEVENS. Based upon his ingenious idea of the validity of the power law in sensory psychology, several attempts were made in the different laboratories engaged in ERA to find clear values for the size of responses versus stimulus intensity. Numerous papers were published about this topic, a list of which can be found in the reference list at the end of this chapter.

Since the entire AER complex consists of many positive and negative peaks, it is obvious that the choice of a given peak and reference level (base line or another neighboring peak) may influence the results drastically. This certainly is one of the major reasons for the conflicting data published in the literature about this topic.

From psychophysical data, values on the order of 0.5 should have been claimed for the exponent, n, of the function $\Psi = \phi^n$, when, for ERA, Ψ is the amplitude and ϕ the stimulus intensity. More specifically, for ERA this formula should read $E = C \cdot (I : I_0)^n$. It was the Erlangen group which started experiments of this type. SPRENG and ICHIOKA proved in 1964 that the dynamic range for electrically elicited pain (canine dens in awake human subjects) was as small as that measured psychophysically by the STEVENS group, while the visual dynamic range measured via the amplitudes of visually evoked averaged responses was much larger (v. LOEWENICH *et al.*, 1967). Vibratory stimuli, on the other hand, lay somewhere between these extremes (FRUHSTORFER, 1966; EHRENBERGER *et al.*, 1965, 1966) and so did the auditory evoked AERs (KEIDEL and SPRENG, 1963; SPRENG and KEIDEL, 1963). It showed furthermore, that the auditory dynamic range was smaller than the visual one and broader than the vibratory one. Finally, this group showed, that responses to gustatory and olfactory stimuli revealed dynamic ranges similar to the ranges of vibratory elicited responses (PLATTIG, 1969; JAUHIAINEN and PLATTIG, 1966; FINKENZELLER, 1966). The problem was very much related to the influence of repetition rate upon the size of potentials. But this topic should be discussed separately.

In 1966 H. DAVIS and ZERLIN published data in which a range of 20 dB in amplitude corresponded to approximately 80 dB above sensation level for a range of 100 dB above the subjective threshold. This yielded an exponent of some 0.2 for the power law and led to the remark – with respect to the data of KEIDEL and SPRENG, 1963 – "as far as our results and his can be compared, they are in reasonable agreement".

The latest available data, however, (SKINNER *et al.*, 1974) confirm experiments performed together with BOB BUTLER in 1969 in Erlangen (BUTLER, KEIDEL, and SPRENG, 1969). Their results are shown in Fig. 37a and are based upon a paper by SPRENG delivered at the London ERA symposion in 1975; Fig. 37b shows a comparison of all data known at present. These figures allows two conclusions: (i) the exponent *n*, when STEVENS's power law is supposed, for a range of at least 50 dB is in the order of 0.2 to 0.3. (ii) It then flattens out over another 50 dB sound pressure level.

Their is some doubt now, whether a log-log plot is meaningful at all for neurophysiological scales like AERs amplitude plots, especially since a semi-log plot at those small slopes fits as well as a log-log plot (DAVIS, 1974; SKINNER *et al.*, 1974; ANTINORO and SKINNER, 1969). Secondly, the AER is an on-effect rather than the response to a permanent auditory event. The response to a permanent stimulus is the perstimulatory DC-potential. Finally, the subjective threshold is considerably influenced by the duration of brief tones up to 180–200 ms (v. BÉKÉSY, 1929; ZWISLOCKI, 1960), while the AER is only influenced by tones up to 30 ms (SKINNER and JONES, 1968; ONISHI and DAVIS, 1968). Nevertheless, it is important to provide an empirical comparison between the two measurements (psychophysical and neurophysiological) (SKINNER *et al.*, 1974). Hence, it is necessary for ERA to measure the dynamic range of its amplitudes versus that of the stimulus and to establish standard comparable conditions for its measurements: N1-P2 or N1 versus baseline (see p. 152). In addition SPRENG in his post-graduate thesis 1970 could show that the dynamic range of perception for all modalities is restricted in general to approximately 30 dB. This might be the reason and explanation as well for the factor of 1.7 which STEVENS found when comparing behavioral matching experiments to perceptual experiments as for the difference of the exponent, *n*, in the psychophysical experiments (0.5) compared to our neurophysiological experiments (0.2–0.3, same factor).

Even in the field of basic neurophysiology of the brains's main functions, great insecurity exists as to how the brain's perceptional function and its behavioral, *i.e.*

motor reaction, act together. To find an explanation for this problem is one of the main goals of the neurophysiology of mentality, especially of the comparison between psychophysics (subjective introversion) and neurophysiology (objective in-

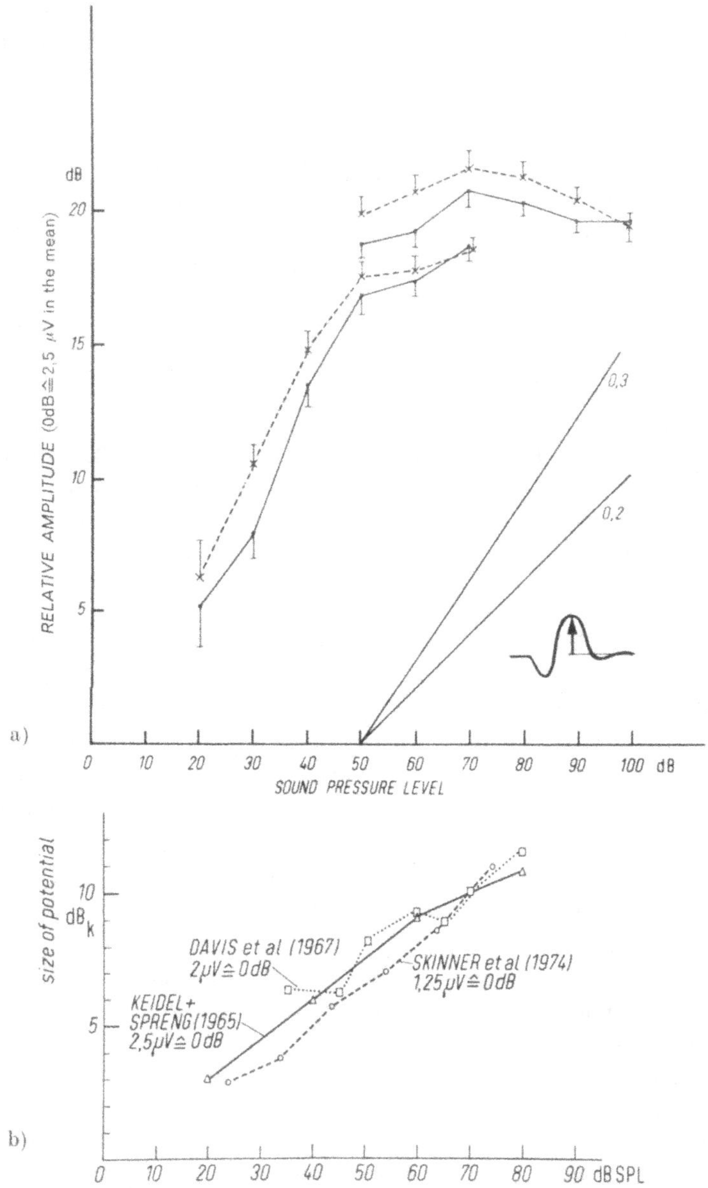

Fig. 37. (a) Intensity function in man, plotted in a log-log scale. The slope for the first 50 dB has an exponent of app. 0.2—0.3 according to STEVENS' power law and then flattens out over 50 dB SPL. (According to BUTLER, KEIDEL, and SPRENG, 1969.) (b) Comparison of most recent data with those of KEIDEL and SPRENG as well as of those of DAVIS and ZERLIN show a fair coincidence. (According to SPRENG, 1975b, 1976)

formation processing). (*E.g.* see SUTTON *et al.*, 1965, 1967). For ERA, certainly three variables in this connection are vigilance, attention, and the state of the subject. They will be discussed later in this chapter.

The break in the intensity function was described in detail by MOORE and ROSE (1969). Based upon their studies, BEAGLEY and KELLOGG (1971) carefully studied the difference of the intensity function for monaural or binaural stimulation. As Fig. 38 shows only in the case of monaural stimulation does the intensity function flatten completely. For binaural stimulation in the high intensity range, it grows still further but with a smaller slope compared to that for small intensities (before the break). Note that this figure is drawn as a semi-log plot. Extensive studies on the problem of intensity functions in general were made by RAPIN, SCHIMMEL, LESTER, TOURK, KRASNEGOR, and POLLAK in 1966. FRANZÉN and OFFENLOCH (1969) confirmed the validity of the log-log plot type of intensity functions discussed above. They clearly obtained exponents, "n", of the power law on the order of 0.5 for the intensity functions of somesthetic evoked responses. This meant, in accordance with the results of the Erlangen-group, a dynamic range about half as broad for tactile stimuli compared to that of auditory stimuli. Correspondingly, the exponents for the power law differ by a factor of two for those two modalities. The broader the intensity and the dynamic range become for a given modality, the less the log-log and semi-log plots differ for mathematical reasons. Therefore, a semi-log plot was claimed to be better fitting for the auditory (DAVIS, 1974) and for the visual (CREUTZFELDT and KUHNT, 1967) modalities. Thus, despite objections concerning the modalities, the useful application of the power law in ERA seems to be confirmed and established. A thorough discussion of the general physiological and even the philosophical implications of those results was written by REENPÄÄ in the "Abhandlungen der Heidelberger Akademie der Wissenschaften" in 1966.

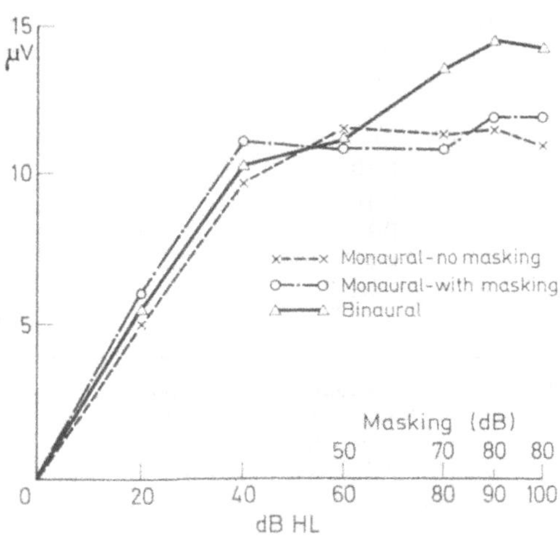

Fig. 38. The "break" in the intensity functions is marked to a complete flat part at high intensities only when monaural stimulation has been administered. For binaural stimuli the function grows even at high intensities but with a smaller steepness. (According to BEAGLEY and KELLOGG, 1971)

4. Interstimulus Interval, Repetition Rates and Their Influence Upon the Size of AERs

During the era of studies in the time domain of the fast early responses of animals in the late fifties, repetition rates of 10 per second were preferably used. Even at that time, however, it was known, that a full recovery time from middle and high intense auditory stimuli would not be smaller than some 5 seconds. For ERA, there was a strong need to shorten the entire measurement procedure of the

Table 1: Exponent n of the power function $R = S^n$. (S a function of repetitionrate.) (a) N_1 versus baseline. (b) N_1 versus P_2 (peak to peak).

	Repetitionrate 1/s	Exponent n of the power function (male)	$\bar{\sigma}$	Correlation coefficient r
a)	1/30	0,28	±0,02	0,9
	1/10	0,23	±0,03	0,8
	1/ 2,5	0,20	±0,02	0,7
	1/ 1	0,12	±0,03	0,4
	2/ 1	0,09	±0,01	0,6
	4/ 1	0,07	±0,03	0,5
	Repetitionrate 1/s	**Exponent n of the power function (female)**	$\bar{\sigma}$	**Correlation coefficient r**
	1/30	0,22	±0,02	0,8
	1/10	0,17	±0,03	0,7
	1/ 2,5	0,14	±0,02	0,7
b)	**Repetitionrate 1/s**	**Exponent n of the power function (male)**	$\bar{\sigma}$	**Correlation coefficient r**
	1/30	0,19	±0,02	0,7
	1/10	0,16	±0,05	0,8
	1/ 2,5	0,12	±0,03	0,6
	1/ 1	0,10	±0,03	0,3
	2/ 1	0,08	±0,03	0,6
	4/ 1	0,06	±0,02	0,4
	Repetitionrate 1/s	**Exponent n of the power function (female)**	$\bar{\sigma}$	**Correlation coefficient r**
	1/30	0,08	±0,02	0,4
	1/10	0,06	±0,05	0,4
	1/ 2,5	0,04	±0,03	0,3

(According to RAU 1968.)

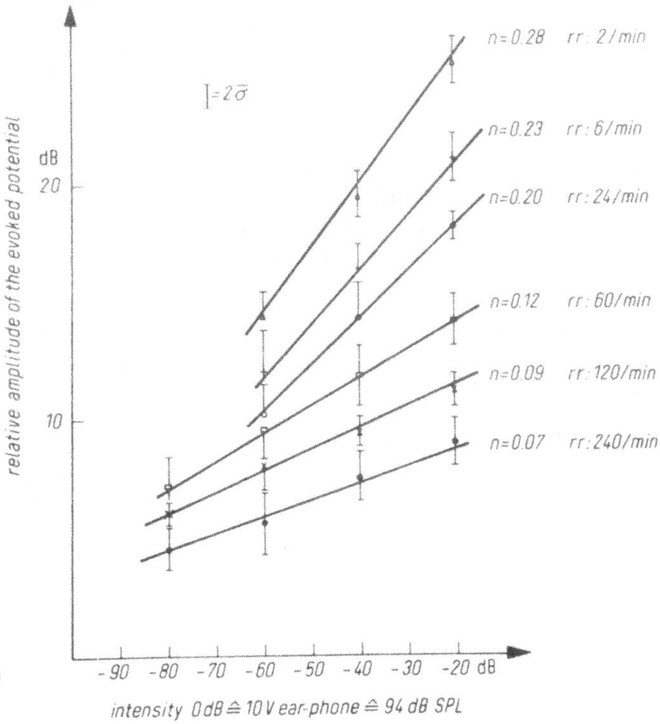

a)

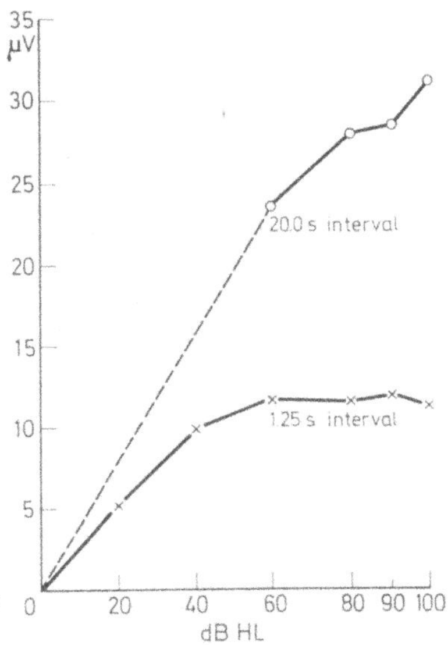

b)

Fig. 39. (a) Intensity-functions in a log-log plot for different repetition rates (as reciprocals of the interstimulus intervals). The exponents are summarized in Table 1. (According to R.-M. Rau, 1968.) (b) Comparable data for the high intensity range above the break in the intensity function (in this case a lone-log plot). (According to Beagley and Kellogg, 1970) delivery of trains of stimuli, mostly of clicks, to a few minutes. Since for meaningful averaging, a number of some 50 stimuli within a train seemed to be optimal (because of the square root law related to size of record versus number of stimuli), a clear tendency to brief, even too brief, interstimulus intervals could be observed. For physiological analysis, interest in experiments with much longer intervals, in other words with very low repetition rates, led to research in this area. One of the first thorough papers concerned with this topic was published by RAU (1968). She was able to demonstrate clearly that the amplitude of P1, N1, P2 was increased when the interstimulus interval was prolonged to some 30 seconds. Figure 39 shows an example of her results based upon 7 subjects, 3 male and 4 female, ranging in age between 20 and 50 years with 405 averaging runs. A run lasted for one, even for one and a half hours. Figure 39a shows a summary of her results. Table 1 of the exponents "n" of the log-log plot completes the reference of her data.

Comparable data for the high intensity range were obtained by BEAGLEY and KELLOGG in 1970. KEIDEL and SPRENG published their data in 1965, preceding

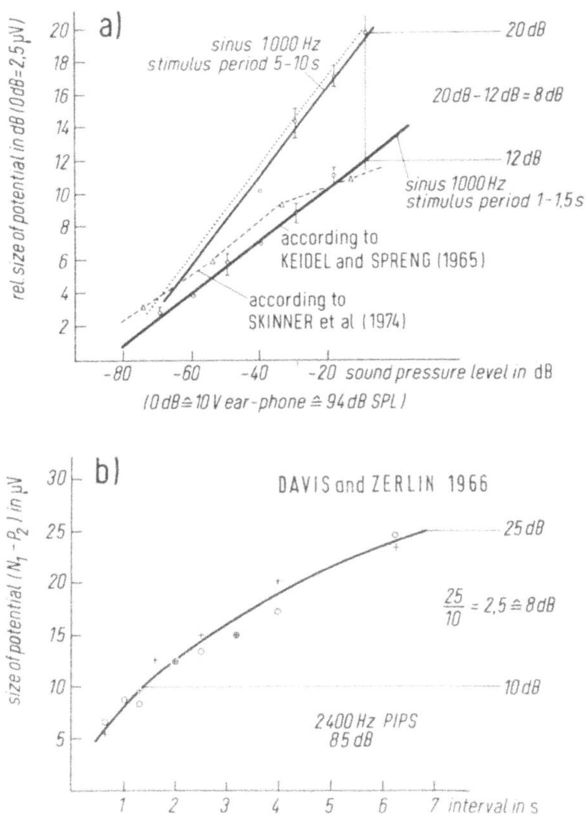

Fig. 39. (c) Comparison of the data of KEIDEL and SPRENG (1965), SKINNER *et al.* (1974) (a) and of DAVIS and ZERLIN (1966) (b), yields full agreement. Note that interval time and repetition rate are connected by an hyperbolic function, since their product is constant. (According to SPRENG, 1975a)

RAU's paper based on their experiments. ABRAHAM and MARSH had already found similar results for the long interstimulus intervals in the *cat* in 1966. Our data were confirmed in 1968 by NELSON and LASSMAN. The St. Louis group (DAVIS, MAST, YOSHIE, and ZERLIN, 1966; ROTHMAN, DAVIS, and HAY, 1970) also came to exactly the same results including the fact, that randomized stimuli result in greater amplitudes of AERs than do periodic ones. A valuable mathematical model of that theory was given by RUCHKIN in 1965. For comparison, finally, in Fig. 39c the data of KEIDEL and SPRENG (1965), DAVIS *et al.* (1966), and of SKINNER *et al.* (1974) are combined. Note that the repetition rate and the interstimulus time as well as the "recovery time" are connected by an hyperbolic function, since the product of interval time and rate is unity.

For practical ERA purposes, one would obtain greatest amplitudes by using long interstimulus intervals. However, to avoid change in the subject's state and tiring of patients some compromise had to be undergone. This led to most suitable repetition rates of one per second to one per two seconds.

5. Latencies of Auditory Evoked Responses

The latencies of the late slow components of the AERs are not only dependent on intensity of the auditory stimuli, but also on the slope of the envelope of tone bursts, if these are used. Another parameter is the location of the electrode (vertex or half-way between vertex and mastoid versus mastoid, see "Mapping"). The vertex reveals shorter latencies, on the order of 6 ms, compared to the more lateral location of the electrode halfway to the mastoid. An example is shown in Fig. 40

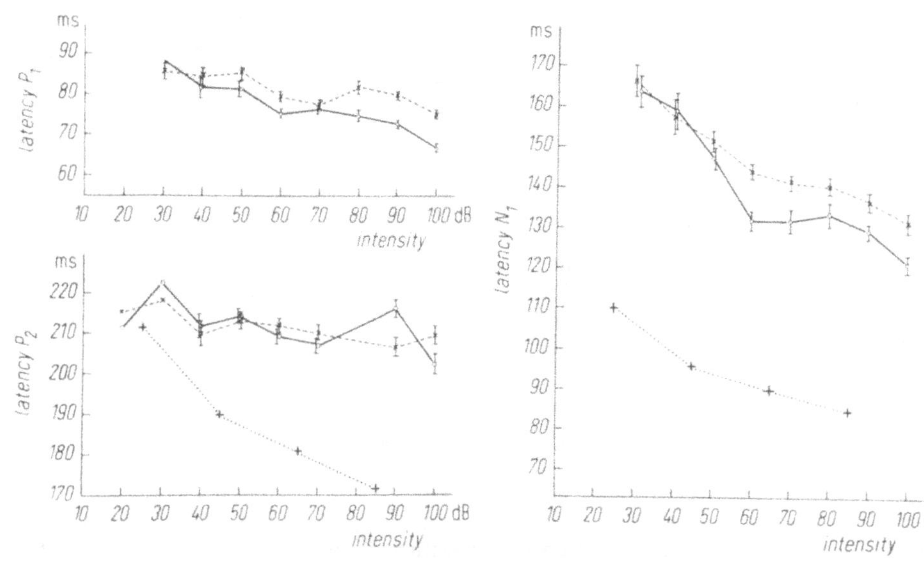

Fig. 40. Latencies of P1, N1, P2 for ipsi-(dashed) and contralateral (solid) stimulation, recorded halfway between vertex-mastoid, (dotted) quick rise time bursts of noise recorded from vertex. (According to SPRENG, 1975a)

for P1, N1 and P2, respectively. The solid lines mean that stimuli were applied contralaterally (terz-filtered 1 kHz tone bursts). Dashed lines resemble responses to ipsilateral stimuli which differ in amplitude only by 1 dB from those elicited contralaterally (BUTLER *et al.*, 1969). Dotted lines mean noise with a steep rise of the envelope and were recorded from the vertex (SPRENG, 1975a).

According to those and similar experiments, the latencies for the main peaks of AERs range as follows: P1 between 60 and 80 ms (P70); N1, between 90 and 140 ms (N120); P2, from 170–225 ms (N210). For N2, the latency is highly dependent upon the filtering used in the amplification channel, because it usually marks the beginning of the perstimulatory DC-response and, hence, can be correctly measured only by means of DC-amplifiers. The dependence of latencies upon the rise (and fall) time of bursts was investigated by ONISHI and DAVIS in 1968. They found that at 45 dB a change of rise time from 3–50 ms yielded an enhancement of latencies on the order of approximately 20 ms.

One important result of measurements on the topic of latencies is that contralateral stimulation is generally accompanied by a clearly shorter latency compared to that of ipsilateral stimuli (BUTLER *et al.*, 1969). RUHM and JANSEN (1969) compared all data available for the latency of N1 when rise time was varied between 10 and 1000 ms with those obtained by ONISHI and DAVIS (1968), and LAMB and GRAHAM (1967). Although the general trend was similar, some numerical differences were still observable. This comparison is shown in Fig. 41.

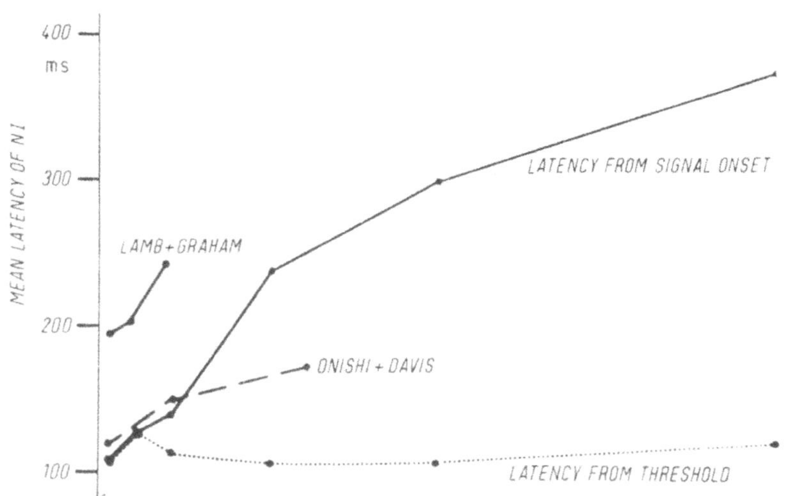

Fig. 41. Dependence of latency for N1 upon the rise time of stimulus onset. Data of their study, measured from threshold, is compared with the same peak measured from signal onset in their and other previous studies at higher intensities. The factor of prolongation of latency when comparing rise times of 1000 ms with those of 10 ms is on the order of 3.5 (360 ms instead of 100 ms). (According to RUHM and JANSEN, 1969)

There is another interesting point in connection with latencies. DAVIS *et al.* in 1972 and 1974, demonstrated that the latencies of N1 and P2 differ slightly for stimuli of four different modalities, especially when auditory and tactile evoked responses are compared. For a given interstimulus interval and sensation level, P2 is more stable in latency, but less stable in amplitude. The stimuli were standardized by adjusting for equal sensation magnitudes and matching to shock at threshold for a muscle twitch. This important result which allows separation of different modalities in the response pattern is shown in Fig. 42.

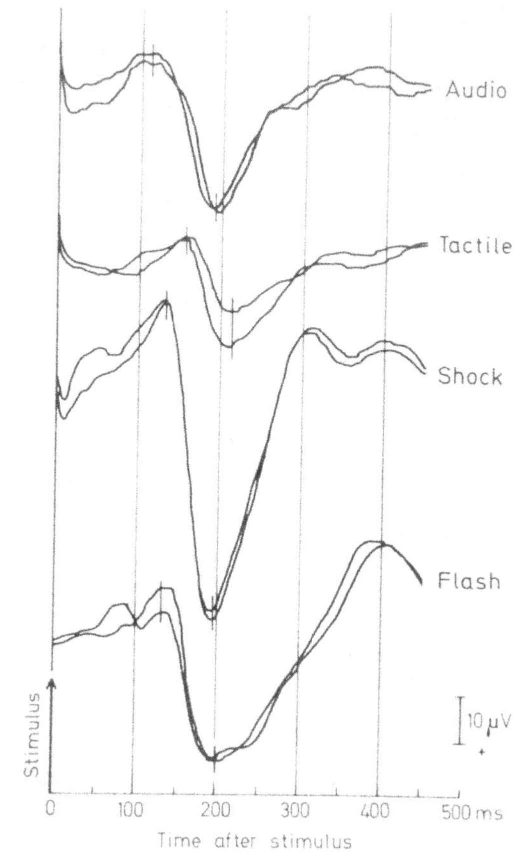

Fig. 42. Superimposed tracings of averaged vertex potentials, reference mastoid, evoked by stimuli ($n = 32$) in four modalities. The latencies differ slightly. The stimuli were adjusted for equal sensation magnitudes. (According to DAVIS *et al*, 1972; DAVIS, 1974)

Sophisticated computer programs for clear separation of even small changes in latencies (and in amplitude) were developed by SPRENG (*e.g.*, 1974a). He also put emphasis upon not only the peak amplitudes but also their latencies for quantitative measurements in clinical ERA. (See especially WIEGAND, BUMM, and SPRENG, 1969.) All related literature is cited in the reference list at the end of this chapter.

That indeed shifts in latencies may be the only significant objective correlate to different states of a subject when significant differences in peak amplitudes fail to occur, could be demonstrated in just one example from many. WANDHÖFER and PLATTIG (1973) and KOBAL *et al.* (1975) reported a decrease of latency of human auditory potentials during *transcendental meditation* (TM). TM is reported as causing evident physiological changes during the state of meditation: decrease of oxygen consumption, of respiratory frequency, of the cardiac output and also a numerical increase of the 8–9 Hz Alpha-waves in the EEG (WALLACE, 1970). BROWN *et al.* (1971) report a few cases of decreased auditory and somesthetic thresholds, and subjective statements by meditators say that sensory perception in general is increased and considerably clearer in TM than before practicing it. To obtain objective correlates to the latter observations KOBAL *et al.* recorded AERs in 15 subjects with experience in TM over a period of 4–47 months. A control group consisted of 15 students (medical and psychology) who had no previous contact with TM. The data were carefully evaluated by a CDC 3300 computer for amplitudes, areas, and latencies with calculation of standard deviation as indicated in Fig. 43a for the measured points of the AERs. Fig. 43b shows the difference

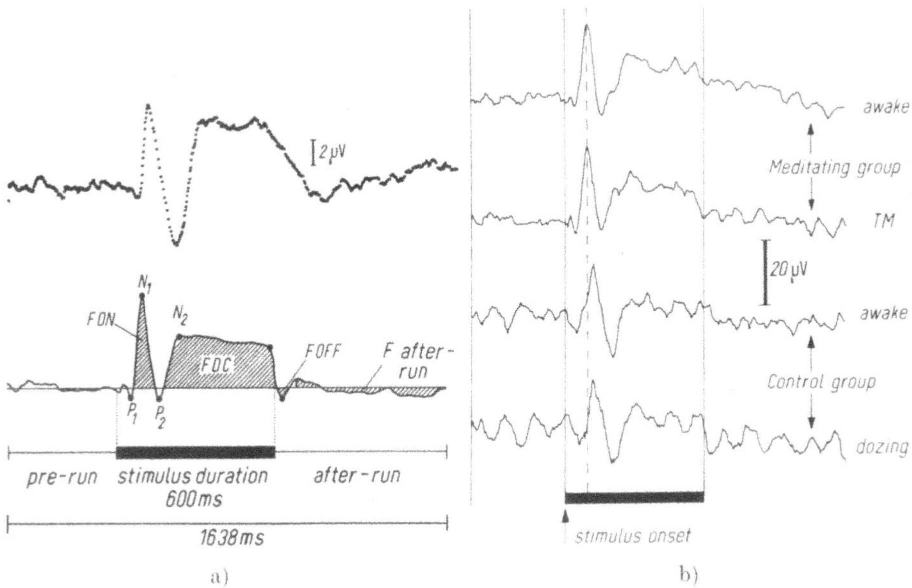

Fig. 43. (a) Computer amplitudes, areas and latencies as indicated in the sketch for transcendental meditating subjects. (b) Only latencies are significantly shorter in the meditating group (for N1) compared to the control group. (According to WANDHÖFER *et al.*, 1976)

between the two groups with and without TM. The results are summarized in Table 2; locations of electrodes are indicated in the left column. Significant differences in amplitudes and in areas could not be found, although a large number of trials was made. The latencies, however, differed significantly in milliseconds, as the Table indicates, (50 dB SPL, 1 kHz, tonebursts, duration 600 ms). In Fig. 43b,

Table 2. Numerical values of latencies computed for meditating (top) and control group (bottom) are clearly shorter for the group with practice in TM. (WANDHÖFER *et al.* 1976)

Meditating group ($n = 15$)

	← awake →						← TM →					
	P_1	s	N_1	s	P_2	s	P_1	s	N_1	s	P_2	s
C_z	*55*	24	*112*	25	*203*	22	*49*	23	*113*	24	*206*	27
P_4	*55*	25	*113*	26	*208*	29	*50*	19	*114*	26	*213*	30
F_4	*55*	22	*113*	24	*203*	26	*49*	23	*117*	28	*212*	26
T_4	*56*	24	*116*	28	*210*	29	*51*	23	*124*	28	*214*	28

Control group ($n = 15$)

	← awake →						← dozing →					
C_z	*70*	13	*126*	9	*214*	15	*71*	16	*131*	11	*222*	16
P_4	*70*	14	*127*	9	*215*	16	*71*	15	*132*	10	*223*	16
F_4	*70*	13	*126*	10	*215*	15	*71*	14	*132*	13	*228*	17
T_4	*72*	13	*128*	10	*222*	18	*72*	15	*134*	12	*234*	16

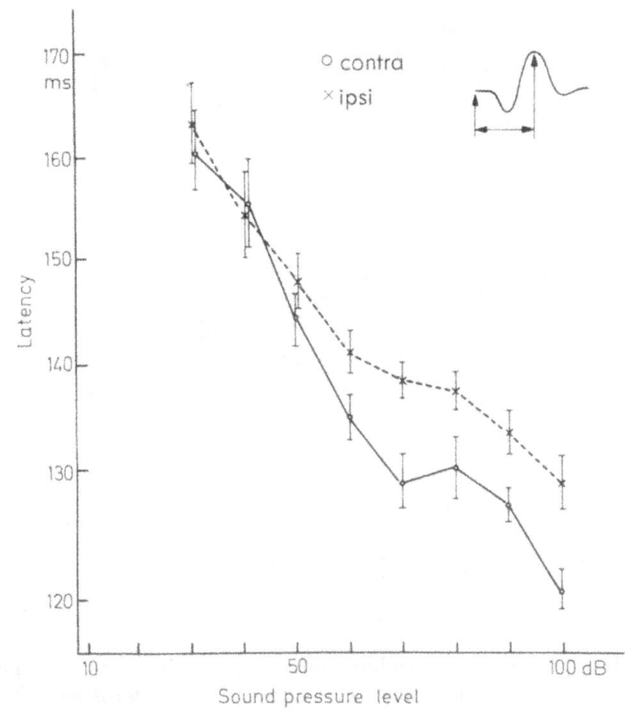

Fig. 44a. Latencies for ipsi- (solid) and contralateral (dotted) stimulation differ clearly, while the difference in amplitude is only small. (According to SPRENG, 1971)

the vertical dotted line is drawn through the peaks N1 of the meditating group, which demonstrates that the respective peaks, N1, of the control group occur about 5–10 ms later from stimulus onset compared to the meditating group. Thus, the results indicate a verification of improved, at least faster sensory perception of the meditating group compared to the control group.

Another example is the observation, that the difference of latencies ipsi-versus contralateral stimulation for N1 can be clearly measured. Both latency curves differ significantly for as much as 10 ms maximally (SPRENG, 1971). This is shown in Fig. 44a. This result is of even more interest for practical ERA, since the difference in amplitudes under those conditions is very small, on the order of 1 dB only (BUTLER *et al.*, 1969) as already mentioned.

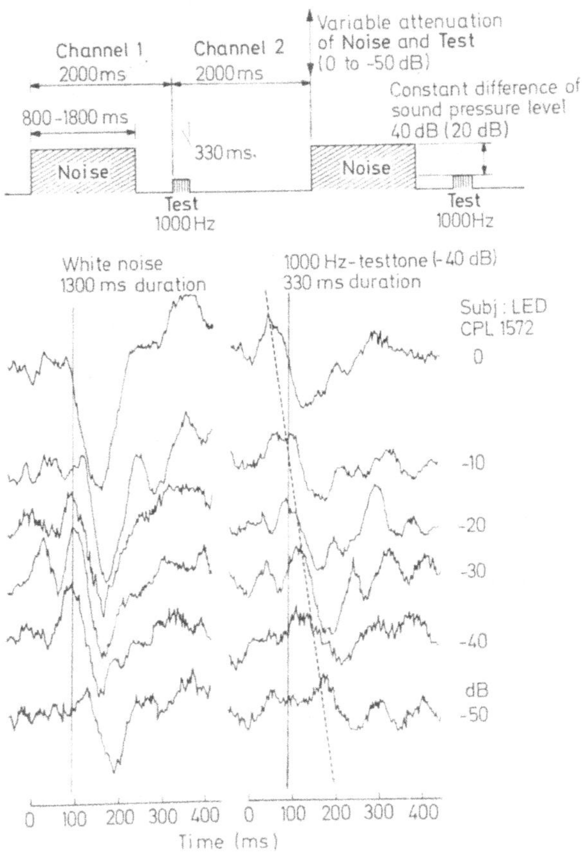

Fig. 44b. Top: Time pattern of a noise burst followed by a tone burst. Bottom: AERs to the noise (left column) and to the tone burst (right column). Parameter is intensity. At high noise intensities the latencies of the tone bursts are shortened (dotted line versus solid line which equals latency of N1 to the tone burst at —40 dB attenuation without preceding noise). In addition the dynamic range of the responses to the tone bursts is enlarged by the preceding noise burst. (According to SPRENG, 1974a)

A last example of possible applications of latency measurements in practical ERA, the abbreviation of latencies to a test tone by a preceding noise burst, might be mentioned (SPRENG, 1974b). His experiments were performed within the context of research contract given by the German Ministry of Internal Affairs with the aim of establishing scales for the annoyance of man by noise (visual and stimuli of other modalities) KEIDEL, SPRENG, PLATTIG, 1972–1976. One result of particular interest was that noise preceding a tone burst shortens the latencies of the response to the bursts of tones considerably and expands the dynamic range of the intensity function. Just one example of an experiment of this type is shown in Fig. 44b (SPRENG, 1974a, b).

6. Frequency Dependence of Amplitudes of AERs

As early as 1965, KEIDEL and SPRENG demonstrated that the amplitudes of AERs to different frequencies differ in that they are largest for 1 kHz, smaller for higher frequencies (BUTLER, 1972b) and also smaller for lower frequencies. The slope of the intensity functions also differs slightly. The difference of the amplitudes for different tonal frequencies, however, is more striking. Reasons for the differences may be: (i) the involvement of more neurons for 1 kHz at a given stimulus intensity, and (ii) a change in the site of cortical origin of the response which might influence the amplitude of a response recorded from a given constant location, for instance the vertex. See also EVANS and DEATHERAGE (1969).

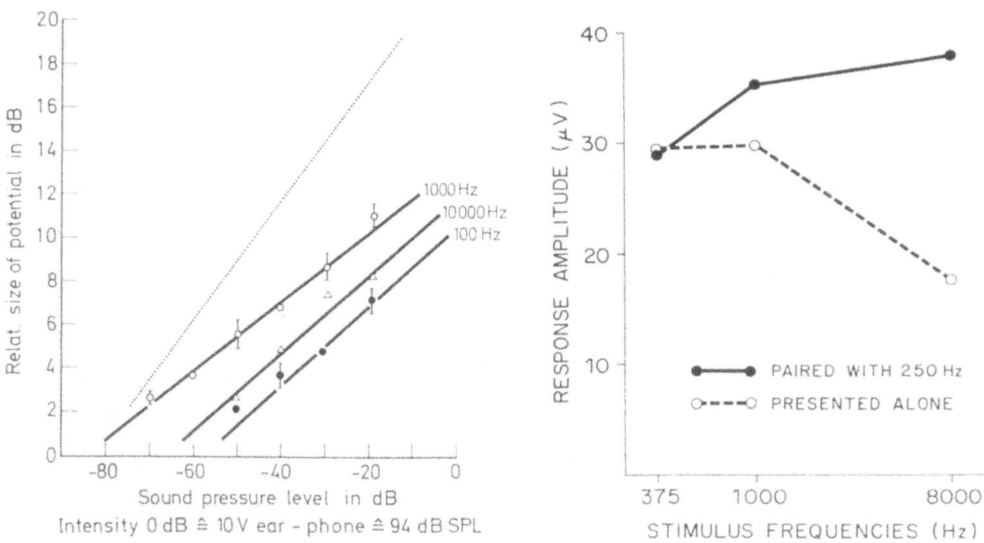

Fig. 45. (a) Fig. 45. (b)

Fig. 45. (a) Frequency dependence of amplitude, N1 of AERs. Those for 1 kHz are greatest for a given intensity (KEIDEL and SPRENG, 1965). (b) Results of BUTLER (1972b) for high frequencies. (c) Comparable results for N1-P2 according to RAPIN, SCHIMMEL, TOURK, KRASNEGOR, and POLLAK (1966)

Similar results, including the low frequency range were gathered by McCandless and Best (1966) and by Davis and Zerlin (1966) and Rapin *et al.* (1966). Examples based on experiments of a) Keidel and Spreng (1965); b) Butler (1972b); and c) Rapin, Schimmel, Tourk, Krasnegor, and Pollak (1966) are reproduced in Fig. 45.

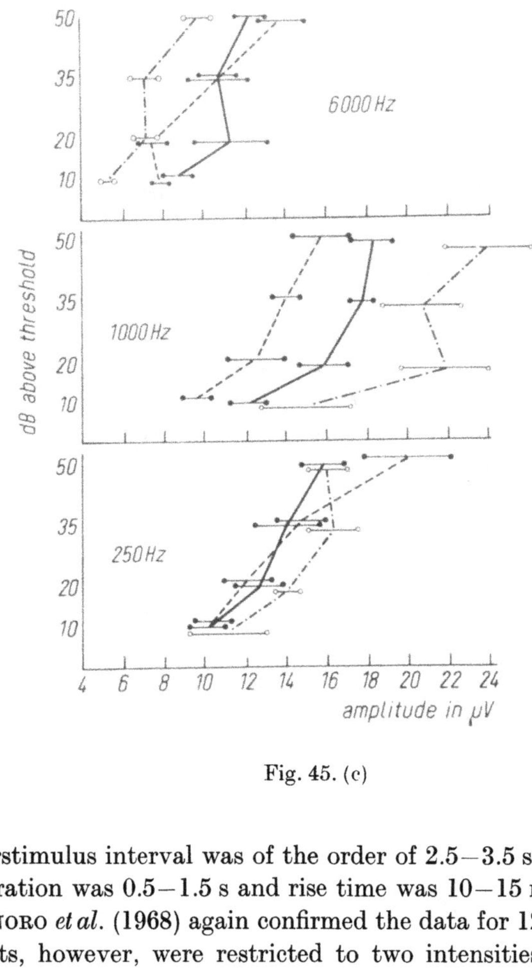

Fig. 45. (c)

The interstimulus interval was of the order of 2.5–3.5 s in their experiments. Stimulus duration was 0.5–1.5 s and rise time was 10–15 ms, to 25 ms, respectively. Antinoro *et al.* (1968) again confirmed the data for 125 Hz to 8 kHz. Their measurements, however, were restricted to two intensities just beneath 60 dB where the frequency dependence is small. They used bursts with durations of 75 ms, intervals of 5 s. Unfortunately, this means some interference of the on- and off-effects. Furthermore, Clynes (eds: Donchin and Lindsley, NASA Washington 1966) could show that *changes* in frequency for a long lasting tone (duration 1 s) lead to an evoked potential. Interestingly enough, this is then the only case, when the stimulus pattern is configurated in such a way that for at least 300 ms, a constant frequency of a sinusoidal tone is delivered, followed by a break to a continuously changing frequency (*e.g.* from 600–860 Hz in 700 ms). In this case, only the break is answered by an evoked potential. It might just be mentioned in this context that the same observation also holds for the stimulus intensity: When a given intensity for 300 ms is obtained followed by a break, where the stimulus intensity rises to a 2.3-fold value in 700 ms, only the break (in intensity in that case) is answered by an AER. CLYNES (1969) labels the phenomenon, the "rest-motion-function" of the CNS. In other words, as mentioned earlier, it is the first derivative to the time in frequency (and in intensity), *i.e.* the *change* in frequency (and intensity) that evokes cortical responses in ERA.

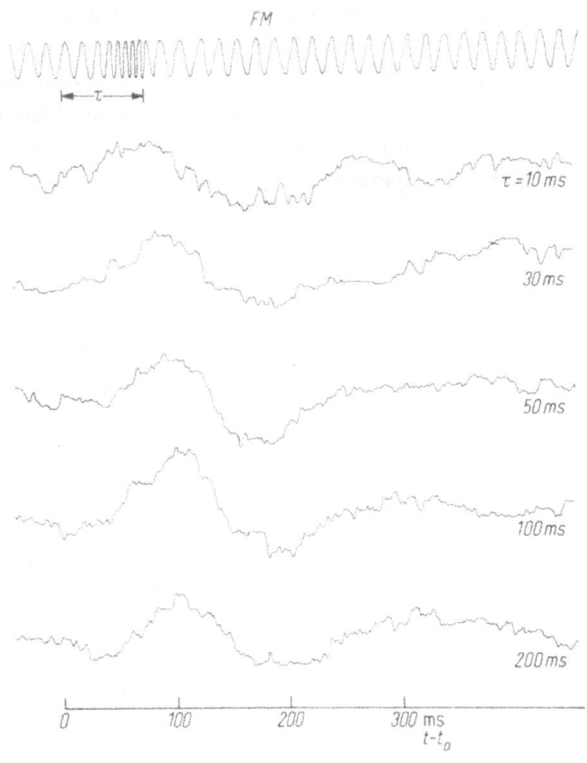

Fig. 46. At an intensity of 60 dB SPL, frequency modulation (300 to 2000 Hz) clearly yields AERs in man. The amplitude of the response has its maximum at durations of FM τ of 50 ms. The latencies for τ ranging between 10 and 200 ms increase slightly with increasing τ. (According to SPRENG, 1974)

In practice, the consequence is that it seems best to use stimulus durations of not less than 300 ms and interstimulus intervals of at least 2 s to obtain the greatest and the clearest responses. For linear and squared frequency modulated stimuli at constant intensities, clear AERs can be obtained. This was demonstrated by SPRENG in 1974. An example of his records is shown in Fig. 46.

7. Off-Responses in ERA

To explore the features of the off-response of the AER more preliminary experiments were performed in only a few laboratories (ONISHI and DAVIS, 1968; KEIDEL and SPRENG, 1963; SPRENG, 1967; GERIN *et al.*, 1968; SPYCHALA *et al.*,

1969; REGAN, 1972). A careful study was presented in 1972 by JOHANNSEN, KEIDEL, and SPRENG. These authors directed their attention to three main features of this off-response, namely, (i) the dependence of its amplitude upon intensity, (ii) the influence of the duration of the preceding tone (or noise) burst, and (iii) the latencies of the off-effect compared to those of the on-response, *i.e.*, the classical AER. A typical example of a series of experiments is shown in Fig. 47.

The authors obtained the following results:

(i) Size of potentials and dependence on stimulus parameters: Slope of intensity function is considerably less than that for the on-responses (increase of size by a factor of 1.5 for 60 dB difference in stimulus intensity). Examples are shown in Fig. 48. When sinusoidal tones are used as stimuli, the size of the off-responses is about 25–45% of that of the on-response measured N_{off}-P_{off}, N1-P2 respectively). For noise as stimuli the same percentage is greater, – on the order of 35–55% (Table 3).

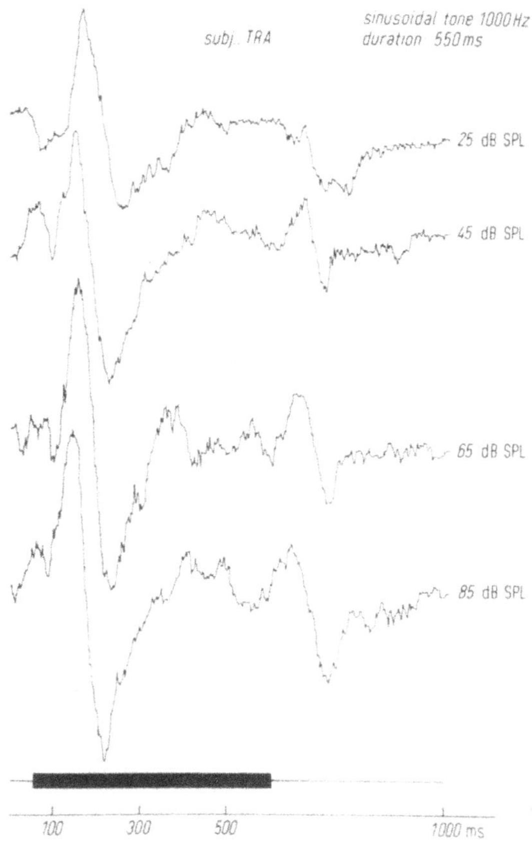

Fig. 47. Off-responses as function of intensity for a tone burst of 550 ms, unfiltered 1 kHz, very short rise and fall time. The effect can be seen at the end of stimulation (black bar). (According to JOHANNSEN, KEIDEL, and SPRENG, 1972)

Table 3a: Latencies in ms measured from end of stimulus to N_{off} 40—70. Mean values out of 18 measurements respectively. Duration of stimuli ranging from 210 ms to 740 ms. Last column overall mean. S: sinusoidal tone 1 kHz, R: noise.

	310 ms		550 ms		740 ms			
(dB)	S	R	S	R	S	R	S	R
15		65,0 ± 12,5		70,2 ± 5		75,0 ± 15		70,1
25	56,7 ± 5		64,5 ± 7,5		70,2 ± 12,5		63,5	
35		58,2 ± 10		67,7 ± 5		62,8 ± 7,5		62,9
45	51,7 ± 7,5		63,7 ± 2,5		62,0 ± 5		58,1	
55		50,0 ± 10		60,2 ± 5		59,5 ± 7,5		56,6
65	43,2 ± 10		58,7 ± 5		49,2 ± 5		50,4	
75		42,7 ± 7,5		49,3 ± 2,5		50,2 ± 10		47,2
85	38,3 ± 5		53,7 ± 2,5		49,2 ± 5		47,1	

Table 3b: Same as (a) but latencies from end of stimulus to P_{off} 120—170.

	310 ms		550 ms		740 ms			
(dB)	S	R	S	R	S	R	S	R
15		161,7 ± 15		123,7 ± 7,5		169,5 ± 10		151,6
25	164,2 ± 10		117,7 ± 10		147,0 ± 10		142,9	
35		177,5 ± 10		125,2 ± 5		159,5 ± 10		154,1
45	183,2 ± 7,5		122,0 ± 7,5		142,7 ± 10		149,3	
55		176,7 ± 7,5		121,2 ± 5		153,7 ± 12,5		150,5
65	145,7 ± 7,5		129,5 ± 5		142,7 ± 10		139,3	
75		171,7 ± 10		118,7 ± 5		139,4 ± 10		143,3
85	159,2 ± 12,5		130,2 ± 5		136,4 ± 7,5		141,9	

(According to JOHANNSEN, KEIDEL and SPRENG 1972.)

(ii) Stimulus duration versus interstimulus interval: Data were obtained for constant interstimulus intervals. Between 300 and 1300 ms duration of stimuli, no dependence of the amplitude of the off-effect on signal duration could be demonstrated.

(iii) The latency of the off-effect decreased with increasing intensity in a manner similar to that of the on-effect. When referred to the point of signal termination, latencies of the off-effect were considerably shorter than those of the on-effect for responses of comparable polarity. For negative components (N_{off}), values varied between 40 and 75 ms, and for positive components (P_{off}) between 100 and 180 ms. See Table 3a and b. There was no detectable $N_{off\,2}$.

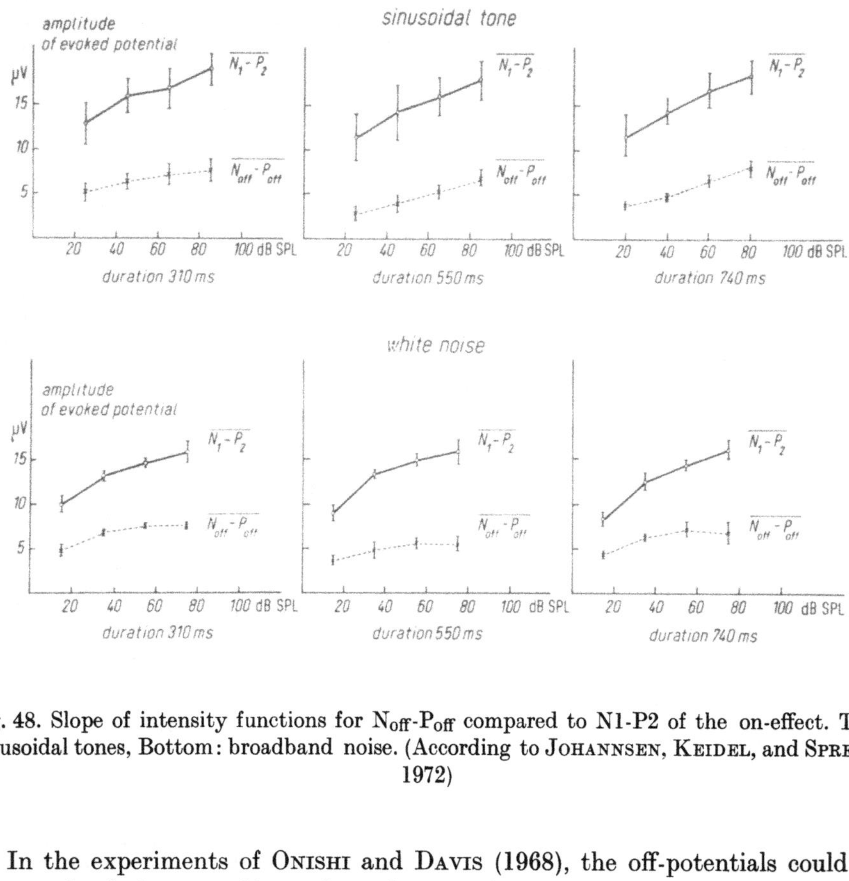

Fig. 48. Slope of intensity functions for N_{off}-P_{off} compared to N1-P2 of the on-effect. Top: Sinusoidal tones, Bottom: broadband noise. (According to JOHANNSEN, KEIDEL, and SPRENG, 1972)

In the experiments of ONISHI and DAVIS (1968), the off-potentials could be measured only in one subject; there the ratio On to Off is 3 : 1 instead of (2–3) : 1 as in JOHANNSEN'S results, which were based upon extensive experiments. However, the difference in latencies N_{off}-P_{off} of 80 ms (ONISHI and DAVIS) agrees fairly well with JOHANNSEN'S 80–120 ms. The latencies, however, for N_{off} (related to end of stimulation) differ for both groups, being 95–105 ms for the Davis group and 40–75 ms for the Erlangen group. The reason is the difference in the fall time of stimuli, ranging from relatively slow to 3 ms for the St. Louis group. It is claimed in the literature that off-effects could be obtained only from preceding stimuli of long duration. SPRENG in 1967, however, showed that even very brief bursts produce an off-effect and, hence, lead to a superimposition of the on and off effects, especially for tone bursts of 50 ms duration. We might suggest that a few discrepancies in the literature be explained, since 50 ms tone bursts are used very frequently in some laboratories (Fig. 49).

Off-effects are highly constant in size and vary intraindividually in latency only slightly.

JÄRVILEHTO and FRUHSTORFER recorded off-responses under some special conditions. A continuous tone (1 kHz, 80 dB above SL) was interrupted for 1 s every 15 seconds. An off-effect was observed which was nearly as large as the normal on-effect under complementary stimulus conditions. The following on-effect looked almost identical to the off at the end of a stimulation but differed in that (i) it had

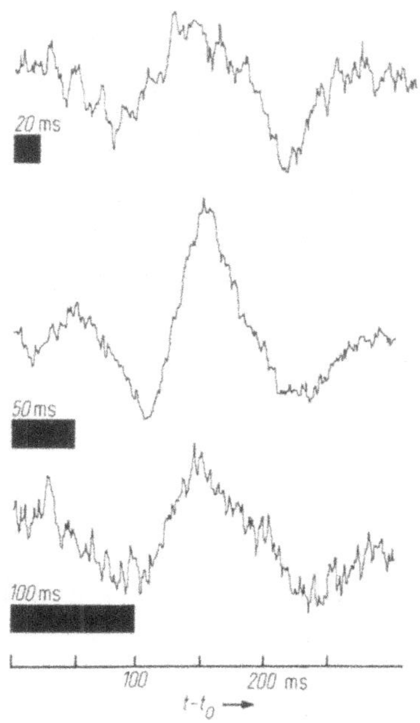

Fig. 49. Superimposition of on and off effect for tone bursts of durations between 20 and 100 ms. By this interaction move parameters for ERA are introduced which complicate the numerical validation of AERs. For instance the increase of amplitude for P1 and N1 relative to P2 is not due to the true intensity dependencies but to the interaction of the on and off effects. [SPRENG, 1975, in KEIDEL (editor), 1975]

an N2 which lacked the normal off-response and (ii) the size of the response related to the normal on-effect (here the response to the begining of pause, bottom trace in Fig. 49, was above 50% in contrast to the usual 35%. As mentioned several times already, the excitability of a membrane, the beginning of depolarization is originated mostly by the differential ratio of the stimulus intensity with a rectifying system. Even to PFLÜGER it was well known, that switching a DC-flow through an ischiadicus nerve on *or* off effects the critical depolarization for both, the on and the off condition and excitation or depolarization. Under these aspects, the polarity sequence of the complex off-response is the same as that of the on-response. No inversion occurs for well known reasons and the same certainly is true for the DC-component, the perstimulatory DC-potential found by DAVID, FINKENZELLER, KALLERT, and KEIDEL, 1969b, c, d, f, 1971; KEIDEL, 1971b, d. It would actually be a miracle, if all other components would behave just opposite to the DC-shift, which is one of the oldest discoveries in neurophysiology. We will go back to this point a bit later in this chapter under the key word "DC-potential".

8. Stimulus Duration and AERs

For the "objective" validation of impulses imbedded in complex sounds, *e.g.* in industry noise, air craft noise and trafic noise, it is important to measure AERs by dependency on brief tonal stimuli. It is known as a first approximation that the auditory system for brief stimuli functions as a mean square root rectifying system

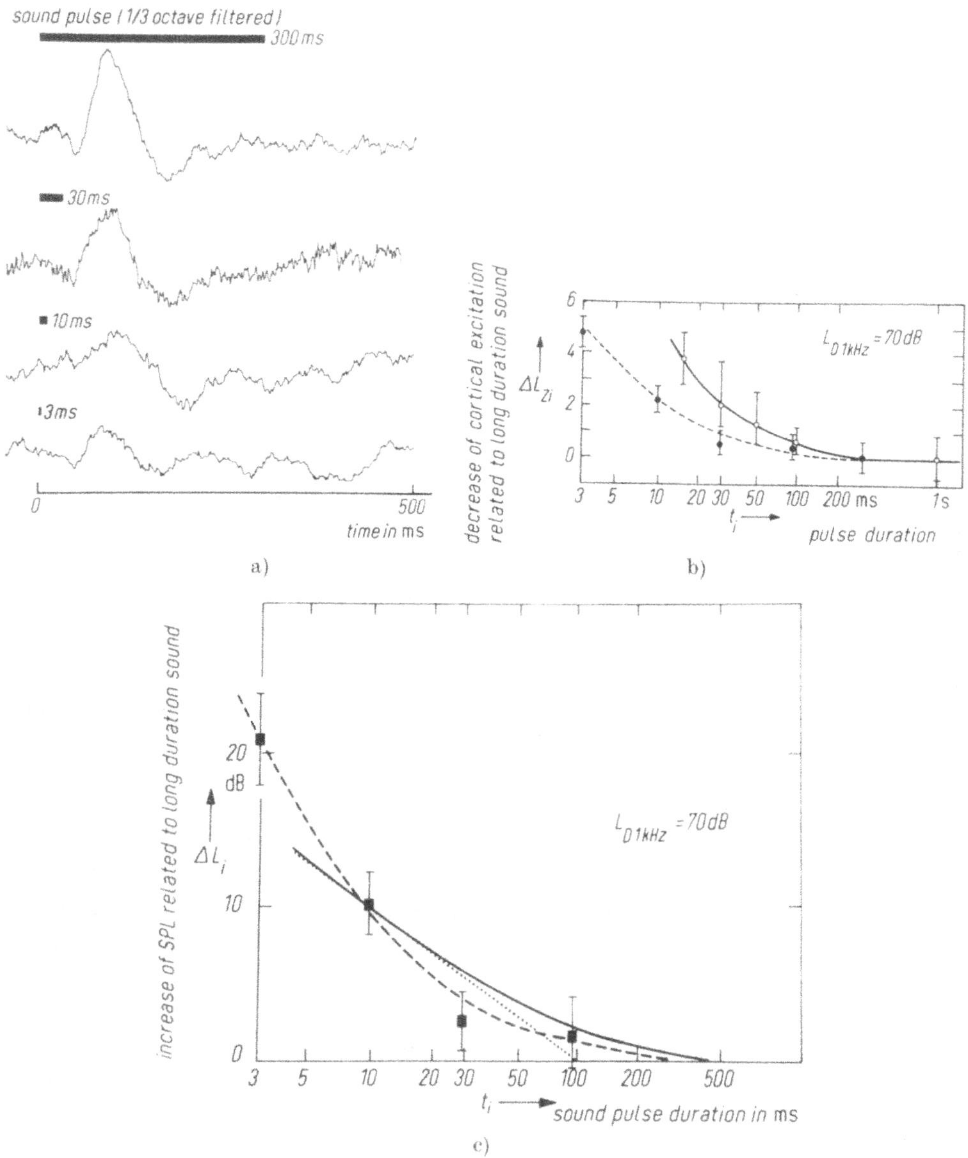

Fig. 50a—c. Amplitude of N1-P2 as function of very brief durations of tone bursts (tone bursts 1 kHz, 70 dB, interstimulus interval 3.5 s). The amplitude, below 200 ms, decreases for a given intensity when the duration time is shortened. (Spreng, 1967, 1975)

with two filter sets arranged sequentially (*e.g.* EVANS and WILSON, 1973). Therefore it was to be expected that AERs would reflect this behavior of the ear and the central part of the auditory system. Psychophysically, this has long been known from v. BÉKÉSY's experiments resulting in the proof for validity up to 180 ms of NERNST's law. Based upon later experiments performed by O. F. RANKE (1955, personal communication) *et al.*, *e.g.* COMMICHAU (1956), KEIDEL (1956) showed that actually the objective loudness increases with stimulus duration in the time domain up to 200 ms according to the equation $E = i \cdot t^{[f(t)]}$ where $f(t) = 1/t$. Thus, if t becomes infinite, the exponent goes to 0 and $t^{[(ft)]}$ becomes 1. Accordingly then, for durations above 200 ms – neglecting the influence of adaptation for the first approximation – the loudness corresponds only to intensity and duration can be neglected. For very short times the factor f equals 2, then 1, then 1/2 (NERNST) and finally 0, as described.

Objective correlates to that experiment can be demonstrated by the ERA too. One series of data is shown in Fig. 50.

As those data show clearly, the size of potentials decreases with duration of stimuli. Here terzfiltered bursts are used so that the influence of off-effects upon the combined potential is smaller than 20% and therefore practically can be excluded. The results are plotted quantitatively in the graph of Fig. 50b (solid line). In Fig. 50c a comparison between psychophysical data (solid) (ZWICKER, 1966) and neurophysiological results (dashed line) is demonstrated.

9. Critical Bandwith in ERA

In his doctoral thesis SPRENG, 1967 by means of AERs performed studies to find the "objective" correlate to STEVENS' and FELDTKELLER's and ZWICKER's subjective "critical bandwith" in man, the latter data being obtained psychophysically. Just one example for such a comparison is shown in Fig. 51.

For the full development of the critical bandwith an integration time of at least 100 ms for the stimuli must be allowed, in agreement with experiments performed by SCHOLL (1961). This explains the lack of results in this topic when shorter stimuli were used (*e.g.* SKINNER and ANTINOVO, 1970). Subjectively, the critical bandwith is 3–4 times greater immediately after stimulus onset compared to the situation after 100–200 ms.

10. Adaptation, Habituation, Vigilance, Attention, Sleep, State of Subjects (Patients) in ERA

In addition to HECHT and WALD, it was particularly RANKE who tried to analyse the basic principles involved in adaptation (1959, KEIDEL post mortem). His differential equation describes and allows to predict precisely the time course of adaptation, during the initial overshoot to an upward step in stimulus intensity, that is, to the "dynamic" and "static" intensity functions before and after the adaptative process has come to an equilibrium. (The "static" curve is therefore flatter compared to the "dynamic" curve which is related to the overshoots). Consequently, his equation smoothly fits the silent period to a downward step of the stimulus intensity. Besides those basic results, he found that during adaptive processes the intensity threshold may adapt in the described sense (*e.g.* increase), but the DL for intensity is improved. This is one criterion for separating it from fatigue. Habituation is a more prolonged process, lasting hours or even days. Acclimatization is a process lasting for weeks, months and even years. On the other hand the peripheral nerve's accommodation is the shortest process in this connection. For ERA, only adaptation and habituation play a role.

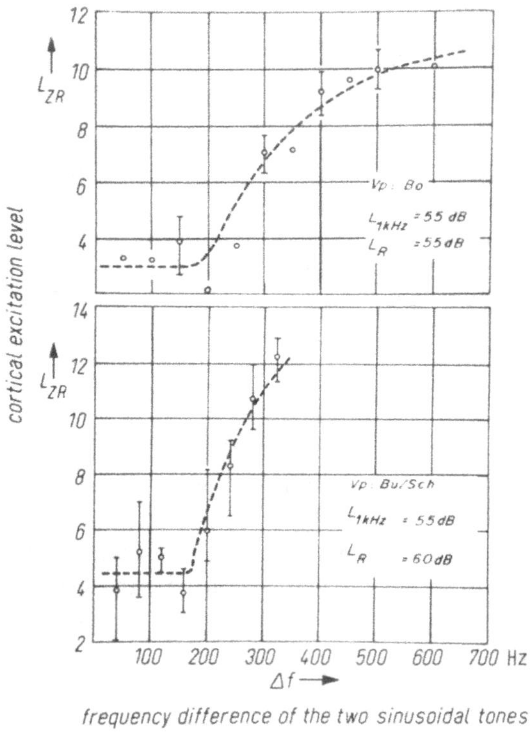

Fig. 51. Comparison of psychophysical data and amplitudes of AERs with mean deviation (solid lines with open circles) 1 for increasing $\triangle f$. The break in the curves at the end of the critical bandwidth is in good agreement with the psychophysical data. (According to SPRENG, 1967, 1975)

An example well illustrates the situation: When averaging is performed in such a way that many trains are averaged within a train of stimuli consisting of 50 repetitive clicks and within each train each first, second, third or n^{th} click is added, the adaptation (or habituation) time curve can be obtained. In this example visual stimuli were used in children and the decrease in amplitude of VERs can clearly be seen (Fig. 52).

Similar records were obtained for the ERA. GOLD and WILPIZESKI in 1966 described the adaptive time curve of evoked auditory potentials in the cat. They confirmed results obtained by KEIDEL, KEIDEL, KIANG, and FRISHKOPF in 1957, which were reported elsewhere in detail (KEIDEL, 1963). BUTLER contributed interesting details to the problem of habituation in 1968 and 1973. STEIN published a model for understanding habituation processes in 1966. STANGE and SODA (1968) could show that the time curve of adaptation was significantly changed in cases of

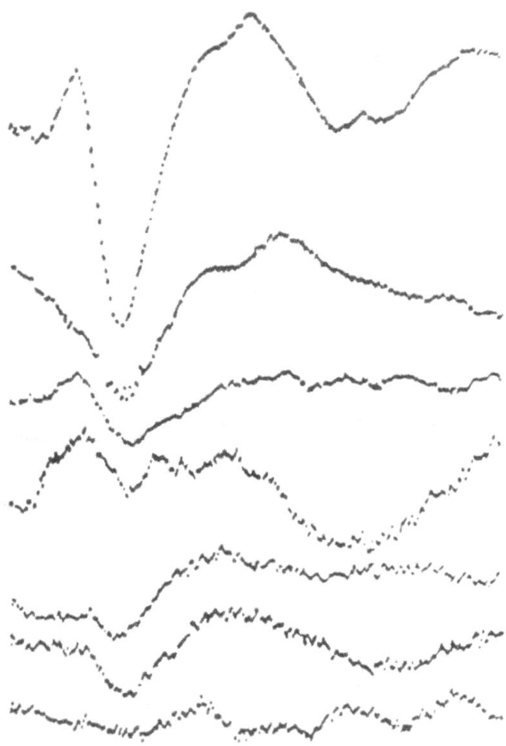

Fig. 52. Adaptation time curve in averaged trains of stimuli when each first, second, third etc. stimulus is added. The top trace belongs to the first, the bottom trace to the last stimulus within the train. Visual stimuli, children. (According to v. LOEWENICH, 1972)

severe hearing loss, after toxic hearing impairment, and in cases of presbyacousis when compared to normal subjects. Their work was based on early research which he performed in 1964 to study the influence of streptomycin and canamycin upon the time curve of adaptation in the auditory nerve. One example is shown in Fig. 53a.

In Fig. 53b a recent study plotting the results as dynamic and static intensity functions is shown for comparison. STANGE's group delivered a great number of important contributions to adaptation measurements in the ENT-hospital.

The differences in the temporal aspects of the time curve of adaptation along the central part of the auditory channel of the cat were described by JAFFE, BOUSTIER, and HAGAMEN in 1969. In the rat, similar trials were performed by HALL

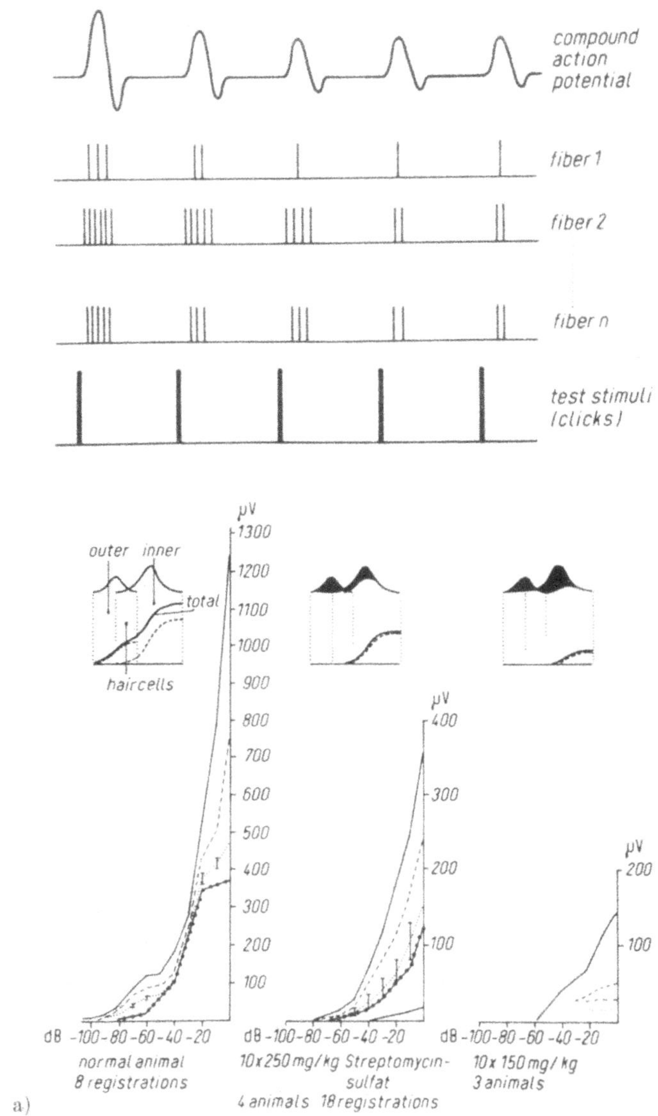

Fig. 53. (a) Basic principle of adaptation in single fibers and in the compound action from KEIDEL (edit. 1975). Bottom: dynamic (steepest, solid) and different static intensity functions on normal cats (left) and on cats treated with Streptomycin (right). Black: poisoned populations. (According to STANGE, SPRENG, and U. O. KEIDEL, 1964.) In general see also HAWKINS. (b) Intensity functions in man's ERA in nonadapted (dashed) and adapted (solid) state. Contralateral stimulation left, ipsilateral right. (According to STANGE, 1971, and STANGE and SODA, 1968)

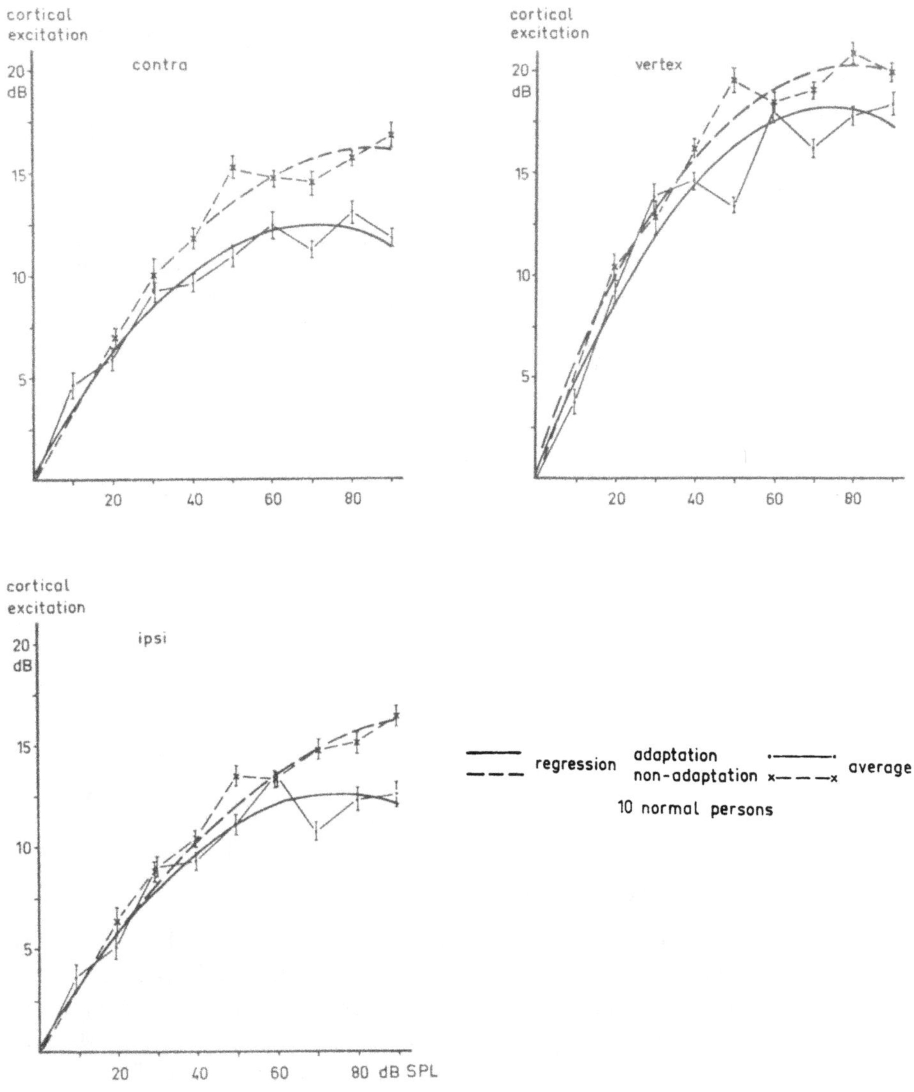

Fig. 53. (b)

in 1968. This author clearly demonstrated that the adaptive process grows, the higher the level for recording within the CNS is choosen. An instructive example is shown in Fig. 54.

This subject with regard to the cat was also discussed by WEINBERGER, GOODMAN, and KITZES in 1969. Auditory habituation at the primary cortex as a function of stimulus rate in the cat was explored by COOK, ELLINWOOD, and WILSON in 1968 and KIMMEL and GOLDSTEIN (1968) dealt with the retention of habituation of the galvani skin reaction (GSR) to visual and auditory stimulation in 1967. Habituative responses to 4 successive blocks of trials, each consisting of 32 stimuli could also be seen in a paper published by ZERLIN and DAVIS (1967).

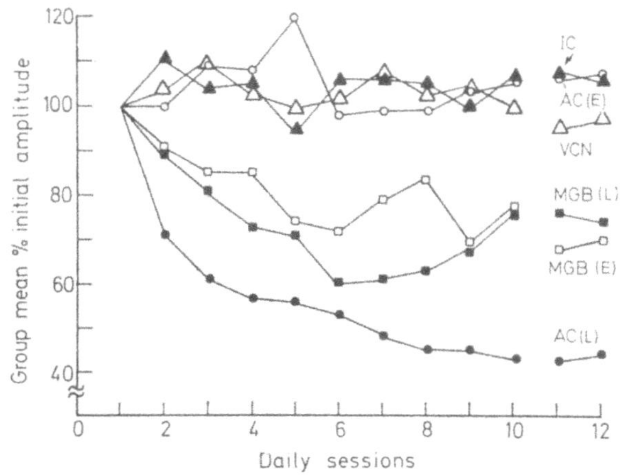

Fig. 54. Time curve of adaptation in the rat. (VCN, ventral cochlear nucleus, IC inferior colliculus, AC (E) early responses cortex, AL (L) late responses cortex, MGB medical geniculate body.) (According to HALL, 1968)

11. Vigilance, Attention, State of Subject

It certainly should be expected that the human waking brain, for the general neurophysiological reasons discussed above (see p. 173ff.), would drastically vary the size of the cortical evoked potential and hence the ERA when changing attention to the different sensory channels or *vigilance* in general (including state of *alertness*). Again, numerous papers have been written about this topic. I would first like to mention an excellent monograph by NÄÄTANEN in 1967 (published by the Finnish Academy of Sciences) which contains a thorough reference list for that time and many interesting papers. The first authors, however, who put emphasis on that point were ZERLIN and DAVIS in 1967 in a paper in which they described the great interindividual (see also DAVIS, 1964) and especially intraindividual variability of the vertex-potential. Figure 55a is an example of a series of successive responses to one and the same stimulus.

Extensive studies on the topic were performed by FRUHSTORFER *et al.* (1969, 1970) and FRUHSTORFER (1971).

Another paper published by H. BAUMANN, R. BAUMANN, GURK, and WOLTER (1968) dealt with electrophysiological studies of central nervous performance during monotony on the cat. Even at that time, they found that the early components were static for alert state, sleep, tired state and deep sleep. They claimed that those responses, in contrast to all other auditory and visual stimuli, showed no significantly different changes in latencies and size when comparing periodic and stochastic stimuli. MAST and WATSON (1968) compared AERs (i) while subjects were reading and (ii) while they were attempting to count auditory signals. They

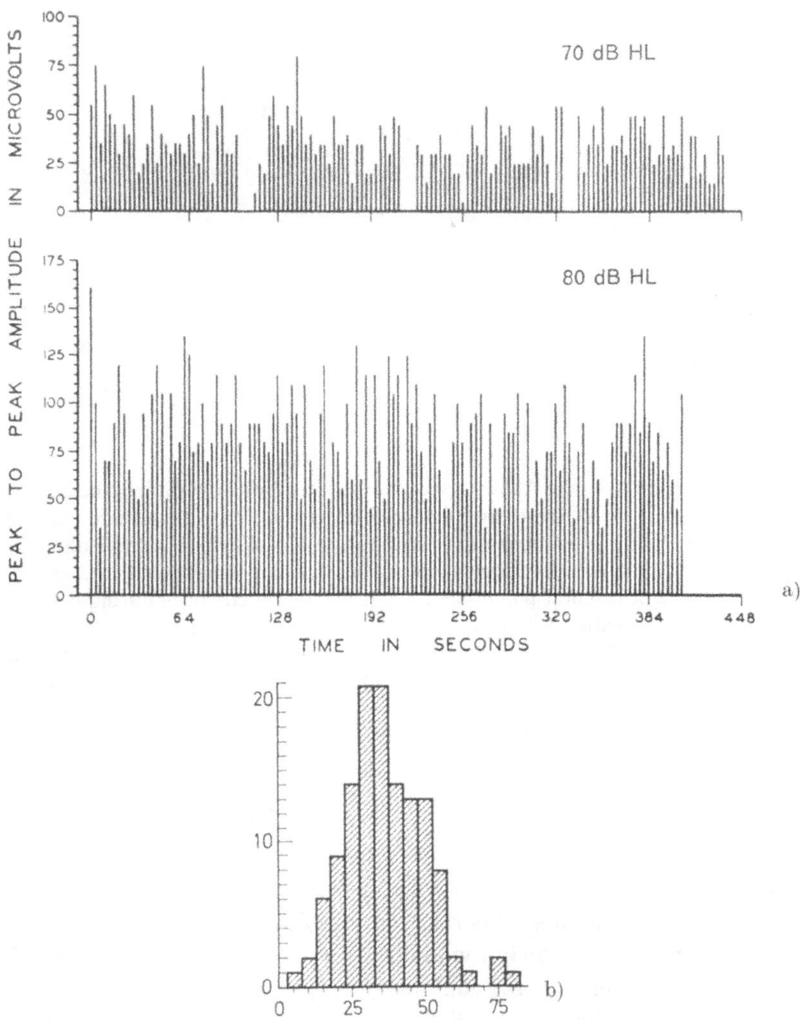

Fig. 55. (a) Individual responses evoked by 1200 H_z tone at 70 and 80 dB hearing level, measured N1-P2 by hand in serial order about 3.2 s, N = 128 in each series. (b) Related combined amplitude histogram. (According to ZERLIN and DAVIS, 1967)

found that the amplitudes of evoked responses to low-detectability auditory stimuli were found to be approximately doubled when the subjects were required to count the number of stimuli as compared to amplitudes recorded when they were reading. The duration of the response was also markedly increased. A beautiful example of this type was reported as early as 1964 by H. DAVIS: He found that the averaged slow response evoked by auditory stimuli (vertex) could usually be enhanced by requiring the listener to make a rather difficult auditory discrimination. In contrast, an easy routine reaction was not effective. Figure 56 shows an example.

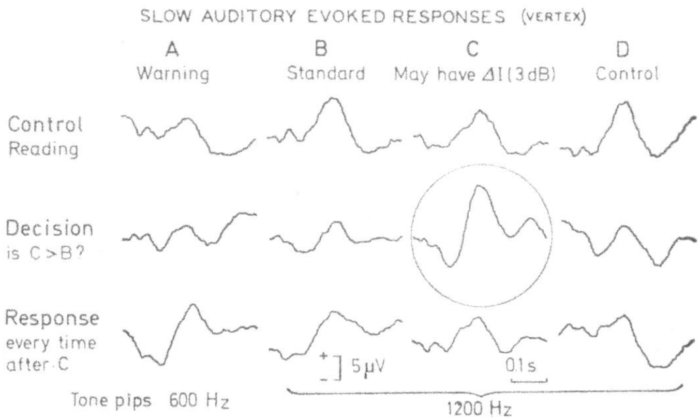

Fig. 56. (a)

Fig. 56. (a) Comparison of size of AERs (vertex) for reading (top) and difficult decision making task (middle). Circling shows the clear enhancement by the difficult decision. (According to DAVIS, 1964.) Note that in these records vertex positive goes *up*. (b) A, sample diagram of the stimulus program with a random sequence of signal and non-signal acoustic clicks and skin stimuli. B-F, records of cerebral potentials evoked by the signal clicks during decision tasks involving either the acoustic (Ac) or the somatosensory (Ss) stimuli. The intervals between successive clicks in the different runs vary from 1007 to 307 ms. The runs were recorded in the order given. The differentiation between signal and non-signal clicks is difficult as their intensity difference is only 5 dB. The "decision" potentials are identified by a star. (According to DEBECKER and DESMEDT, 1971)

ROTH, KOPELL, and BERTOZZI in 1970 studied the average evoked response to prerecorded sentences and monosyllables in ten subjects. Attention and non-attention conditions (listening, ignoring) produced differences in the wave forms. They were idiosyncratic to the individual subject, usually appearing in the N1-P2 region. Sense and nonsense words could not be distinguished. Similar results were found by YOUNG and SPRENG in 1973 (unpublished data). BURIAN on the other hand found clear differences in the CNV behavior to spoken words when they made sense to the subject (1969). KLINGER in 1973 studied variations of amplitudes of AERs dependent upon the subjective information content of stimuli and upon the state of fatigue. He found a significant decrease of the amplitude of AER by fatigue. The amplitude, furthermore, was significantly smaller for contingent stimulus triggering compared to uncorrelated triggering. BÜCHELE and SEILER (1973) could prove that the perstimulatory DC-component of AERs depended markedly upon the alertness, vigilance, attention and concentration for a given task. In these case of fatigue, they found significant *greater* DC-shifts of the perstimulatory type. In sleep, this DC-response was decreased for barbiturate-elicited sleep more rapidly than for natural sleep. The classical P1-N1-P2 responses were influenced significantly less.

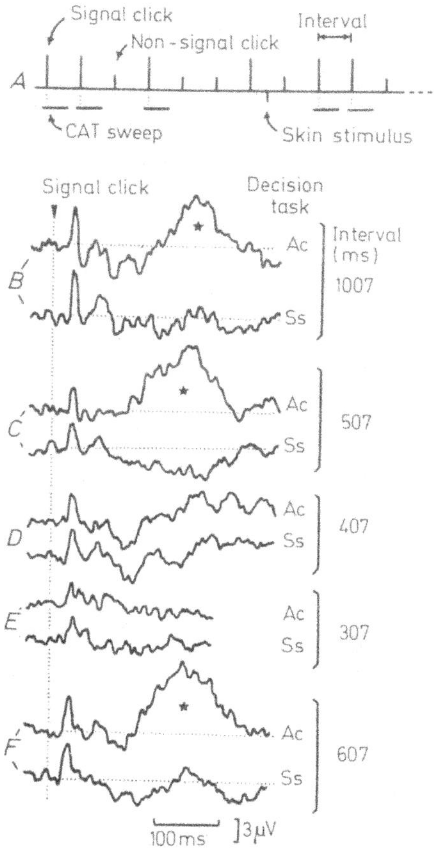

Fig. 56. (b)

12. Sleep, Anesthesia, Sedation

Changes in the auditory input in wakefulness and during the synchronized and desynchronized stages of sleep in the cat were explored in 1964 by BAUST, BERLUCCHI, and MORUZZI. These experiments were extended by WINTERS, MORI, SPOORER, and KADO in 1967. The latter authors studied the correlation of reticular and cochlear multiple unit activity with auditory evoked responses during wakefulness and sleep. They came to the following conclusions: "their studies involved a correlation of the cochlear nucleus and midbrain reticular formation multiple unit activity with EEG and auditory evoked responses during wakefulness and sleep. The basal level of reticular unit activity decreased from wakefulness to slow wave sleep but was highest during rhombencephalic sleep. On the other hand, the basal level of the cochlear nucleus unit activity did not change during wakefulness or sleep. The amplitude of the evoked responses in the cochlear nucleus, reticular formation and assoziation cortex all were largest during slow wave sleep, smaller during wakefulness, and smallest during rhombencephalic sleep. The findings suggest that the input stimulus is modulated at a level peripheral to the cochlear nucleus presumably by reticular influence on this system."

Subject 21. (Night 1) 21 year old woman, vertex-occiput

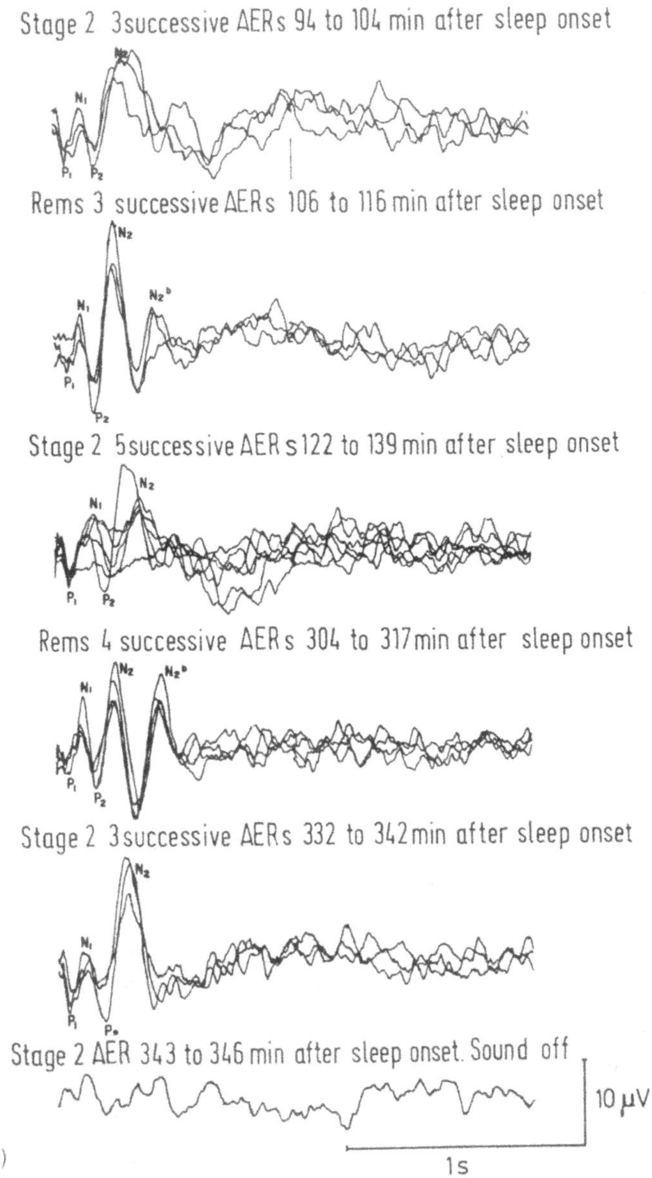

Fig. 57. (a)

Fig. 57. (a) Alternations of stage 2 and REM sleep in adult. Amplitude of N2 remains large during REM in this subject. (b) Transition from REM to stage 2 sleep in a child. Wave N2 shows less variability and larger amplitude during REM sleep. (According to ORNITZ *et al.*, 1967)

The variability of the auditory averaged evoked response during sleep and dreaming in children and *adults* was studied by ORNITZ, RITOO, CARR, PANMAN, and WALTER in 1967, 1969. An example of their results is shown in Fig. 57a for an adult woman and in Fig. 57b for a child of three and a half years.

Subject 6. 3 years 5 month old girl vertex-occiput

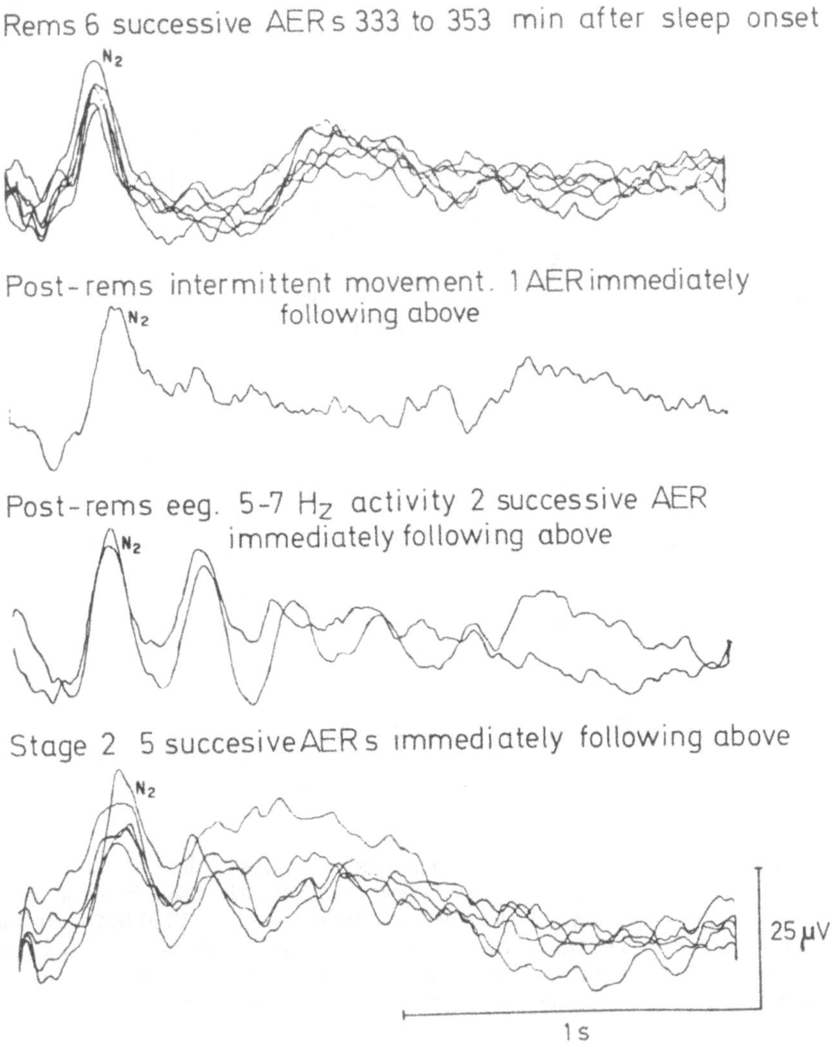

Fig. 57. (b)

These authors find a marked interindividual variability in the amplitude of N2 during REM sleep. Latencies were shorter during REM sleep than during stage 2. The latency of N2 in the children was significantly shorter than in adults during stage 2, but there was no corresponding difference during REM sleep. Younger children showed just one single positive deflection before N2 instead of before

P1-N1-P2 as in adults. Within REM sleep in all subjects over 19 months, the AER was smaller during the bursts of ocular activity than during ocular quiescence. The authors related that result to the concept of a phasic inhibition distinct from tonic inhibitory effects and associated with the phasic excitation manifested by ocular activity during REM sleep.

OSTERHAMMEL, DAVIS, WIER, and HIRSH (1973) presented a paper in which the typical patterns of AERs during the different stages of sleep were shown (Fig. 58).

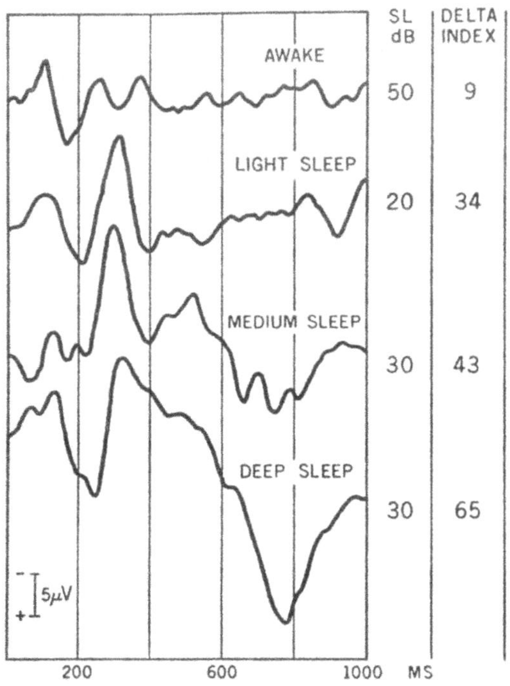

Fig. 58. AERs of an adult subject for awake and different stages of sleep as indicated. The N90-P170 complex appears in the upper tracing (awake). P200-N320 is seen in the second. In the third, a clear N320 appears with little or no P200. Deep sleep shows P200-N320 with N320 prolonged to a very prominent late positive wave. There is also a suggestion of a late positive swing at 600 ms in the third tracing. The delta index during each collection is shown in the second volume at the right. (According to OSTERHAMMEL, DAVIS, WIER, and HIRSH, 1973)

PFURTSCHELLER (1970) discussed the changes in the AERs (and in the EEG) during extracranial polarization as used for electrically induced sleep.

Finally, BURNS, BORBÉLY, and HALL in 1967 presented a fine three-dimensional record of the sliding averages of click-evoked potentials recorded at the vertex with scalp electrodes from a sleeping human subject. Clicks were presented continuously every 3 seconds (Fig. 59).

Investigations of AERs of mentally retarded children were performed by Taguchi, Goodman, and Brummitt (1970) and in adults with mental retardation by Nodar and Graham (1967). The differences in comparison to normal subjects were small. In mongoloid children, the amplitudes were considerably larger than usual.

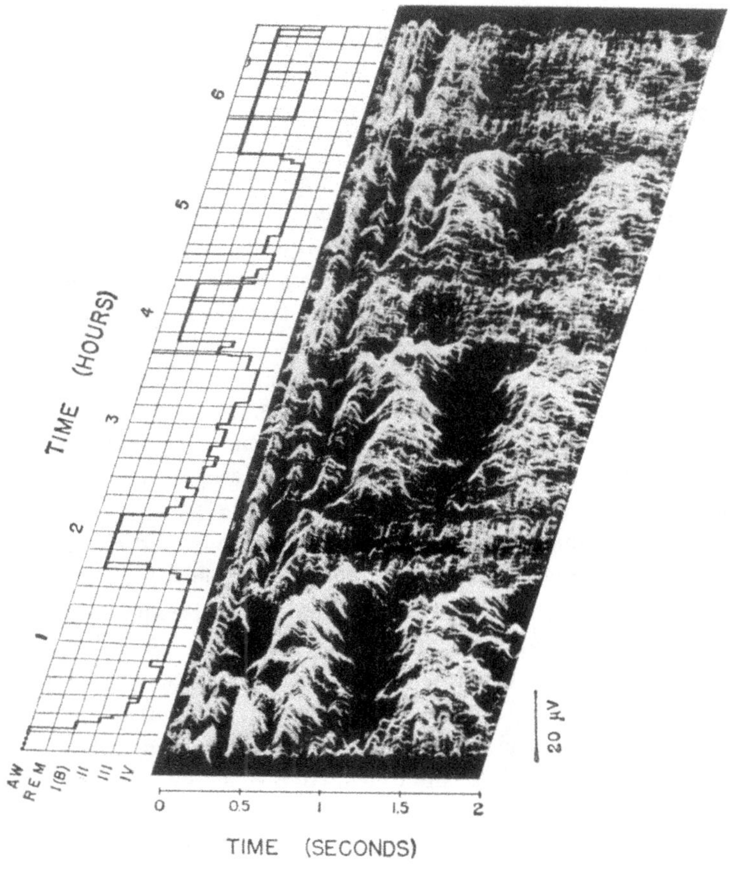

Fig. 59. Sliding averages of AER in man (vertex) from a sleeping subject. RR 1 per 3 seconds. State of sleep indicated on left. (According to Burns, Borbély, and Hall, 1967)

Effects of verbal association on averaged auditory evoked responses were first described by Burian (1969) with specially considering given to how the size and the temporal pattern of the negative contingent variation would be influenced by speech. More recently, Lenhardt (1973) found significantly different averaged audioelectroencephalic responses to verbal association similar to those results in the visual system which were described by Begleiter, Gross, and Kissin (1967). That intramodal selective attention would influence the size of NCV and the power spectra of EEG was described by Donchin and Cohen in detail (1967).

13. Intermodal Interaction

That intermodal interaction may occur in man when recording AERs was published as early as 1962 at the Leyden International Congress by SPRENG and KEIDEL. Since then quite a few papers have been written dealing with that problem, although knowledge about the precise underlying neurophysiological mechanisms which cause the intermodal interaction is still lacking.

Intermodal interactions between somatic and visual auditory responses in the thalamus of the cat based upon microelectrode studies were described by HOTTA and KAMEDA (1963). HOTTA and TERASHIMA (1965) also reported about audiovisual interaction and its correlation with cortical stimulation in the lateral thalamus. These authors found good agreement of their data with ALBE-FESSARD'S and BUSER'S experimental evidence for multisensory convergence at the cellular level in the postmedial thalamic region (centrum medianum and adjacent structures) from visual and auditory stimulation with a predominance of convergence of somatic afferent origin. They proposed that peripheral sensory systems project to the cerebral cortex through the medial thalamus. There is experimental evidence (PURPURA *et al.*, 1962, 1963) for the existence of intrathalamic connections between these two parts of the thalamus. Hence, their data might at least partially explain the phenomenon of multisensory intermodal interaction in AERs. Interaction of sound and light in the related evoked potentials was reported by CIGÁNEK (1966), ALLISON (1962); crossmodality interaction of light plus tones by GUTH (1967). By far the most thorough study on this topic, however, was again published by the Davis group at St. Louis. (DAVIS, 1971; HAY and DAVIS, 1971; DAVIS, OSTERHAMMEL, WIER, and GJERDINGEN, 1972; ROTHMAN, DAVIS, and HAY, 1970.) Their main result has already been described in this chapter (see Fig. 42). It might be emphasized here that the most prominent differences in size and latency is that of N2 when comparing responses to stimuli of different modalities. This might be even more striking if DC-records would be available in the future. According to DAVIS and his coworkers the reduced amplitude of the second response of a pair, expressed as percentage of its corresponding reference response, measures the interaction. This depression occurred intramodally to pairs of responses (interval 0.5 s) but was significantly less with crossmodal than with intramodal pairs. For crossmodal depression of the second response, the amplitude was 64% of the reference response, while for intramodal pairs the, second response was 39%. Clear cross-modality interactions were also found by ROTHMAN *et al.* (1970) for shock and auditory stimuli, with the same depression in amplitude. Finally, the paper of DEBECKER and DESMEDT (1966) should also be mentioned in this connection, although it has already been discussed in this chapter. The interaction between visual and auditory evoked DC-potentials in man was discussed and published at a meeting in 1969 by DAVID, FINKENZELLER, KALLERT, and KEIDEL. Their results will be described in the context of the perstimulatory DC-response.

14. Relation to Psychophysics

It was especially SUTTON who gave out a very informative survey entitled "The specification of psychological variables in an average evoked potential experiment" as a series of papers dealing with the problems on this topic. Here, in a neurophysiological chapter, it is certainly not the place to go into details. Thus, only topics or titles will be cited: Information delivery and the sensory evoked potential (SUTTON, TUETING, ZUBIN, and JOHN, 1967); relationship between pre-stimulus negative shifts and post-stimulus components of the averaged evoked potential (TUETING and SUTTON, 1972); sensory, conceptual and emotional components of the evoked response to sound stimuli in man (SUTTON, BRAREN, ZUBIN, and JOHN, 1965); the sensitivity of the evoked potential to psychological variables (SUTTON, 1970a); correspondence between psychological and physiological thresholds (SUTTON, 1970b); quantitative evoked potential correlates of the probability of events (TUETING, SUTTON, and ZUBIN, 1971); information delivery and the sensory evoked potential (SUTTON, TUETING, ZUBIN, and JOHN, 1967); evoked-potential correlates of stimulus uncertainty (SUTTON, BRAREN, ZUBIN, and JOHN, 1965); recent eddies in brain currents (SUTTON, 1968). There are other interesting papers in this field such as by DEBECKER, DESMEDT, and MANIL (corrélations psychologiques des potentials évoqués cérébraux, 1965). BOSTOCK and JARVIS (1970) reported about the relationship between simple auditory reaction time and form of the AER. The amplitude and latency of a wave of around 250 ms (N2) were found to relate very strongly to the speed of reaction time. HALL and MARK published a paper "Fear and the modification of acoustically evoked potentials during conditioning" in 1967. There still exist, however, marked differences in the interpretation of the data in this field. DONCHIN and SUTTON (1970) in a paper entitled: "the psychological significance" of evoked responses refer to a paper by CLARK, BUTLER, and ROSNER (1969) and conclude with the statement: "In summary, CLARK *et al.* failed to present convincing evidence of a dissociation between sensation and evoked responses." In brief, if one considers the high degree of complexity of the human awake brain, there is just not enough data at present to close the existing gap between psychology and neurophysiology. As one example of good agreement between psychophysical and neurophysiological data SPRENG (1975) may be cited (Fig. 60).

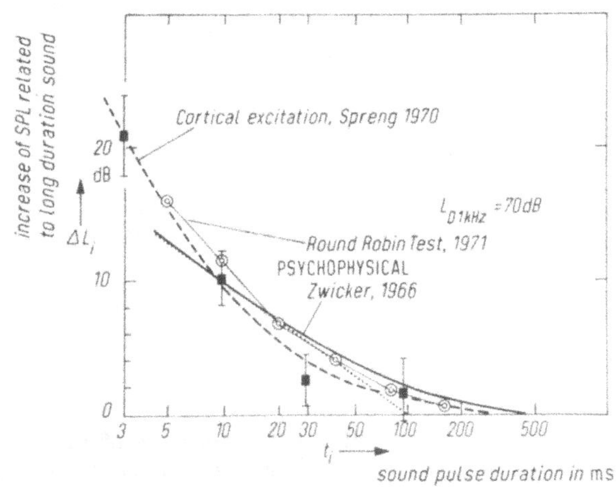

Fig. 60. Round Robin test, psychophysical data of ZWICKER and neurophysiological data obtained by means of ERA are plotted as size of SPL versus duration of a tone burst. (According to SPRENG, 1975)

15. Newborns, Children, Sedation

Studies of newborns, children and the effects of sedation covered in the chapter by DAVIS; hence they need not be discussed here. Just one additional survey article may be mentioned, entitled "Electroencephalographical Audiometry of the New-Born" by KEIDEL, INNITZER, NEUHÄUSER, and PLATTIG (1973), presented at Montreux in 1972. All clinical papers in ERA, which are numerous, are listed as references either in Professor DAVIS' chapter or at the end of that chapter. An excellent review about sedation was given by DAVIS at the Vienna symposium of the IERA Study Group in 1971, published in 1972 (Sedation of Young Children for Electric Response Audiometry – The ERA-Newsletters).

C. Perstimulatory DC-Response (Potential Shift - PSS)

In the first part of this chapter, the cat's perstimulatory DC-potential shift was described. The slow potential changes after N2 or even beginning with N2 and lasts only as long as the tonal or noise stimulus. We have already mentioned that

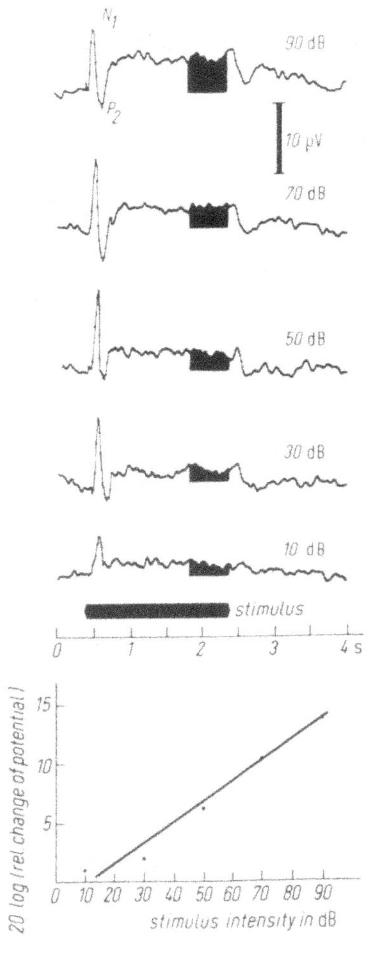

Fig. 61a. Dependence of the perstimulatory DC-response upon intensity. The black rectangular area is computed and plotted versus intensity in the bottom figure. (According to DAVID, FINKENZELLER, KALLERT, and KEIDEL, 1969—1971)

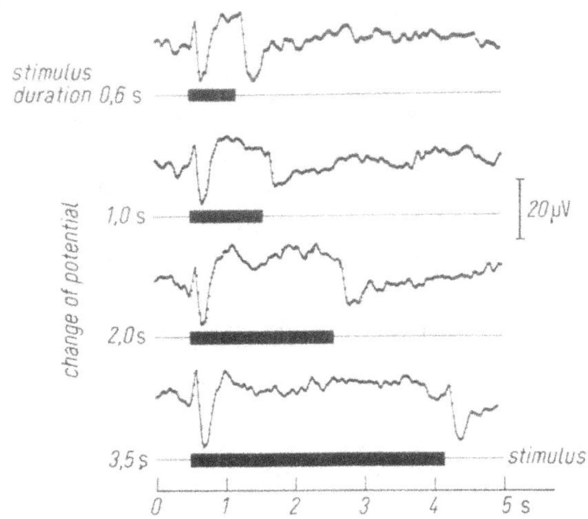

Fig. 61 b. Dependence of the perstimulatory DC-component upon duration of stimuli. (According to DAVID, FINKENZELLER, KALLERT, and KEIDEL, 1969—1971)

to avoid interaction between the on- and off-effect, 300 ms duration is recommanded for the auditory stimulus. In this series of experiments, however, performed by the Erlangen group (KEIDEL, 1971 b, 1972 a, 1974 a; DAVID, FINKENZELLER, KALLERT, KEIDEL, 1969 b, 1969 c, 1969 d, 1969 f, 1971), longer stimuli approximately 2 s, were used to study the perstimulatory DC-potential. In Fig. 61, the dependence of those potentials upon the stimulus intensity is shown. They may stay constant for seconds. This series corresponds to parallel experiments performed in the cat (see Fig. 17). At the end of each average, a clear off-effect can be seen.

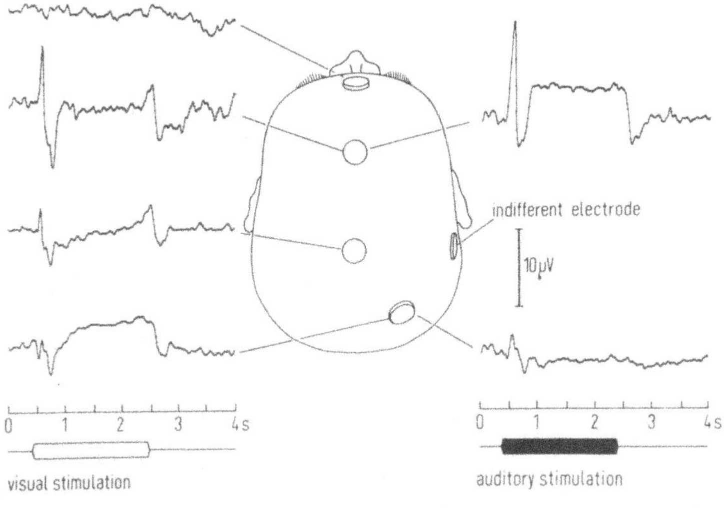

Fig. 62. Mapping experiments for the perstimulatory DC-component show clearly that the response is greatest at occiput electrode location for visual stimulation and above vertex for auditory stimuli. This is in good agreement with KOEHLER'S *et al.* classical experiments. (According to DAVID, FINKENZELLER, KALLERT, and KEIDEL, 1971)

Similarly in Fig. 61b it is demonstrated, that the duration of the response increases with the length of auditory stimuli.

Figure 62 shows mapping experiments of the DC-response. Visual stimuli produce the greatest perstimulatory DC-changes at the occiput, while the auditory DC-response is clearly greatest at the vertex. A simple relation between the classical AER's size and the amplitude of the DC-component does not exist, neither for the on-effect nor for the off-response, as can be seen in the figure.

Similarly, as already described for AERs, the cross-modal interaction in the DC-component also causes depression of the size of potential when any other modality is stimulated. This is demonstrated in Fig. 63a and b. In each case, the

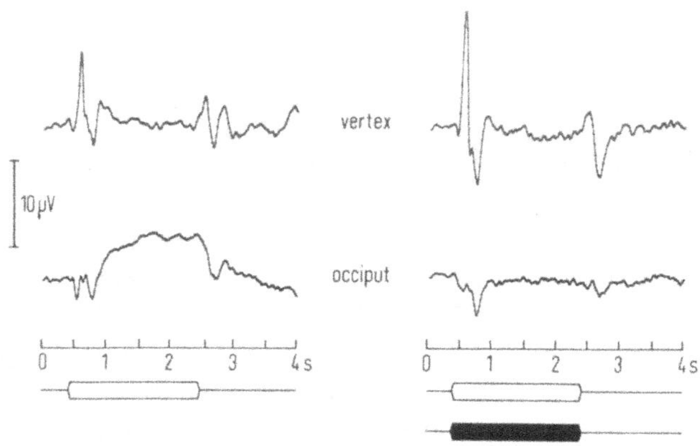

Fig. 63. (a) visual stimulation — visual and auditory stimulation

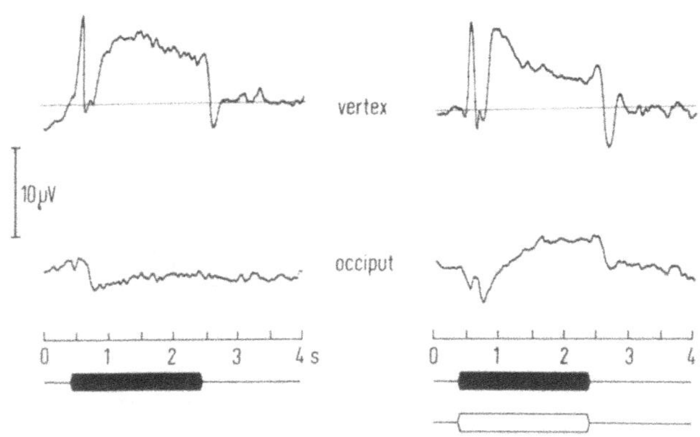

Fig. 63. (b) auditory stimulation — auditory and visual stimulation

Fig. 63. (a) Cross-modal interaction of visual (left) and auditory (right) stimulation. Some sort of depression of the original response occurs, in the record shown, at the occiput electrode. (b) Same as (a), but interaction of auditory (left) and visual stimulation (right). Again depression of the DC component (at vertex). The temporal pattern of depression here is mirror-imaged to the DC-component arising at occiput, when the visual stimulus is added. (According to David, Finkenzeller, Kallert, and Keidel, 1971) additional crossmodal stimulation is added. The result of that procedure is shown in the right column. (According to DAVID, FINKENZELLER, KALLERT, and KEIDEL, 1971.)

The temporal pattern, in contrast to that of NCV, is, furthermore, analogous to an increasing or decreasing type of stimulus. It especially decreases from a marked N2 when the shape of the auditory stimulus is linearly or exponentially decreasing during its duration of some seconds.

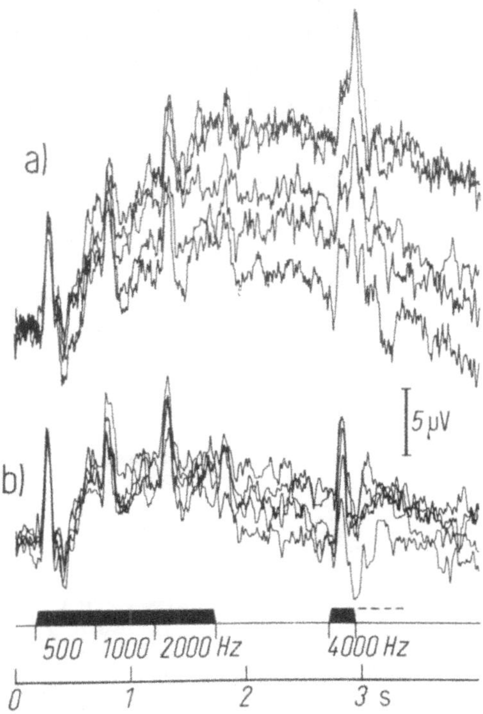

Fig. 64. (a) NCV plus perstimulatory DC-shift (PSS). The subject had the task to pay attention to the following imperative stimulus. (b) The 4 kHz stimulus was neglected. Thus, the perstimulatory DC-shift without the NCV can clearly be seen. (According to FINKENZELLER and KEIDEL, 1975a, b)

Finally, to separate the perstimulatory DC-component from WALTER's NCV in Fig. 64, each of 5 averages are compared. In case a), the subject draws its attention to a consecutive imperative stimulus (2.5 s after stimulus onset), top; in case b), the subject gives no notice to the second stimulus (bottom). In case a), the second tone was expected; in case b), it wasn't. Thus, case b) represents the perstimulatory DC-component alone. Case a) is a composition of the perstimulatory DC-shift and the negative contingent variation. (FINKENZELLER and KEIDEL, 1975a, b.) Also, the difference between the two negative DC-components, the expectancy wave and the perstimulatory wave, could be clearly separated by the same authors. Details about the late DC-component may be read in the original papers.

D. Objective v. Békésy Audiometry by Means of ERA

Finkenzeller (1969 to 1975) made an attempt to obtain all data necessary for objective v. Békésy audiometry in the following way: Using tone bursts of 250 ms duration he varied the interstimulus interval from 8 s to zero (Fig. 65). Thus, all components if ERA could be obtained including the PSS (perstimulatory DC-shift). Then, by an enlarged time scale, one could study the change of N1 and P2 under this variation in detail. The experiments revealed the fact that N1 consists of two components N1a and N1b. Only N1a is present in the 2nd to the nth response as can be seen in the right column of Fig. 65. Moreover P2 fades completely with the sequence of stimuli within a train of bursts. Finally, the PSS is built with stimulus repetition, up to a level of negativity which stays at approximately at the level of N1 (second last traces to bottom in the right column of Fig. 65).

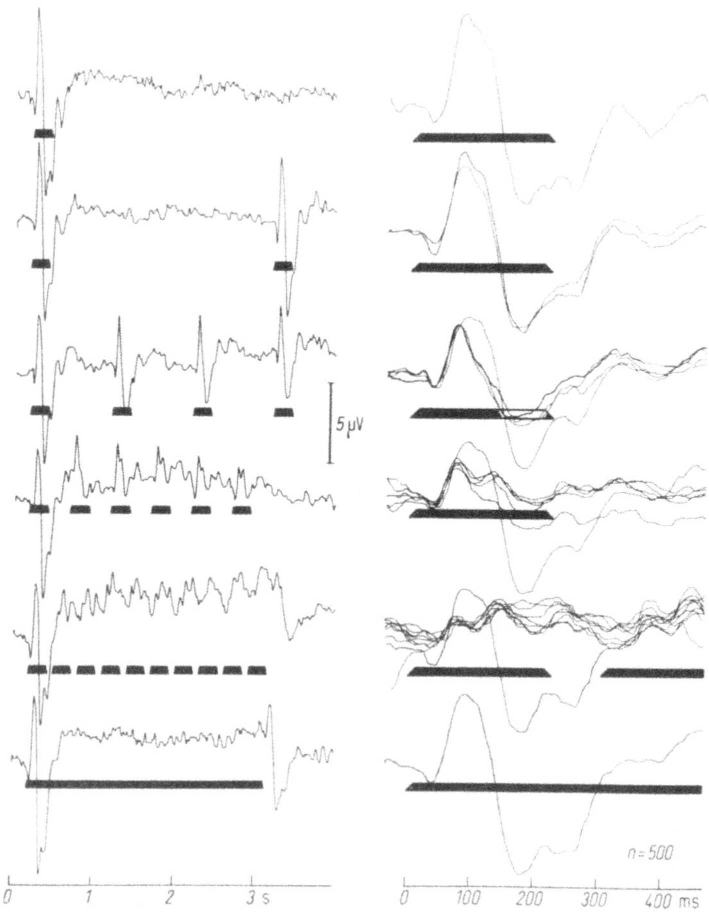

Fig. 65. AERs to trains of tone bursts of 250 ms duration each. The PSS is built up with decreasing interstimulus intervals (increasing repetition rate). N1 consists of two parts, the first of which (N1a) remains, while N1b fades from top to bottom, right column. P2 disappears completely; in place of P2 PSS reaches a negativity comparable to that of N1; adult human subjects. (According to Finkenzeller and Keidel, 1975b)

Based upon the fact that the AERs are due to changes of stimulus parameters rather than to steady conditions (sensitivity to the differential ratio plus the fundamental stimulus parameters; proportional-differential-function; "PD"-transient-function), it was, therefore, possible to obtain as a respond to *steps* in intensity *and* frequency as well as the on-effect, as in the increasing PSS described before. Results are shown in Fig. 66a und b for intensity steps and frequency steps, respectively. Note the marked increase in the perstimulatory DC-shift (PSS) (complete DC-amplification).

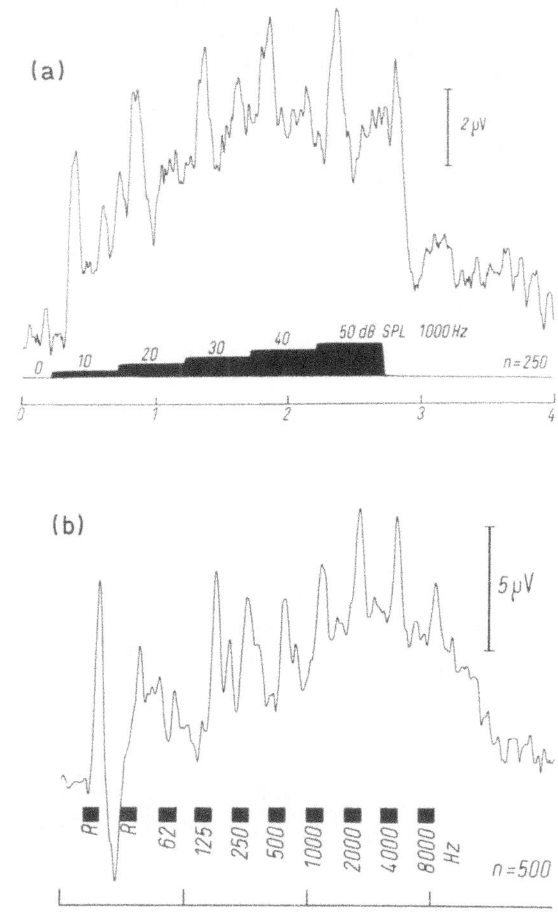

Fig. 66. (a) AERs to steps of intensity; full DC-amplification, therefore considerable PSS. (b) Same for steps in frequency at a constant intensity. (According to same authors as in Fig. 65)

If one plots the two traces of Fig. 66a and b perpendicularly, a three dimensional trace results which is shown in Fig. 67a; Fig. 67b represents a model where one axis means frequency, the second axis intensity and the third axis the (negative) amplitudes of all combined responses for all interesting frequencies and intensities from threshold to 60 dB SPL. The single averages are plotted in Fig. 67c for comparison.

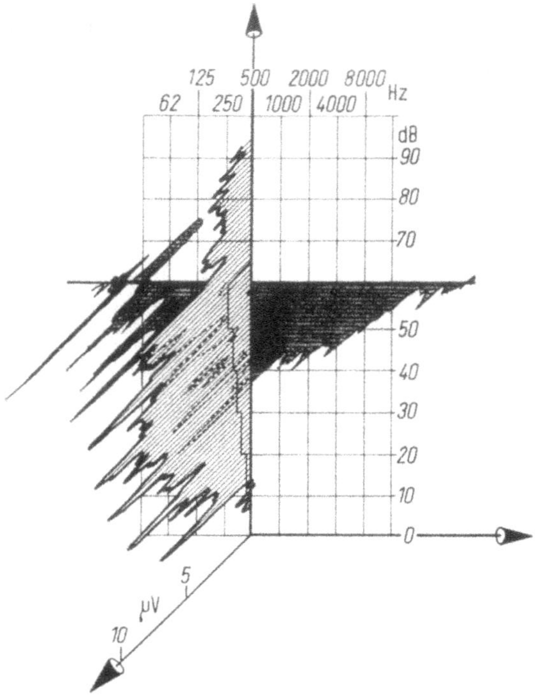

Fig. 67. (a)

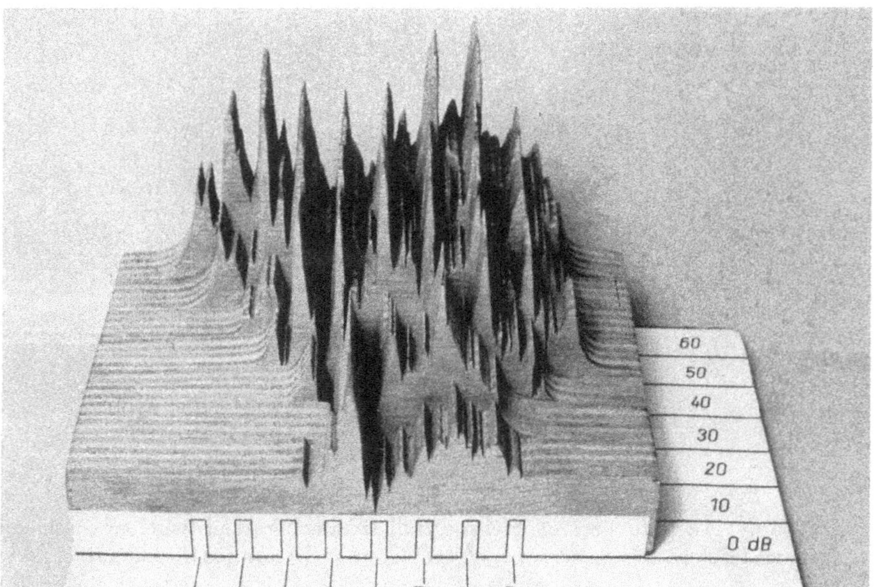

Fig. 67. (b)

Fig. 67. (a) One intensity response curve (Fig. 66a) and one frequency response average (Fig. 66b) are plotted three dimensionally as in conventional audiometry. Third ordinate is size of AERs. (b) Photograph of a model based on a complete run through all interesting stimulus-parameters. All responses are averages, which can be seen as single traces in Fig. 67c. (According to same authors as Fig. 65)

Thus, if the three dimensional model is viewed in the two directions of intensity (Fig. 68a) and frequency (Fig. 68b), all information about the intensity and frequency function of a given subject is availabe at a glance.

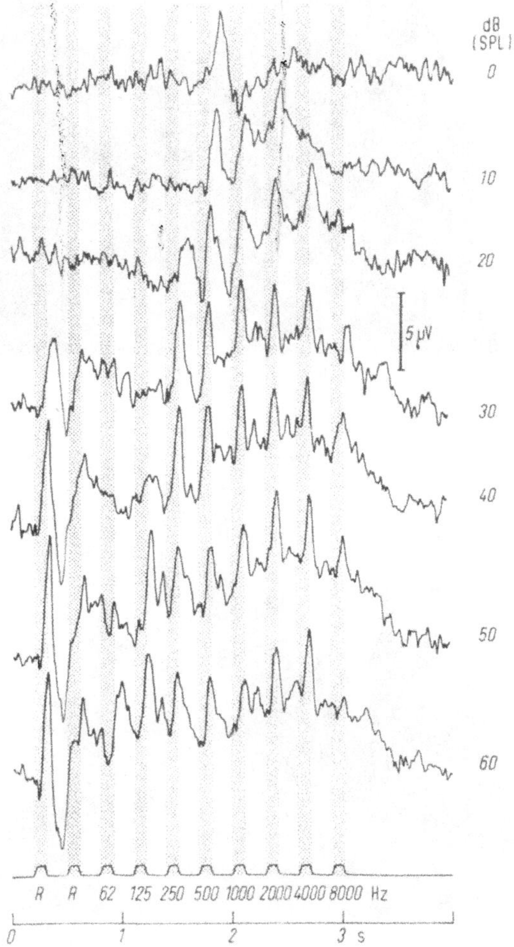

Fig. 67. (c)

Finally, most interestingly for ERA, a view of the model from the amplitude direction yields a very clear picture of an "objective" v. Békésy-audiogram as a typical threshold curve for a normal hearing adult subject (Fig. 68c). What is shown as a wooden model can easily be plotted by any small computer. To record AERs with this technique was the goal of Finkenzeller and Keidel in 1975 (paper given at the London symposium of the IERA study group).

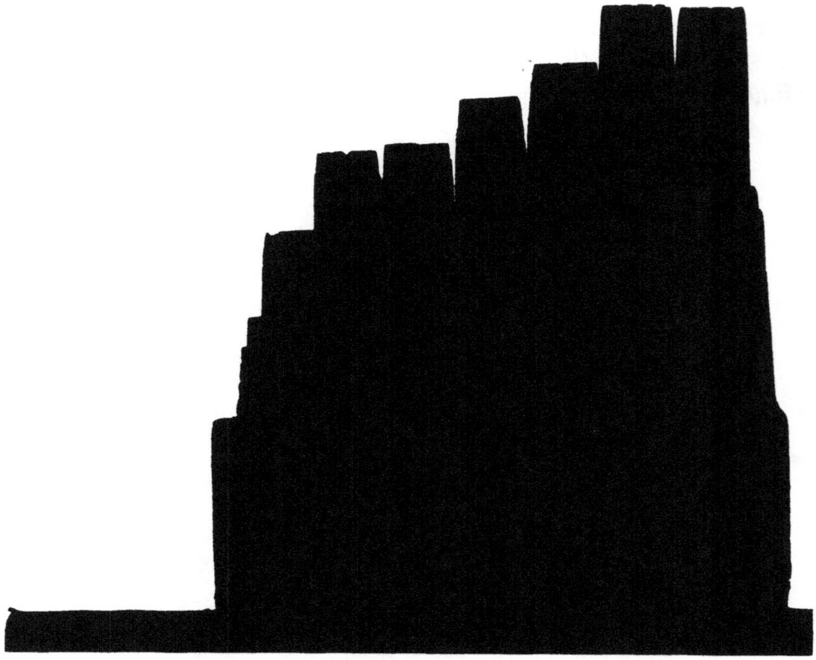

Fig. 68. (a)

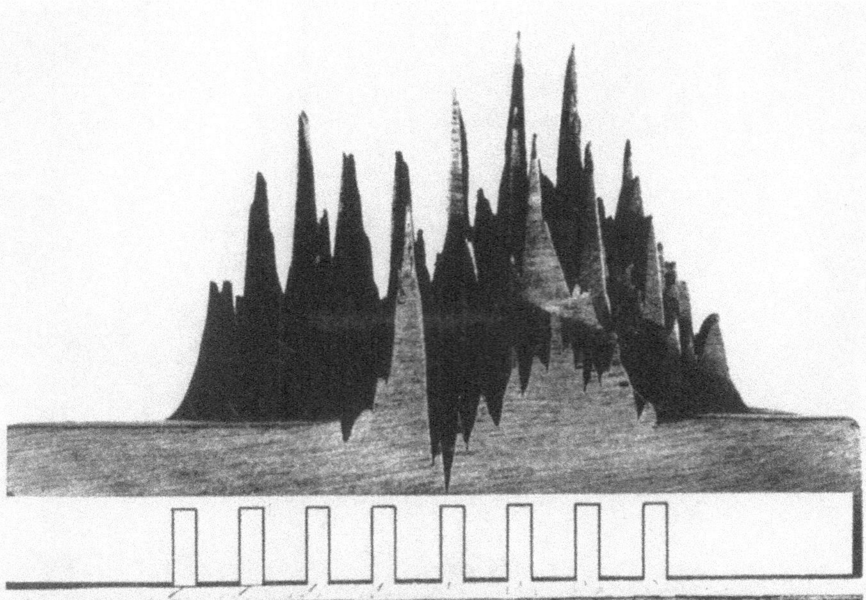

Fig. 68. (b)

Fig. 68. (a) Shadow-picture (silhouette) of the model revealing the intensity-function of the subject. b) Same as (a), but frequency-function. (c) View of the model from the amplitude direction gives the threshold-curve in the frequency-intensity area as is convenient for the conventional v. Békésy-audiometry which is measured psychophysically. Those diagrams might be plotted by a small computer. They are the neurophysiological correlates to the subjective audiograms. (According to FINKENZELLER and KEIDEL, 1975b)

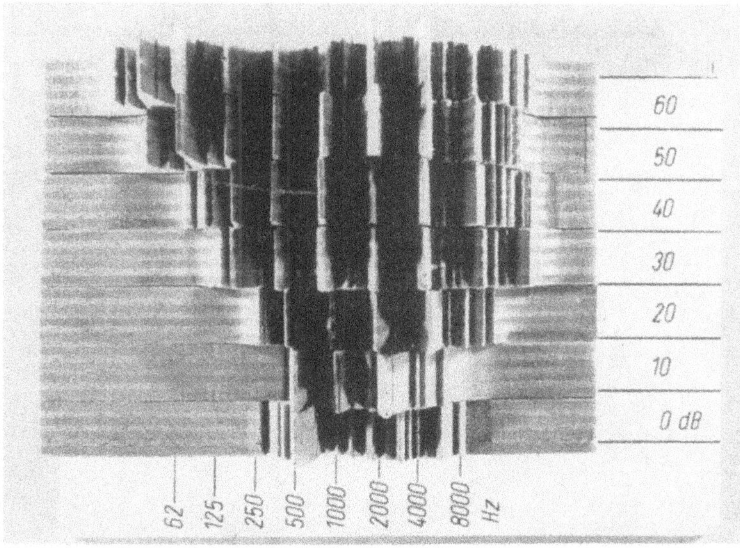

Fig. 68. (c)

E. Electrocochleography, Early Response, BERA

The first attempts to record Electrocochleograms in man were performed by YOSHIE, OHASHI, and SUZUKI in 1967. The electrodes were located as needles within the external meatus, and, hence, the amplitudes of the responses, although already consisting of N1 and N2, were small and could be obtained only at high intensities (brief clicks of 0,5 ms duration). The Bordeaux group (ARAN *et al.*, 1968 to 1975; ARAN and PORTMAN, 1972; PORTMAN *et al.*, 1967–1973) then succeeded in recording larger amplitudes with reliable and reproducible results by situating transtympanal electrodes on the promontorium. ARAN and PORTMAN developed their technique during the last decade to such a perfection that clear diagnosis even in difficult cases could be obtained. SALOMON improved YOSHIE's technique without surgical procedures and also produced a high degree of clinical application for the ECG. SOHMER and FEINMESSER, 1967, 1972, 1973, based upon older data of GALAMBOS, developed recording techniques with high rates of repetitions of stimuli (1967–1975) from the mastoid and were able to record not only the compound action potential of the auditory nerve, but also the brain stem responses with up to 5 negative peaks after stimulation. KESHINASHVILI *et al.* (1972), using alternating rarefaction and condensation clicks introduced their technique in ENT hospitals in their country. SPRENG and KEIDEL (1967, 1970, 1971), KEIDEL and SPRENG (1970) and KEIDEL (1971c, 1973) recorded with a plastic prothesis sitting on the hard palate; this technique, however, although yielding relatively great amplitudes, was not really useful in the clinic. They, therefore, later went over to SOHMER's technique in combination with classical ERA, as will be described later. In the meantime, numerous papers have been published about that topic. Excellent review articles were written by SCHULMAN-GALAMBOS and GALAMBOS (1975) about BERA and by EGGERMONT *et al.* about ECG (see especially the chapter by EGGERMONT in this volume on the handbook).

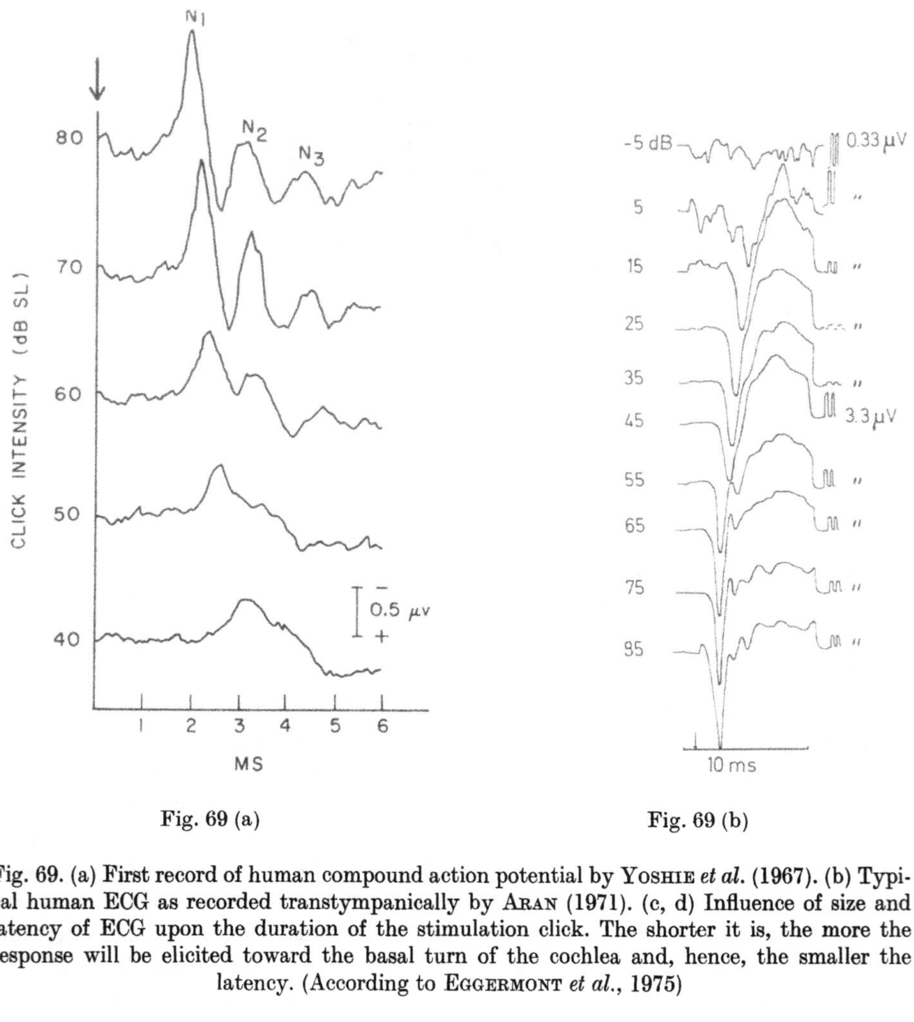

Fig. 69 (a) Fig. 69 (b)

Fig. 69. (a) First record of human compound action potential by YOSHIE *et al.* (1967). (b) Typical human ECG as recorded transtympanically by ARAN (1971). (c, d) Influence of size and latency of ECG upon the duration of the stimulation click. The shorter it is, the more the response will be elicited toward the basal turn of the cochlea and, hence, the smaller the latency. (According to EGGERMONT *et al.*, 1975)

At first glance the physiological analysis of what is recorded in the ECG seems easy, since it means the well known compound action potential is recorded often in the animal with N1 and N2, which was first labelled by DAVIS. But when considering this problem more carefully, it turns out to be very complex, if one includes the recent data of the Dutch group (EGGERMONT, ODENTHAL, SPOOR up to 1975). They also recorded the summating potential and – as ELBERLING and SALOMON (1971) do – put emphasis upon the fact that the time necessary for the traveling wave inside the human cochlea to reach the first turn makes the choice of stimulus duration and hence its fundamental frequency decisive for the pattern and latency of the ECG. Examples of this very important progress in the analysis of ECG are shown in Fig. 69a, b, c and d as records of Yoshie, Aran, and Eggermont. In their data the influence of the stimulus frequency can clearly be seen.

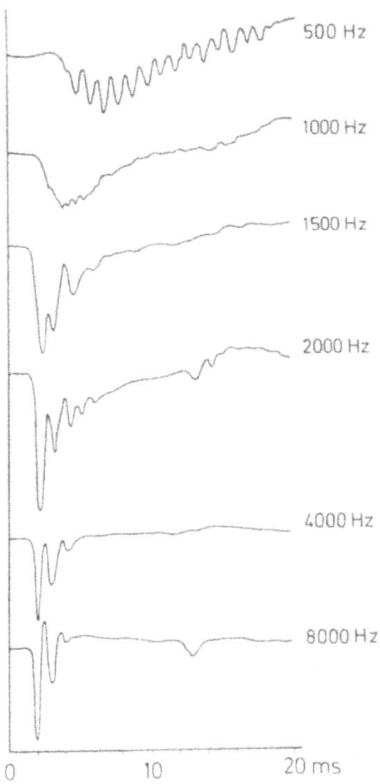

Fig. 69 (c)

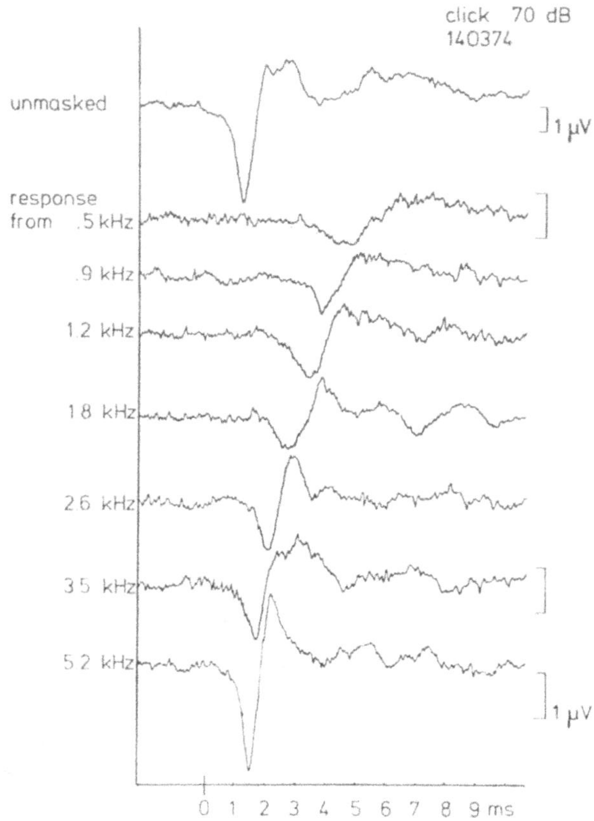

Fig. 69 (d)

In the meantime, an excellent clinical monograph about ECG was written by Aran in 1971. When including masking experiments, other problems arise, in so far that we know now both from morphological data (Spoendlin, 1973, 1975) and from neurophysiological evidence Kiang (1965), Evans (see Chapter 1, second part of this handbook volume V) that 95% of all available and contributing fibers to the compound ECG originate from *inner* hair cells. Furthermore, the outer hair cells seem to act as amplifiers for the inner ones, and, based upon some unknown mechanisms, either due to the hydrodynamics or to the neurophysiology of the first order, single fibers, improve the slope of the tuning curves of the auditory nerve considerably compared to that of the basilar membrane (Kiang, 1965). A survey of the problem is shown in Fig. 70.

In addition, the early responses, which probably originate in the brainstem with latencies between 6 and maximally 30 ms, being partially of myogenic and partially of neurogenic origin, began to play an important role in the ERA, since they were relatively stable despite the state of alertness, sleep, attention and even the degree of anesthesia of the subject, which made them very applicaple for clinical use. They have already been described in this chapter and are discussed in detail in GALAMBOS' paper about BERA (1975). They were studied carefully in man by GOLDBERG (personal communication, 1971) and recently by GERULL *et al.*

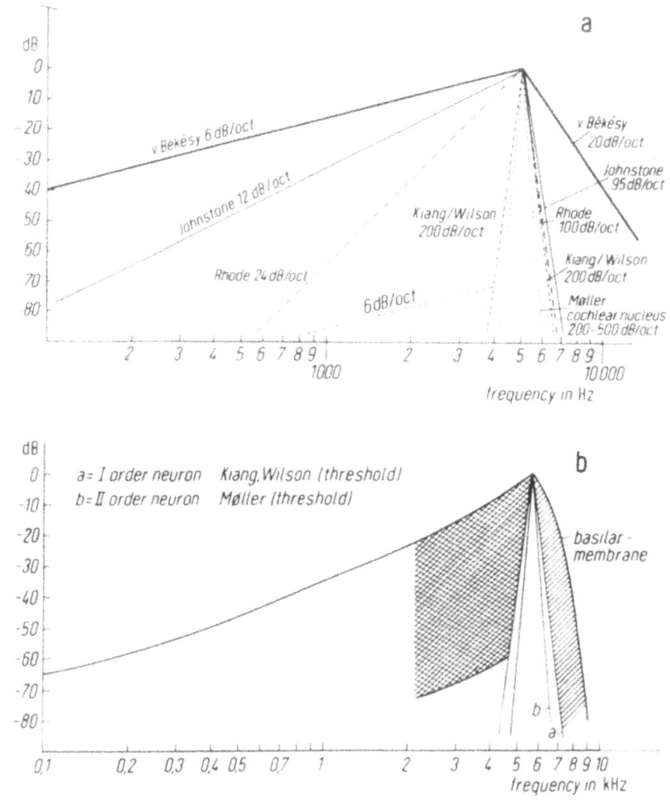

Fig. 70. Improvement of the slope of the tuning curves of the first order neuron compared to that of the basilar membrane. (According to KEIDEL, 1974a, 1975b)

(1973) and by THEISSING JR. (1970). Since their origin within the brain stem still needs further explanation, and since DAVIS in his chapter as well as EGGERMONT and ZÖLLNER and STANGE deal with this matter, only two examples of brain stem responses are shown in Fig. 71a, b.

Further details are omitted in this chapter. A full list of reports is given in References.

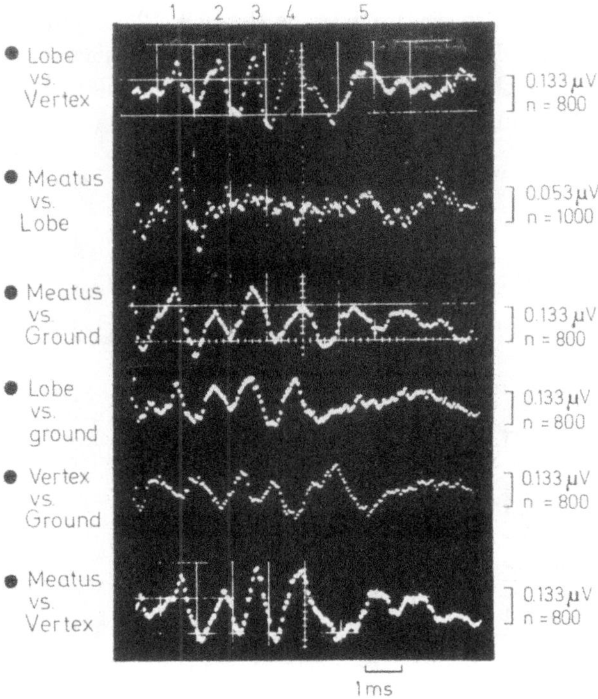

Fig. 71. (a)

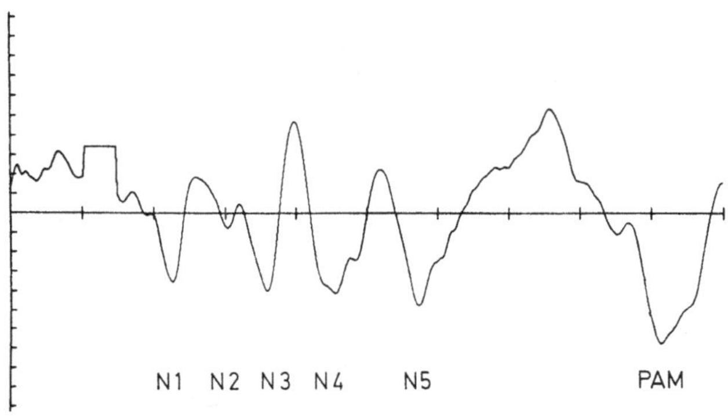

Fig. 71. (b)

Fig. 71. (a) Brain stem responses. Records are taken from mastoid. The different peaks are influenced differently by brain stem lesions. (According to SOHMER and FEINMESSER, 1973.) (b) Records showing the brain stem responses. (According to THORNTON, 1975)

F. Combined Simultaneous Record of ECG, BERA, ERA and PSS

GESTRING, BURIAN, and INNITZER in 1973 (Bordeaux) reported about a combined record of early and late responses to auditory stimuli in man based on one logarithmic time scale as abscissa. At RUBEN'S symposium in 1974 (New York), a similar technique was described (see symposium volume to be published). The goal of the Erlangen group was the simultaneous record on three time scales (8 ms; 40 ms; 2 s) by means of a special program on the PDP 12 computer (Fig. 72) of all available physiological data from the auditory channel. This was reported at the London symposium of the ERA Study Group in 1975; earlier work was reported in Budapest in 1971 and in Dundee in 1970.

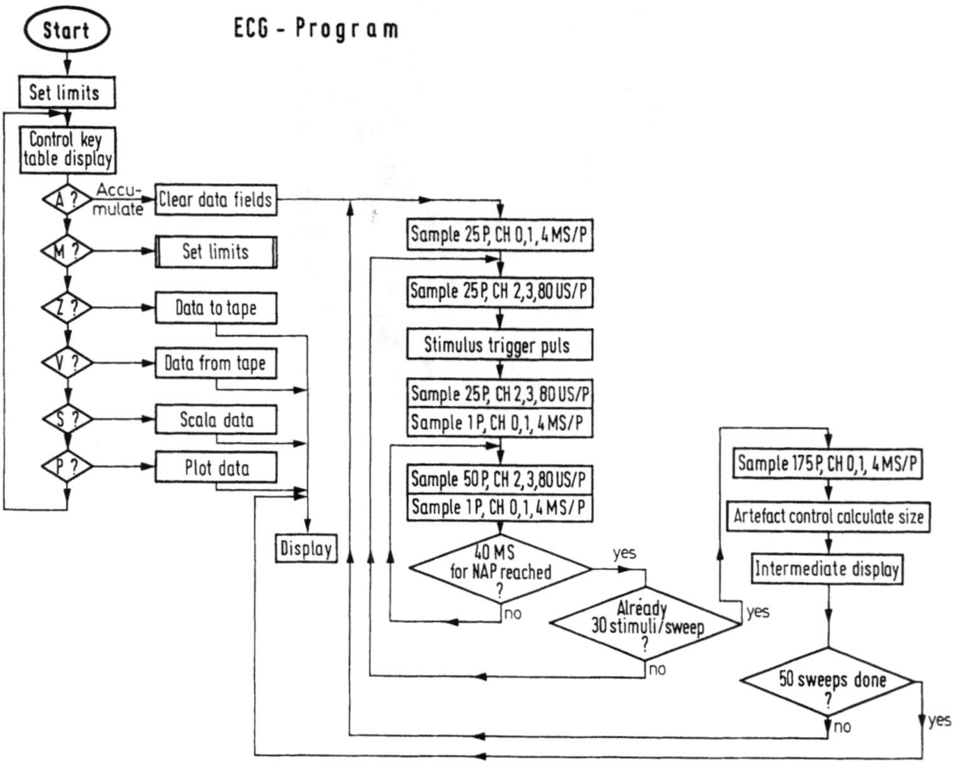

Fig. 72. Program for simultaneous recording of ECG, BERA, ERA and PSS, labelled ECG 7. This program was written for the PDP 12 by FINKENZELLER (1975)

Usually the display on the cathode ray screen or the plot by the plotter was on a 40 ms (left section) plus a 2 s (right section) basis. A sense switch allowed for change to the 8 or 10 ms display, as shown in Fig. 73a and b for a typical record.

Trains of filtered clicks (0.5 ms) were used as stimuli. Each train consisted of 30 clicks with 40 ms interstimulus intervals. Two additional seconds for full recovery were allowed. The program furthermore provided the setting of limits for potential size to omit all possible types of artifacts. Thus, the numbers at the top indicate the numbers of admitted and omitted responses for controll. Full DC-amplification was used for the ERA and PSS section, broadband amplification for the ECG and BERA section. Electrode location was at both mastoids and the

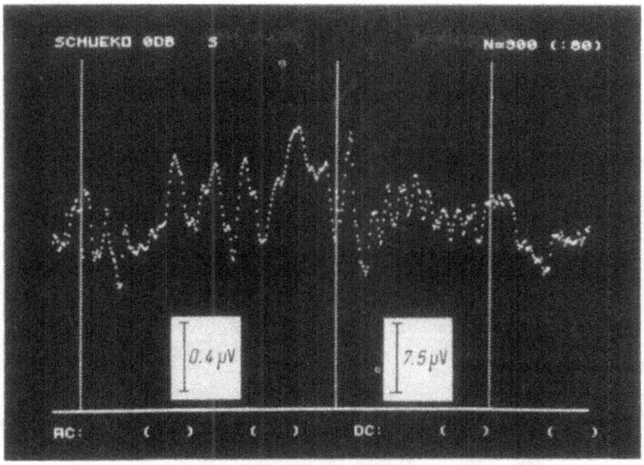

Fig. 73. (a)

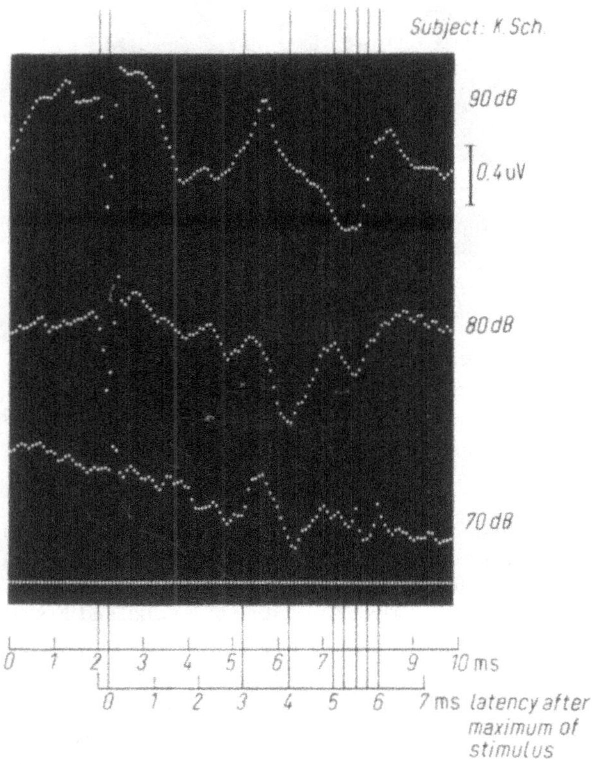

Fig. 73. (b)

Fig. 73 (a) Display of data obtained by the program ECG 7. 40 ms after stimulus onset between first and second cursor, 1.2 s between second and third cursor. Preceding a brief perstimulatory period. After the third cursor, a 700 ms post stimulus period. ECG's brain stem responses can be seen in the left section, N1, P2, N2 and PSS in the right section (with Alpha-rhythm). In the poststimulatory section, the off-response is visible. (b) Same record, enlarged time scale for ECG observation. (Both according to KEIDEL and FINKENZELLER, 1975) vertex, left partition of the display contralateral versus ipsilateral mastoid, right partition vertex versus contralateral partition. Two more additional records demonstrate the interindividual variation (Fig. 74a und b).

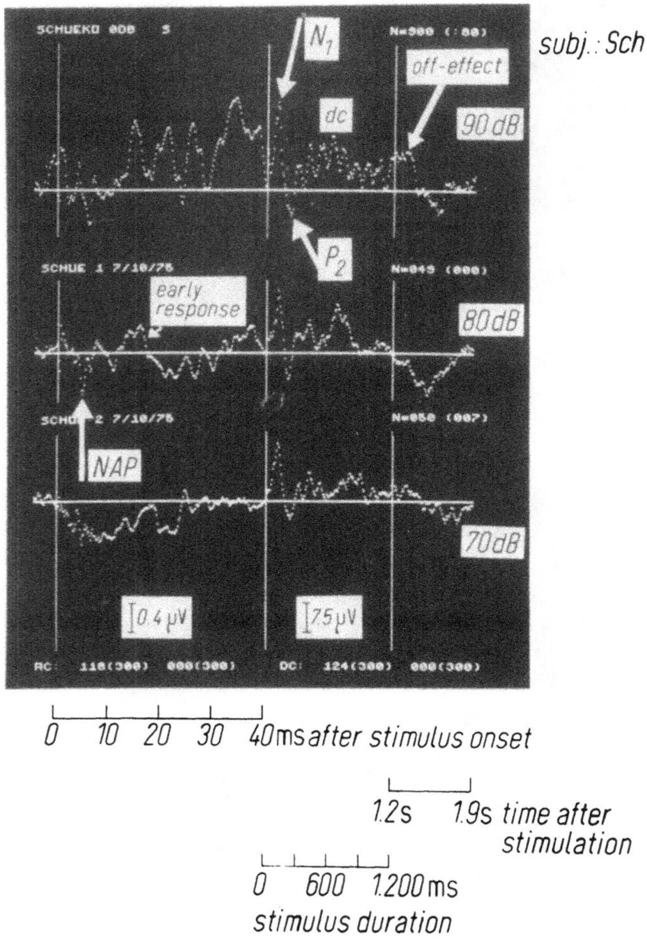

Fig. 74. (a)

Fig. 74a—c. Typical record of one subject. (b) and (c) records of two subjects, early responses with greatly different responses. In (b) and (c) the ECG's are relatively small and the brain stem responses, especially the first ones at 4; 5.5; 6 ms latency are relatively large because of the broadband filtering (1 Hz to 3 kHz). (According to KEIDEL and FINKENZELLER, 1975)

An additional program allowed the computation of the running average of N1 and P2 of the classical AERs as well as the running correlation to the mean size and pattern averaged over hours (Fig. 75). The running average of N1 stayed at a stable value, while the running average for P2 had a clear trend to level out with time, revealing an overshooting recovery after a pause of 10 min. Accordingly, the running correlation (top), because of the behavior of P2, had a clear tendency to go from greater values of r to smaller values with increasing time of stimulation. Records were taken from the vertex KEIDEL and FINKENZELLER (1975).

The "objective" correlate to the SISI-test is shown in Fig. 76 as one example of clinical application.

There is certainly no need to emphasize the possible application in the clinic and the overall advantage of that type of recording from the intact human skull.

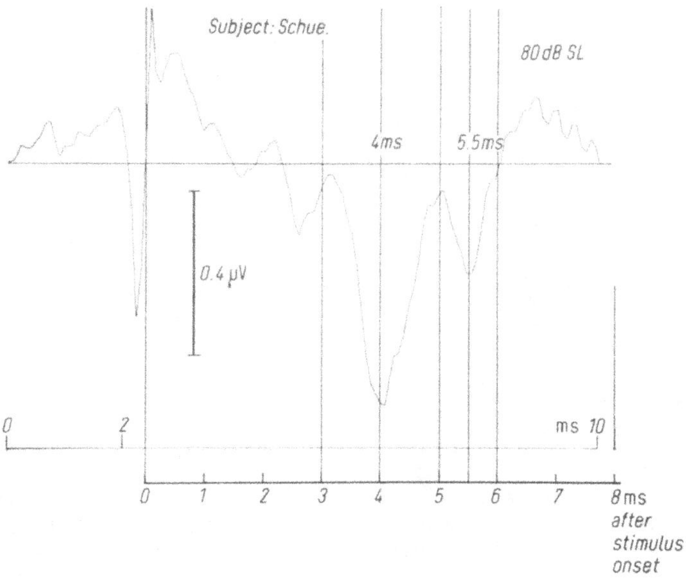

Fig. 74. (b)

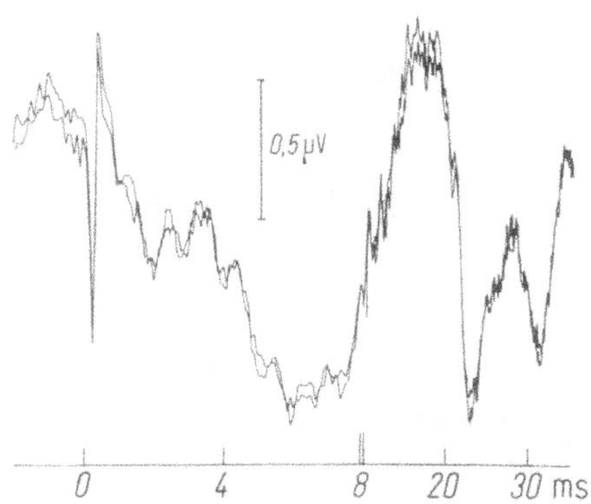

Fig. 74. (c)

Finally, the reader's attention should be draw to some monographs about the neurophysiology of Evoked Responses of the auditory system: Cobb and Morocutti (1967), Regan (1968), Aran (1971), Eggermont *et al.* (1974), Theissing Jr. (1970), Keidel (1975b). Furthermore it is a pleasure for the reviewer to be informed that Professor Davis, the head of the St. Louis group, is in the process of writing a monograph on this topic which may be published in 1976.

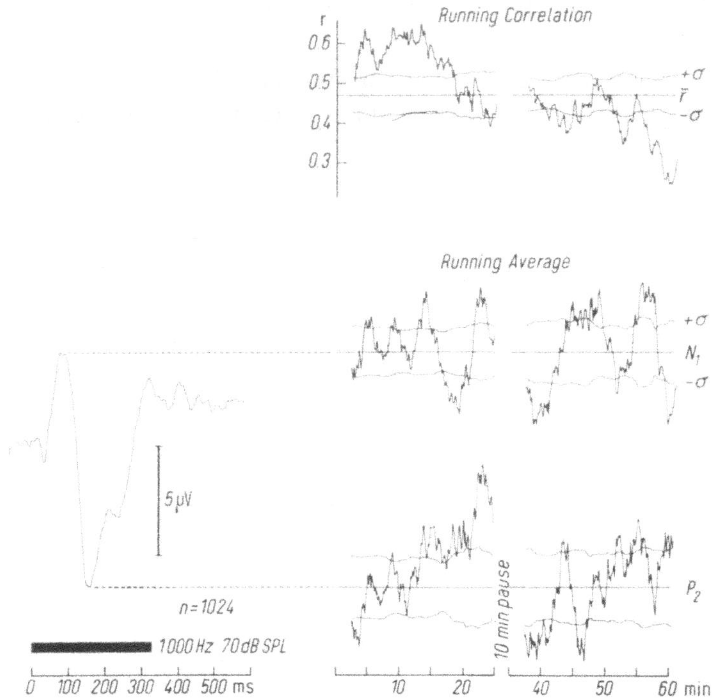

Fig. 75. Running average and running correlation with the mean average of 2 hours record time reveal a stable size of N1 and a trend of P2 to level off with time. A pause of 10 min allows the running average of P2 to recover. (According to KEIDEL and FINKENZELLER, 1975)

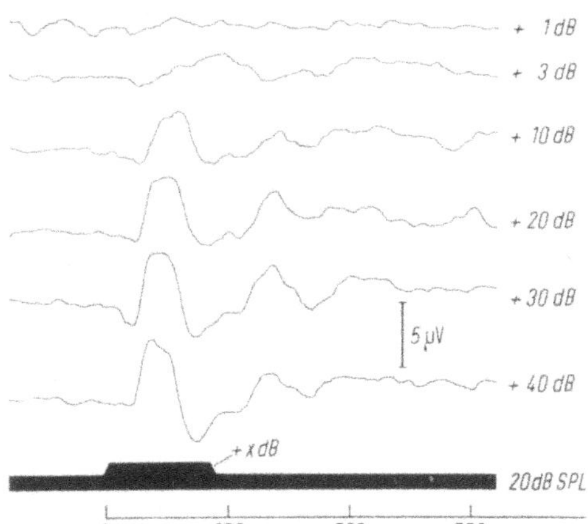

Fig. 76. "Objective" SISI-test. Threshold for the difference limen of intensity can be recorded by means of ERA between 1 dB and 3 dB. This is in full agreement with the results obtained from the SISI-test. (According to FINKENZELLER, 1975)

Aknowledgements

The author wishes to thank Mr. BURIAN and his wife for all drawings and photographs, Mrs. FRÖHLICH for typing the manuscript, Dr. KALLERT and Miss FÖRSTEL for help in compiling the reference list and last but not least Miss CHRISTENSON for help in looking through the manuscript from the point-of-view of the English language.

References

ABDELMOUMÈNE, M., BESSON, J.-M., ALÉONARD, P.: Neurophysiologie. Effets des anesthésiques sur le contrôle cortical de la polarisation des fibres afférentes primaires chez le Chat. C. R. Acad. Sci. (Paris) **265**, 1138—1140 (1967), Série D.

ABRAHAM, F. D., MARSH, J. T.: Amplitude of evoked potentials as a function of slow presenting rates of repetitive auditory stimulation. Exp. Neurol. **14**, 187—198 (1966).

ABRAHAMS, V. C.: Some factors affecting the form of averaged evoked potentials. J. Physiol. (Lond.) **185**, 60—61 (1966).

ABRAHAMS, V. C., LANGWORTH, E. P.: The contribution of background electrical activity to the form of averaged evoked potentials in chloralose anesthetized cats. Exp. Neurol. **18**, 253—266 (1967).

ADAMO, N. J., KING, R. L.: Evoked responses in the chicken telencephalon to auditory, visual, and tactile stimulation. Exp. Neurol. **17**, 498—504 (1967).

ADES, H. W.: A secondary acoustic area in the cerebral cortex of the cat. J. Neurophysiol. **6**, 59—63 (1943).

ADEY, W. R., BUCHWALD, N. A., LINDSLEY, D. F.: Amygdaloid, pallidal and peripheral influences on mesencephalic unit firing patterns with reference to mechanisms of tremor. Electroenceph. clin. Neurophysiol. **12**, 21—40 (1960).

ADEY, W. R., DUNLOP, C. W., SUNDERLAND, S.: A survey of rhinencephalic interrelations with the brain-stem. J. comp. Neurol. **110**, 173—204 (1958).

ADEY, W. R., LINDSLEY, D. F.: On the role of subthalamic areas in the maintenance of brainstem reticular excitability. Exp. Neurol. **1**, 407—426 (1959).

ADEY, W. R., SEGUNDO, J. P., LIVINGSTON, R. B.: Corticifugal influences on intrinsic brainstem conduction in cat and monkey. J. Neurophysiol. **20**, 1—16 (1957).

ADRIAN, H. O., GOLDBERG, J. M., BRUGGE, J. F.: Auditory evoked cortical potentials after lesions of brachium of inferior colliculus. J. Neurophysiol. **29**, 456—466 (1966).

AITKIN, L. M.: Medial geniculate body of the cat: responses to tonal stimuli of neurons in medial division. J. Neurophysiol. **36**, 275—283 (1973).

AITKIN, L. M., WEBSTER, W. R.: Medial geniculate body of the cat: organization and responses to tonal stimuli of neurons in the ventral division. J. Neurophysiol. **35**, 365—380 (1972).

AKIYAMA, Y., SCHULTE, F. J., SCHULTZ, M. A., PARMELEE, A. H.: Acoustically evoked responses in premature and full term newborn infants. Electroenceph. clin. Neurophysiol. **26**, 371—380 (1969).

ALBE-FESSARD, D., FESSARD, A.: Thalamic integrations and their consequences at the telencephalic level. In: MORUZZI, G., FESSARD, A., JASPER, H. H. (Eds.): Brain Mechanisms. Progress in Brain Research, Vol. 1. Amsterdam: Elsevier 1963.

ALBE-FESSARD, D., GILLETT, E.: Convergences d'afférences d'origines corticale at périphérique vers le centre médian du chat anesthésié ou éveillé. Electroenceph. clin. Neurophysiol. **13**, 257—269 (1961).

ALLISON, T.: Recovery functions of somatosensory evoked responses in man. Electroenceph. clin. Neurophysiol. **14**, 331—343 (1962).

AMASSIAN, V. E.: Studies on organization of a somesthetic association area, including a single unit analysis. J. Neurophysiol. **17**, 39—58 (1954).

ANDERSEN, P.: Rhythmic 10/sec activity in the Thalamus. In: PURPURA, D. P., YAHR, M. D. (Eds.): The Thalamus. New York-London: Columbia University Press 1966.

ANDERSEN, P., BROOKS, C. MCC., ECCLES, J. C.: Electrical responses of the ventro-basal nucleus of the thalamus. In: BARGMANN, W., SCHADÉ, J. P. (Eds.): Progress in Brain Research, Vol. 5. Amsterdam: Elsevier 1964a.

ANDERSEN, P., SEARS, T. A.: The ventro-basal nucleus of the thalamus: potential fields, synaptic transmission and excitability of both presynaptic and postsynaptic components. J. Physiol. (Lond.) **174**, 348—369 (1964b).

ANTINORO, F., SKINNER, P. H.: The effects of frequency on the auditory evoked response. J. Aud. Res. **8**, 119—123 (1968).

ANTINORO, F., SKINNER, P. H., JONES, J. J.: Relation between sound intensity and amplitude of the AER at different stimulus frequencies. J. acoust. Soc. Amer. **46**, 1433—1436 (1969).

ARAN, J.-M.: L'Électro-Cochléogramme. I. Principe et Technique. Les Cahiers C.F.A., No. 12, 3—45 (1971). (Compagnie Francaise d'Audiologie.)

ARAN, J.-M.: L'Électro-Cochléogramme. II. Résultats. Les Cahiers de la C.F.A., No. 13, 49—98 (1971). (Compagnie Francaise d'Audiologie.)

ARAN, J.-M.: L'Électro-Cochléogramme. III. Essai d'Interprétation. Les Cahiers de la C.F.A., No. 14, 101—128 (1972). (Compagnie Francaise d'Audiologie.)

ARAN, J.M., PORTMANN, M.: L'électrocochléogramme. J. franç. Oto-rhino-laryng. **21**, 211 (1972).

ARDUINI, A., MANCIA, M., MECHELSE, K.: Slow potential changes elicited in the cerebral cortex by sensory and reticular stimulation. Archives ital. Biol. **95**, 127—138 (1957).

ASANUMA, H.: Microelectrode studies on the evoked activity of a single pyramidal tract cell in the somato-sensory area in cats. Jap. J. Physiol. **9**, 94—105 (1959).

BAER, K. E. VON: Die Abhängigkeit unseres Weltbilds von der Länge unseres Moments. Reden gehalten in wissenschaftlichen Versammlungen. St. Petersburg, 1864, Verlag der Kaiserlichen Hofbuchhandlung H. Schmitzdorff. Neudruck erschienen als Beiheft zu Band 3/1962 der Grundlagenstudien aus Kybernetik und Geisteswissenschaft. Quickborn bei Hamburg. Verlag Schnelle 1962.

BAN, T., INOUE, K., OZAKI, S., KAWASHIMA, K., YOSHIOKA, T.: Cerebral cortical potential evoked by hypothalamic stimulation in cat. Med. J. Osaka Univ. **7**, 859—864 (1957).

BARLOW, J. S.: An electronic method for detecting evoked responses of the brain and for reproducing their average waveforms. Electroenceph. clin. Neurophysiol. **9**, 340—343 (1957).

BARLOW, J. S., BRAZIER, M. A. B.: Correlation studies of brain potentials. Ruar. Progr. Rep., MIT Cambridge, April 15, 79—82 (1955).

BARNET, A. B., LODGE, A.: Click evoked EEG responses in normal and developmentally retarded infants. Nature (Lond.) **214**, 252—255 (1967).

BATINI, C., MORUZZI, G., PALESTINI, M., ROSSI, G. F., ZANCHETTI, A.: Effects of complete pontine transections on the sleepwakefulness rhythm: the midpontine pretrigeminal preparation. Arch. ital. Biol. **97**, 1—12 (1959).

BAUMANN, H., BAUMANN, R.: Zur Frage einer spezifischen Signalverarbeitung der Formatio reticularis und ihrer Beziehung zur kortikalen evozierten Aktivität. Acta biol. med. germ. **19**, 961—983 (1967).

BAUMANN, H., BAUMANN, R., GURK, CH., WOLTER, F.: Electrophysiological studies of central nervous performance during monotony. Electroenceph. clin. Neurophysiol. **24**, 259—273 (1968).

BAUST, W., BERLUCCI, G., MORUZZI, G.: Changes in the auditory input in wakefulness and during the synchronized and desynchronized stages of sleep. Arch. ital. Biol. **102**, 657—674 (1964).

BEAGLEY, H. A., KELLOGG, S. E.: Amplitude of the auditory evoked response at high intensities. Sound **4**, 86—90 (1971).

BECK, A.: Die Bestimmung der Lokalisation der Gehirn- und Rückenmarksfunktionen vermittelst der elektrischen Erscheinungen. Zbl. Physiol. **4**, 473—476 (1890).

BEGLEITER, H., GROSS, M. M., KISSIN, B.: Evoked cortical responses to affective visual stimuli. Psychophysiology **3**, 336—344 (1967).

BEGLEITER, H., PLATZ, A.: Evoked potentials: Modifications by classical conditioning. Science **166**, 769—771 (1969).

BÉKÉSY, G. VON: Zur Theorie des Hörens. Über die eben merkbare Amplituden- und Frequenzänderung eines Tones. Die Theorie der Schwebungen. Phys. Z. **30**, 721—745 (1929).

BÉKÉSY, G. VON: Experiments in hearing. New York: McGraw Hill Comp. 1960.

BENNING, C. D., KARNAHL, TH., STANGE, G.: ERA-Kennlinien und Latenzen bei 15 normalhörenden Kleinkindern. Arch. klin. exp. Ohr-, Nas.- u. Kehlk.-Heilk. **201**, 222—230 (1972).

BENNING, C., STANGE, G.: Das Verhalten peripherer und zentraler akustischer Reizantworten des Meerschweinchens unter Sinustonbeschallung. Arch. klin. exp. Ohr-., Nas.- u. Kehl.-Heilk. **199**, 529—533 (1971).

BERLUCCHI, G., MUNSON, J. B., RIZZOLATTI, G.: Auditory-evoked responses in cats with teno. tomized middle ear muscles during sleep. Pflügers Arch. ges. Physiol. **292**, 80—82 (1966)-

Berlucchi, G., Munson, J. B., Rizzolatti, G.: Changes in click-evoked responses in the auditory system and the cerebellum of free-moving cats during sleep and waking. Arch. ital. Biol. **105**, 118—135 (1967).

Berlucchi, G., Munson, J. B., Rizzolatti, G.: Click-evoked responses in cats with tenotomized middle ear muscles during sleep and waking. Electroenceph. clin. Neurophysiol., Supp. 26 "The Evoked Potentials", 1967.

Besson, J.-M., Abdelmoumène, M., Aléonard, P.: Neurophysiologie, Répartition des aires corticales contrôlant l'inhibition présynaptique chez l'animal éveillé et anesthésié. C. R. Acad. Sci. (Paris) **265**, 1412—1414 (1967), Série D.

Bickford, R. G.: Application of central averaging. Ann. N. Y. Acad. Sci. (1963).

Bickford, R. G., Jacobson, J. L., Galbraith, R. F.: A new audio motor system in man. Eastern association of electroencephalographers No. 7. Electroenceph. clin. Neurophysiol. **15**, 922 (1963).

Bickford, R. G., Jacobson, J. L., Cody, D. T. R.: Nature of average evoked potentials to sound and other stimuli in man. Ann. N. Y. Acad. Sci. **112**, 204—223 (1964).

Bignall, K. E.: Effects of subcortical ablations on polysensory cortical responses and interactions in the cat. Exp. Neurol. **18**, 56—67 (1967).

Bignall, K. E.: Auditory input to frontal polysensory cortex of the squirrel monkey: Possible pathways. Brain Res. **19**, 77—86 (1970).

Boakes, R. J., Kerkut, G. A., Munday, K. A.: Effect of hypothermia on cortical evoked potentials. Life Sci. **6**, 457—459 (1967).

Bonvallet, M., Bloch, V.: Bulbar control of cortical arousal. Science **133**, 1133—1134 (1961).

Borbély, A. A.: Changes in click-evoked responses as a function of depth in auditory cortex of the rat. Brain Res. **21**, 217—247 (1970).

Bostock, H., Jarvis, M. J.: Changes in the form of the cerebral evoked response related to the speed of simple reaction time. Electroenceph. clin. Neurophysiol. **29**, 137—145 (1970).

Botte, M. C., Cocholle, R.: Mise en évidence d'asymétries auditives par une méthode psychoacoustique et par l'enregistrement des potentiels évoqués auditifs. Rev. Acoustique **27**, 227—230 (1973).

Bowsher, D., Mallart, A., Petit, D., Albe-Fessard, D.: A bulbar relay to the centre median. J. Neurophysiol. **31**, 288—300 (1968).

Brazier, M. A. B.: A study of the late response to flash in the cortex of the cat. Acta physiol. pharmacol. neerl. **6**, 692—714 (1957).

Bremer, F.: Étude oscillographique des réponses sensorielles de l'aire acoustique corticale chez le chat. Arch. int. Physiol. **53**, 53—103 (1943).

Bremer, F.: Les aires auditives de l'écorce cérébrale. Cours International d'Audiologie Clinique, Mardo 12-Février 1952.

Bremer, F., Dow, R. S.: The acoustic area of the cerebral cortex in the cat. A combined oscillographic and cytoarchitectonic study. J. Neurophysiol. **2**, 308—318 (1939).

Brooks, V. B.: Some factors governing sensory convergence in the cat's motor cortex. Studies in Physiology. New York-Berlin-Heidelberg: Springer 1965.

Brooks, V. B., Enger, P. S.: Spread of directly evoked responses in the cat's cerebral cortex. J. gen. Physiol. **42**, 761—777 (1959).

Brown, F. M., Stewart, W. S., Blodgett, J. T.: EEG kappa rhythmus during transcendental meditation and possible perceptual threshold changes following. Proc. Kentucky Acad. Sci. Richmond 1971.

Büchele, U., Seiler, C. F.: Die reizkorrelierte Gleichspannungsantwort (RGA) akustisch evozierter Potentiale und ihre Abhängigkeit von Vigilanz und Aufmerksamkeit. H.N.O. (Berl.) **22**, 114—117 (1974).

Bullock, T. H., Grinnell, A. D., Ikezono, E., Kameda, K., Katsuki, Y., Nomoto, M., Sato, O., Suga, N., Yanagisawa, K.: Electrophysiological studies of central auditory mechanisms in cetaceans. Z. vergl. Physiol. **59**, 117—156 (1968).

Bumm, P., Johannsen, H. S., Spreng, M., Wiegand, H. P.: Zur Registrierung langsamer Rindenpotentiale bei rotatorischer Reizung des Menschen. Ärztl. Forsch. **24**, 59—62 (1970).

Burdick, J. A., Sugerman, A. A., Goldstein, L.: The application of regression analysis to quantitative electroencephalography in man. Psychophysiology **3**, 249—254 (1967).

BURIAN, K.: Evoked response audiometry (ERA) — ein objectives Hörprüfungsverfahren. H.N.O. (Berl.) **17**, 353—358 (1969).

BURIAN, K., GESTRING, G. F.: Die EEG-Computer-Audiometrie: eine objektive Hörprüfungsmethode. Image **1**, 11—15 (1968).

BURKE, R. E., NELSON, P. G.: Synaptic activity in motoneurons during natural stimulation of muscle spindles. Science **151**, 1088—1091 (1966).

BURKE, W., SEFTON, A. J.: Discharge patterns of principal cells and interneurones in lateral geniculate nucleus of rat. J. Physiol. (Lond.) **187**, 201—212 (1966).

BURKE, W., SEFTON, A. J.: Recovery of responsiveness of cells of lateral geniculate nucleus of rat. J. Physiol. (Lond.) **187**, 213—229 (1966).

BURKE, W., SEFTON, A. J.: Inhibitory mechanisms in lateral geniculate nucleus of rat. J. Physiol. (Lond.) **187**, 231—246 (1966).

BURNS, S. K., BORBÉLY, A. A., HALL, R. D.: Evoked potentials: Three-dimensional display. Science **157**, 457—459 (1967).

BUSER, P., BORENSTEIN, P.: Réponses corticales secondaires à la stimulation sensorielle chez chat curarizé non anaesthesié. Electroenceph. clin. Neurophysiol. Suppl. **6**, 89—108 (1957).

BUSER, P., BORENSTEIN, P.: Réponses somesthésiques, visuelles et auditives, recueillies au niveau du cortex associatif suprasylvien chez le chat curarisé non anesthésié. Electroenceph. clin. Neurophysiol. **11**, 285—304 (1959).

BUSER, P., BORENSTEIN, P., BRUNER, J.: Étude des systèmes associatifs visuels et auditifs chez le chat anesthésié au chloralose. Electroenceph. clin. Neurophysiol. **11**, 305—324 (1959).

BUTLER, R. A.: Effect of changes in stimulus frequency and intensity on habituation of the human vertex potential. J. acoust. Soc. Amer. **44**, 945—950 (1968).

BUTLER, R. A.: The auditory evoked response to stimuli producing periodicity pitch. Psychophysiology **9**, 233—237 (1972a).

BUTLER, R. A.: Frequency specificity of the auditory evoked response to simultaneously and successively presented stimuli. Electroenceph. clin. Neurophysiol. **33**, 277—282 (1972b).

BUTLER, R. A.: The influence of spatial separation of sound sources on the auditory evoked response. Neuropsychologia **10**, 219—225 (1972c).

BUTLER, R. A.: The cumulative effects of different stimulus repetition rates on the auditory evoked response in man. Electroenceph. clin. Neurophysiol. **35**, 337—345 (1973).

BUTLER, R. A., KEIDEL, W. D., SPRENG, M.: An investigation of the human cortical evoked potential under conditions of monaural and binaural stimulation. Acta oto-laryng. (Stockh.) **68**, 317—326 (1969).

BUTLER, R. A., KLUSKENS, L.: The influence of phase inversion on the auditory evoked response. Audiology **10**, 353—357 (1971).

BUTLER, R. A., SPRENG, M., KEIDEL, W. D.: Stimulus repetition rate factors which influence the auditory evoked potential in man. Psychophysiol. **5**, 665—672 (1969).

CALLAWAY, E.: Averaged evoked responses in psychiatry. J. nerv. ment. Dis. **143**, 80—94 (1966).

CALVET, J., THIEFFRY, M.: Analyse statistique des activités électrocorticales à type de fuseaux. J. Physiol. (Paris) **58**, 485—486 (1966).

CASPERS, H.: Die Beeinflussung der corticalen Gleichspannung durch sensible und sensorische Reize beim wachen, frei beweglichen Tier. Pflügers Arch. ges. Physiol. **272**, 53—54 (1960/61).

CASPERS, H., SCHULZE, H.: Die Veränderungen der corticalen Gleichspannung während der natürlichen Schlaf-Wach-Perioden beim freibeweglichen Tier. Pflügers Arch. ges. Physiol. **270**, 103—120 (1959).

CELESIA, G. G., BROUGHTON, R. J., RASMUSSEN, T., BRANCH, CH.: Auditory evoked responses from the exposed human cortex. Electroenceph. clin. Neurophysiol. **24**, 458—466 (1968).

CHALOUPKA, Z.: Comparison of the reproduction of cortical auditory responses to rhythmic acoustical stimulation in various species of mammals (dog, cat, rabbit, guinea-pig). Activ. nerv. sup. (Praha) 8, 176—177 (1966).

CHALOUPKA, Z., VOZEH, F., CHARLIER, M.: Cortical evoked potentials in dependence on different levels of nutrition. Activ. nerv. sup. (Praha) **11**, 283—284 (1969).

CHATRIAN, G. E., PETERSEN, M. C., LAZARTE, J. A.: Responses to clicks from the human brain: some depth electrographic observations. Electroenceph. clin. Neurophysiol. **12**, 479—489 (1960).

Chow, K. L., Randall, W., Morrell, F.: Effect of brain lesions on conditioned cortical electropotentials. Electroenceph. clin. Neurophysiol. **20**, 357—369 (1966).

Ciganek, L.: Evoked potentials in man: interaction of sound and light. Electroenceph. clin. Neurophysiol. **21**, 28—33 (1966).

Ciganek, L.: A comparative study of visual, auditory and somatosensory EEG responses in man. Exp. Brain Res. **4**, 118—125 (1967).

Clark, D. L., Butler, R. A., Rosner, B. S.: Dissociation of sensation and evoked response by a general anaesthetic in man. J. comp. physiol. Psychol. **68**, 315—319 (1969).

Coats, A. C., Dickey, J. R.: Nonsurgical recording of human auditory nerve action potentials and cochlear microphonics. Ann. Otol. (St. Louis) **79**, 844 (1970).

Cobb, W., Morocutti, C.: The evoked potentials. Electroenceph. clin. Neurophysiol. Suppl. **26**, (1967).

Cody, D. T. R., Bickford, R. G.: Cortical audiometry; an objective method of evaluating auditory acuity in man. Proc. Mayo Clin. **40**, 273—287 (1965).

Collard, M., Conraux, C., Picart, P., Greiner, G. F., Rohmer, F.: Recherche de potentiels évoqués d'origine vestibulaire chez l'homme. Rev. neurol. **117**, 218—221 (1967).

Commichau, R.: Adaptationszustand und Unterschieds-Schwellenenergie für Lichtblitze. Z. Biol. **108**, 145—160 (1956).

Cook, J. D., Ellinwood, E. H. Jr., Wilson, W. P.: Auditory habituation at primary cortex as a function of stimulus rate. Exp. Neurol. **21**, 167—175 (1968).

Cooper, R., Winter, A. L., Crow, H. J., Grey Walter, W.: Comparison of subcortical, cortical and scalp activity using chronically indwelling electrodes in man. Electroenceph. clin. Neurophysiol. **18**, 217—228 (1965).

Cowen, M. A.: Some higher functional correlates of the transcephalic d. c. circuit. Psychiat. Quart. **42**, 409—429 (1968).

Cowen, M. A., Ross, J.: Some biochemical factors that modify the transcephalic dc potential. Psychophysiology **4**, 90—98 (1967).

Cowen, M. A., Ross, J., McDonald, R.: Some aspects of the transcephalic dc circuit. Psychophysiology **4**, 207—215 (1967).

Creutzfeldt, O., Lux, D., Nacimiento, A. C.: Intracelluläre Reizung corticaler Nervenzellen im motorischen Cortex der Katze. Pflügers Arch. ges. Physiol. **278**, 68 (1963).

Creutzfeldt, O. D., Kuhnt, U.: The visual evoked potential: Physiological, developmental and clinical aspects. Electroenceph. clin. Neurophysiol. Suppl. **26**, 29—41 (1967).

Creutzfeldt, O., Rosina, A., Ito, M., Probst, W.: Visual evoked response of single cells and of the EEG in primary visual area of the cat. J. Neurophysiol. **32**, 127—139 (1969).

Dagnino, N., Favale, E., Loeb, C., Manfredi, M.: Sensory transmission in the geniculostriate system of the cat during natural sleep and arousal. J. Neurophysiol. **28**, 443—456 (1965).

David, E., Finkenzeller, P., Spreng, M.: Komplexe akustisch evozierte Potentiale der wachen Katze (implantierte Elektroden-AI). Pflügers Arch. ges. Physiol. **291**, 45 (1966).

David, E., Finkenzeller, P., Kallert, S., Keidel, W. D.: Reizfrequenzkorrelierte ,,untersetzte" neuronale Entladungsperiodizität im Colliculus inferior und im Corpus geniculatum mediale. Pflügers Arch. **309**, 11—20 (1969a).

David, E., Finkenzeller, P., Kallert, S., Keidel, W. D.: Reizkorrelierte Gleichspannungsänderungen der primären Hörrinde an der wachen Katze. Pflügers Arch. **306**, 281—289 (1969b).

David, E., Finkenzeller, P., Kallert, S., Keidel, W. D.: Akustisch ausgelöste Gleichspannungspotentiale am Menschen. Pflügers Arch. **307**, 137 (1969c).

David, E., Finkenzeller, P., Kallert, S., Keidel, W. D.: Akustischen Reizen zugeordnete Gleichspannungsänderungen am intakten Schädel des Menschen. Pflügers Arch. **309**, 362—367 (1969d).

David, E., Finkenzeller, P., Kallert, S., Keidel, W. D.: Wechselwirkung zwischen optisch und akustisch ausgelösten Gleichspannungspotentialen am Menschen. Pflügers Arch. **312**, 131 (1969e).

David, E., Finkenzeller, P., Kallert, S., Keidel, W. D.: Interaction between visually and auditorily evoked DC-potentials in man. In: Drischel, H., Tiedt, N. (Eds.): Biokybernetik, Band III. Jena: VEB Gustav Fischer 1971.

DAVID, E., FINKENZELLER, P., KALLERT, S., KEIDEL, W. D.: Korrelationsanalyse von gemittelten und ungemittelten evozierten Potentialen. Kybernetik **9**, 22—26 (1971).

DAVIS, H.: Enhancement of evoked cortical potentials in humans related to a task requiring a decision. Science **145**, 182—183 (1964).

DAVIS, H.: Validation of evoked-response audiometry (ERA) in deaf children. Int. Audiology—Audiologie Internationale **5**, 77—81 (1966).

DAVIS, H.: Averaged-evoked-response EEG audiometry in North America. Acta oto-laryng. (Stockh.) **65**, 79—85 (1968).

DAVIS, H.: Evoked response audiometry. Trans. Amer. Acad. Ophthal. Otolaryng. **74**, 1236—1237 (1970).

DAVIS, H.: Interactions of tactile and electric stimuli with auditory V potentials. Arch. klin. exp. Ohr-, Nas.- u. Kehlk.-Heilk. **198**, 108—109 (1971).

DAVIS, H.: Sedation of young children for ERA. ERA, 18th Issue, December 1971.

DAVIS, H.: Is ERA ready for routine clinical use? Arch. klin. exp. Ohr.-, Nas.- u. Kehlk.-Heilk. **198**, 2—8 (1971).

DAVIS, H.: Sedation of young children for electric response audiometry (ERA). (Summary of a symposium.) Transactions, Released August 1972.

DAVIS, H.: Sedation of young children for electric response audiometry (ERA). Summary of a symposium. Audiology **12**, 55—57 (1973).

DAVIS, H.: Classes of auditory evoked responses. Audiology **12**, 464—469 (1973).

DAVIS, H.: Relations of peripheral action potentials and cortical evoked potentials to the magnitude of sensation. In: MOSKOWITZ, H. R., SCHARF, B., STEVENS, J. C. (Eds.): Sensation and measurement. Dordrecht-Holland/Boston-USA: D. Reidel Publ. Comp. 1974.

DAVIS, H.: Electric response audiometry, with special reference to the vertex potentials. In: KEIDEL, W. D., NEFF, W. D. (Eds.): Handbook of sensory physiology, Vol. V/3. Berlin-Heidelberg-New York: Springer 1976.

DAVIS, H., DAVIS, P. A., LOOMIS, A. L., HARVEY, E. N., HOBART, G.: Electrical reactions of the human brain to auditory stimulation during sleep. J. Neurophysiol. **2**, 500—514 (1939).

DAVIS, H., ENGEBRETSON, M., LOWELL, E. L., MAST, T., SATTERFIELD, J., YOSHIE, N.: Evoked responses to clicks recorded from the human scalp. Ann. N. Y. Acad. Sci. **112**, 224—225 (1964).

DAVIS, H., HIRSH, S. K., SHELNUTT, J., BOWERS, C.: Further validation of evoked response audiometry (ERA). J. Speech Res. **10**, 717—732 (1967).

DAVIS, H., MAST, T., YOSHIE, N., ZERLIN, S.: The slow response of the human cortex to auditory stimuli: recovery process. Electroenceph. clin. Neurophysiol. **21**, 105—113 (1966).

DAVIS, H., NIEMOELLER, A. F.: A system for clinical evoked response audiometry. J. Speech Dis. **33**, 33—37 (1968).

DAVIS, H., OSTERHAMMEL, P. A., WIER, C. C., GJERDINGEN, D. B.: Slow vertex potentials: interactions among auditory, tactile, electric and visual stimuli. Electroenceph. clin. Neurophysiol. **33**, 537—545 (1972).

DAVIS, H., YOSHIE, N.: Human cortical response to auditory stimuli. Physiologist **6**, 164 (1963).

DAVIS, H., ZERLIN, S.: Acoustic relations of the human vertex potential. J. acoust. Soc. Amer. **39**, 109—116 (1966).

DAVIS, P. A.: Effects of acoustic stimuli on the waking human brain. J. Neurophysiol. **2**, 494—499 (1939).

DEBECKER, J., DESMEDT, J. E.: Rate of intermodality switching disclosed by sensory evoked potentials averaged during signal detection tasks. J. Physiol. (Lond.) **185**, 52—53 P (1966).

DEBECKER, J., DESMEDT, J. E.: Cerebral Evoked potential correlates in forced-paced tasks. Nature (Lond.) New Biol. **234**, 118—120 (1971).

DEBECKER, J., DESMEDT, J. E., ECTORS, M.: Etude des potentiels évoqués chez l'homme. Arch. int. Physiol. Biochim. **75**, 353—354 (1967).

DEBECKER, J., DESMEDT, J. E., MANIL, J.: Corrélations psychologiques des potentiels évoqués cérébraux. J. Physiol. (Paris) **57**, 595 (1965).

DELGADO, J. M. R.: Prolonged stimulation of brain in awake monkeys. J. Neurophysiol. **22**, 458—475 (1959).

DERBYSHIRE, A. J., DRIESSEN, G. J., PALMER, C. W.: Technical advances in the analysis of single, acoustically evoked potentials. Electroenceph. clin. Neurophysiol. **22**, 476—481 (1967).

DESMEDT, J. E., DEBECKER, J.: The somatosensory cerebral evoked potentials of the sleeping human newborn. In: CLEMENTE, C. D., PURPURA, D. P., MAYER, F. E. (Eds.): Sleep and the maturing nervous system. New York: Academic Press 1972.

DESMEDT, J. E., DEBECKER, J., MANIL, J.: Mise en évidence d'un signe électrique cérébral associé à la détection par le sujet, d'un stimulus sensoriel tactile. Bull. Acad. Méd. Belg. **5**, 887—936 (1965).

DESMEDT, J. E., MANIL, J.: Somatosensory evoked potentials of the normal human neonate in REM sleep, in slow wave sleep and in waking. Electroenceph. clin. Neurophysiol. **29**, 113—126 (1970).

DESMEDT, J. E., MANIL, J., CHORAZYNA, H., DEBECKER, J.: Potentiel évoqué cérébral et conduction corticipète pour une volée d'influx somesthésique chez le nouveau-né normal. C. R. Soc. Biol. **161**, 205 (1967).

DESMEDT, J. E., NOËL, P.: Average cerebral evoked potentials in the evaluation of lesions of the sensory nerves and of the central somatosensory pathway. In: DESMEDT, J. E. (ed.): New developments in electromyography and clinical neurophysiology. Basel: Karger 1973.

DEZA, L., EIDELBERG, E.: Development of cortical electrical activity in the rat. Exp. Neurol. **17**, 425—438 (1967).

DONCHIN, E.: A multivariate approach to the analysis of average evoked potentials. IEEE Transa. Bio-Med. Eng. **13**, 131—139 (1966).

DONCHIN, E., COHEN, L.: Averaged evoked potentials and intramodality selective attention. Electroenceph. clin, Neurophysiol. **22**, 537—546 (1967).

DONCHIN, E., LINDSLEY, D. B.: Average evoked potentials. Washington, D.C.: NASA SP-191 1966.

DONCHIN, E., SUTTON, S.: The psychological significance of evoked responses: A comment on CLARK, BUTLER, and ROSNER. Commun. Behavioral Biol. 5, 111—114 (1970).

DORMONT, J. F., MASSION, J.: Étude topographique des relations entre le cortex cérébral et le noyau ventrolatéral. J. Physiol. (Paris) **59**, 233 (1967).

DOWNMAN, C. B. B., WOOLSEY, C. N., LENDE, R. A.: Auditory areas I, II and Ep: Cochlear representation, afferent paths and interconnections. Bull. Johns Hopkins Hosp. **106**, 127—142 (1960).

DUMERMUTH, G.: Electronic data processing in pediatric EEG research. Neuropädiatrie **4**, 349—374 (1971).

DUMERMUTH, G., HUBER, P. J., KLEINER, B., GASSER, T.: Numerical analysis of electroencephalographic data. IEEE Trans. Audio Electroacoustics AU-**18**, 404—411 (1970).

DUNLOP, C. W., WEBSTER, W. R., RODGER, R. S.: Amplitude changes of evoked potentials in the auditory system of unanesthetized cats during acoustic habituation. J. Aud. Res. **6**, 47—66 (1966).

DUNLOP, C. W., ITZKOWIC, D. J., AITKIN, L. M.: Tone-burst response patterns of single units in the cat medial geniculate body. Brain Res. **16**, 149—164 (1969).

DUSTMAN, R. E., BECK, E. C.: Long-term stability of visually evoked potentials in man. Science **142**, 1480—1481 (1963).

EGGERMONT, J. J.: Analog modelling of cochlear adaptation. Kybernetik **14**, 117—126 (1973).

EGGERMONT, J. J.: Basic principles for electrocochleography. Acta otolaryng. (Stockh.) Suppl. **316**, 7—16 (1974).

EGGERMONT, J. J.: Electrocochleography and recruitment. IV. Biennial Symposium der International ERA Study Group, London 28.—30.7. 1975a. To be submitted to the Ann. Otol. (St. Louis).

EGGERMONT, J. J.: Summating potentials in electrocochleography: Relation to hearing pathology. IV. Biennial Symposium der International ERA Study Group, London 28.—30.7. 1975b.

EGGERMONT, J. J.: Compound action potential responses to tonebursts in the human and guinea pig cochlea. IV. Biennial Symposium der International ERA Study Group, London 28.—30.7. 1975c. To be submitted to JASA.

EGGERMONT, J. J.: Cochlear adaptation: A theoretical description. Biol. Cybernetics **19**, 181—189 (1975d).

EGGERMONT, J. J., ODENTHAL, D. W.: Methods in electrocochleography. Acta oto-laryng. (Stockh.) Suppl. **316**, 17—24 (1974).

EGGERMONT, J. J., ODENTHAL, D. W., SCHMIDT, P. H., SPOOR, A.: Electrocochleography. Basis principles and clinical application. Acta oto-laryng. (Stockh.) Suppl. **316** (1974a).

EGGERMONT, J. J., SPOOR, A., ODENTHAL, D. W.: Frequency specificity of tone-burst electrocochleography. To be published in: RUBEN, ELBERLIN, SALAMON (eds.): Proc. electrocochleography conference. New York: 1974b.

EHRENBERGER, K., SCHÖNE, W., SPRENG, M.: Corticogramme der somatischen Rinde SI der Katze bei beidseitiger vibratorischer Reizung der Schnurrhaare. Pflügers Arch. ges. Physiol. **286**, 159—170 (1965).

EHRENBERGER, K., FINKENZELLER, P., KEIDEL, W. D., PLATTIG, K. H.: Elektrophysiologische Korrelation der Stevensschen Potenzfunktion und objektive Schwellenmessung am Vibrationssinn des Menschen. Pflügers Arch. ges. Physiol. **290**, 114—123 (1966).

ELBERLING, C., SALOMON, G.: Electrrical potentials from the inner ear in man, in response to transient sounds generated in a closed acoustic system. Rev. Laryng. (Bordeaux) Suppl. **691** (1971).

ELLINWOOD, E. H. JR., COOK, J. D., WILSON, W. P.: Periodic evoked response amplitude fluctuation in the auditory cortex as a function of changing interaural stimulus intervals. Brain Res. **9**, 59—70 (1968).

EULER, C. VON, GREEN, J. D., RICCI, G.: The role of hippocampal dendrites in evoked responses and after-discharges. Acta physiol. scand. **42**, 87—111 (1958).

EVANS, E. F., WILSON, J. P.: The frequency selectivity of cochlea. In: MØLLER, A. R. (ed.): Basic mechanisms in hearing. New York-London: Academic Press 1973.

EWERTSEN, H. W., BIRK-NIELSEN, H.: Social hearing handicap index. Audiology **12**, 180—187 (1973).

FELDMAN, S., HEIDE, C. S. VAN DER, PORTER, R. W.: Evoked potentials in the hypothalamus. Amer. J. Physiol. **196**, 1163—1167 (1959).

FELDTKELLER, R., ZWICKER, E.: Das Ohr als Nachrichtenempfänger. Stuttgart: Hirzel 1956.

FINKENZELLER, P.: Gemittelte EEG-Potentiale bei olfactorischer Reizung. Pflügers Arch. ges. Physiol. **292**, 76—80 (1966).

FINKENZELLER, P.: Die Mitteilung von Reaktionspotentialen. Kybernetik **6**, 22—44 (1969).

FINKENZELLER, P., DAVID, E., KALLERT, S., KEIDEL, W. D.: Die Aussagekraft gemittelter Potentiale. Pflügers Arch. **307**, 136 (1969).

FINKENZELLER, P., KEIDEL, W. D.: Eigenschaften akustisch evozierter Potentiale bei Gleichspannungsregistrierung. Arch. Oto-Rhino-Laryng. **207**, 508 (1974).

FINKENZELLER, P., KEIDEL, W. D.: Correlates of auditory perception in averaged perstimulatory EEG-DC-recordings. Communication at the second symposium of the Study Group for Methodology in Electroencephalography from 30.4.—4.5. 75 in Vevey, Switzerland.

FINKENZELLER, P., KEIDEL, W. D.: Evoked potentials to evaluate the perception of complex sounds. IV. Biennial Symposium der International ERA Study Group in London, 28.—30.7. 1975b. To be published in: International Audiology.

FISHMAN, M. C., MICHAEL, C. R.: Integration of auditory information in the cat's visual cortex. Vision Res. **13**, 1415—1419 (1973).

FLACH, M., SEIDEL, P.: Mikrophonpotentiale (MP) des menschlichen Ohres. Arch. klin. Ohr.-, Nas.- u. Kehlk.-Heilk. **190**, 229—243 (1968).

FLECHSIG, P. E.: Die Leitungsbahnen im Gehirn und Rückenmark des Menschen. Leipzig: W. Engelmann 1876.

FLEISCHL VON MARXOW, E.: Mittheilung, betreffend die Physiologie der Hirnrinde. Zbl. Physiol. **4**, 537—540 (1890).

FOX, M. W.: The effects of short-term social and sensory isolation upon behavior, EEG and averaged evoked potentials in puppies. Physiol. Behav. **2**, 145—151 (1967).

FRANZÉN, O., OFFENLOCH, K.: Evoked response correlates of psychophysical magnitude estimates for tactile stimulation in man. Exp. Brain Res. 8, 1—18 (1969).

FREEMAN, W. J.: Relations between unit activity and evoked potentials in prepyriform cortex of cats. J. Neurophysiol. **31**, 337—348 (1968).

FRENCH, J. D., HERNANDEZ-PEON, R., LIVINGSTON, R. B.: Projections from cortex to cephalic brainstem (reticular formation) in monkey. J. Neurophysiol. **18**, 74—95 (1955).

FRITZSCH, G. T., HITZIG, E.: Über die electrische Erregbarkeit des Großhirns. Arch. v. Reichert u. DuBois-Reymond **1870**, 300—332. Referiert in: Centralbl. med. Wiss. **9**, 132 (1871).

FROMM, G. H., BOND, H. W.: The relationship between neuron activity and cortical steady potentials. Electroenceph. clin. Neurophysiol. **22**, 159—166 (1967).

FRUHSTORFER, H.: Der Einfluß von Reizfolgefrequenz, Reizanzahl und Reizort auf die Intensitätsabhängigkeit vibratorisch ausgelöster corticaler Antworten beim Menschen. Dissertation, Erlangen 1966.

FRUHSTORFER, H.: Habituation and dishabituation of the human vertex response. Electroenceph. clin. Neurophysiol. **30**, 306—312 (1971).

FRUHSTORFER, H., BERGSTRÖM, R. M.: Human vigilance and auditory evoked responses. Electroenceph. clin. Neurophysiol. **27**, 346—355 (1969).

FRUHSTORFER, H., SOVERI, P., JÄRVILEHTO, T.: Short-term habituation of the auditory evoked response in man. Electroenceph. clin. Neurophysiol. **28**, 153—161 (1970).

GALAMBOS, R.: The human auditory evoked response. In: MOSKOWITZ, H. R., SCHARF, B., STEVENS, J. C. (eds.): Sensation and measurement. Dordrecht-Holland/Boston-USA: D. Reidel 1974.

GALAMBOS, R., MYERS, R. E., SHEATZ, G. C.: Extralemniscal activation of auditory cortex in cats. Amer. J. Physiol. **200**, 23—28 (1961).

GASTAUT, H.: Some aspects of the neurophysiological basis of conditioned reflexes and behavior. In: WOLSTENHOLME, G. E. W., O'CONNOR, C. M. (eds.): Ciba foundation symposium on the neurological basis of behavior. Boston: Little, Brown and Co. 1958.

GEISLER, C. D.: Electrical responses to acoustic clicks in monkeys. Quart. Progr. Rep. No. 53, MIT Cambridge, April 15, 184—187 (1959).

GEISLER, C. D.: Electrical responses to acoustic clicks recorded from human scalp. Quart. Progr. Rep. No. 57, MIT Cambridge, April 15, 137—143 (1960).

GEISLER, C. D., FRISHKOPF, L. S.: Development of the K-complex with sleep. Quart. Progr. Report, MIT Cambridge, July 15, 148—150 (1957).

GEISLER, C. D., FRISHKOPF, L. S., BROWN, R. M.: The early response to clicks in awake subjects. Quart. Progr. Rep. MIT Cambridge, July 15, 144—148 (1957).

GEISLER, C. D., FRISHKOPF, L. S., ROSENBLITH, W. A.: Extracranial responses to acoustic clicks in man. Science **128**, 1210—1211 (1958).

GERIN, P., MORGON, A., CHARACHON, D., MUNIER, F., PERNIER, J., ARNAL, D., LEBRETON, M. F.: Une methode d'audiometrie objective — l'audiometrie electroencephalographique. J. franç. Oto-rhino-laryng. **17**, 547—595 (1968).

GERKEN, G. M., NEFF, W. D.: Experimental procedures affecting evoked responses recorded from auditory cortex. Electroenceph. clin. Neurophysiol. **15**, 947—957 (1963).

GERULL, G., GIESEN, M., MROWINSKI, D., RUDOLPH, N.: Audiologie und Phoniatrie. Untersuchung eines frühen, von der Kopfhaut ableitbaren Potentials für die objektive Audiometrie. H.N.O. (Berl.) **20**, 339—343 (1972).

GERULL, G., GIESEN, M., MROWINSKI, D., RUDOLPH, N.: Properties of an early AER of 6—10 ms latency. IIIrd Symposium of the International Electric Response Audiometry Study Group, 10.—12. Sept. 1973 in Bordeaux.

GERULL, G., GIESEN, M., MROWINSKI, D., RUDOLPH, N.: Klinischer Einsatz verschiedener ERA-Verfahren zur Untersuchung von Funktionsstörungen der Hörbahn. Laryng. Rhinol. **54**, 671—676 (1975).

GESTRING, G. F., BURIAN, K., INNITZER, J.: Computer sweep-splitting for simultaneous ECOG and ERA display. IIIrd Symposium of the International Electric Response Audiometry Study Group, 10.—12. September 1973, Bordeaux.

GOLD, A., WILPIZESKI, C. R.: Studies in auditory adaptation: II. Some effects of sodium salicylate on evoked auditory potentials in cats. Laryngoscope **76**, 674—685 (1966).

GOLDBERG, J. M., NEFF, W. D.: Frequency discrimination after bilateral section of the brachium of the inferior colliculus. J. comp. Neurol. **116**, 256—290 (1961).

GOLDRING, S., O'LEARY, J. L.: Cortical d. c. changes incident to midline thalamic stimulation. Electroenceph. clin. Neurophysiol. **9**, 577—584 (1957).

GOLDRING, S., O'LEARY, J. L.: Pharmacological dissolution of evoked cortical potentials. Fed. Proc. **19**, 612—618 (1960).

GOLDRING, S., SHEPTAK, P., KARAHASHI, Y.: Averaged responses from association areas in waking cat. Electroenceph. clin. Neurophysiol. **23**, 241—247 (1967).

GOLDSTEIN, M. H. JR., KIANG, N. Y. S.: Responses at the auditory cortex to repetitive stimuli. Quart. Progr. Rep. MIT Cambridge, April 15, 135—139 (1957).

GRAZIANI, L. J., WEITZMAN, E. D., VELASCO, M. S. A.: Neurologic maturation and auditory evoked responses in low birth weight infants. Pediatric **41**, 483—494 (1968).

GROSS, M. M., BEGLEITER, H., TOBIN, M., KISSIN, B.: Changes in auditory evoked response induced by alcohol. J. nerv. ment. Dis. **143**, 152—156 (1966).

GUMNIT, R. J.: D. C. Potential changes from auditory cortex of cat. J. Neurophysiol. **23**, 667—675 (1960).

GUMNIT, R. J.: The distribution of direct current responses evoked by sounds in the auditory cortex of the cat. Electroenceph. clin. Neurophysiol. **13**, 889—895 (1961).

GUMNIT, R. J., GROSSMAN, R. G.: Potentials evoked by sound in the auditory cortex of the cat. Amer. J. Physiol. **200**, 1219—1225 (1961).

GUTH, S. L.: Patterning effects with compound stimuli. J. comp. physiol. Psychol. **63**, 480—485 (1967).

HAIDER, M.: Erwartungswirkung, Antizipation und corticale evozierte Potentiale. Electroenceph. clin. Neurophysiol. 88, 167—168 (1965).

HAIDER, M.: Corticale evozierte Potentiale, Vigilanz und Aufmerksamkeit. In: HECKHAUSEN, H.; herausgegeben im Auftrage der Deutschen Gesellschaft für Psychologie. (Hrsg.): Bericht über den 24. Kongreß der Deutschen Gesellschaft für Psychologie. Göttingen: Verlag für Psychologie, Dr. C. J. Hogrefe 1965.

HAIDER, M., SPONG, P., LINDSLEY, D. B.: Attention, vigilance, and cortical evoked-potentials in humans. Science **145**, 180—182 (1964).

HAIDER, M., GROLL, E., STUDYNKA, G.: Orientierungs- und Bereitschaftspotentiale bei unerwarteten Reizen. Exp. Brain Res. **5**, 45—54 (1968).

HÄKKINEN, V., FRUHSTORFER, H.: Correlation between spontaneous activity and auditory evoked responses in the human EEG. Acta neurol. scand. **43**, Suppl. 31, 160—161 (1967)

HALL, R. A., RAPPAPORT, M., HOPKINS, H. K., GRIFFIN, R.: Tobacco and evoked potential. Science **180**, 212—214 (1973).

HALL, R. D.: Habituation of evoked potentials in the rat under conditions of behavioral control. Electroenceph. clin. Neurophysiol. **24**, 155—165 (1968).

HALL, R. D., MARK, R. G.: Fear and the modification of acoustically evoked potentials during conditioning. J. Neurophysiol. **30**, 893—910 (1967).

HARLY, S., NEERGAARD, E. B., HARBO, A., BLEGVAD ANDERSEN, O., ELBRØND, O.: Registration of acoustically evoked vertex potentials with unconventional averaging technique. Acta oto-laryng. (Stockh.) **263**, 242—244 (1970).

HASSMANNOVÁ, J., SPECTOR, I.: Relations fonctionnelles entre relais acoustique (G. M.) et claustrum. J. Physiol. (Paris) **59**, 427—428 (1967).

HASSMANNOVÁ, J., MYSLIVEČEK, J.: Maturation of the primary cortical response to stimulation of medial geniculate body. Electroenceph. clin. Neurophysiol. **22**, 547—555 (1967).

HAWKINS, J. E. JR.: Disturbances of vestibular function produced in animals by streptomycin. Fed. Proc. **6**, 125 (1947).

HAWKINS, J. E. JR.: Cochlear signs of streptomycin intoxication. J. Pharmacol. exp. Ther. **100**, 38—44 (1950).

HAWKINS, J. E. JR.: The Ototoxicity of Hydrostreptomycin. Transactions of the 10th Conference on the Chemotherapy of Tuberculosis (Streptomycin Conference), held on 25. to 28. Jan. 1951 at the Fulton County Medical Society, Atlanta Georgia.

HAY, I. S., DAVIS, H.: Slow cortical evoked potentials: Interactions of auditory, vibro-tactile and shock stimuli. Audiology **10**, 9—17 (1971).

HENINGER, G. R., MCDONALD, R. K., GOFF, W. R., SOLLBERGER, A.: Diural Variations in the cerebral evoked response and EEG. Arch. Neurol. **21**, 330—337 (1969).

HERMANS, J., EGGERMONT, J. J., HAGEDOOREN, J., ODENTHAL, D. W.: Probabilistic differential diagnosis of auditory dysfunction on the basis of electrocochleography. Meth. inform. Med. **14**, 87—95 (1975).

HILGER, J. A., BOIES, L. R. JR., ROTH, N. A.: Percutaneous recording of cochlear microphonics in cats. Arch. Otolaryng. **82**, 591—593 (1965).

HILLYARD, S. A., GALAMBOS, R.: Effects of stimulus and response contingencies on a surface negative slow potential shift in man. Electroenceph. clin. Neurophysiol. **22**, 297—304 (1967).

HIRSCH, J.-C.: Électrophysiologie. Variations selon les modalités d'enregistrement de l'électrocorticogramme d'un gyrus cortical isolé. C. R. Acad. Sci. Paris **263**, 778—780 (1966), Série D.

HIRSCH, J.-C., HIRSCH, J.-F., LANDAU-FEREY, J., HUGUENARD, P., SCHERRER, J.: Modifications du tracé électrique du cortex isolé par les anesthésiques. J. Physiol. (Paris) **59**, 429 (1967).

HIRSH, S. K.: Vertex potentials associated with an auditory discrimination. Psychon. Sci. **22**, 173—175 (1971).

HOFFMAN, J. P., WALKER, J. V. JR., WOLIN, L. R., KADOYA, S., MASSOPUST, L. C. JR.: Evoked responses in the auditory cortex of the cebus monkey. J. Aud. Res. **9**, 89—99 (1969).

HOLM, C., STANGE, G.: Pathologische ERA-Kennlinien als Kriterien zur Wirkungsweise von Hörtrainern. Arch. klin. exp. Ohr.-, Nas.- u. Kehlk.-Heilk. **202**, 471—476 (1972).

HOLM, C., STANGE, G.: Überschwellige ERA-Befunde als therapeutische Basis zur Versorgung innenohrgeschädigter Kinder. H.N.O. (Berl.) **21**, 163—166 (1973).

HOLMES, O., SHORT, A. D.: Correlation between evoked potentials and spontaneous activity in the cortex cerebri of rats. J. Physiol. (Lond.) **204**, 84P (1969).

HORN, G., HILL, R. M.: Effect of removing the neocortex on the response to repeated sensory stimulation of neurones in the mid-brain. Nature (Lond.) **211**, 754—755 (1966).

HORVATH, F., BUSER, P.: Facteurs affectant la répartition corticale des fuseaux évoqués chez le chat. J. Physiol. (Paris) **58**, 534 (1966).

HORVATH, R. S.: Variability of cortical auditory evoked response. J. Neurophysiol. **32**, 1056—1063 (1969).

HOTTA, T., KAMEDA, K.: Interactions between somatic and visual or auditory responses in the thalamus of the cat. Exp. Neurol. 8, 1—13 (1963).

HOTTA, T., TERASHIMA, S.: Audiovisual interaction and its correlation with cortical stimulation in the lateral thalamus. Exp. Neurol. **12**, 146—158 (1965).

HOUCHIN, J.: Cortical potentials evoked by pairs of peripheral stimuli. J. Physiol. (Lond.) **204**, 75—77P (1969).

HRBEK, A., HRBKOVA, M., LENARD, H.-G.: Somato-sensory, auditory and visual evoked responses in newborn infants during sleep and wakefulness. Electroenceph. clin. Neurophysiol. **26**, 597—603 (1969).

HUGELIN, A., BONVALLET, M.: Tonus cortical et controle de la facilitation motrice d'origine reticulaire. J. Physiol. (Paris) **49**, 1171—1200 (1957).

HUTT, S. J., HUTT, C., LENARD, H. G., BERNUTH, H. v., MUNTJEWERFF, W. J.: Auditory responsivity in the human neonate. Nature (Lond.) **218**, 888—890 (1968).

IRWIN, D. A., KNOTT, J. R., MCADAM, D. W., REBERT, C. S.: Motivational determinants of the contingent negative variation. Electroenceph. clin. Neurophysiol. **21**, 538—543 (1966).

JACOBSON, J. L., CODY, D. T., LAMBERT, E. H., BICKFORD, R. G.: Physiological properties of the postauricular responses (sonomotor) in man. Physiologist **7**, 167 (1964).

JAFFE, S. L., BOURLIER, P. F., HAGAMEN, W. D.: Adaptation of evoked auditory potentials: A midbrain through frontal lobe map in the unanesthetized cat. Brain Res. **15**, 121—136 (1969).

JANE, J. A., MASTERTON, R. B., DIAMOND, I. T.: The function of the tectum for attention to auditory stimuli in the cat. J. comp. Neurol. **125**, 165—192 (1965).

JÄRVILEHTO, T., FRUHSTORFER, H.: Differenciation between slow cortical potentials associated with motor and mental acts in man. Exp. Brain Res. **11**, 309—317 (1970).

JÄRVILEHTO, T., FRUHSTORFER, H.: Is the sound-evoked DC potential a contingent negative variation? Electroenceph. clin. Neurophysiol., Suppl. **33**, 105—108 (1973).

JAUHIAINEN, T.: Objektiivinen audiometria. Eripainos Akustinen Aikakauslehti **4**, 12—13 (1966).

JAUHIAINEN, T., PLATTIG, K. H.: Reizsynchrone langsame Rindenpotentiale beim Menschen nach elektrischer Reizung der Zunge. Pflügers Arch. ges. Physiol. **289**, R 27 (1966).

JEWETT, D. L., ROMANO, M. N., WILLISTON, J. S.: Human auditory evoked potentials: Possible brain stem components detected on the scalp. Science **167**, 1517—1518 (1970).

JOHANNSEN, H. S., KEIDEL, W. D., SPRENG, M.: Der Einfluß von Intensität und Dauer der Beschallung auf den Off-Effekt des akustisch evozierten Potentials. Arch. klin. exp. Ohr.-, Nas.- u. Kehlk.-Heilk. **201**, 208—221 (1972).

JUNG, R., KORNHUBER, H. D., DAFONESCA, J. D.: Multisensory convergence on cortical neurons. In: MORUZZI, G., FESSARD, A., JASPER, H. H. (eds.): Brain mechanisms. Progress in brain research, Vol. 1. Amsterdam-London-New York: Elsevier 1963.

KADO, R. T., ADEY, W. R.: Electrode problems in central nervous monitoring in performing subjects. Ann. N. Y. Acad. Sci. **148**, 263—278 (1968).

KALLERT, S.: Über die Reizantwort einzelner Zellen im Corpus geniculatum mediale der Katze bei Untersuchung mit Mikroelektroden. Dissertationsarbeit, Erlangen 1972.

KALLERT, S.: Telemetrische Mikroelektrodenuntersuchungen am Corpus geniculatum mediale der wachen Katze. Habilitationsschrift, Erlangen 1973.

KALLERT, S., DAVID, E., FINKENZELLER, P.: Reizintensitätsabhängige Aktivitätsänderungen einzelner Neurone in den höheren Kerngebieten der spezifischen Hörbahn. Pflügers Arch. ges. Physiol. **297**, R 29 (1967).

KALLERT, S., DAVID, E., FINKENZELLER, P., KEIDEL, W. D.: Two different neuronal discharge periodicities in the acoustical channel. In: PLOMP, R., SMOORENBURG, G. F. (eds.): Frequency analysis and periodicity detection in hearing. Leiden: A. W. Sijthoff 1970.

KARNAHL, TH., BENNING, C. D.: Effect of sedation upon evoked response audiometry: Amplitude and latency vs sound pressure level. Arch. klin. exp. Ohr.-, Nas.- u. Kehlk.-Heilk. **201**, 181—188 (1972).

KARNAHL, TH., STANGE, G.: Ergebnisse bei der Standardisierung der Electric Response Audiometry (ERA). Arch. klin. exp. Ohr.-, Nas.- u. Kehlk.-Heilk. **202**, 452—457 (1972).

KARNAHL, TH., BENNING, C.-D., STANGE, G.: Akustisch evozierte, aus dem EEG gemittelte Potentiale beim Erwachsenen unter dem Einfluß von Sedativa und Psychopharmaka. Dtsch. med. Wschr. **97**, 1102—1103 (1972).

KARNAHL, TH., BENNING, C.-D., STANGE, G.: Acoustically evoked, EEG-derived potentials in adults under the influence of sedatives and psychoactive drugs. Germ. Med. **2**, 101—102 (1972).

KARNAHL, TH., SPRENG, M., STANGE, G.: Calculations of ERA-potentials (CAT 1000 and PDP-12). Rev. Laryng. **95**, 554—559 (1974).

KAUFMAN, L., PRICE, R.: The detection of cortical spike activity at the human scalp. IEEE Trans. Bio-Med. Eng. Vol. BME-14, 84—90 (1967).

KEIDEL, W. D.: Vibrationsreaction. Der Erschütterungssinn des Menschen. Erlanger Forschungen, Reihe B: Naturwissenschaften, Bd. 2. Erlangen: Universitätsbund 1956.

KEIDEL, W. D.: Periphere und corticale Komponenten der Adaptation bei Reizung des Ohres und der Haut der Katze mit Impulsfolgen. Pflügers Arch. ges. Physiol. **268**, 34—35 (1958).

KEIDEL, W. D.: Rankes Adaptationstheorie. Z. Biol. **112**, 411—425 (1961).

KEIDEL, W. D.: Nachrichtenübermittlung und Nachrichtenverarbeitung in Organismen. Vortrag auf Einladung der Carl-Friedrich-von-Siemens-Stiftung, München-Nymphenburg 1962a.

KEIDEL, W. D.: Elektronisch gemittelte langsame Rindenpotentiale des Menschen bei akustischer Reizung. Collegium ORLAS in Athen, 16.—21.9. 1962b.

KEIDEL, W. D.: Kybernetische Systeme des menschlichen Organismus. (Hrsg.: Arbeitsgemeinschaft für Forschung des Landes Nordrhein/Westf.). Westdeutscher Verlag, Köln und Opladen: **118**, 31—71 (1963a).

KEIDEL, W. D.: Tuning between central auditory pathways and the ear. IEEE Transactions on Military Electronics MIL-7, 131—143 (1963b).

KEIDEL, W. D.: Physiologie der Hautsinne. In: MARCHIONINI, A. (Hrsg.): Handbuchartikel. Ergänzungsband zu Jadassohn: Handbuch der Dermatologie. Berlin-Heidelberg-New York: 1963c.

KEIDEL, W. D.: Rindenpotentiale beim Menschen und Hörvermögen. Tagung der Deutschen Audiologen in Bremen, 5.—8. 3. 1964a.

KEIDEL, W. D.: Audiometric aspects and multisensory power functions of electronically averaged slow evoked cortical responses in man. Tagung des Collegium ORLAS in Würzburg, 30. 8.—3. 9. 1964b (gemeinsame mit SPRENG, M.).

KEIDEL, W. D.: Objective audiometry in man. 7th International Congress of Audiology in Copenhagen, 25.—28. 8. 1964c.

KEIDEL, W. D.: Biophysical aspects of auditory information processing. International Biophysics Meeting at Paris, June 1964d.

KEIDEL, W. D.: Kybernetische Leistungen des menschlichen Organismus. Elektrotechn. Z. **24**, 769—808 (1964f).

KEIDEL, W. D.: Die Physiologie der Informationsverarbeitung. Pflügers Arch. ges. Physiol. **281**, 5—7 (1964g).

KEIDEL, W. D.: Neuere Ergebnisse der Physiologie des Hörens. Arch. Ohr.-, Nas.- u. Kehlk.-Heilk. **185**, 548—575 (1965).

KEIDEL, W. D.: Electrophysiology of vibratory perception. In: NEFF, W. D. (ed.): Contributions to sensory physiology, Vol. 3. New York-London: Academic Press 1968.

KEIDEL, W. D.: Informationsphysiologische Aspekte des Hörens. Studium Generale **22**, 49—82 (1969).

KEIDEL, W. D.: Neuere Ergebnisse der akustischen Informationsverarbeitung. In: Präsidium der Deutschen Gesellschaft für experimentelle Medizin. (Hrsg.): Ergebnisse der experimentellen Medizin, Bd. 3. Berlin: VEB Verlag Volk und Gesundheit 1970.

KEIDEL, W. D.: Information processing in the higher parts of the auditory pathway. In: Proceedings of the International Union of Physiological Siences, Volume VIII. (Ed.: German Physiological Society, Munich 1971a). XXV. International Congress, Munich 1971.

KEIDEL, W. D.: What do we know about the human cortical evoked potential after all? Arch. klin. exp. Ohr.-, Nas.- u. Kehlk.-Heilk. **198**, 9—37 (1971b).

KEIDEL, W. D.: The use of quick correlators in electro-cochleography both in oto-audiography (OAG) and in neuro-audiography (NAG). In: PORTMANN, G. (Ed.): Rev. Largng. Supplémentum 1971c.

KEIDEL, W. D.: D.C.-potentials in the auditory evoked response in man. Acta oto-laryng. (Stockh.) **71**, 242—248 (1971d).

KEIDEL, W. D.: The dc-potential in the human cortical evoked response, a new contribution to the objective audiometry. J. franç. Oto-chino-laryng. **21**, 153—158 (1972a).

KEIDEL, W. D.: Intermodale Spezifität elektrophysiologischer Reizkorrelate. In: JANZEN, R., KEIDEL, W. D., HERZ, A., STEICHELE, C. (Hersg.): Schmerz. Grundlagen — Pharmakologie — Therapie. Stuttgart: Georg Thieme 1972b.

KEIDEL, W. D.: The use of fast correlators in electro-cochleography in man. In: TAYLOR, W. (ed.): Disorders of auditory function. London-New York: Academic Press 1973.

KEIDEL, W. D.: Recent advances in information processing within the auditory system. In: KEIDEL, W. D., HÄNDLER, W., SPRENG, M. (Hrsg.): Kybernetik und Bionik — Cybernetics and bionics. München: Olbenbourg 1974a.

KEIDEL, W. D.: Information processing in the higher parts of the auditory pathway. In: ZWICKER, E., TERHARDT, E. (eds.): Psychophysical models and physiological facts in hearing. Berlin-Heidelberg-New York: Springer 1974b.

KEIDEL, W. D.: Anatomische und kommunikationstheoretische Grundlagen des Gehörs. In: KEIDEL, W. D. (Hrsg.): Physiologie des Gehörs. Stuttgart: Georg Thieme 1975a.

KEIDEL, W. D.: Physiologie des Gehörs. Stuttgart: Georg Thieme 1975b.

KEIDEL, W. D.: Slow potentials, in man to voluntary motor intentions, computed by autocorrelation. In preparation (1976).

KEIDEL, W. D., KEIDEL, U. O., KIANG, N. Y. S., FRISHKOPF, L. S.: Time course of adaptation of evoked responses from the cat's somesthetic and auditory systems. Quart. Progr. Rep. Massachusetts Inst. Technol. RLE **48**, 121—124 (1958).

KEIDEL, W. D., SPRENG, M.: Elektronisch gemittelte langsame Rindenpotentiale des Menschen bei akustischer Reizung. Acta oto-laryng. (Stockh.) **56**, 318—328 (1963).

KEIDEL, W. D., SPRENG, M.: Objektive Audiometrie. Arbeitstagung Deutscher Audiologen in Erlangen am 9.—10. 4. 1965.

KEIDEL, W. D., SPRENG, M.: Neurophysiological evidence for the Stevens power function in man. J. acoust. Soc. Amer. **38**, 191—195 (1965).

KEIDEL, W. D., SPRENG, M.: Computed audio-encephalograms in man (a technique of objective audiometry). Int. Audiology **4**, 56—60 (1965).

KEIDEL, W. D., SPRENG, M.: Recent status results and problems of objective audiometry in man. 1st Part. J. franç. Oto-rhino-laryng. **14**, 45—53 (1970).

KEIDEL, W. D., ENGELEN, S., RIX, R.: Versuch einer systemtheoretischen Erklärung des Alpha-Rhythmus im menschlichen Elektroencephalogramm. Naturwissenschaften **58**, 91—93 (1971).

KEIDEL, W. D., INNITZER, J., NEUHÄUSER, G., PLATTIG, K.-H.: Electroencephalographical audiometry of the new-born. J. franç. Oto-rhino-laryng. **22**, 671—683 (1973).

KEIDEL, W. D., FINKENZELLER, P.: Simultaneous computation of ECG, early response and ERA. IV. Biennial Symposium der International ERA Study Group in London, 28.—30. 7. 1975, to be published in: International Audiology.

KEIDEL, W. D., KALLERT, S.: Auditory nervous system. In: HARRISON, D. F. N., HINCHCLIFFE, R. (eds.): Scientific basis of otolaryngology. London: William Heinemann Medical Books Ltd. (to be published).

KERN, E. B., CODY, D. T. R., BICKFORD, R. G.: Neurogenic components of the averaged response evoked by clicks in guinea pigs. Mayo Clin. Proc. **44**, 886—899 (1969).

KERN, E. B., CODY, D. T. R., BICKFORD, R. G.: Vertex-response thresholds to pure tones in guinea pigs. Arch. Otolaryng. **90**, 79—89 (1969).

KEY, B. J.: Effect of lysergic acid diethylamide on potentials evoked in the specific sensory pathways. Brit. med. Bull. **21**, 30—35 (1965).

KHECHINASHVILI, S. N., KEVANISHVILI, Z. SH., KADJAIA, O. A.: Evoked potentials of the auditory system in man. Sechenov physiol. J. U.S.S.R. **58**, 527—533 (1972).

KIANG, N. Y. S.: Discharge patterns of single fibres in the cats' auditory nerve. Res. Monogr. 35. Cambridge: MIT Press 1965.

KIANG, N. Y. S., CRIST, A. H., FRENCH, M. A., EDWARDS, A. G.: Postauricular electric response to acoustic stimuli in humans. Quart. Progr. Rep. No. 68, MIT Cambridge, January 15, 218—225 (1963).

KIANG, N. Y. S., GOLDSTEIN, M. H. JR.: Evoked cortical responses and anesthesia. Ruart. Progr. Rep. MIT Cambridge, July 15, 142—144 (1957).

KIANG, N. Y. S., PEAKE, W. T.: Studies of the auditory nervous system by using combined acoustic and electric stimulation. Quart. Progr. Rep. MIT Cambridge, January 15, 124—128 (1958).

KIANG, N. Y. S., SANDEL, T. T.: Cortical "off" responses to bursts of noise in unanesthetized cats. Quart. Progr. Rep. MIT Cambridge, July 15, 139—142 (1957).

KIETZELL, H. R. VON: Vibratorisch evozierte Hirnrindenpotentiale bei wachen Katzen. Dissertation, Erlangen 1971.

KIMMEL, H. D., GOLDSTEIN, A. J.: Retention of habituation of the GSR to visual and auditory stimulation. J. exp. Psychol. **73**, 401—404 (1967).

KITASATO, H.: The change in the surface negative cortical response during nembutal anesthesia and firing level of neurons in the cortex of rabbit. Jap. J. Physiol. **15**, 71—91 (1965).

KLASS, D. W.: Central association of electroencephalographers. Electroenceph. clin. Neurophysiol. **15**, 720—725 (1963).

KLEE, M. R., OFFENLOCH, K., TIGGES, J.: Cross-correlation analysis of electroencephalographic potentials and slow membrane transients. Science **147**, 519—521 (1965).

KLINGER, K.-P.: Amplitudenvariationen akustisch evozierter Potentiale in Abhängigkeit von der Signalinformation und belastungsbedingter Ermüdung. Int. Z. angew. Physiol. **31**, 269—278 (1973).

KLINKE, R., FRUHSTORFER, H., FINKENZELLER, P.: Evoked responses as a function of external and stored information. Electroenceph. clin. Neurophysiol. **25**, 119—122 (1968).

KLIVINGTON, K. A., GALAMBOS, R.: Resistance shifts accompanying the evoked cortical response in the cat. Science **157**, 211—213 (1967).

KOBAL, G.: Amplituden und Latenzen evozierter Hirnpotentiale nach elektrischer Zungenreizung beim Menschen in Abhängigkeit von der Ableiteposition. Dissertation, Erlangen 1973.

KOBAL, G., WANDHOEFER, A., PLATTIG, K.-H.: EEG power spectra and auditory evoked potentials in transcendental meditation (TM). Pflügers Arch. **359**, R96 (1975).

KÖHLER, W., HELD, R., O'CONNELL, D. N.: An investigation of cortical currents. Proc. Amer. Phil. Soc. **96**, 290—330 (1952).

KÖHLER, W., WEGENER, J.: Currents of the human auditory cortex. J. cell. comp. Physiol. **45**, Suppl. 1, 1955.

KÖHLER, W., NEFF, W.D., WEGENER, J.: Currents of the auditory cortex in the cat. J. cell. comp. Physiol. **45**, Suppl. 1, 1—24 (1955).

KÖHLER, W., O'CONNELL, D.N.: Currents of the visual cortex in the cat. J. cell. comp. Physiol. **49**, Suppl. 2, 1—43 (1957).

KORNHUBER, H.H., DEECKE, L.: Hirnpotentialänderungen bei Willkürbewegungen und passiven Bewegungen des Menschen: Bereitschaftspotential und reafferente Potentiale. Pflügers Arch. ges. Physiol. **284**, 1—17 (1965).

KORNMÜLLER, A.E.: Bioelektrische Erscheinungen architektonischer Felder. Eine Methode der Lokalisation auf der Großhirnrinde. Dtsch. Z. Nervenheilk. **130**, 44—60 (1933).

KRYTER, K., ADES, H.: Studies on the function of the higher acoustic nervous centers in the cat. Amer. J. Psychol. **56**, 501—536 (1943).

LA GRUTTA, V., AMATO, G., MILITELLO, L.: The responsiveness of acoustic area after stimulation of the caudate nucleus. Experimentia (Basel) **26**, 259—260 (1970).

LAMB, L.E., GRAHAM, J.T.: Influence of signal variables on evoked response to sound. J. Speech Res. **10**, 257—267 (1967).

LANDAU, W.M., BISHOP, G.H., CLARE, M.H.: Analysis of the form and distribution of evoked cortical potentials under the influence of polarizing currents. J. Neurophysiol. **27**, 788—813 (1964).

LARSSON, L.-E.: Correlation between the psychological significance of stimuli and the magnitudes of the startle blink and evoked EEG potentials in man. Acta physiol. scand. **48**, 276—294 (1960).

LEHMANN, D., FENDER, D.H.: Component analysis of human averaged evoked potentials: dichoptic stimuli using different target structure. Electroenceph. clin. Neurophysiol. **24**, 542—553 (1968).

LEHNHARDT, E.: Audiometrische Topodiagnostik im Hirnstamm. Z. Laryng. Rhinol. **52**, 11—21 (1973).

LENARD, H.G., BERNUTH, H. VON, HUTT, S.J.: Acoustic evoked responses in newborn infants: The influence of pitch and complexity of the stimulus. Electroenceph. clin. Neurophysiol. **27**, 121—127 (1969).

LETTICH, E., MARGERISON, J.H.: The use of data from low frequency analysis to illustrate serial EEG changes in depressed patients during tratment with iproniazid. J. ment. Sci. **106**, 1111—1114 (1960).

LEVONIAN, E.: Evoked potential in relation to subsequent alpha frequency. Science **152**, 1280—1282 (1966).

LIBET, B., KAHN, J.B. JR.: Steady potentials and neurone activity in mammals. Fed. Proc. **6**, 152 (1947).

LICKEY, M.E., FOX, S.S.: Localization and habituation of sensory evoked DC responses in cat cortex. Exp. Neurol. **15**, 437—454 (1966).

LILLY, J.C., CHERRY, R.B.: Surface movements of click responses from acoustic cerebral cortex of cat: leading and trailing edges of a response figure. J. Neurophysiol. **17**, 521—532 (1954).

LINDSLEY, D.F., MORTON, T.H., ZAROODNY, T.: Effects of subthalamic stimulation on sensory-evoked potentials in the reticular formation and cortex. Exp. Neurol. **17**, 439—450 (1967).

LINDSLEY, D.F., ZAROODNY, T., MORTON, T.H.: Effects of subthalamic lesions on sensory-evoked potentials in the reticular formation and sensorimotor cortex. Exp. Neurol. **17**, 210—220 (1967).

LOEWENICH, V. VON: Leistungsfähigkeit und Grenzen elektroencephalographischer Hörprüfung bei Säuglingen und Kleinkindern. Mschr. Kinderheilk. **118**, 400—403 (1970).

LOEWENICH, V. VON: Methodische Voraussetzungen zur diagnostischen Verwertung auditorisch evozierter Potentiale bei Kleinkindern und Säuglingen. Pädiat. Fortbildk. Praxis **34**, 39—48 (1972).

LOEWENICH, V. VON, FINKENZELLER, P.: Reizstärkenabhängigkeit und Stevenssche Potenzfunktion beim optisch evozierten Potential des Menschen. Pflügers Arch. ges. Physiol. **293**, 256—271 (1967).

LOFTUS-HILLS, J. J., JOHNSTONE, B. M.: Auditory function, communication, and the brain-evoked response in anuran amphibians. J. acoust. Soc. Amer. **47**, 1131—1138 (1970).

LOMBROSO, C. T., MERLIS, J. K.: Suprasylvian auditory responses in the cat. Electroenceph. clin. Neurophysiol. **9**, 301—308 (1957).

LOW, M. D., BORDA, R. P., KELLAWAY, P.: Contingent negative variation in rhesus monkeys: An EEG sign of a specific mental process. Percept. Motor Skills **22**, 443—446 (1966).

LOW, M. D., BORDA, R. P., FROST, J. D. JR., KELLAWAY, P.: Surface-negative, slow-potential shift associated with conditioning in man. Neurology **16**, 771—782 (1966).

MAGNI, F., MORUZZI, G., ROSSI, G. F., ZANCHETTI, A.: EEG arousal following inactivation of the lower brain-stem by selective injection of barbiturate into vertebral circulation. Arch. ital. Biol. **97**, 33—46 (1959).

MAJKOWSKI, J.: Wplyw niszczenia dróg sluchowych kota na oroces uczenia się odowiedzi na bodźce dźwiękowe. Rozpr. Wydz. Nauk. med. pol. Akad. Nauk **9**, 59—108 (1964).

MAJKOWSKI, J., MORGADES, P. P.: Primary auditory evoked potentials after section of brachium of the inferior colliculus. Electroenceph. clin. Neurophysiol. **27**, 587—593 (1969).

MANIL, J., DESMEDT, J.-E., DEBECKER, J., CHORAZYNA, H.: Les potentiels cérébraux évoqués par la stimulation de la main chez le nouveau-né normal. Rev. Neurol. **117**, 53—61 (1967).

MARCZYNSKI, T. J., ROSEN, A. J., HACKETT, J. T.: Post-reinforcement electrocortical synchronization and facilitation of cortical auditory evoked potentials in appetitive instrumental conditioning. Electroenceph. clin. Neurophysiol. **24**, 227—241 (1968).

MARK, R. G., HALL, R. D.: Acoustically evoked potentials in the rat during conditioning. J. Neurophysiol. **30**, 875—892 (1967).

MARSH, J. T., WORDEN, F. G.: Auditory potentials during acoustic habituation: Cochlear nucleus, cerebellum and auditory cortex. Electroenceph. clin. Neurophysiol. **17**, 685—692 (1964).

MASSOPUST, L. C. JR., WOLIN, L. R., KADOYA, S.: Evoked responses in the auditory cortex of the squirrel monkey. Exp. Neurol. **21**, 35—40 (1968).

MAST, T. E.: Short-latency human evoked responses to clicks. J. appl. Physiol. **20**, 725—730 (1965).

MAST, T. E., WATSON, C. S.: Attention and auditory evoked responses to low-detectability signals. Percept. Psychophys. **4**, 237—240 (1968).

MCADAM, D. W., IRWIN, D. A., REBERT, C. S., KNOTT, J. R.: Conative control of the contingent negative variation. Electroenceph. clin. Neurophysiol. **21**, 194—195 (1966).

MCCANDLESS, G. A., BEST, L.: Summed evoked responses using pure-tone stimuli. J. Speech Res. **9**, 266—272 (1966).

MENDEL, M. I., GOLDSTEIN, R.: The effect of test conditions on the early components of the averaged electroencephalic response. J. Speech Res. **12**, 344—350 (1969).

MENDEL, M. I., GOLDSTEIN, R.: Stability of the early components of the averaged electroencephalic response. J. Speech Res. **12**, 351—361 (1969).

MEULDERS, M., GYBELS, J., BERGMANS, J., GEREBTZOFF, M. A., GOFFART, M.: Sensory projections of somatic, auditory and visual origin to the cerebral cortex of the sloth (Choloepus hoffmanni Peters). J. comp. Neurol. **126**, 535—546 (1966).

MILLER, G. A.: The magical number seven, plus-or-minus two. Some limits of our capacity for processing information. Psychol. Rev. **63**, 81—97 (1956).

MILLICHAP, J. G., EGAN, R. W., HART, Z. H., STURGIS, L. H.: Auditory perceptual deficit correlated with EEG dysrhythmias. Neurology **19**, 870—872 (1969).

MIMURA, K., SATO, K., OZAKI, T., HONDA, N., MASUYA, S.: On the physiological significance of the EEG changes caused by sonic stimulation. Electroenceph. clin. Neurophysiol. **14**, 683—696 (1962).

MOLNAR, C. E., WEISS, T. F.: Repetitive cortical responses to acoustic clicks. Quart. Progr. Rep. No. 57, MIT Cambridge, April 15, 143—150 (1960).

MONOD, N., GARMA, L.: Auditory responsivity in the human premature. Biol. Neonate **17**, 292—316 (1971).

MONTANDON, P. B., MEGILL, N. D., KAHN, A. R., PEAKE, W. T., KIANG, N. Y. S.: Recording auditory-nerve potentials as an office procediure. Ann. Otol. **84**, 2—10 (1975).

MONTANDON, P. B., SHEPARD, N. T., MARR, E. M., PEAKE, W. T., KIANG, N. Y. S.: Auditory-nerve potentials from ear cannals of patients with otologic problems. Ann. Otol. **84**, 164—173 (1985).

MOORE, E. J. II, ROSE, D. E.: Variability of latency and amplitude of acoustically evoked responses to pure tones of moderate to high intensity. Int. Audiol. 8, 172—181 (1969).

MORI, K., WINTERS, W. D., SPOONER, C. E.: Comparison of reticular and cochlear multiple unit activity with auditory evoked responses during various stages induced by anesthetic agents. II. Electroenceph. clin. Neurophysiol. **24**, 242—248 (1968).

MORRELL, F.: An anatomical and physiological analysis of electrocortical conditioning. Proc. IV. Congr. Int. Electroenceph., Brussels, 377—391 (1957).

MORRELL, F.: Some electrical events involved in the formation of temporary connections. In: Henry Ford Hospital Symposium: Reticular formation of the brain. Boston: Little, Brown and Co. 1958.

MORRELL, F., BARLOW, J. S., BRAZIER, M. A. B.: Analysis of conditioned repetitive response by means of the average response computer. Recent Advanc. Biol. Psychiat. **2**, 123—137 (1960)

MORRELL, F., JASPER, H. H.: Electrographic studies of the formation of temporary connections in the brain. Electroenceph. clin. Neurophysiol. 8, 201—215 (1956).

MORRELL, F., NAQUET, R., GASTAUT, H.: Evolution of some electrical signs of conditioning: Part I. Normal cat and rabbit. J. Neurophysiol. **20**, 574—587 (1957).

MORRELL, L. K., MORRELL, F.: Evoked potentials and reaction times: A study of intra-individual variability. Electroenceph. clin. Neurophysiol. **20**, 567—575 (1966).

MORUZZI, G., MAGOUN, H. W.: Brain stem reticular formation and activation of the EEG. Electroenceph. clin. Neurophysiol. **1**, 455—473 (1949).

MOSKOWITZ, H. R., SCHARF, B., STEVENS, J. C.: Sensation and measurement. Papers in honor of S. S. Stevens. Dordrecht-Holland/Boston-USA: D. Reidel 1974.

NÄÄTÄNEN, R.: Selective attention and evoked potentials. Ann. Acad. Sci. fenn. Sarja-Ser. B, Nide-Tom. **151** (1967).

NAKAHAMA, H.: Cerebral response of anterior sigmoid gyrus to ipsilateral posterior sigmoid stimulation in cat. J. Neurophysiol. **22**, 573—589 (1959).

NARIKASHVILI, S. P.: Association area of the cerebral cortex and its interaction with the sensory zones. Zh. vyssh. nerv. Deyat. Pavlova **19**, 110—123 (1969) Russ.

NEERGAARD, E. B., HARLY, S.: Instrumentation for acoustically evoked potentials using a photographic averaging technique. Acta oto-laryng. (Stockh.) **263**, 145—146 (1970).

NEFF, W. D.: On the relationships between physical, physiological, and psychological variables. In: ROSENBLITH, W. A. (ed.): Sensory communication. New York: MIT Press 1961.

NELSON, D. A.: Human auditory electrical responses. Reviews of scientific literature 1970 continuing Education Program American Academy of Ophthalmology and Otolaryngology, 1971. S. 81—97.

NELSON, D. A., LASSMAN, F. M.: Effects of intersignal interval on the human auditory evoked response. J. acoust. Soc. Amer. **44**, 1529—1532 (1968).

NIAUSSAT, M.-M.: Audiométrie comparée, par potentiel évoqué auditif et par réflexe de Preyer de souris normales et de souris sensibles à la crise audiogène. C. R. Soc. Biol. (Paris) **163**, 2503 (1969).

NIEDER, P. C., RANDALL, W.: Sound-evoked potentials in neocortex of unanesthetized opossum. Science **144**, 429—430 (1964).

NIEDER, P. C., STROMINGER, N. L.: Evoked potentials in auditory cortex after bilateral transection of the brachium of the inferior colliculus in the cat. J. Neurophysiol. **28**, 1185—1194 (1965).

NODAR, R. H., GRAHAM, J. T.: An investigation of auditory evoked responses of mentally retarded adults during sleep. Electroenceph. clin. Neurophysiol. **25**, 73—76 (1968).

NOËL, P., DESMEDT, J. E.: Les potentiels évoqués cérébraux dans l'hémiplégie infantile. Revue E. E. G. (Paris) **2**, 189—194 (1972).

OCHS, S., CLARK, F. J.: Tetrodotoxin analysis of direct cortical responses. Electroenceph. clin. Neurophysiol. **24**, 101—107 (1968).

OCHS, S., CLARK, F. J.: Interaction of direct cortical responses — a possible dendritic site of inhibition. Electroenceph. clin. Neurophysiol. **24**, 108—115 (1968).

ODENTHAL, D. W., EGGERMONT, J. J.: Clinical electrocochleography. Acta oto-laryng. (Stockh.) Suppl. **316**, 62—74 (1974).

OJEMANN, G. A., HENKIN, R. I.: Steroid dependent changes in human visual evoked potentials. Life Sci. **6**, 327—334 (1967).

ONISHI, S., DAVIS, H.: Effects of duration and rise time of tone bursts on evoked V potentials. J. acoust. Soc. Amer. **44**, 582—591 (1968).

ORNITZ, E. M., RITVO, E. R., CARR, E. M., PANMAN, L. M., WALTER, R. D.: The variability of the auditory averaged evoked response during sleep and dreaming in children and adults. Electroenceph. clin. Neurophysiol. **22**, 514—524 (1967).

ORNITZ, E. M., RITVO, E. R., TANGUAY, P. E., WALTER, R. D.: EEG spikes and the averaged evoked response to clicks and flashes. Electroenceph. clin. Neurophysiol. **27**, 387—391 (1969).

ORNITZ, E. M., LEE, J. C. M., TANGUAY, P. E., SIVERTSEN, B., WILSON, C.: The effect of stimulus interval on the auditory evoked response during sleep in normal children. Electroenceph. clin. Neurophysiol. **33**, 159—166 (1972).

OSTERHAMMEL, P. A., DAVIS, H., WIER, C. C., HIRSH, S. K.: Adult auditory evoked vertex potentials in sleep. Audiology **12**, 116—128 (1973).

OWENS, E.: Audiologic evaluation in cochlear versus retrocochlear lesions. Acta oto-laryng. (Stockh.) Suppl. **283** (1971).

PÁSZTOR, E., TOMKA, I., DEÁK, GY.: The effect of local cerebral hypothermia on the electrocorticogram and on experimental epileptic activity. J. Neurosurg. **23**, 49—53 (1965).

PEREZ-BORJA, C., TYCE, F. A., MCDONALD, C., UIHLEIN, A.: Depth electrographic studies of a focal fast response to sensory stimulation in the human. Electroenceph. clin. Neurophysiol. **13**, 695—702 (1961).

PETŘEK, J., GOLDA, V., LISONĚK, P.: Changes in cortical acoustic responses in cats during long-lasting rhythmical stimulation. Activ. nerv. sup. (Praha) **9**, 284—286 (1967).

PETŘEK, J., GOLDA, V., LISONĚK, P.: Relation between cortical acoustic evoked responses and amplitude of the EEG. Activ. nerv. sup. (Praha) **9**, 289—290 (1967).

PETŘEK, J., GOLDA, V., LISONĚK, P.: Changes in EEG and cardiac activity elicited by irregularly repeated acoustical stimulation in intact animals and in cats with bilateral orbital ablation. Activ. nerv. sup. (Praha) **11**, 273 (1969).

PFURTSCHELLER, G.: Änderungen in der evozierten und spontanen Hirnaktivität des Menschen bei extracranialer Polarisation. Z. ges. exp. Med. **152**, 284—293 (1970).

PICTON, T. W., HILLYARD, S. A., KRAUSZ, H. I., GALAMBOS, R.: Human auditory evoked potentials. I: Evaluation of components. Electroenceph. clin. Neurophysiol. **36**, 179—190 (1974).

PIMONOW, L.: La parole synthétique et son application dans la correction auditive. Ann. Télécommun. **20**, 151—187 (1965).

PLATTIG, K. H.: Über den elektrischen Geschmack. Reizstärkeabhängige evozierte Hirnpotentiale nach elektrischer Reizung der Zunge des Menschen. Z. Biol. **116**, 161—211 (1969).

PODVOLL, E. M., GOODMAN, S. J.: Averaged neural electrical activity and arousal. Science **155**, 223—225 (1967).

POLIAKOVA, A. G.: Origin of the early component of the evoked response in the association cortex of the cat. Electroenceph. clin. Neurophysiol. **32**, 129—138 (1972).

PORTMANN, M., ARAN, J. M.: Relations entre pattern cochléographique et pathologie retrolabyrinthique. Acta oto-laryng. (Stockh.) **73**, 190—196 (1972).

PORTMANN, M., ARAN, J. M., LE BERT, G.: Électro-cochléogramme en dehors de toute intervention chirurgicale. Acta oto-laryng. (Stockh.) **65**, 105 (1968).

PORTMANN, M., ARAN, J. M., LAGOURGE, P.: Testing for recruitment by electrocochleography. Ann. Otol. **82**, 36—43 (1973).

PORTMANN, M., LE BERT, G., ARAN, J. M.: Potentiels cochléaires obtenues chez l'homme en dehors de toute intervention chirurgicale. Rev. Laryngol. (Bordeaux) 88, 157—164 (1967).

PORTMANN, M., NEGREVERGNE, M.: Apport de l'electrocochleographie dans l'examen audiometrique de l'enfant. Rev. Laryngol. **94**, 359—379 (1973).

PRIBRAM, K. H., SPINELLI, D. N., KAMBACK, M. C.: Electrocortical correlates of stimulus response and reinforcement. Science **157**, 94—96 (1967).

PURPURA, D. P., COHEN, B.: Intracellular recording from thalamic neuron during recruiting responses. J. Neurophysiol. **25**, 621—635 (1962).

PURPURA, D. P., POOL, J. L., RANSOHOFF, J., FRUMIN, M. J., HOUSEPIAN, E. M.: Observations on evoked dendritic potentials of human cortex. Electroenceph. clin. Neurophysiol. **9**, 453—459 (1957).

PURPURA, D. P., SHOFER, R. J.: Intracellular recording from thalamic neurons during reticulocortical activation. J. Neurophysiol. **26**, 493—505 (1963).

RAAB, D., ADES, H.: Cortical and midbrain mediation of a conditioned discrimination of acoustic intensities. Amer. J. Psychol. **59**, 59—83 (1946).

RANKE, O. F.: Physiologie des Gehörs. In: TRENDELENBURG, W., SCHÜTZ, E. (Hrsg.): Lehrbuch der Physiologie. Berlin-Göttingen-Heidelberg: Springer 1953.

RAPIN, I.: Evoked responses to clicks in a group of children with communication disorders. Ann. N. Y. Acad. Sci. **112**, 182—203 (1964).

RAPIN, I., GRAZIANI, L. J.: Auditory-evoked responses in normal, brain-damaged, and deaf infants. Neurology **17**, 881—894 (1967).

RAPIN, I., SCHIMMEL, H., TOURK, L. M., KRASNEGOR, N. A., POLLAK, CH.: Evoked responses to clicks and tones of varying intensity in waking adults. Electroenceph. clin. Neurophysiol. **21**, 335—344 (1966).

RAU, R. M.: Über die Abhängigkeit der objektiv ermittelten Intensitätsfunktion des menschlichen Gehörs von der Tonfolgefrequenz. Arch. klin. exp. Ohren-, Nas.- u. Kehlk.-Heilk. **190**, 133—145 (1968).

REENPÄÄ, Y.: Axiomatische Darstellung des phänomenal-zentralnervösen Systems der sinnesphysiologischen Versuche Keidels und Mitarbeiter. S.-B. Heidelberger Akad. Wissensch. Math.-naturwiss. Kl. 5. Abh. S. 235—247. Berlin-Heidelberg-New York: Springer 1966.

REGAN, D.: Evoked potentials and sensation. Perception & Psychophys. **4**, 347—350 (1968).

REGAN, D.: Evoked potentials in psychology, sensory physiology and clinical medicine. London: Chapman and Hall Ltd. 1972.

RÉMOND, A.: Level of organization of evoked responses in man. Ann. N. Y. Acad. Sci. **112**, 143—159 (1964).

RHOTON, A., GOLDRING, S., O'LEARY, J. L.: Comparison of direct cerebral and cerebellar cortical responses in the cat. Amer. J. Physiol. **199**, 677—682 (1960).

RIETVELD, W. J.: The occipitocortical response to lightflashes in man. Acta physiol. pharmacol. neerl. **12**, 373—407 (1963).

RIETVELD, W. J., TORDOIR, W. E. M.: The influence of flash intensity upon the visual evoked response in the human cortex. Acta physiol. pharmacol. neerl. **13**, 160—170 (1965).

RIETVELD, W. J., TORDOIR, W. E. M., HAGENOUW, J. R. B.: Influence of attentiveness, of vigilance task difficulty, and of habituation on cortical evoked responses and on artifacts. Acta physiol. pharmacol. neerl. **14**, 18—37 (1966).

ROBINSON, B. W.: Head-mounted electrode platform: Construction and error analysis. Physiol. Behavior **2**, 455—457 (1967).

ROSEN, A. J., MARCZYNSKI, T.: Effects of alpha-methyl-meta-tyrosine on operant behavior, auditory evoked potentials and postreinforcement electrocortical synchronization in the cat. Physiol. Behavior **2**, 413—419 (1967).

ROSENZWEIG, M. R., ROSENBLITH, W. A.: Responses to successive auditory stimuli at the cochlea and at the auditory cortex. Gen. appl. Psychol. Monogr. **67**, 1 (1953).

ROTH, J. G., MACPHERSON, C. H., MILSTEIN, V.: The use of carbon electrodes for chronic cortical recording. Electroenceph. clin. Neurophysiol. **21**, 611—615 (1966).

ROTH, W. T., KOPELL, B. S., BERTOZZI, P. E.: The effect of attention on the average evoked response to speech sounds. Electroenceph. clin. Neurophysiol. **29**, 38—46 (1970).

ROTHENBERG, S., DAVIS, H.: Auditory evoked response in chinchilla: Application to animal audiometry. Perception & Psychophys. **2**, 443—447 (1967).

ROTHMAN, H. H.: Effects of high frequencies and intersubject variability on the auditory-evoked cortical response. J. acoust. Soc. Amer. **47**, 569—573 (1970).

ROTHMAN, H. H., DAVIS, H., HAY, I. S.: Slow evoked cortical potentials and temporal features of stimulation. Electroenceph. clin. Neurophysiol. **29**, 225—232 (1970).

RUCHKIN, D. S.: An analysis of average response computations based upon aperiodic stimuli. IEEE Trans. Bio-Med. Eng. Volume BME-12, 87—94 (1965).

RUCHKIN, D. S., JOHN, E. R.: Evoked potential correlates of generalization. Science **153**, 209—211 (1966).

RUDOMIN, P., MALLIANI, A., ZANCHETTI, A.: Microelectrode recording of slow wave and unit responses to afferent stimuli in the hypothalamus of the cat. Arch. ital. Bio. **103**, 90—118 (1965).

RUHM, H., WALKER, E. JR., FLANIGIN, H.: Acoustically-evoked potentials in man: Mediation of early components. Laryngoscope **77**, 806—822 (1967).

RUHM, H. B., JANSEN, J. W.: Rate of stimulus change and the evoked response: I. Signal rise-time. J. Auditory Res. **3**, 211—216 (1969).

SAKABE, N., ARAYAMA, T., SUZUKI, T.: Human fetal evoked response to acoustic stimulation. Acta oto-laryng. Suppl. **252**, 29—36 (1969).

SALOMON, G.: Electric response audiometry (ERA) based on rank correlation. Audiology **13**, 181—194 (1974).

SALOMON, G., BECK, O., ELBERLING, C.: The role of sedation in ERA from the vertex. Audiology **12**, 150—166 (1973).

SANCES, A. JR., LARSON, S. J., JACOBS, J. E.: Electronarcosis and evoked cortical responses. Science **141**, 733—735 (1963).

SATO, K.: On the transforming action related to the threshold, chronaxie and accommodation constant of a living excitable system. Jap. J. Physiol. **9**, 327—335 (1959).

SATO, K., OZAKI, T., MIMURA, K., YAMAMOTO, Y., MASUYA, S., HONDA, N.: The effects of auditory stimulation on the electroencephalogram. — In the sight of frequency power spectra and frequency characteristics. Proc. VIIth Ann. Meet. Jap. EEG Soc. and XIth Ann. Meet. Jap. EMG Soc. 1958.

SATO, K., OZAKI, T., MIMURA, K., MASUYA, S., HONDA, N.: On the frequency response of EEG activity obtained by the intermittent click stimulation. Proc. VIIIth Ann. Meet. Jap. EEG Soc. and XIIth Ann. Meet. Jap. EMG Soc. Held in Hirosaki on July 6th and 7th, 1959.

SATO, K., OZAKI, T., MIMURA, K., MASUYA, S., HONDA, N., NISHIKAWA, T., SONODA, T.: On the physiological significance of the average time- and frequency-patterns of the electroencephalogram. Electroenceph. clin. Neurophysiol. **13**, 208—215 (1961).

SATO, K., MIMURA, K., SATA, H., OCHI, N., ISHINO, T.: On random fluctuations in EEG and evoked potentials. Jap. J. Physiol. **21**, 167—185 (1970).

SATTERFIELD, J. H.: A system for selection of responses for averaging. Electroenceph. clin. Neurophysiol. **21**, 86—88 (1966).

SAUNDERS, J. C.: Cochlear nucleus and auditory cortex correlates of a click stimulus-intensity discrimination in cats. J. comp. physiol. Psychol. **72**, 8—16 (1970).

SAYERS, B. MCA., BEAGLEY, H. A.: Objective evaluation of auditory evoked EEG responses. Nature (Lond.) New Biol. **251**, 608—609 (1974).

SAYERS, B. MCA., BEAGLEY, H. A., HENSHALL, W. R.: The mechanism of auditory evoked EEG responses. Nature (Lond.) New Biol. **247**, 481—483 (1974).

SCHEIBEL, M. E., SCHEIBEL, A. B.: Coupling a sensory artefact to the brain. Nature (Lond.) **213**, 605—606 (1967).

SCHMIDT, P. H., EGGERMONT, J. J., ODENTHAL, D. W.: Study of Menière's disease by electrocochleography. Acta oto-laryng. (Stockh.) Suppl. **316**, 75—84 (1974).

SCHMIDT, P. H., SPOOR, A.: The place of electrocochleography in clinical audiometry. Acta oto-laryng. (Stockh.) Suppl. **316**, 5—6 (1974).

SCHOLL, H.: Das dynamische Verhalten des Gehörs im Bereich der Hörschwellen. Dissertation, T.H. Stuttgart 1961.

SCHULMAN-GALAMBOS, C., GALAMBOS, R.: Recording the brainstem evoked response: A manual. IV. Biennial Symposium of the International ERA Study Group, 28.—30. 7. 1975 in London.

SCHWARTZ, M., SHAGASS, C.: Effect of different states of alertness on somatosensory and auditory recovery cycles. Electroenceph. clin. Neurophysiol. **14**, 11—20 (1962).

SCHWARTZ, M., HALL, O. W.: Selected trial averaging of sensory evoked brain responses. Electroenceph. clin. Neurophysiol. **23**, 480—482 (1967).

SEM-JACOBSEN, C. W., PETERSEN, M. C., DODGE, H. W., LAZARTE, J. A., HOLMAN, C. B.: Electroencephalographic rhythms from the depths of the parietal, occipital and temporal lobes in man. Electroenceph. clin. Neurophysiol. **8**, 263—278 (1956).

SHEVRIN, H., RENNICK, P.: Cortical response to a tactile stimulus during attention, mental arithmetic and free associations. Psychophysiology **3**, 381—388 (1967).

SKINNER, P. H., ANTINORO, F.: Critical-band theory and the auditory-evoked slow-ware V potential. J. acoust. Soc. Amer. **48**, 557—560 (1970).

SKINNER, P. H., ANTINORO, F., SHIMOTA, J.: An evaluation of linear extrapolation to threshold in electroencephalic response audiometry. J. Aud. Res. **12**, 26—31 (1974).

SKINNER, P. H., JONES, H. C.: Effects of signal duration and rise time on the auditory evoked potential. J. Speech Res. **11**, 301—306 (1968).

SMITH, M. C.: Stimulus-response compatibility and parallel response selection. Canadian J. Psychol./Rev. Canad. Psychol. **21**, 496—502 (1967).

SMITH, M. C.: Theories of the psychological refractory period. Psychol. Bull. **67**, 202—213 (1967).

SOHMER, H., FEINMESSER, M.: Cochlear action potentials recorded from the external ear in man. Ann. Otol. **76**, 427—435 (1967).

SOHMER, H., FEINMESSER, M.: Routine use of electrocochleography (cochlear audiometry) on human subjects. Audiology **12**, 167—173 (1973).

SOHMER, H., FEINMESSER, M., BAUBERGER-TELL, L., LEV, A., DAVIS, S.: Routine use of electrocochleography in infants with uncertain diagnosis. Ann. Otol. **81**, 72 (1972).

SPARKS, D. L., POWELL, E. W.: Interaction of evoked potentials in the anterior thalamus of the cat. Electroenceph. clin. Neurophysiol. **20**, 470—474 (1966).

SPECKMANN, E.-J., CASPERS, H.: Les modifications du potentiel continu cortical pendant l'arrêt respiratoire. Rev. Neurol. **117**, 5—19 (1967).

SPECKMANN, E.-J., CASPERS, H.: Verschiebungen des corticalen Bestandpotentials bei Veränderungen der Ventilationsgröße. Pflügers Arch. **310**, 235—250 (1969).

SPIEGEL, E. A., SZEKELY, E. G., MOFFET, R.: Cortical responses to rotation. I. Responses recorded after cessation of rotation. Acta oto-laryng. (Stockh.) **66**, 81—88 (1968),

SPIEGEL, E. A., EGYED, J., SZEKELY, E. G.: Cortical responses to rotation. II. Responses recorded at the onset of rotation from the second somatic sensory and posterior areas. Acta oto-laryng. (Stockh.) **66**, 261—272 (1968).

SPOENDLIN, H.: The innervation of the cochlear receptor. In: MØLLER, A. R. (ed.): Basic mechanisms in hearing. New York-London: Academic Press 1973.

SPOENDLIN, H.: Neuroanatomical basis of cochlear coding mechanisms. Audiology **14**, 383—407 (1975).

SPONG, P., HAIDER, M., LINDSLEY, D. B.: Selective attentiveness and cortical evoked responses to visual and auditory stimuli. Science **148**, 395—397 (1965).

SPOOR, A.: Apparatus for electrocochleography. Acta oto-laryng. (Stockh.) Suppl. **316**, 25—36 (1974).

SPRENG, M.: Über die Messung der Frequenzgruppe und der Integrationszeit des menschlichen Gehörs durch vom Schall abhängige Hirnspannungen längs der Kopfhaut. Dissertation, Stuttgart 1967.

SPRENG, M.: Problems in objective cerebral audiometry using short sound stimulation. Int. Audiol. — Audiol. Internationale **8**, 424—429 (1969).

SPRENG, M.: Objektivierende Messungen am Schmerzsinn des Menschen. Habilitationsschrift, Erlangen 1970.

SPRENG, M.: Small computers in evoked response audiometry (ERA). Arch. klin. exp. Ohr.-, Nas.- u. Kehlk.-Heilk. **198**, 50—70 (1971).

SPRENG, M.: Artefact recognition and diazepam in electric response audiometry. Audiology **12**, 137—149 (1973).

SPRENG, M.: Neuere Hinweise zu ERA und ECOG — aus physiologischer Sicht. Arch. Oto-Rhino-Laryng. **206**, 191—215 (1974a).

SPRENG, M.: Objective electrophysiological measurements of ear-characteristics, intelligibility of vowels and judgement of the stage of attention. Proceedings of the 31. Aerospace Medical Panel Meeting, Neapel 1974. AGARD publication, AGARD-CPP-152 A6, A6-10 (1974b).

SPRENG, M.: Langsame Rindenpotentiale, objektive Audiometrie und Psychoakustik. In: KEIDEL, W.D. (Hrsg.): Physiologie des Gehörs. Stuttgart: Georg Thieme 1975a.

SPRENG, M.: Short sound stimulation and temporal integration model of evoked responses. Biennial Symposium of the International ERA Study Group, London 1975b.

SPRENG, M.: Grenzen der sensorischen Informationsverarbeitung des Menschen. Naturwissenschaften (in press) (1976).

SPRENG, M., KEIDEL, W.D.: Human evoked cortical responses to auditory stimuli: interaction, time course of adaptation, influence of stimuli parameters. In: DUYFF, J.W. (ed.): Abstracts of free communications, films, and demonstrations presented at the XXIInd international congress of physiological sciences, Leyden. Int. Congr. Ser. 48. Excerpta Medica Foundation, Amsterdam 1962 (S. 1010).

SPRENG, M., KEIDEL, W.D.: Neue Möglichkeiten der Untersuchung menschlicher Informationsverarbeitung. Kybernetik **1**, 243—249 (1963).

SPRENG, M., KEIDEL, W.D.: Objektive Audiometrie. Pflügers Arch. ges. Physiol. **281**, 82 (1964).

SPRENG, M., ICHIOKA, M.: Langsame Rindenpotentiale bei Schmerzreizung am Menschen. Pflügers Arch. ges. Physiol. **279**, 121—132 (1964).

SPRENG, M., KEIDEL, W.D.: Separierung von Cerebroaudiogramm (CAG), Neuroaudiogramm (NAG) und Otoaudiogramm (OAG) in der objektiven Audiometrie. Arch. klin. exp. Ohr.-, Nas.- u. Kehlk.-Heilk. **189**, 225—246 (1967).

SPRENG, M., KEIDEL, W.D.: Recent status results and problems of objective audiometry in man. 2nd Part. J. franç. Oto-Rhino-Laryng. **19**, 55—60 (1970).

SPRENG, M., KEIDEL, W.D.: Problems of simple averaging of electro-physiological recordings and the use of additional methods. In: PORTMANN, G. (ed.): Revue de Laryngologie, Suppl. Bordeaux: 1971.

SPRENG, M., BUMM, P., KEIDEL, W.D., WIEGAND, H.P.: Elektrophysiologische Untersuchungen am peripheren Teil des menschlichen Ohres unter Benützung geeigneter Rechnerprogramme. Pflügers Arch. **307**, R 134 (1969).

SPYCHALA, P., ROSE, D.E., GRIER, J.B.: Comparison of the "On" and "Off" characteristics of the acoustically evoked response. Int. Audiology **3**, 416 (1969).

STANGE, G.: The relation between functional parameters of subjective and objective audiometry. Arch. klin. exp. Ohr.-, Nas.- u. Kehlk.-Heilk. **198**, 85—101 (1971).

STANGE, G.: The effect of sedative agents in psychotropic drugs on acoustically evoked responses. Arch. klin. exp. Ohr.-, Nas.- u. Kehlk.-Heilk. **201**, 294—308 (1972).

STANGE, G.: Diagnostik überschwelligen Hörvermögens bei innenohrgeschädigten Kindern mittels ERA. H. N. O. (Berl.) **21**, 83—87 (1973).

STANGE, G., SODA, T.: Quantitative Untersuchungen zur Hörschwelle, Adaptation und Lautheitsempfindung am gesunden und hörgeschädigten Menschen mittels der „Objektiven Audiometrie". Arch. klin. exp. Ohr.-, Nas.- u. Kehlk.-Heilk. **190**, 210—228 (1968).

STANGE, G., HOLM, C.: Gemittelte zentrale akustische Reizantworten — eine Erweiterung pädaudiologischer Gesichtspunkte ?. H. N. O. (Berl.) **18**, 27—28 (1970).

STANGE, G., SPRENG, M., KEIDEL, U.O.: Die Wirkung von Streptomycinsulfat auf Erregung und Adaptation der Haarzellen des Cortischen Organs. Pflügers Arch. ges. Physiol. **279**, 99—120 (1964).

STARZL, T.E., WHITLOCK, D.G.: Diffuse thalamic projection system in monkey. J. Neurophysiol. **15**, 449—468 (1952).

STEIN, L.: Habituation and stimulus novelty: A model based on classical conditioning. Psychol. Rev. **73**, 352—356 (1966).

STEINBUCH, K.: Automat und Mensch. Heidelberger Taschenbücher, Bd. 81. Berlin-Heidelberg-New York: Springer 1971.

STEVENS, S.S.: Neural events and the psychophysical law. Science **170**, 1043—1050 (1970).

STEVENSON, G.C., COLLINS, W.F., RANDT, C.T., SAURWEIN, T.D.: Effects of induced hypothermia on subcortical evoked potentials in the cat. Amer. J. Physiol. **194**, 423—426 (1958).

SUGA, N.: Echo-location and evoked potentials of bats after ablation of inferior colliculus. J. Physiol. (Lond.) **203**, 707—728 (1969).

SUTTON, S.: Recent eddies in brain currents. Bull. Atomic Sci. **24**, 23—27 (1968).

SUTTON, S.: The specification of psychological variables in an average evoked potential experiment. In: DONCHIN, E., LINDSLEY, D. B. (eds.): Average evoked potentials. Washington, D. C.: NASA SP-191 1969.

SUTTON, S.: Correspondence between psychological and physiological thresholds. Presented to Amer. Psychol. Ass. Miami 1970.

SUTTON, S.: The sensitivity of the evoked potential to psychological variables. Presented at meeting of EEG Soc., Washington, D. C. 1970.

SUTTON, S., BRAREN, M., ZUBIN, J., JOHN, E. R.: Evoked-potential correlates of stimulus uncertainty. Science **150**, 1187—1188 (1965).

SUTTON, S., TUETING, P., ZUBIN, J., JOHN, E. R.: Information delivery and the sensory evoked potential. Science **155**, 1436—1439 (1967).

SUZUKI, H., TAIRA, N.: Regional difference of the direct cortical response. Jap. J. Physiol. **8**, 365—377 (1958).

SUZUKI, H., TAIRA, N.: An analysis of direct cortical response. Tohoku J. exp. Med. **70**, 1—10 (1959).

SUZUKI, T.: Problems in electric response audiometry (ERA) during sedation. Audiology **12**, 129—136 (1973).

SUZUKI, T., ASAWA, I.: Evoked potential of waking human brain to acoustic stimuli. Acta oto-laryng. (Stockh.) **48**, 508—515 (1957).

SUZUKI, T., ORIGUCHI, K.: Averaged evoked response audiometry (ERA) in young children during sleep. Acta oto-laryng. (Stockh.) Suppl. **252**, 19—28 (1969).

SYMMES, D., ANDERSON, K. V.: Reticular Modulation of higher auditory centers in monkey. Exp. Neurol. **18**, 161—176 (1967).

TAGUCHI, K., PICTON, T. W., ORPIN, J. A., GOODMAN, W. S.: Evoked response audiometry in newborn infants. Acto oto-laryng. (Stockh.) Suppl. **252**, 5—17 (1969).

TAGUCHI, K., GOODMAN, W. S., BRUMMITT, W. M.: Evoked response audiometry in mentally retarded children. Acta Otolaryng. **70**, 190—196 (1970).

TEAS, D. C., KIANG, N. Y-S.: Evoked cortical responses as a function of state variables. Quarterly Progress Report No. 63, MIT Cambridge, October 15, 171—176 (1961).

TEAS, D. C., KIANG, N. Y. S.: Evoked Responses from the auditory cortex. Exp. Neurol. **10**, 91—119 (1964).

THEISSING, J.: Objektive Hörprüfung im Kindesalter. Akt. Oto-Rhino-Laryng. **4**, 1—38 (1970).

THOMPSON, R., SINDBERG, R.: Auditory response fields in association and motor cortex of cat. J. Neurophysiol. **23**, 88—105 (1960).

THOMPSON, R. F., PATTERSON, M. M.: Bioelectric recording techniques. Part B: Electroencephalography and human brain potentials. New York-London: Academic Press 1974.

THORNTON, A. R. D.: Distortion of averaged post-auricular muscle responses due to system bandwidth limits. Electroenceph. clin. Neurophysiol. **39**, 195—197 (1975).

THORNTON, A. R. D.: The diagnostic potential of surface recorded electrocochleography. Brit. J. Audiology **9**, 7—13 (1975).

THORNTON, A. R. D.: The measurement of surface-recorded electrocochleographic responses. Scand. Audiol. **4**, 51—58 (1975).

THORNTON, A. R. D.: Statistical properties of surface-recorded electrocochleographic responses. Scand. Audiol. **4**, 91—102 (1975).

TOMAN, W.: Einführung in die Allgemeine Psychologie. Bd. I: Biologische Grundlagen, Wahrnehmung, Gedächtnis, Intelligenz. Freiburg: Rombach 1973a.

TUETING, P., SUTTON, S.: The relationship between pre-stimulus negative shifts and post-stimulus components of the averaged evoked potential. In: KORNBLUM, S. (ed.): Attention and performance IV. New York: Academic Press 1972.

TUETING, P., SUTTON, S., ZUBIN, J.: Quantitative evoked potential correlates of the probability of events. Psychophysiology **7**, 385—394 (1971).

TUNTURI, A. R.: Statistical analysis of afferent potential in the auditory cortex. Am. J. Physiol. **213**, 597—612 (1967).

UTTAL, W. R.: Evoked brain potentials: Signs or codes? Perspect. Biol. Med. **10**, 627—639 (1967).

VATTER, O., MÜLLER, J., RISCHMAUI, B.: Das DC-Potential des Schädels und seine Beziehungen zum EEG. Elektromedizin **13**, 89—98 (1968).

VATTER, O., RISCHMAUI, B.: DC-Potentiale der Hirnrinde. Naturwissenschaften **54**, 286 (1967).

VAUGHAN, H. G. JR., RITTER, W.: The sources of auditory evoked responses recorded from the human scalp. Electroenceph. clin. Neurophysiol. **28**, 360—367 (1970).

VERZEANO, M., DILL, R. C., VALLECALLE, E., GROVES, P., THOMAS, J.: Evoked responses and neuronal activity in the lateral geniculate. Experientia (Basel) **24**, 696—698 (1968).

WALLACE, R. K., BENSON, H., WILSON, A. F.: A wakeful hypometabolic physiologic state. Amer. J. Physiol. **221**, 795—799 (1971).

WALTER, W. GREY: The convergence and interaction of visual, auditory and tactile responses in human nonspecific cortex. Ann. N. Y. Acad. Sci. **112**, 320—361 (1964).

WALTER, W. GREY, COOPER, R., ALDRIDGE, V. J., MCCALLUM, W. C., WINTER, A. L.: Contingent negative variation: An electric sign of sensorimotor association and expectancy in the human brain. Nature (Lond.) **203**, 380—384 (1964).

WANDHÖFER, A., PLATTIG, K.-H.: Stimulus-linked dc-shift and auditory evoked potentials in transcendental meditation (TM). Pflügers Arch. **343**, R 79 (1973).

WANDHÖFER, A., KOBAL, G., PLATTIG, K.-H.: Decrease of latency of human auditory evoked potentials during transcendental meditation (TM). In preparation (1976).

WEBSTER, W. R., AITKIN, L. M.: Evoked potential and single unit studies of neural mechanisms underlying the effects of repetitive stimulation in the auditory pathway. Electroenceph. clin. Neurophysiol. **31**, 581—592 (1971).

WEINBERGER, N. M., GOODMAN, D. A., KITZES, L. M.: Is behavioral habituation a function of peripheral auditory system blockade? Cummun. Behav. Biol. Part A, **3**, 111—116 (1969).

WIEGAND, H. P., BUMM, P., SPRENG, M.: Extracranial gemessene Ohrcharakteristiken und gestörte Informationsaufnahme. Pflügers Arch. **307**, 134 (1969).

WIESENDANGER, M., TARNECKI, R.: Der tonische Einfluß der Pyramidenbahn auf corticale evoked potentials. Helv. physiol. Acta **23**, C111—C112 (1965).

WILLIAMS, H. L., TEPAS, D. I., MORLOCK, H. C. JR.: Evoked responses to clicks and electroencephalographic stages of sleep in man. Science **138**, 685—686 (1962).

WILLIAMS, H. L., MORLOCK, H. C. JR., MORLOCK, J. V., LUBIN, A.: Auditory evoked responses and the EEG-stages of sleep. Ann. N. Y. Acad. Sci. **112**, 172—181 (1964).

WILSMANN, K.: Evozierte Hirnrindenpotentiale nach Schmerzreizung am Zahn der Katze. Dissertation, Erlangen 1969.

WINTERS, W. D., MORI, K., SPOONER, C. E., KADO, R. T.: Correlation of reticular and cochlear multiple unit activity with auditory evoked responses during wakefulness and sleep. I. Electroenceph. clin. Neurophysiol. **23**, 539—545 (1967).

WOOLSEY, C. N.: Organization of cortical auditory system: A review and a synthesis. In: RASMUSSEN, G. L., WINDLE, W. F. (eds.): Neural mechanisms of the auditory and vestibular systems. Springfield, Ill.: C. C. Thomas 1960.

WOOLSEY, C. N., WALZL, E. M.: Topical projection of nerve fibers from local regions of the cochlea to the cerebral cortex of the cat. Johns Hopk. Hosp. Bull. **71**, 315 (1942).

WORDEN, F. G., MARSH, J. T.: Frequency-following (microphonic-like) neural responses evoked by sound. Electroenceph. clin. Neurophysiol. **25**, 42—52 (1968).

WORDEN, F. G., MARSH, J. T., ABRAHAM, F. D., WHITTLESEY, J. R. B.: Variability of evoked auditory potentials and acoustic input control. Electroenceph. clin. Neurophysiol. **17**, 524—530 (1964).

YOSHIE, N.: Auditory evoked responses in man recorded by scalp electrodes. Excerpta Medica International Congress Series No. 113, 418—419 (1965).

YOSHIE, N.: Auditory nerve action potentials in man recorded from the external auditory meatus. Audiology **9**, 129—131 (1966).

YOSHIE, N.: Adaptation of the AP in man. Audiology **3**, 274—275 (1967).

YOSHIE, N.: Auditory nerve action potential responses to clicks in man. Laryngoscope **78**, 198—215 (1968).

YOSHIE, N., OHASHI, T.: Auditory nerve action potentials in man. Jap. J. Otol. Tokyo **70**, 920—931 (1967).

YOSHIE, N., OHASHI, T.: Clinical use of cochlear nerve action potential responses in man for differential diagnosis of hearing losses. Acta oto-laryng. (Stockh.) Suppl. **252**, 71—87 (1969).

YOSHIE, N., OHASHI, T., SUZUKI, T.: Non-surgical recording of auditory nerve action potentials in man. Laryngoscope **77**, 76—85 (1967).

YOSHIE, N., OKUDAIRA, T.: Myogenic evoked potential responses to clicks in man. Acta oto-laryng. (Stockh.) Suppl. **252**, 89—103 (1969).

ZERLIN, S., DAVIS, H.: The variability of single evoked vertex potentials in man. Electroenceph. clin. Neurophysiol. **23**, 468—472 (1967).

ZERLIN, S., NAUNTON, R. F.: Early and late averaged electroencephalic responses at low sensation levels. Audiology **13**, 366—378 (1974).

ZÖLLNER, CH., KARNAHL, TH.: Elektrokochleographisches Potentialmuster, an verschiedenen Ableitungsorten registriert. Laryng. Rhinol. **54**, 681—688 (1975).

ZSCHOCKE, St., SPECKMANN, E.-J.: Verschiebungen des corticalen Bestandpotentials durch Veränderungen der Ventilationsgröße bei verschiedenen CO_2-Ausgangsdrucken. Pflügers Arch. ges. Physiol. **297**, R 40 (1967).

ZVONAR, M., ZVONAR-KUHNDL, B., ODENTHAL, D. W.: Anaesthesia and sedation for electrocochleography. Acta oto-laryng. (Stockh.) Suppl. **316**, 37—38 (1974).

ZWICKER, E.: Über psychologische und methodische Grundlagen der Lautheit. Acustica 8, 237 (1958).

ZWICKER, E.: Ein Beitrag zur Lautstärkemessung impulshaltiger Schalle. Acustica **17**, 11—22 (1966).

ZWISLOCKI, J.: Analysis of some auditory characteristics. J. acoust. Soc. Amer. **32**, 1046—1060 (1960).

Chapter 5

Clinical Experiences with Evoked Response Audiometry

F. ZÖLLNER and G. STANGE, Freiburg (Germany)

With 16 Figures

Contents

I. Introduction

Early diagnosis of impaired hearing and evaluation of remaining residual hearing are important in planning effective therapy for all patients and, particulary, for children. This chapter will be concerned primarily with clinical experiences with children.

With the exception of the vestibular system, hearing is the most important sensory system for establishing the first contacts between the organism and its environment. As early as in the four-month-old fetus, the vestibular tracts are myelinated; the acoustic pathways are myelinated after six months; the optical tracts do not receive their myelin sheaths until the fourth month after birth (JOPPICH and SCHULTE, 1968). Thus, the fetus reacts to acoustic stimuli while still in the womb (the startle response) and is born with an almost completely established acoustic sensory system. The child's emotional development, which is at first linked to the differentiation of noises and later to the learning of speech, can proceed without hearing only haltingly and incompletely. Therefore, it has been important for the scientist to find new methods of testing the hearing ability of infants.

The routine methods that have been used were either based on producing unlearned responses such as startle, withdrawal orienting or awakening, or on conditioned responses such as those in play-audiometry; the latter require collaboration on the part of the child.

The methods dependent on unlearned responses can only be applied with stimuli well above the threshold of hearing. Therefore, they are useful as screening tests but not as accurate measures of degree of hearing impairment. The second kind of tests, based on learned responses, permits an assessment of auditory threshold; the accuracy of the assessment depends on the maturity and willingness for collaboration of the child. In any event, the responses obtained in both kinds of tests that have been routinely used are dependent not only on the condition of the auditory but also on other neural pathways and on the general condition of the child and his emotional development. Moreover, it is only possible to establish the presence of either normal hearing or a pathological auditory threshold; we can get no information about the supraliminal function of hearing until more elaborate audiometric tests can be performed.

Direct objective measurement of the capability of the entire acoustic system from peripheral end-organ to the cortex, isolated and without consideration of reflex paths of other modalities, is of high scientific value. The electrically evoked response audiometry (ERA) has made possible the desired objective measurement; in recent years, it has been given thorough clinical tests. Without active collaboration of the child, ERA allows isolated evaluation of the auditory end-organ (cochleography) and testing of more general function by recording responses of the central nervous system. The method requires appropriate electronic equipment and critical application by a trained staff. ERA techniques continue to be developed (although they now give reliable results) surpassing any measurements obtained by methods formerly used. They give new insights into pathology of the acoustic system.

To show best the significance and value of the ERA method as used under clinical conditions, the possibilities and limiations of other procedures will be reviewed briefly.

Even in the last months of pregnancy, distinct reactions of the fetus in the womb to sound stimuli were shown by Peiper (1924). Fleischer (1955) was able to eliminate errors caused by reflexes of the mother by measuring at the same time the maternal movements as well as those of the fetus. Serial tests of early-deliveries, from the sixth month of gestation on, confirmed the ability of the immature child to react to acoustic stimuli. Mounier-Kuhn reported reflexes in 79% and Grisanti and Priolisi in 86% of early-deliveries when they were exposed to sounds at intensities of 80—100 dB.

With mature newborn children, definite reactions are only attainable by exposure to strong sound stimuli; responses cannot be produced immediately after birth in all children.

Kussmaul, in 1859, assumed that all children were born deaf and that hearing began to function gradually. Genzmer (1873) reported that he was able repeatedly to bring about definite acoustical reactions. Systematic research was carried out by Canestini and Stubbs, and a number of other investigators. With the help of a gong, which had an intensity of 126–133 dB, Fröding (1960) noticed positive auropalpebral reflexes in 96.1% of 2000 children when they were tested 1/2 hr post partum. Systematic studies by Suzuki (1965) showed that such high intensities were not necessary and that distinctly recognizable reactions could be obtained with intensities of 40–90 dB, most frequently at 70–80 dB, using pure tones as well as other sounds. In most cases, reactions consisted of a blinking of the eyelid, a jerking of the body, and a sudden deep intake of breath. It was possible to register these signs with the help of electrodes attached near the eyelids, with pneumatic belts and measurement of galvanic skin responses.

Serial tests on newborn children up to the 8th day were carried out by Mounier-Kuhn (1969) who used different noise stimuli, such as whistles, bells, and drums;

definite reactions (grimaces, laughing, sucking movements and trunk- and limb-movements) were observed in 83% of the infants examined.

Readiness for reaction develops rather quickly after birth. Relke and Frey (1966) observed absence of response to loud sounds in 10.8% of infants one hour after birth, but only in 5.2% in 3-month-old infants. De Reynier (1969), likewises noticed this fast development of response to sound; he believed that from 6 month, on extreme impairment of hearing could be separated from normal hearing capability with the help of tests of reflex responses.

In addition to general observations of awake and freely moving children, a number of techniques requiring special equipment and recording methods have been used. Biesalski (1969) made use of a particular arrangement of loudspeakers on the child's bed; he named the method "Baby-Bed-Audiometry". Wedenberg (1963), Rosenau (1962), and Jakobi (1965) observed the reactions of the calmly sleeping child to sounds of different intensities. Kumpf (1971) made detailed measures of changes in breathing when a child was exposed to acoustic stimuli. With the help of a microphone fixed to the child's neck, he registered the changes of the breathing sound when the child was exposed to wide band noise. He found that with the sudden onset of supraliminal noise, respiration became stronger; starting with a weak sound stimulus and gradually increasing intensity, a brief interruption or weakening of the breathing sound occurred when the auditory threshold was reached. Thus, an acoustic reception threshold could be established even in 2-year-old children. This very subtle method cannot always be used successfully. Particular difficulties arise with restless children; they have to be calmed down with drugs (one of the best is Dehydropenzperidol). The use of drugs, however, influences the results of the hearing tests.

Reliable objective results were expected using a measure of changes in galvanic skin resistance in response to acoustic stimuli. Strong sensory stimuli, including sounds, produce secretion of sweat on hands and feet. Bordley *et al.* (1948) were the first to use this response as an objective hearing test. In order to avoid using excessive sound intensities, they used a conditioning procedure, sound accompanied by electrical shock applied to the skin. With this method, the auditory threshold of adults and of children (ages 10 and older) can be measured objectively within 25 dB. According to Lüscher and Kusen (1958), this method has many sources of error. Changes in skin resistance accompany changes in affective state. It is not possible to condition children who refuse to cooperate. On the whole this method has not proved as satisfactory as once was hoped.

An objective measurement of the auditory threshold may be obtained by recording responses of middle-ear muscles (acoustic reflex) – without collaboration of the child, even under anaesthesia – through the use of instruments that measure changes in the impedance of the middle-ear. Metz (1946) was the first to use the so-called "Schusterbrücke" to record the acoustic reflex. The response is elicited by sound stimuli of 70–90 dB above threshold.

In summary, we can say that all of the above-mentioned tests of hearing for children in early infancy have definite limitations. For practical use in the future, they will be applied primarily to exclude deafness and, in some cases, to obtain an estimate of a pathological auditory threshold. When additional audiometric tests are not possible, little can be said about residual hearing.

In the fellowing sections, it will be seen that the use of Evoked Response Audiometry enables us to overcome many of the limitations of the methods that have been used in the past to assess the hearing of infants, young children, or others, whose hearing cannot be tested by standard audiometric methods.

In addition, a combined record of all electrophysiological phenomena obtainable by simultaneous registrations, ranging from N_1 to the early components of the classical ERA-potential shift, and including the perstimulating DC-shift, as described by KEIDEL, may enable us to gain new clinical knowledge concerning the functioning of the different sections of the acoustic system.

II. Fundamental Aspects of Evoked Response Audiometry for Clinical Use

The history of the development of the Evoked Response Audiometry and Electrocochleography is competently and thoroughly covered by DAVIS in another chapter of this handbook. The technique of measurement is described extensively in the same chapter by DAVIS, and the physiological principles in another by KEIDEL.

In the following sections of this chapter, the recent status of the pathophysiological observations and their practical use for clinical work will be reported in detail and critically discussed.

Corresponding to experiments with animals, where biopotentials can be picked up from cochlea to cortex, which are correlated in intensity and frequency with stimuli (first, ROSENBLITH and ROSENZWEIG, 1951), research of the last 20 years tried to discover and record – without surgery – these acoustically evoked biopotentials in human subjects as well. BERGER (1938), in Jena, observed characteristic changes in the EEG when hearing was stimulated, the so-called "K-complex", but the latter was not useful for objective audiological tests (MARCUS *et al.*, 1949; PEARL *et al.*, 1953; DERBYSHIRE and MCDERMOTT, 1958; THEISSING, 1970). The statistically dispersing activity of the resting EEG and the repeated onset of muscle potentials do not permit derivation of acoustically evoked biopotentials from cochlea and central pathways. According to DAWSON (1947 m) acoustically evoked potentials can also be made visible in man, if the relationship of signal (acoustically evoked biopotential) to the electrically recorded response (EEG, muscle potential) in the EEG is improved by averaging. Thus, GEISLER *et al.* (1958) using click-stimulation, and KEIDEL and SPRENG 1963 with long-lasting tone-stimulation as well as DAVIS and YOSHIE 1963, were able, by using a computer, to demonstrate acoustically evoked biopotentials in awake persons with intact skull, amplitude of the responses being dependent on intensity. On the basis of these studies, a number of research teams started to make use of the computer to average the time-locked evoked responses to acoustic stimuli and to relate the results to those which were already known from experiments with animals.

A. Peripheral Acoustic Biopotentials

Peripheral acoustic biopotentials, cochlear microphonics and nerve action potentials of the acoustic nerve, have been demonstrated in human beings by direct recording from an electrode planted at the round window in the open middle

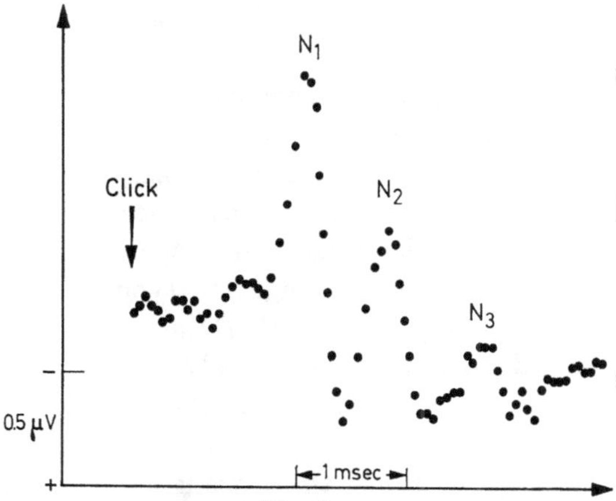

Fig. 1a

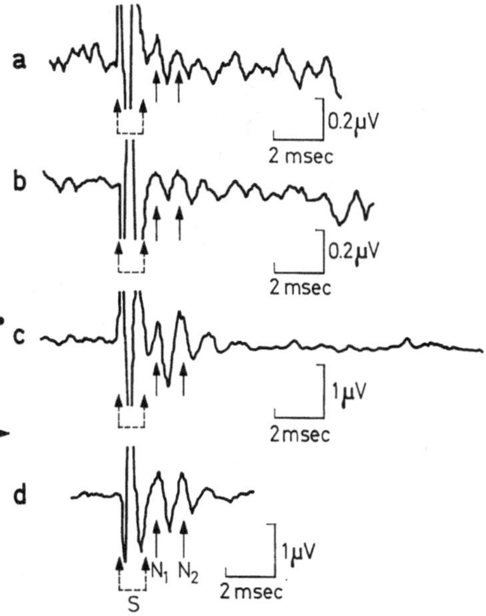

Fig. 1b

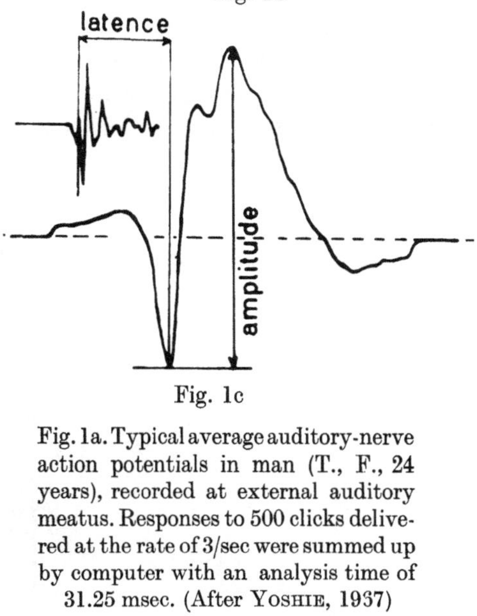

Fig. 1c

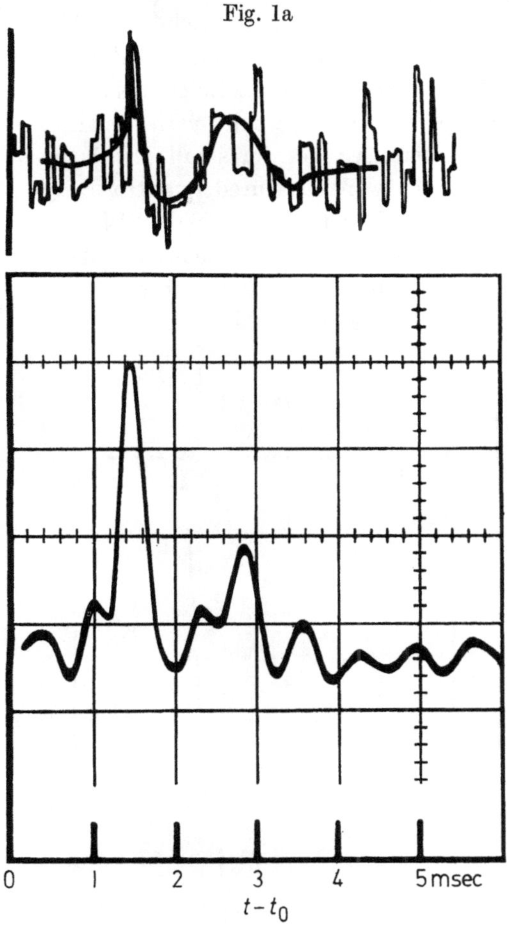

Fig. 1d

Fig. 1a. Typical average auditory-nerve action potentials in man (T., F., 24 years), recorded at external auditory meatus. Responses to 500 clicks delivered at the rate of 3/sec were summed up by computer with an analysis time of 31.25 msec. (After YOSHIE, 1937)

Fig. 1b. Average neural responses to click stimuli (compound action potential of the acousticnerve in man), recorded from a patient with small tympanic membrane perforation. Click intensity 115 dB SPL; (a) active electrode at ear lobe, (b) active electrode at remnant of tympanic membrane, (c) active electrode within middle-ear cavity through perforation, average of 500 clicks, (d) same as (c), click polarity reversed. (Acc. to SOHMER and FEINMESSER, 1967)

Fig. 1c. Amplitude and latency of compound action potential of acoustic nerve through tympanic membrane in man. (Acc. to ARAN, 1971)

Fig. 1d. Average neural responses to click stimuli in man (upper trace) compared with compound action potential of the acoustic nerve in cats (round window, — lower trace). (Acc. to SPRENG and KEIDEL, 1967) ear (Lempert *et al.*, 1947; Ruben *et al.*, 1961). By means of computer technique and by locating the electrodes in the external auditory meatus (Yoshie *et al.*, 1967; Sohmer and Feinmesser, 1967) on the hard palate (Spreng and Keidel, 1967) and in the eustachian tube (Stange, 1967) it has been possible to demonstrate an intensity dependent nerve action potential in awake persons in response to acoustic stimuli. With a fine needle, which was moved through the tympanic membrane towards the round window, Portmann and Aran (1971) as well as Sohmer and Feinmesser (1967) have obtained numerous physiological and pathophysiological data by examination of the nerve action potentials of the acoustic nerve (Fig. 1a–d). It was also possible, in the supraliminal field, to show the characteristic curves of the compound action potentials of the acoustic nerve in potentials of the acoustic nerve in normal and in hearing impaired children. The dependence of the latency of the nerve action potential on stimulus intensity could be quantitatively recorded. Figure 2 shows the characteristic curves of the nerve action potentials of a normal hearing person and of a child with impaired hearing (Aran, 1971). In the diagrams, we distinctly see (in small print) the amplitudes of the nerve action potentials, which were measured quantitatively These potentials decrease when stimulus intensity is reduced. At 50 dB SPL, the normal characteristic curve shows the double-peaks (Fig. 2a), which had earlier been seen in animal experiments, where at the same time the responses of two different sensory cell populations (external and internal hair cells) could be shown,

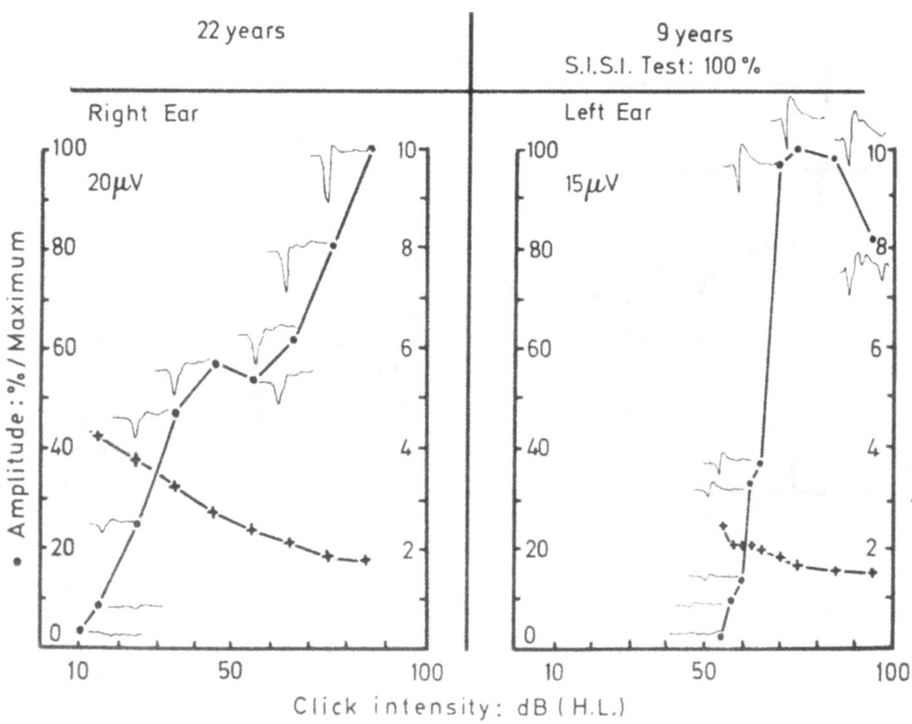

Fig. 2a. Comparison of the input/output amplitude and latency curves for a normal hearing patient (22 years old) and a child (9 years old) with hearing loss and recruitment. (Acc. to Aran, 1971)

when the animals were poinsoned by Streptomycine (STANGE *et al.*, 1964; STANGE *et al.*, 1966). The latency is shortened with rising stimulation intensity; this may be seen in the same diagram. For comparison, a corresponding diagram is shown for a 9-year-old child with impaired hearing on the right (Fig. 2b). You can distinctly see the shift of threshold and the steep course of the characteristic curve, in the sense of a recruitment, with a descent of this characteristic curve at 70 dB SPL in the normal region with nearly normal latency of the evoked potential. If one disregards the fact that for the procedure in which an electrode is inserted into the middle ear, the ear drum must be pierced and variations in the position of the electrode are unavoidable, this procedure not only appears to be the most advanced in its development for clinical purposes, but it may well prove to have even greater value in future clinical work (PORTMANN *et al.*, 1973).

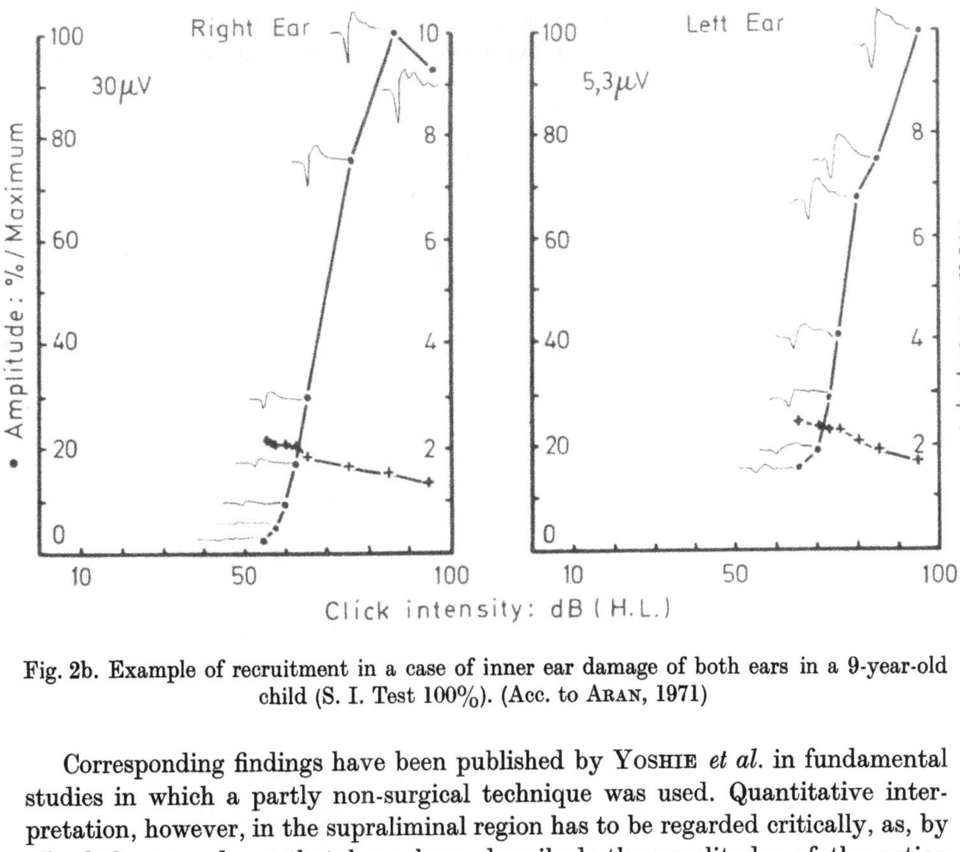

Fig. 2b. Example of recruitment in a case of inner ear damage of both ears in a 9-year-old child (S. I. Test 100%). (Acc. to ARAN, 1971)

Corresponding findings have been published by YOSHIE *et al.* in fundamental studies in which a partly non-surgical technique was used. Quantitative interpretation, however, in the supraliminal region has to be regarded critically, as, by all of the procedures that have been described, the amplitudes of the action potentials amount at best to 20 μV with 90 dB SPL. For the supraliminal sphere in hearing impaired children with acoustic recruitment, this method may also be quantitatively sufficiently reliable, but interpretation of results becomes difficult if a hearing defect exists with only low amplitudes of nerve action potentials to supraliminal stimuli. It is rather interesting to see that, in all the literature on this topic, only scarce information is given about characteristic curves of nerve action potentials following the shifting of threshold. In addition, it must be said that electrocochleography registers the peripheral part only of the acoustic system and, therefore, cannot give sufficient information about location and functioning of an impaired hearing ability. It remains to be seen, whether the programs for larger computers, that have been demonstrated by SPRENG at the 1st International ERA Symposion (1970) in Freiburg (West Germany) will bring quantitatively better results for clinical use.

B. Fast Responses

By extra-cranial recording from the intact human skull acoustically evoked potentials of different latencies can be seen. Recording between electrodes on pinna auris and vertex, we find an acoustic response of five waves within a time sphere of the peak latencies from 1.5–7.0 msec. LEV and SOHMER (1972) assigned these five different acoustically evoked waves to different sites of the acoustic pathways; they based their interpretation upon animal experiments with direct pick-up from different levels of the hearing pathway and upon tests with adults and children with recording from extra-cranial electrodes. Figure 3a shows a

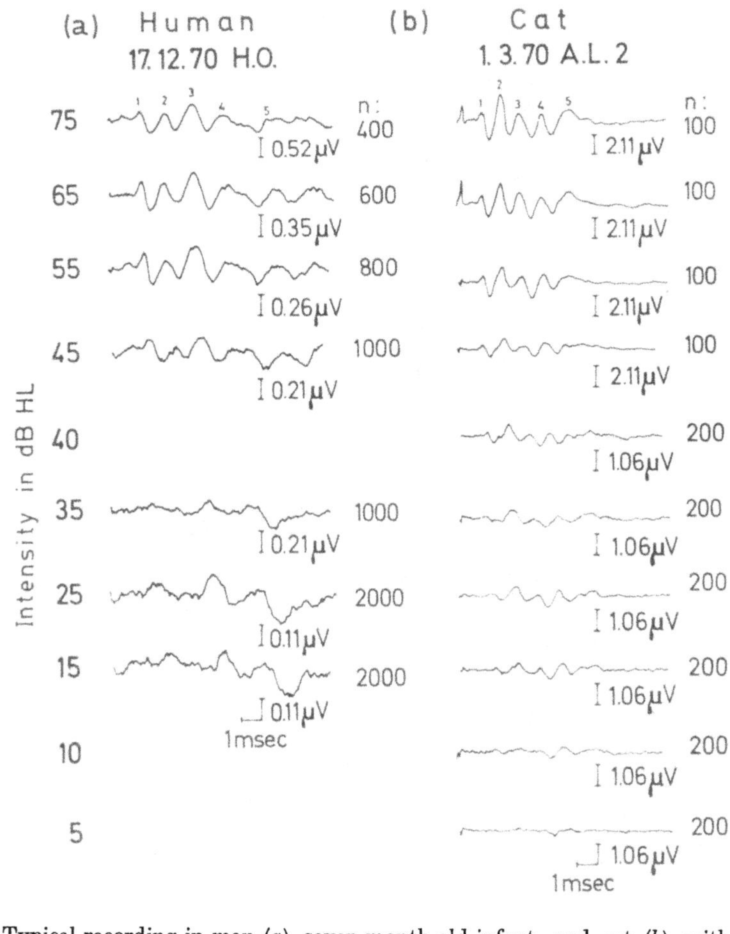

Fig. 3a. Typical recording in man (*a*), seven-month-old infant, and cat (*b*), with pinna and vertex electrodes. The stimulus is always given at the beginning of the trace. In this and subsequent figures, pinna negativity is shown. The number of averaged responses (N) is calculated from equal numbers of condensation and rarefaction clicks. (Acc. to LEV and SOHMER, 1972)

comparison between responses from scalp electrodes in a normal hearing person and the direct recording from the acoustic pathways of the cat. The first wave, with a latency of about 1.5 msec, may correspond to the activity in the cochlear nerve; the second wave, with a latency of 2.5 msec, may originate in the cochlear nucleus; the third, with a latency of 3.5 msec, may be the acoustic response of the nucleus olivarius superior; and the fourth and fifth waves, with latencies of about 4.8 msec and 7.0 msec, may be derived from the colliculus inferior. As acoustic stimuli, clicks with 75 dB SPL condensation-clicks 10/sec were used. Averaging was done by CAT 1000. Number N of evoked responses averaged was 1000 in human beings, 200 in cats. One can speculate that by this mode of derivation and with further knowledge about these five acoustic responses a more exact diagnosis of damage in the auditory parts of the central nervous system may become possible.

Potentials were recorded extracranially also by Terkildsen *et al.* (1973); stimuli were condensation and rarefaction tone pips. You will observe that both A and B (Fig. 3b) contain cochlear microphonics and neurogenic responses. If A and B are added, only the neurogenic response remains; if they are subtracted, it is the cochlear microphonics that are seen.

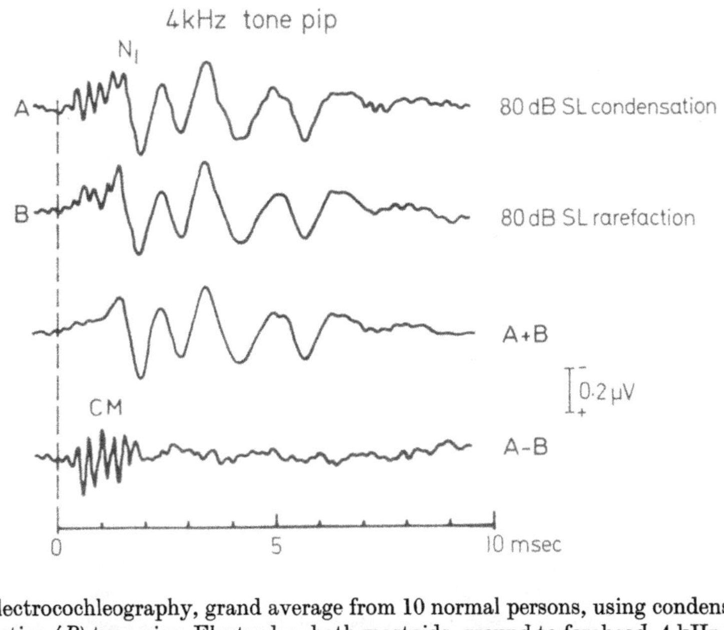

Fig. 3b. Electrocochleography, grand average from 10 normal persons, using condensation (*A*) and rarefaction (*B*) tone pips. Electrodes: both mastoids, ground to forehead. 4 kHz tone pips, repetition 10/sec. (Acc. to Terkildsen *et al.*, 1973)

Another short latency potential evoked by acoustic stimulus in human subjects was demonstrated by Müller and Stange (1970) at the Austrian ENT-Congress in Vienna. This potential appears under 1000-fold averaging after stimulation with clicks and recording from the mastoid tragus; it has a negative peak at 13–14 msec after onset of ipsilateral stimulation (Fig. 4a). The size and shape of the response is dependent on the intensity of the stimulation. It is interesting that the response can be registered only within a narrowly confined region, at a distance

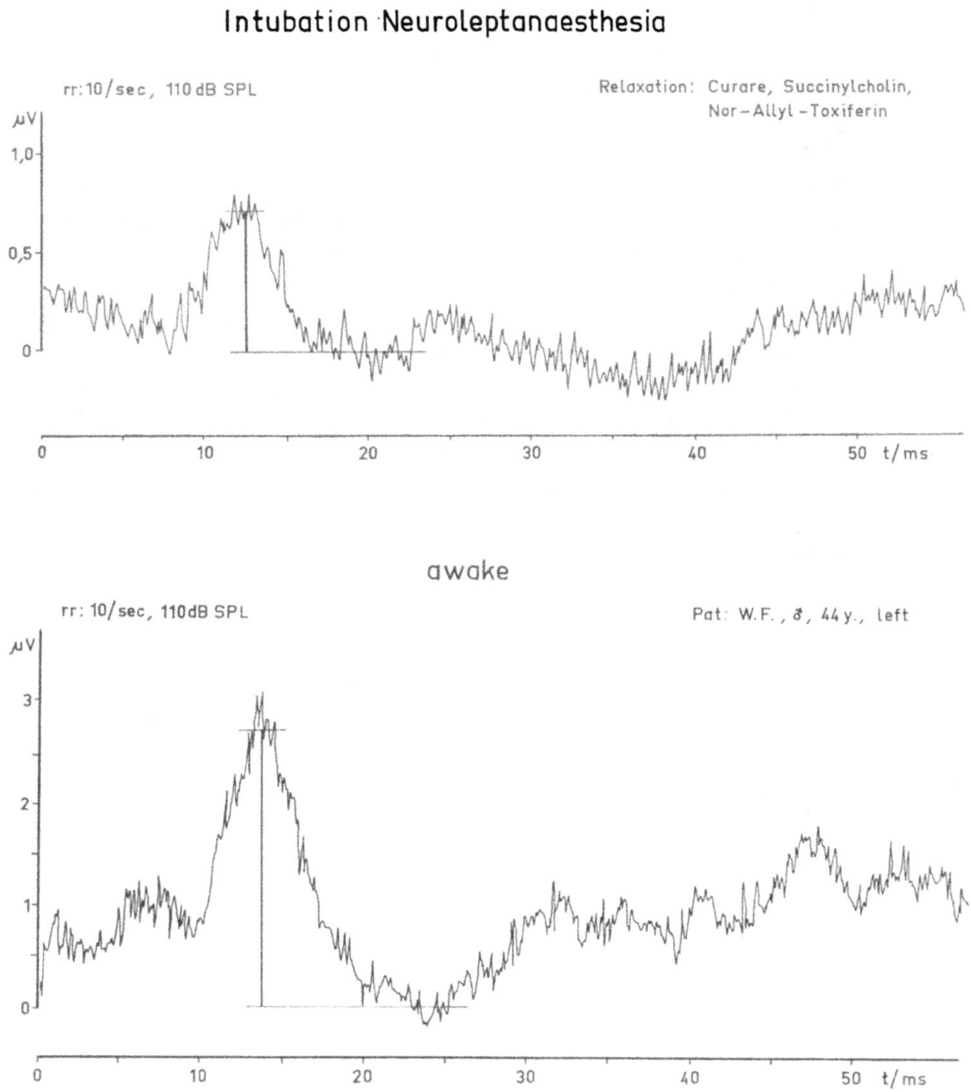

Fig. 4a. 1000-fold averaged acoustically evoked responses of an adult before stapedectomy (upper trace) with active electrode at a narrowly confined area of the mastoid, and with the indifferent electrode above the tragus. Acoustic stimulation: 90 dB SPL, clicks 10/sec, duration: 200 μsec. In the upper trace of the same adult, the same potential with complete relaxing anesthesia, intubation, and artifical respiration. One clearly recognizes that this potential is considerably smaller in its amplitude, but nevertheless distinctly visible. (After STANGE and KARNAHL, 1973)

of 2 cm dorsally and 1 cm cranially from the external auditory meatus. Over an adjacent area the response becomes gradually weaker, and, within a circumference of about 3 cm of the principal location, the response cannot be recorded any longer. Figure 4b shows the course of the characteristic curve of the response in 5 normal hearing adults. You can observe that first responses can be obtained at

30 dB above threshold. Then the characteristic curve bends sharply at 20–30 dB SPL above threshold. It then takes a steep course with rising stimulus intensity. In order to be certain that this has a neurogenic component, the acoustically evoked potential was also taken from a patient under intubation-anaesthesia, complete muscular relaxation and artificial respiration. The first clinical data were

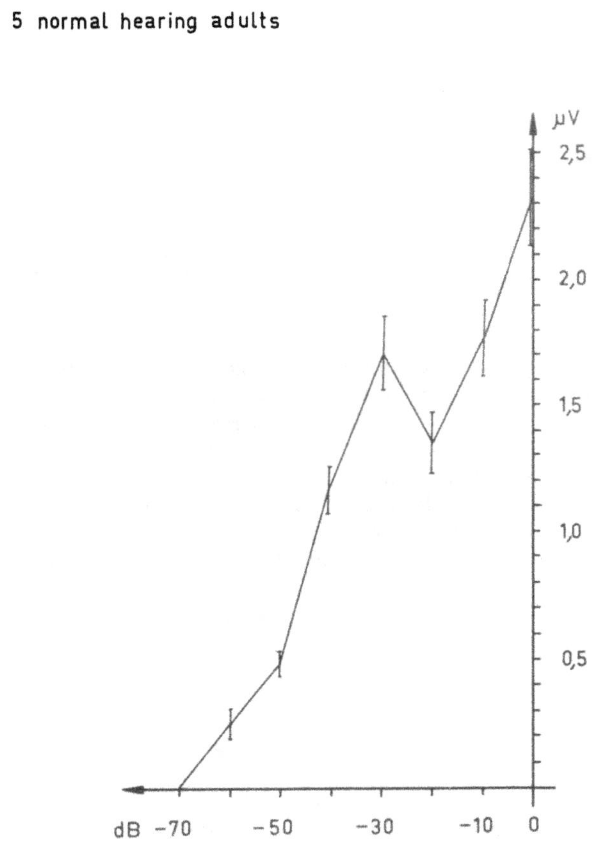

Fig. 4b. Course of characteristic curves of a 1000-fold averaged, acoustically evoked response in 5 normal-hearing test persons. — 1 vertical bar = 1 $\bar{\sigma}$

obtained in 12 patients who had undergone a stapedectomy (Fig. 4c) and in adults with inner-ear damage. In those patients with stapes graft and excision of the M. stapedius, the characteristic curve of the evoked response corresponds to the subjective tone-audiogram, according to hearing ability before and after surgery. In the patients with inner ear damage, a diminution of the early evoked response appears, with curves becoming flatter, and corresponding to the characteristic curves of the late potentials (120 msec) and to the subjective hearing test. Further studies with these acoustic biopotentials in children and other more advanced clinical studies of patients with inner ear damage or after stapedectomy have not yet been made (for detailed information, see STANGE and KARNAHL, 1974).

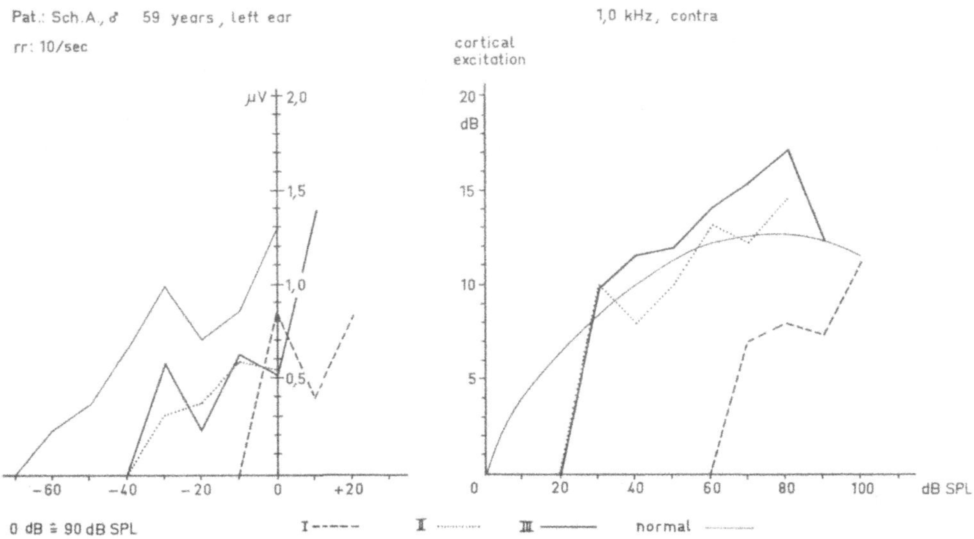

Fig. 4c. In all diagrams, we have as a parameter, hearing ability, that is to say, the responses of the acoustically evoked biopotentials, before and after stapedectomy. I ---- before surgery, II .... 15 days after surgery, ------- 30 days after surgery. Upper diagrams: left-course of the earlier (13 msec), right: — of the later (110 msec) acoustically evoked biopotentials. In the characteristic curves, a postoperative tendency towards normalisation can distinctly be seen. Lower diagrams: speech and tone audiograms of a patient who had undergone a stapedectomy; before and after surgery. Hatched lengthwise: hearing gain, which can clearly be correlated to the responses of the earlier and later potentials. (After STANGE and KARNAHL, 1974)

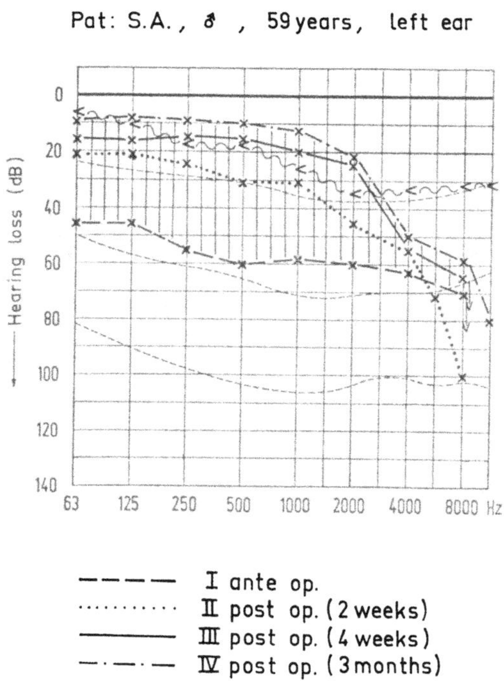

Fig. 4c

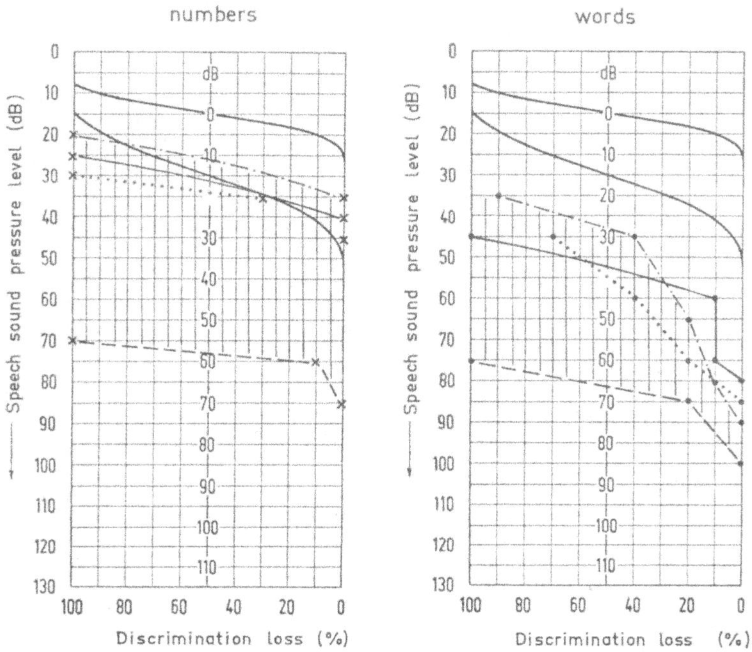

Fig. 4c

Another acoustically evoked response having a negative peak latency of 15 msec after onset of stimulation was reported by THEISSING (1969). It is characteristic of this potential that it can only be recorded from a narrowly confined place at the contralateral temporal lobe under relaxation anesthesia of Stages I and II. In Fig. 5a, you will notice the dependence on intensity of this acoustically evoked response under short pure-tone stimulation of 32 msec duration. It is possible to approach the threshold of human hearing within 10 dB. Figure 5b shows that the characteristic curve obeys the WEBER-FECHNER law for all stimulation frequencies. In deaf persons, this potential cannot be reproduced. Further clinical experiences by THEISSING (1969, 1970) have not yet been reported.

When comparing both of these early evoked responses, the first described by STANGE *et al.*, with derivation from the ipsilateral mastoid and with a latency of 13 msec, and the second (THEISSING, 1969) picked up from the contralateral temporal scalp with a peak latency of 15 msec, we might expect to find a characteristic curve of the earlier 13 msec response more or less comparable to that of the acoustic nerve in animals and a characteristic curve of the 15 msec response substantially more like the characteristic curve of the acoustically evoked response that can be picked up in an anaesthetized animal with an electrode directly on the auditory cortex. It appears that there are two different, extra-cranial potentials, which can be derived from man's uninjured skull; the first representing the activity in the higher centres of the central auditory pathways, whereas the second represents the activity of the auditory cortex. Only further studies on hearing impaired children and adults may definitely prove the clinical value of these acoustically evoked responses. Here, we have of course to consider that this could only be due to the influence of the neurogenic components of the acoustic responses by muscular origin, though the muscles were under complete relaxation.

The last of the "fast" acoustically evoked responses in human subjects are those having a peak latency of 20–80 msec. As BORSANY reported in 1964, these responses disappear almost entirely after relaxation, and only a very small potential with 15 msec peak latency remains, probably the response that THEISSING

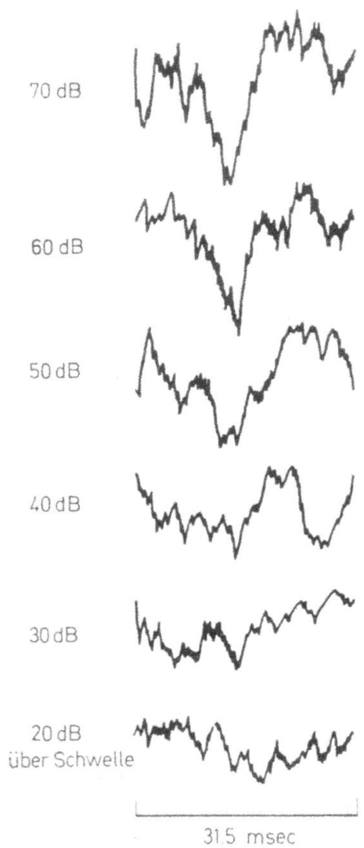

Fig. 5a

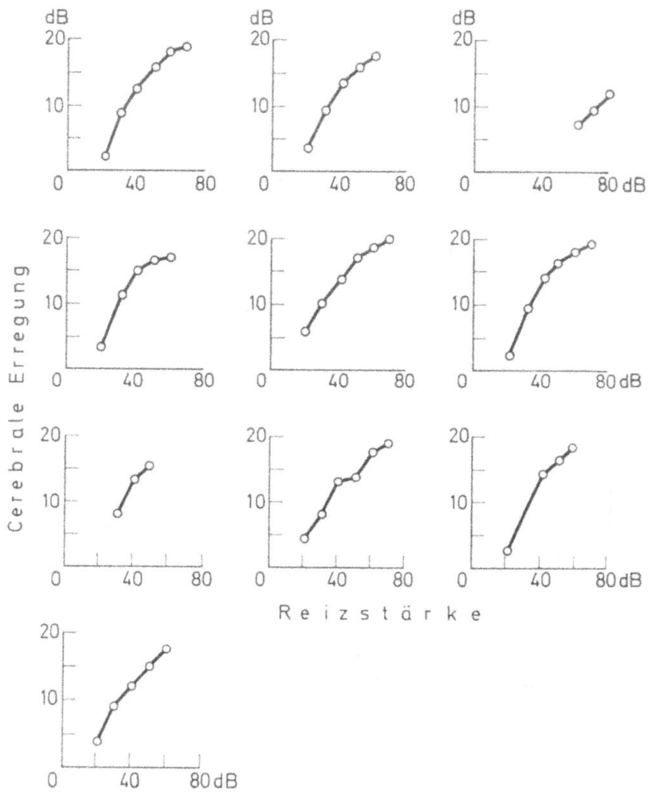

Fig. 5b

Fig. 5a. Acoustic evoked responses of man under relaxation anaesthesia; (average of 3000 responses; trace: 32 msec, positive maximum 15 msec). (Acc. to THEISSING, 1970)

Fig. 5b. Dependency on stimulation intensity of the amplitude of the acoustic evoked response in 10 normal hearing persons (double logarithmic scale). (Acc. to THEISSING, 1970)

recently examined more thoroughly. It is interesting that BORSANY did not recognize this residual potential. These acoustically evoked potential oscillations have mostly been regarded by other authors, too, as myogenic reflex potentials and were thought unsuitable for diagnosis of hearing damage (BICKFORD *et al.*, 1964; BORSANY, 1964; DAVIS, 1965; WALKER *et al.*, 1964; KEIDEL and SPRENG, 1965, and others). During prolonged acoustic stimulation, however, and while fast asleep, this component is preserved with invariable amplitudes and latencies.

The sounder the sleep, the more this potential diminishes. Corresponding results by MENDEL and GOLDSTEIN (1971) are shown in Fig. 6. One could imagine that under these conditions of stimulation and registration the early myogenic component could also be involved in cases of very difficult and severely brain injured children, in order to establish fundamentally whether acoustic perception happens at all. But also with this method of continuous registration during natural sleep extensive studies have not yet been made.

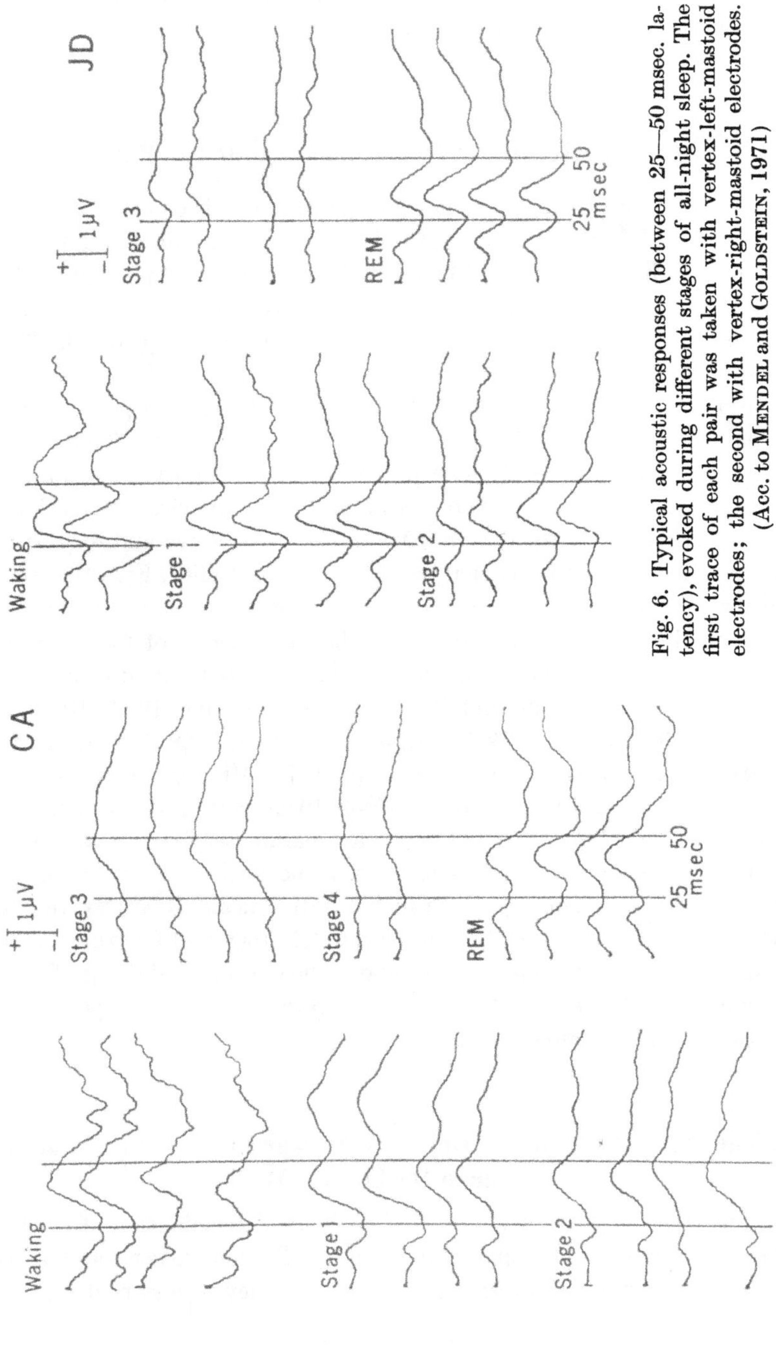

Fig. 6. Typical acoustic responses (between 25—50 msec. latency), evoked during different stages of all-night sleep. The first trace of each pair was taken with vertex-left-mastoid electrodes; the second with vertex-right-mastoid electrodes. (Acc. to MENDEL and GOLDSTEIN, 1971)

Only the future can show whether these early acoustic biopotentials will give us valuable data for clinical use. Recent studies of early acoustic potentials may indeed bring new aspects; unfortunately, sufficient clinical studies have not yet been made. Until now, only those experiments with registration of compound action potentials of the acoustic nerve have been thoroughly studied (Portmann and Aran, 1971; Yoshie and Ohashi, 1969; Sohmer and Feinmesser, 1972), as well as registration procedure with cochlear microphonics for clinical diagnosis (Yoshie and Yamaura, 1969). Certainly, the results hitherto obtained will yield further valuable revelations for clinical use.

C. The Acoustically Evoked Slow Central Responses

The slow components of the acoustic responses have been studied most extensively. They can be picked up from the intact human scalp. The latency of the negative peak is between 90 and 150 msec. The peak latency of N_1 (90–150 msec) occurs in the normal hearing adult only. For children and patients with impaired hearing, much longer peak latencies for N_1 have been registered. Therefore, participants at the "Round Table Conference" of the 1st. International ERA-Symposium (1970) in Freiburg agreed to take not only N_1 for a point of reference, but to look for N_1 also between the latency times of 100 and 300 msec (Davis, 1971). The first appearance of these potentials under increasing sound pressure and the application of two or three stimulation frequencies are used by most authors as a criterion for the determination of an "objective auditory threshold" and for the detection of an eventual impaired hearing ability. For other scientists, the auditory threshold, dependent on the frequency alone, is not sufficient; they also measure the supraliminal sphere, *i.e.* the dependency of the amplitudes of these acoustically evoked potentials on stimulation intensity, in order to get the characteristic curve (Keidel and Spreng, 1965; Stange, 1966; Beagley and Knight, 1966/1967; Spreng, 1967; Stange and Soda, 1968; Stange and Holm, 1970; Beagley and Kellog, 1971; Stange, 1971; Müller and Stange, 1971; Stange, 1972/1973; Karnahl and Benning, 1972; Benning *et al.*, 1972; Holm and Stange, 1972/1973). As a third important parameter for critical examination of the acoustically evoked slow potentials, some authors indicate the time of latency, mostly with reference to the first negative peak. Beagley and Knight (1966/1967), Theissing (1967), Stange (1968), Burian and Gestring (1969 and 1971), Benning *et al.* (1972) have pointed out the enormous shifting of the acoustical response after beginning of stimulation, up to 300–400 msec peak latency of N_1 in patients with impaired hearing.

1. The Importance of the Objective Measurement of the Auditory Threshold for Clinical Work

Most investigators have been satisfied with the determination of the auditory threshold by using evoked response audiometry. By comparing standard behavioral audiometry with evoked response audiometry, they believe that we now have the possibility of an objective diagnosis of hearing impairment. LOWELL *et al.* (1961) presented the first comparative measurements (objective/subjective) in normal hearing and hearing impaired persons. These authors pointed out the usefulness of the method and its value for clinical use. DAVIS (1965) showed the dependence of the averaged acoustic biopotentials on age and underlined their wide dispersion range in children. He, too, could observe a possibility for error of only $\pm$ 10 dB when compared to the subjective threshold; this finding has been confirmed by other investigators. Ample clinical cases of normal-hearing, cerebrally injured and deaf children were presented with reliable objective and subjective measurements of threshold by RAPIN and GRAZIANI (1967). A number of other researchers have reported extensive clinical studies of hearing impaired children (DAVIS, 1966; BURIAN *et al.*, 1969; ENGEL and YOUNG, 1969; SHARRARD, 1969, 1971; STANGE and HOLM, 1970; BARNET, 1971; BEAGLEY, 1971; BURIAN and GESTRING, 1971; MORGON *et al.*, 1971, and others). A suitable method for clinical use in view of a more exact definition of the threshold by way of interaction of sensory stimuli, was indicated by BURIAN *et al.* (1968). With acoustic-optical interaction of two sensory stimuli, favourable results were obtained, and still better results with acoustic-acoustical interaction. In difficult children, such a tone-tone interaction with constant stimulation interval, as shown in Fig. 7a, is certainly a valuable help for objective measurement of threshold. Also rather helpful for a more precise and exact definition of the threshold are the difference-

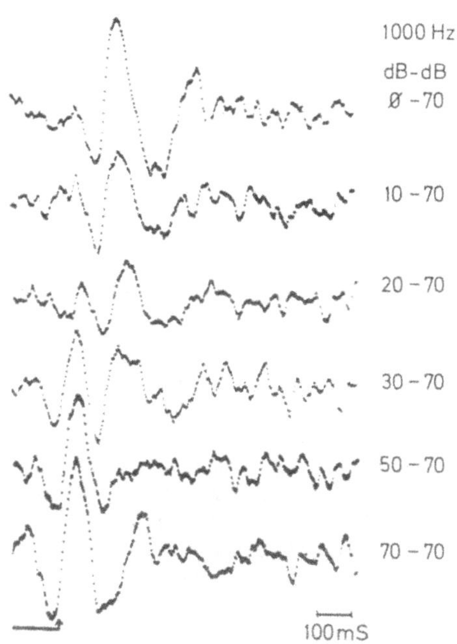

Fig. 7a. Tone-tone interaction under constant stimulation interval and increasing intensity of the early stimulation for exact determination of threshold. The first stimulation occurs in all modes of testing at the beginning of the time of analysis, the secound stimulus after 130 msec (Acc. to BURIAN *et al.*, 1968)

amplitude histograms, as described by SPRENG (1971) (Fig. 7b). SUZUKI and TAGUCHI (1965) as well as DAVIS *et al.* (1965, 1966) noticed that the objective threshold has higher values in younger children. BARNET and GODWIN (1965) reported the first results of audiometry on new-born children; auditory thresholds were 35–40 dB higher than in juveniles. Recently, MATHIS and GRAF (1972) have given a clear survey of the present state of threshold-audiometry with new-borns. In their report the most important findings of earlier authors are represented in tabulated form. SPRENG (1967), ONISHI and DAVIS (1968), and SPRENG (1969) drew particular attention to the importance of the ascending flank and to the duration of the tone bursts used as stimuli.

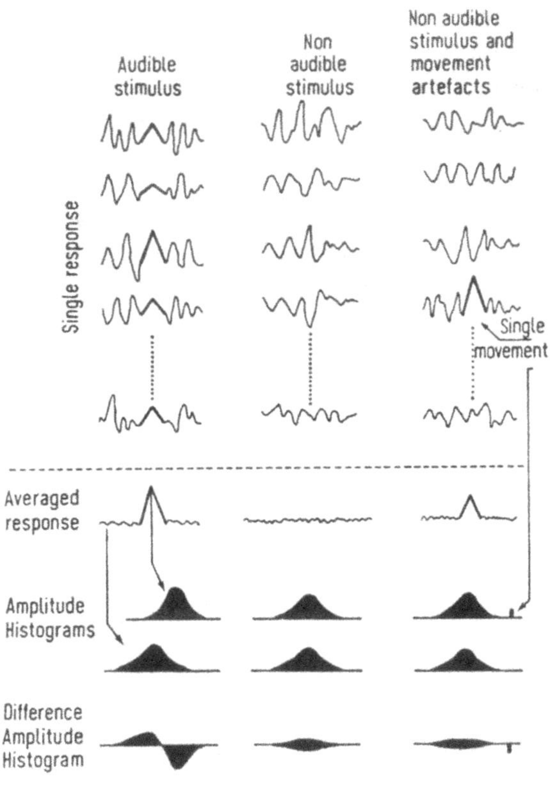

Fig. 7b. Determination of threshold by amplitude-difference-histogram. (Acc. to KEIDEL and SPRENG, 1971). Left column: an audible stimulus evokes feeble hidden responses in each registration. Therefore, the amplitude histograms for the two time points of the averaged result (origin of long arrows) show clearly separate peaks. As a consequence, the difference of both amplitude histograms has an asymmetrical shape. Central column: if no audible stimulus exists and no single response appears, the amplitude histograms of the same time points are quite similar; therefore, the amplitude-difference-histogram looks more symmetrical or shows zero. The averaged result is identical with the rest of the EEG. Right column: if no audible stimulus exists and no single hidden response appears except one, or a few large responses like voltage oscillations, caused f. i. by movement artefacts, the average result shows a response (non-stationary noise). But the symmetrical shape of the amplitude difference histogram with one or a few separate counts indicates subthreshold stimulation and averaged result caused by one single movement (take notice of the arrows)

In summary, and without naming all authors and describing their discoveries, we may say that evoked response audiometry has brought very satisfying clinical results, probably in new-borns, but for certain in children and adults. There are surprisingly few authors who refer to the difficulties with restless and cerebrally damaged children; these difficulties will be dealt with in the last section of this chapter, entitled: "Evoked Response Audiometry under Sedation". All the findings of evoked response audiometry show very clearly that, with this method alone, an exact statement on the dynamics of hearing, *i.e.* the functioning of the acoustic sensory system in the supraliminal sphere, cannot be made. Acoustic sensory modalities, as perception of loudness, adaptation, recruitment and discrimination, cannot be examined with evoked response audiometry alone. Furthermore,

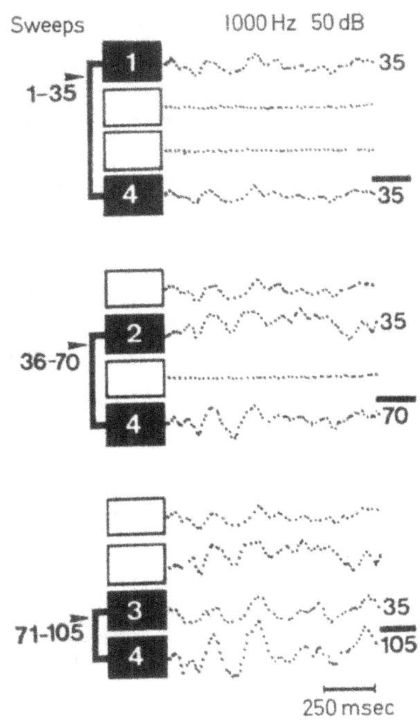

Fig. 8a. Multiple-channel-write-out method. (Acc. to Burian and Gestring, 1971)

it is not possible to differentiate between right and left acoustic sensory pathways solely by recording from the vertex. Therefore, several investigators have used the synchronous, multi-channel technique of recording (Burian and Gestring, 1971; Stange, 1971; Müller and Stange, 1971). With multi-channel pick-up at different sites simultaneously, it has been possible to recognize responses to acoustic stimuli close to the threshold and to differentiate between the right and left sides of the auditory system. Examples of records made by Burian and Gestring (1971) and by Stange (1971, 1973) are shown in Fig. 8a and b. These records indicate how valuable such synchronous multi-channel techniques of pick-up and registration can be.

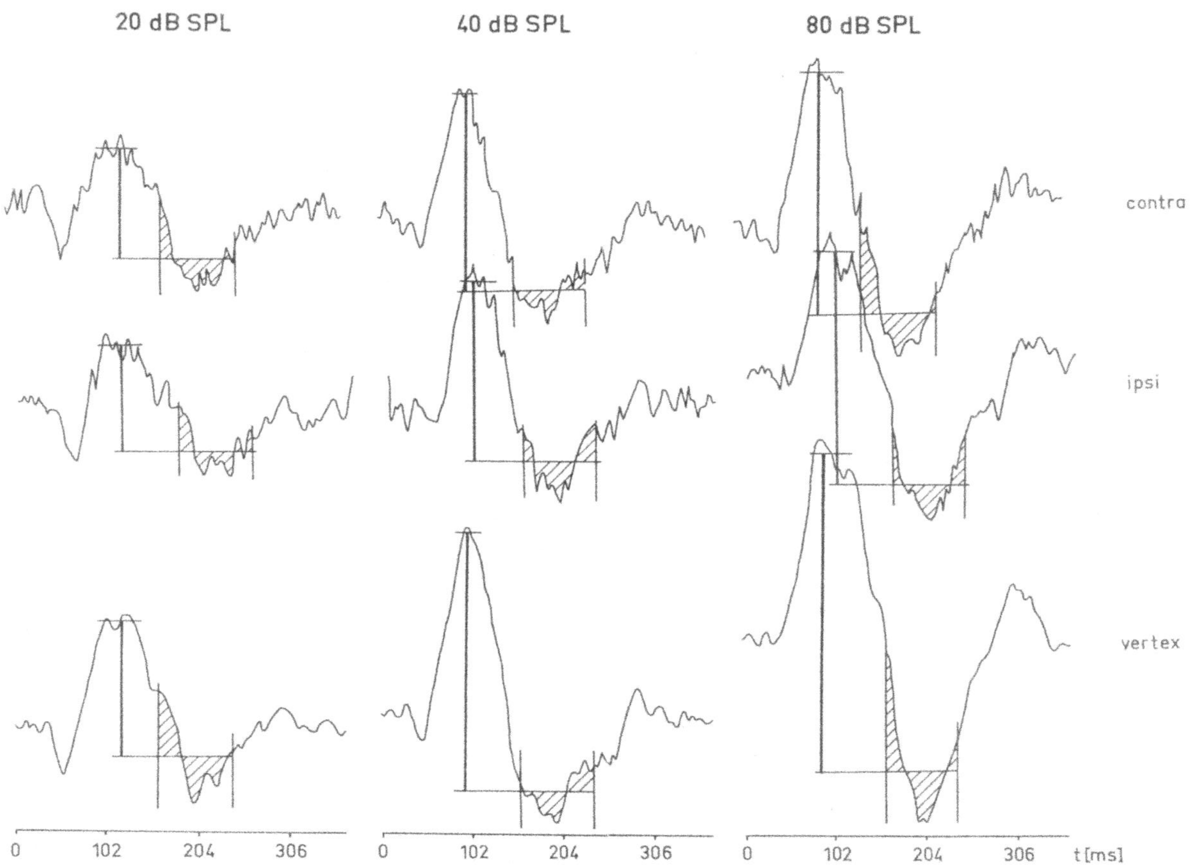

Fig. 8b. Contralateral, ipsilateral and vertex registrations, simultaneously with 20 dB SPL (on the left), 40 dB SPL (in the middle) and 80 dB SPL (on the right). Ordinate: amplitude of acoustic electrical responses; abscissa: time (msec) after onset of acoustic stimulation. (Acc. to Stange, 1971)

2. Evoked Response Audiometry in the Supraliminal Sphere

In order to understand quantitatively the dynamics of hearing disbilities, we have to perform supraliminal measurements. KEIDEL and SPRENG were the first to point out the relationship of amplitude of evoked response and intensity of acoustic stimulation, and, for the range of middle frequencies in particular, they were able to demonstrate and prove a dependence of the intensity function equivalent to the subjectively measured and calculated power function according to STEVENS. BEAGLEY and KNIGHT (1967) realized its usefulness; later STANGE and SODA (1968). All these authors obtained and reported ample clinical data about hearing disabilities which were until then only subjectively noticed. The course of the ERA-characteristic curves for adults can be correlated with hearing defects (STANGE and SODA, 1968; STANGE, 1971; MÜLLER and STANGE, 1971). Likewise, in children a more exact knowledge of dynamics and function of the affected acoustic sensory pathways, right and left separately, became possible. Thereby, the field of pedaudiological diagnosis expands, thus making easier (or even possible) a pedaudiological therapy either by training or by the use of protheses (STANGE and HOLM, 1970; HOLM, 1971; STANGE, 1971; BENNING *et al.*, 1972; STANGE, 1973; HOLM and STANGE, 1972, 1973).

In order to obtain a comparison between normal hearing and affected hearing, the ERA-characteristic curves in the supraliminal sphere have to be recorded from an adequate sample of normal hearing children.

Two points are of the greatest importance for exact quantitative measurements of hearing ability in the supraliminal sphere:

1. the acoustic stimulation program has to be standardized;

2. the evaluation of the amplitudes of the evoked potentials has to be carried out giving consideration to the level of electrically recorded cerebral activity.

Quantitative statements may then become possible about hearing disabilities in the supraliminal sphere and a comparison may be made between normal physiological and pathophysiological data. The acoustic stimulation program has to be set up with consideration of the fundamental papers by SPRENG (1967), ONISHI and DAVIS (1968), and SPRENG (1969). These studies clearly showed the importance of an exact definition of rise and fall time as well as duration of tone-bursts used in evoked response measurements. STANGE and SODA developed an acoustic stimulus program that was always alike and that contained statistically distributed tone-bursts with rise and fall times of 25 msec and plateau duration of 500 msec. They obtained very good clinical results. The stimulation program and the CAT-computer were triggered together. Thus, a comparison between normal and impaired hearing became possible in the supraliminal sphere. According to KEIDEL and SPRENG (1965), a state of adaptation of the acoustic system can be measured by inserting short intervals between tone-bursts; a nonadapted state, by inserting long intervals between the tonebursts. In this way, an impaired ability of adaptation may be observed (STANGE, 1966; STANGE and SODA, 1968; STANGE and HOLM, 1971; STANGE, 1971; MÜLLER and STANGE, 1971; HOLM and STANGE, 1973). Nevertheless, we cannot be sure, in clinical conditions, whether there is impaired adaptation (KEIDEL, 1963, 1966) or a functional disorder of habituation (Butler, 1968). For evaluation of the acoustic evoked response, a calculation of the whole area of potentials with the help of computers seems to be the best measure, as Spreng (1971), Stange and Karnahl (1973), and Karnahl *et al.* (1973) have shown in their studies of patients with impaired hearing. However, only a few clinical research scientists have available computers large enough for computations of this kind.

The calculation of amplitudes in relation to registration trace under conversion of the found values into cerebral excitation level in dB, as given by Spreng (1967), therefore, proved to be clinically very useful indeed for Stange *et al.* during these last years. Thus, from 1966–1972 they could gather ample clinical material by testing adults and children in the supraliminal sphere. Corresponding changes of the characteristic curves, for instance, in a sort of recruitment, an adaptation disorder or a diminution of the dynamics in the supraliminal sphere could be made use of therapeutically. In a lager number of adults with inner ear damage, for example, whose tone-audiograms differed from their speech audiograms, the ability of understanding speech being reduced, together with a lack of discrimination, a severe adaptation disorder, on the one hand, and a very flat characteristic curve on the other, was by this method ascertained. After many weeks of intensive inner ear therapy (Stange, 1969), the characteristic curves in the supraliminal sphere in relation to steepness and adaptation could be normalized, whereafter speech audiograms corresponded to tone audiograms. It is natural that these patients had much more facility in understanding every-day language. Corresponding details about this therapy with children will be reported later.

Figure 9a now shows the calculation procedure, as proposed by Spreng (1967). Figure 9b illustrates the importance of this calculation in an examination of a 6-month-old child. Figure 8b gives an example of registration with a 3-channel simultaneous pick-up at the contra- and ipsilateral side and at the vertex with rising sound pressure; the increase of the amplitudes can be distinctly seen. Figure 9d shows the characteristic curves of the supraliminal sphere with contra- and ipsilateral recording and from the vertex for the adapted and nonadapted state of the acoustic system (Müller and Stange, 1971). These characteristic curves for the adapted and non-adapted state of the acoustic system are valid for normal hearing adults at 1.0 kHz. Corresponding characteristic curves were reported by Beagley and Knight (1966, and 1967) (Fig. 9c). The dependency of these characteristic curves on stimulus intensity was reported for the first time by Benning *et al.* (1972). They tested 15 normal hearing children, 3–6 years of age. It was clearly seen that a difference exists between the characteristic curves of adults and those of children, and that, with increasing stimulation frequency, the characteristic curves become flatter (Fig. 10).

The observation that the shape of the characteristic curves depends on frequency of the stimulus is particulary important for children and for their eventual hearing prostheses as well as for their therapeutic speech training (Stange and Holm, 1970; Stange, 1971; Holm, 1971; Holm and Stange, 1972; Benning *et al.* 1972; Holm and Stange 1973). We have already referred to the importance of the shifting of the threshold in infants. We shall now show measurements in the supraliminal sphere for 3 and 6 month-old children, compared to 3–6 year-old children and to normal hearing adults; differences in the characteristic curves can

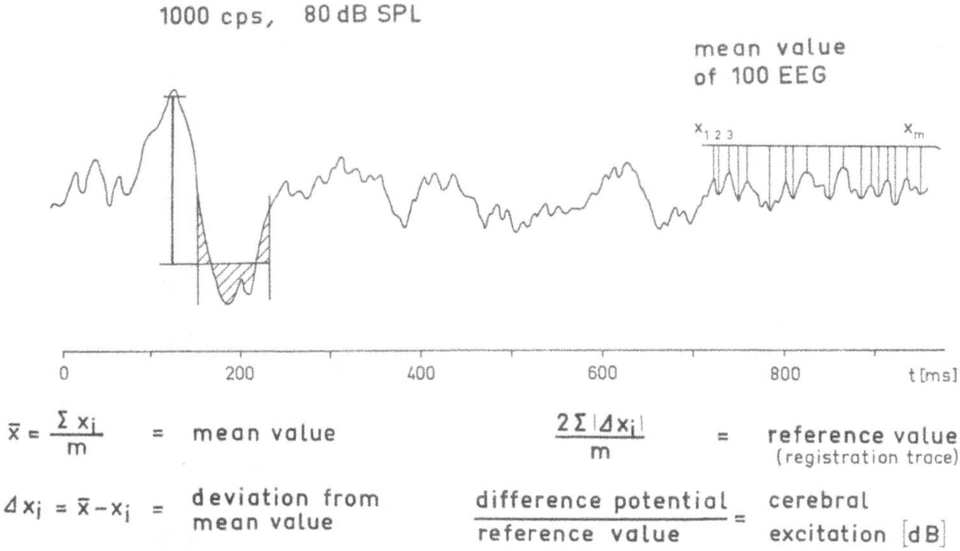

Fig. 9a. Calculation of amplitudes of the acoustically evoked responses, (Acc. to SPRENG, 1967; STANGE, 1971)

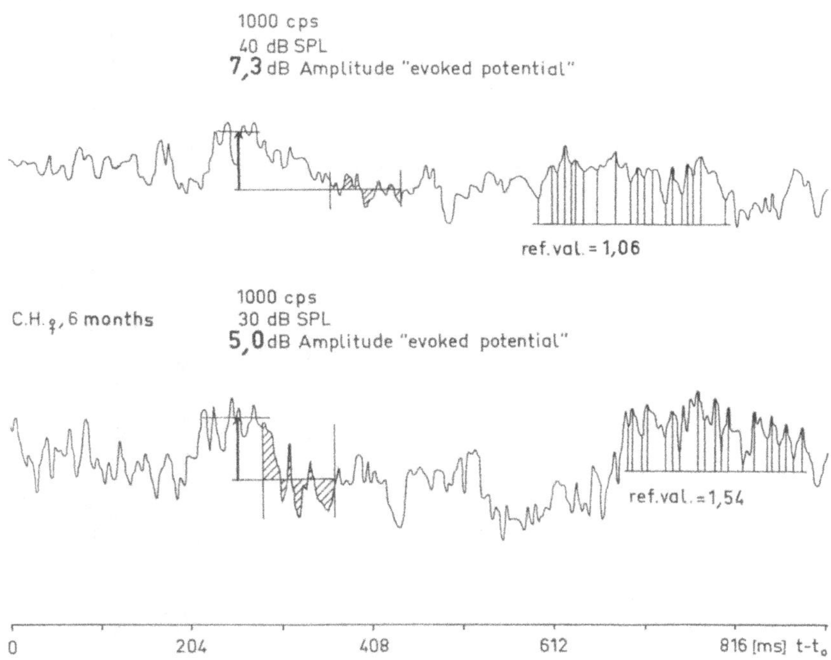

Fig. 9b. Importance of calculation of acoustically evoked responses for quantitative discrimination (a hearing impaired 6-month-old infant). At first glance, the response in the lower registration trace seems to be the larger one; but actually in terms of cortical excitation in dB its value is lower (5.0 dB cortical excitation) than that of the potential registered in the upper trace (7.3 dB cortical excitation); this result is due to the different reference values on which the calculated registrations are based. (STANGE, 1971)

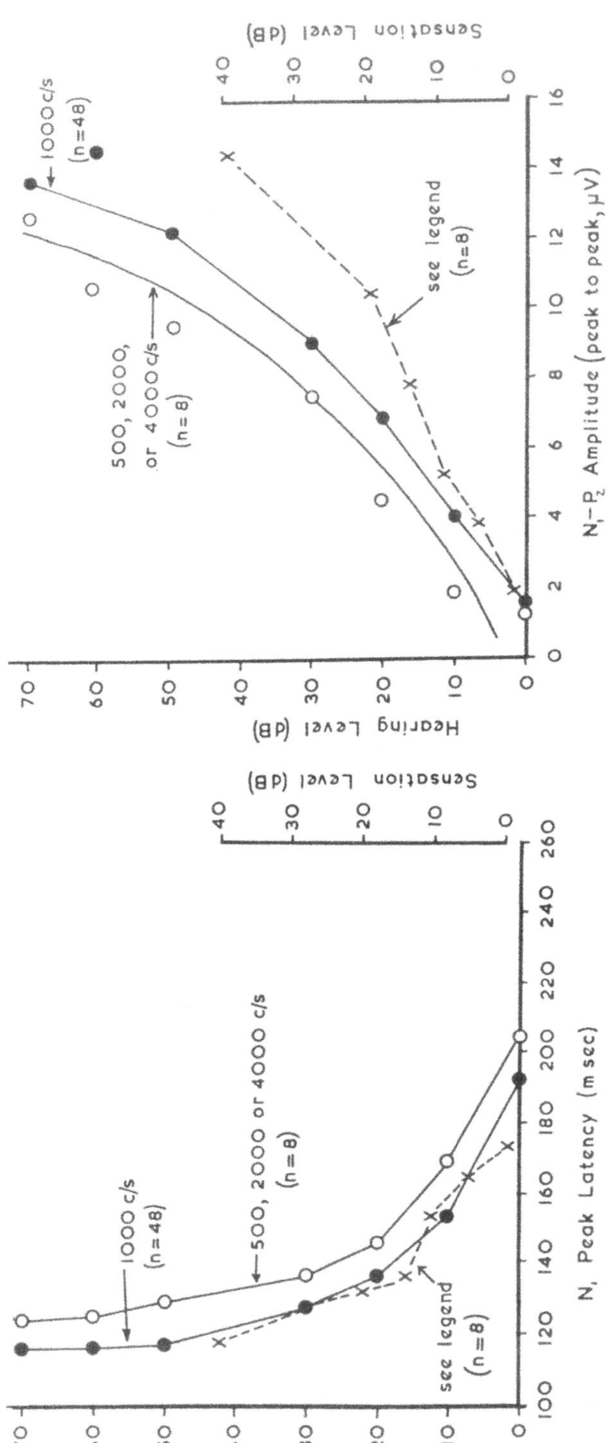

Fig. 9c. Amplitudes (top) and latencies (bottom) of ERA: dependency on frequency and intensity of tone. (Acc. to BEAGLEY and KNIGHT, 1966, 1967.) o------o main experiment with 1000 cps at different hearing levels, O------O other frequencies at various hearing levels, x------x experiment with 1000 cps at sensation levels

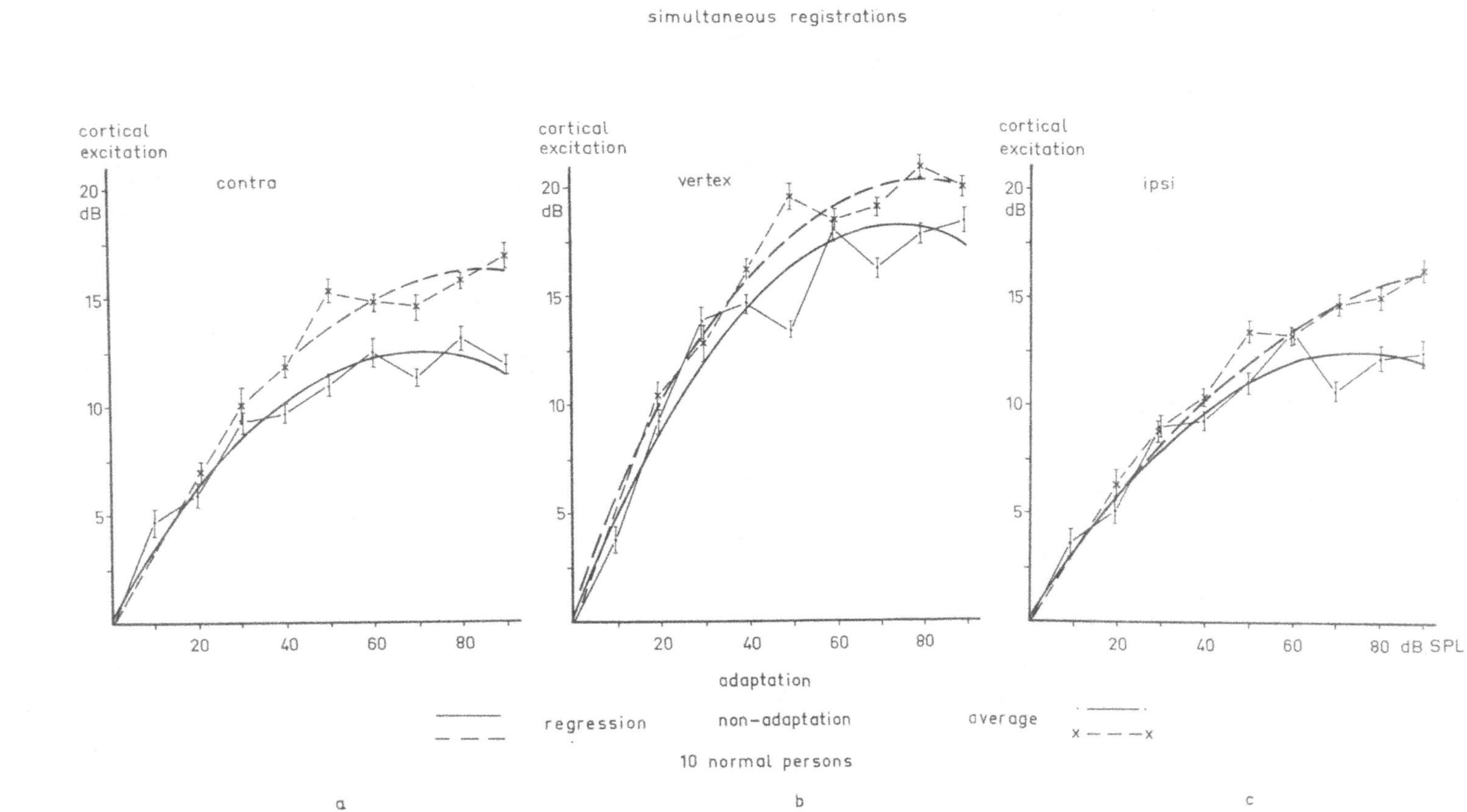

Fig. 9d. ERA-characteristic curves (1000 kHz, 11 normal hearing adults); relation between sound pressure level (abscissa) and level of cortical excitation (ordinate), when simultaneously picked-up with small Beckman-electrodes. The continuous lines represent the regression in the non-adapted stage; the dotted lines, those in the adapted stage. The standard error is shown as a vertical line at each point. a: contralateral pick-up, b: vertex pick-up, c: ipsilateral pick-up. (For detailed interpretation see Müller and Stange, 1971)

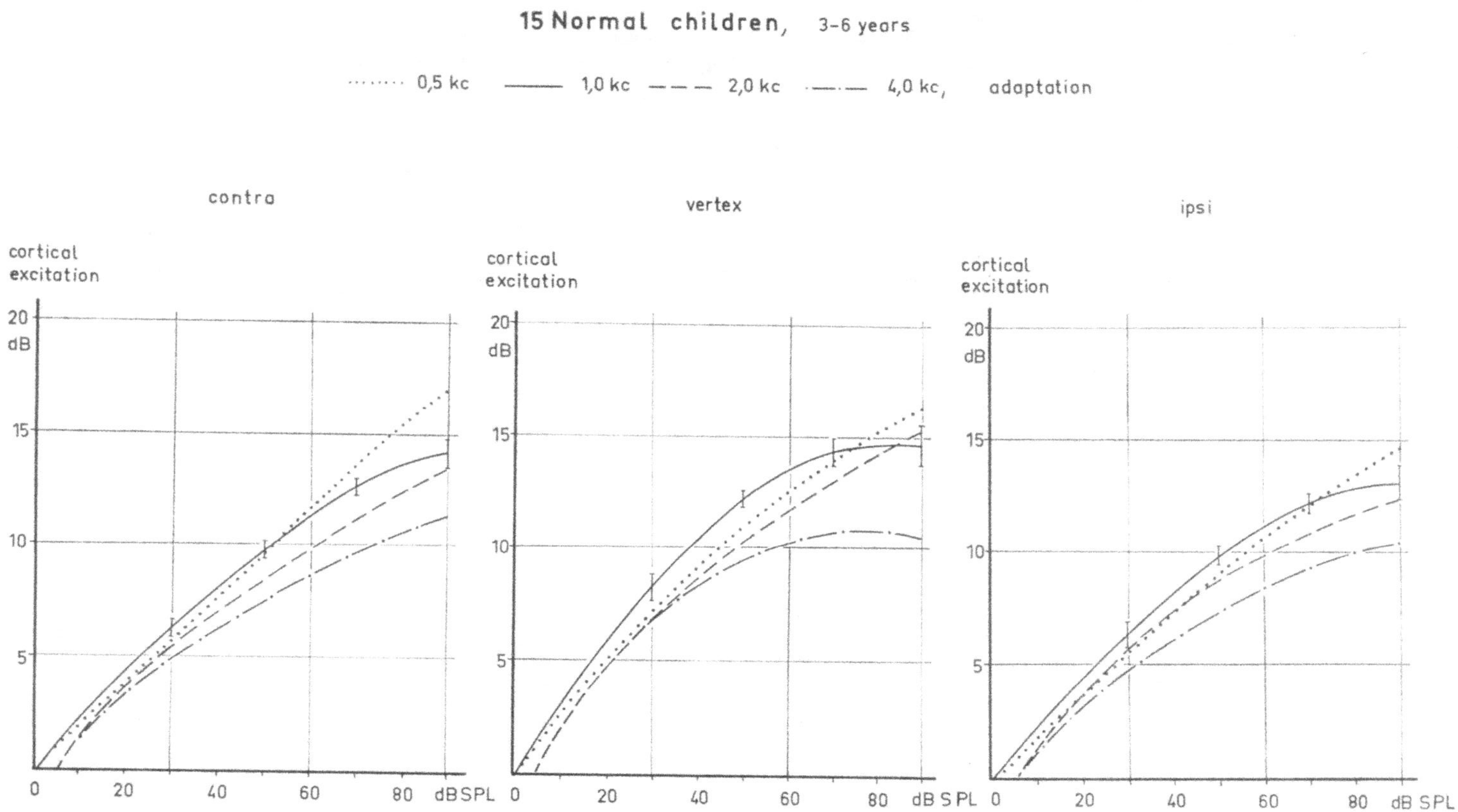

Fig. 10. ERA-characteristic curves of 15 normal hearing children (3—6 years); measured frequencies: 0.5, 1.0, 2.0, and 4.0 kHz. The curves are different from the characteristic curves of adults (see Fig. 9d). (Acc. to BENNING *et al.*, 1972)

be distinctly seen. Figure 11a shows recorded examples of a 3-month-old girl, while Fig. 11b represents the corresponding characteristic curves. You will note the steepness of the characteristic curves of 3-month-old infants. It has not been possible to record with a higher SPL than 50 dB as the children then start to cry. The shifting of threshold of about 20 dB with the subsequent very steep characteristic curve of the 3-month-old child is very clearly seen. In 3–6 year-old children,

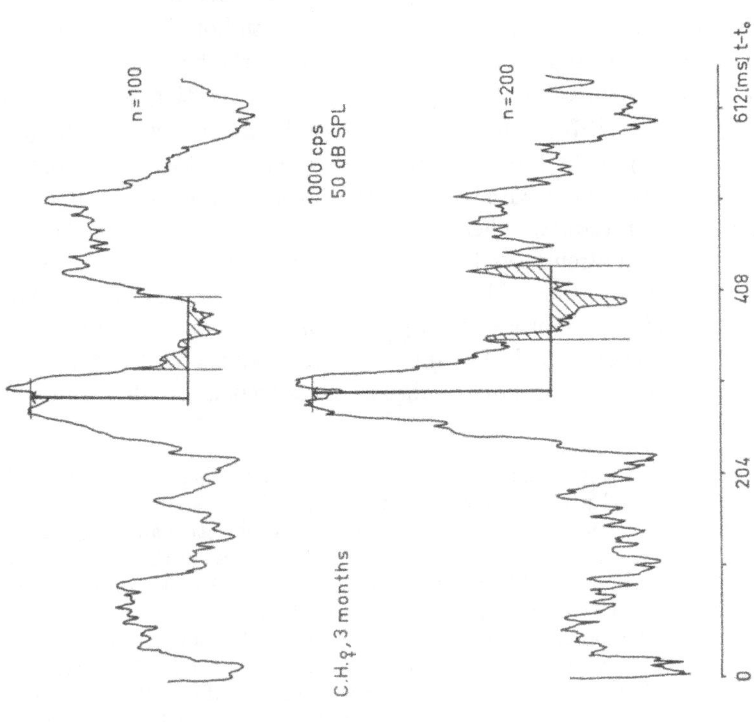

Fig. 11a. Acoustically evoked potentials at the cortex of a three-month-old infant. Upper trace: $n = 100$; lower trace: $n = 200$

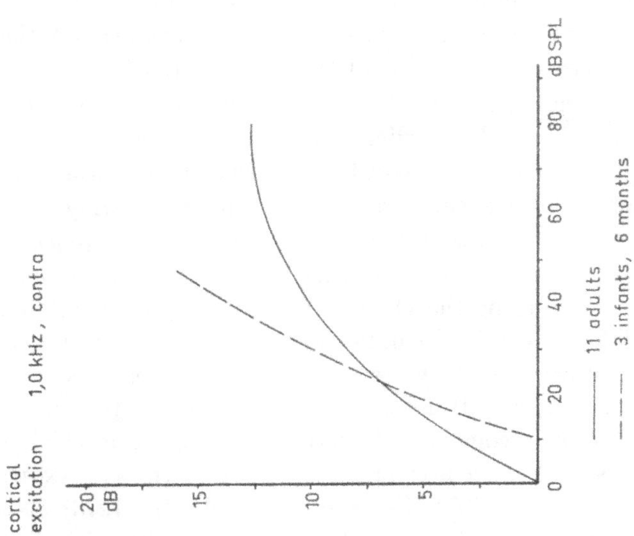

Fig. 11b. Characteristic curves of normal-hearing children; - - - - - - 6 months; ——— 25-years (11 adults)

the characteristic curves more closely approach those of adults. Observation of these characteristic ERA curves is necessary if functional defects in the supraliminal sphere are to be recorded in infants at an early stage. Of further importance, especially for detecting the evoked response, is the knowledge of the dependency of the latency times of peak N_1 on SPL and frequency. BEAGLEY and KNIGHT (1966, 1967) reported the first reliable data in the physiological field, as shown in Fig. 9c. It is interesting to note that, for the frequencies of 500, 2000, and 4000 Hz, there is no difference in the latency of evoked responses, whereas we have shorter latency times for a stimulus of 1000 Hz. The extension of the latencies of N_1 under low stimulation intensities was confirmed by BENNING *et al.* (1972), these authors found shorter latencies for N_1 than BEAGLEY and KNIGHT.

Only an exact knowledge and the most careful observance of the technical data about stimulation and recording make a narrow physiological dispersion range in the supraliminal sphere possible, and only then can a comparison be made between physiological hearing ability and impaired hearing.

During recent years, teamwork between paedaudiologists, otoneurologists and communication-engineers on the basis of data obtained from sensory physiology have shown how important the clinical diagnosis of the supraliminal sphere, especially for children, can be for drawing therapeutical consequences. Particularly in the field of paedaudiology, results so far have been most prolific. In cooperation with KEIDEL and HOLM and STANGE were able to reach therapeutic conclusions for the most complicated hearing impairments in children. Reports about some of these cases have been made in medical journals (STANGE and HOLM, 1970; HOLM, 1971; STANGE, 1971; HOLM and STANGE, 1972, 1973). As an illustration of the use of ERA, a brief report will be given here difficult cases of children who were examined with both subjective and objective audiometry. For these children, it was not possible to give an exact diagnosis of their hearing damage by means of the usual subjective and (partly) objective testing procedures, such as listed by THEISSING (1970). The data for the two children are representative of the results obtained for about 100 children. All of them were thoroughly diagnosed in the supraliminal sphere with Evoked Response Audiometry and with paedaudiological testing procedures. Their different hearing disabilities were correspondingly treated. The children have been selected for illustration here for two reasons: first, they had been examined previously in other clinics, but it had not been possible to provide appropriate therapy on the basis of measurements obtained by the usual paedaudiological examination methods; secondly, they are typical of the frequently recurring hearing disturbances that are rather difficult to diagnose correctly.

Such different and contradictory diagnoses as "autism", "abnormal behaviour", "mental retardation", "normal hearing" and "audiometrical test impossible" had been made of a 6-year-old girl at other institutions. After repeated subjective and objective audiometry, we discovered that the was suffering from a symmetrical inner-ear deafness of the U-type (Fig. 12a). After thorough examination, the child's EEG, intelligence and behaviour proved to be without pathological findings. The objective auditory threshold curves measured with ERA corresponded to the subjective ones, but they were in relation to hearing loss about 20—40 dB better. For 0.25 kHz, the supraliminal ERA characteristic curves yielded a cortical excitation of only about 5 dB with a dynamic range of 60 dB; the course of the ERA characteristic curves was too flat compared with the normal curve, without substantial side difference between right and left acoustic system. The ERA characteristic curves of 1.0 kHz ran steep and with different dynamic range, on the right side it was lower comprising 40 dB, whereas it ranged within an area of 60 dB on the left side. Cortical excitation on the right was lower, on the left higher and with rising stimulation intensity higher than normal. At 4.0 kHz and with contralateral derivation, ERA characteristic curves corresponded on the right by 1/3, on the left by more than 2/3 to the normal curve, with about the same dynamic range of 40—50 dB (Fig. 12b). If latency times — enormously extended latency at 1.0 kHz, partly also at 0.25 kHz for N_1 of the right acoustic pathway — are included in our critical examination of the child's hearing ability, the discrepancy in the functioning of the acoustic systems will be realized in spite of the courses of the ERA characteristic curves, which do not always show this difference so distinctly. Functioning of the left acoustic canal seems to correspond more to the physiological standard than the right one. Only a multifactored supraliminal analysis of the whole acoustic system can result in satisfactory information about pathological function and adequate therapeutic measures. The stereophonic hearing aid was to be applied with identically adjusted hearing aids according to the subjective audiogram. Our attempt met with the child's refusal and with an obviously worsened comprehension of speech. By different adjustment of the AVC and PC and monaural application separately for the right and left ear, an equally good hearing and understanding could be obtained. According to the supraliminal ERA findings (characteristic curve and latency times) ear-training was carried through with hearing aids individually adjusted for each ear. In this case, we desisted from the use of linear, *i.e.* in their frequency scarcely variable stereo-hearing-trainers. Only intensive hearing training under special pedagogical guidance made stereophonic utilization of both differently functioning acoustic canals in this inner ear damaged child possible.

The second example is that of a three-year-old boy, who, on account of recurring bronchitis since infancy, had received repeated doses of streptomycine. In the meantime, diagnoses about his hearing ability ranged from normal hearing to deafness. Subjective audiograms showed a symmetrical residual hearing (Fig. 13a). The use of a stereophonic hearing-aid had been refused by the child. A diagnostic and therapeutic attempt with his own hearing-aids as well as with stereophonic ear-trainers did not bring the expected hearing gain. The ERA threshold curve corresponds approximately to the subjectively found values (Fig. 13a). Here, as is often the case, the objective threshold values are better, and the curves do not suggest a U-shaped course. As we can see in Fig. 13b, the ERA curves have a much steeper course than those of a patient with normal hearing. Cortical excitation on the left side, under high stimulation intensities, for 0.5, 1.0, and 4.0 kHz meets the normal value, while the curves for the right ear do not average more than 2/3 of the normal values. The ERA curves seem to have a similar course; they prove, however, that the right ear and the left ear offer a different (on the left better than on the right) dynamic range to be corrected by hearing prostheses, that can be measured by the supraliminal cortical excitation. If we now include the latency times for N_1, as shown in the upper part of Fig. 13c, into our critical examination, we see that these latencies have the same course as the normal curves, but they seem to be much shorter, and the right side seems to differ from the left. These curves now explain the child's refusal of two identically adjusted hearing aids, *i.e.* his rejection of the synchronous signal on both sides in the stereophonic hearing trainers.

As has been reported in earlier studies, there are kinds and degrees of hearing loss in children which, for an optimal therapy, require variable ear trainers, as the "SUVAG II" of GUBERINA or the compensation trainer of LAFON (HOLM and STANGE, 1972). Because of the ERA-findings, the behaviour of supraliminal dynamics and latency of the acoustic system, this case was treated with the help of the "SUVAG II"-ear trainer. On account of its characteristics, the steepness of the high and low pass filter, it was possible to eliminate in the beginning the frequencies that were disagreeable for the child; in the course of further therapy, this frequency region was improved in its functional performance by correcting the filter's steepness. Only then, and with the help of individual hearing aids, the child was able to understand speech without further problems.

When considering the supraliminal ERA-findings, the importance of the acoustic adaptation or habituation has to be pointed out. A merely different adaptation behaviour of both sensory pathways can make a successful use of

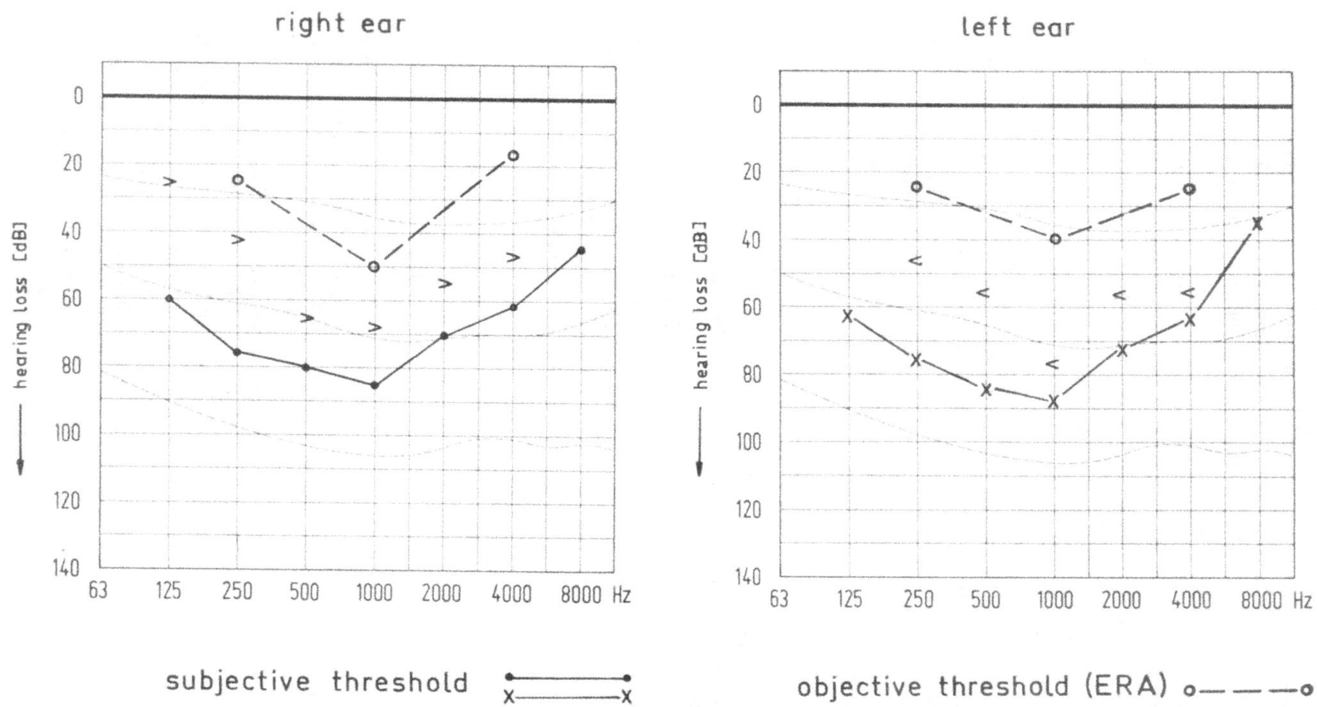

Fig. 12a. Subjective and objective threshold curves of a 6-year-old girl with inner ear damage

---

Fig. 12b. ERA-characteristic curves for frequencies of 0.25, 1.0, and 4.0 kHz of the same 6-year-old girl as in Fig. 12a, with synchronous 3-channel contralateral, ipsilateral derivation and pick-up at the vertex. The thin, broken lines in frequency specific shape represent ERA-standard curves for children (see interpretation)

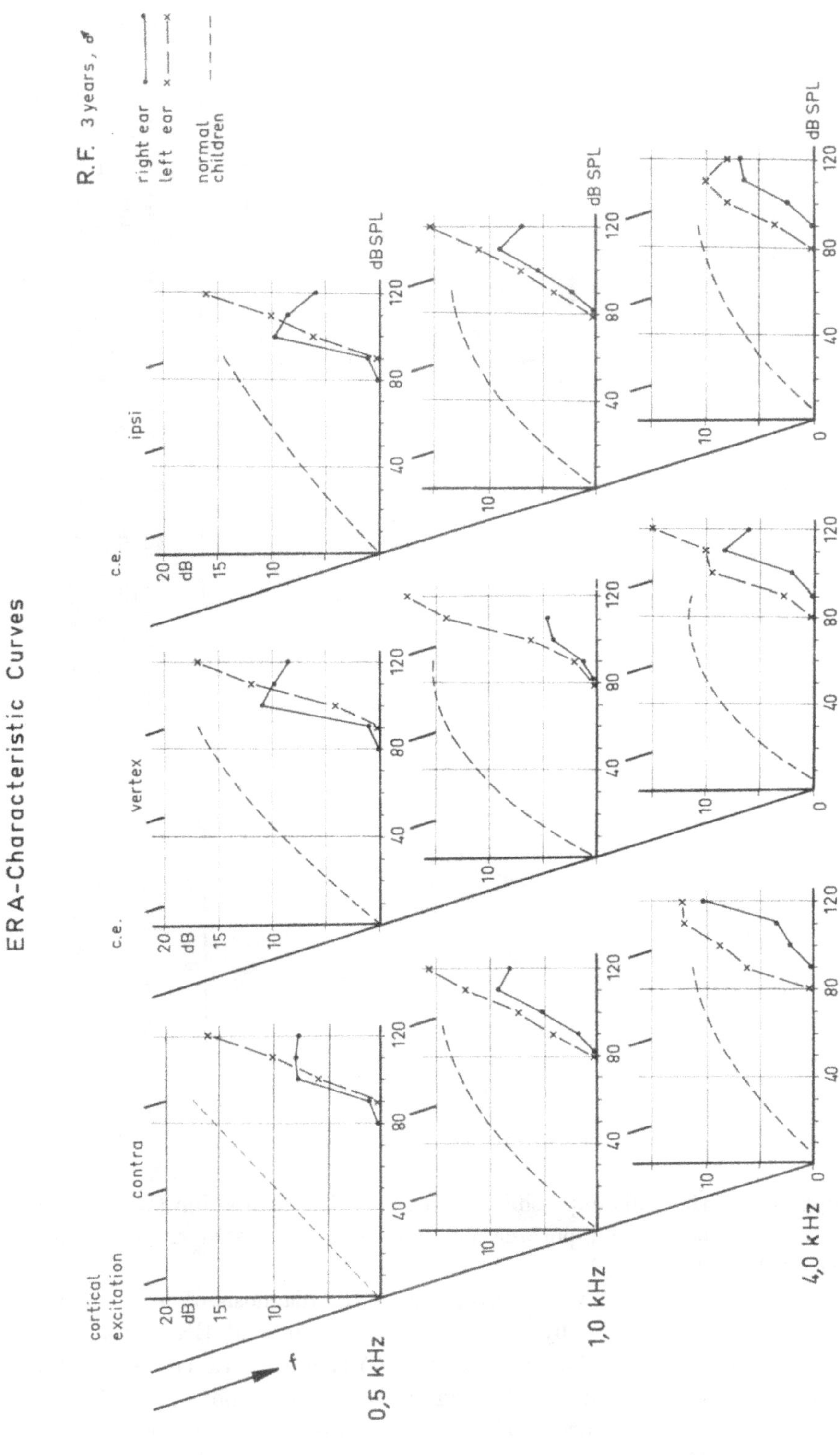
ERA-Characteristic Curves
R.F. 3 years, ♂
right ear
left ear
normal children
cortical excitation
contra
c.e.
vertex
c.e.
ipsi
dB SPL
0,5 kHz
1,0 kHz
4,0 kHz
f

Fig. 12b

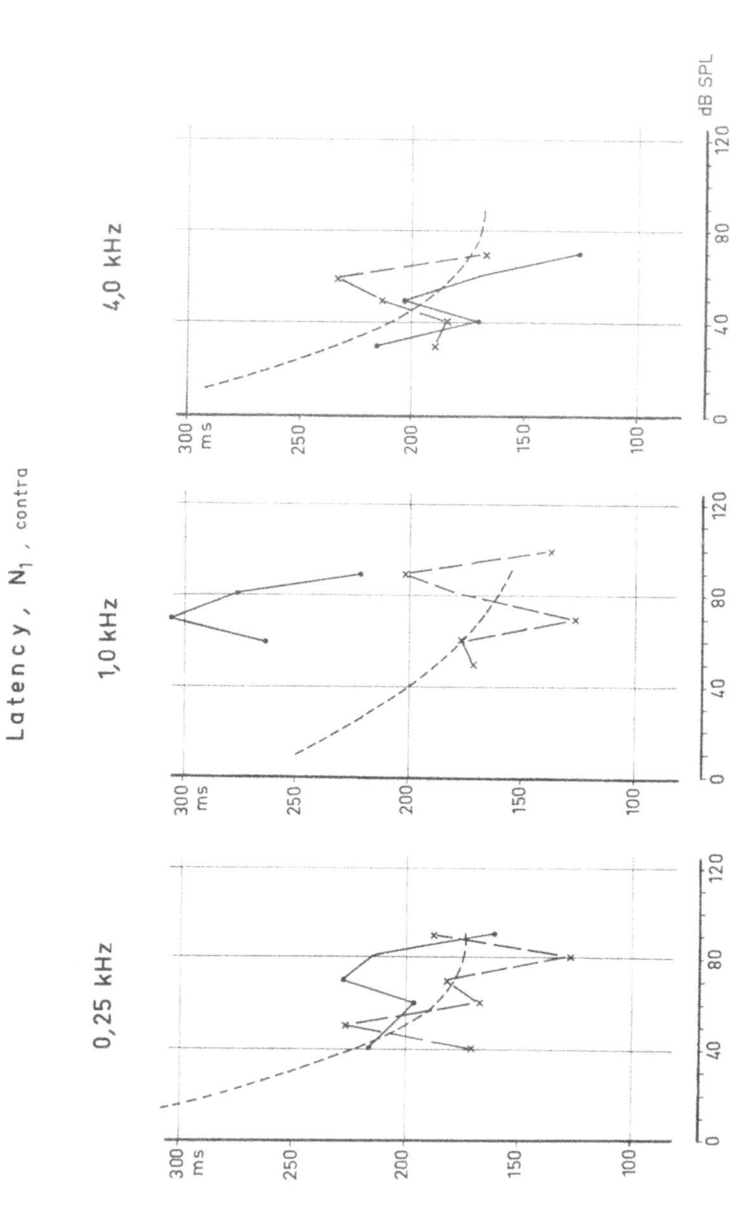

Fig. 12c. Latency behaviour of the acoustically evoked potential of the same girl as in (a) and (b), for frequencies of 0.25, 1.0, and 4.0 kHz. The thin, broken lines show the frequency specific standard latency. (Acc. to BENNING *et al.*, 1972). The latency behaviour of the central biopotential that was registered at the left acoustic sensory pathway corresponds considerably more to the standard, especially at 1.0 kHz, than that registered atthe right sensory pathway

stereophonic hearing aids impossible. At the 1st ERA-Symposiun (1970) in Freiburg (West Germany) the importance of adaptation was pointed out and discussed (STANGE, 1971; HOLM, 1971).

From the studies of STANGE (1973) during the diagnosis of more than 100 inner ear damaged children by application of supraliminal ERA, it has been possible to show typical pathophysiological ERA characteristic curves for amplitudes and latencies of N_1. In the left diagram of Fig. 14, we observe the following pathophysiological ERA curves of hearing impaired children (SPRENG, 1967; STANGE, 1971). This illustration does not reproduce actual results in their averaged form, but schematically shows the pathophysiological ERA curves as they are found in inner ear damaged children who have a shift of threshold. Here the curve *N* represents the physiological course for 1.0 kHz. The curve *I* shows the same course after shift of threshold. At first, the course of curve *II* reproduces the standard at some dB levels, but it then bends steeply down towards lower values. The course of curve *III* shows, with an only slightly increased sound intensity, recruitment with subsequent steepness of the characteristic curve. This means that with a greater sound intensity, the amplitudes are far above normal. The course of curve *III* may also be bending down towards normal values when compensation of loudness has been attained. Finally, curve *IV* becomes a rather flat following the shifting of the threshold, which means that only small amplitudes appear. The diagram of Fig. 14 presents, on the right, the typical courses for latency at N_1. The curve *N* shows the typical course for 15 normal- hearing children. The other four curves (*a*, *b*, *c*, *d*) represent the latency times of acoustically evoked potentials in hearing impaired children as they can be observed again and again. Thus, the curve "*a*", in the supraliminal sphere, shows a course quite similar to the normal one. In many of the children with impaired hearing, no shifting of latency of the evoked potentials in the supraliminal sphere has taken place. The curve "*b*" shows that the latencies for N_1 are remarkably lengthened, but the course of these curves, depending on the intensity of stimulation, corre-

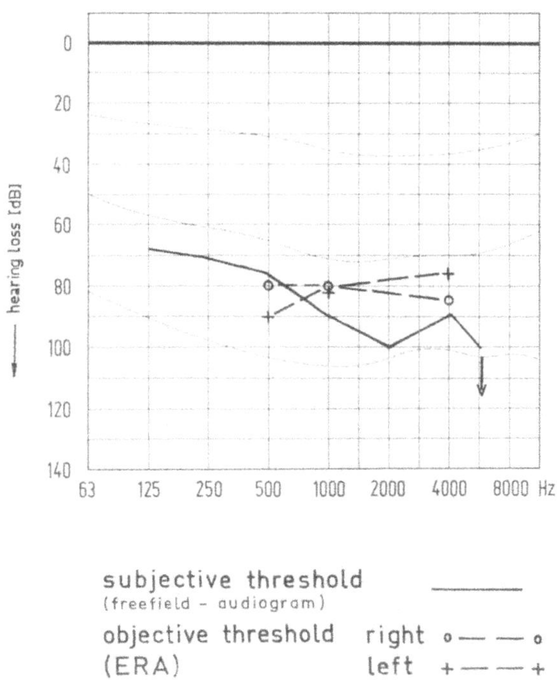

Fig. 13a—c. Subjective and objective auditory threshold curves: (a): ERA-characteristic curves: (b) and latency behaviour: (c) compared with contralaterally measured ERA-characteristic curves in a 3-year-old boy with inner ear damage caused by streptomycine. Parameter and symbols as in Fig. 12a—c (see further interpretation)

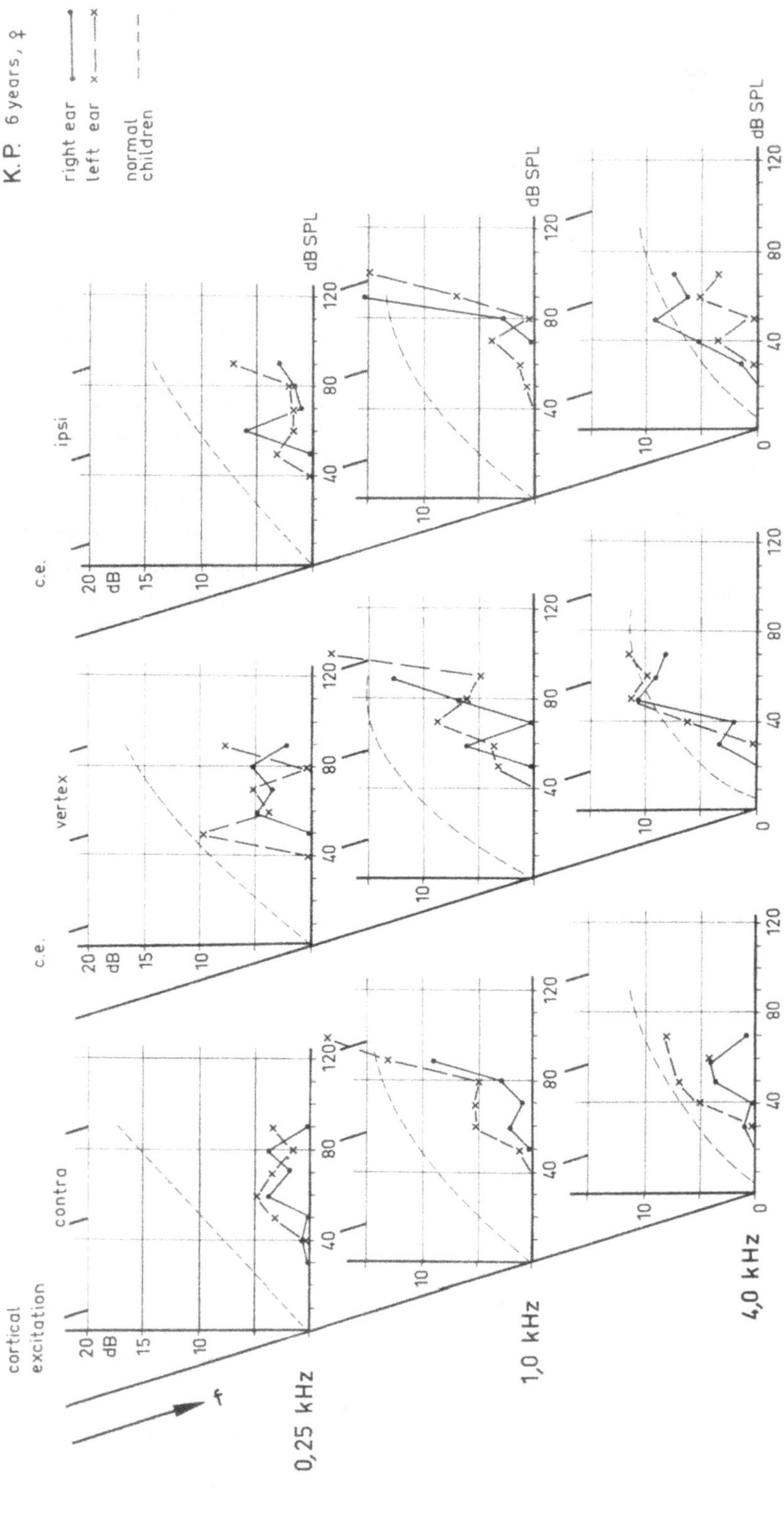
ERA-Characteristic Curves
K.P. 6 years, ♀
right ear
left ear
normal children
cortical excitation
contra
c.e.
vertex
c.e.
ipsi
dB
dB SPL
0,25 kHz
1,0 kHz
4,0 kHz
f

Fig. 13b

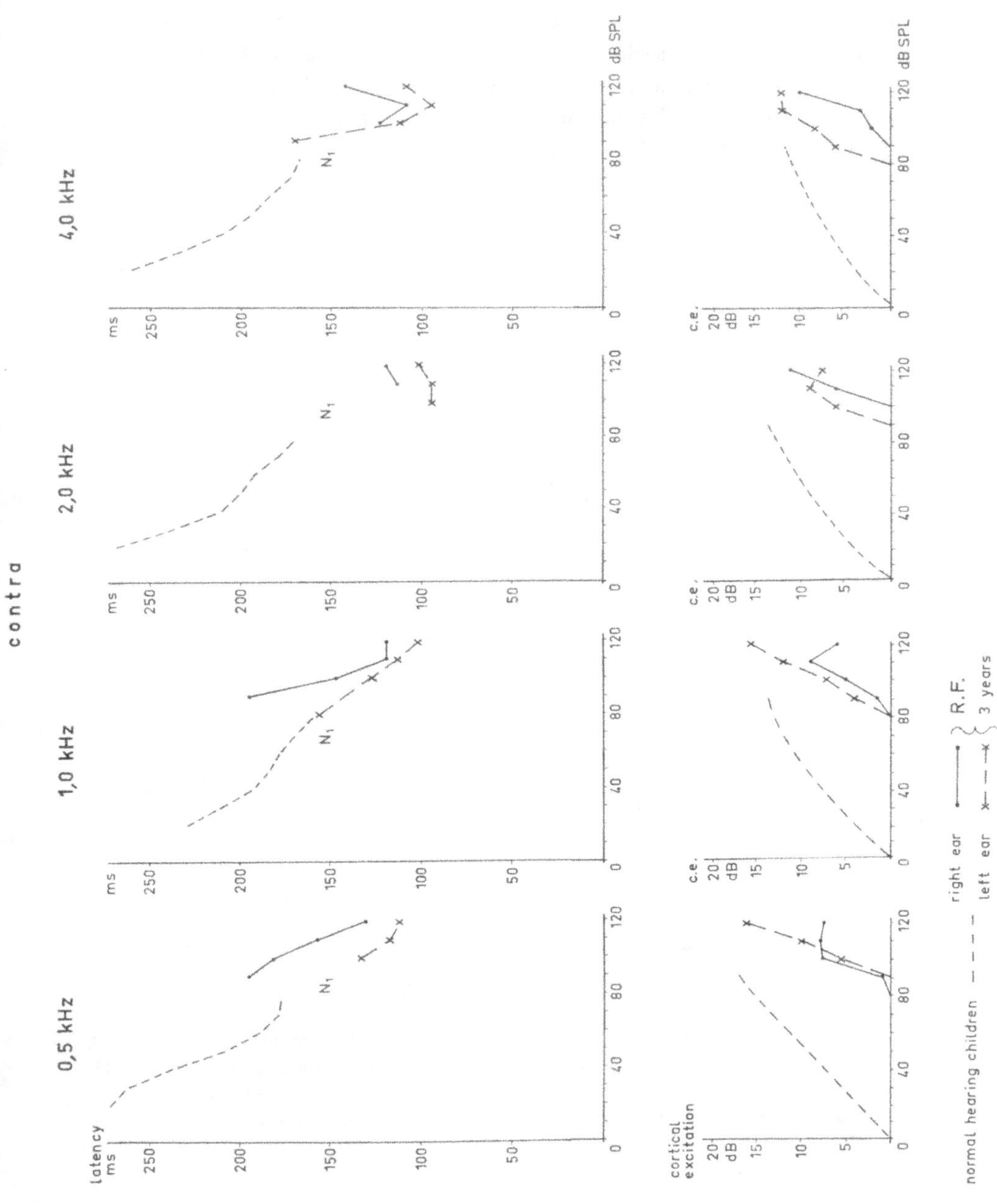

Fig. 13c

sponds to normal. Curve "*c*" illustrates the fact that remarkably lengthened latencies occur with lower stimulation intensities, but these latencies approximate the norm under higher intensities. Curve "*d*", which appears rather seldom, is U-shaped; this means that, in the supraliminal sphere, the latencies correspond to the standard in the central region of stimulation intensity; under higher and lower stimulation intensities, latencies are remarkably lengthened. These different latency times in children with impaired hearing make an evaluation of supraliminal hearing ability extraordinarily difficult. Especially, the curves of the latencies "*c*" and "*d*" require repeated derivations; the use of synchronous three-channel derivation- and recording technique, as described above, facilitates the task. A correlation of paedaudiological test results with these typically pathophysiological ERA curves has been tried but has not yet given exact and detailed causal connections (Holm and Stange, 1971, 1972).

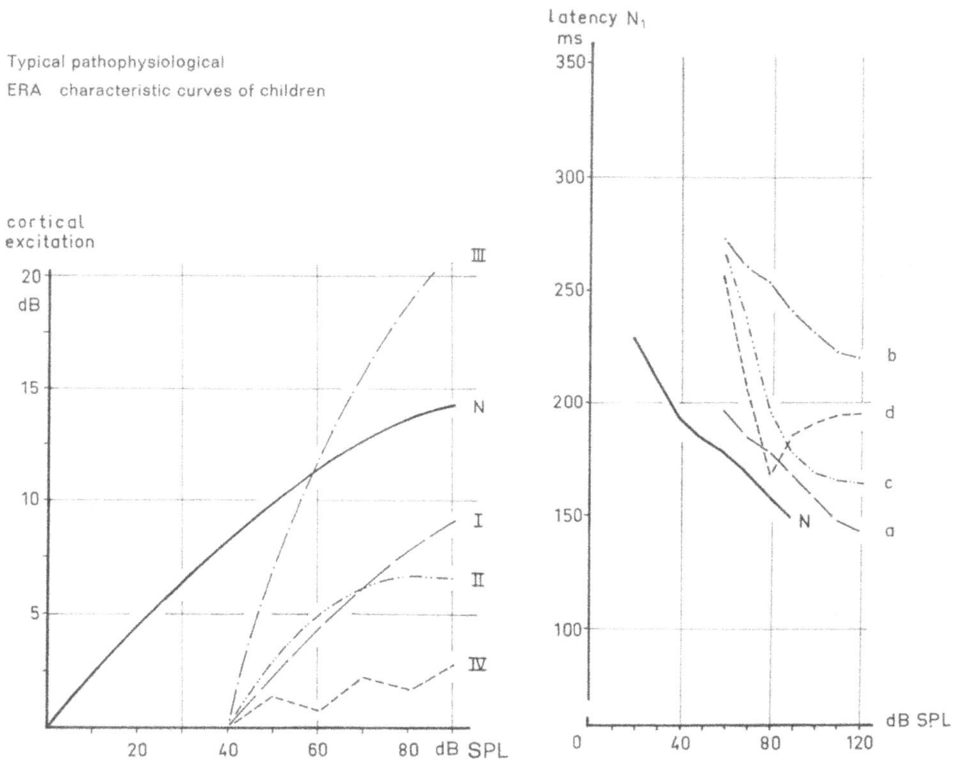

Fig. 14. Typical pathophysiological ERA-characteristic curves (diagram on the left) and ERA-latency curves (diagram on the right), whose courses could be seen again and again (in the recurrence acc. to I-IV and a—c) in more than 100 children with inner ear damage. (Stange, 1973.) In all of the children, ear training with hearing aids and, thereby, development of the faculty of speech could be obtained after supraliminal ERA-diagnosis. (Acc. to Holm and Stange, 1973.) — See detailed discussion

When studying paedaudiological and ERA literature, one gets the impression that the future of Evoked Response Audiometry in cases of inner ear damaged children does not seem to lie in the measuring of auditory thresholds but in the examination of responses to supraliminal stimuli. According to the recommendation of Biesalski and Holm (1966), the physician is under obligation to both the inner ear damaged child and to his parents to make use of Evoked Response Audiometry in all difficult and problematical cases.

III. Evoked Response Audiometry under Sedation

As optimal recording conditions with ERA are only possible with calm and awake patients, it is very important to select the appropriate sedative drugs to be given to children who are to be examined. First reviews of relevant data were given at the 2nd International ERA-Symposion in Vienna (Austria) (1971) (ERA-Newsletter, 1971), summarizing papers by BEAGLEY (1971), SALOMON (1971), SPRENG (1971), STANGE (1971), SUZUKI (1965), and Proceedings of the Round Table Discussion, moderated by DAVIS – (Participants: BEAGLEY, GESTRING, SALOMON, SPRENG, STANGE). Figures 15 and 16 show results obtained by BEAGLEY *et al.* (1972) and by STANGE *et al.* (1972); their results were in agreement with those of other participants in the symposion. All agreed that the promethacines (English: "Phenergen", German: "Atosil") seem to be most suitable for Evoked Response Audiometry (BEAGLEY, 1972; SALOMON, 1972; STANGE, 1972) and that they cause the least changes and diminutions of the potentials. Figure 15a gives the results by BEAGLEY *et al.* (1972) which were obtained after administering Phenergen. Figure 15b shows the respective average values of four normal hearing persons (STANGE, 1972). Every single curve represents the result of 12 registrations recorded during 4 hrs. Figure 15b has to be interpreted as follows: the diagram indicates the results for 70 dB SPL with contralateral, vertex,

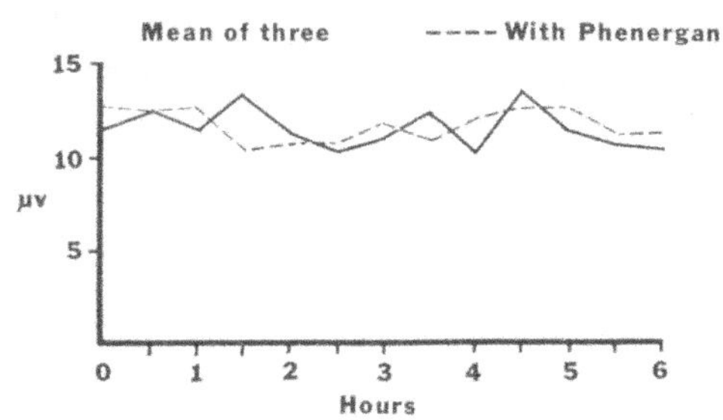

Fig. 15a. The diagram shows the averaged evoked response amplitudes with 70 dB HL, 1.0 kHz in three young adult volunteers over a period of $6^1/_2$ hrs. Continuous line ——— without Promethacine, Dashed line ------ with Promethacine (Phenergen, 25 mg/man, 15 mg/woman, per os). (Acc. to BEAGLEY *et al.*, 1972)

and ipsilateral pick-up. The vertical lines always represent 1σ. At the same time, the dispersion range is identical for measurements taken under medication of without any such influence. When comparing the range of dispersion under Atosil (Promethacine 0.8 mg/kg), Valium (Diazepam 0.3 mg/kg) and Mandrax (a combination of methaqualone and diaphenylhydramine hydrochloride; 1 tabl. containing 250 mg + 50 mg), no difference could be observed. The curves referring to the influence of drugs run below the standard curve for 70 dB SPL, and are not dependent on the location of the scalp electrode. The curve under the influence of Atosil comes closest to the standard curve, that has been reported by BEAGLEY *et al.* (Fig. 15a). The curve after administering Valium runs below that for Atosil, but approaches again the standard

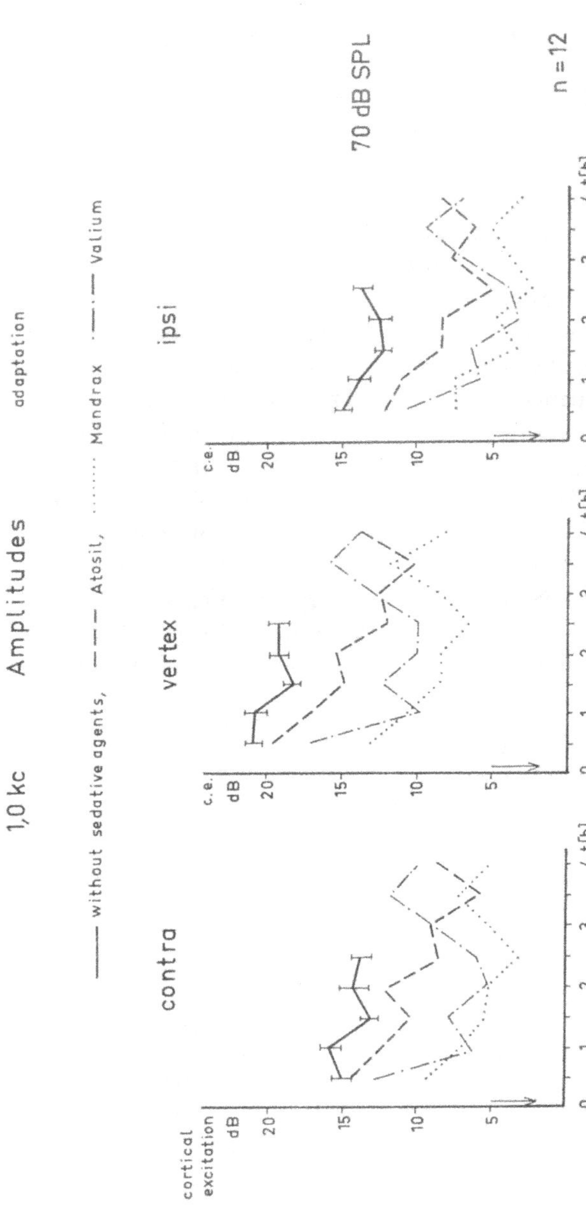

Fig. 15b. This diagram represents the averaged evoked response amplitude to a 70 dB SPL 1 kHz tone (pick-up contralateral, vertex and ipsilateral) in four young adult volunteers, over a period of 4 hrs. Continuous line —— without sedative agents, Broken line ------ with Promethacine (ATOSIL®) 0.8 mg/kg, given orally). (For further description see STANGE, 1972)

curve, $2^1/_2$ hrs after medication. The Mandrax curve runs lowest; thus the curve of Atosil is the most favourable one. This result becomes still more obvious if the averaged amplitudes are indicated above sound pressure level as ERA characteristic curves (see STANGE, 1972). It is again evident that Atosil has the least influence when compared to Valium and Mandrax. Reproducible results can be obtained with Atosil at near threshold sound pressure levels.

The standard deviation of average values under sedation is shown in Fig. 16. In this diagram, the standard deviations are related to the average values, on the

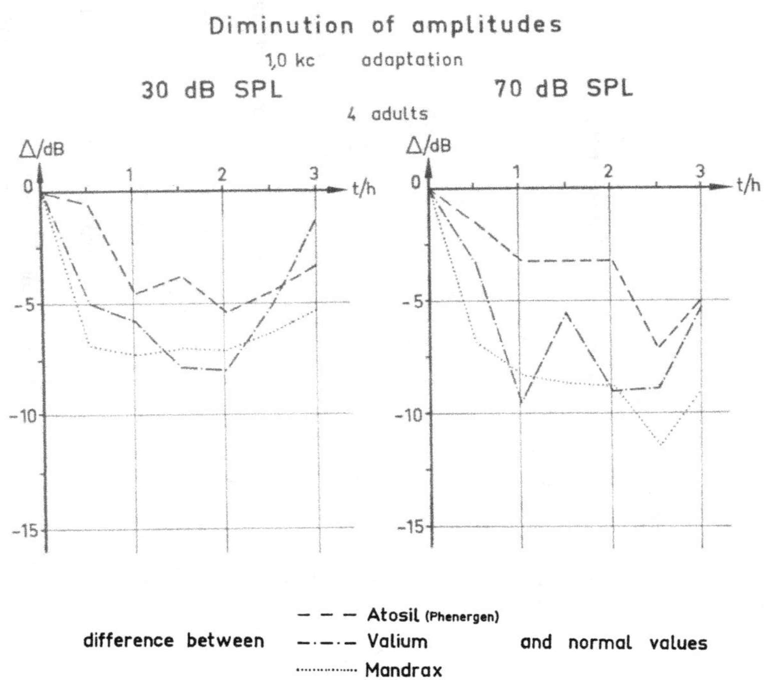

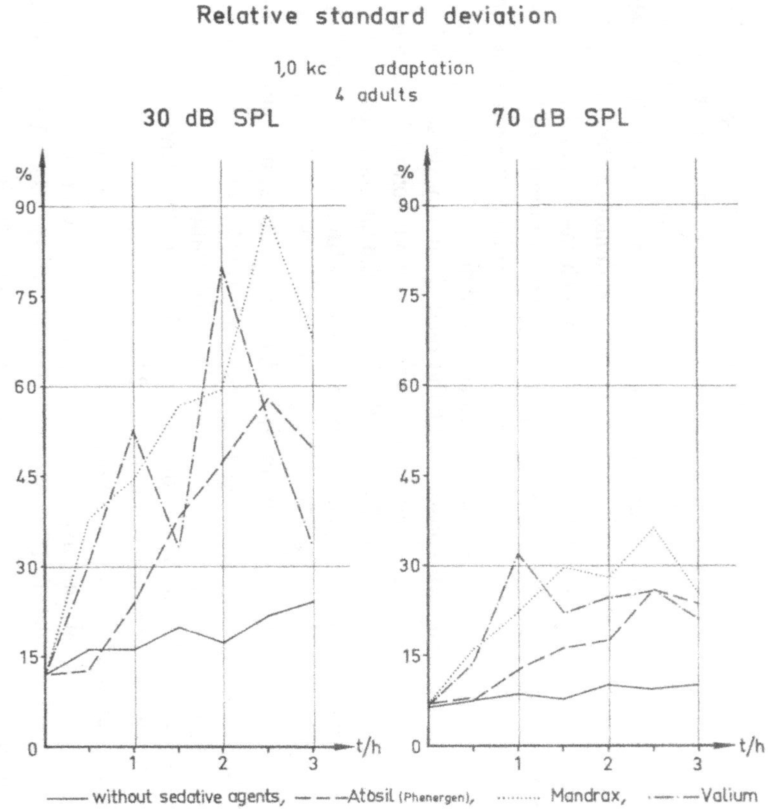

Fig. 16. Acoustically evoked potentials in 4 persons with normal hearing: in absence of drugs: ———, under the influence of Promethacine: ------ under the influence of Diazepam: .-.-.-.-. under the influence of Mandrax: ...., related to time (1 kHz, adapted state of the acoustic system). a = averaged difference between normal and drug-influenced potential amplitudes, b = average of relative measurement error (%). (Acc. to KARNAHL *et al.*, 1972)

left for 30 dB SPL and on the right for 70 dB SPL. Calculation is only made for N_1 (above) and P_2 (below), on account of the amplitude between these two peaks. Relative standard deviations are at first calculated for each pick-up and then averaged, because of the minor changes of the standard deviations within each peak of the contra-, ipsilateral, and vertex recording, as demonstrated in Fig. 16, and because of the partly non-existent amplitudes, which means infinite latency. Thus, each data-point for the drugs is based on a maximum number of 36 values. Each point or solid line is composed of 48 values, because this control examination was carried out with 4 persons. One recognizes again for both sound pressure levels the very good temporal constancy of the related latency deviation while testing without sedation (solid line): relative standard deviation of N_1 amounts at 30 dB SPL to (5.5 $\pm$ 1%) and at 70 dB SPL to (4.6 $\pm$ 0.6%); for P_2 the relative standard deviation is nearly independent of examination time. At 30 dB SPL, it amounts to about 4.5% and, at 70 dB SPL, to about 3.8%. — If medication is given, the largest dispersion appears in N_1 at 30 dB SPL. Here, standard deviation or standard error of the average value oscillates for N_1 between 0% and almost 18%, and for P_2 between 0% and 12%. At 70 dB SPL, standard error varies for N_1 between 5% and 11% and for P_2 only between 3% and 6%. Under sedation with Promethacine, registration during nearly 2 hrs is possible.

The above examples have shown that the Evoked Response Audiometry under sedation is problematical and may give rather dangerously erroneous results. Without an exact and detailed knowledge about the drugs used, ERA under sedation should not be carried out. The careful use of promethacines apparently gives satisfactory results with little or no threshold shift although some diminution (about 20%) in amplitude of evoked responses.

References

Aran, J. M.: L'électro-cochléogramme. I. Principe et technique. Les Cahiers de la C.F.A., No. 12, Paris 1971.

Aran, J. M.: L'électro-cochléogramme. II. Résultats. Les Cahiers de la C.F.A., No. 13, Paris 1971.

Aran, J. M.: The electrocochleogram. Arch. klin. exp. Ohr.-, Nas.- u. Kehlk.-Heilk. **198**, 128—141 (1971).

Barnet, A. B.: Evoked response audiometry in 241 normal and hearing impaired children under three years. Arch. klin. exp. Ohr.-, Nas.- u. Kehlk.-Heilk. **198**, 154—157 (1971).

Barnet, A. B., Goodwin, R. S.: Averaged evoked electroencephalographic responses to click in the human newborn. Electroenceph. clin. Neurophysiol. **18**, 441—450 (1965).

Beagly, H. A.: The role of ERA in the diagnosis of receptive aphasia. Arch. klin. exp. Ohr.-, Nas.- u. Kehlk.-Heilk. **198**, 152—153 (1971).

Beagly, H. A., Forteen, A. M., Gordon, A. G.: Clinical experience of evoked response testing with sedation. Sound **6**, 8—13 (1972).

Beagly, H. A., Kellog, S. E.: Comparison of evoked response and subjective auditory thresholds. Int. Audiol. **8**, 345—353 (1969).

Beagly, H. A., Kellog, S. E.: Amplitude of the auditory evoked response at high intensities. Sound **4**, 86—90 (1971).

Beagly, H. A., Knight, J. J.: Changes in auditory evoked response with intensity. Rep. Inst. Laryng. Otol. **17**, 263—275 (1966/67).

Benning, C. D., Karnahl, Th., Stange, G.: ERA-Kennlinien und Latenzen bei 15 normalhörenden Kleinkindern. Arch. klin. exp. Ohr.-, Nas.- u. Kehlk.-Heilk. **201**, 222—230 (1972).

BERGER, H.: Das Elektroencephalogramm des Menschen. Nova Acta Leopoldina NF. 6, No. 38 (1938).

BIESALSKI, P.: Fachärztliche Untersuchung hörgeschädigter Säuglinge und Kleinkinder. Hörgeschädigte Kinder **1**, 6—8 (1966).

BIESALSKI, P.: Durchführung und Beurteilung der Säuglingsaudiometrie. In La surdité du premier age, pp. 164—170. Besancon 1969.

BIESALSKI, P., HOLM, C.: Pädaudiologische Therapie als klinischer Aufgabenbereich. Z. Laryng. Rhinol. **45**, 52—60 (1966).

BIESALSKI, P., LEITNER, H.: Weitere klinische Erfahrungen mit der Electric-Response-Audiometrie (Audio EEG) bei hörgeschädigten Kindern. Arch. klin. exp. Ohr.-, Nas.- u. Kehlk.-Heilk. **199**, 551—552 (1971).

BICKFORD, R. G., JACOBSON, J. L., CODY, D. T. R.: Nature of average evoked potentials to sound and other stimuli in man. In: Kathmann, Whipple (Eds.): Sensory evoked response in man Ann. N. Y. Acad. Sci. **112**, 204—223 (1964).

BORDLEY, J. E.: An evaluation of the psychogalvanic skin-resistance-technic in audiometry. Laryngoscope (St. Louis) **66**, 1162 (1956).

BORDLEY, J. E., HARDY, W. G., RICHTER, C. P.: Audiometry with use of galvanic skin-resistance response. Bul. Johns. Hopk. Hosp. **82**, 569 (1948).

BORSANYI, J. S.: Some aspects of auditory evoked potentials in man. Ann. Otol. (St. Louis) **73**, 61—71 (1964).

BURIAN, K., GESTRING, G. F.: Discrepancies between subjective and objective acoustic thresholds. Arch. klin. exp. Ohr.-, Nas.- u. Kehlk.-Heilk. **198**, 73—82 (1971).

BURIAN, K., GESTRING, G. F., HRUBY, S.: Die Interaktion sensorischer Reize im Rahmen der objektiven Hörschwellenbestimmung. Arch. klin. exp. Ohr.-, Nas.- u. Kehlk.-Heilk. **192**, 116—123 (1968).

BURIAN, K., GESTRING, G. F., HRUBY, S.: Clinical experience with the EEG-Computer audiometry. Int. Audiol. 8, 633—638 (1969).

BUTLER, R. A.: Effect of changes in stimulus frequency and intensity on habituation of the human vertex potential. J. acoust. Soc. Amer. **44**, 945—950 (1968).

BUTLER, R. A., KEIDEL, W. D., SPRENG, M.: An investigation of the human cortical evoked potential under conditions of monaural and binaural stimulation. Acta oto-laryng. (Stockh.) **68**, 317—326 (1969).

CANESTRINI, S.: Über das Sinnesleben des Neugeborenen. Monographien aus dem Gesamtgebiet der Neurologie und Psychiatrie, Heft 5, Berlin: Springer 1913.

DAVID, E., FINKENZELLER, P., KALLERT, S., KEIDEL, W. D.: Korrelationsanalyse von gemittelten und ungemittelten evozierten Potentialen. Kybernetik **9**, 22—26 (1971).

DAVIS, H.: Slow cortical response evoked by acoustic stimuli. Acta oto-laryng. (Stockh.) **59**, 179—185 (1965).

DAVIS, H.: Validation of evoked response audiometry (ERA) in deaf children. Int. Audiol. **5**, 77—81 (1966).

DAVIS, H.: Is ERA ready for routine clinical use? Arch. klin. exp. Ohr.-, Nas.- u. Kehlk.-Heilk. **198**, 2—8 (1971).

DAVIS, H., HIRSH, S. K., SHELNUTT, J., BOWERS, J. and BOWERS, C.: Further validation of evoked response audiometry (ERA). J. Speech. Hear. Res. **10**, 717—732 (1967).

DAVIS, H., YOSHIE, N.: Human cortical response to auditory stimuli. Physiologist **6**, 164 (1963).

DAVIS, H., ZERLIN, S.: Acoustic relations of the human vertex potentials. J. acoust. Soc. Amer. **39**, 109—116 (1966).

DAWSON, G. D.: Cerebral responses to electrical stimulation of peripheral nerve in man. J. Neurol. Neurosurg. Psychiat. **10**, 134—140 (1974).

DERBYSHIRE, A. J., McDERMOTT, M.: Further contrictions to the EEG methode of evaluation auditory function. Laryngoscope (St. Louis) **68**, 558—570 (1958).

ENGEL, R., YOUNG, N. B.: Calibrated pure tone audiograms in normal neonates based on evoked electroencephalographic responses. Neuropädiatrie **1**, 149—160 (1969).

EPPSTEIN, A., SCHILL, A.: Electrodermal responses and tolerance thresholds for pure tones. Acta oto-laryng. (Stockh.) **66**, 417—432 (1968).

ERA: I. International Symposion 1970 in Freiburg i. Br. (West Germany). Arch. klin. exp. Ohr.-, Nas.- u. Kehlk.-Heilk. **198**, 1—361 (1971).

ERA: II. International Symposion 1971 in Vienna (Austria) (Ed.): K. Burian. ERA-newsletter 18th issue, pp. 2—68, Vienna, December 1971.

Finkenzeller, P.: Die Mitteilung von Reaktionspotentialen. Kybernetik **6**, 22—44 (1969).

Fleischer, K.: Untersuchungen zur Entwicklung der Innenohrfunktion. Z. Laryng. Rhinol. Otol. **34**, 733—739 (1955).

Fröding, C. A.: Acoustic investigation of newborn infants. Acta oto-laryng. (Stockh.) **52**,(1960) 31—40.

Geisler, C. H., Frishkopf, L. S., Rosenblith, W. A.: Extracranial responses to acoustic clicks in man. Science **128**, 1210 (1958).

Genzmer, A.: Untersuchungen über die Sinneswahrnehmungen des neugeborenen Menschen (zitiert bei Fröding) (1873).

Holm, C.: Discussion of the paper of Stange on the I. International Symposion of the ERA-Club. Arch. klin. exp. Ohr.-, Nas.- u. Kehlk.-Heilk. **198**, 101—(1971).

Holm, C., Stange, G.: Pathologische ERA-Kennlinien als Kriterien zur Wirkungsweise von Hörtrainern. Arch. klin. exp. Ohr.-, Nas.- u. Kehlk.-Heilk. **202**, 452—457 (1972).

Holm, C., Stange, G.: l-Importance des lignes de stimulation-excitations évoqueés acoustiques pour la discrimination de la parole chez l'enfant. J. franz. Oto-rhino-laryng. **21**, 665—670 (1972).

Holm, C., Stange, G.: Überschwellige ERA-Befunde als therapeutische Basis zur Versorgung innenohrgeschädigter Kinder. H. N. O. (Berl.) **21**, 163—168 (1973).

Jakobi, H.: Erfahrungen mit der Kinderaudiometrie. Arch. klin. exp. Ohr.-, Nas.- u. Kehlk.-Heilk. **169**, 383 (1956).

Joppich, G., Schulte, F. J.: Neurologie des Neugeborenen. Berlin-Heidelberg-New York Springer 1968.

Karnahl, Th., Benning, C. D.: Effect of sedation upon evoked response audiometry: amplitudes and latency vs sound pressure level. Arch. klin. exp. Ohr.-, Nas.- u. Kehlk.-Heilk. **201**, 181—188 (1972).

Karnahl, Th., Spreng, M., Stange, G.: Calculation of ERA-potentials. Rev. Laryng. (Bordeaux) **95**, 554—559 (1974).

Karnahl, Th., Stange, G.: Ergebnisse bei der Standardisierung der "Electric Response Audiometry" (ERA). Arch. klin. exp. Ohr.-, Nas.- u. Kehlk.-Heilk. **202**, 452—457 (1972).

Keidel, W. D.: Anatomie und Elektrophysiologie der zentralen akustischen Bahnen. In: Berendes, Link, Zöllner (Eds.): Handbuch der HNO-Heilkunde, Bd. III/3, pp. 2013—2098, Stuttgart: Thieme Verlag 1966.

Keidel, W. D.: What do we know about the human cortical evoked potential after all? Arch. klin. exp. Ohr.-, Nas.- u. Kehlk.-Heilk. **198**, 9—37 (1971).

Keidel, W. D.: DC-potentials in the auditory evoked response in man. Acta oto-laryng. (Stockh.) **71**, 242—248 (1971).

Keidel, W. D., Spreng, M.: Elektronisch gemittelte Rindenpotentiale des Menschen bei akustischer Reizung. Acta oto-laryng. (Stockh.) **56**, 318—328 (1963).

Keidel, W. D., Spreng, M.: Neurophysiological evidence for the Stevensshe power function in man. J. acoust. Soc. Amer. **38**, 191—195 (1965).

Keidel, W. D., Spreng, M.: Computed audio-encephalogram in man. A technic of objective audiometry. Int. Audiol. **4**, 56—60 (1965).

Keidel, W. D., Spreng, M.: Audiometry aspects and multisensory power functions of electronically averaged evoked cortical responses in man. Acta oto-laryng. (Stockh.) **59**, 201—208 (1965).

Keidel, W. D., Spreng, M.: Recent status results and problems of objective audiometry. J. franc. oto-rhino-laryng. **19**, 45—53 (1970).

Kottmeier, G., Heimann, G.: Versuche der Objektivierung von Reizwahrnehmungen an schlafenden Kindern. Arch. klin. exp. Ohr.-, Nas.- u. Kehlk.-Heilk. **186**, 298—308 (1966).

Kumpf, W.: Zur Methodik der Hörschwellenbestimmung. H. N. O. (Berl.) **19**, 209—211 (1971).

Kussmaul, A.: Untersuchungen über das Seelenleben des neugeborenen Menschen (zitiert bei Fröding) (1859).

Lempert, J., Meltzer, P. E., Wever, E. G., Lawrence, M.: The cochleogram and its clinical application: a preliminary report. Arch. oto-laryng. **45**, 61—67 (1947).

LEMPERT, J., MELTZER, P. E., WEVER, E. G., LAWRENCE, M.: The cochleogram and its clinical application: concluding observations. Arch. oto-laryng. **51**, 307—311 (1950).

LEV, A., SOHMER, H.: Sources of averaged neural responses recorded in animal and human subjects during cochlear audiometry (Electro-Cochleogram). Arch. klin. exp. Ohr.-, Nas.- u. Kehlk.-Heilk. **201**, 79—90 (1972).

LOEWENICH, V. VON: Methodische Voraussetzungen zur diagnostischen Verwertung auditorisch evozierter Potentiale bei Kleinkindern und Säuglingen. Paediatr. Fortbildungsh. „Praxis" **34**, 39—48 (1972).

LOWELL, E. L., WILLIAMS, C. F., BALLINGER, R. M., ALVIG, D. P.: Measurement of auditor threshold with a special purpose analog computer. J. Speech. Hear. Res. **4**, 105—112 (1961).

LÜSCHER, E., KUSEN, E.: Die psychogalvanische Hautaudiometrie. Arch. klin. exp. Ohr.-, Nas.- u. Kehlk.-Heilk. **172**, 286—298 (1958).

MARCUS, R. E., GIBBS, E. L., GIBBS, E. A.: Electroencephalographyin the diagnosis of hearing loss in the very young child. Dis. nerv. Syst. **10**, 170—173 (1949).

MATHIS, A., GRAF, K.: Die elektrische Reaktionsaudiometrie (ERA) beim Neugeborenen. Arch. klin. exp. Ohr.-, Nas.- u. Kehlk.-Heilk. **201**, 231—240 (1972).

MENDEL, M. J., GOLDSTEIN, R.: Effect of sleep on the early components of the averaged electroencephalographic response. Arch. klin. exp. Ohr.-, Nas.- u. Kehlk.-Heilk. **198**, 110—115 (1071).

MENDEL, M. J., GOLDSTEIN, R.: Early components of the averaged encephalographic response to constant level clicks during all night sleep. J. Speech. Hear. Res. **14**, 829—840 (1917).

METZ, O.: The acoustic impedance measured on normal pathologica ears. Acta oto-laryng. (Stockh.) **63**, 1—18 (1946).

MORGON, A., CHARACHON, D., GENIN, P.: Electroencephalographic audiometry for young children. Arch. klin. exp. Ohr.-, Nas.- u. Kehlk.-Heilk. **198**, 144—150 (1971).

MOUNIER-KUHN, P., MORGON, A., CHARACHON, D.: Travaux et enquêtes de l'Institut d'audiophénologie de Lyon. La Surdité du Premier Age, Editor Camponovo, Besanson, 123—146 (1969).

MÜLLER, G., STANGE, G.: The input-output function of the slow auditory evoked potential in contralateral, ipsilateral and vertex recordings. Arch. klin. exp. Ohr.-, Nas.- u. Kehlk.-Heilk. **198**, 116—126 (1971).

MÜLLER, G., STANGE, G.: Ein frühes akustisch evoziertes Potential am Menschen. Mschr. Ohrenheilk. **105**, 166 (1971).

ONISHI, S., DAVIS, H.: Effects of duration and rise time of tone bursts on evoked v potentials. J. acoust. Soc. Amer. **44**, 582—591 (1968).

PEARL, E. R., GALAMBOS, R., GLORIG, A.: The estimation of hearing threshold by electroencephalography. Electroenceph. clin. Neurophysiol. **5**, 501—512 (1953).

PEIPER, A.: Sinnesempfindungen des Kindes vor seiner Geburt. Mschr. Kinderheilk. **29**, 236—241 (1924).

PORTMANN, M., ARAN, J. M.: Electro-cochléographie sur le nourisson et le jeune enfant. Acta oto-laryng. (Stockh.) **71**, 253—261 (1971).

PORTMANN, M., ARAN, J. M., COSTE, Ch.: Experimental vertification in animals concerning some aspects of human electro-cochleographic pathology. Acta oto-laryng. (Stockh.) 1973 **75**, 132—142 (1973).

RAPIN, J., GRAZIANI, L. J.: Auditory evoked potentials in normal, brain damaged and deaf infants. Neurology (Minneap.) **17**, 881—894 (1967).

RELKE, W., FREY, M. H.: Höruntersuchungen bei Neugeborenen mittels Reflexaudiometrie. Z. Laryng. **45**, S. 707—720 (1966).

ROSENBLITH, W. A., ROSENZWEIG, M. R.: Electrical responses to acoustic clicks: influence of electrode location in cats. J. acoust. Soc. Amer. **23**, 583—588 (1951).

ROSENAU, H.: Die Schlafbeschallung. Z. Laryng. Rhinol. **41**, 194—208 (1962).

RUBEN, R. J., LIEBERMANN, T. A., BORDLEY, J. E.: Some observations on cochlear potentials and nerve action potentials in children. Laryngoscope (St. Louis) **72**, 545—554 (1962).

RUBEN, R. J.: Cochlear potentials as a diagnostic test in deafness. In: Graham, A. B. (Ed.): Sensory neural hearing process and disorders, p. 313. Boston: Little Brown and Co. 1967.

DE REYNIER, J. P.: Etude systématique de l'audition dans un Service de prématurés: A propos du dépistage des réactions auditives du nouveau-né, du prématuré et du bébé âgé de 2 à 6 mois. — Colloque Internationale Camponovo. In: La Surdité du Premier Age, pp. 195—210. Besanson 1969.

SALOMON, G., BECK, O., ELBERLING, C.: The role of sedation in ERA from the vertex. Audiology **12**, 150—166 (1973).

SHARRARD, G. A. W.: Evoked responses — introductory studies on their relationship to the perception of language. J. Laryng. **83**, 947—958 (1969).

SHARRARD, G. A. W.: The auditory evoked potentials of language disordered children. Arch. klin. exp. Ohr.-, Nas.- u. Kehlk.-Heilk. **198**, 158—166 (1971).

SOHMER, H., FEINMESSER, H.: Cochlear action potentials recorded from the external ear in man. Ann. Otol. Rhinol. Laryng. **76**, 427—435 (1967).

SOHMER, H., FEINMESSER, H.: Cochlear and cortical audiometry. Israel J. Med. Sci. **6**, 219—223 (1970).

SOHMER, H., FEINMESSER, H.: Routine use of electrocochleography (cochlear audiometry) on human subjects. Audiology **12**, 167—173 (1973).

SPRENG, M.: Über die Messung der Frequenzgruppe und der Integrationszeit des menschlichen Gehörs durch vom Schall abhängige Hirnspannungen längs der Kopfhaut. Doctor Thesis, TH Stuttgart, 1967.

SPRENG, M.: Problems in objective cerebral audiometry using short sound stimulation. Int. Audiol. **8**, 424—429 (1969).

SPRENG, M.: Small computers in evoked response audiometry (ERA). Arch. klin. exp. Ohr.-, Nas.- u. Kehlk.-Heilk. **198**, 50—70 (1971).

SPRENG, M.: Artefact recognition and Diazepam in electric response audiometry. Audiology **12**, 137—149 (1973).

SPRENG, M., KEIDEL, W. D.: Separierung von Cerebroaudiogramm (CAG), Neuroaudiogramm (NAG) und Otoaudiogramm (OAG) in der Objektiven Audiometrie. Arch. klin. exp. Ohr.-, Nas.- u. Kehlk.-Heilk. **189**, 225—246 (1967).

SPRENG, M., KEIDEL, W. D.: Recent status results and problems of objective audiometry in man. J. franc. Oto-rhino-laryng. **19**, 55—60 (1970).

STANGE, G.: Behandlungsergebnisse bei Hörstürzen. Arch. klin. exp. Ohr.-, Nas.- u. Kehlk.-Heilk. **194**, 538—544 (1969).

STANGE, G.: The relation between functional parameters of the subjective and objective audiometry. Arch. klin. exp. Ohr.-, Nas.- u. Kehlk.-Heilk. **198**, 85—101 (1971).

STANGE, G.: Résultats cliniques d'une audiométrie objective chez le nouveau-né et le jeune enfant. In: Lafon, C. (Ed.): La surdité du premier âge, pp. 240—251. Besançon: Editions Camponovo 1971.

STANGE, G.: The effect of sedativa agents in psychotropic drugs on acoustically evoked responses. Arch. klin. exp. Ohr.-, Nas.- u. Kehlk.-Heilk. **201**, 294—308 (1972).

STANGE, G.: Diagnostik überrchwelligen Hörvermögens bei innenohrgeschädigten Kindern mittels ERA. H.N.O. (Berl.) **21**, 83—87 (1973).

STANGE, G., HOLM, C.: Gemittelte zentrale akustische Reizantworten — eine Erweiterung pädandiologischer Gesichtspunkte? H.N.O. (Berl.) **18**, 27—28 (1970).

STANGE, G., HOLZ, E., TERAYAMA, Y., BECK, Chl.: Korrelation biochemischer, morphologischer und elektrophysiologischer Untersuchungsergebnisse des akustischen Systems. Arch. klin. exp. Ohr.-, Nas.- u. Kehlk.-Heilk. **186**, 229—246 (1966).

STANGE, G., KARNAHL, Th.: Clinical results of the ERA-characteristic curves by means of the computer PDP 12. Exerpta Medica, Int. Congr. Ser. **276**, 287—288 (1973).

STANGE, G., KARNAHL, Th.: Early (15 msec) and late (100 msec) acoustic responses in patients suffering from otosclerosis, before and after stapedectomy. III. International Congress of Rev. Laryng. (Bordeaux) **96**, — (1975). **96**, — (1975).

STANGE, G., SODA, T.: Quantitative Untersuchungen zur Hörschwelle, Adaptation und Lautheitsempfindung am gesunden und hörgeschädigten Menschen mittels „Objektiver Audiometrie". Arch. klin. exp. Ohr.-, Nas.- u. Kehlk.-Heilk. **190**, 210—228 (1968).

STANGE, G., SPRENG, M., KEIDEL, W. D.: Die Wirkung von Streptomycinsulfat auf Erregung und Adaptation des Cortischen Organs. Pflügers Arch. ges. Physiol. **279**, 99—120 (1964).

STEVENS, S. S.: The psychophysics of sensory function. In: Rosenblith, W. A. (Ed.): Sensory communication. New York: J. Wiley 1961.

STUBBS: The effect of the factors of duration, intensity, and pitch of sound stimulation upon the responses of newborn infants. Univ. Iowa, Stud. Child. Welfare **9**, 77—135 (1960).

SUZUKI, T., TAGUCHI, K.: Cerebral evoked responses to auditory stimuli in waking man. Ann. Otol. (St. Louis) **74**, 128—139 (1965).

TERKILDSEN, K.: Clinical application of impedance measurement with a fixed frequency technique. Int. Audiol. **3**, 147—155 (1964).

TERKILDSEN, K., OSTERHAMMEL, P., HUIS IN'T VELD, F.: Electrocochleography with a far field technique. Scand. Audiology **2**, 141—148 (1973).

THEISSING, J.: Klinische Möglichkeiten und Ergebnisse der Objektiven Audiometrie mit Computertechnik. Arch. klin. exp. Ohr.-, Nas.- u. Kehlk.Heilk. **187**, 612—620 (1966)

THEISSING, J.: Untersuchungen zur Bedeutung des Zeitfaktors in der Objektiven Audiometrie. Z. Laryng. Rhinol. Otol. **46**, 648—651 (1967).

THEISSING, J.: Über Beziehungen von Computeraudiogrammen und konventionellen Audiogrammen. Z. Laryng. Rhinol. Otol. **46**, 455—460 (1967).

THEISSING, J.: Objektive Audiometrie in Narkose. Arch. klin. exp. Ohr.-, Nas.- u. Kehlk.-Heilk. **194**, 455—460 (1969).

THEISSING, J.: Objektive Hörprüfung im Kindesalter. Aktuelle Oto-Rhino-Laryngologie **4**, 1—39 (1970).

THEISSING, J.: Praktische Möglichkeiten der Objektiven Computer-Audiometrie. H.N.O. (Berl.) **19**, 123—127 (1971).

WALKER, J. C., JACOBSON, J. L., CODY, D. T. R.: Comparison of cerebral and myogenic components of the averaged responses to sound stimulation. Electroenceph. clin. Neurophysiol. **17**, 456 (1964).

WEDENBERG, E.: Objective auditory tests on non-cooperative children. Int. Audiol. (Leiden) **2**, 108—114 (1963).

YOSHIE, N.: Clinical cochlear response audiometry by means of an average response computer: non-surgical technique and clinical use. Rev. Laryng. (Bordeaux) Suppl. 646—672 (1971)

YOSHIE, N., OHASHI, T.: Clinical use of cochlear nerve action potential responses in man for differential diagnosis of hearing losses. Acta oto-laryng. (Stockh.) **252**, 71—87 (1969).

YOSHIE, N., OHASHI, T., SUZUKI, T.: Non-surgical recording of auditory nerve action potentials in man. Laryngoscope (St. Louis) **77**, 76—85 (1967).

YOSHIE, N., YAMAURA, K.: Cochlear microphonic responses to pure tones in man recorded by a non surgical method. Acta oto-laryng. (Stockh.) **252**, 37—69 (1969).

Chapter 6

Hearing and Equilibrium in Renal Failure

M. E. WIGAND, Erlangen, Germany

With 10 Figures

Contents

I. Introduction

There is widespread consensus in the nephrologic literature that patients with uremia often suffer from dizziness and vertigo, less frequently from deafness (BRIGHT, 1836; RAYER, 1840; ROSENSTEIN, 1894; MORF, 1897; VOLHARD, 1931; SCHREINER, and MAHER, 1961). In so far as these symptoms are due to a coincident otitis media with subsequent labyrinthitis, they will not be dealt with, here; neither will we refer to the uremic neuro-encephalopathy or diffuse vascular lesions, both of which are often considered as the primary sources of auditory symptoms in terminal renal failure (GRAHE, 1924; STRÜMPELL-SEYFARTH, 1930; VOLHARD, 1931; MATHES-CURSCHMANN, 1947; HEYMAN *et al.*, 1951; BEANEY, 1964; BROD, 1964; SARRE, 1967; HEINTZ, 1968).

For the knowledge of the pathophysiology of the inner ear, every detailed observation or measurement of cochleo-vestibular disturbances in clinical or experimental uremia may be of particular interest. Only few data exist on the frequency of such disturbances. GRAHE (1924) observed hearing losses in 27 out of 33 patients with chronic nephritis, but the losses were hardly perceived by the patients. Impairments of equlibrium were much less frequent and did not correlate with the deafness. BEANEY (1964) detected only one hearing loss among 262 kidney diseases, but he noted 5 cases of vestibular irritation. RANSOME *et al.* (1966) could not find any pertinent evidence in the literature between 1945 and 1966; in their own research, they recorded slight high tone losses in 3 out of 6 uremic patients who were not dialysed. YASSIN *et al.* (1966, 1970a, b) reported the highest incidence of hearing deficit in cases of renal disorder: Only 13% of 73 cases of nephritis revealed no signs of hearing disorder; of 114 cases 57% showed an increased and 15% a reduced caloric response of the vestibular apparatus.

Apparently the frequency of cochleo-vestibular disorders in uremia is dependant of the kind of renal disease and of the definition of the terminal renal insufficiency. To the term of uremia — which was, according to SARRE (1967), introduced 1840 by PIORRY and L'HÉRITIER — we subscribe a clinical entity which is induced by an acute or chronic renal failure and is characterized by the retention of urinary components in the blood, usally accompanied by a reduction of water excretion.

The developing intoxication influences the different organs, and the breakdown of the "milieu interne" can be inferred from metabolic disturbances, most prominent in the derangement of the water and electrolyte balance (TRAUT and JUTZLER, 1970). The regulations of volume and osmolarity fail, followed by extra- and intracellular space shifts. The sodium concentration of the plasma is usually lowered (Hyponatremia); the total balance is positive. On the other hand, we find a rise of potassium concentration in the phase of oligo- and anuria with development of neuromuscular threshold reduction, leading to muscle itching, cardiac arrhythmia, and ventricular waving. Other transmineralisation processes concern calcium and phosphorus; metabolic acidosis will follow to end in the decompensation of the acidbase balance.

According to TYLER (1970) the sensorineural symptomatology of chronic renal failure is grouped into *encephalopathy* (confusion; lethargy; obtundation; myoclonus; fasciculations; convulsions; stupor; mental changes ranging from depression to schizophrenia), *neuromuscular irritability* (asterixis, which coincides with a synchronous lapse of electrical activity in the EMG, due to a periodic inhibition of the spinal motor neurone pool arising from a supraspinal level; metabolic tremor), and *cranial nerve signs* (uremic amaurosis; sixth-nerve palsy, probably the result of small vascular infarctions in the brain stem). Deafness and vestibular disorders are only occasionally reported.

Spontaneous complaints of the uremic patients are seldom. Only if asked, they admit slowly progressive deafness, sometimes tinnitus. Acute hearing losses in uremia (BEANEY, 1964) are exceptions. Often the perception of only the high frequencies is reduced together with occurrence of speech discrimination loss (GRAHE, 1924). Vertigo, dizziness, and nausea are more frequent; however, the type of unsystemical vertigo prevails, which could, without specific vestibular testing, be interpreted as central intoxication. TYLER (1968) frequently observed nystagmus, but of fluctuating intensity and of evanescent character.

The fact that many patients with chronic pyelonephritis are accustomed to analgetic drugs containing phenacetine and receive streptomyces antibiotics over a long period has embarrassed the attribution of these symptoms to a pathophysiological concept. Every audiometrical evaluation has to take these concomitant noxes into consideration; the same is the case with acute hearing drops following hemodialysis.

II. Morphologic Similarities between the Nephron and the Labyrinth

In a synopsis of uremic deafness and the terminal nephrogen failure of water and electrolyte balance in uremia, some morphologic analogies invite further examination. In particular the stria vascularis, which plays a prominent part in the production of inner ear fluids and in the maintenance of the physiological electrolyte pattern offers many a question. The establishment of different electrolyte gradients, for instance in the endolymph the highest potassium concentration (140 mEq/l) of a body extracellular fluid, requires enormous energies to achieve the ion transport.

In comparison of the stria with the micromorphology of the kidney some strikingly similar features challenge further investigations:

1) As early as 1851, Corti pointed to the close contact of the capillary network of the stria vascularis to its epithelium, which mirrors the fine architecture of the nephron. Electron microscopy has recently revealed the direct contiguity of the stria capillaries and the chromophile cells (SPOENDLIN, 1967).

2) The basal membrane, always present among Bowman's capsule and the capillary endothelium at the glomerulum and around proximal tubular cells, is also visible around the capillaries of the stria. It is considered as the (ultra-) filter of the primary urine.

3) The discontinuity of the endothelial plasma, known as "pores" of the glomerular cells, can be encountered at the stria capillaries as "pinocytotic vesicles", which open to both the capillary lumen and the basal membrane.

4) The structures concerned with transport of water always exhibit an obvious intraplasmatic folding (PEASE, 1956, "basal labyrinth" of RUSKA *et al.*, 1957), which was meticulously described for the renal tubules by THOENES (1961, 1965). It is also clearly visible at the stria vascularis epithelia (SMITH, 1957), and RAUCH (1964) assumed, on the basis of its particular arrangement at the capillary front of the chromophile cells, that the stria is mainly resorptive in function (Fig. 1).

5) But independant of its more resorptive or secretory (SPOENDLIN, 1967) activity, the clustering of numerous mitochondria at the basis of the chromophile cell tentacles reminds one of the very similar distribution of mitochondria at those sites of the renal tubules which show plasmatic folds.

6) The concentration of SH-radicals in both the proximal tubules and the stria vascularis, demonstrated histochemically by BARNETT and SELIGMANN (1954) and by MÜSEBECK and SCHÄTZLE (1963), was concordantly interpreted as the occurrence of carboanhydrase by RAUCH (1964).

7) Experimental evidence was given by QUICK *et al.* that also an immunological relationship exists between the kidney and the ear: the serum of goats or rabbits, sensitized against stria vascularis tissue of rats or guinea pigs, induced immunofluorescence of epithelial structures of the distal convoluted tubules, while antiglomerular antibody reacted with vascular elements of both stria and spiral ligament.

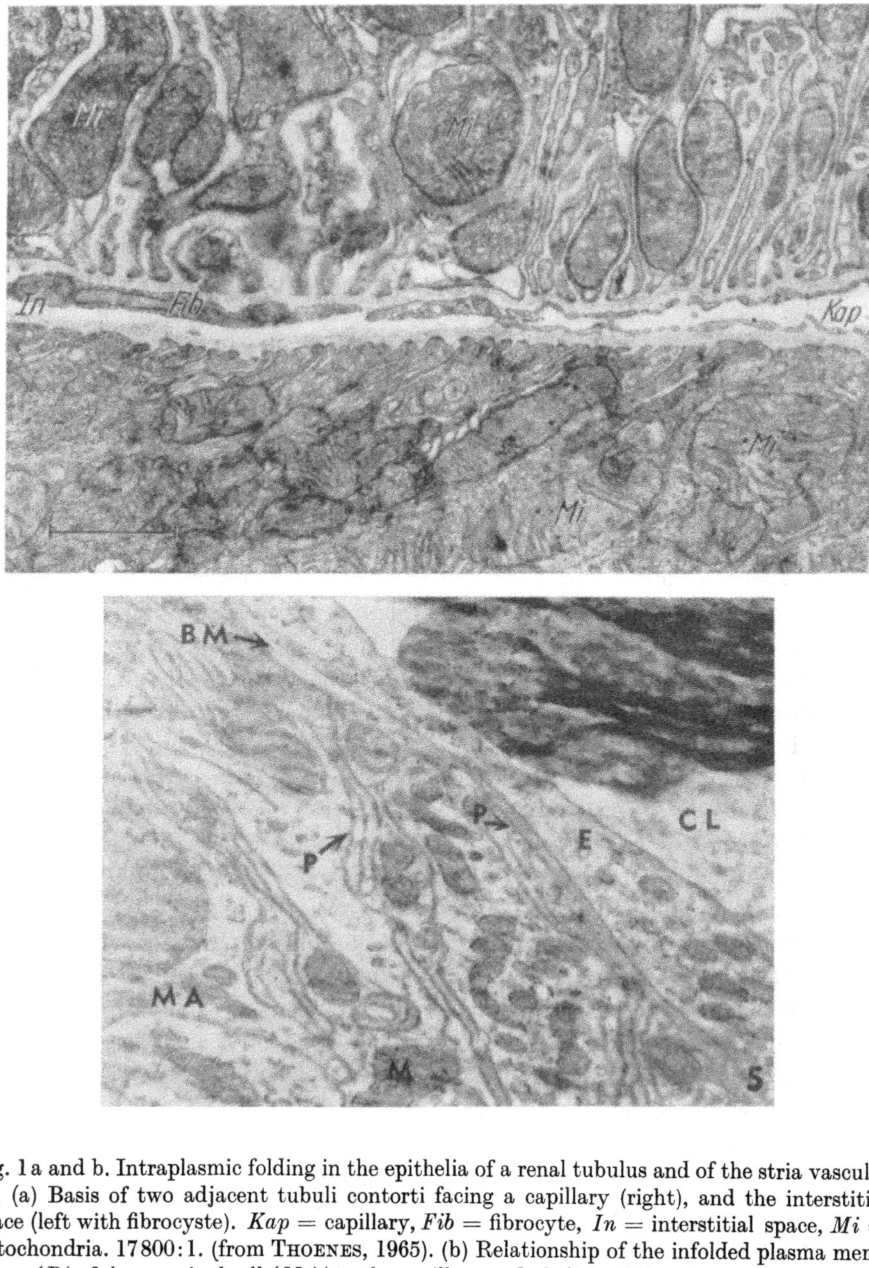

Fig. 1a and b. Intraplasmic folding in the epithelia of a renal tubulus and of the stria vascularis. (a) Basis of two adjacent tubuli contorti facing a capillary (right), and the interstitial space (left with fibrocyste). *Kap* = capillary, *Fib* = fibrocyte, *In* = interstitial space, *Mi* = mitochondria. 17800:1. (from THOENES, 1965). (b) Relationship of the infolded plasma membrane *(P)* of the marginal cell *(MA)* to the capillary endothelium *(E)*. *CL* = capillary lumen, *BM* = basement membrane, *M* = mitochondria. 22800:1. (from C. A. SMITH, 1957)

These concomitant morphological features in structures which are involved in water and electrolyte transport offered possibilities of studying parallel pathophysiological traits in transport disorders. The parallel intoxicability of the kidneys and the inner ear by classes of substances such as antibiotics, diuretics, ouabain and others fit into this concept. Also, hereditary diseases with both renal and auditory deficiencies are interesting in this respect.

III. Hereditary Oto-Renal Syndromes

A. Alport's Syndrome

The coincidence of progressive sensorineural deafness with terminal nephritis on a hereditary basis has been called *Alport*-syndrome since 1961 (WILLIAMSON). First reports emphasized the familiarly renal insufficiency (SAMUELSON, 1874; DICKINSON, 1875; TYSON, 1881; KIDD, 1882). The historical background is given by NIETH (1968), ARENBERG (1967), and TURNER (1970). HURST (1923) first mentioned, but ALPORT (1927) recognized the significant correlation between renal disease and deafness, and pointed to the probably dominant inheritance. Later, the parallel visual impairment by spherophakia, cataract, and lenticonus were noticed by SOHAR (1954) and ARNOTT *et al.* (1966). Facultative symptoms were malformations of the urinary tract and osseous lesions of the fingers (BRAUN *et al.*, 1962; MINDER *et al.*, 1965a, b). While in the female members of the families sometimes only a moderate proteinuria without impairment of the kidney function is combined with slight deafness, the malignant course in the masculine members of the kindred is often fatal in the 3rd decade with death in uremia.

With hematuria as the initial principal finding, at various stages of the disease proteinuria, pyuria, cylindruria and aminoaciduria may occur (WALLACE and JONES *et al.*, 1960; SCHAFER *et al.*, 1962; MINDER *et al.*, 1965b). Hypertension sometimes is marked (GREGG and BECKER, 1963; MILLER *et al.*, 1970). Occasionally, the deafness precedes the nephritis (MILLER *et al.*, 1970). Neurological symptoms, such as EEG abnormalities, were reported by GUERRIER and DÉJEAN (1964), GOETZ *et al.* (1965), FISCHER *et al.* (1970).

Laboratory data have revealed disturbances of the aminoacid metabolism, especially for proline, hydroxyproline, glycine (WALLACE and JONES, 1960; MINDER *et al.*, 1965a, b). Aminoaciduria was noted by MINDER *et al.* (1965b), ONISAWA *et al.* (1965), DUBACH *et al.* (1966), SCRIVER *et al.* (1961). A common transport system for renal tubular reabsorption is shared by the amino acids proline, hydroxyproline and glycine (SCRIVER *et al.*, 1964), which might be disturbed. Hyperprolinemia was observed by DUBACH *et al.* (1966). OHLSSON *et al.* (1963) found increased excretion of alanine, glutaminic acid, histidine, threonine, but no serum amino acid correlation was obtained. NIETH (1959) found valine besides cystine in considerable amounts in the urine. CASSADY *et al.* (1965) reported a statistically significant decrease in serum alpha lipoproteine. Glycosuria was present in the families studied by NIETH (1959) and BERLYNE (1962). Several unaffected members of a family with Alport's disease had diabetes mellitus (CRAWFURD *et al.*, 1968).

In end stages of the disease, the frequently atrophic kidneys reveal the features of chronic glomerulonephritis, together with the characteristics of pyelonephritis, and interstitial nephritis. In young people the pathologic picture may resemble glomerulonephritis, while that in older patients has usually been pyelonephritis (TURNER, 1970). KRICKSTEIN *et al.* (1966) showed that the lesions of the renal parenchyme were a definite pathologic entity, different from glomerulonephritis with pyelonephritis or interstitial nephritis superimposed. PERKOFF *et al.* (1958) and CRAWFURD *et al.* (1968) stressed the appearance of prominent yellow linear streaks, which microscopically consisted of rows of lipid-filled foam cells (KRICKSTEIN *et al.*, 1966). The cells probably contained fat, mucopolysaccharids, phospholipids, cholesterol and phosphatides. Interstitial lymphocytic infiltrates and foam cells were often reported as typical (WHALEN *et al.*, 1961; KONIGSMARK, 1969). The occurrence of foam cells was, nevertheless, not pathognomic for Alport's syndrome (WHALEN *et al.*, 1961), but no other single renal disease had foam cells with the same consistency, quantity and distribution (KRICKSTEIN *et al.*, 1966).

A frequent morphologic feature resembles interstitial nephritis with initially no involvement of the glomerula (KONIGSMARK, 1969) while VAN BUCHEM and BEETSTRA (1965) interpreted the findings of their renal biopsies over 10 years as the primary disorder to be located in the distal tubules. Slight basement thickening and hyalinized glomeruli were noted by PERKOFF *et al.* (1958) and by GOETZ *et al.* (1965).

B. Audiological Evaluation in Alport's Disease

Sensorineural hearing loss has been the prominent feature of the hearing component of Alport's disease throughout the family reports in the last 40 years (TURNER, 1970). In some families, it may be present at birth (FLOWER, 1964), in others it occurs during infancy (MAMOU, 1966; FISCHER *et al.*, 1970), although it usually becomes manifest in the second decade in the male and later in the female (TURNER, 1970). There is a wide range of the familial expression and penetrance of the hearing deficit: 0% (OHLSSON, 1963), 10% (CHAPPELL and KELSEY, 1960), 34,6% (JOHNSON and HAGAN, 1965), 87,5% (SOHAR, 1954, 1956), 100% (COHEN *et al.* 1961). ALPORT, who reported on 14 members of a kindred, found that 11 were hard of hearing; he stated that nerve deafness may exist in individuals who otherwise are healthy. This was confirmed by CRAWFURD and TOGHILL (1968).

On the other hand, many family members with nephritis will show close to normal audiological findings (CASSADY *et al.*, 1965; TURNER, 1970). As a rule, deafness is more common among the affected males. 19 of 20 patients of GRAHAM (1959) that were hard of hearing, were males. In CASSADY's series, 55% of the affected males showed deafness as compared to 39% of the affected females.

Two different types of audiometric curves are prevalent in ALPORT's disease: a "descending" and a "trough-shaped" type (GOLDBLOOM *et al.*, 1957). FLOWER (1964) stated that all of his audiograms appeared reasonably similar with average, speech range, pure-tone losses between 25 and 45 dB, the slope of the curves sometimes nearly identical in close relatives. Other investigators have reported dips at 4096 cps (STEPHENS and PERKOFF, 1951) or an isolated drop at 6000 cps (TURNER, 1970). DUBACH *et al.* (1962) showed trough-shaped curves with 50 dB losses within the speech range, without a loss greater than at 4000 cps. Also KLOTZ (1959) reported a sensorineural hearing loss with maximum loss at 2048 cps, but he was able to follow the progressive loss from a trough-shaped curve to a descending curve in a 15-year-old boy.

An opposite kind of progressive hearing deficit is even more frequent: GREGG and BECKER (1963) and GEKLE *et al.* (1969) published follow-up studies which documented the development of trough-shaped audiograms from slightly descending slopes of the hearing curve (Fig. 2).

The small air-bone gap shown in Fig. 2 was not interpreted as conductive hearing loss. Several authors have noted, however, the occurrence of mixed hearing losses (ARENBERG *et al.*, 1967) with a history of old, difficult to treat perforated ear drums. This is consistent with findings of CASSADY *et al.* (1965) and KRICKSTEIN *et al.* (1966). Also the family studied by FLOWER (1964) had a strong history of allergy, and the hearing losses reported seemed to be associated with frequent earaches, draining ears etc. POLI (1955) and OHLSSON (1963) stressed the unusually high incidence of severe otitis media in Alport's syndrome.

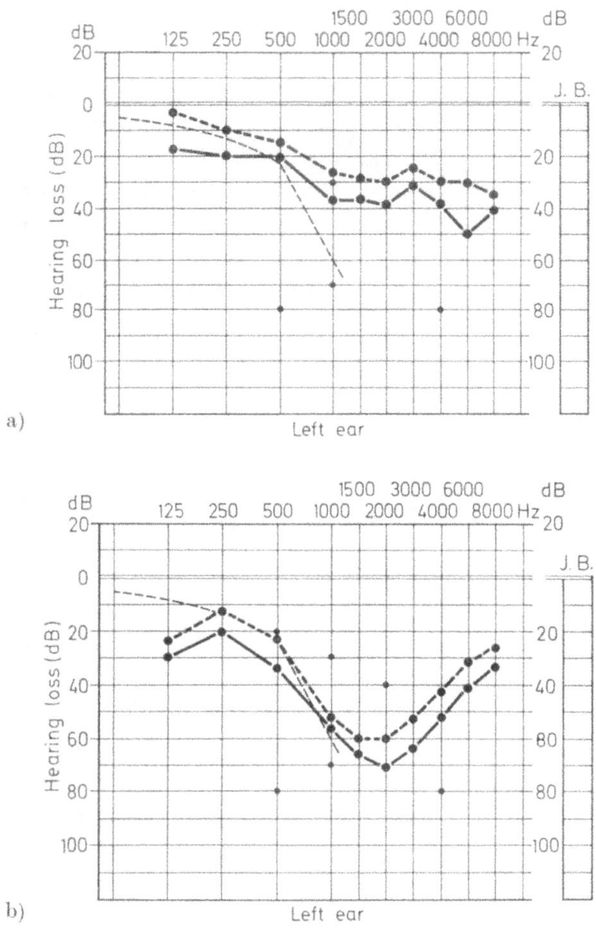

Fig. 2a and b. *Alport*-Syndrome. Development of a trough-shaped threshold curve *(B)* out of a descending curve *(A)* within three years. (From GEKLE *et al.*, 1969). (a) Pure tone audiogram of patient H.-D. W., kindred Nr. 41, June 2, 1961 (●------● bone conduction, ●——● air conduction, ······ vibration theshold). (b) Pure tone audiogram of patient H.-D. W., kindred Nr. 41, December 7, 1964

In most cases, the hearing loss in Alport's disease is bilateral, almost symmetrical. Unilateral deafness is exceptional (POLI, 1955; GEKLE *et al.* 1969). MILLER *et al.* (1970) did audiometric examinations of 5 patients from 4 kindreds; the patients had severe neurosensory hearing losses. He also used speech discrimination test, tone decay test, SISI-test, and Békésy audiometry. From his data, it became obvious that the hearing loss in all of his patients was due to a lesion in the end-organ of the auditory system. His results confirmed the observation of JOHNSON and HAGAN (1965) who had, on the basis of short increment sensitivity index (SISI) and type II v. Békésy tracings greater than 50%, localized the lesion audiometrically to the cochlea. In addition, by the use of tonal decay tests, he ruled out retrocochlear involvement.

C. Vestibular Function in Alport's Disease

While PERRIN (1964) had mentioned nystagmus as an ocular symptom in Alport's disease, SUZUKI *et al.* (1964) and GOETZ *et al.* (1965) recorded normal vestibular function in the caloric test. One patient of MILLER's *et al.* (1970) complained of short attacks of vertigo. In this patient, as well as in 3 others, there was no spontaneous or positional nystagmus. Results of caloric examination using Frenzelglasses were within normal limits in both ears. However, electronystagmographic recording of eye movements, evaluating ten nystagmoid beats with the

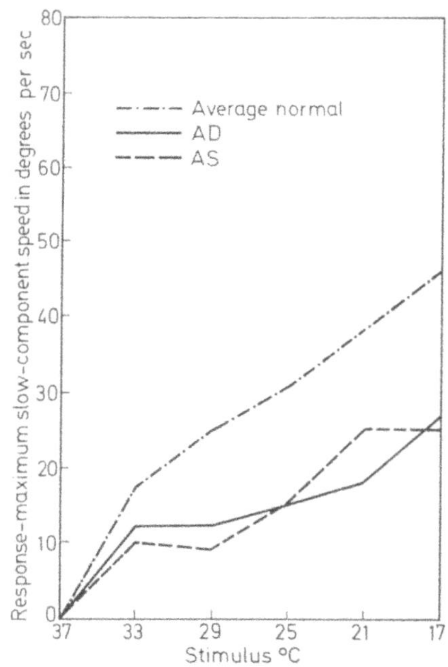

Fig. 3. Thermal vestibulogram summary in *Alport's* syndrome. Note flattening of response vs stimulus line. [From MILLER *et al.*, 1970]

highest slow-velocity phase (SPV), revealed bilateral decreased caloric response: 10,5°/sec compared to expected normal of 26°/sec. Thermal vestibulometry displayed a lower intensity of nystagmus at each temperature than the expected normal average (Fig. 3). No vestibular fatigue was present. This pattern is known for end-organ hair-cell disease.

D. Temporal Bone Histopathology in Alport's Disease

Compared to the vast clinical literature on Alport's syndrome there are only few morphologic investigations of the inner ear (PERKOFF *et al.*, 1958; GOLDBLOOM *et al.*, 1959; NIETH, 1959; WHALEN *et al.*, 1961; DUBACH and GSELL, 1962; GREGG and BECKER, 1963; OHLSSON, 1963; WOOD and KNIGHT, 1966; ARENBERG and JOHNSSON, 1967; CRAWFURD and TOGHILL, 1968; LACHHEIN *et al.*, 1968; WINTER *et al.*, 1968; FUJITA and HAYDEN, 1969; MILLER *et al.*, 1970).

Histological sections showed no significant sensory cell loss or any significant pathology (NIETH, 1959; WHALEN *et al.*, 1961; FUJITA and HAYDEN, 1969) or failed to give a definite explanation for the hearing loss (OHLSSON, 1963). Others found complete absence of the organ of Corti (CRAWFURD and TOGHILL, 1968); traces of the tectorial membrane could be seen only in the apical turn. MILLER *et al.* (1970) observed a shrunken, hyalinized and collapsed tectorial membrane, while any recognizable hair cells and supporting cells were absent. GREGG and BECKER (1963) reported degeneration of the stria vascularis and hair cells in the basal coil in one patient. Cyst-like vesicle formation in the spiral ligament of each basal turn and under each utricular macule was reported by CRAWFURD and TOGHILL (1968), WINTER *et al.* (1968), and MILLER *et al.* (1970). Ganglion cell population and number of nerve fibres appeared to be normal (GREGG and BECKER, 1963; MILLER *et al.*, 1970) or reduced in number (MINDER *et al.*, 1965a, b; DUBACH *et al.*, 1966; WINTER *et al.*, 1968). CRAWFURD and TOGHILL (1968) noted macrophage foam cells in the saccus endolymphaticus, but they were doubtful about the significance of this finding. All of the authors agree as to the absence of inflammatory reactions or exudate.

E. Genetics

According to MILLER *et al.* (1970) more than 90 kindreds have been reported to date, but the mode of inheritance of this syndrome is still controversial (*c. f.* COHEN *et. al.*, 1961; ARENBERG, 1967; NIETH, 1968). While PERKOFF *et al.* (1951) and STEPHENS and PERKOFF (1951) favored the idea of a dominant, partial sex-linked transmission, GRAHAM (1969), who had noted an abnormal sex-ratio, postulated an early loss of heterozygous males in intrauterine life, and decided that the mode of inheritance was a sex-influenced, autosomal, dominant trait, more severe in males. SHAW and GLOVER (1961) suggested that the trait for renal dysfunction and hearing loss is inherited as an autosomal dominant with non-random segregation and preferential association of the autosome carrying the gene with the X-chromosome.

F. Comment on Alport's Disease

The coincidence of chronic nephritis, leading to endstage kidney failure, with progressive sensorineural hearing loss in Alport's disease is based on inherited factors. Dysfunction of the hearing and equilibrium organs may be localized in the inner ear (JOHNSON and HAGAN, 1965), and the point of lesion may be sought, according to the sparse information, in the sensory cells or the stria vascularis. Deafness and dysequilibrium are not always concomitant with nephritis, nor correlated with the degree of kidney failure. It remains obscure, whether the renal intoxication will lead to secondary lesion of the predisposed inferior structures of the labyrinth (CRAWFURD and TOGHILL 1968). GUERRIER and DÉJEAN (1964) suggested such a noxious influence of the nephritis on the capillaries of the inner ear. The lack of otherwise typical uremic, neurologic symptoms in Alport's disease fits into this concept.

G. Other Hereditary Oto-Renal Syndromes

Some observations of malformations of the genito-urinary tract in Alport's disease lead to the description of genito-urinary tract abnormalities in general concomitant with otologic disorders (HILSON, 1957; TAYLOR, 1965). Another related syndrome is the familial occurrence of muscle wasting, nephritis, and deafness reported by LEMIEUX and NEEMEH (1967) and by HANSON *et al.* (1970); this syndrome is possibly a variant of Alport's disease because of related symptoms in the families. Other syndromes, conveying one or the other characteristic of Alport's disease but different from the heredobiologic standpoint, are the familial hyperprolinemia described by SCHAFER *et al.* (1962), the dominant urticaria, amyloidosis, nephritis, and hearing loss (MUCKLE and WELLS 1962), and the recessive renal, genital, and middle-ear anomalies reported by WINTER *et al.* (1968). Also the syndromes of familial lipodystrophy associated with hearing loss (SENIOR and GILLIS, 1964) should be mentioned here.

IV. The Inner Ear in Uremia

A. Hearing in Endstage Kidney Failure

Cochlear manifestations of uremic intoxication would preferably be studied in patients with end stage kidney failure not due to hereditary nephritis but occurring in the course of acquired glomerulonephritis and pyelonephritis. In contrast to the above-mentioned clinical familial disorder with deafness as a symptom of uremia, almost no audiological data are hitherto available in the literature. YASSIN *et al.* (1970a) have reported an audiometric examination of 114 cases of renal insufficiency; they classified the observed neurosensory hearing losses into 5 groups, according to GULICK (Table 1). Their figures gave an impression of the frequency of moderate to very severe deafness in uremic patients, but there was no comment on the possible influence of age, other diseases, or abuse of drugs on the hearing ability in this group of patients.

Table 1. Frequency of hearing loss in uremia (after YASSIN *et al.*, 1970)

Group	Category		No. of cases	Percentage
0	No hearing	loss	9	12,7
I	Mild	deafness	9	12.7
II	Moderate	deafness	22	30.9
III	Severe	deafness	19	26.8
IV	Very Severe	deafness	12	16.9

WIGAND *et al.* (1971) corrected the auditory thresholds of their 60 cases of endstage kidney failure for sex and age, according to SCHMIDT. Their material comprised only patients with a glomerular filtration rate (GFR) of less than 15 ml/min, a serum creatinine level of more than 3 mg-%, and a nonprotein nitrogen of 50 mg-% or more. The average hearing loss showed a steady increment toward the higher acoustic frequencies (Fig. 4A). Only a few of the patients in this group were hard of hearing; their age ranged from 16 to 68 years. From the division into four subgroups with four different primary diseases, it was concluded that the observed hearing losses seemed to be independant of the kind of renal disease – *e.g.* glomerulonephritis, pyelonephritis, or vascular involvement (Fig. 4B).

a)

b)

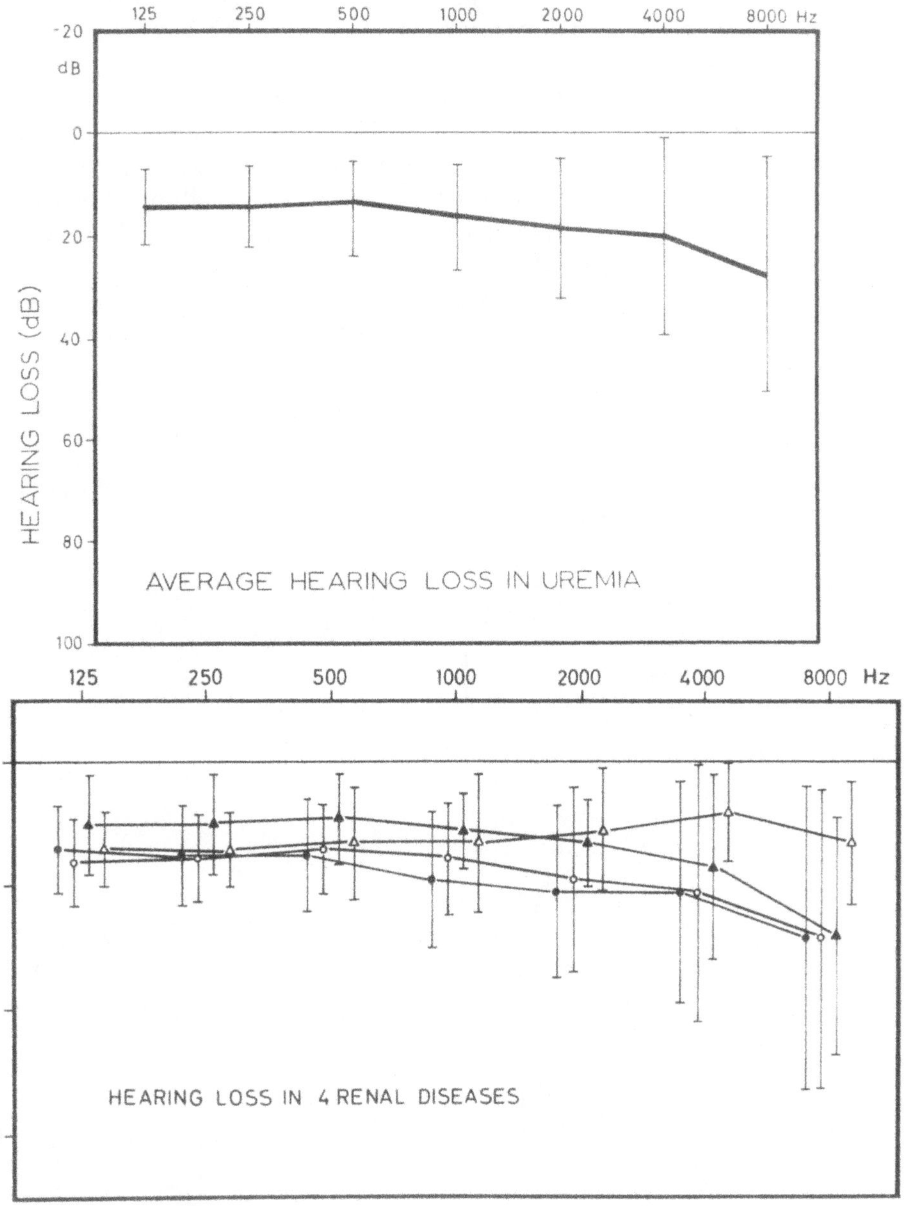

Fig. 4a and b. Influence of uremia on pure tone thresholds. (a) Average hearing threshold of 60 patients with end stage kidney failure. (b) No significant difference of threshold shift in 4 different groups of renal diseases. ● = Pyelonephritis (n = 50); ○ = Glomerulonephritis (n = 45); ▲ = Cystic degeneration (n = 16); △ = Diabetic glomerulosclerosis (n = 6). [From Wigand *et al.*, 1972]

Compared to other uremic patients, hearing losses were not markedly higher in patients with pyelonephritis despite the fact that the latter used potentally ototoxic drugs such as phenacetine or streptomycine (Fig. 4 B).

BERGSTROM *et al.* (1973) found sensorineural hearing losses in about 43% of a group of 224 pre-end-stage and end-stage renal patients. They, however, attributed 80% of these cochlear deficiencies to ototoxic drugs, noise exposures, presbyacousis, mumps, genetic disorders, and otosclerosis, while the rest remained obscure with regard to etiology.

Following the therapeutic course of uremic patients, some cases of remission of hearing loss could be observed. YASSIN *et al.* (1970a) reported 80% improvement in cases of acute renal failure, whereas, in chronic cases, only 52.4% were improved. Audiometric tests revealed improvement of auditory thresholds in seven patients with chronic nephritis, when the renal functions had been definitely restored by kidney transplantation (MITSCHKE *et al.*). ODA *et al.* (1974), on the other hand, attributed significant hearing losses in 43 out of 290 patients, treated by hemodialysis and renal transplant, directly to the therapy of the kidney problems.

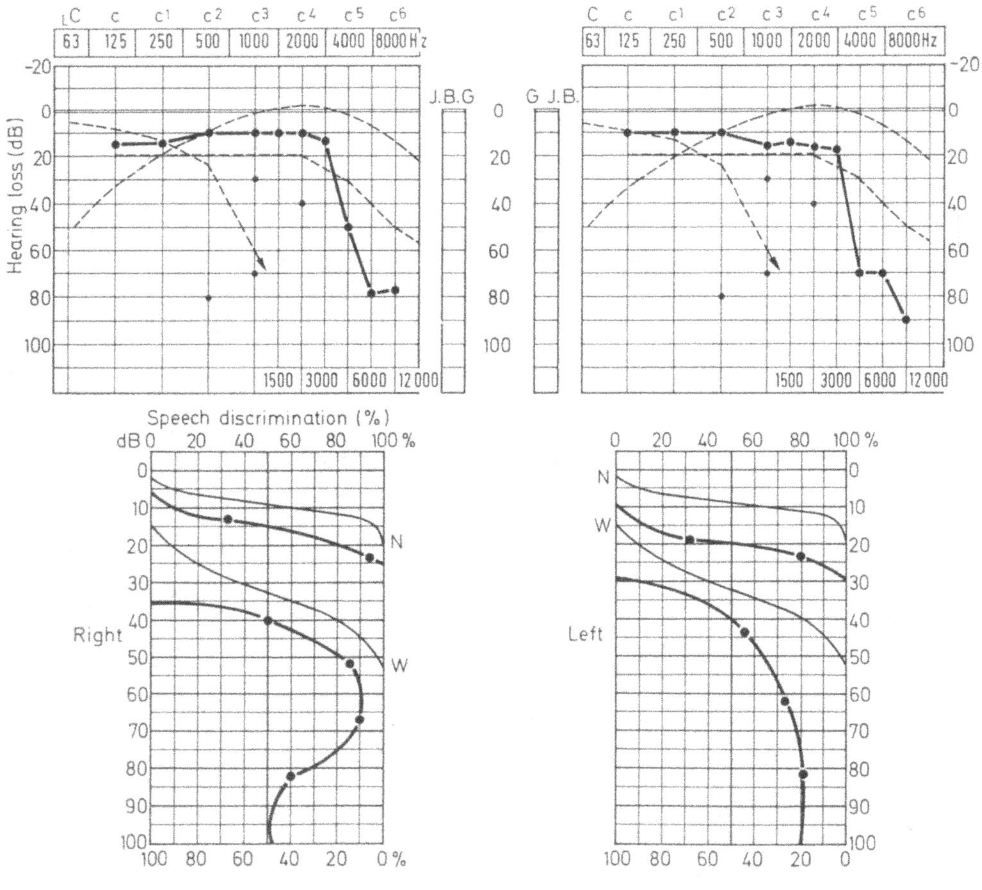

Fig. 5. Pure tone threshold (above) and speech perception threshold (below) of a 17 years old patient with uremia. Notice the occurrence of discrimination loss in the right ear in spite of only slightly reduced tone perception up to 3000 cps. [From WIGAND *et al.*, 1971]

Testing speech perception in uremic patients revealed unequal results: Very often speech perception was slightly or not reduced, but, in other cases, the discrimination curve showed a course („Glockenkurve"), which may be typical for intracochlear lesions, the discrimination score depending on the range of frequency perception in the audiogram (Fig. 5). Recruitment tests always evidenced cochlear affection (YASSIN *et al.*, 1970a).

B. Vestibular Function in Endstage Kidney Failure

In contrast to frequent reports of vertigo and vomiting as symptoms of uremic intoxication (TYLER, 1968), there is very little information on the pathophysiology of the peripheral vestibular system and optomotoric coordination available. Forty-two (= 36.8%) of 114 cases of uremia complained of vertigo (YASSIN *et al.*, 1970b). Spontaneous nystagmus was observed in 5 of 16 examined uremic patients; 6 patients showed abnormal positional reactions (WIGAND *et al.*, 1972). GRAHE (1924), who detected imbalance of the equilibrium in 56% of his uremic patients, ascribed the disorders to a lesion of the central vestibular nuclei.

With respect to caloric excitability, there are two different types of response. Of the 114 cases of YASSIN *et al.* (1970b) of renal disease 65 (57%) showed hyperexcitable labyrinths, whereas 17 (15%) showed variable degrees of canal paresis. Acute kidney failure had a higher incidence of hyperexcitability than chronic renal failure. WIGAND *et al.* (1971) found no increased caloric response in 16 uremic patients, but normal (14 cases) or reduced (2 cases) values.

C. Inner Ear Function in Uremia Correlated with Plasma Electrolytes and GFR

YASSIN *et al.* (1970a) were the first to correlate plasma electrolytes with the degree of auditory threshold shift and caloric response in 71 uremic patients.

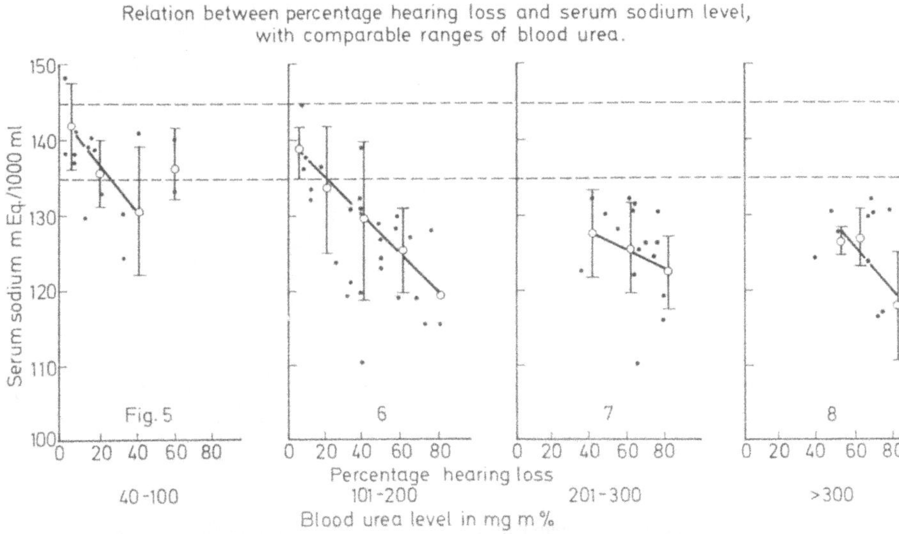

Fig. 6. Correlation between hearing loss and hyponatremia in uremia. [From YASSIN *et al.*, 1970a]

They found a direct relationship to the hyponatremia, which was independent of the level of blood urea (Fig. 6). WIGAND *et al.* (1971, 1972) confirmed the correlation plasma sodium concentration to uremic hearing loss, while they could not find similar relationships with potassium, blood nitrogen and creatinine (Fig. 7). The correlation of the glomerular filtration rate (GFR) to the threshold shift of an 8000 Hz tone, which resulted in a coefficient 0.52, conveyed the impression that the severity of the water transport inhibition was linked with the hearing impairment rather than with a disturbance of the protein metabolism.

Also, TYLER's (1968) observation that neurologic disorders in renal function, represented by electroencephalographic abnormalities, could not be correlated with any single electrolyte would point to a particular nature of the neurosensory hearing loss in uremic patients. Sometimes the EEG showed marked improvement in the face of stable abnormal blood chemistries; in this group, the serum potassium/serum calcium ratio was the most important parameter. But MEENTS (1972) was unable to detect significant potassium, calcium, and creatinine abnormalities in his group of deaf uremic patients.

In an attempt to refer the vestibular affections of 114 uremic patients to plasma electrolyte abnormalities, YASSIN *et al.* (1970b) reported a direct relation-

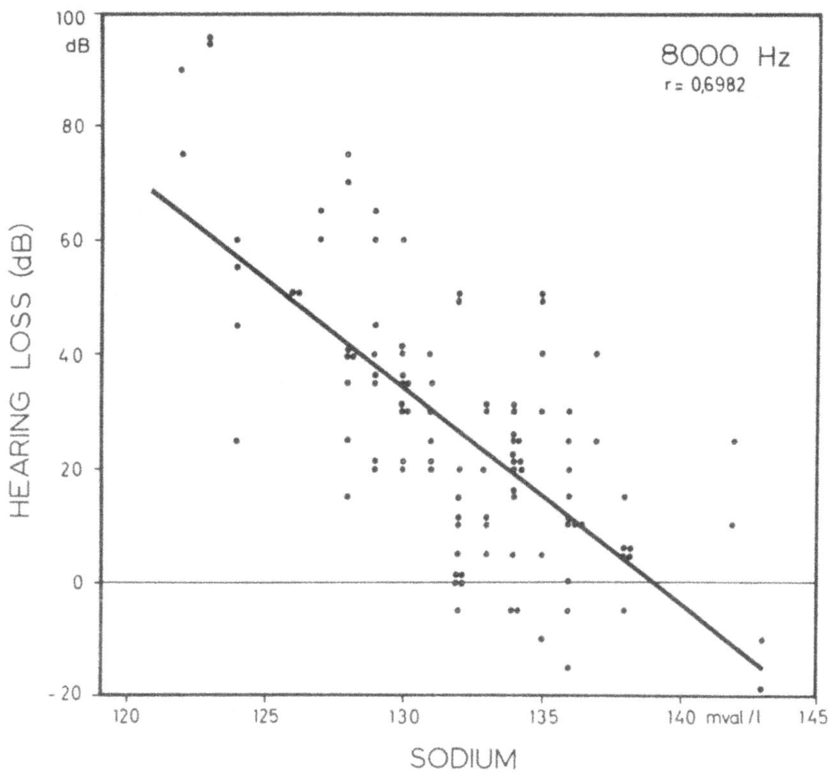

Fig. 7a

Fig. 7a—c. Correlation between hearing loss in uremia and plasma sodium (a), plasma creatinine (b), and glomerular filtration rate (c). [From WIGAND *et al.*, 1971]

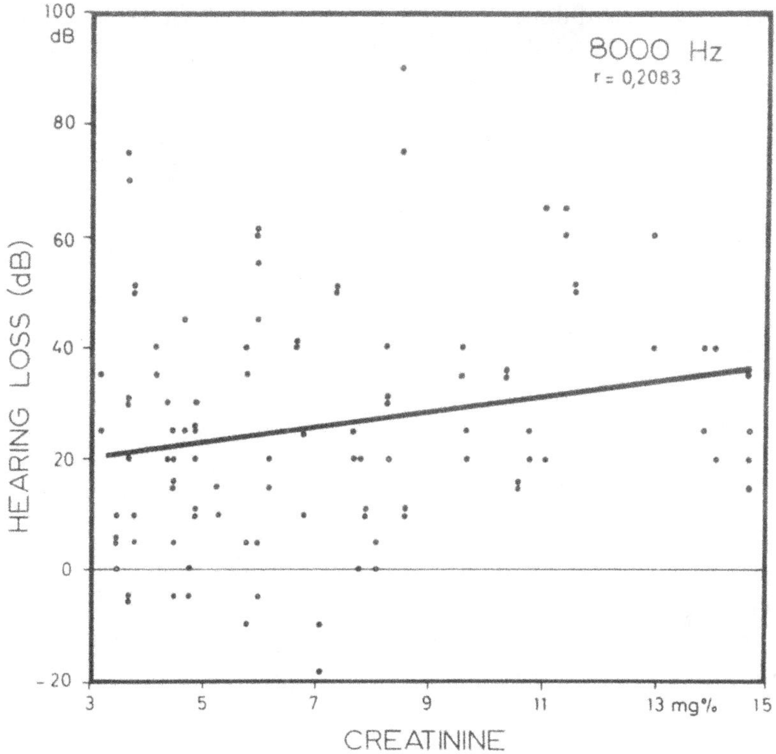
8000 Hz
r = 0,2083
HEARING LOSS (dB)
100 dB
80
60
40
20
0
-20
3
5
7
9
11
13 mg%
15
CREATININE

Fig. 7b

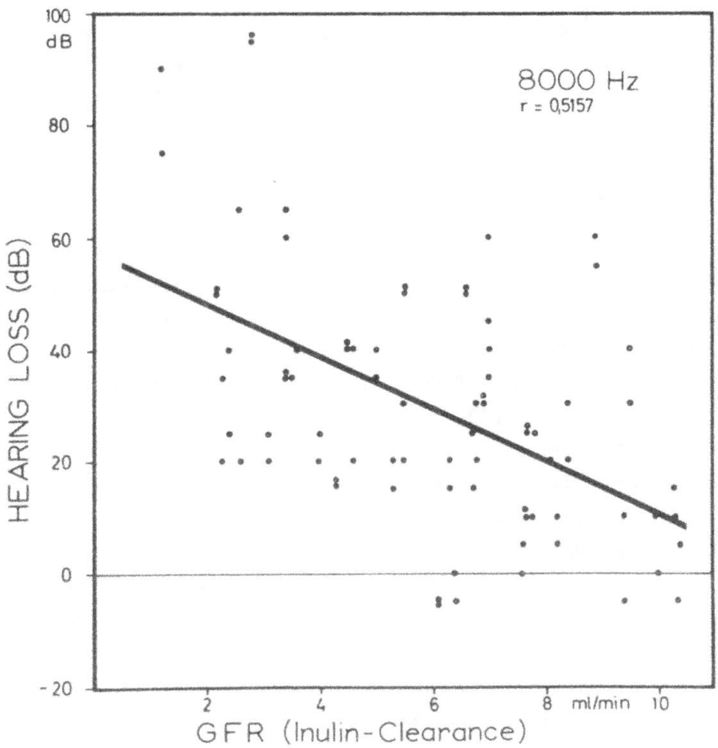
8000 Hz
r = 0,5157
HEARING LOSS (dB)
100 dB
80
60
40
20
0
-20
2
4
6
8 ml/min
10
GFR (Inulin-Clearance)

Fig. 7c

ship between the increased duration of caloric response and the level of hyponatremia (Fig. 8). Similar correlative studies on serum potassium, blood hemoglobin, sex, or age showed no definite relation.

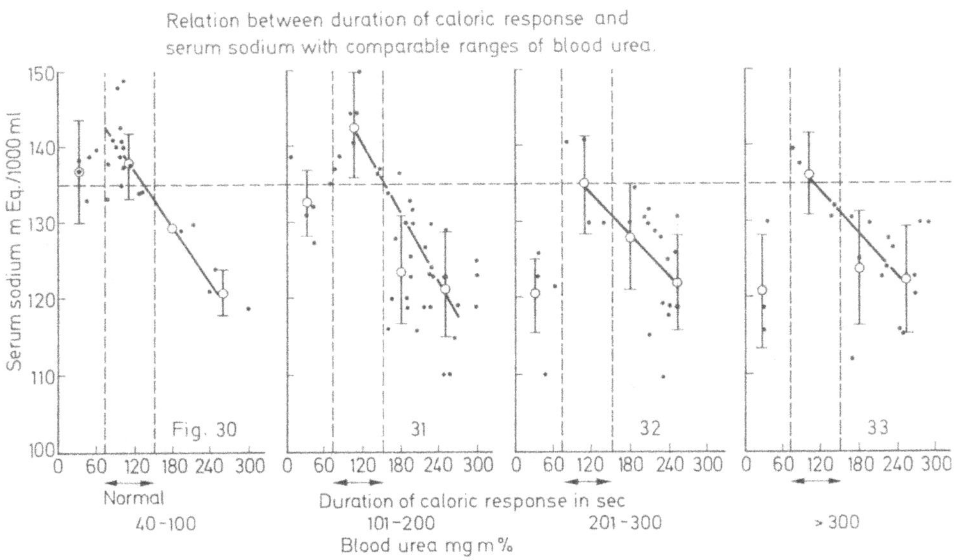

Fig. 8. Correlation between the caloric response of the vestibular organ to hyponatremia in patients with uremia. [From YASSIN *et al.*, 1970b]

D. Morphology of the Inner Ear in Uremia

Sparce information is available on morphologic changes of inner ear structures in uremia. SCHWARTZE (1869) emphasized the occurrence of hemorrhage in the cochlea. DIEULAFOYE (1877) reported local edema and extravasate, ROSENSTEIN (1894) suggested, and LYNCH (1912) found swelling of the auditory nerve, and accepted the hypothesis, that undulating hearing losses were due to fluctuations of uremic edema. In a series of 18 temporal bones of uremic patients, GRAHE (1924) could not detect any degenerative feature of the organ of Corti or of the peripheral vestibular apparatus. The spiral and vestibular ganglia and the eighth nerve showed no pathological abnormalities. Also BERGSTROM *et al.*, who recently examined 10 temporal bones of patients died with uremia, were unable to describe an inner ear pathology typical of renal disease. KELEMEN could verify regular labyrinthine structures in a fetus, which had to be removed for severe maternal nephritis with uremic intoxication.

A spiral ligament band, partitioning the beginning of the scala vestibuli, and spongy spiral ligament changes were found by GUSSEN in a patient who had received a renal transplant, and was maintained on immunosuppressive therapy for four years.

V. Ototoxic Side Effects of Diuretic Drugs in Uremia

The above-mentioned morphologic similarities between the kidneys and the organ of Corti are paralleled by a particular vulnerability of both sense organs to groups of substances which hence are potentially nephrotoxic and ototoxic. Among other drugs, *e. g.* chinine, phenacetine, streptomyces antibiotics, some diuretics have recently focussed attention on ototoxic side-effects, but not always could other influences be ruled out, such as the uremia itself or combination therapy with other ototoxic drugs.

A. Ethacrynic Acid

(2,3 dichloro-4-(2-methylene butyryl) phenoxy-acetic acid)

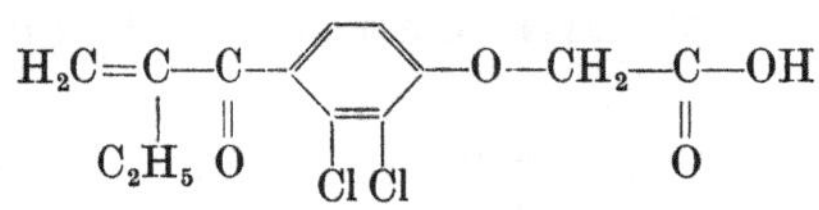

Acute hearing loss due to ethacrynic acid was first observed by Maher and Schreiner (1965) in one of 38 patients with refractory edema after intravenous injection of the drug. Transient high tone depression (30—40 dB) was also reported by Schneider and Becker (1966) in 5 cases of renal impairment receiving oral or i. v. doses of ethacrynic acid (50—700 mg a day). Severe tinnitus preceded and accompanied the hearing loss, but the specific lack of vertigo and nausea was not in harmony with a concept of a disturbed electrolyte balance in the inner ear fluids. Deafness from ethacrynic acid without renal insufficiency was noted by Schmidt and Friedmann (1967), and, after a single dose of 50 mg, by Matz and Naunton (1968). Pillay *et al.* (1969) emphasized that the deafness could be permanent; this finding was confirmed by Mathog and Klein (1969) and by Meriwether *et al.* (1971); the latter investigators underlined the absence of vestibular symptoms.

In cats, daily doses of 20 to 30 mg/kg of ethacrynic acid induced complete loss of cochlear responses within 15 min after injection; full recovery took from 6 to 8 h. Sometimes, the hearing failed to recover (Matz and Naunton, 1968). Similar data were reported on the depression of cochlear microphonics and action potentials in cats using tone burst stimuli of 2000 and 8000 Hz. The minimal dose that caused any alteration was 10 mg/kg i. v.; a cumulative effect was observed. Rapid depression of cochlear microphonic and action potential responses was also demonstrated by Silverstein and Yules (1971). Also marked reduction of the endolymphatic dc potential without recovery was seen in guinea pigs 1 h after injection of 25 mg/kg of ethacrynic acid (Dilling *et al.*). The influence of the dosage on the cochlear microphonic response was studied in guinea pigs by Kohonen *et al.* (1970) and by Jung and Machold (1970), in dogs by Goldmann *et al.* (1973). Similar changes of the endocochlear potential with respect to the dosis were reported by Prazma *et al.* (1972), while depression of the evoked cortical responses was described by Walloch *et al.* (1974). Parallel depressant effects on the cochlear N_1 potential in cats were studied by Brown.

The caloric response of the vestibular system of cats was reduced to 50% of its normal value by intravenous application of ethacrynic acid. This effect was very rapid and only transient (LEVINSON *et al.*).

Morphologic changes after application of ethacrynic acid were reported by MATZ and NAUNTON (1968) and by MATZ *et al.* (1969); outer hair cell losses occurred in the first 20 mm of the basal coil of a patient with poor renal and hepatic function receiving a single dose of 50 mg. This finding was confirmed by MATHOG *et al.* (1970) and FEDERSPIL and MAUSEN in animal experiments. In an electron microscopic evaluation, QUICK and DUVAL (1970) could not only provide further details on degenerative changes of the outer hair cells, but the most striking changes were confined to the stria vascularis: intra- and extracellular edema, destruction of intermediate cells, and elongation of tentacles of marginal cells. This was confirmed by BOSHER *et al.* (1973) and CRIFO (1973). No morphological changes could be seen in the endolymphatic sac or the vestibular labyrinth. Severe intercellular edema and cystic changes of the stria were also found by SILVERSTEIN and YULES (1971).

The diuretic effect of ethacrynic acid is based on its ability to bind sulfhydryl groups of renal cellular proteins (KOMORN and CAFRUNY, 1964), resulting in inhibition of tubular sodium reabsorption. The ototoxic mechanism is unknown; possible factors have been discussed by F. D. SCHWARTZ *et al.* (1970), COHN (1973), BOSHER *et al.* (1973), and DON BROWN (1973). WILSON and JUHN (1970) measured markedly elevated K (13.5 mEq/l compared to 6.0 mEq/l in the control group) in the perilymph of guinea pigs following the injection of 50 mg/kg of ethacrynic acid over 48 h. The sodium concentration in the perilymph was not significantly altered, nor in the serum or cerebrospinal fluid. One speculation was that ethacrynic acid ototoxicity might result from the inhibition of a cochlear duct membrane ATPase. The time course of the reduction of ATP and phosphocreatine levels in the stria vascularis of guines pigs, however, was not correlated to that of the endolymphatic potential depression following intoxication with ethacrynic acid (THALMANN *et al.*). KAKU *et al.* (1973) detected a moderate decrease of respiratory enzyme activities in the outer hair cells of guinea pigs after doses of more than 70 mg/kg. SILVERSTEIN and YULES (1971) stated that a small transient rise in endolymph sodium concentration after application of 30 mg/kg ethacrynic acid could not be responsible for the observed cochlear potential depression because the inner ear fluid composition was normal at the time of the cochlear microphonic reduction. They recorded a moderate change of glucose concentration in both endolymph and perilymph due to hyperglycemia.

COHN *et al.* (1971), on the other hand, detected profound changes in the composition of the endolymph of dogs after the administration of ethacrynic acid; there were no marked reactions in the perilymph. They speculated that the drug may interfere with a specific ion transport system, as it does in other biological systems.

COHN (1973) recently emphasized that the effects are species specific. At human dose levels of 1 mg/kg marked changes were observed only in the dog, while in the cat and guinea pig endolymph electrolytes did not change consistently. Even between different animals within the same species there are large variabilities of sensitivity to ethacrynic acid (PRAZMA).

B. Furosemide

(4-chlor-N-[2-furylmethyl]-5-sulfamoyl-anthranilic acid)

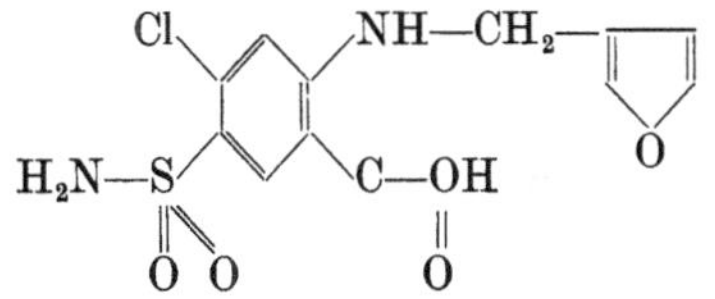

HEIDLAND *et al.* (1969) drew attention to transient hearing losses in patients with end-stage kidney failure receiving high intravenous doses (1000—2000 mg a day) of furosemide. Audiological studies revealed sudden drops up to 50—70 decibels, which were most prominent at 2000—4000 Hz and recovered within a few hours (WIGAND and HEIDLAND, 1969, 1970; HEIDLAND and WIGAND, 1970). The sudden losses occurred even in patients with normal hearing thresholds (Fig. 9).

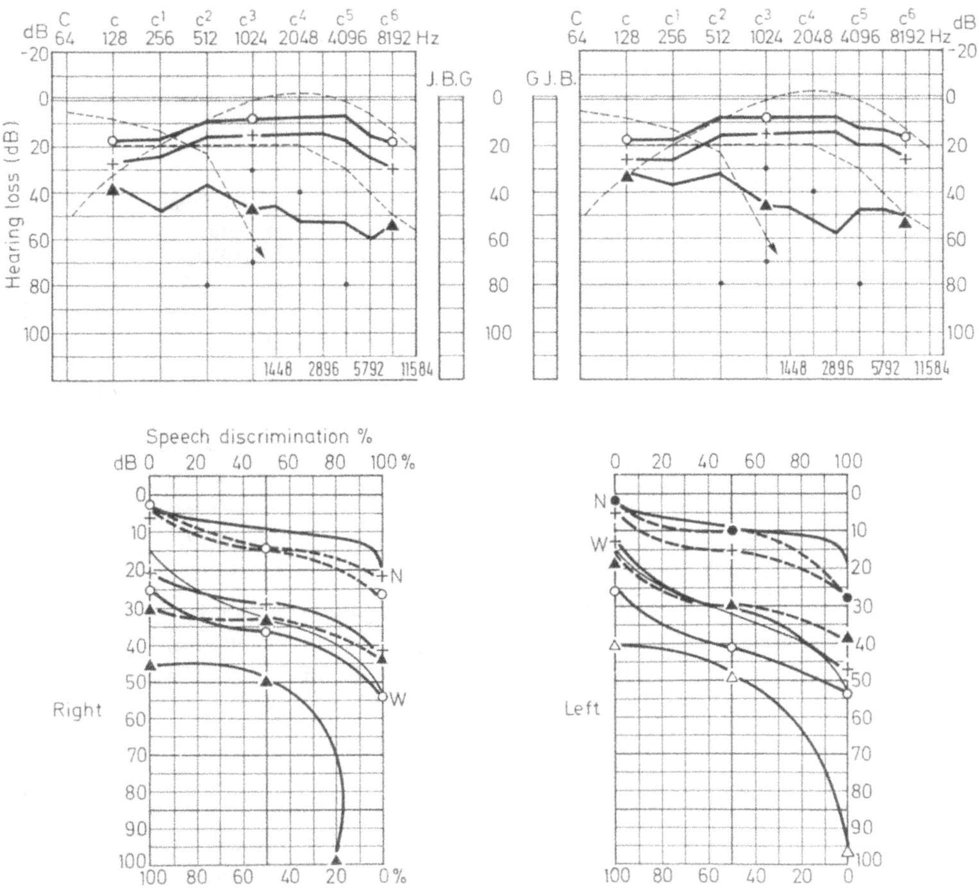

Fig. 9. Acute transient hearing loss after intravenous application of 1000 mg furosemide within 40 min. Pure tone thresholds (above) before o, immediately after the injection ▲, and 1 h later +. Speech reception thresholds (below) show discrimination loss of 20% in the right ear. [From HEIDLAND *et al.*, 1970]

The average threshold shift of 16 patients is given in Fig. 10. Oral and protracted application did not provoke any reaction. The intravenous infusion of PAH, a substance with similar physico-chemical properties and transport characteristics in the renal tubule (HADJU and HÄUSSLER, 1964; GAYER, 1965; DEETJEN, 1966) was without effect.

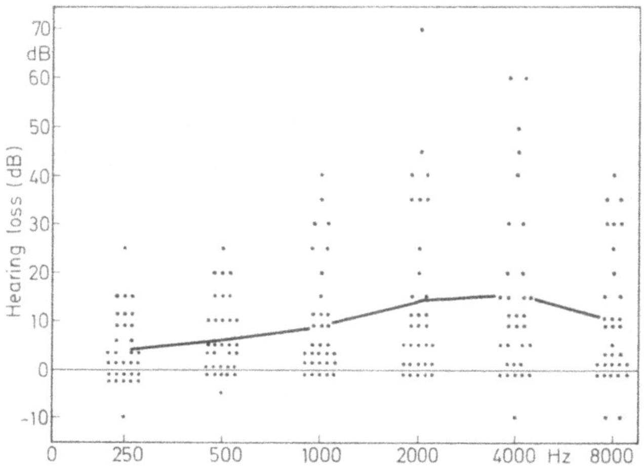

Fig. 10. Acute transient hearing loss after intravenous application of 1000 mg furosemide within 40 min in 16 patients with uremia. The average threshold shift is most marked in the frequencies 2000 and 4000 cps. [From HEIDLAND *et al.*, 1970]

Recording the round window responses in guinea pigs, JUNG (1970) examined the effect of the perfusion of the perilymphatic space with different concentrations of furosemide ranging from 4 to 300 mg-%; he reported nonlinear depressions. Intravenous injections of 10 mg/kg furosemide in cats produced an immediate reduction of cochlear microphonics and action potentials, followed by complete recovery within one hour (MATHOG *et al.*, 1970). Nystagmus responses to caloric stimulation observed in cats after injection of furosemide (about 20 mg/kg) were not significantly different from those of control animals. Enzyme histochemical investigations of the organ of Corti by HAUBRICH and SCHÄTZLE (1970) failed to reveal prominent alterations in the stria except a slight decrease of activity of different enzymes but an increase of acid phosphatase in the spiral sulcus. Even the administration of high doses (200 mg/kg) did not produce visible changes in the histocochleograms of guinea pigs (FEDERSPIL and MAUSEN).

C. Other Diuretics

No inner ear reactions were observed after administration of the osmodiuretics *Mannit* (HEIDLAND and WIGAND, 1970; WIGAND and HEIDLAND, 1970) and *Urea* (JUNG and MACHOLD, 1970), while reduction of cochlear microphonics in guinea pigs was evident after perfusion of the cochlea with *Mefruside* (JUNG and MACHOLD, 1970). Enzyme histochemical alterations were noted after the application of *Diamox* and *Aldactone* by HAUBRICH and SCHÄTZLE (1970).

VI. Interpretation of Cochleo-Vestibular Deficiency in Renal Disorders

On the pathogenesis of cochleo-vestibular disturbances in end-stage kidney failure only speculative considerations are available at the present time. From the above compiled data, it can be concluded that there exist hearing losses due to uremic intoxication, and that a nephro-cochlear relationship, at the same time, renders the organ of Corti more vulnerable to other ototoxic influences. Nothing could be revealed of the reversiblity of the uremic deafness, and no certainty exists as to the point of lesion within the peripheral or central auditory system. The same must be said about vestibular symptoms.

According to the well-known uremic neuro-encephalopathy the existence of circulating noxious substances such as to inhibit the enzyme phosphofructokinase (Tyler, 1968) or to disturb the pentosephosphate cyclus by inhibiting the enzyme transketolase (Lange *et al.*, 1971) or others can be assumed. A comprehensive survey on the present concepts of central nervous intoxication by uremia is provided by the 1970 Symposium on Uremic Toxins held at Monterey, California. Hennemann *et al.* (1971) renewed older suspicions on derivatives of the amino acid metabolism in uremia when they reproduced derangement of sodium transport activity in guinea pigs by i. v. injections of methylguanidine.

Perhaps more than one transport mechanism is involved: examining the salivary electrolyte characteristics of uremic patients Kreusser *et al.* (1971) observed changes of mono- and divalent ions which represented a general disturbance of transport mechanisms across membranes in uremia. They suggested a pathological distribution of intra- and extracellular sodium concentration which may be deleterious also to the electro-chemical activity of the organ of Corti. It must be emphasized, however, that a derangement of the electrolyte balance within the plasma is not necessarily correlated with a dysequilibrium beyond the borders of the blood/csf-barrier (Prill, 1969); that which is true for the central nervous system may well be valid for the functions of the inner ear.

References

Alport, A. C.: Hereditary familial congenital haemorrhagic nephritis. Brit. med. J. **1927** *I*, 504—506

Arenberg, I. K.: Alport's syndrome: hereditary nephropathy, neurosensory hearing loss, and ocular abnormalities: a review. Univ. Mich. med. Cent. J. **33**, 278—285 (1967).

Arenberg, I. K., Dodson, V. N., Falls, H. F., Stern, S. D.: Alport's syndrome: re-evaluation of the associated ocular abnormalities and report of a family study. J. Pediat Ophthal. 4, 21 (1967)

Arenberg, I. K., Johnsson, L. G., Ritter, F. N.: Alport's syndrome: sensorineural hearing loss and hereditary nephropathy, cit. after Arenberg (1967).

Arnott, E. J., Crawfurd, M. D., Toghill, P. J.: Anterior lenticonus and Alport's syndrome. Brit. J. Ophthal. 50, 390—403 (1966).

Barnett, R. J., Seligman, A. M.: Histochemical demonstration of protein bound sulfhydryl and disulfide groups of protein. J. nat. Cancer Inst. **14**, 769 (1954).

BEANEY, G. P. E.: Otolaryngeal problems arising during the management of severe renal failure. J. Laryng. **78**, 507—515 (1964).

BERGSTROM, L. V., JENKINS, P., SANDO, I., ENGLISH, G. M.: Hearing loss in renal disease; clinical and pathological studies. Ann. Otol. **82**, 555—576 (1973).

BERLYNE, G. M.: Familial Nephritis. Manchester med. Gaz. **41**, 26 (1962).

BOSHER, S. K., SMITH, C., WARREN, R. L.: The effect of ethacrynic acid upon the cochlear endolymph and stria vascularis, a preliminary report. Acta oto-laryng. (Stockh.) **75**, 184—191 (1973).

BRAUN, F. C., BAYER, J. F.: Familial nephrosis associated with deafness and congenital urinary tract anomalies in siblings. J. Pediat. **60**, 33 (1962).

BRIGHT, R.: Cases and observations illustrative of renal disease accompanied by the secretion of albuminous urine. Guy's Hosp. Rep. **1**, 338—379 (1836).

BROD, J.: Die Nieren. Physiologie, klinische Physiologie und Klinik. Berlin: VEB Verlag Volk und Gesundheit 1964.

BROWN, R. D.: Cochlear N_1 depression produced by the sodium salts of ethacrynic acid and its cysteine adduct. Neuropharmacology **12**, 967—974 (1973).

CASSADY, G., BROWN, K., COHEN, M., DEMARIA, W.: Hereditary renal dysfunction and deafness. Pediatrics **35**, 967 (1965).

CHAPPEL, J. A., KELSEY, W. M.: Hereditary nephritis. Amer. J. Dis. Child **99**, 401—407 (1960).

COHEN, M. M., CASSADY, G., HANNA, B. L.: Genetic study of hereditary renal dysfunction with associated nerve deafness. Amer. J. hum. Genet. **13**, 379—389 (1961).

COHN, E. S.: Ethacrynic acid. Arch. Otolaryng. **97**, 300 (1973).

COHN, E. S., GORDES, E. H., BRUSILOW, S. W.: Ethacrynic acid effects on the composition of cochlear fluids. Science **171**, 910—911 (1971).

CORTI, A.: Recherches sur l'organe de l'ouie des mammifères. Z. wiss. Zool. **3**, 109—169 (1851).

CRAWFURD, M. D., TOGHILL, P. J.: Alport's syndrome of hereditary nephritis and deafness. Quart. J. Med. **37**, 563—576 (1968).

CRIFO, S.: Ototoxicity of sodium ethacrynate in the guinea pig. Arch. Oto-Rhino-Laryng. **206**, 27—38 (1973).

DEETJEN, P.: Micropuncture studies of diuretics in rats. Proc. 3rd Int. Congr. Nephrology, Washington 1966 (Basel-New York 1967), S. 250.

DICKINSON, W. H.: Disease of the kidney, characterized by albuminuria. In: Albut's, a system of medecine, Vol. **4**, 352. New York; McMillan 1875.

DIEULAFOYE, G.: France méd. **24**, 122 (1877), zit. n. KELEMEN (1957).

DILLING, J. M., NAKASHIMA, T., SNOW, J. B. JR.: Effect of ethacrynic acid on endolymphatic dc potential. Arch. Otolaryng. 98, 183—186 (1973).

DON BROWN, R.: Ototoxicity caused by ethacrynic acid and furosemide. Minerva otorinolaring. **22**, 213—221 (1973).

DUBACH, U. C., GSELL, O.: Alport's syndrome. Lancet 1962 I, 159.

DUBACH, U. C., MINDER, F. C., ANTENER, I.: Familial nephropathy and deafness: First observation of a family and close relatives in Switzerland. Helv. med. Acta **33**, 36—43 (1966).

FEDERSPIL, P., MAUSEN, H.: Experimentelle Untersuchungen über die Ototoxizität eines starken Salidiuretikums (Ethacrynsäure). Mschr. Ohrenheilk. **107**, 256—263 (1973).

FEDERSPIL, P., MAUSEN, H.: Experimentelle Untersuchungen zur Ototoxicität des Furosemids. Res. exp. Med. **161**, 175—184 (1973).

FISCHER, W., FRITZSCHE, S., SCHUBEL, F., WURSTER, U.: Alport-Syndrom. Neurologische und psychiatrische Betrachtungen. Med. Welt (Stuttg.) **21**, 2058—2060 (1970).

FLOWER, R. M.: Familial coincident renal disease and hearing loss. J. Speech Dis. **29**, 329—333 (1964).

FUJITA, S., HAYDEN, R. C.: Alport's syndrome; temporal bone report. Arch. Otolaryng. **90**, 453—466 (1969).

GAYER, J.: Die renale Excretion des neuen Diureticums Furosemid. Klin. Wschr. **43**, 898 (1965).

GEKLE, D., ESSLER, H., BRUNNER, H.: Familiäre Nephropathie und Schallempfindungsschwerhörigkeit (Alport-Syndrom). Arch. Kinderheilk. **178**, 290—302 (1969).

GOETZ, O., KARL, H. J., DATTENBERG, I.: Familiäre Hämaturie und Innenohrschwerhörigkeit. Z. Kinderheilk. **94**, 63—97 (1965).

GOLDBLOOM, R, B., FRASER, F. C., WAUGH, D., ARANOVITCH, M., WIGGLESWORTH, D.: Hereditary renal disease associated with nerve deafness and ocular lesions. Pediatrics **20**, 241—252 (1957).

GOLDBLOOM, R. B., HABERFELDE, G. C.: Hereditary nephritis: report of a kindred. New Engl. J. Med. **261**, 734 (1959).

GOLDMAN, W. J., BIELINSKI, T. C., MATTIS, P. A.: Cochlear microphonic potential response of the dog to diuretic compounds. Toxicol. appl. Pharmacol. **25**, 259—266 (1973).

GRAHAM, J. B.: Hereditary chronic kidney disease: an alternative to partial sex linkage in the Utah kindred. Amer. hum. Genet. **11**, 333 (1959).

GRAHE, K.: Hör- und Gleichgewichtsstörungen bei Nephritis. Z. Hals-Nas.-Ohrenheilk. 8, 375—471 (1924).

GREGG, J. B., BECKER, S. J.: Concomitant progressive deafness, chronic nephritis, and ocular lens disease. Arch. Ophthal. **69**, 293—299 (1963).

GURRIER, Y., DÉJAN, Y.: Le syndrome familial néphropathie-surdité. Rev. Laryng. **85**, Suppl. 925—935 (1964).

GUSSEN, R.: Scala vestibuli partition with deafness and renal disease. Ann. Otol. Rhinol. **82**, 871—875 (1973).

HANSON, P. A., FARBER, R. E., ARMSTRONG, R. A.: Distal muscle wasting, nephritis, and deafness. Neurology **20**, 426—434 (1970).

HAJDU, P., HÄUSSLER, A.: Untersuchungen mit dem Salidiuretikum 4-Chlor-N-(2-furylmethyl) -5-sulfanylanthranylsäure. Arzneimittel-Forsch. **14**, 709—710 (1964).

HAUBRICH, J., SCHÄTZLE, W.: Zur Frage histochemischer Veränderungen der Meerschweinchenschnecke unter dem Einfluß von Diuretica. Arch. klin. exp. Ohr.-, Nas,- u. Kehlk. Heilk. **196**, 319-324 (1970).

HEIDLAND, A., KLÜTSCH, K., MOORMANN, A., HENNEMANN, H.: Möglichkeiten und Grenzen hochdosierter Diuretikatherapie bei hydropischer Niereninsuffizienz. Dtsch. med. Wschr. **94**, 1568—1574 (1969).

HEIDLAND, A., WIGAND, M. E.: Einfluß hoher Furosemiddosen auf die Gehörfunktion bei Urämie. Klin. Wschr. **48**, 1052—1056 (1970).

HEIDLAND, A., HENNEMANN, H., WIGAND, M. E.: Dosiswirkung und optimale Infusionsgeschwindigkeit hoher Furosemidgaben bei terminaler Niereninsuffizienz. 4. Symposium über Nephrologie, Freiburg 1970. Edit. R. KLUTHE, Stuttgart: G. Thieme (1971).

HEINTZ, R.: Nieren-Fibel für Klinik und Praxis. Stuttgart: Thieme 1968.

HENNEMANN, H., BLOEMERTZ, B., HEIDLAND, A.: Studies on natriuretic properties of methylguanidine. Z. exp. Med. (1972).

HEYMANN, A., PATTERSON, J. L., JONES, R. W.: Cerebral circulation and metabolism in uremia. Circulation **3**, 558—563 (1951).

HILSON, D.: Malformations of the ears as a sign of malformations of the genito-urinary tract. Brit. med. J. **1957 II** 785.

HURST, A.: Hereditary familial congenital hemorrhagic nephritis, occurring in sixteen individuals in three generations. Guy's Hosp. Rep. **73**, 368 (1923).

JOHNSON, W. J., HAGAN, P. J.: Hereditary nephropathy and loss of hearing. Arch. Otolaryng. **82**, 166—172 (1965).

JUNG, W., MACHOLD, W.: Zum Einfluß von Salidiuretica auf die Cochlea-Mikrophonpotentiale beim Meerschweinchen. Arch. klin. exp. Ohr.-, Nas.- u. Kehlk. Heilk. **196**, 307—314 (1970).

JUST, L., SCHIECHE, M., WEIGL, E.: Das Syndrom familiärer erblicher Nephropathie mit Innenohrschwerhörigkeit (Alport-Syndrom). Med. Welt (Stuttg.) **40**, 2340—2344 (1967).

Kaku, Y., Farmer, J. C. Jr., Hudson, W. R.: Ototoxic drug effects on cochlear histochemistry. Arch. Otolaryng. **98**, 282—286 (1973).

Kelemen, G. F.: Embryonaler Ohrbefund nach operativer Entfernung wegen mütterlicher Nephritis. Mschr. Ohrenheilk. **91**, 136—145 (1957).

Kidd, J.: The inheritance of Bright's disease of the kidney. Practitioner **29**, 104 (1882).

Klotz, R. E.: Congenital hereditary kidney disease and hearing loss: a case history. Arch. Otolaryng. **69**, 560—562 (1959).

Kohonen, A., Jauhiainen, T., Tarkkanen, J.: Experimental deafness caused by ethachrynic acid. Acta otolaryng. (Stockh.) **70**, 187—189 (1970).

Komorn, R. M., Cafruny, E. J: Ethacrynic acid: diuretic property coupled to reaction with sulfhydryl groups of renal cells. Science **143**, 133 (1964).

Konigsmark, B. W.: Hereditary deafness in man. New Engl. J. Med. **281**, 827—832 (1969).

Kreusser, W., Heidland, A., Hennemann, H., Knauf, H., Wigand, M. E.: Speichelelektrolyte und Flußrate bei terminaler Niereninsuffizienz. Arch. klin. exp. Ohr.-, Nas.- u. Kehlk. Heilk. **199**, 614—618 (1971).

Krickstein, H. I., Gloor, F. J., Balogh, K.: Renal pathology in hereditary nephritis with nerve deafness. Arch. Path. **82**, 506—517 (1966).

Lachhein, L., Kemnitz, P., Büttner, H., Thal, W., Witkowski, R.: Erbliche Nephritis mit Innenohrschwerhörigkeit (Alport-Syndrom). Dtsch. med. Wschr. **93**, 1891—1896 (1968).

Lange, K., Lonergan, E. T., Semar, M., Sterzel, R. B.: Transketolase inhibition as a mechanism in uremic neuropathy. 1. Internat. Urämie-Symposium über Pathogenese, Stoffwechsel, Klinik und Ernährung, Freiburg 1971 (in press).

Lederer, L.: Die Erkrankungen des Gehörorgans in ihren Beziehungen zu Erkrankungen des Stoffwechsels etc. In: A. Denker, O. Kahler's Handb. Hals-Nasen-Ohrenheilk. VI, I. Teil, S. 654. Berlin: J. Springer 1926.

Lemieux, G., Neehmeh, J. A.: Charcot-Marie-Tooth disease and nephritis. Canad. med. Ass. J. **97**, 1193 (1967).

Levinson, R. M., Capps, M. J., Mathog, R. H.: Ethacrynic acid, furosemide, and vestibular caloric responses. Ann. Otol. **83**, 223—229 (1974).

Lynch, R. C.: Otologic signs in general diseases. New Orleans Med. Surg. J., July 1912, ref. Internat. Zbl. Ohrenheilk. **11**, 18 (1913).

Maher, J. F., Schreiner, G. E.: Studies on ethacrynic acid in patients with refractory edema. Ann. intern. Med. **62**, 15—29 (1965).

Mamou, H.: Maladie périodique familiale avec néphropathie et surdité. Sem. Hop. Paris **42**, 3363—3366 (1966).

Matthes, M., Curschmann, H.: Lehrbuch der Differentialdiagnose Innerer Krankheiten. 12. Aufl. Berlin-Göttingen-Heidelberg: Springer 1947.

Mathog, R. H., Klein, W. J.: Ototoxicity of ethacrynic acid and aminoglycoside antibiotics in uremia. New Engl. J. Med. **280**, 1223—1224 (1969).

Mathog, R. H., Thomas, W. G., Hudson, W. R.: Ototoxicity of new and potent diuretics. A preliminary study. Arch. Otolaryng. **92**, 7—13 (1970).

Matz, G. J., Beal, D. D., Krames, L.: Ototoxicity of ethacrynic acid. Arch. Otolaryng. **90**, 152—158 (1969).

Matz, G. J., Naunton, R. F.: Ototoxic drugs and poor renal function. J. Amer. med. Ass. **206**, 2119 (1968).

Meents, O.: Gehör- und Gleichgewichtsfunktion bei Urämie und unter hochdosierter Furosemidtherapie. Inauguraldissertation, Würzburg 1972.

Meriwether, W. D., Mangi, R. J., Serpick, A. A.: Deafness following standard intravenous dose of ethacrynic acid. J. Amer. med. Ass. **216**, 795—798 (1971).

Miller, G. W., Joseph, D. J., Cozad, R. L., McCabe, B. F.: Alport's syndrome. Arch. Otolaryng. **92**, 419—436 (1970).

MINDER, F. C., DUBACH, U. C., ANTENER, I.: Hereditäre Nephropathie mit Schwerhörigkeit. Z. klin. Chem. **158**, 601 (1965a).

MINDER, F. C., DUBACH, U. C., ANTENER, I.: Familiäre Nephropathie und Schwerhörigkeit: erste Beobachtung in der Schweiz. Helv. med. Acta **32**, 404—405 (1965b).

MITSCHKE, H., SCHMIDT, P., KOPSA, ZAZGORNIK, J.: Effekt der Nierentransplantation auf die urämische Hörstörung. Dtsch. med. Wschr. **98**, 2445—2447 (1973).

MORF, J.: Die Krankheiten des Ohres beim acuten und chronischen Morbus Brightii. Z. Ohrenheilk. **30**, 313—343 (1897).

MUCKLE, T. J., WELLS, M.: Urticaria, deafness, and amyloidosis: a new heredo-familial syndrome. Quart. J. Med. **31**, 235—248 (1962).

MÜSEBECK, K., SCHÄTZLE, W.: Die Verteilung der Sulfhydryle und der Disulfide in der Meerschweinchenschnecke. Arch. Ohr.-, Nas.- u. Kehlk. Heilk. **181**, 75 (1963).

MUIROW, P. J.: Hereditary nephritis: Report of a kindred. Amer. J. Med. **35**, 737—748 (1963).

NIETH, H.: Beitrag zum Syndrom der hereditären Hämaturie, Nephropathie und Schwerhörigkeit. Verh. Dtsch. Ges. inn. Med. **65**, 664—667 (1959).

NIETH, H.: Hereditäre und endemische Nephropathien vorwiegend interstitieller Lokalisation. In: SCHWIEGK, H. C. ED.: Handb. Inn. Med. VIII. Nierenkrankheiten, Teil 2, S. 909—941. Berlin-Heidelberg-New York: Springer 1968.

ODA, M., PRECIADO, M. C., QUICK, C. A., PAPARELLA, M. M.: Labyrinthine pathology of chronic renal failure in patients treated with hemodialysis and kidney transplantation. Laryngoscope **84**, 1489—1506 (1974).

OHLSSON, L.: Congenital renal disease, deafness, and myopia in one family. Acta med. scand. **174**, 77 (1963).

ONISAWA, J., SATO, H., SUZUKI, Y.: Paediat. Univ. Tokyo **11**, 9 (1965), cit. n. CRAWFURD and TOGHILL (1968).

PAPARELLA, M., WINTER, L.: Sensorineural deafness in children. Trans. Amer. Acad. Ophthal. Otolaryng. **72**, 782—788 (1968).

PEASE, D. C.: Infolded basal plasma membranes found in epithelia noted for their water transport. J. Biophys. Biochem. Cytology **2**, Suppl. 203—208 (1956).

PERKHOFF, G, T., NUGENT, C. A., DOLOWITZ, D. A., STEPHENS, F. E., CARNES, W., TYLER, F. H.: Follow-up study of hereditary chronic nephritis. Arch. intern. Med. **102**, 733 (1958).

PERKOFF, G. T., STEPHENS, F. E., DOLOWITZ, D. A., TYLER, F. H.: A clinical study of hereditary interstitial pyelonephritis. Arch. intern. Med. **88**, 191—200 (1951).

PERRIN, D.: Alport's syndrome. Ann. Oculist. **197**, 329 (1964).

PILLAY, V. K. G., SCHWARTZ, F. D., AIMI, K., KARK, R. M.: Transient and permanent deafness following treatment with ethacrynic acid in renal failure. Lancet **1969**, 77—79.

PIORRY, L'HERITIER: Traité des altérations du sang. Paris 1840, cit. n. SARRE (1967).

POLI, M.: Nephropathie médicale bilaterale familiale à evolution chronique. Helv. med. Acta **22**, 109 (1955).

PRAZMA, J., THOMAS, W. G., FISCHER, N. D., PRESLAR, M. J.: Ototoxicity of the ethacrynic acid. Arch. Otolaryng. **95**, 448—456 (1972).

PRAZMA, J., THOMAS, W. G.: Ethacrynic acid. Reply. Arch. Otolaryngol. **97**, 300 (1973).

PRILL, A.: Die neurologische Symptomatologie der Niereninsuffizienz. Schriftenreihe Neurologie, Neurology Series, Vol. 2. Berlin-Heidelberg-New York: Springer 1969.

QUICK, C. A., DUVALL, A. J.: Early changes in the cochlear duct from ethacrynic acid: An electronmicroscopic evaluation. Laryngoscope **80**, 954—965 (1970).

QUICK, C. A., FISH, A., BROWN, C.: The relationship between cochlea and kidney. Laryngoscope **83**, 1469—1482 (1973).

RANSOME, J., BALLANTYNE, J. C., SHALDON, S., BOSHER, S. K., HALLPIKE, C. S.: Perceptive deafness in subjects with renal failure treated with hemodialysis and polybrene: a clinicopathological study. J. Laryng. **80**, 651—677 (1966).

RAUCH, S.: Biochemie des Hörorgans. Stuttgart: Thieme 1964.

Rayer: Traité des maladies des reins, 1840, cit. n. Lederer (1926).

Rosenstein,: Nierenkrankheiten, 4. Aufl., 1894, cit. n. Lederer (1926).

Ruska, H., Moore, D. H., Weinstock, J.: The base of the proximal convoluted tubule cells of rat kidney. J. Biophys. Biochem. Cytol. 2, 249—254 (1957).

Samuelsson, F.: Über hereditäre Nephritis und über den Hereditätsbegriff im allgemeinen. Virchows Arch. path. Anat. **59**, 257 (1874).

Sarre, H.: Nierenkrankheiten. Physiologie, Pathophysiologie, Untersuchungsmethoden, Klinik und Therapie, 3. Aufl. Stuttgart: Thieme 1967.

Schafer, I. A., Scriver, C. R., Efron, M. L.: Familial hyperprolinemia, cerebral dysfunction and renal anomalies occurring in a family with hereditary nephropathy and deafness. New Engl. J. Med. **267**, 51 (1962).

Schmidt, P. H.: Presbyacusis. Internat. Audiol. Suppl. 1 (1967).

Schmidt, P., Friedman, I. S.: Adverse effects of ethacrynic acid. N. Y. St. J. Med. **67**, 1438—1442 (1967).

Schneider, W. J., Becker, E. L.: Acute transient hearing loss after ethacrynic acid therapy. Arch. intern. Med. **117**, 715—717 (1966).

Schreiner, G. E., Maher, J. F.: Uremia: Biochemistry, pathogenesis, and treatment. Springfield, Ill.: Ch. Thomas 1961.

Schreiner, L.: Klinische und histologische Untersuchungen zum Alport-Syndrom. Arch. klin. exp. Ohren-, Nas.- u. Kehlk. Heilk. **191**, 618—622 (1968).

Schwartz, F. D., Pillay, V. K. G., Kark, R. M.: Ethacrynic acid: its usefulness and untoward effects. Amer. Heart J. **79**, 427—428 (1970).

Schwartz, G. H., David, D. S., Riggio, R. R., Stenzel, K. H., Rubin, A. L.: Ototoxicity induced by furosemide. New Engl. J. Med. **282**, 1413—1414 (1970).

Schwartze, H.: Ein Fall von Bluterguß in die Paukenhöhle bei Morbus Brightii. Arch. Ohrenheilk. **4**, 12—14 (1869).

Scriver, C. R., Schafer, I. A., Efron, M. E.: New renal tubular amino acid transport system and new hereditary disorder of amino acid metabolism. Nature (Lond.) **192**, 672 (1961).

Scriver, C. R.: Evidence for a renal tubular amino acid transport system common to glycine, L-proline, and hydroxy-L-proline. J. clin. Invest. **40**, 1080 (1961).

Scriver, C. R.: Renal tubular transport of proline, and glycine in health and in familial hyperprolinemia. J. clin. Invest. **43**, 374 (1964).

Senior, B., Gillis, S. S.: The syndromes of total lipodystrophy and of partial lipodystrophy. Pediatrics **33**, 593—612 (1964).

Shaw, R. F., Glover, R. A.: Abnormal segregation in hereditary renal disease with deafness. Amer. J. hum. Genet. **13**, 89—97 (1961).

Silverstein, H., Yules, R. B.: The effect of diuretics on cochlear potentials and inner ear fluids. Laryngoscope **81**, 873—888 (1971).

Smith, C. A.: Structure of the stria vascularis and the spiral prominence. Ann. Otol. **66**, 521—536 (1957).

Sohar, E.: Heredofamilial syndrome characterized by renal disease, inner ear deafness, and ocular changes. Harefuah **47**, 161 (1954).

Sohar, E.: Renal disease, inner ear deafness and ocular changes: new heredo-familial syndrome. Arch. intern. Med. **97**, 627—630 (1956).

Spoendlin, H.: Vascular stria. In: Iurato, S.: Submicroscopic structure of the inner ear. Oxford-London-New York: Pergamon Press 1967.

Stephens, F. E., Perkoff, G. T.: Partially sex-linked dominant inheritance of interstitial pyelonephritis. Am. J. hum. Genet. **3**, 303 (1951).

Strümpell-Seyfarth: Lehrbuch der speziellen Pathologie und Therapie der inneren Krankheiten, 29. u. 30. Aufl., II. Band, S. 14. Leipzig: F. C. W. Vogel (1930).

Sturtz, G. S., Burke, E. C.: Hereditary hematuria, nephropathy, and deafness; preliminary report. New Engl. J. Med. **254**, 1123—1126 (1956).

SUZUKI, Y., KANZAKI, J.: Alport's syndrome of familial kidney disease with deafness. J. Oto-Rhino-Laryng. Soc. Jap. **67**, 1175 (1964).

Symposium on uremic toxins. Guest Editors: WELT, L. G., BLACK, H. R., KRUEGER, K. K. Monterey, Calif. (1970). Arch. intern. Med. **126**, 733—910 (1970).

TAYLOR, W. C.: Congenital deformity of the ears and kidneys. Canad. Med. J. **93**, 107 (1965).

THALMANN, R., KUSAKARI, J., MIYOSHI, T.: Dysfunctions of energy releasing and consuming processes of the cochlea. Laryngoscope **83**, 1690—1712 (1973).

THOENES, W.: Die Mikromorphologie des Nephron in ihrer Beziehung zur Funktion. Klin. Wschr. **39**, 504—518; 827—839 (1961).

THOENES, W.: Transportwege in den Harnkanälchen der Säugerniere. In: Funktionelle und morphologische Organisation der Zelle. Sekretion und Exkretion, S. 315—341. Berlin-Heidelberg-New York: Springer 1965.

TRAUT, G., JUTZLER, G. A.: Urämie. Klinik und Therapie. Fortschr. Med. 88, 227—230 (1970).

TURNER, J. S., JR.: Hereditary hearing loss with nephropathy (Alport's syndrome). Acta Otolaryngol. Suppl. **271**, 1—26 (1970).

TYLER, H. R.: Neurologic disorders in renal failure. Amer. J. Med. **44**, 734—748 (1968).

TYLER, H. R.: Neurologic disorders seen in the uremic patient. Arch. intern. Med. **126**, 781—786 (1970).

TYSON, J.: A treatise on Bright's disease and diabetes. Philadelphia: Lindsay and Blakiston 1881.

VAN BUCHEN, F., BEETSTRA, A.: Hereditary renal disease associated with deafness: Alport's syndrome. Proc. Kon. Ned. Akad. Wet. Ser. C **68**, 350 (1965).

VOLHARD, F.: Die Urämie. In: Die doppelseitigen hämatogenen Nierenerkrankungen. Handb. Inn. Med. Bd. VI, 1, 2. Aufl. Berlin: Springer 1931.

WALLACE I. R., JONES, I. H.: Familial glomerulonephritis and amino-aciduria. Lancet **1960** *I*, 941.

WALLOCH, R. A., ANTHONY, J., GIBBONS, N.: Depression of the evoked cortical potential by ethacrynic acid. Laryngoscope **84**, 256—266 (1974).

WHALEN, R. E., HUANG, S., PESCHEL, E.: Hereditary nephropathy: deafness and renal foam cells. Amer. J. Med. **31**, 171—186 (1961).

WIGAND, M. E., HEIDLAND, A.: Ototoxic side-effects of high doses of furosemide in patients with uremia. IV. Internat. Congr. Nephrology, Stockholm, 1969. Postgrad. med. J. **47**, April 1971, Suppl. 54—56.

WIGAND, M. E., HEIDLAND, A.: Akute, reversible Hörverluste durch rasche, hochdosierte Furosemidinfusionen bei terminaler Niereninsuffizienz. Arch. klin. exp. Ohr.-, Nas.- u. Kehlk. Heilk. **196**, 314—319 (1970).

WIGAND, M. E., MEENTS, O., HEIDLAND, A.: Cochleovestibuläre Störungen bei Patienten mit terminaler Niereninsuffizienz IV. Symposium über Niereninsuffizienz, Innsbruck, 1971. Edit. P. v. DITTRICH, F. SKRABAL. Friedberg: C. Bindernagel, 1971.

WIGAND, M. E., MEENTS, O., HENNEMANN, H., HEIDLAND, A.: Kochleo-vestibuläre Störungen bei Urämie in Beziehung zum Elektrolytstoffwechsel und Glomerulumfiltrat. Schweiz. med. Wschr. **102**, 477—482 (1972).

WILLIAMSON, D. A. J.: Alport's syndrome of hereditary nephritis with deafness. Lancet 1961 *II*, 1321—1323.

WILSON, K. S., JUHN, S. K.: The effect of etharcrynic acid on perilymph Na and K (Preliminary report). Pract. oto-rhino-larnyg. **32**, 279—287 (1970).

WINTER, L. E., CRAM, B. M., BANOVETZ, J. D.: Hearing loss in hereditary renal disease. Arch. Otolaryng. **88**, 238—241 (1968).

WOOD, J. J., KNIGHT, L. W.: A family with Alport's syndrome of hereditary nephritis and deafness. Med. Mschr. **20**, 227—235 (1966).

YASSIN, A., BADRY, A., FATT-HI, A.: The relationship between electrolyte balance and cochlear disturbances in cases of renal failure. J. Laryng. **84**, 429—435 (1970a).

YASSIN, A., BADRY, A., FATT-HI, A.: The role of electrolyte balance on vestibular disturbances. in case of renal failure. J. Laryng. **84**, 437—442 (1970b).

YASSIN, A., SAFWAT, F., FATT-HI, A.: Ear, nose and throat manifestations in cases of renal failure treated by dialysis, hemodialysis, and peritoneal dialysis. Ann. Otol. **75**, 192—201 (1966).

Chapter 7

Community Response to Noise

W. K. CONNOR and W. RUDMOSE, Austin, Texas (USA)

With 8 Figures

Contents

I. Introduction

In the last two decades, community noise has become a problem of major dimensions in many countries. Increasing numbers of people are exposed to noise generally present in their residential and working environments; the level of this general noise has risen steadily along with the state of machine technology, especially in the transportation field. In response to the problem, research has been undertaken to study the effects of noise on man, to identify factors affecting human response both of individuals and of groups, to establish relevant criteria, and to devise means of alleviation. A great deal of useful knowledge has been amassed, but a both comprehensive and accurate understanding of community response to noise has not been attained, nor is this goal well within present reach. A dominant reason for this is the complexity of the subject. The statistical nature of the problem is self-evident; the greater difficulty, however, lies in the number of independent variables necessary to delineate some modes of response with even moderate certainty. Furthermore, investigations purporting to examine the subject in its fullest context are necessarily of an epidemiological nature and to undertake them, resources of unusual magnitude are necessary. Because of the latter fact and the public character of community noise problems, most research in this area has been performed or sponsored by governmental agencies. This is reflected in the references in this chapter. The largely pragmatic nature of the research that has been done and the fact that much of it deals only with noise from specific sources, such as aircraft, place obvious limitations on the contribution of research results to a fundamental understanding of the basic problem, community response to noise.

This chapter will deal exclusively with community noise, defined here as noise to which members of the community as a whole are generally and indiscriminately exposed. In this context, any sizable group of individuals in a specific geographical area, whether or not this group has a unique political or other social structure, will be called a community. A community could thus be a neighborhood for which exposure to particular noise sources is the major point of commonality.

It should be pointed out that individual response to community noise is an inseparable aspect of community reaction. However, since individual response may be strongly conditioned by social factors or socially reinforced psychological factors, the response manifested by the community as a whole cannot properly be considered as simply the sum of individual responses. This will be demonstrated in later portions of this chapter.

II. Sources of Community Noise

Surveys have assessed the relative disturbance due to different community noise sources; these also attest to the multiplicity of significant sources, particularly in urban areas. Table 1 gives the percentage of people disturbed by different sources in a general survey made in London in 1961—1962. Similar data

Table 1. Percentage of people disturbed by various sources of noise in 1961—1962 London survey (Wilson, 1963) $N = 1{,}400$

Source	When at home	When outdoors	When at work
Road traffic	36	20	7
Aircraft	9	4	1
Trains	5	1	—
Industry/Construction works	7	3	10
Domestic/Light appliances	4	—	4
Neighbors' impact noise	6	—	—
Children	9	3	—
Adult voices	10	2	2
Wireless/TV	7	1	1
Bells/Alarms	3	1	1
Pets	3	—	—
Other	—	—	—

are shown in Table 2 for three large U.S. cities and in Table 3, for two smaller cities. The survey samples included in Table 3 were in areas particularly exposed to aircraft noise. From the data of these three tables, it appears that road vehicles are the primary source of noise disturbance in the areas represented. Noises produced by other human beings and by a wide variety of other sources are significant but of less importance. Those sources which produce the greatest disturbance are not necessarily those which are the subject of the highest levels of public reaction. For example, an airport or other establishment under the control of known agencies is a more likely object of complaint than traffic noise in general.

It is notable in Table 1 that less disturbance from almost all sources was reported when away from home, the perhaps obvious exception being "Industry/Construction works" when at work.

Table 2. Percentage mention as first source of bother of various noise sources in Boston, Los Angeles, and New York City (Bolt *et al.*, 1967) $N = 259$

Source	Percentage mention
Traffic	15.4
Children/neighbors	13.9
Other	6.2
Planes	5.4
Animals	5.0
Sirens/horns	3.9
Industry	2.7
Sonic boom	2.3
Motorcycles	2.3
Passersby	2.3
Trains	0.8
(Not bothered)	39.8

Table 3. Mean annoyance (on a 0-4 scale) with various sources of community noise in Chattanooga and Reno neighborhoods exposed to aircraft operations (Connor and Patterson, 1972) $N = 1{,}960$

Source	Mean annoyance
Trucks and autos	0.8
Aircraft operations	1.5
Neighborhood children	0.5
Dogs and other pets	1.3
People	0.2
Motorcycles and hot rods	1.8
Trains	0.1
Sirens	1.0
Construction	0.3
Lawnmowers and garbage collection	0.5
Sonic boom	1.2

Community disturbance due to noise in non-urban areas has borne little scientific investigation, perhaps because the magnitude of the problem and the numbers of people affected are small. A survey in Norway provided the results of Table 4. The rank ordering in importance of the four noise sources listed is the same for both urban and rural samples and, furthermore, is similar to that found in the British and American studies cited above. However, the percentage of persons annoyed is much lower in the rural sample than in the urban.

It will be readily appreciated that the effects of noise from different sources upon communities and their individual inhabitants will not be the same, even at identical sound levels. For example, aircraft noise may interfere with conversation and induce apprehensive fear, while equally disturbing sounds produced by neighbors may be interpreted mainly in terms of loss of privacy. Because of these differences, it is often appropriate to employ different measures of noise exposure and sets of non-acoustical parameters when studying reaction on other than a gross scale. Various exposure measures and other response-related parameters will be presented later in this chapter.

Table 4. Percentage of persons annoyed by various noise sources according to a Norwegian survey (Gallup, 1968) $N = 1{,}600$

Source	Urban	Rural	All
Motor vehicles	20	11	17
Aircraft	4	1	3
Railroads	5	1	4
Neighbors	6	3	5

III. Patterns of Reaction

The terms reaction and response will be used synonymously to refer to a state or action resulting directly or indirectly from a noise stimulus. The word "reaction" often carries more adverse connotations in popular usage, but since noise is unwanted sound, it is reasonable to assume that any response will be unfavorable. Community reaction includes both the responses of individuals exposed to the general noise environment and concerted aggregate reaction within the community; investigations may be, and have been, conducted on both levels. Responses may be either latent or overt.

The fundamental latent individual reaction to noise stimuli is annoyance. Annoyance is the state of being disturbed or irritated, particularly by a specific set of repeated stimuli. It is a conscious subjective reaction which can be quantitatively assessed, given appropriate instruments. Scaling techniques are discussed under "Disturbance and Annoyance". For most noise stimuli, annoyance is the most immediate and fundamental response mode. The degree of annoyance is not a function only of the acoustical stimulus; it depends also upon the pattern of disturbance, the perceptual content of the stimulus, and various attitudes. Thus, the annoyance of individuals may vary widely under identical exposure conditions. The term "annoyance" is occasionally applied to the noise parameter, such as perceived noise level, being used to describe the stimulus and to predict human reaction. This usage should be discouraged because it confuses stimulus and response. The distinction between the two is particularly important because noise exposure values alone are rather poor predictors of ensuing annoyance.

The initial overt response is normally complaint. This may be in the form of discussion among peers, telephone calls to authorities presumed responsible, or letters to officials or to editors of publications. In some cases, this reaction becomes chronic. In a community around a major airport, it was observed that 35—53% of the monthly telephone complaints were from persons who registered more than one complaint (CONNOR, 1971, unpublished). The factors predisposing toward chronic complaint behavior are not known.

Complaint, as well as more complex reaction modes such as formal petitions, group demonstrations, and legal suits, may well take place on an organized basis as well as on the part of individuals. The vehicle may be either an existing organizational structure such as a community council or citizens' league or an *ad hoc* group.

The following model was postulated for response to one class of community noise (NIXON and HUBBARD, 1965):

$$\text{Stimulus} \rightarrow \text{Interference} \rightarrow \text{Annoyance} \rightarrow \text{Reaction} \rightarrow \text{Complaint.}$$

To this succession could be added the more vigorous forms of reaction. The pattern proposed by NIXON and HUBBARD appears to hold for most community reaction situations. However, a study of reaction to sonic boom suggests that, for that special type of stimulus, interference of activities must be preceded by the formation of negative attitudes regarding the source, supersonic aircraft. These negative attitudes are in turn associated with cost of housing (TRACOR, 1970a).

The progression from annoyance to successively stronger forms of reaction is positively related to the level of noise exposure, but this relationship becomes increasingly indistinct with reaction beyond the annoyance stage; other factors condition response. Thus, a simple stimulus-response model is inadequate for describing community reaction. The improved response model shown in Fig. 1

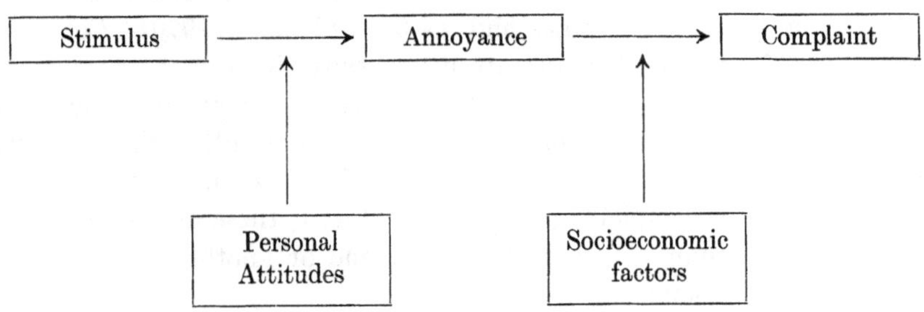

Fig. 1. Noise response model

includes nonacoustical mediating factors and is generally in agreement with results of research performed to date. The preponderance of this research has been in connection with aircraft noise, but the results of studies concerned with other types of noise are not inconsistent with the model. Some of the attitudinal factors which are believed to influence noise annoyance are as follows (BORSKY, 1969b):

1. Feelings about the necessity or preventability of the noise.
2. Feelings of the importance of the noise source and the value of its primary functions.
3. Extent to which there are other things disliked in the residential environment.
4. Belief in the effect of noise on general health.
5. Extent to which fear is associated with the noise.
6. Other variables.

In a study of reaction to aircraft noise, the attitudinal variables which, in conjunction with noise exposure, were the best predictors of annoyance are the following, in order of importance (Tracor, 1970b):

1. Fear of aircraft crashes.
2. Susceptibility to noise irritation in general.
3. Willingness to adapt to increased noise.
4. Belief in misfeasance by authorities responsible for aircraft operations.
5. Feelings concerning the importance of the local airport and air transportation in general.

The first two items may well be related to fundamental psychological predispositions, while the latter three are more in the nature of opinion and more likely to be mutable. Indeed, some success at reducing annoyance due to both motor vehicle and aircraft noise by attitudinal influences has been reported (Sörensen, 1970). It is notable that personal or demographic factors such as age, sex, income, and occupation have essentially no effect on annoyance (McKennell, 1963; Borsky, 1961; Jonsson, 1964). Thus, annoyance may be regarded as the product of noise exposure and the attitudinal set of the subject individual.

The transition from annoyance to complaint, like that from exposure to annoyance, involves strong mediating factors. It is well-known that complaint, at least by an individual, tends to require a certain level of annoyance, but that of all persons at that level, only a fraction ever complain (McKennell, 1963, 1970; Tracor, 1970b; Connor and Patterson, 1972; Wilson, 1963). The fraction may range from as low as 5% to as high as 32% (Tracor, 1970b; Connor and Patterson, 1972). In another aircraft noise study, it was observed that the complainants represented about 11% of the population at a given annoyance level (McKennell, 1963). The effect on complaint, of factors other than annoyance, has not been well validated; various studies have indicated involvement of somewhat different sets of complaint predictors. In Fig. 1, these are denoted "socioeconomic factors"; many of these belong in one or another of the following categories (Borsky, 1969a):

1. Knowledge of where to complain and to whom.
2. Belief in the effectiveness of a complaint.
3. Level of annoyance.
4. Effectiveness of local organizations.
5. Influence of other major problems, personal or local.

The first two items tend to be related to a person's social status, articulateness, and political orientation. The individual who is conversant with institutional structures and channels of communication, who possesses superior intellectual and verbal resources, and who can enlist the support of influential persons and organizations is most inclined to complaint, given the impetus, since he can readily gain a hearing and can presume some possibility of remedial action. The person who has none of these attributes has little incentive save desperation and is more likely to remain frustrated and silent. Not supprisingly, these circumstances devolve upon rather basic socioeconomic indicators. A comparison of complainants and noncomplainants annoyed by noise in the vicinity of Heathrow (London) Airport indicated that the former were higher in occupational status, had received longer education, had houses of higher value, were more likely to be members of organizations, and were more active politically; they were, however, no more annoyed than noncomplainants at a given level of noise exposure (McKENNELL, 1963). A study of reaction to sonic booms revealed that complainants liked their areas as well as noncomplainants, were equally sensitive to noise in general, and had higher levels of education and income; the complainants were less convinced of the importance of aviation and of the necessity of a supersonic transport but more often had some ties with the aviation industry (BORSKY, 1965). In communities around large U.S. airports, complainants were found to be older, more highly educated, and more affluent than noncomplainants; complainants also were less annoyed by potentially irritating sounds and by neighborhood noises other than that of aircraft (TRACOR, 1970b). It seems certain that, in the main, those who complain are not hypersensitive or neurotic individuals; they are highly annoyed persons who have the means and the will to express their discontent. The evidence of the last cited study suggests that such active expression may suppress noise annoyance except that which is the subject of complaint.

As might be surmised from the foregoing discussion, the level or probability of complaint cannot be accurately predicted in a given case from noise exposure information alone. It is often possible, on the basis of past experience, to stipulate noise exposure levels for similar situations which will give reasonable assurance of no significant overt reaction from a community; however, it may be found that other communities are quite tolerant of much higher noise levels. The span of uncertainty is equivalent to at least 10 dB in effective level, making the problems of regulation and noise control difficult without some insight into the nonacoustical factors that contribute to response of a community. The quantitative assessment of community reaction is treated in a subsequent section entitled "Prediction of Reaction".

Reaction beyond complaint has not been studied systematically in specific connection with noise, although there are numerous examples of organized opposition and of legal suits. Such behavior is probably less related to the psychoacoustical aspects of the situation than to political and legal considerations. The following conditions are believed to be most conducive to threatened or actual legal action:

1. Moderate or higher annoyance.
2. Lack of other recourse (such as complaint) or unlikelihood of favorable response.
3. Existence of a probable cause of action.
4. Reasonable assurance of success.

IV. Measurement of Annoyance

Noise can produce a variety of deleterious effects in a community. Potentially, at least, these effects range from loss of hearing and interference with conversation or other auditory communication to disturbance of sleep, rest, or mental activity. Conscious community reaction at either the individual or group level appears to be based mainly upon auditory interference and disturbance of various normal activities. The first effect is readily related to the physical characteristics of noise, expressed in terms of speech interference level (BERANEK, 1954; WEBSTER, 1965) or articulation index (FRENCH and STEINBERG, 1947; KRYTER, 1962), but the second effect, activity disturbance, tends to be strongly affected by individual attitudes regarding the source of noise as well as its acoustical aspects. These attitudes typically have to do with the perceived importance or value of the noise-producing activity, the appropriateness of the levels or exposure patterns produced, and the possibility of danger to life or property.

Since annoyance is the fundamental component of community exposure, the ability to measure it is of great importance. This is difficult to do indirectly from data concerning overt response, such as complaint, because of extraneous factors affecting such responses. Either these factors must be systematically accounted for (which is not feasible with present knowledge), or considerable uncertainty in the results must be accepted. Direct measurement of annoyance is therefore preferable; it may be performed by means of social surveys in which community residents are interviewed and their responses to a series of questions are recorded. The design of the questionnaire to be used and the selection of the population sample to be interviewed are special problems which must be carefully dealt with in order to insure accurate results (BORSKY, 1969b). If the object is merely to assess the distribution of annoyance in a community, a random sample, sufficient in size to provide the desired confidence limits, may be drawn. If, as is more often the case, the data are to be used for research, the usual procedure is to distribute the sample evenly with respect to the most accessible annoyance-related variable, noise exposure, at the same time attempting to obtain reasonably good distributions based on demographic factors such as income and race, as estimated from census data. Usually, it is not possible in a real population to approximate ideal representation with respect to all salient variables.

The survey questionnaire is constructed so as to elicit the desired information without biasing the respondent in the process, either directly or through the interviewer. The techniques may include any or all of the following:

1. Description of the survey in vague terms (for example, "A study of community attitudes") without revealing the specific area of interest.
2. Use of many peripheral or even irrelevant questions.
3. Impartial language.
4. Use of general or "open" questions.
5. Programmed questioning whereby the asking of some questions is contingent upon certain answers to previous questions.

The particular questions on which annoyance assessment is based are those concerning the fundamental effects of community noise that have been identified previously, *i.e.*, auditory interference and disturbance of activities. The latter may subsume the former, the result being a list of typical activities, for each of which the respondent is asked to express the degree of disturbance caused by the noise in question. A specific question might be, "Does the noise of aircraft interfere with your conversation very much, moderately, a little, or not at all?" (WILSON, 1963).

Alternatively, the respondent may indicate the degree of disturbance nonverbally on some sort of physical scale (TRACOR, 1970b).

A number of alternative procedures may be employed to construct a scale of annoyance from questionnaire data regarding disturbance of activities. In two of the earlier large surveys concerned with community reaction to noise, scales were formulated according to the scalogram technique of GUTTMAN (BORSKY, 1961; MCKENNELL, 1963). Both of the foregoing references contain discussions of this technique as applied to the formation of noise annoyance scales. In this cumulative scaling process, the various activities disturbed are ordered and their respective responses scored in such a way that they conform maximally to an ideal scale type. Such a scale type is one in which an attribute for one item inexorably implies the same attribute for all items lower in the scale. The procedures for establishing the hierarchical ranking and scoring, as well as validity criteria, have been extensively treated in the literature (GUTTMAN, 1947; GUTTMAN, 1950). A survey of community annoyance around London (Heathrow) Airport provides an example (MCKENNELL, 1963). Respondents were first asked if the noise of aircraft bothered them very much, moderately, a little, or not at all. They were then asked if the noise ever (a) awakened them, (b) interfered with listening to television or radio, (c) made the house vibrate or shake, (d) interfered with conversation, or (e) interfered with or disturbed any other activity, or bothered, annoyed, or disturbed them in any other way, and were asked in each case to what extent, according to the five categories given above. The Guttman technique, applied to these responses for all respondents in the survey, established the hierarchical order shown in Table 5 and dichotomized the response categories for each question for a (0, 1) scoring; the result met the required coefficient of reproducibility and secondary criteria. According to the order given in Table 5, disturbance of listening to television or radio for a prototypical resident implies disturbance of conversation and sleep as well as general bother. The higher on the scale an individual is, the greater he is annoyed.

MCKENNELL also constructed simpler scales by scoring 1 for each activity disturbed to any extent whatever and by scoring responses on a (0, 1, 2) basis and found that annoyance ratings thus obtained correlated highly ($r > 0.9$) with the original GUTTMAN scale values. He concluded that there was little if any statistical advantage in using the more sophisticated approach. MCKENNELL also found that the correlation of self-ratings (the responses to the initial question) with the

Table 5. GUTTMAN scale for disturbances in London (Heathrow) airport survey (MCKENNELL, 1963)

Ranking	Disturbance	Percent annoyed
1	Various activities	6
2	House vibration	18
3	TV/Radio listening	28
4	Conversation	41
5	Sleeping	57
6	Aircraft noise bother	86

GUTTMAN values was good (r = 0.78). Similar conclusions were reached following a second survey of the same area (MIL RESEARCH, 1971).

In a later U.S. survey, a comparison was made between the scale of Table 5 and scales based upon data obtained in four American cities (TRACOR, 1970b). The latter are given in Table 6. The similarity between the two sets of results is close, considering the six years time span between the surveys and the fact that responses were obtained using entirely different questionnaires. The one significant difference is the exchanging of scale position of "sleeping" and "TV/radio listening", the former being a less prevalent and more serious form of disturbance in the U.S. This difference might well be of cultural origin.

Table 6. GUTTMAN scales for aircraft noise disturbances in four U.S. cities (TRACOR, 1970b)

	Chicago		Dallas		Denver		Los Angeles	
Ranking	Disturbance	Annoyed (%)	Disturbance	Annoyed (%)	Disturbance	Annoyed (%)	Disturbance	Annoyed (%)
1	Various activities	4	Various activities	5	Various activities	3	Various activities	7
2	Sleeping	24	Sleeping	22	Sleeping	19	Sleeping	35
3	House vibration	44	Conversation	40	House vibration	31	House vibration	60
4	Conversation	51	House vibration	49	TV/Radio listening	36	Conversation	66
5	TV/Radio listening	56	TV/Radio listening	52	Conversation	37	TV/Radio listening	68
6	Aircraft noise bother	65	Aircraft noise bother	67	Aircraft noise bother	49	Aircraft noise bother	80

Using GUTTMAN scale ratings as a standard, the self-ratings as obtained in the British studies would appear quite adequate for general assessments of annoyance or for similar indicators which might be of interest, such as the "dissatisfaction" scale used in connection with traffic noise (GRIFFITHS and LANGDON, 1968) or the "interference" scale applied to sonic boom reaction (NIXON and HUBBARD, 1965). It is presumed that such self-ratings would be obtained in the course of a carefully structured interview, as no assurance of their validity under other circumstances is available. For research purposes, however, these ratings may not be quite reliable enough. There is then a need for a rating scheme intermediate in complexity between the single question and the time-consuming GUTTMAN procedure. The value of the latter seems to lie in replication, that is, in the fact that it is based upon a series of questions rather than a single question. This concept, combined with simplicity of scoring, leads to the "summated rating" approach of LIKERT (LIKERT, 1932; EDWARDS, 1957).

In the summated rating technique, a series of responses concerning a particular attribute or dimension, such as disturbance, are scored identically and then summed to obtain a composite rating. In certain studies of annoyance due to aircraft noise (TRACOR, 1970b; CONNOR and PATTERSON, 1972), respondents were asked to indicate the degree to which this noise bothered each of the following activities:

1. Eating.
2. Sleeping.
3. Reading or concentration.
4. Listening to records or tapes.
5. Telephone usage.
6. Relaxing outdoors.
7. Relaxing indoors.
8. Face to face conversation.
9. TV or radio reception.

The degree of bother or disturbance was scored on a range of 0—5, giving a summated range (for all nine activities) of 0—45. It was found that the nine items listed formed a valid GUTTMAN scale for individual city samples. However, this is not a necessary condition; only reasonable care in the selection of categories, so that they are comprehensive and mutually exclusive, appears to be necessary.

Annoyance scales can also be constructed by factor analysis of groups of variables or disturbance items according to established techniques (THURSTON, 1947; BLALOCK, 1960). This process detects or confirms the association of a set of particular items along a common dimension. This combination of items is called a factor and is usually assigned a specific name on the basis of its component variables. The degree of association of each component with the factor is measured by the factor loadings, for which some minimum criterion is specified; the coefficient to be used for each variable in a linear equation expressing the dimension or attribute of the factor is given by the standardized weights. The loadings and weights for an aircraft noise annoyance factor are shown in Table 7 (HAZARD, 1968). A scale of annoyance R is given by

$$R = \sum_{i=1}^{8} b_i \, x_i$$

where b_i is the standardized weight and x_i is the individual score for the i th variable.

Table 7. Components of annoyance factor (HAZARD, 1968)

Variable	Item	Factor loading	Standardized weight
x_1	Perception of neighbors being annoyed	0.80	0.25
x_2	Disturbance of activities	0.78	0.25
x_3	Perception of city-wide annoyance	0.62	0.21
x_4	Complaint potential	0.58	0.19
x_5	Willingness to adapt to more noise	—0.52	—0.17
x_6	Past annoyance	0.50	0.19
x_7	Perception of increase in air traffic	0.46	0.13
x_8	Moved because of noise	0.44	0.12

Another application of factor analysis is the evaluation of the unidimensionality of the disturbance items in a summated rating scale, such as the one previously discussed, and the determination of their relative weights. It is certainly conceivable that a given degree of disturbance of one activity might contribute more to general annoyance than the same disturbance of another, in which case appropriate weightings should be assigned rather than scoring each activity identically. Table 8 gives the results of this analysis. The weights indeed vary over a ratio of about two to one. It was found that annoyance scores calculated using these weights correlated very highly with the summated rating scores ($r = 0.97$), leading to the conclusion that factor analytic techniques were not justified in this case (CONNOR and PATTERSON, 1972).

Table 8. Factor loadings and weights of activities disturbed by aircraft noise (CONNOR and PATTERSON, 1972)

Activity disturbed	Factor loading	Standardized weight
Relaxing indoors	0.78	0.18
Relaxing outdoors	0.76	0.14
Face to face conversation	0.80	0.20
Telephone usage	0.77	0.17
Sleeping	0.69	0.10
Listening to records or tapes	0.70	0.11
TV or radio reception	0.59	0.09
Reading or concentration	0.74	0.14
Eating	0.63	0.14

From the foregoing evidence, it can be concluded that noise annoyance due to disturbance of activities admits of quite reliable measurement using relatively simple procedures. From the analyses employing statistical techniques designed for much more difficult problems in measurement, it would appear that most reasonably constructed scales will give practically identical results. This is a fortunate circumstance, since it happens to apply also to noise exposure variables, thus permitting ready exploration of the attitudinal factors mediating the relationship of annoyance and exposure.

V. Measurement of Noise Exposure

Considerable effort has been expended in the past two decades in the formulation of noise exposure measures applicable to communities. Meaningful measures, which is to say, measures closely related to observed response, are obviously needed for purposes of planning, legislation, assessment, regulation, and research. In most cases, a particular approach to exposure measurement has been developed exclusively for a certain class of noise sources; this has been especially true of aircraft and traffic noise. The prevalence of disturbance from those particular sources has certainly influenced this circumstance, but the character of the noise itself has also helped determine the fundamental measurement approach. For example, aircraft noise is conveniently characterized as a series of discrete events (flyovers) and thus the natural basic parameters are the number of such events and some basic measure of a single flyover. These are in fact the fundamental parameters of aircraft noise exposure measures such as the composite noise rating (CNR), noise exposure forecast (NEF), and noise and number index (NNI), each of which is described below. Traffic noise, which is more continuous yet varying in level, is more readily characterized by standard statistical measures such as those used to form the traffic noise index (TNI) and noise pollution level (L_{NP}).

Another consideration in the development of noise exposure ratings, perhaps not often recognized, is the existing state of instrumentation technology. Convenient quantitative acoustical measurements became a reality in the twentieth century (with the development of the vacuum tube); more recently, the successive introductions of the octave band analyzer, the statistical level analyzer, and the real-time third octave band analyzer have permitted progressively more sophisticated and more rapid handling of acoustical signals. The modern digital computer should be included in this list for its contributions to real-time analysis and its capability in efficiently processing vast amounts of data. Examination of the various exposure measures considered in this section will reveal that each tends to take advantage of instrumentation readily available at the time and place of origin.

In an earlier section, it was stated that the effects of noise upon human activity are so varied that a comprehensive evaluation must necessarily include multiple measures of exposure. There has been no research performed to date, however, in which an entire matrix of effects and exposure parameters has been systematically investigated. Such are the difficulties in an endeavor of this kind that the tendency has been rather to formulate generalized single measures of both exposure and response, even though the correlation between these is relatively poor. Thus, all of the exposure measures discussed below are of the generalized single rating type. (Specific measures of speech interference and hearing damage risk are not described here, since the former is rarely an isolated community concern and the latter only peripherally so; both are discussed extensively in the preceding chapter.)

All community noise exposure rating schemes take into account, albeit in different ways, the following physical variables:

1. Amplitude. This intensive attribute of sound is normally expressed in terms of a weighted sound level or a computed perceived noise level.

2. Frequency. The frequency content of sound is incorporated either implicitly by the use of standard weightings or explicitly through spectral analysis, the latter usually in octave or third-octave frequency bands.

3. Temporal pattern. As appropriate for different types of noise, time parameters may include the duration of an event, the number of events per hour or day, the specific time of occurrence, the statistical time variation of level, and the rise time or peak factor of impulsive stimuli. Also included are functions for temporal summation and integration.

It is apparent that the above parameters may vary widely in a given community; therefore, it is usual to determine noise exposure values at a number of locations and to construct geographical equal-exposure contours in order to represent a particular exposure pattern. Fig. 2 is one example of noise exposure

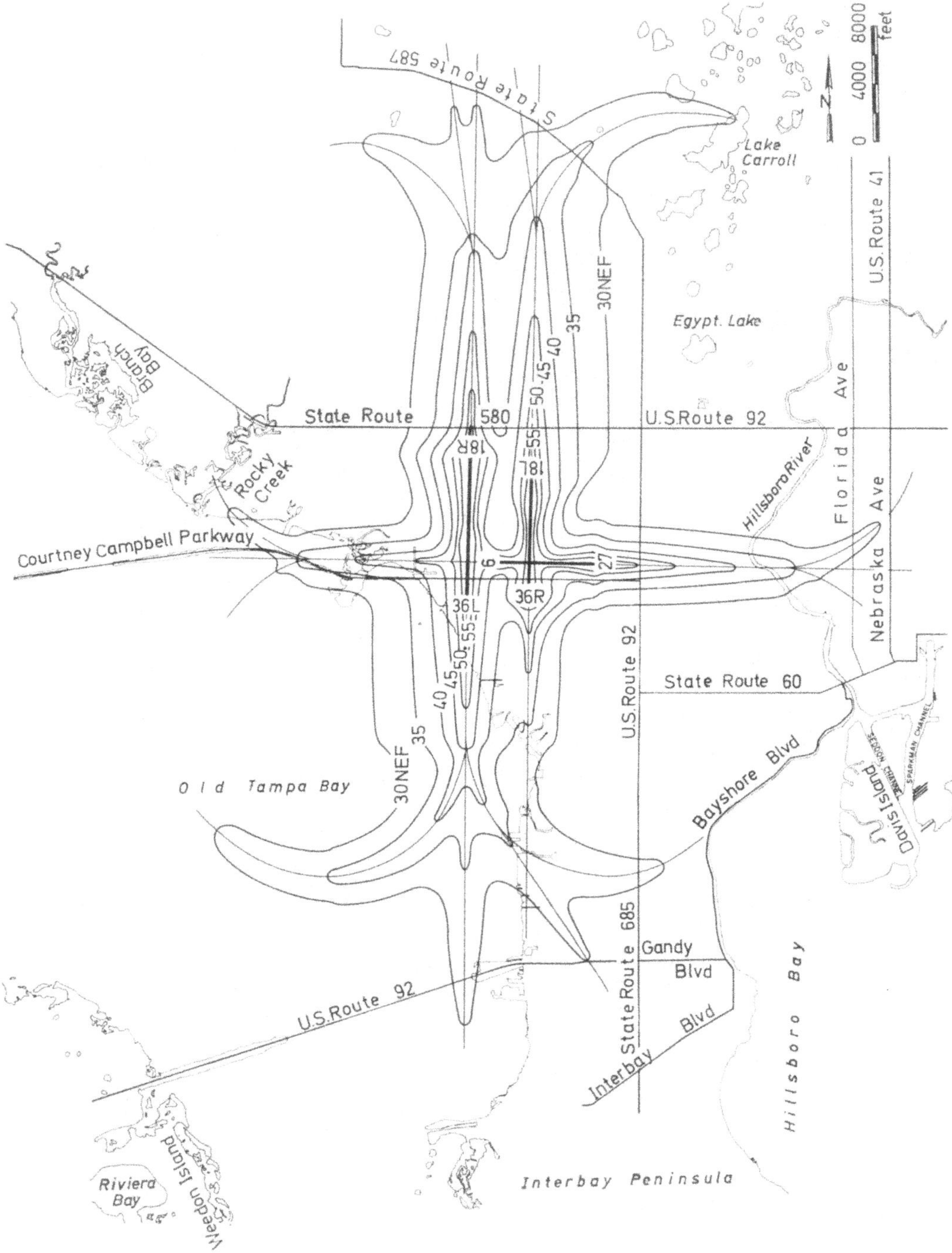

Fig. 2. Noise exposure forecast (NEF) contours around an airport (BISHOP and SIMPSON, 1970)

contours (in terms of Noise Exposure Forecast values) superimposed on an airport community.

Although the fundamental variables listed above are physically measurable acoustical entities, their import in connection with community exposure and response is essentially psychological. Thus, the determination of frequency characteristics is useful because of variations in subjective response with frequency and with spectral shape, and specification of time of day, because normal activities and associated noise sensitivity vary with the hour. The fundamental psychophysical measures in terms of which community exposure may be expressed on an instantaneous, single event, or other short-term basis are weighted sound level, loudness level, and perceived noise level. Each may be measured according to several different procedures, but they all tend to be rather closely related, especially for the same category of noise sources.

Weighted sound level or correctly, sound level, is sound pressure level (measured in decibels with respect to a reference mean-square sound pressure) when the sound signal has been subjected to a standardized frequency weighting. The best known such weightings are the A, B, and C weightings of the sound level meter (IEC, 1965; ANSI, 1971). Two other weightings, the D and the N, both have the inverse shape of the 40 noy contour (KRYTER and PEARSONS, 1964). The D weighting has a value of zero at 1 kHz, however, while the N has a value of + 7 dB at that frequency so that, with the latter, direct readings give an approximation of perceived noise levels. (Before the naming of the D weighting, it was referred to by some writers as the N characteristic, so some confusion between the two exists in the literature.) The frequency characteristics of these weightings are shown in Fig. 3. Various other characteristics have been suggested for special

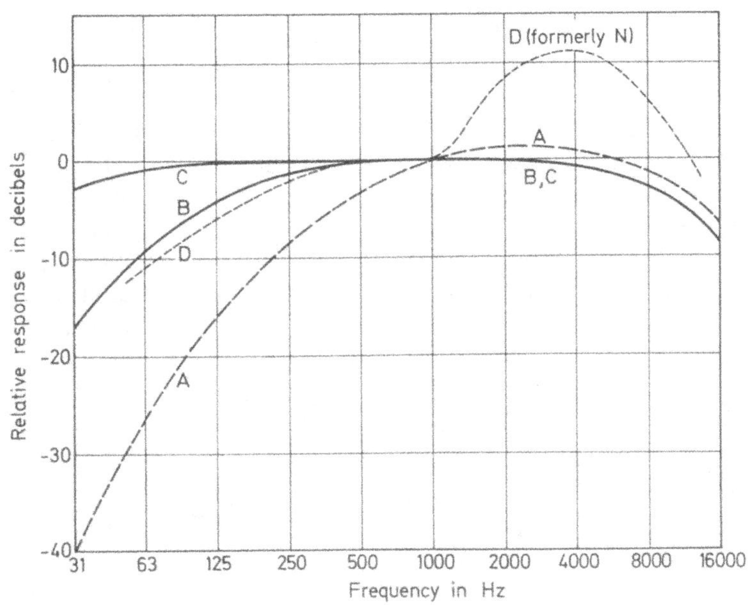

Fig. 3. Frequency response of standard weightings

purposes but have not been generally adopted. Notable among these is the E-weighting recently proposed by STEVENS, which provides an approximation of perceived level in decibels (STEVENS, 1972). It has become conventional (though not strictly proper) to associate the weighting used with the unit of measurement. Thus, sound level data taken with the A characteristic may be expressed in units of dB(A) or dBA. Weighted levels are used as measures of human response largely on the basis of their good agreement, within limits, with more complex measures, especially when dealing with a single type of noise. They are particularly appropriate for community noise evaluations because of this fact and also because their simplicity permits allocation of measurement resources toward the more difficult aspects of the noise environment, such as temporal and spatial patterns.

Loudness is a fundamental psychoacoustical attribute forming a ratio scale, *i.e.*, one on which the absolute subjective "magnitudes" of different sounds are correctly expressed. The unit is the sone and the loudness of a pure tone of 1 kHz and a sound pressure level of 40 dB re 2×10^{-5} N/m^2 is assigned the value of one sone. The loudness level of any sound is uniquely related to its loudness and is equal numerically to the sound pressure level of a 1 kHz tone judged to be equally loud; it is expressed in phons. Various procedures have been devised for calculating the loudness of sounds from frequency band data in order to obtain an approximation of direct judgment estimations, taking into account level, frequency, and inhibition or masking effects. The most generally known of these are the methods of ZWICKER (1960) and of STEVENS (1956, 1961, 1972). Both are the subject of standards (ISO, 1967; ANSI, 1968). Recently, a new procedure (Mark VII) for calculating loudness was proposed by STEVENS, associated with which is a new scale, perceived level, analogous to loudness level but yielding values approximately 8 dB lower (STEVENS, 1972).

Loudness and loudness level have been used, but not extensively, for rating of community noise. However, perceived noisiness and perceived noise level, which employ the STEVENS approach to loudness computation, have seen extensive development and application in that area. The concept of perceived noisiness was originally developed for evaluation of aircraft noise (KRYTER, 1959); it has since been more generally applied. Although perfectly analogous to their loudness counterparts, the parameters of perceived noisiness (measured in units called noys) and perceived noise level (measured in perceived noise decibels, abbreviated PNdB) were devised as measures not simply of the magnitude or subjective intensiveness of sound but of its unwantedness or unacceptability. The latter attributes are perceptual and are thought to be influenced by attitudes toward a sound and its source and by affectual meanings and connotations. Accordingly, in judgment tests for noisiness, subjects are typically asked to rate or compare sounds on the basis of how acceptable, disturbing, or preferable they would be if heard regularly a number of times a day in the home.

The full implications of the perceived noisiness concept and the distinction between it and loudness are not yet well understood. In one study involving human judgments of a variety of sounds, for example, it was concluded that noisiness and unacceptability may be independent attributes and also that, without the usual detailed instructions to the subject, ratings of noisiness and loudness produce nearly identical valuations (KERRICK *et al.*, 1968). In earlier tests of loudness and annoyance judgments of bands of noise, no significant difference was observed (SPIETH, 1956). The same result was obtained when specific loudness and noisiness instructions were given subjects in similar experiments (PARNELL *et al.*, 1967). In another psychoacoustical investigation which utilized samples of aircraft flyover noise, it was found that loudness level computed according to the STEVENS Mark VI method (1961) provided better agreement with subjective comparison judgments than did any other measure tested, including perceived noise level, provided that a correction for discrete frequency components was made (LITTLE and MABRY, 1969).

The present value of perceived noisiness may reside less in the ultimate validity of the basic concept than in the extensive modifications and improvements which have been made in the procedures for using it in noise rating systems. These modifications include corrections for the effects of pure tone or discrete frequency content (LITTLE, 1961; KRYTER and PEARSONS, 1963, 1965), effective duration of a noise event (KRYTER and PEARSONS, 1963; OLLERHEAD, 1968; LITTLE and MABRY, 1969; PEARSONS and BENNETT, 1969), and other attributes such as Doppler shift and onset time. A fuller treatment of variables affecting perceived noisiness is given in the preceding chapter and in publications of KRYTER (1968, 1970). Specific perceived noise level computation procedures to be applied to aircraft noise have been standardized (ISO, 1966; ARP, 1964).

Comparisons have been made of perceived noise levels and weighted sound levels for aircraft flyover noise (BISHOP, 1967; TRACOR, 1970b) and for road vehicle passby noise (HILLQUIST, 1967; PEARSONS and HORONJEFF, 1967). Other investigations have been made of the correlation of subjective estimations of aircraft and of other noise with these various physical measures (KRYTER and PEARSONS, 1963; HECKER and KRYTER, 1968; OLLERHEAD, 1968, 1971). On the basis of such studies, it is apparent that the following approximations can be made:

$$\left.\begin{aligned} \mathrm{PNL} &\cong \mathrm{L(N)} \\ \mathrm{PNL} &\cong \mathrm{L(D)} + 7 \\ \mathrm{PNL} &\cong \mathrm{L(A)} + 12 \end{aligned}\right\} \quad \text{Valid for aircraft flyovers and certain other classes of noise}$$

where PNL is perceived noise level computed from band sound pressure levels (without discrete frequency corrections) and L(X) is X-weighted sound level, all in decibels. The standard deviations associated with such approximations are on the order of 2 decibels, which is of the same order of magnitude as that normally encountered in related psychophysical experiments. For other variants of perceived noise level, or of restricted classes of noise (such as landing noise for large fan-jet aircraft), conversion constants slightly different from those used above may provide improved accuracy. Weighted sound level data are thus quite adequate for most community noise measurement purposes. Computed perceived noise levels employing the currently most appropriate corrections are preferred, however, when the greatest available accuracy in assessing the noise of a particular aircraft is required.

The subjective valuation of impulsive sounds such as sonic booms is a special problem. In early studies, the single acoustical parameter used to characterize the signature of a sonic boom was the peak acoustic pressure (pressure exceeding atmospheric) measured in pounds per square foot (psf) (BROADBENT and ROBINson, 1964; Stanford Research Institute, 1967). Below values of 1.0—1.5 psf, booms were found to be relatively mild. However, overpressure alone is a relatively poor predictor of subjective response. Other significant characteristics of the boom waveform include the initial rise time, duration, and secondary transients (Shepherd and Sutherland, 1968). By computing loudness level from the Fourier transform of the boom signature, good agreement with subjective judgments can be obtained (Johnson and Robinson, 1967, 1969). Although this procedure was developed specifically for sonic booms, it can probably be employed advantageously for evaluation of other impulsive sounds.

The various measures described above are applicable to noise which is steady in level or to discrete noise events. In connection with community response, however, it is normally desirable to consider noise exposure on a long-term basis. Although substantial response to a particularly obnoxious single event or short exposure period can occur, the majority of community noise problems are associated with chronic exposure conditions. Thus, procedures have been developed for expressing cumulative exposure over long periods or due to a succession of noise events. Such procedures are generally based upon the fundamental short-term or event measures discussed above and formulated according to actual observations of community response.

The exposure measures presented below were developed for the most part for particular classes of noise, one important exception being the "noise pollution level" of Robinson (1969a). Their fundamental components, in addition to the basic noise measure, are an algorithm for summation or integration over time and certain secondary elements, such as time of day and variability of noise level, which are believed to influence response. The intent in each case is to obtain ratings which will predict community response as well as possible.

The noise rating procedure of Rosenblith and Stevens (1953) represents the first comprehensive scheme for assessing community noise in relation to probable overt response. This procedure is notable in that it has continued in use to the present and in that it incorporated essentially all the physical variables which have proven to be important. The latter are accounted for in somewhat rudimentary fashion because of the instrumentation of the day, which caused measurements to be limited largely to manual readings of octave band sound pressure levels.

The first step in performing an assessment according to the noise rating procedure is to compare the measured octave band spectrum with the level rank contours shown in Fig. 4. The level rank of the noise in question is the alphabetical designation of the highest zone into which any portion of the spectrum extends. The level rank is then increased or decreased a certain number of steps equal to the sum of a series of correction numbers representing the effects of the following factors:

1. Spectrum character (presence of pure tones).
2. Peak factor (impulsiveness of the noise).
3. Repetitive character (temporal pattern).
4. Level of background noise.
5. Time of day.
6. Adjustment to exposure (adaptation).
7. Other factors (psychosociological).

Table 9 presents a summary of the correction numbers recommended by ROSENBLITH and STEVENS. No specific corrections were provided for item 7. above, as this was considered a matter requiring individual judgment. The level rank adjusted according to the appropriate correction numbers is called the noise rating and is used to predict community response as discussed in the next section.

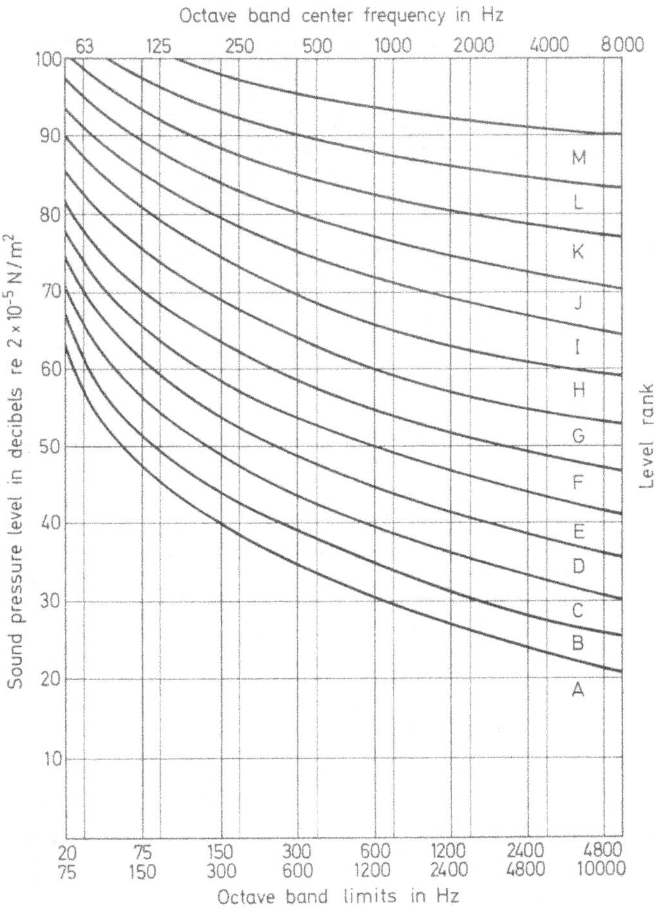

Fig. 4. Noise level rank contours (after ROSENBLITH and STEVENS, 1953)

There are certain aspects of the ROSENBLITH and STEVENS noise rating method which distinguish it from most of the more recent exposure formulations. The adjustment for background noise operates in such a way as to make the final noise rating in essence a differential between the noise in question and that produced by extraneous sources. That ultimate community response correlates best with such a differential has not been confirmed, and most subsequent exposure measures have dealt with noise levels on an absolute rather than relative basis. A factor for adaptation has also been discarded. This effect certainly does obtain, but there are counterinfluences, and the dynamics of community response under changing exposure conditions are not understood; hence meaningful corrections cannot be formulated.

Table 9. Correction numbers to be applied to level rank to obtain noise rating (ROSENBLITH and STEVENS, 1953)

Influencing factor	Possible conditions	Correction number
Spectrum character	Continuous	0
	Pure tone components	1
Peak factor	Continuous	0
	Impulsive	1
Repetitive character (20—30 second exposures assumed)	Continuous or more than 60 exposures per hour	0
	10—60 exposures per hour	—1
	1—10 exposures per hour	—2
	4—20 exposures per day	—3
	1—4 exposures per day	—4
	Less than one exposure per day	—5
Background noise	Very quiet suburban area	1
	Suburban area	0
	Residential urban area	—1
	Urban area near some industry	—2
	Area of heavy industry	—3
Time of day	Daytime only	—1
	Nighttime	0
Adjustment to exposure	No previous exposure	0
	Considerable exposure	—1
	Extreme conditions of exposure	—2

The next evolved community exposure measure was the Composite Noise Rating (CNR) developed specifically for prediction of community reaction to aircraft noise (BOLT *et al.*, 1964). The method is based upon air traffic projections, although it can be adapted for use with actual measurement data. The CNR measure is comprised of the following:

1. A flyover noise rating for each type of aircraft involved, in terms of maximum perceived noise level computed from octave band data (no discrete frequency corrections).

2. A time of day weighting according to which a flyover at night (2200—0700 h) is assigned an equivalent level about 13 dB higher than that of a daytime flyover.

3. An algorithm for the combined effect of many flyover events based upon energy summation over one day.

The cited 1964 document presents a simplified step by step procedure, whereby, CNR contours can be produced for an entire airport community. Values at a specific site may be computed as follows (TRACOR, 1970b):

The partial CNR for a particular class of operation j, *i.e.*, for flyovers which produce the same maximum perceived noise level PNL_j at the site is given by

$$CNR_j = PNL_j + 10 \log_{10} (N_{Dj} + 20\, N_{Nj}) - 12,$$

where N_{Dj} and N_{Nj} are respectively the numbers of daytime and nighttime occurrences. The combined CNR for all classes of operation is then

$$CNR = 10 \log_{10} \sum_j \text{antilog}\,(CNR_j/10).$$

CNR values are normally computed for daily events averaged over a year.

The Noise Exposure Forecast (NEF) may be regarded as a further development of the CNR measure, as it contains the same fundamental elements. The differences are employment of an effective perceived noise level (EPNL), which incorporates corrections for discrete frequency components and flyover duration, as the basic noise measure, a slight change in time of day correction, and a different additive constant (Bishop and Horonjeff, 1967; Galloway and Bishop, 1970). The NEF formulation may be expressed as follows, using the terminology employed above for the CNR:

$$NEF_j = EPNL_j + 10 \log_{10} (N_{Dj} + 16.7\, N_{Nj}) - 88$$

$$NEF = 10 \log_{10} \sum_j \text{antilog}\,(NEF_j/10).$$

In both CNR and NEF measures, the $(10 \log_{10} N)$ factor for the temporal summation of events is the same as it would be if one wished to obtain the sum of acoustic energies of the events. This must be accepted as coincidence, since the human ear is not an energy-sensing mechanism, but it is a computational convenience and also is consistent with the short-term effect of flyover duration. Other possibilities have been suggested, however. One is the $\bar{Q}$ measure developed in Germany (Bürck *et al.*, 1965). This may be expressed

$$\bar{Q} = (10q/3) \log_{10} [(1/T) \sum_k 10^{(3Q_K/10q)} \cdot \tau_k]$$

where Q_k is the level (weighted level or computed loudness level) during a period of duration τ_k (for a flyover, defined as the period during which the level is within 10 dB of maximum), T is the total period of observation, and q is a variable constant. The last may take values from 2—8. If the value is 3, the entire expression reduces to a computation of the mean acoustic energy for the period of observation. It has been suggested that $q > 3$ be used for short, intense noise events; and $2 < q < 3$, for lower levels and prolonged exposure (Rathé and Muheim, 1968). A value of 4 was used in one study of traffic noise (Lang, 1965) producing a $(13.3 \log_{10} N)$ summation of noise events.

It may be noted that the measure $\bar{Q}$ does not incorporate a day-night correction as did the previous examples; in general, inclusion of this correction is an American practice. Exposure measures developed elsewhere are normally used for separate evaluations for different periods of the day, without special correction or adjustment; the latter are considered separately in terms of community effects and criteria. This holds for the Noise and Number Index (NNI) developed specifically in connection with aircraft noise around London (Heathrow) Airport (MCKENNELL, 1963; MIL RESEARCH, 1971); this rating is given by

$$\text{NNI} = \text{APNL} + 15 \log_{10} \text{N} - 80,$$

where APNL is the energy-mean perceived noise level and N is the total number of aircraft flyovers for the period in question. The NNI measure differs from the CNR and NEF in that it accounts for each class of operation twice, in its respective contributions to APNL and N, but at differing rates (10 log and 15 log), and in the coefficient of 15 in the temporal summation term.

Of an entirely different nature is the traffic noise index (TNI) (GRIFFITHS and LANGDON, 1968; GRIFFITHS, 1968). The TNI is computed from the statistical distribution of A-weighted sound levels accumulated over daytime, nighttime, or 24-h periods. It is given by

$$\text{TNI} = 4\,(L_{10} - L_{90}) + L_{90} - 30,$$

where L_{10} and L_{90} are the levels exceeded 10% and 90% of the time, respectively.

Each of the preceding exposure measures has been largely associated with a particular category of noise — industrial, traffic, aircraft, etc. — although in some cases the fundamental methodology has been extended for the sake of greater generality. The disparity of these various measures and the apparent need for a universally applicable noise rating scale led to the development of the rating known as noise pollution level (L_{NP}) (ROBINSON, 1969a). This measure may be expressed

$$\text{L}_{\text{NP}} = L_{eq} + 2.56\,\sigma$$

where L_{eq} is the energy-mean level over the period of time under consideration (and thus is identical to $\bar{Q}$ for $q = 3$), σ is the standard deviation of the level over that period, and 2.56 is a provisionally assigned constant. The basic level parameter used to determine L_{eq} and σ may be either perceived noise level or weighted sound level. Noise pollution level is purported to subsume the measures $\bar{Q}$, NNI, and TNI described above; however, the evidence for its validity is based largely upon secondary analyses of previous studies, no direct investigation having yet been reported.

The various measures of aircraft noise exposure given above, although distinguishable in their treatment of fundamental variables, tend to be highly correlated with one another in real situations. GALLOWAY and BISHOP discuss the similarities and differences of these and less well-known exposure measures in historical detail. Fig. 5 presents their comparison of CNR, NEF, NNI, and $\bar{Q}$ as a function of the number of operations per day (GALLOWAY and BISHOP, 1970). In order to permit such a comparison, it was necessary to make certain reasonable assumptions; therefore, the relationships shown are approximate.

A comparison of three aircraft noise ratings as computed from actual survey data is given in Table 10. These data were obtained in American cities containing large airports and represent a range of 80 to over 130 CNR units (TRACOR, 1970b). If a linear relationship is assumed, the following approximations were found to hold

$$\text{CNR} \cong \text{NEF} + 72$$

$$\text{CNR} \cong \text{NNI} + 56.$$

In view of the importance of the "number correction" ($K \log N$) in the various exposure ratings, or the corresponding summation or integration procedure, it should be noted that recent analyses demonstrate that the correlation of exposure

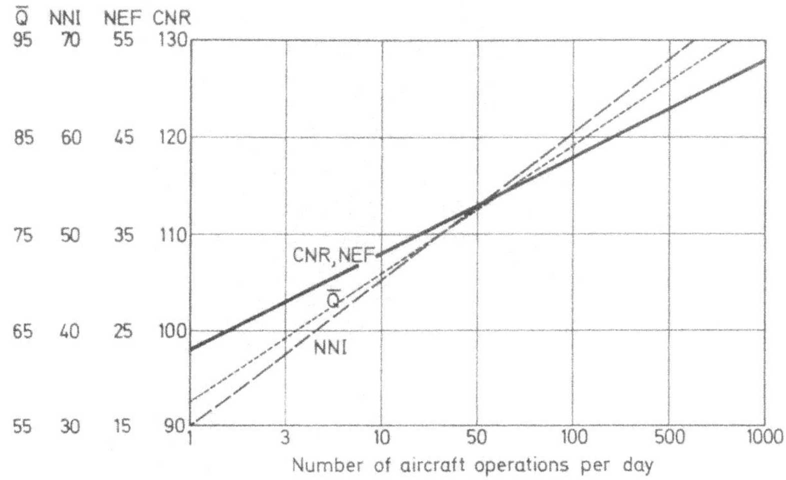

Fig. 5. Comparison of CNR, NEF, NNI, and $\bar{Q}$ for maximum flyover level of 110 PNdB and effective flyover duration of 10 sec (110 EPNdB for NEF) (GALLOWAY and BISHOP, 1970)

with measured annoyance is very insensitive to the form of this correction. This may be seen in the results of American investigations shown in Table 11. These correlation coefficients suggest that a lower rather than a higher weighting than that corresponding to energy summation is appropriate (CONNOR and PATTERSON, 1972).

A re-examination of the survey data upon which the measure NNI was based and a second investigation produced somewhat similar conclusions regarding the number correction. The original study was hampered by the fact that the corre-

Table 10. Correlations between aircraft noise exposure measures (TRACOR, 1970b)

	CNR	NNI	NEF
CNR	1.00	0.99	0.90
NNI	—	1.00	0.88
NEF	—	—	1.00

Table 11. Correlation of annoyance with CNR computed with various number corrections (CONNOR and PATTERSON, 1972)

Number correction	1969 Survey (N = 2,912)	1970 Survey (N = 1,960)
5 log N	0.43	0.27
10 log N	0.41	0.25
15 log N	0.40	0.22
20 log N	0.40	0.22

lation between APNL and N ($r = 0.70$) was substantially higher than that between annoyance and either variable or, for that matter, between annoyance and NNI ($r = 0.46$) (MCKENNELL, 1963). In a second survey of the same area in 1967, it was found that a lower coefficient for the number correction produced the best correlation with annoyance ($r = 0.43$). Furthermore, use of a linear rather than logarithmic form of the number variable produced an even higher correlation ($r = 0.46$) (MIL RESEARCH, 1971). Though annoyance increases with the number of exposure events, from survey data, little else can be said concerning this increase.

A standard for evaluating general community noise was recently adopted following several years of deliberation (ISO, 1971). The procedure for noise assessment is based upon the energy-mean level L_{eq}, which is a particular variant of $\bar{Q}$; the A-weighting characteristic is specified. The energy-mean level is computed by

$$L_{eq} = 10 \log_{10} \sum_i g_i \, 10^{(L_i/10)}$$

where g_i is the fraction of the total time period of interest during which the level L_i prevails and the summation is to be made over all levels present. Corrections are to be added to L_{eq} as specified in Table 12. These corrections are derived largely from those of the earlier ROSENBLITH and STEVENS procedure, as comparison with Table 9 will show.

A detailed exposition of certain other exposure formulations which are less well known and which in many cases are simply variants of those presented above is not deemed necessary. Such measures include the noise rating (NR) curves, derived from the ROSENBLITH and STEVENS system, used as the basis for draft ISO standards, the rating method of British Standard 4142, the weighted noise exposure level (WECPNL) developed by the International Civil Aviation Organization (ICAO), and a number of national ratings. Those who wish to delve into the intricacies and nuances of these and other measures are referred to the previously cited work of GALLOWAY and BISHOP (1970) and to ROBINSON (1969b).

Table 12. Corrections to be added to L_{eq} (ISO, 1971)

Factor	Condition	Correction (dB)
Time of day	Day	0
	Evening	5
	Night	10—15
Peak factor	Continuous	0
	Impulsive	5
Spectrum character	Continuous	0
	Audible tone components	5
Type of district	Rural residential, hospital, recreational	0
	Suburban residential	5
	Urban residential	10
	Urban residential with business, industry, or main roads	15
	City	20
	Heavy industry	25

To summarize: a number of procedures for the assessment of community noise exposure have been developed, the objective being prediction of one or more modes of response. Of those listed above, only $\overline{Q}$ and L_{NP} have any pretense to generality beyond a single category of noise source, and none has very high predictive power, as will be seen in the following section. A need obviously still exists for further development. To that end, the following criteria for an ideal noise exposure measure are suggested:

1. The measure should be based entirely upon established or at least credible psychophysical functions.

2. The measure should predict response with the greatest possible accuracy and should be of the greatest simplicity compatible with that requirement.

3. The measure should quantify the relative effects of noise from different sources as well the combined effect.

4. The measure should not be constrained by instrumentation limitations, as present technology can remove this constraint.

VI. Prediction of Reaction

The ultimate purpose of community noise exposure measurement is to predict or explain response. In this section the reaction expected on the basis of each noise exposure measure previously presented will be described and the relationships between predictor and predicted variables will be examined.

The procedure of ROSENBLITH and STEVENS (1953) produces a noise rating in alphabetic notation which may be applied to the chart in Fig. 6 to determine

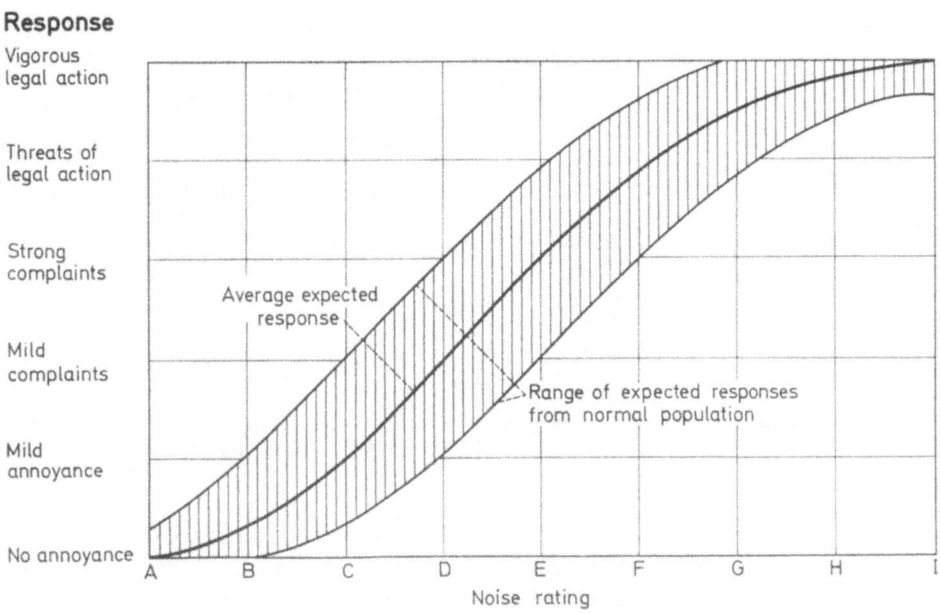

Fig. 6. Expected community response as a function of noise rating (ROSENBLITH and STEVENS, 1953)

the average and expected range of response for a community as a whole. The original document presents a summary of eleven case histories which generally support the prediction chart insofar as overt reactions (complaints, threats, and legal action) are concerned. Where the procedure of ISO R. 1996 (1971) is used to assess community noise, the corrected L_{eq} noise rating is compared to a basic criterion level of 35—45 dBA, the precise value of the latter to be selected according to known local circumstances. Reaction is then estimated according to Table 13.

Table 13. Estimated community response to noise (ISO, 1971)

Amount by which noise rating level exceeds criterion level in dBA	Estimated community response	
	Category	Description
0	None	No observed reaction
5	Little	Sporadic complaints
10	Medium	Widespread complaints
15	Strong	Threats of community action
20	Very strong	Vigorous community action

Fig. 7 shows the expected range of reaction for $\bar{Q}$, NNI, and CNR ratings as well as a number of points representing actual community "case histories" (KRYTER, 1968).

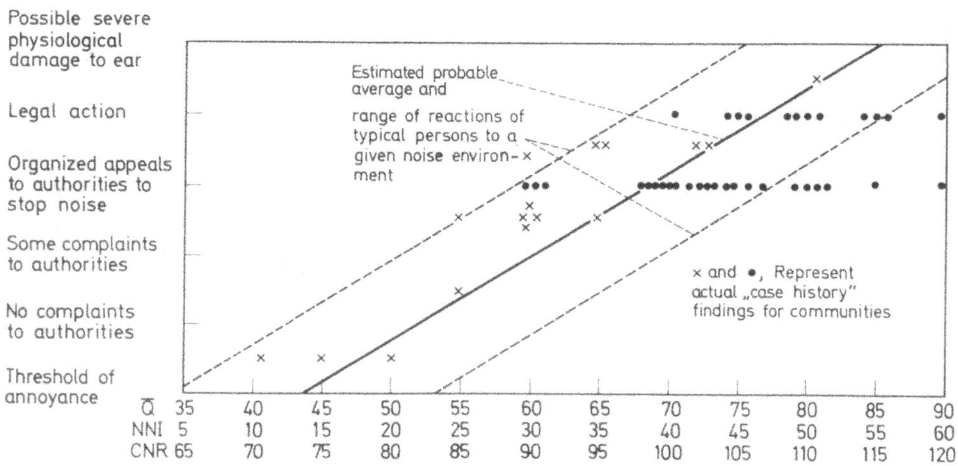

Fig. 7. Relationship between reactions and noise ratings, with case history data. Fifty daily occurrences of the noise are assumed for the NNI measure (KRYTER, 1968)

Fig. 8 shows three different ratings of annoyance from two sources, as a function of CNR. It is notable that annoyance and unacceptability both begin at CNR 70 and that the latter and high annoyance are essentially parallel functions. The percentage of highly annoyed, H, is given approximately by

$$H = 1.6\,(\mathrm{CNR} - 85).$$

For various measures utilized, especially in connection with aircraft noise in the community, the following ranges of expected reaction are specified (GALLOWAY and BISHOP, 1970; WILSON, 1963):

CNR	< 100	Essentially no complaints; some interference of activities by noise.
	100–115	Vigorous complaint and concerted group action.
	> 115	Repeated, vigorous complaints and concerted group action probable.
NEF	< 30	Some noise complaints and noise interference of activities possible.
	30–40	Vigorous repeated complaint and concerted group action possible.
	> 40	Serious noise problems probable.
NNI	30–45	"Unreasonable level" and high annoyance for nighttime exposure.
	50–60	"Unreasonable level" and high annoyance for daytime exposure.

The expected modes and intensities of reaction for CNR and NEF are based primarily upon observations of overt response in actual communities. Those for NNI are based upon social survey data as well and reflect consideration of aircraft noise in the context of other potential community problems and disadvantages;

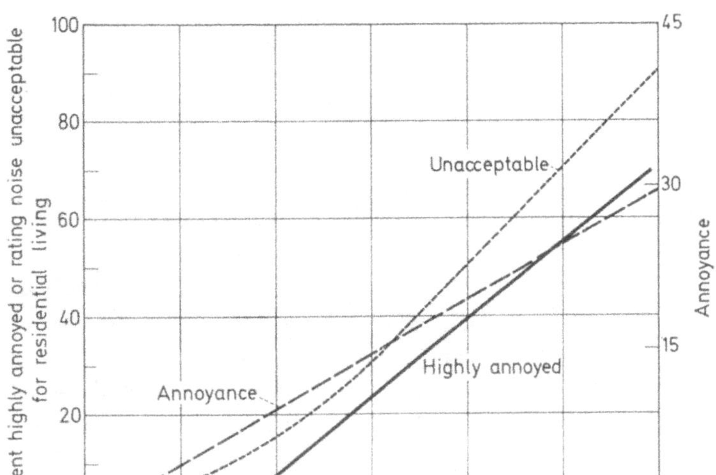

Fig. 8. Estimates of reaction *vs* exposure. Percent highly annoyed and annoyance are regression lines based on survey data related to aircraft noise. ("Highly annoyed" represents a value of 21 or greater on a 0—45 scale.) (CONNOR and PATTERSON, 1972.) Percent unacceptable ratings are estimates of attitudes to be expected from non-fear-provoking noise derived from various sources (KRYTER, 1970)

at the upper tolerable limit, noise from aircraft becomes the dominant reason for residents wanting to move from the area, the main thing they would like to change in their living environment, etc.

On the basis of the direct results of a survey relating to road traffic noise, the expected median dissatisfaction with the noise on a scale of 1—7, for certain values of the traffic noise index (TNI), is as follows (GRIFFITHS and LANGDON, 1968):

TNI	Median dissatisfaction score
56—58	1.8
74	3.5
90	5.3

A similar table for the störindex $\bar{Q}$ was derived from a study of traffic noise in Vienna (LANG, 1965). The results apply specifically to daytime conditions, and the levels are those measured indoors with open windows. The author suggests that, in the evening and at night (1800—0600 h), the same reaction would be observed at 5 dB lower levels and that the exterior levels would be approximately 5 dB higher than those cited. The observed disturbance conditions in the survey sample were as follows:

$\bar{Q}$	Condition
<40	100% not disturbed
45—50	50% not disturbed
50—55	moderate disturbance
>50	over 50% strongly disturbed

Inasmuch as the above two studies did not purport to establish general prediction schemes or limits of tolerance, they should not be relied on for these without some reservation. However, the results are indicative of expected reaction.

Limited information is available concerning reaction to sonic booms, partly because there are no regularly exposed communities in which to observe response. Communities in the USA which have been exposed to series of supersonic flights were subjected to intensive public relations programs prior to and during exposure, making it impossible to obtain unbiased response. On the basis of laboratory experiments, it was found that sonic booms of 1.9 psf overpressure were judged about as annoying as flyover noise of 110 PNdB maximum level; these values were believed to represent the upper limit of acceptability (BROADBENT and ROBINSON, 1964). In sonic boom field experiments it was found that 26% of the subjects rated the boom environment between less than "just acceptable" and "unacceptable" when subjected to about 10 booms per day at a median nominal peak overpressure of 1.7 psf; about 14% gave this rating at 4—8 booms per day and 1.2 psf (Stanford Research Institute, 1967). Thus, some degree of reaction can be expected when booms in the 1—2 psf range occur, but the extent of this reaction and the effect of boom characteristics other than peak overpressure are not known.

From the foregoing, it is apparent that the range of expected reaction, as predicted by accepted community noise exposure measures, is quite wide. Typically this range is 10—15 exposure units of the logarithmic or decibel type. The uncertainty represented can be diminished by consideration of nonacoustical factors and the relationship of individual response to total community reaction. The variation in annoyance from one individual to another under the same exposure conditions is a fundamental area of uncertainty. Table 14 shows the correlation of different exposure measures with individual annoyance. It is apparent, from the coefficients, that noise exposure is not a very good predictor of individual response. There are also indications of the fact, mentioned in the previous section, that such correlations do not make a good test of the relative predictive power of different exposure measures.

Table 14. Correlation of community noise exposure measures with measured individual response (various investigators)

Investigator	Types of noise	Exposure measure	Response index	Correlation coefficient
GRIFFITHS (1968)	Traffic	TNI	Dissatisfaction	0.29
		$\bar{Q}$	Dissatisfaction	0.18
McKENNELL (1963)	Aircraft	NNI	Annoyance	0.46
BOLT *et al.* (1965)	Aircraft	(PNL + 10 log N)	Annoyance	0.457
(McKENNELL data)		(PNL + 15 log N)	Annoyance	0.463
TRACOR (1970b)				
Sample I	Aircraft	CNR	Annoyance	0.37
		NNI	Annoyance	0.34
		NEF	Annoyance	0.32
Sample II	Aircraft	CNR	Annoyance	0.49

Evidence of the mediating effect of other variables, particularly psychological ones, upon the relationship between exposure and individual annoyance is based largely upon studies of reaction to aircraft noise involving community surveys. In such studies, the survey data were used to construct a number of attitudinal scales as well as an annoyance scale. Analysis of the combined set of variables is complicated by the fact that some attitudinal variables are merely alternative expressions of annoyance and that most significant variables tend to be intercorrelated (McKENNELL, 1968). Nevertheless, it is from these analyses that much of the existing information concerning individual annoyance has been derived.

The variable known as "fear" was identified early as perhaps the most important mediating variable in aircraft noise annoyance (BORSKY, 1961). The scale of fear is typically constructed from interview questions relating to perception of excessively low overflights, likelihood of crashes in the neighborhood, etc. The relationship of fear to exposure and annoyance was examined quantitatively in both British and American studies (McKENNELL, 1968; TRACOR, 1970b). In both cases, fear alone was a better predictor of annoyance than was noise exposure, although the correlation decreased if exposure was held constant. The following raw correlations were obtained:

Source	McKENNELL (1968)		TRACOR (1970b)	
Variable	Annoyance	Exposure	Annoyance	Exposure
Exposure	0.43	1.00	0.43	1.00
Fear	0.52	0.28	0.62	0.37

The patterns for the two studies are notably similar in view of the fact that different survey instruments and scale constructions were used. Fear was slightly less salient in the British study. (The exposure measure for the British work was NNI; for the American, CNR.) Use of exposure and fear as the two predictors in a linear model yielded a correlation of 0.65 for the American data (CONNOR, unpublished).

By increasing the number of predictor variables, the correlation between predicted and observed annoyance can usually be improved. One may use a linear predictive equation, *i.e.*, of the form

$$A = \sum_i \beta_i X_i + \text{constant},$$

where A is the predicted annoyance, X_i is the ith predictor variable, and β_i is a coefficient or weight; or a nonlinear model, one general form of which is

$$A = \sum_i \sum_j \alpha_{ij} X_i + \text{constant},$$

where an independent weighting α_{ij} is provided for each value $_j$ which X_i may take. Some idea of the potential of additional variables and nonlinear models may be had from the following correlations of predicted and measured annoyance:

Prediction scheme	Source	
	McKENNELL (1968)	TRACOR (1970b)
Exposure alone	0.43	0.37
Linear model, 8—9 predictor variables	0.49	0.67
Nonlinear model, 8 predictor variables	—	0.78

The predictors used in the American case were fear of aircraft crashing, general susceptibility to noise irritation, distance of residence from the center of the airport, willingness to adapt to increased noise, noise exposure (CNR), city of residence, belief in misfeasance by authorities in connection with the aircraft noise problem, and feelings about the importance of the local airport and of air transportation in general. McKENNELL's nine predictors were not explicitly stated but apparently included fear of aircraft crashing, number of things disliked about the neighborhood, annoyance from noise other than aircraft, and general attitude toward noise, among others.

It is important to note that, although such variables as social class, income, education, and house value were investigated in various British and American studies dealing with aircraft noise, in no case did these prove to be strongly related to annoyance. In a study of reaction to road traffic noise, however, an indication that socioeconomic status affected annoyance was found (GALLOWAY *et al.*, 1969). It would seem that different sets of predictors may be required to best describe annoyance due to different noise sources.

The effects upon annoyance of national differences, adaptation, background noise level, and being indoors or outdoors all have been explored but are in need of more accurate definition. In a study of reaction to traffic noise in Italy and Sweden, carefully designed to minimize experimental differences, a significant variation in response, apparently traceable to cultural characteristics, was observed (JONSSON *et al.*, 1968).

In the noise assessment procedure of ROSENBLITH and STEVENS (1953), a downward adjustment in effective noise exposure of up to 10 dB was specified for previous conditioning exposure; this adjustment was omitted from the procedure of ISO R 1996 (1971). In studies of reactions to aircraft noise, no apparent decrease in reaction with length of residence in the noise-affected area was observed (BORSKY, 1961). It has been suggested that a sort of "natural selection" in the vicinity of large airports may occur whereby the adjacent population tends to have a higher proportion of "imperturbables" than the community as a whole, but this effect has not been systematically investigated.

Observations regarding the effect of background noise level upon reaction to a specific stimulus are contradictory. BORSKY (1961) found that persons in quiet areas were less annoyed with aircraft noise than those in noisy environments. In the second London airport survey, higher ambient levels were associated with less aircraft noise annoyance (MIL RESEARCH, 1971). BOTTOM and WATERS (no date) observed a higher response to aircraft noise at low levels of road traffic noise. ROBINSON (1969b) suggests that, when the intruding noise is much louder than the existing noise, the absolute level of the former is likely the decisive factor, but when the differential is small the excess is the likely determinant.

In field tests involving judgments by both indoor and outdoor subjects, it is generally found that the former will give ratings similar to those of the latter at substantially lower levels, as if they were making a mental correction for the attenuation provided by the building. Typically this "correction" is somewhat less than the actual attenuation provided. In one experiment involving aircraft noise, for example, the actual attenuation was 24 dBA, while judgments of "intrusiveness" differed by 18 dBA for indoor and outdoor subjects; judgments of "noisiness" differed by 14—15 dBA (BOWSHER *et al.*, 1966). For sonic boom, the difference is considerably less owing to the decreased attenuation by building structures of this type of acoustical signal (Stanford Research Institute, 1967; JOHNSON and ROBINSON, 1967). It would appear that persons indoors may judge outdoor sounds in terms of some preconceived idea of indoor-outdoor differences rather than according to the performance of a particular structure. When noise exposure values were corrected for actual house attenuation in one study, the correlation of individual annoyance with exposure decreased from 0.49 to 0.25 (TRACOR, 1970b).

The prediction of complaint is difficult. A high degree of annoyance is practically a necessary condition for complaint, but it is by no means a sufficient condition. Various predisposing factors were listed earlier under Patterns of Reaction. Using a nonlinear predictive scheme with no less than seventeen independent variables, a correlation of 0.52 was obtained for complaint due to aircraft noise (TRACOR, 1970b). A number of social variables were significant, including ethnicity, household size, occupation, organizational involvement, and house cost.

In a large population, it is possible to relate the percentage of complainants to the percentage of highly annoyed persons, at least with respect to aircraft noise (CONNOR and PATTERSON, 1972). The relationship, which appears to hold for a range of highly annoyed up to at least 65%, is given by

$$H = 14.3\sqrt{C}$$

where H and C are, respectively, the percentages of highly annoyed and of complainants. The mathematical nature of this relationship suggests that, given a highly annoyed individual, the existence of other such persons is a further incentive toward complaint.

It should be mentioned that complaint regarding aircraft noise is a seasonal phenomenon in northern cities of the USA, and perhaps elsewhere. In one case, the proportion of yearly complaints received in a summer month average about 17%, while for other months of the year, the average is about 2%. The factors responsible for this behavior are as yet unknown (CONNOR and PATTERSON, 1972).

No procedures for accurately predicting community reaction more severe than complaint have to date been formulated. It is generally accepted that organized opposition, legal action, and other such manifestations are normally preceded by severe annoyance and perhaps complaint, but what other conditions and interactions are involved remains to be determined.

VII. Modification of Reaction

In most studies of community reaction to noise, one basic motivation has been to learn what might be done to alleviate disturbance and annoyance. Aside from the obvious but not always attainable step of significantly reducing the noise exposure itself, the most promising area for such attempts appears to be altering the sociopsychological characteristics or attitudes which earlier were shown to be closely related to annoyance.

Practical experiments on modification of attitudes have been conducted in the last few years in Sweden. In laboratory studies of reactions to motor vehicle noise, it was found that by categorizing vehicles as "useful" and "non-useful", subject responses could be definitely biased at a given sound level (CEDERLÖF *et al.*, 1963). In further laboratory experiments, three groups of subjects were exposed respectively to positive, neutral, and negative statements regarding aircraft and motor vehicle noise. The subjects were than exposed to identical sets of noise samples and asked to estimate the degree of disturbance each would cause in a residential situation. The percentages estimating "great annoyance" were as follows:

Statement bias	Aircraft (%)	Motor vehicles (%)
Positive	14	27
Neutral	36	41
Negative	59	75

Subsequently, a field study concerned with the noise of military aircraft was performed in which half the respondent sample was subjected to positive influences through a biased questionnaire, positive information regarding the survey itself, and a presentation book. The proportion of persons greatly bothered was 23% in the influenced group and 46% in the control group. Similar results (12% and 24%) were obtained regarding awakening by aircraft noise. A follow-up survey three years later showed that the effect had persisted (35% and 62% very bothered) to a high degree. It is not known to what extent these effects can be induced under other circumstances. The investigators found a smaller change in annoyance at higher noise levels and suggest that such manipulation is most feasible at intermediate levels of exposure (SÖRENSEN, 1970).

References

ANSI S3.4-1968: Procedure for the computation of loudness of noise. New York: American National Standards Institute, Inc., 1968.

ANSI S1.4-1971: Specification for sound level meters. New York: American National Standards Institute, Inc., 1971.

BERANEK, L. L.: Acoustics. New York: McGraw-Hill Inc., 1954.

BISHOP, D. E.: Frequency spectrum and time duration descriptions of aircraft flyover noise signals. Report DS-67-6, Federal Aviation Administration, U.S. Department of Transportation, May 1967.

BISHOP, D. E., HORONJEFF, R. D.: Procedures for developing noise exposure forecast areas for aircraft flight operations. Technical Rept. DS-67-10, Contract No. FA67WA-1705. Van Nuys, Calif.: Bolt, Beranek and Newman, Inc., 1967.

BISHOP, D. E., SIMPSON, M. A.: Noise exposure forecast contours for 1967, 1970, and 1975 operations at selected airports. Rept. FAA NO-70-8, U.S. Dept. of Transportation, September 1970.

BLALOCK, H. M., JR.: Social statistics. New York: McGraw-Hill, Inc., 1960.

BOLT, BERANEK, NEWMAN, Inc.: Land use planning with respect to aircraft noise. AFM 86-5, TM5-365, NAVDOCKS P-98, U.S. Department of Defense, 1 October 1964.

BOLT, BERANEK, NEWMAN, Inc.: Noise environment of urban and suburban areas. Federal Housing Administration, U.S. Department of Housing and Urban Development, January 1967.

BORSKY, P. N.: Community reactions to air force noise, Parts 1 and 2. Rept. No. TR 60-689, Contract AF 41(657)-79, National Opinion Research Center, University of Chicago, Chicago, 1961.

BORSKY, P. N.: Community reactions to sonic booms in the Oklahoma City area, I and II. Rept. AMRL-TR-65-37, AD 613 620, Wright-Patterson Air Force Base, Ohio, 1965.

Borsky, P. N.: Effects of noise on community behavior. In: Ward, W. D., Fricke, J. E. (Eds.): Noise as a public health hazard. American Speech and Hearing Association, Washington, D.C., 187—201, 1969a.

Borsky, P. N.: The use of social surveys for measuring community response to noise environment. Presented at Symposium on Acceptability Criteria for Transportation Noise, Seattle, Washington, 26—28 March 1969b.

Bottom, C. G., Waters, D. M.: A social survey into annoyance caused by the interaction of aircraft noise and traffic noise. TT 7102, Department of Transport Technology, Loughborough University of Technology, G.B. (no date).

Bowsher, J. M., Johnson, D. R., Robinson, D. W.: A further experiment on judging the noisiness of aircraft in flight. Acustica **17**, 245—267 (1966).

Broadbent, D. E., Robinson, D. W.: Subjective measurements of the relative annoyance of simulated sonic bangs and aircraft noise. J. Sound Vib. **1**, 162—174 (1964).

Bürck, W., Grützmacher, M., Meister, F. J.: Fluglärm: „Seine Messung und Bewertung, seine Berücksichtigung bei der Siedlungsplanung, Maßnahmen zu seiner Minderung". Gutachten erstattet im Auftrage des Bundesministeriums für Gesundheitswesen, Göttingen, 1965.

Cederlöf, R., Jonsson, E., Kajland, A.: Annoyance reactions to noise from motor vehicles. An experimental study. Acustica **13**, 270—279 (1963).

Connor, W. K., Patterson, H. P.: Community reaction to aircraft noise around smaller city airports. National Aeronautics and Space Administration, CR-2104, August 1972.

Edwards, A. L.: Scalogram analysis. In: Techniques of attitude scale construction, pp. 193—198. New York: Appleton-Century Crofts, Inc., 1957.

French, N. R., Steinberg, J. C.: Factors governing the intelligibility of speech sounds. J. acoust. Soc. Amer. **19**, 90—119 (1947).

Galloway, W. J., Clark, W. E., Kerrick, J. S.: Highway noise, measurement, simulation, and mixed reactions. National Cooperative Highway Research Program, Rept. 78, Highway Research Board, 1969.

Galloway, W. J., Bishop, D. E.: Noise exposure forecasts: Evolution, evaluation, extensions, and land use interpretations. FAA-NO-70-9, U.S. Department of Transportation, August 1970.

Gallup (Norwegian Gallup Institute): No title. Oslo Aftenposten, 22 July 1968, cited in Urban Traffic Noise, Organization for Economic Cooperation and Development, Paris, 1971.

Griffiths, I. D.: A note on the traffic noise index and the equivalent sound level. J. Sound Vib. **8**, 298—300 (1968).

Griffiths, I. D., Langdon, F. J.: Subjective response to road traffic noise. Building Research Station, Current Paper 37/68, Ministry of Public Building and Works, Garson, Watford, Herts, England, 1968.

Guttman, L.: The Cornell technique for scale and intensity analysis. Educ. Psychol. Measmt. **7**, 247—280 (1947).

Guttman, L.: The basis for scalogram analysis. In: Studies in social psychology in World War II, Vol. IV. Measurement and prediction. Princeton University 1950.

Hazard, W. R.: Community reactions to aircraft noise, public reactions, in NASA SP-189, 661—672, October 1968.

Hecker, M. H. L., Kryter, K. D.: Comparisons between subjective ratings of aircraft noise and various objective measures. FAA NO-68-33, April 1968.

Hillquist, R. K.: Objective and subjective measurement of truck noise. Sound and Vibration **1**, 8—13 (1967).

IEC-179: Specification for precision sound level meters. International Electrotechnical Commission. International Standards Organization, 1, Rue de Varembé, Geneva, Switzerland, 1965.

ISO R.507-1966 (E): Procedure for describing aircraft noise around an airport. International Standards Organization, 1, Rue de Varembé, Geneva, Switzerland, 1966.

ISO R.532: Procedure for calculating loudness level. International Standards Organization, 1, Rue de Varembé, Geneva, Switzerland, 1967.

ISO R.1996: Assessment of noise with respect to community response. International Standards Organization, 1, Rue de Varembé, Geneva, Switzerland, May 1971.

Jonsson, E.: Annoyance reactions to external environmental factors in different sociological groups. Acta Soc. **7**, 229—263 (1964).

Johnson, D. R., Robinson, D. W.: On the subjective evaluation of sonic bangs. Acustica **18**, 241—258 (1967).

Johnson, D. R., Robinson, D. W.: Procedure for calculating the loudness of sonic bangs. Acustica **21**, 307—318 (1969).

Jonsson, E., Kajland, A., Paccagnella, B., Sörensen, S.: Annoyance reactions to traffic noise in Italy and Sweden. Karolinska Institutet, University of Stockholm and University of Ferrara, 1968.

Kerrick, J. S., Nagel, D. C., Bennett, R. L.: Multiple ratings of sound stimuli. J. acoust. Soc. Amer. **45**, 1014—1017 (1969).

Kryter, K. D.: Scaling human reactions to the sound from aircraft. J. acoust. Soc. Amer. **31**, 1415—1429 (1959).

Kryter, K. D.: Methods for the calculation and use of the articulation index. J. acoust. Soc. Amer. **34**, 1689—1697 (1962).

Kryter, K. D., Pearsons, K. S.: Some effects of spectral content and duration on perceived noise level. J. acoust. Soc. Amer. **35**, 866—883 (1963).

Kryter, K. D., Pearsons, K. S.: Modification of noy tables. J. acoust. Soc. Amer. **36**, 394—397 (1964).

Kryter, K. D., Pearsons, K. S.: Judged noisiness of a band of random noise containing an audible pure tone. J. acoust. Soc. Amer. **38**, 106—112 (1965).

Kryter, K. D.: Concepts of perceived noisiness, their implementation and application. J. acoust. Soc. Amer. **43**, 344—361 (1968).

Kryter, K. D.: The effects of noise on man. New York and London: Academic Press, 1970.

Lang, J.: Verkehrslärm-Messung und Darstellung. Paper F35, Proc. 5th Int. Cong. on Acoustics, Liège, 1965.

Likert, R.: A technique for the measurement of attitudes. Arch. Psychol. **140**, (1932).

Little, J. W.: Human response to jet engine noises. Noise Control **7**, 11—13 (1961).

Little, J. W., Mabry, J. E.: Empirical comparisons of calculation procedures for estimating annoyance of jet aircraft flyovers. J. Sound Vib. **10**, 71—80 (1969).

McKennell, A. C.: Aircraft noise annoyance around London (Heathrow) airport. U. K. Government Social Survey Rept. SS. 337, Cmnd. 2056. London: Her Majesty's Stationery Office, 1963.

McKennell, A. C.: Methodological problems in a survey of aircraft noise annoyance. Statistician **19** (1968).

McKennell, A. C.: Noise complaints and community action. In: Chalupnik, J. D. (Ed.): Transportation noises pp. 228—244. Seattle, Washington: University of Washington Press, 1970.

Mil Research Ltd.: Second survey of aircraft noise annoyance around London (Heathrow) airport. Prepared for Social Survey Division on behalf of the Department of Trade and Industry. London: Her Majesty's Stationery Office, 1971.

Nixon, C. W., Hubbard, H. H.: Results of the USAF-NASA-FAA flight program to study community responses to sonic booms in the greater St. Louis area. Tech. Note D-2705, National Aeronautics and Space Administration, Washington, D.C., May 1965.

Ollerhead, J. B.: Subjective evaluation of general aviation aircraft noise, FAA NO-68-35, AD 673-982. Huntsville, Ala.: Wyle Laboratories, Inc., 1968.

Ollerhead, J. B.: An evaluation of methods for scaling aircraft noise perception. Rept. CR-1883, National Aeronautics and Space Administration, October 1971.

Parnell, J. E., Nagel, D. C., Parry, H. J.: Growth of noisiness for tones and bands of noise at different frequencies. Tech. Rept. DS 67-21, Federal Aviation Administration, U.S. Department of Transportation, December 1967.

Pearsons, K. S., Horonjeff, R. D.: Category scaling judgment tests on motor vehicle and aircraft noise. Rept. DS 67-9, Federal Aviation Administration, U.S. Department of Transportation, July 1967.

PEARSONS, K. S., BENNETT, R. L.: The effects of temporal and spectral combinations on the judged noisiness of aircraft sounds. Rept. NO 69-3, Federal Aviation Administration, U.S. Department of Transportation, June 1969.

RATHÉ, E. J., MUHEIM, J.: Evaluation methods for total noise exposure. J. Sound Vib. **7**, 108 (1968).

ROBINSON, D. W.: The concept of noise pollution level. NPL Aero Rept. AC 38, National Physical Laboratory, Teddington, Middlesex, England, 1969a.

ROBINSON, D. W.: An outline guide to criteria for the limitation of urban noise. NPL Aero Rept. AC 39, National Physical Laboratory, Teddington, Middlesex, England, 1969b.

ROSENBLITH, W. A., STEVENS, K. N., Staff of BOLT, BERANEK and NEWMAN, Inc.: Handbook of acoustic noise control, Vol. II. In: Noise and man. Rept. WADC TR 52-204, Wright-Patterson Air Force Base, Ohio, June, 1953.

SHEPHERD, L. J., SUTHERLAND, W. W.: Relative annoyance and loudness judgments of various simulated sonic boom waveforms. NASA Contract NAS1-6193, Lockheed California Company, Burbank, California, 1968.

Society of Automotive Engineers, Inc., ARP 865: Definitions and procedures for computing the perceived noise level of aircraft noise, 1964.

SÖRENSEN, S.: On the possibilities of changing the annoyance reaction to noise by changing the attitudes to the source of annoyance. Nordisk Hygienisk Tidskrift, Supplementum 1, Stockholm, 1970.

SPIETH, W.: Annoyance threshold judgments of bands of noise. J. acoust. Soc. Amer. **28**, 872—877 (1956).

Stanford Research Institute, Sonic boom experiments at Edwards Air Force Base. Interim Rept., National Sonic Boom Evaluation Office, Arlington, Virginia, 28 July 1967.

STEVENS, S. S.: Calculation of the loudness of complex noise. J. acoust. Soc. Amer. **28**, 807—832 (1956).

STEVENS, S. S.: Procedure for calculating loudness: Mark VI. J. acoust. Soc. Amer. **33**, 1577—1585 (1962).

STEVENS, S. S.: Perceived level of noise by Mark VII and decibels (E). J. acoust. Soc. Amer. **51**, 575—601 (1972).

THURSTON, L. L.: Multiple-factor analysis: A development and expansion of the vectors of mind. Chicago: University of Chicago Press, 1947.

TRACOR, Inc.: Public reactions to sonic booms. National Aeronautics and Space Administration, CR-1665, September 1970a.

TRACOR, Inc.: Community reaction to airport noise. National Aeronautics and Space Administration, Vol. I: CR-1761, Vol. II: CR-111316, 1970b.

WEBSTER, J. C.: Speech communications as limited by ambient noise. J. acoust. Soc. Amer. **37**, 692—699 (1965).

WILSON, A. H.: Noise. London: Her Majesty's Stationery Office, 1963.

ZWICKER, E.: Ein Verfahren zur Berechnung der Lautstärke. Acustica **10**, 304 (1960).

Chapter 8

Habituation and Attention in the Auditory System

TERENCE W. PICTON, STEVEN A. HILLYARD, and ROBERT GALAMBOS, La Jolla, California (USA)

With 21 Figures

Contents

I. Introduction

This chapter[1] surveys some current experimental evidence regarding the neurophysiological basis of habituation and attention in the auditory system. The principal focus is upon electrophysiological studies in man although a number of relevant animal studies will also be reviewed.

Human and animal subjects each have their own distinct advantages for the study of the neural mechanisms of auditory behavior. Animal electrophysiology allows more exact delineation of the underlying neuronal and synaptic processes, but is unfortunately much less exact in the depth of available psychological correlation. Habituation involves a relatively simple experimental paradigm and its mechanisms can therefore be readily studied in animals. Human subjects, however, offer marked advantages for the study of attention, since satisfactory operational definitions of the construct "attention" in terms of reliable, unambiguous behavioral measures are hard to come by for sub-humans. Furthermore, distinguishing between brain events associated with the selective processing of sensory information and the so-called "non-specific" brain processes accompanying alerting and arousal, which may alter stimulus inputs and response propensities in an unselective fashion, is simpler in man.

Use of human subjects for electrophysiological investigation imposes a limitation in that the brain sources of scalp-recorded electrical responses can only be inferred. We will point out, however, that reliable correlations can be demonstrated between particular categories of human brain potentials, having well-defined scalp distributions, and concurrent psychophysical indices of selective attention and habituation. Given these facts, it does not seem untowardly optimistic to predict, as we do, that these specific potentials will come to be identified with psychologically defined stages of sensory processing and, thus, provide evidence for or against particular hypotheses regarding the structure of selective information processing in the human brain.

II. The Human Auditory Evoked Potential (AEP)

A. Early Components

An abrupt sound evokes in the auditory pathways a characteristic series of potentials that can be recorded from the scalp using computer averaging techniques. The evoked action potential of the eighth nerve to a click has been recorded from the cochlear promontory in the middle ear (Yoshie and Ohashi, 1969; Portmann and Aran, 1971), from the external auditory meatus (Yoshie, 1968; Coats and Dickey, 1970), and even from the earlobe (Sohmer and Feinmesser,

[1] Submitted September, 1973

1967). The components of this response are a pair of waves labelled "n_1" and "n_2" (Fig. 1a). The first wave no doubt represents activation of cochlear nerve fibers; the n_2 wave might represent a secondary discharge of the cochlear nerve or far-field conduction from the cochlear nucleus. Vertex-mastoid and vertex-earlobe recordings also exhibit click-evoked potentials from the auditory nerve and nuclei of the brainstem (JEWETT and WILLISTON, 1971), as illustrated in Fig. 1b. Following these authors, the successive components of the human brainstem evoked response are labelled I—VII. There is strong evidence that Wave I represents the far-field of the summed action potential of the cochlear nerve, while the succeeding waves originate from the brainstem auditory nuclei and pathways (JEWETT and WILLISTON, 1971; LEV and SOHMER, 1972; PICTON *et. al.*, 1974).

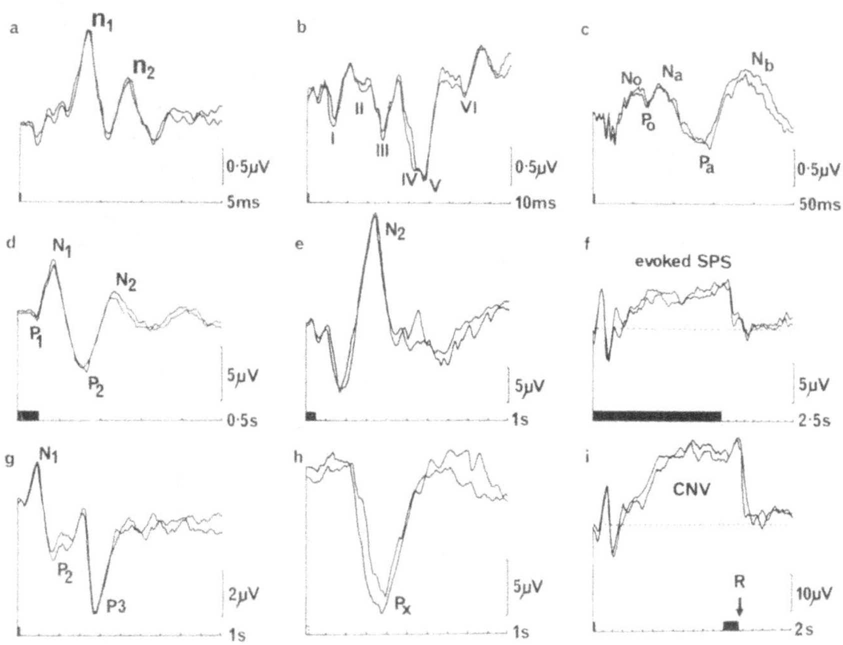

Fig. 1a—i. A pastiche of potentials recorded from the human brain in response to sound. (a) Auditory nerve response to a 55dB click, recorded from an electrode in the skin of the auditory meatus near the tympanic membrane. Each tracing is the average of $N = 256$ responses. (b) Brainstem evoked response to a 60dB click, recorded from vertex to mastoid electrodes. $N = 2048$. (c) Middle latency evoked response to a 60dB click, recorded from vertex-mastoid electrodes. $N = 1024$. (d) Vertex potential to a 60dB 1kHz toneburst, recorded from vertex-mastoid electrodes. $N = 128$. Subject was awake. (e) Vertex potential to a 50dB 1kHz toneburst from vertex-mastoid electrodes. $N = 64$. Subject was drowsy. (f) Slow potential shift evoked during a 50 dB 1K Hz tone burst lasting 1.6 seconds. N=64. (g) Late positive component (P 3) in the evoked potential to a detected fainter "signal" in an ongoing train of nonsignal stimuli. $N = 128$. (h) Response following a detected omitted click in a regular train of clicks presented once every 1.1 sec. $N = 64$. (i) After a warning click and prior to a tone that the subject must terminate by making a motor response (R) there develops a slow negative shift — the Contingent Negative Variation. $N = 12$. In all records negativity of the initial electrode relative to the second is displayed as an upward deflection

B. "Middle Latency" Components

Numerous laboratories have reported that a well-defined sequence of "middle latency" (8—50 msec) waves follows the early brainstem evoked response to a click in the vertex-mastoid recording (GEISLER *et al.*, 1958; BORSANYI and BLANCHARD, 1964; RAPIN, 1964; MAST, 1965; GOLDSTEIN and RODMAN, 1967; RUHM *et al.*, 1967; GOFF *et al.*, 1969). The degree to which these scalp-recorded waves (Fig. 1c), designated N_o, P_o, N_a, P_a, and N_b by the GOLDSTEIN group, may represent the activation of the primary auditory cortex is uncertain since they show (except for N_a) little resemblance to what can be recorded directly from primary cortex at operation (CELESIA and PULETTI, 1971). The widespread scalp distribution of the mid-latency components (PICTON *et al.*, 1974) suggests that they may be derived from either broad zones of association cortex (*cf.* primate studies of BIGNALL and IMBERT, 1969), or from deep sensory structures such as the thalamus.

It is within this latency range of 8—50 msec that potentials arising from evoked reflex contraction of the scalp musculature may seriously contaminate the records (CODY and BICKFORD, 1969; BICKFORD, 1972). Distinguishing the intra-cranially generated potentials from those of myogenic origin can be accomplished by manipulating muscle tension in the course of evoked potential studies and by separately mapping the scalp topographies of the two classes of phenomena (PICTON *et al.*, 1974a).

C. Long-Latency Components: the Auditory Vertex Potential

A series of late waves in the AEP (50—250 msec) are prominent and easily recorded (Fig. 1d). These waves, the auditory "vertex potential", are consistently recorded in the great majority of subjects, have been designated as P_1, N_1, P_2, and N_2 (DAVIS and ZERLIN, 1966; RAPIN *et al.*, 1966), and are maximally distributed over frontal cortex, being largest at the vertex (GOFF *et al.*, 1969; KOOI *et al.*, 1971; PICTON *et al.*, 1974a). Homologous components have been recorded directly from the frontal cortex of lower primates (HARDIN and CASTELLUCI, 1970) and man (WALTER, 1964a and b). Unlike the early and middle latency waves, the vertex potential is markedly altered with changes in alertness or arousal, with the N_2 component increasing dramatically during drowsiness and sleep (Fig. 1e) (WILLIAMS *et al.*, 1962).

The early, middle and late waves of the AEP may be conveniently illustrated by plotting the entire sequence on log-log axes (Fig. 2). This "typical" representation is a grand average derived from measurements of a large number of subjects in our laboratory and it corresponds closely with the componentry described by others (PICTON *et al.*, 1974a).

D. Auditory-Evoked Slow Potential Shifts

Following the N_1-P_2-N_2 complex that is evoked by the onset of a continuous auditory stimulus (such as a steady tone), D.C. recordings show a vertex-negative baseline shift which lasts for the duration of the stimulus (Fig. 1f). The cessation of the tone elicits N_1 and P_2 waves similar to those of the "on-response" (ROSE and MALONE, 1965; CLYNES, 1969). The source of the auditory slow potential shift in man is unknown, although KÖHLER and WEGENER (1955) proposed that it derived from surface negativity of the primary auditory cortex, which is consistent with results obtained in animals (GUMNIT, 1960; DAVID *et al.*, 1969). KEIDEL (1971) has reviewed evidence for the cortical generation of these sensory evoked baseline shifts, their utility in evoked response audiometry, and their inter-modality interactions.

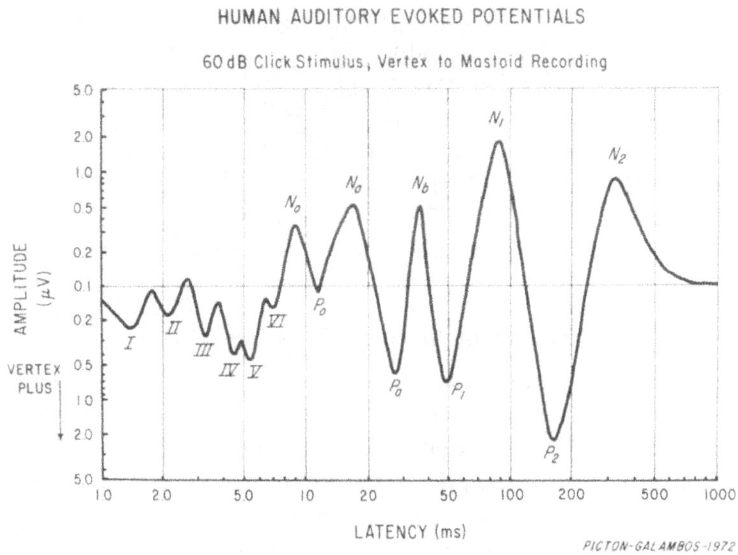

Fig. 2. The characteristic sequence of components in the human auditory evoked potential plotted on log-log coordinates (PICTON *et al.*, 1974a)

E. "Event-Related" Potentials during Attention and Perception

The event-related potentials shown in Fig. 2 are "evoked" in the sense that their latency and amplitude are controlled mainly by the stimulus and not the subjective state of the listener. Two additional classes of electrical events seem, however, to be largely independent of the physical parameters of the triggering stimuli and to reflect instead the subject's attentiveness, expectancies and decision-making vis-a-vis the stimulus. Such event-related potentials have been termed "endogenous" (SUTTON *et al.*, 1965), in that they index psychological processes that are "released" by (and time-locked to) a stimulus only as a function of its meaning and significance.

1. Late Positive "P 3" Wave

A long-latency positive wave, designated the P_3 component, occurs in a variety of situations wherein a stimulus event delivers task-relevant or significant information to which a decision is made. The P_3 is elicited some 300 msec or more (hence the alternate "P_{300}" label) after a subjectively interesting or novel stimulus (WALTER, 1965; RITTER *et al.*, 1968), correct and incorrect feedback cues (TEUTING *et al.*, 1970; SQUIRES *et al.*, 1973a), detected signals in a train of non-signals (see Fig. 1g) (RITTER and VAUGHAN, 1969; SMITH *et al.*, 1970), detected threshold level signals (HILLYARD *et al.*, 1971), and cues for motor reaction (WILKINSON and MORLOCK, 1967; KARLIN *et al.*, 1970). The amplitude of the P_3 is relatively independent of stimulus parameters and may even be triggered by the omission of a stimulus in an ongoing train (KLINKE *et al.*, 1968; PICTON *et al.*, 1974b), thereby emphasizing its endogenous character. The endogenous positive wave following an omitted stimulus is termed "P_x" in Fig. 1h because it is not a member of a sequence of positive waves in this circumstance; in all known respects, however, including scalp topography, temporal relation to decision, and effects of attention, the P_x appears to be equivalent to P_3 (PICTON *et al.*, 1974b). The scalp distribution of P_3 is much broader than that of the N_1-P_2 and has a more posterior maximum (VAUGHAN and RITTER, 1970; RITTER *et al.*, 1972; PICTON and HILLYARD, 1974). The brain source for the P_3 has not been identified, but its diffuse and posterior topography is consistent with the suggestion that it represents widespread activity of association cortex (RITTER *et al.*, 1972).

2. Contingent Negative Variation (CNV)

Following a warning stimulus and prior to a subsequent perceptual or motor act there develops a slow negative shift of the electro-cortical baseline which has been called the Contingent Negative Variation or CNV (WALTER *et al.*, 1964). The CNV, illustrated in Fig. 1i, precedes the motor response or perceptual decision made to a second stimulus only as long as the subject remains alert and actively engaged in the task; in some circumstances the amplitude of the CNV has been found to vary roughly with the degree of attention devoted to the task (TECCE, 1972). The CNV is most prominent over the anterior scalp (maximum at the vertex) and has been recorded directly from frontal cortex of primate (LOW *et al.*, 1966; BORDA, 1970; DONCHIN *et al.*, 1971; REBERT, 1972) and human (WALTER, 1964b) subjects.

III. Habituation

A. Defining Characteristics

1. Habituation

Habituation can be defined as a decline in the magnitude or probability of a response upon repetition of the eliciting stimulus. Habituation functions to prevent the needless stereotyped response to repeating stimuli, and thereby "helps to ensure the serial variety of reaction" (SHERRINGTON, 1906, p. 222).

Habituation usually connotes a change in central nervous system activity, being differentiated, therefore, from sensory adaptation and receptor fatigue. Other defining properties (THOMPSON and SPENCER, 1966) include stimulus specificity, which may be very narrow in some cases, and an inverse relation to interstimulus interval and stimulus intensity (although the latter point has become controversial — DAVIS and WAGNER, 1968).

2. Dishabituation

A phenomenon usually associated with habituation and occasionally considered as a necessary characteristic of the habituation process is dishabituation. Here a stimulus that does not elicit the response being habituated, when presented during the habituation process, returns the strength of the response to or toward its prehabituation level. Habituation is defined by some as a response decrement that can be dishabituated in this way, in contrast to "rate-effects" which cause response decrements that are not subject to dishabituation. THOMPSON and his co-workers (THOMPSON and SPENCER, 1966; GROVES and THOMPSON, 1970) on the other hand, have argued elegantly that dishabituation is consequent upon a separate "sensitization" process that is superimposed upon the decrement of habituation. In support of this hypothesis they point out that a dishabituating stimulus often strengthens a response that has not yet been habituated.

3. Rate Effects

Any stimulus-evoked neural or behavioral response will decrease in magnitude as the inter-stimulus interval encroaches upon the refractory period of the mediating neural pathways. It is important to distinguish these response decrements from those in which the additional mechanisms of "habituation" may operate. In practice this distinction may prove most difficult, since for rapid rates of stimulation rate effects and habituation effects may be superimposed and interactive. One important basis for distinguishing between the two processes is that rate effects typically stabilize rapidly over the first few stimuli, leaving the response at a sustained plateau level thereafter, whereas habituation usually entails a long-term progressive decline in responsiveness. Habituation may also take place with inter-stimulus intervals longer than that of the refractory period, which should preclude any rate effects. It is also possible to define rate effects as being less sensitive to dishabituation than is "true" habituation. An example of rate effects in the evoked potential from the human auditory nerve is shown in Fig. 3; this summed action potential persists unchanged indefinitely at stimulus

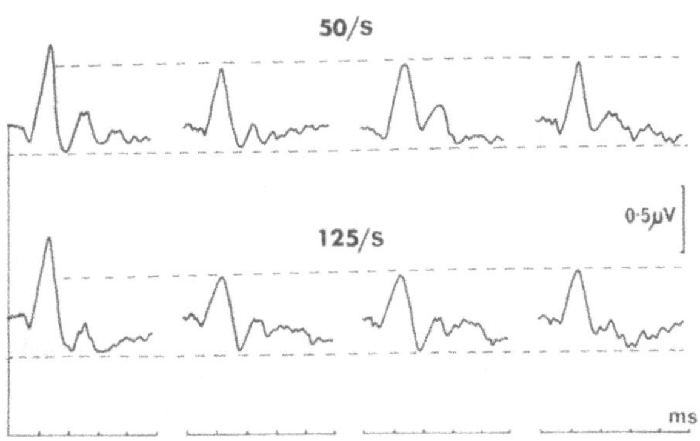

Fig. 3. Rate effects in human auditory nerve response. Bursts of 45dB SL clicks lasting 100 msec. were presented every two seconds for a total of 512 bursts. Within each burst the click repetition rate was 50Hz (top) and 125Hz (bottom). The four tracings from left to right are the averaged auditory nerve responses ($N = 512$) to the first, second, third and fourth responses in the burst. Time markers indicate milliseconds

repetition rates below about 10 Hz, but at higher rates there is a decrement in amplitude after the initial response which plateaus immediately.

B. Neurophysiological Studies of Habituation in Animals

1. Relative Stability of Lemniscal Responses

Early reports of evoked potential decrements during habituation at the level of the cochlea (GERSHUNI *et al.*, 1960) and the cochlear nucleus (HERNANDEZ-PEON *et al.*, 1957; MARSH *et al.*, 1961) have been effectively criticized because fluctuations in the acoustic input to the cochlea were not ruled out (see WORDEN, 1966, 1973). Subsequent studies that have carefully controlled the acoustic variability have shown that evoked potentials in the lower brainstem auditory nuclei remain stable under long-term continuous stimulation (MARSH and WORDEN, 1964; WICKELGREN, 1968c; HALL, 1968; IRVINE and WEBSTER, 1972). No evidence of habituation was seen below the medial geniculate relay, and the initial positive component of the auditory cortex also remained stable provided that the animal's state of arousal was maintained (WICKELGREN, 1968a). Secondary components of the auditory cortex response, however, have been found to show marked habituation (COOK *et al.*, 1968).

A series of careful studies by WEBSTER (1971) has shown rate effects in the absence of habituation for evoked responses in the brainstem auditory nuclei of cats: when stimuli were presented at rates greater than one per second, there was a decline in the response over the first several stimuli which became stable thereafter. The magnitude of the rate-dependent decrement at cochlear nucleus and inferior colliculus was increased by systemic barbiturate, suggesting that the decrement had resulted from reduced synaptic efficiency in the primary auditory pathway rather than from a multi-synaptic inhibitory system vulnerable to barbiturate (WEBSTER and AITKIN, 1971). These authors argued that these response decrements represent "rate effects", not habituation, on the grounds that they were insensitive to stimulus intensity, did not dishabituate, and were absent at slow repetition rates.

There is, then, a reasonable consensus that auditory habituation is not mediated early in the analysis of auditory input. Dissenting reports include the study of BUNO *et al.* (1966), who reported habituation and dishabituation of the auditory nerve action potential and of the cochlear microphonic to repeated click or tone-pip stimulation in the guinea pig, despite paying close attention to acoustic stimulus control. They failed to find such habituation in animals with sectioned olivo-cochlear bundles, and suggested that efferent inhibition via this tract might be the underlying mechanism. However, since electrical stimulation of the olivo-cochlear bundle causes enlargement of the cochlear microphonic as the nerve response is depressed (FEX, 1959), it is difficult to attribute concurrent decreases in both to efferent activity. Since the over-riding majority of evoked potential studies do indicate a high degree of stability of transmission of the auditory lemniscal system, one is tempted to resort to species differences as an explanation for these guinea pig results reported by BUNO *et al.*

Recent studies of evoked multiple-unit discharge in the lower auditory nuclei have also revealed clear evidence of habituation (BUCHWALD and HUMPHREY,

1972a). In the course of habituation and dishabituation trials there were small changes (15% or less) in the evoked multiple unit discharge from the brainstem auditory nuclei of awake paralyzed cats. In decerebrated cats, however, the response decrements with habituation were far more striking (up to 45%) (BUCHWALD and HUMPHREY, 1972b). These effects developed in the absence of any change in the cochlear microphonic at the round window and were unaffected by strychnine blockade of post-synaptic inhibition, suggesting that recurrent or intrinsic inhibitory control of nervous transmission was not a major factor. BUCHWALD and HUMPHREY, therefore, surmised that depression of synaptic transmission in specific pathways involving the cochlear nucleus was responsible for this habituation. The difference between the habituation patterns in intact and in decerebrate cats seems to implicate some higher process which in the intact animal may act to stabilize the analysis of incoming auditory information in the primary or classical auditory system.

2. Habituation in the Reticular Activating System

Evoked electrical responses in the extralemniscal (or, as we shall call it, the secondary auditory system) have, in general, been found to exhibit marked habituation. Click-evoked potentials in the brainstem reticular formation have onset latencies similar to those in the lemniscal pathway but last much longer (STARZL *et al.*, 1951). Upon stimulus repetition they decline progressively in amplitude while lemniscal responses remain constant (FRENCH *et al.*, 1953). Single unit activity in the reticular formation also undergoes marked habituation, even with long inter-stimulus intervals (BELL *et al.*, 1964; HORN and HILL, 1964; HIRANO *et al.*, 1970; GROVES *et al.*, 1970), and the evoked unit responses may recover spontaneously after a period of silence, upon shifting to a different stimulus (specificity), or with injection of a novel stimulus into an ongoing train (sensitization/dishabituation). These single unit phenomena are paralleled by behavioral studies showing that reticular formation activity correlates with habituation of orienting eye movements in response to repeated sounds (WEINBERGER *et al.*, 1969) and that habituation of the startle response to an acoustic stimulus is lacking in rats with bilateral lesions of the midbrain reticular formation (CAPPS and STOCKWELL, 1969).

3. The Arousal and Orienting Responses

The brainstem and thalamic reticular formations also mediate sound-evoked arousal and orienting responses: combined autonomic, electrophysiological and cognitive reactions to unexpected or novel stimuli. These are often considered to be two variants of one type of response: the generalized orienting response, or tonic arousal reaction, and the localized orienting response, or phasic arousal reaction (see LYNN, 1966 for review). For the sake of simplicity we shall refer to the generalized response as arousal and the localized as orienting. The arousal response is the change in state of an animal (for example, from sleep to waking) brought about by the presentation of an intense stimulus. Associated with this behavioral change there is a generalized alteration of the electroencephalogram from large, slow rhythmic activity to a rapid, low voltage discharge, an effect that seems to be mediated by the rostropontine reticular formation (MORUZZI, 1972) and to indicate cortical neuronal desynchronization (ELUL, 1966). A series of classic experiments with cats (SHARPLESS and JASPER, 1956) demonstrated that this arousal response to a loud tone habituated to zero within about 30 presentations and was specific to the stimulus frequency. Neither the time course nor the specificity of habituation was substantially altered after ablation of the auditory and surrounding cortex, but severing the auditory pathway at the brachia of the inferior colliculus both elevated the threshold for the EEG arousal response and increased the speed of its habituation.

The orienting reaction was first described in terms of an investigatory "What is it?" response to a novel and potentially significant stimulus (PAVLOV, 1927). With it come two distinctive changes in the EEG — a local desynchronization in the modality-specific cortex, probably mediated by the thalamic reticular formation (JASPER, 1960), and a burst of hippocampal theta rhythm (LISSAK and GRASTYAN, 1960; BENNET and GOTTFRIED, 1970). Unlike the arousal response to a more intense signal, the orienting reaction often fails to appear upon the first occurrence of the stimulus but may do so after repetition; with further stimulation the response may then habituate, although it is less susceptible to habituation and more stimulus-specific than the arousal response. Human EEG studies of the orienting reaction have most often used visual or somatic stimuli, since their primary cortices are more accessible to scalp recording than the auditory. Upon repetition of a visual stimulus the EEG desynchronization becomes localized to occipital cortex and then finally disappears; this habituation is stimulus specific, since the desynchronization returns if the stimulus is decreased in intensity (SOKOLOV, 1960).

C. Habituation of the Human Auditory Evoked Potential

1. Early and Middle-Latency Responses

As shown in Fig. 4, the "early" (0—8 msec) and "middle" (8—50 msec) latency components of the click-evoked potential do not change appreciably during prolonged stimulation. Like the auditory nerve action potential (Fig. 3) they exhibit rate effects (PICTON et al., 1974a) but not progressive habituation, thereby resembling the evoked responses in the auditory brainstem of animals.

Unfortunately, evoked potentials generated in the primary auditory cortex do not seem to manifest themselves clearly in scalp recordings. When recorded from man at operation, however, auditory cortex responses show the initial positive components to remain relatively stable under repeated stimulation, beyond a refractory period of several hundred msec (PULETTI and CELESIA, 1970).

2. Habituation of the Auditory Vertex Potential

The N_1-P_2 waves of the auditory vertex potential are the only components of the AEP to decline systematically over a session of repetitive stimulation. They show both short-term and long-term habituation. Short-term effects can be examined by presenting short trains of stimuli with relatively long intervals between the trains and then averaging evoked responses according to their ordinal position in the train (Figure 5, top).

At rates greater than 0.1/sec the auditory vertex response declines in amplitude over the first several stimuli and then tends to remain relatively stable; with intervals of 10 sec between stimuli there is no significant short term habituation (RITTER *et al.*, 1968; FRUHSTORFER and BERGSTROM, 1969; FRUHSTORFER *et al.*, 1970). ROTHMAN *et al.* (1970) have shown that the size of the evoked potential varies with the interval preceding the stimulus and to a lesser degree with the interstimulus intervals before that; on this basis, they were able to predict the vertex potential amplitude at many different rates of stimulation.

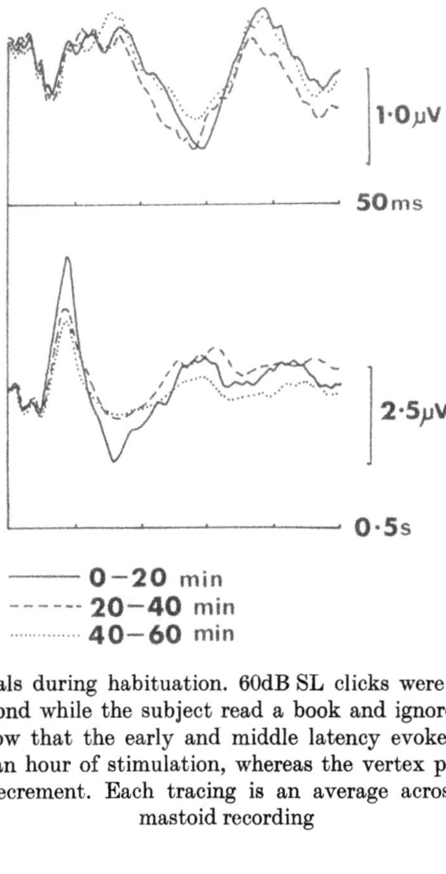

Fig. 4. Evoked potentials during habituation. 60dB SL clicks were presented continuously at a rate of once a second while the subject read a book and ignored the auditory stimuli. The upper tracings show that the early and middle latency evoked potential components are stable throughout an hour of stimulation, whereas the vertex potential (lower tracings) shows a progressive decrement. Each tracing is an average across 1024 stimuli. Vertex-mastoid recording

FRUHSTORFER (1971) reported that the amplitude of the initial response to a train of clicks was strongly dependent upon the subject's attentiveness. We have confirmed this by having subjects count the number of clicks in each train; this markedly accentuates a positive wave at about 300 msec latency (P_3) in the AEP to the first click (Fig. 6). This P_3 component, which is more fully discussed later in this chapter, seems to be associated with making a stimulus-related decision: here, the decision to begin counting.

OHMAN and LADER (1972) found that attending to a repeating auditory stimulus (in order to make a quick motor response thereto) enhanced the evoked potential amplitude, but there was still a decrement with stimulus repetition.

This effect is not present in Fig. 6 (*i.e.* the EP's at train Positions 2 and 6 are not changed by attention); this difference is probably due to the difference in the attentive task — in our case the task (counting) was relatively easy.

Long-term habituation of the vertex potential, characterized by a slow and progressive decline in amplitude, is difficult to assess since any change in the subject's level of alertness may obscure the habituation process. Drowsiness, for instance, is associated with a diminution of the N_1 wave but an enormous aggrandizement of the N_2 wave (Fig. 7) (Williams *et al.*, 1962; Weitzman and Kremen, 1965). When the level of alertness is maintained reasonably constant, long-term habituation of the vertex potential amplitude clearly develops (Fig. 5, bottom)

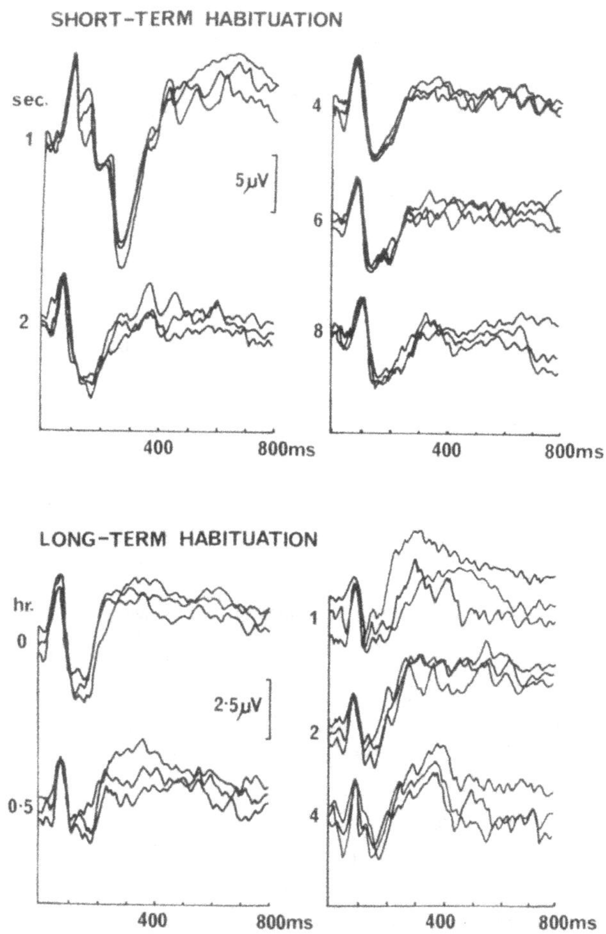

Fig. 5. Short and long term habituation of the human vertex potential. Short term habituation: A train of ten 60dB SL clicks at a rate of 1/sec was presented every minute and evoked responses for each position of the train were averaged over 64 such trains. Numbers indicate serial position of response within the train. Long-Term habituation: 60 dB SL clicks were presented continuously at a rate of 1/second for four hours. Responses were averaged over 128 clicks beginning at the designated times after the commencement of the clicks

and is largely completed within the first half-hour of stimulation (Roeser and Price, 1969). Townsend and his colleagues (personal communication) report habituation of responses to loud tone pips over 15 h of presentation at 28-sec

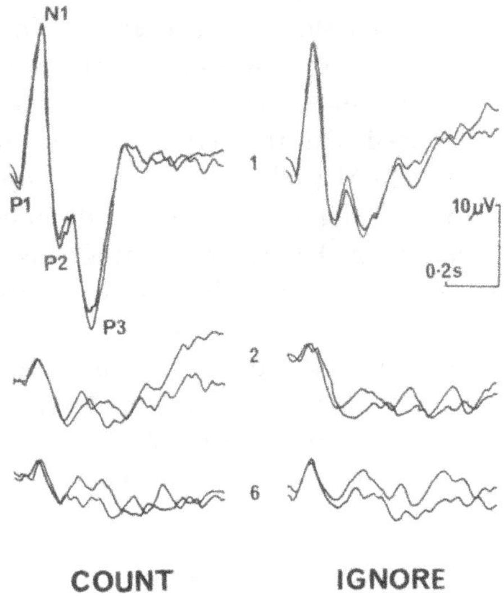

Fig. 6. Effects of attentiveness upon short-term habituation. The subject was presented every 30 sec with trains of seven or eight 60dB SL clicks at a rate of 1/sec under one of two conditions. In the "count" condition (left column) he had to count the number of clicks in each train, and in the "ignore" condition (right column) he read a book. Each tracing is the average of 20 responses with the numbers indicating the serial position of the click within the train

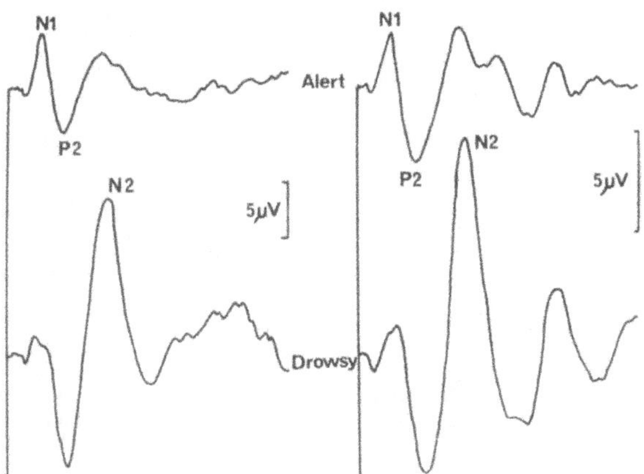

Fig. 7. Modification of the vertex potential during drowsiness. The evoked potentials on the left are to a 70dB SL 1kHz tone presented once every two seconds. Each tracing is the average of 64 responses. Subject B.M. The evoked potentials on the right are to a 60dB SL click presented once every second. Each tracing is the average of 1024 responses. Subject J.S.

intervals, the response returning to prominence when the subject falls asleep. Although falling asleep does change a previously habituated auditory response, continuation of the stimulus during sleep may again result in response decrement (FIRTH, 1972). In a recent study, DAVIS and HENINGER (1972) failed to obtain long-term habituation of the vertex potential to loud (96 dB) noise bursts, despite a clear habituation of the accompanying reflex eyeblink response, and they concluded that the behavioral response was dissociable from the brain response. It is not clear, however, to what extent the corneo-retinal potential artifact from the eyeblink may have summed with the vertex potential and masked its habituation. The consensus remains that there is a slow progressive habituation of the vertex potential with repetition of the auditory stimulus.

The amount of habituation of the vertex potential depends upon the rate of delivery of the stimulus (DAVIS et al., 1966; NELSON and LASSMAN, 1968; MILNER, 1969; ROTHMAN et al., 1970) as well as on its duration and intensity. Lengthening the duration of a repeated toneburst enhances the decrement in the vertex potential (WEBER, 1970), as does increasing the stimulus intensity (Fig. 8b compares the short-term habituation to 30 versus 60 dB SL tone bursts). This dependence of habituation upon stimulus intensity might explain why ROSE and

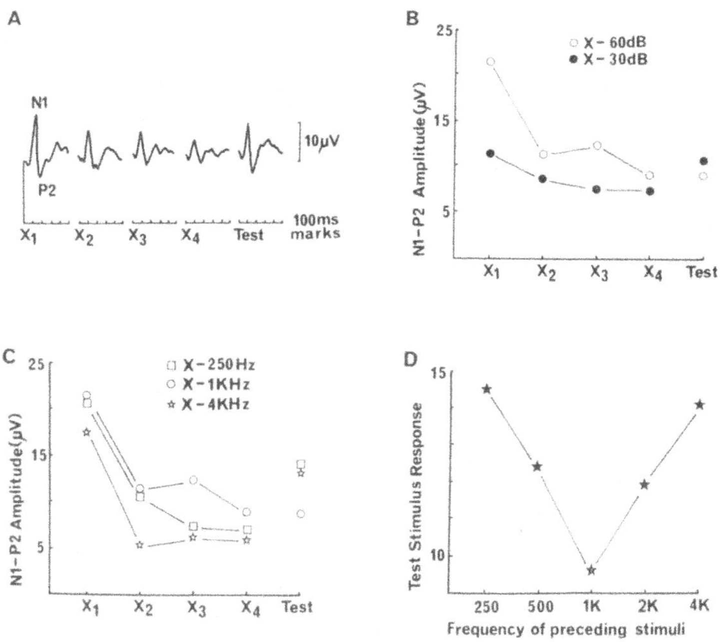

Fig. 8a—d. Specificity of habituation. A train of four tonebursts (X1—4) each lasting one second and occurring every two seconds was followed by a 1kHz toneburst test stimulus. Such a train was presented to a reading subject once a minute. (a) Illustrates $N1$-$P2$ components when x=2kHz. Each tracing is the average of 25 responses obtained from vertex-mastoid electrodes. (b) Amplitudes of $N1$-$P2$ components for different intensities of X when all stimuli are 1kHz. (c) Amplitudes of $N1$-$P2$ components for different frequencies of X when all stimuli are 60 Phon in loudness. (d) Amplitude of $N1$-$P2$ component evoked by 1kHz test stimulus as a function of the frequency of the habituating stimulus (X)

Ruhm (1966) did not observe any substantial long-term decrements using low intensity clicks.

In summary, the vertex potential declines in amplitude with stimulus repetition. This change has some characteristics of a rate-effect: the major decrement occurs after the first stimulus and the effect is highly sensitive to interstimulus interval. It also, however, shows some definite properties of a true habituation process with a progressive decline over a longer time period.

3. Specificity of Vertex Potential Habituation

The habituation of the human vertex potential has been extensively studied as to its stimulus specificity. To the extent that the vertex potentials are generated by common nonspecific neuronal systems, cross-modality interactions should occur. Initial reports by Walter (1964a) and Hay and Davis (1971) indicated that the temporal recovery of the auditory vertex potential was little affected by interposed visual or somatic stimuli. However, a more thorough study by Davis *et al.* (1972) revealed some cross-modality interactions, such that a preceding flash or shock reduced the auditory vertex potential by some 30—40%, as compared to 60% with a prior auditory stimulus. Thus, the vertex potential has a certain degree of modality specificity, but there is a generalization of recovery interval effects across modalities.

Butler has studied the specificity of the vertex potential to different stimulus attributes within the auditory modality by presenting test stimuli at a slow rate (0.2 Hz) after several intervening habituating stimuli. He found that habituation was specific to the spatial position (Butler, 1972a) and frequency (Butler, 1968, 1972b), but not the periodicity pitch of the stimulus (Butler, 1972c). Butler suggested that stimuli differing in frequency and localization attributes activated distinctive but overlapping neuronal populations in the course of producing the vertex potential. He also found that increasing the intensity of the intervening stimuli decreased the vertex response to the test stimulus until the intervening became louder than the test, whereupon no further reductions ensued (Butler, 1968). This was explained by postulating that the intervening stimulus activated all possible "habituable" neural units when it reached the intensity of the test and further increases merely activated neurons unresponsive to the test stimulus.

We have confirmed the frequency specificity of the auditory vertex potential using a somewhat different paradigm: once each minute a train of four tonebursts at a given frequency, spaced one second apart, was followed by a 60 dB, 1000 Hz test stimulus (Fig. 8a). The decline in the vertex response during the 4 tonebursts was sharply specific to stimulus frequency, since the difference in frequency between the repetitive and test tones largely determined the amplitude of the vertex potential to the latter (Fig. 8 c and d).

4. Dishabituation of the Vertex Potential

The injection of an unexpected stimulus into a train of habituating stimuli does not result in significant dishabituation of the average evoked response. Indeed the evoked response to the dishabituating stimulus is smaller than if it were presented alone — there is some generalization of the habituation (FRUHSTORFER, 1971). The response to the unexpected stimulus, however, has a late positive component by which it differs from the habituated response (RITTER *et al.*, 1968; ROTH, 1973). Since averaging techniques are used however, one wonder, how unexpected the dishabituating stimuli are and how quickly any dishabituating effect might itself habituate.

Using shocks injected in trains of tone pips we have also failed to demonstrate dishabituation of the auditory vertex potential (Fig. 9). However, a sustained dishabituation response may be obtained by asking the subject to attend to the stimuli in order to detect occasional small alterations in their tonal frequency. This result recalls the reappearance of the orienting response by instructions to attend to the presented signals (LURIA and HOMSKAYA, 1970), and suggests that dishabituation may amount to shifting attention back to the repetitive stimulus. If this is so, the mechanism of human auditory habituation may be the same as that of sustained selective inattention; in other words, habituation and attention may be, in part, inverse aspects of the same process.

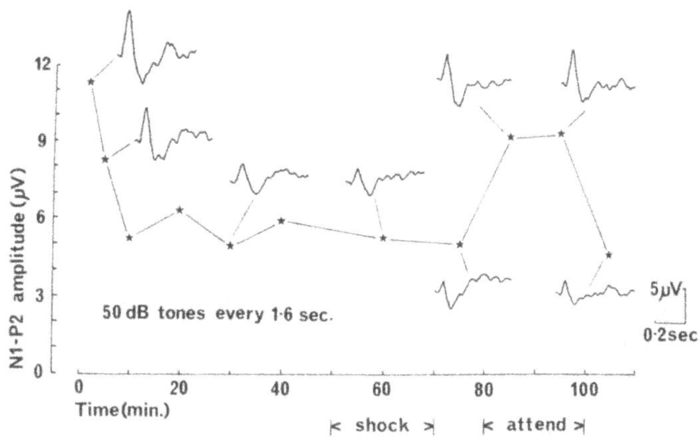

Fig. 9. Habituation and dishabituation of the auditory vertex potential. 50dB SL 50 msec tones were presented every 1.6 sec to an alert subject reading a book. The injection of noxious median nerve shock stimuli every 10—20 sec into the ongoing auditory sequence caused no change in the auditory evoked potential. Asking the subject to stop reading and attend to the auditory stimuli so as to detect small frequency changes (which had been occurring all along) caused a marked enhancement of the vertex potential. Each tracing represents the average of 256 responses except the first which is the average of 128

5. Evoked Slow Potential Shifts

One of the physiological concomitants of the stimulus-provoked arousal reaction is a generalized negative baseline shift at the cortical surface (CASPERS, 1963). Similar prolonged negative shifts may be elicited by electrical stimulation of the brainstem and thalamic reticular formation (ARDUINI, 1958). Novel auditory stimuli evoke, in addition, a negative slow potential shift localized to the auditory cortex (GUMNIT, 1960), which habituates at a slower rate than the generalized cortical baseline shift (LICKEY and FOX, 1966). Slow potential shifts evoked by sound stimuli have also been recorded at the vertex in man, and these potentials habituate upon stimulus repetition (KÖHLER and WEGENER, 1955). See Fig. 10.

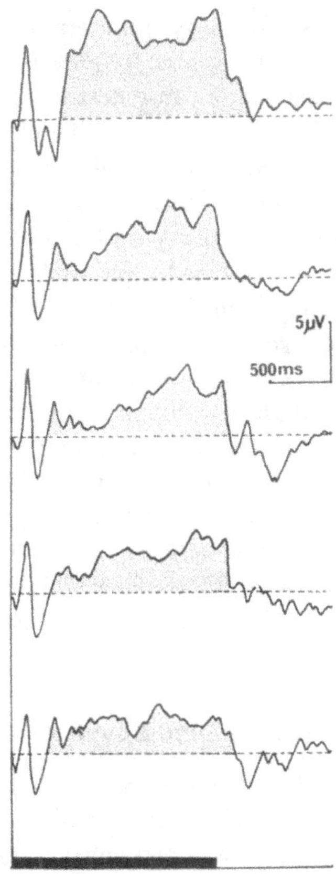

Fig. 10. Habituation of the auditory evoked slow potential shift. Trains of five 1kHz 1.6 sec tonebursts occurring at a rate of 0.25 Hz were presented every minute. Evoked potentials were averaged (over 100 presentations) for each successive position in the train (top to bottom). Subject was reading

D. Theories of Habituation

1. Efferent Control Theories

One widely disseminated proposal for the mechanism of habituation has been that incoming auditory activity is gated at peripheral levels under the control of the reticular formation (HERNANDEZ PEON, 1960; LIVINGSTON, 1959) or the "corticofugal control system" (DESMEDT, 1960, 1962), so that non-significant inputs are prevented from entering the afferent pathways. While efferent inhibition of auditory impulses does indeed exist (*e.g.* GALAMBOS, 1956), there is no solid evidence that such efferent inhibition mediates habituation.

What then is the function of the efferent auditory system? We suspect it represents a feedback system for the analysis of incoming auditory information, but that instead of being under "central" control (the significance of the stimulus to the animal) its action is determined by the acoustic properties of the stimulus. Olivo-cochlear fibers, for example, are discharged by moderately intense acoustic stimulation (FEX, 1962, 1963). Also, contralaterally applied sound can affect the discharge of cochlear neurons evoked by ipsilateral tonal stimulation: when the contralateral tone is at the neuron's center frequency no effect is noted, but tones of slightly higher or lower frequency cause a striking inhibition (KLINKE *et al.* 1969). How much of this effect is due to activity of the crossed olivo-cochlear bundle and how much to acoustically evoked efferent activity from higher centers projecting to the cochlear nucleus (PFALZ, 1962) is unsettled. However, it certainly seems that the efferent auditory pathway subserves some frequency resolving function: disrupting the crossed olivo-cochlear pathway results in impairment of frequency discrimination (CAPPS and ADES, 1968). The efferent pathway may also assist in the resolution of intensity information. Cochlear nerve fibers have a limited range — approximately 30 dB in the cat — and the thresholds tend to be around 0—20 dB SL, thus leaving uncertain how the coding of intensity information for loud signals or signals in noise is accomplished (KIANG, 1968). The efferent pathway might raise the threshold of certain auditory nerve fibers such that their range would then encompass the higher intensity sounds (NIEDER and NIEDER, 1970; WIEDERHOLD, 1970). Cutting the olivo-cochlear bundle impairs signal-in-noise discriminations which are performed at relatively high intensity levels (DEWSON, 1968; TRAHIOTIS and ELLIOT, 1970).

2. Decreased Synaptic Efficiency Theories

This type of theory can be traced to SHERRINGTON (1906) who attributed the decrement in reflex strength with stimulus repetition to a synaptic "fatigue". The concept of progressive synaptic depression has recently been reformulated by SHARPLESS (1964), THOMPSON and SPENCER (1966), HORN (1967), and SEGUNDO and BELL (1970) and has received impressive neurophysiological support from studies of the gill withdrawal reflex of *Aplysia* (KUPFERMAN *et al.*, 1970, CASTELLUCCI *et al.*, 1970) and of the leg flexion reflex of the spinal cat (GROVES and THOMPSON, 1970).

In *Aplysia* the EPSP in the motor neuron sub-serving gill withdrawal decreases in size with repetitive stimulation of an afferent nerve. This effect was not due to adaptation of the afferent nerve or to a cumulative post-synaptic inhibitory process, since it was not altered by hyper-polarization of the cell membrane beyond the equilibrium potential of the IPSP. Accordingly, CASTELLUCI *et al.* ascribed this habituation to a decrease in synaptic efficiency and distinguished its mechanism from that of dishabituation, produced by an unknown facilitatory input to the cell (possibly heterosynaptic facilitation; KANDEL and TAUC, 1965). Dishabituating stimuli in these preparations were found to enhance non-habituated EPSPs (CAREW *et al.*, 1971) and were therefore considered as "sensitizing" rather than simply a relieving of the habituation process.

In reviewing their work with the leg flexion reflex in the cat, GROVES and THOMPSON (1970) described a habituating system having properties very similar to the *Aplysia* gill reflex. They proposed that some of the synapses in the flexion reflex pathway become less effective as a stimulus is repeated; in other words, the habituating property is intrinsic to this type of synapse. A habituating synapse may also be sensitized by a "state system" that is activated by a strong or novel stimulus, and this activation itself also habituates upon repetition of the sensitizing stimulus. Studying single units of the spinal cord, GROVES and THOMPSON described three basic kinds of responses: the non-plastic response that remains stable upon stimulus repetition; the habituating response, which declines as a stimulus is repeated; and the sensitizing response which initially increases and then begins to decline after a few stimuli. These latter types of units were said to be influenced by a "state system" which in intact animals most likely comes under the control of higher centers.

GROVES and LYNCH (1972) have recently extended these concepts to cover the habituating properties of sensory neurons in the brainstem. They proposed that habituation of the reticular activating system is largely effected by the parvicellular "associational" neurons of the brainstem reticular formation, which undergo habituation and sensitization similar to that described for spinal interneurons. They also point to the intimate anatomical connections between these reticular neurons and the hippocampus and frontal lobe which have been implicated in many forms of habituation.

3. Memory Comparison Theories

In order to account for the stimulus specificity of habituation, various "memory-comparison" or "model-making" theories have been proposed. The essential feature of these hypotheses is that sensory data reaching the cerebral cortex is compared with stimulus information held in memory, presumbably in the form of an active cell assembly called a "neuronal model" (SOKOLOV, 1960, 1963a and b) or a "gnostic unit" (KONORSKI, 1967). In SOKOLOV's formulation, stimulus repetition leads to the forging of a highly specific neuronal model in the cortex, and when the anticipated stimulus that "fits" the model occurs, an efferent inhibition is applied to the collateral transmission of sensory impulses into the reticular arousal system. If a stimulus is so novel as not to fit with any available model, the reticular formation is no longer inhibited and an orienting response is triggered. The orienting response activates the cortex, as evidenced by EEG desynchronization, thereby permitting a new model or gnostic unit to be formed to receive the new stimulus. Habituation is thus considered to be cortical inhibition of the reticular arousal response upon stimulus repetition.

It has recently been proposed on the basis of microelectrode recordings that it is the hippocampus which registers incoming information, encodes it into a "model", and thereby controls the activity of the reticular formation to prevent orientation to familiar signals (VINOGRADOVA, 1970). A novel stimulus which finds no appropriate model in the so-called "extrapolatory" (memory) neurons elicits inhibition of a population of hippocampal cells which normally hold the reticular arousal response in check. In keeping with this concept, REDDING (1967) has shown that hippocampal stimulation decreases the auditory cortical evoked potential, which may be enhanced by reticular stimulation. It has also been suggested that the hippocampus functions to inhibit learned behavior (KIMBLE, 1967), with the release of motor behavior accompanied by a burst of rhythmic hippocampal theta waves (VANDERWOLF, 1970). This suggests that the hippocampus functions in general as an inhibitor of inappropriate perceptual and motor responses, with theta activity signifying their disinhibition. Different frequencies of hippocampal theta (ELAZAR and ADEY, 1967; LOPES da SILVA and KAMP, 1969) could reflect the disinhibition of separate cell populations which control the various aspects of sensory and motor behavior.

The comparator theory accounts well for the triggering of the orienting response to an omitted stimulus in a habituation paradigm: when an expected stimulus is not forthcoming, the discordance between stimulus and neuronal model results in reticular activation and orientation. Additional mechanisms must exist, however, for habituating the cortical arousal response, since auditory-evoked EEG desynchronization still habituates after complete ablation of the auditory cortex (SHARPLESS and JASPER, 1956). This effect might be explained by postulating a decline of synaptic efficiency in brainstem reticular neurons driven by simple tonal stimuli, with a superimposed cortical (comparator) system to encode a higher order of stimulus specificity.

E. Summary of Auditory Habituation Mechanisms

From the animal and human evidence reviewed above a tentative picture of the salient neural mechanisms underlying auditory habituation can be formulated. The initial synapses of the auditory lemniscal pathways are, like those of the spinal cord, relatively immune to habituation although displaying those refractory period phenomena known as rate effects. The interneurons of the reflex pathways which branch off the lemniscal route habituate to a greater or lesser degree and are subject to sensitization by neurons of the reticular formation. Thus the auditory reflexes organized within the brainstem, such as the startle, cardiac and middle ear muscle responses, probably habituate along lines similar to those proposed by GROVES and THOMPSON for the flexion reflex. The efferent auditory system does not appear to participate in habituation of auditory input but rather acts as part of a feedback system controlled by the acoustic properties of the stimulus and improves the resolution of sensory information. The reticular formation, as well as sensitizing the brainstem auditory reflexes, activates the cerebral cortex as evidenced by the arousal and orienting responses.

The properties of the auditory vertex potential in man, as revealed by studies of intra- and cross-modal interaction and habituation, indicate that it represents a combination of both lemniscal and non-specific-reticular influences upon the frontal association cortex. The habituation of cortical activation as indexed by the vertex potential may be inferred to result from two processes: first, the input to the reticular formation from the lemniscal pathway, which habituates directly; and second, a cortico-reticular path that inhibits reticular activation when a repeating stimulus comes to be expected or loses its importance, and disinhibits it when attention is required to the signal.

IV. Attention

A. Concepts of Selective Attention

Selective attention is defined as a central nervous system function that allows perceptual or motor responses to be made selectively to one aspect of a total stimulus configuration in preference to others; competing, "irrelevant" messages are either partially or completely rejected from perceptual experience and control over behavior. By virtue of their selective influence upon sensory processing, attentional processes are to be distinguished from generalized activation, alerting, mobilization, arousal, excitability, and the like, which influence a broad spectrum of sensory inputs non-selectively.

James (1890) differentiated between two varieties of attention — passive and active. Passive attention involves the inquisitory orientation reaction to an unexpected or novel stimulus, whereas active attention involves the directed examination of a particular expected sensory message. Active attention is mediated by a variety of mechanisms, among which James identified "the accommodation and adjustment of the sensory organs; and the anticipatory preparation from within of the ideational centres concerned with the object to which the attention is paid" (p. 434).

Within the past two decades attentional processes have come under renewed psychological and neurophysiological scrutiny. Prior to this, experiments tended to follow the behavioristic *Zeitgeist*, with only one stimulus presented and one response required; the need to postulate an intervening selective process was thus obviated and the stimulus-response connection became the basic tenet of psychology. The striking selectivity of perception that was revealed in such complex multi-stimulus tasks as the binaural listening paradigm of Cherry (1953), however, made the examination of attentional processes mandatory.

1. Levels of Stimulus Selection

Current psychological approaches to the problem of selective perception generally entail a series of "information processing" stages, which may include: an initial sensory feature analysis, a short-term memory or "buffer store" of input, a perceptual and semantic content analysis during which specific objects and events are recognized, and a decision system for selecting those stimuli most worthy of response. The simplest conceptual approach to selective attention has been to postulate a "filter" which blocks or attenuates the processing of some categories of stimuli more than others. Broadbent (1958) initially proposed that such a filter was situated rather peripherally, blocking the sensory message (from, say, the unattended ear during dichotic listening) immediately after the buffer storage stage. Treisman, however, placed the filter somewhat more centrally, allowing some perceptual analysis (but not verbal content analysis) to precede the filtering operation (Treisman, 1964; Treisman and Geffen, 1967). Theories by Selfridge (1959) and Deutsch and Deutsch (1963), in contrast, have asserted that all sensory inputs are fully analyzed for content and significance before any selection takes place. Treisman (1969) has categorized these "early" and "late" conceptions of stimulus selection in terms of: "selection of inputs" (analagous to a peripheral filter), "selection of analyzer" (for analysis of the stimulus along particular physical or conceptual dimensions), "selection of targets" (specific target stimuli are recognized), and "selection of outputs" (attachment of responses to some of the fully analyzed stimuli).

In BROADBENT's (1971) more recent formulation, he distinguishes between two fundamental modes of stimulus selection, termed "stimulus set" and "response set". Stimulus-set attention operates by selectively blocking or attenuating some sensory "channels" more than others, a channel being defined as a stimulus category possessing a simple attribute (*e.g.* pitch, color, spatial position) or falling upon a contiguous receptor surface (*e.g.* one ear or one retinal locus). The response set mode operates after this attenuator and involves the serial comparison of more or less analyzed stimulus patterns against a set of memory representations ("templates", "categories" or "dictionary units") for the selected target stimuli. A matching of stimulus to template leads to recognition and selective response. This response set concept recalls again JAMES' (1890) view of attention as "the creation of an imaginary duplicate of the object in the mind, which shall stand ready to receive the outward impression as if in a matrix" (p. 439).

Under normal circumstances, human attentive strategy requires the interaction of both modes of attention. At the celebrated "cocktail party", for example, it is necessary to establish a stimulus set which favors the location and pitch of the attended speaker's voice, and a succession of anticipatory response sets to recognize the ongoing stream of words. In such situations, however, when stimulus set mechanisms direct attention to one channel, a highly "biased" response set (such as for one's own name) may still permit the recognition of that stimulus spoken over a different channel.

The response set idea has been elaborated in various cybernetic or "analysis by synthesis" theories of perception (MILLER *et al.*, 1960; LIBERMAN *et al.*, 1963; NEISSER, 1967; HOCHBERG, 1970; MACKAY, 1970). This type of theory asserts that sensory information is attended to (and recognized) on the basis of its matching internal stimulus analogs which are generated in advance according to the subject's expectancy or "best guess" as to what the stimulus will be and continually "updated" by comparison to the actual sensory input. A succession of templates may, thus, be generated until a satisfactory match has been achieved. The subject makes and perceives a model of the world that is compared to and revised with his sensory input; what is not well encoded in such a model must go unattended.

B. Physiological Correlates of Auditory Attention in Man

1. Stability of Cochlear and Brainstem Responses

We have studied the behavior of the early and middle latency waves of the click-evoked potential during a task where attention is directed towards a repetitive sequence of clicks in order to detect (and count) an occasional, slightly fainter click (PICTON *et al.*, 1971; PICTON and HILLYARD, 1974). Attending to the clicks does not alter either the cochlear nerve response (Fig. 11) or the brainstem and mid-latency waves (Fig. 12) evoked by the "standard", higher intensity click; the control records are made when the subject ignores the click by reading or doing mental arithmetic. These results indicate that the auditory input is analyzed in a relatively stable fashion for the first 40—50 msec, regardless of the direction of attention. In these experiments, the stability of the early evoked potential components to attentional manipulation contrasted with the substantial changes occurring in the vertex potential.

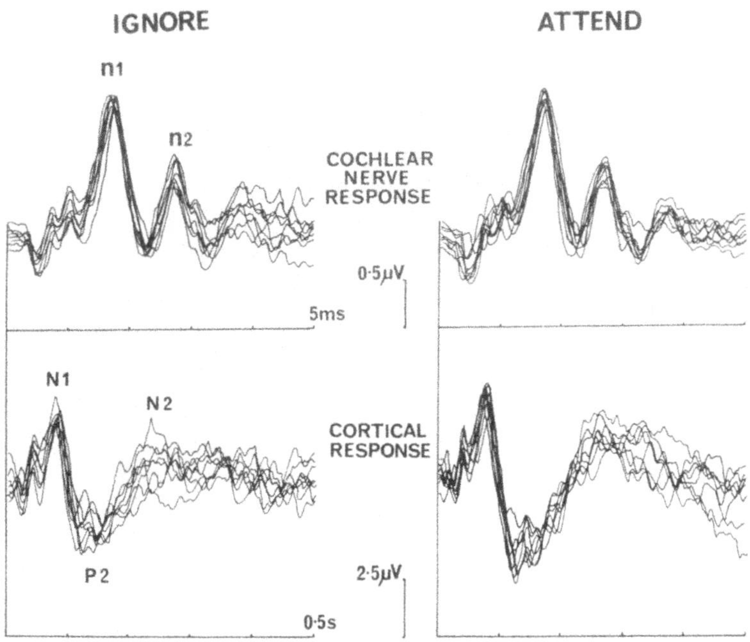

Fig. 11. Effects of attention at cochlea and cortex. 55dB SL clicks were presented every 1.3 sec. In the "attend" condition the subject was asked to count the number of faint 51dB SL clicks occurring occasionally in the ongoing train. In the "ignore" condition the subject read a book. Cochlear nerve responses were recorded from an electrode in the external auditory meatus and cortical responses were recorded from vertex mastoid electrodes. Each tracing represents the average of 256 responses. (Based on Picton *et al.*, 1971)

2. The Auditory Vertex Potential

A large number of studies are in agreement that the amplitude of the vertex potential, usually measured as the N_1-P_2 peak to peak amplitude, is increased when attention is shifted towards an auditory stimulus (Davis, 1964; Gross *et al.*, 1965; Wilkinson and Morlock, 1967; Keating and Ruhm, 1971; Picton *et al.*, 1971; Picton and Hillyard, 1974) (Figs. 11 and 12). While it is possible that these effects upon the vertex potential reflect selectivity of attention, the experiments are open to criticism since they did not control for possible differences in non-selective arousal or alertness between the attending and ignoring conditions. Such differences in the subject's overall state might have produced AEP differences that were independent from any selective attention effect. It seems unlikely, however, that differences in arousal (wakefulness) existed between attend and ignore conditions, because the evoked potential signs of lowered arousal — mainly an increase in N_2 amplitude — should have overshadowed the N_1-P_2 effects that were observed.

In order to obviate any possible effect that tonic arousal level might have on the AEPs, other experiments presented auditory stimuli in alternation with some other stimulus while the subject attended to one and ignored the other. Again, when attention was directed towards the auditory stimulus, the N_1-P_2 measure of the vertex potential was typically enhanced (Spong *et al.*, 1965; Satterfield, 1965; Debecker and Desmedt, 1966; Sheatz and Chapman, 1969). In these experiments, however, the occurrence of relevant (attended) and irrelevant (ignored) stimuli was predictable, and thus subjects might have altered their state of arousal phasically in anticipation of the known stimulus. Using long time constant amplifiers, Naatanen (1967) showed that in such experiments

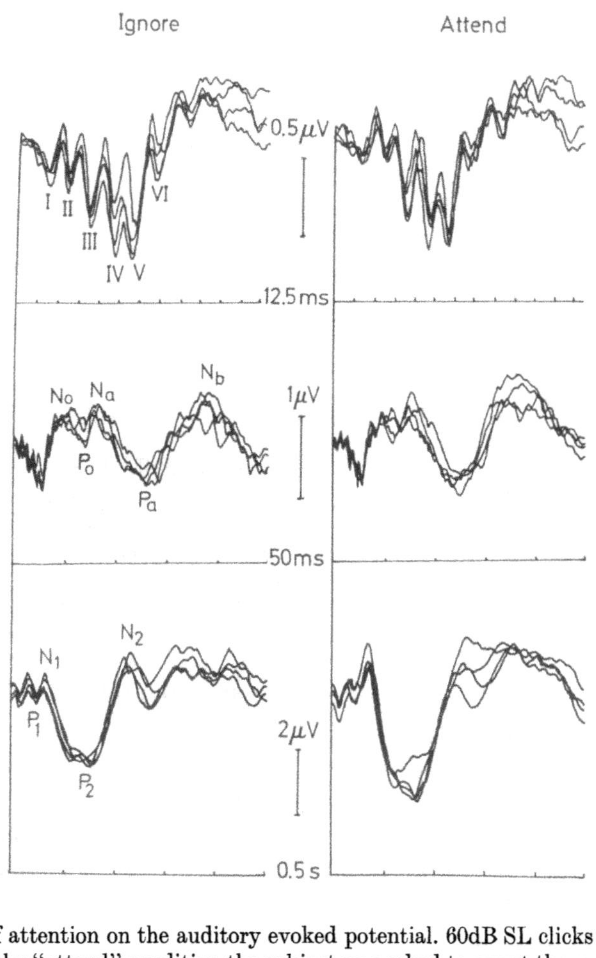

Fig. 12. Effects of attention on the auditory evoked potential. 60dB SL clicks were presented every second. In the "attend" condition the subject was asked to count the number of fainter signals occasionally occurring in the ongoing train. In the "ignore" condition the subject read a book and disregarded the click stimuli. Evoked potentials were recorded from vertex to mastoid electrodes and averaged using three separate time scales. Each tracing of the four replicated tracings represents the average of 1024 responses. (Picton and Hillyard, 1974)

there was a slowly waxing and waning negativity (CNV) over the vertex area, with a maximum amplitude occurring at the time of delivery of the relevant stimuli. Thus he reasoned that changes in AEPs may not reflect selective perception but rather the "non-specific and preparatory arousal and activation preceding relevant stimuli". In accordance with this postulate, the effect of attention upon the auditory vertex potential disappeared when relevant and irrelevant stimuli were presented in a randomized order making any differential preparatory state impossible (NAATANEN, 1967; HARTLEY, 1970; SMITH *et al.*, 1970). However, these randomized stimuli were presented at rates slow enough to permit subjects to attend indiscriminately and non-selectively to both relevant and irrelevant stimuli. To quote HARTLEY (1970): "Stimuli are presented at such a slow rate that it is well within the subject's capacity to handle the information on both channels should they wish to do so, even if experimental instructions do not require it".

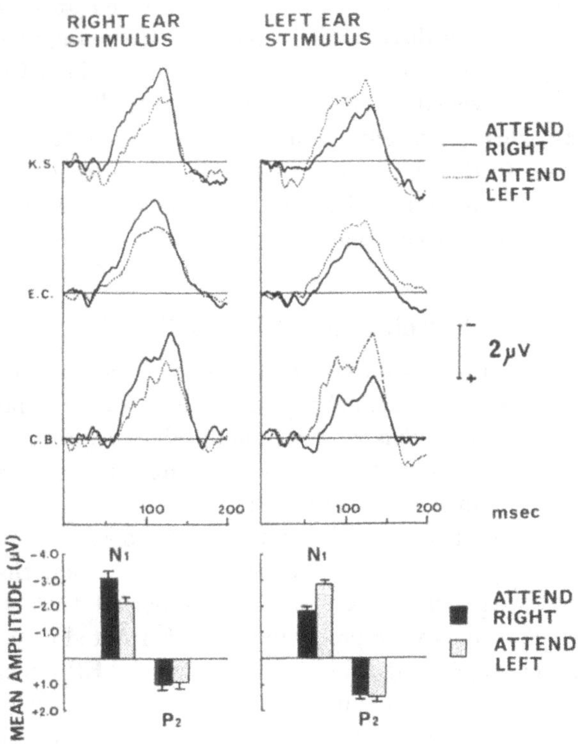

Fig. 13. Effects of selective binaural attention on the auditory evoked potential. A random sequence of 800Hz tones were presented to the right ear and a concurrent series of 1500Hz tones to the left such that it was impossible to predict either the timing of the next stimulus or the ear to which it was presented. An occasional stimulus was a signal of higher frequency (840Hz on right and 1560Hz on left). Subjects attended to one ear at a time and counted the number of signals occurring in that ear. Each tracing represents the average response of 1024 stimuli presented to each ear under attend-right (solid line) or attend-left (dotted line) conditions. Bar graphs give the mean and standard error for 10 subjects of the baseline-peak amplitudes of $N1$ and $P2$ evoked via each ear under each attention condition. (HILLYARD *et al.*, 1973)

Wilkinson and Lee (1972) also reasoned that slow rates of stimulus delivery might not succeed in "forcing" the subjects to attend selectively, and accordingly presented a random sequence of three types of tone pips differing in frequency at a rapid rate (every 300—1760 msec). They found that counting one of the three stimuli enhanced its evoked N_1-P_2 component by about 10%, an effect the authors attributed to an augmentation of P_2 by a D.C. baseline shift subsequent to signal recognition, rather than to selective attention.

Following up this line of investigation, we presented relevant and irrelevant auditory stimuli over two separate channels (the two ears) at such a high rate and level of difficulty as to restrict attention to one channel at a time. A substantial enhancement (30—50%) of the N_1 wave occurred when attention was confined to one ear's input in both a binaural click-pattern discrimination (Picton *et al.*, 1971) and frequency discrimination (Hillyard *et al.*, 1973). Results of the latter experiment are shown in Fig. 13: tones of two different frequencies were presented rapidly (every 100—800 msec) and unpredictably to the two ears while the subject attended to one ear at a time and detected an occasional shift in frequency that was barely discernable. This attention manipulation resulted in a reciprocal enhancement of the N_1 wave to stimuli in the attended ear and a decrement in the N_1 evoked by contralateral stimuli. This effect upon N_1 was attributed to "stimulus set" attention directed towards the stimuli in the attended ear. The conclusion of a decade of controversy then seems to be that the amplitude of the vertex potential does indeed reflect the direction of the subject's selective attention independently from whatever effects may ensue from non-selective changes of state.

3. Specificity of the Vertex Potential

The foregoing experiments provide evidence that the auditory vertex potential is larger when a sensory channel has been selected by a stimulus set mechanism. There are also indications that its amplitude, waveform and topography may reflect in part the subsequent cognitive, linguistic, or attribute analysis performed on the stimulus. Wood *et al.* (1971) found that the interhemispheric symmetry of the vertex potential was shifted more towards the left (dominant) hemisphere when a signal was analyzed for linguistic content than for its pitch. Morrell and Salamy (1971) have similarly reported that auditory vertex potentials to speech sounds were predominantly distributed over the hemisphere dominant for speech, suggesting that an asymmetrical AEP somehow reflects the hemispheric specialization for language processing. An alternative interpretation of these effects, however, was proposed by Matsumiya *et al.* (1970), who concluded that the difficulty of making a discrimination determined the asymmetry of the AEP more so than did its verbal content. Finally, Gardiner and Walter (1969) have reported that the waveform of the AEP by a tone pip is slightly different when its frequency rather than its intensity is being discriminated. This evidence suggests that the vertex potential may reflect the type of selectivity of processing which Treisman has termed "selection of the analyzer".

An intriguing experiment by Weinberg *et al.* (1970) suggests that the vertex potential may have a substantial "endogenous" character, being determined in part by the subject's expectancy of which stimulus will be perceived, whether or not it actually occurs. Their subjects pressed a lever one way or the other denoting whether or not they expected to hear a click; if a click was expected but not presented, an "emitted" potential was recorded from intracerebral and extradural electrodes in frontal cortex which resembled that evoked by an actual click. While it was not established that these emitted potentials were completely equivalent to the actual AEP, the suggestion that the vertex potential represents in part the subject's hypothesis of which stimulus should occur might mean that the cybernetic perceptual operations described above are amenable to physiological study.

The magnitude and distribution of the vertex potential is thus determined by several conditions: the physical attributes of the stimulus, the direction of selective attention, and the type of content analysis performed on the signal.

4. The Contingent Negative Variation (CNV)

If a subject anticipates the occurrence of a stimulus that will require his attention and/or motor response, a negative slow potential shift (CNV) develops prior to the signal and returns to baseline thereafter (WALTER *et al.*, 1964). Subsequent studies by WALTER (1965) made it clear that the CNV occurs prior to interesting or informative stimuli which command attention, and he suggested that the CNV served as an electrocortical sign of "expectancy", of which motor preparation was a special case. It has been well documented since WALTER's pioneering studies that these negative slow potentials occur in conjunction with motor acts without sensory stimuli and with sensory discriminations without motor response. This raises the fundamental question of whether "the CNV" is a unitary and generalized phenomenom or whether it can be subdivided into classes of slow potentials specific to particular psychological operations (CANT and BICKFORD, 1967).

The pre-motor "readiness potential" (KORNHUBER and DEECKE, 1965) can be examined alone by having a subject respond on his own volition, rather than to any external signal, and by computer averaging both backwards and forwards from the motor response. For about a second prior to a finger movement a slow negative baseline shift of 5—10 μV (the readiness potential) builds up, having a scalp distribution overlying both pre- and post-central gyri and slightly larger over the Rolandic cortex contralateral to the moving joint (GILDEN *et al.*, 1966; GERBRANDT *et al.*, 1973). Following the readiness potential is a sharp negative-positive complex which may well represent the somatosensory evoked potential to the joint movement (GERBRANDT *et al.*, 1973). Prior to spontaneous speech the readiness potential is largest over the frontal lobe of the dominant hemisphere (MCADAM and WHITAKER, 1971). It has not been established whether the readiness potential is generated by the specific patterned neuronal activity responsible for initiating the movement or by some other aspect of cortical function. MCADAM and SEALES (1969) found that when demands are placed upon the spontaneous movement the readiness potential is greatly enhanced, suggesting that it increased with the subject's motivation. However, since this incrementing of the readiness potential by task demands was bilaterally symmetrical, it might be interpreted as a separate slow potential component reflecting the arousal properties of the task which is summated upon the asymmetrical readiness potential.

A purely sensory CNV or expectancy wave has been observed in numerous types of tasks, prior to stimuli which require a perceptual discrimination, a decision, attentive examination, or when they deliver significant information without an immediate motor response (*e.g.* Faidherbe and Deliege, 1968; Donchin *et al.*, 1972). The CNV is now widely recognized as an active ingredient in practically all attention/evoked potential paradigms in which stimuli can be anticipated beforehand, and its modes of interaction with the AEP have become a subject of hot debate (Karlin, 1970; Teuting and Sutton, 1972). The amplitude of the perceptual CNV depends upon the interest value or motivational quality of the stimulus (Cohen and Walter, 1966), the sex of the subject (Knott and Peters, 1973), the meaningfulness of the information (Picton and Low, 1971; Weinberg, 1972), and the difficulty of the perceptual task (Low *et al.*, 1967).

A number of studies have examined the question of whether the size of the CNV prior to a perceptual task is related to the accuracy or selectivity of the subsequent decision or discrimination. From these reports one can only conclude that the relationship of the CNV to perceptual accuracy, when present, is small and inconsistent. In a series of signal detection tasks, Hillyard (1969) and Hillyard *et al.* (1971) found that CNVs preceding correct threshold stimulus detections were slightly larger than before incorrect judgments. In a highly similar task, however, Paul and Sutton (1972) obtained no such relation between CNV amplitude and correctness of decisions. In an auditory intensity discrimination, Wilkinson and Haines (1970) observed a correlation over time between CNV amplitude and percent correct judgments; on the other hand, Jarvilehto and Fruhstorfer (1970) found no such correlation in a similar paradigm. Using visual discriminanda, larger CNVs were reported to precede correct decisions (McAdam and Rubin, 1971; Cohen, 1973), but these reports can be balanced against the negative results obtained in two types of auditory frequency discriminations (Jenness, 1972; Delse *et al.*, 1972).

In the Delse *et al.* report, moreover, females were found to have larger CNVs (on one block of trials) preceding *incorrect* perceptual judgements. The small amplitude of the feminine CNVs, however, suggests an interpretation of this "paradoxical" CNV effect, and perhaps some of the aforementioned negative results, in terms of variations of a "baseline" D.C. level upon which CNVs may be superimposed (Knott and Irwin, 1967). It has been reported that females show relatively smaller CNVs under stressful circumstances than do males (Knott and Peters, 1973; Low and Swift, 1971), which could have resulted from an increased negativity of a hypothetical resting D.C. baseline in the more stressed females, so that their CNVs "saturated" against a ceiling voltage. Thus, a relaxation of the subject might reduce the resting negativity and permit a larger phasic CNV to occur, but in conjunction with poorer perceptual performance.

This hypothetical D.C. baseline factor could be responsible for the generally poor association between the CNV and behavioral measures (Hillyard, 1973). Another consideration is that a highly attentive subject is likely to have a large CNV on each trial (or a highly negative tonic D.C. baseline), small variations of which would not relate to perceptual acuity. On the other hand, a subject who is drowsy or uninvolved and makes an inconsistent effort from trial to trial will have large variations in CNV amplitude which ought to be correlated with performance. Given these complicating factors and the unresolved inconsistencies among published reports, it seems premature to conclude that the CNV indexes any selective processes (such as attention) in anticipation of a task signal.

Despite its questionable psychological specificity, there is growing evidence that CNVs are task-specific in their scalp topography and, inferentially, in their cerebral generators. JARVILEHTO and FRUHSTORFER (1970) reported that the CNV associated with an auditory discrimination is more frontally localized than that associated with motor preparation, and that the classical (warn-respond) CNV seemed to represent a combination of these two phenomena. The CNV preceding a visual discrimination is reportedly distributed more posteriorly than that prior to an auditory discrimination (COHEN, 1973; SYNDULKO, 1972). Figure 14 illustrates a distributional analysis of CNVs preceding sensory and motor tasks. Prior to an auditory discrimination the CNV is largest fronto-centrally,

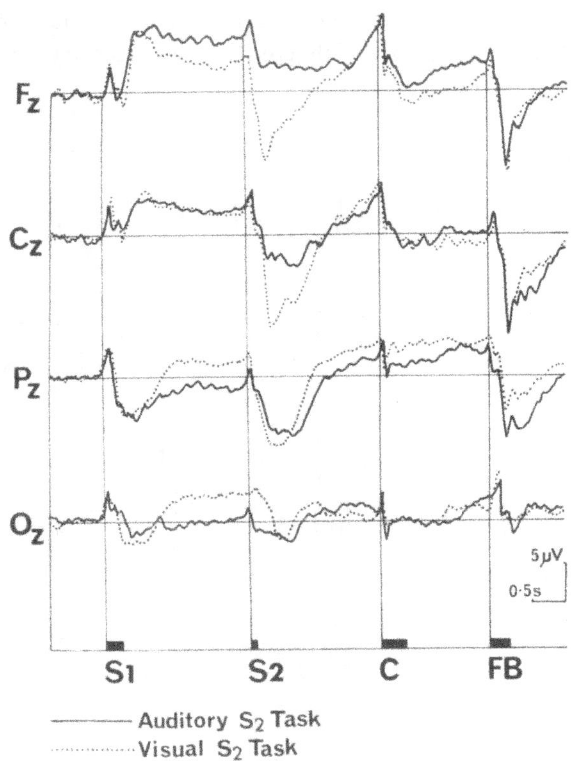

Fig. 14. Slow potential shifts during perceptual tasks. A visual stimulus ($S1$) informed the subject on each trial whether a visual or an auditory task was to be performed at $S2$. The visual task was the recognition of a tachistoscopically presented number; the auditory task was the discrimination of a tonal frequency. The subject then responded at an auditory command signal (C) and received visual feedback (FB) as to whether or not he was correct. Responses were obtained at several scalp locations so as to compare the scalp distribution of the slow potentials during auditory (continuous line) and visual (dotted line) tasks. Each tracing represents the average of 40 trials. D.C. amplification

but before a visual discrimination it is more widerspread, with a posterior focus of negativity: in preparation for a motor response (to stimulus "C") the CNV was maximum at the vertex, as reported by COHEN (1969). Individual subjects were found to display variants on this pattern of topography. Whether the greater frontal negativity of the pre-auditory CNVs reflects selectivity of attention or a more diffuse general excitability of frontal neurons remains to be determined. It may well turn out, however, that the CNV distribution provides a "map" of the cortical areas involved in a particular preparatory activity, without signifying anything of the detailed information processing occurring within those regions (HILLYARD, 1973).

5. Late Positive Component (P_3)

The long latency (300—500 msec) positive wave known as the P_3 was described first by WALTER (1965), following a complex, "semantic" stimulus and by SUTTON *et al.* (1965), after a feedback cue which resolved the subject's uncertainty. In a subsequent study, SUTTON *et al.* (1967) established the important principle that P_3 is triggered at the point in time when significant or task-relevant information is delivered, whether delivered by the intensity of a cue or by its

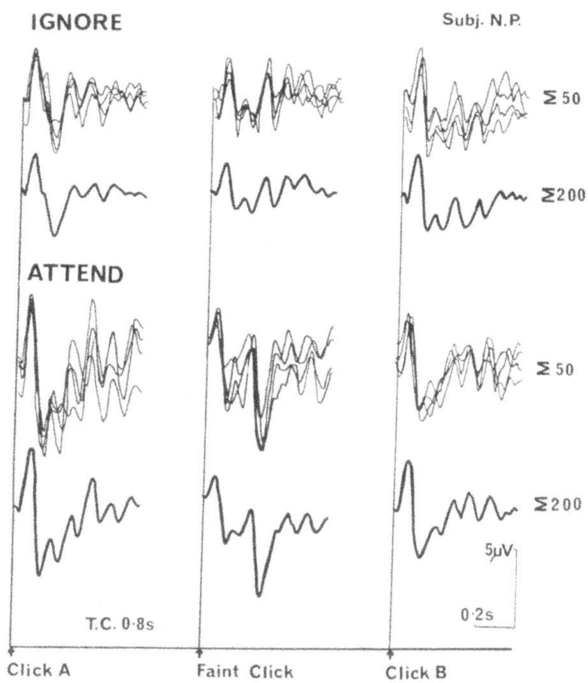

Fig. 15. Evoked potentials following a detected "target" signal. Clicks were presented every 1.3 sec and occasionally the intensity of one was decreased slightly. Averaged evoked responses are shown to the standard clicks immediately preceding (A) and following (B) the faint click and to the faint click itself under conditions of "ignore" (subject reading) and "attend". For each evoked response four averages over 50 epochs are superimposed and the overall average is shown beneath (PICTON *et al.*, 1974b)

presence or absence. An auditory discrimination experiment of RITTER and VAUGHAN (1969) indicated, moreover, that only the delivery of some of the task-relevant stimuli elicited the P_3 component. They presented tone pips at one per 3 sec, some of which (about one in ten) were slightly fainter "signals" which the subject listened for; a P_3 wave was elicited only after the correctly identified signals, and not after the "standard" intensity tone pips. RITTER and VAUGHAN (1969) interpreted this P_3 as a sign of an orientation reaction towards the target signal and a "cognitive evaluation" of it.

Numerous studies have subsequently verified that a P_3 wave is triggered by an occasional "target" stimulus that is being searched for among an equal or greater number of non-target stimuli. The P_3 elicited upon the detection of a slightly fainter target click in the vigilance paradigm described previously is shown in Fig. 15 (attend condition). No P_3 component is discernable for the standard intensity clicks preceding (A) or following (B) the target. In Fig. 16 the comparison is made between AEPs to standard versus signal clicks for the early, middle, and long-latency recordings in another subject, in both attend and inattend conditions. Paying attention does not influence any component prior to

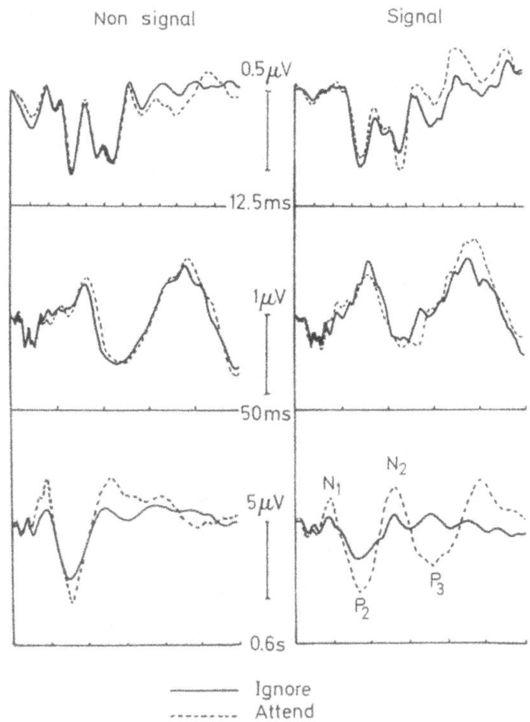

Fig. 16. Evoked potentials to "standard" and "signal" stimuli. Clicks were presented every second and could be either "standard" (60dB SL) or "signal" (50dB SL). In the "attend" condition the subject counted the number of signal stimuli which occurred as approximately 20% of the clicks. In the "ignore" condition he read a book. Evoked potentials in each condition were recorded over three separate time epochs. The effects of attention are limited to the late components of the evoked potential. (PICTON and HILLYARD, 1974)

the N_1-P_2 complex, which is augmented for both signal and standard click in the attend condition. The P_3, however, only follows the attended signals.

The P_3 wave is also elicited upon the detection of a signal that is near threshold in intensity (Hillyard, 1969; Hillyard et al., 1971; Squires et al., 1973b). The amplitude of P_3 grows with the subject's level of confidence (rated on an eight point scale) that he heard the signal, and is small or absent for equally confident reports of signal absence (correct rejections). In a similar threshold level signal detection paradigm, Paul and Sutton (1972) found that the P_3 on

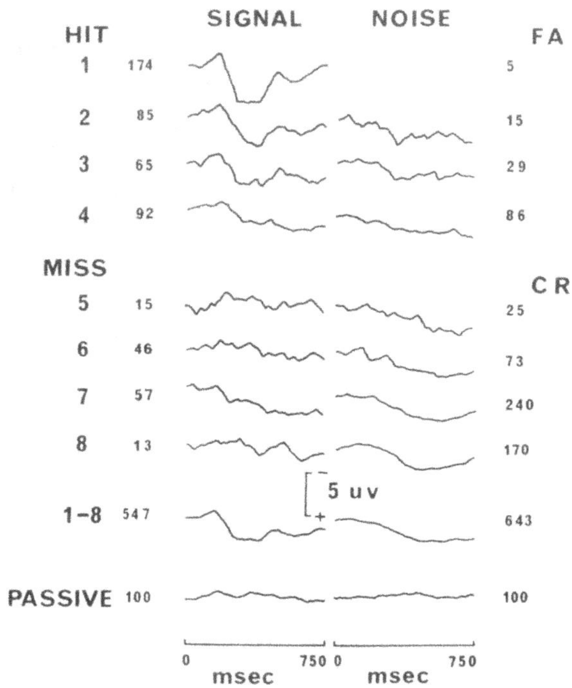

Fig. 17. Confidence rating and magnitude of $P3$ to detected threshold stimuli. Following a warning flash subject was presented with a threshold level 50 msec 1kHz tone in noise with a probability of 0.5. After a delay subject reported as to whether or not he heard the stimulus along a 1—8 confidence scale; 1 meaning high confidence about the presence of a signal and 8 meaning high confidence about its absence. Responses could therefore be grouped into hits, misses, false alarms and correct rejections. A passive control evoked potential was also recorded while the subject read a book and ignored the stimuli (Squires et al., 1973b)

Hits (correct detections) increased as the decision criterion was experimentally elevated; this was also interpreted as resulting from a higher confidence or certainty in the Hit decisions which had to surpass a raised decision criterion. The scalp distribution of the P_3 wave which accompanies detection of a threshold level tone pip is shown in Fig. 18 in comparison with that of the N_1-P_2 waves evoked by a much louder (but unattended) tone pip in the same subject. The P_3 has a much broader amplitude distribution laterally and posteriorly, indicating that it is not simply a delayed P_2 wave but a separate component having a different cerebral source. A similarly widespread and posterior topography has been reported for the P_3's evoked in the orientation (VAUGHAN and RITTER, 1970) and omitted stimulus (PICTON *et al.*, 1974b) paradigms.

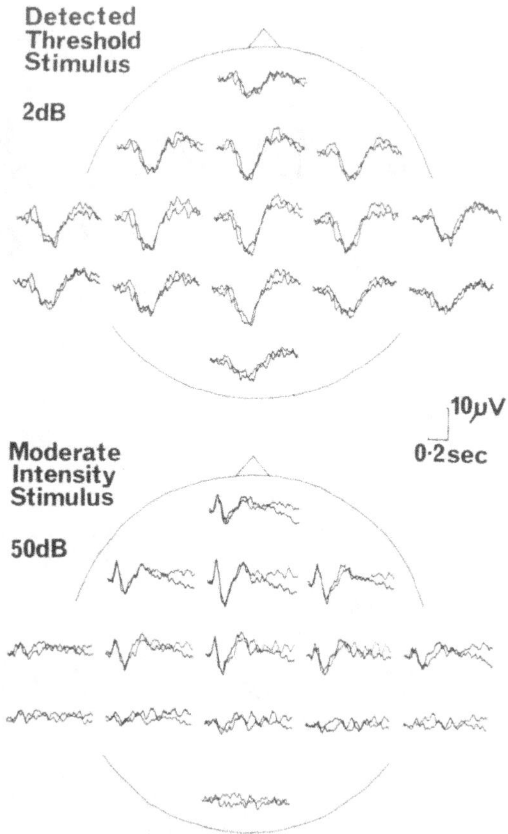

Fig. 18. $N1$-$P2$-$P3$ scalp distributions. The upper part of the figure shows the distribution of the large positive wave following a correctly detected threshold stimulus in a signal detection task. Each tracing represents the average of 30 responses. The lower portion of the figure represents the $N1$-$P2$ components of the auditory evoked potential to a moderate intensity toneburst that the subject is ignoring. Each tracing is the average of 60 responses. All responses were obtained using a chest reference electrode

The endogenous nature of the P_3 is emphasized when the "target" stimulus to be detected is the occasional omission of a stimulus from a repetitive train (KLINKE *et al.*, 1968; BARLOW, 1969; PICTON *et al.*, 1974b). As seen in Fig. 19, the P_3 is largest when the subject is actively counting the omissions, but is still present (in a delayed and attenuated form) when the clicks are being ignored, suggesting that the reading subject is still "registering" the target stimuli (see also RITTER *et al.*, 1968; ROTH, 1973). The P_3 wave has also been observed following the detection of a wide variety of target stimuli including:

clicks among a series of spoken words (SMITH *et al.*, 1970) one visual pattern or color amongst others (HARTER and SALMON, 1972), shifts of pitch in a series of tone pips (HILLYARD *et al.*, 1973; WILKINSON and LEE, 1972), a letter which completes a word (SHELBURNE, 1972), noise bursts amidst clicks and flashes (FORD *et al.*, 1973) and many others.

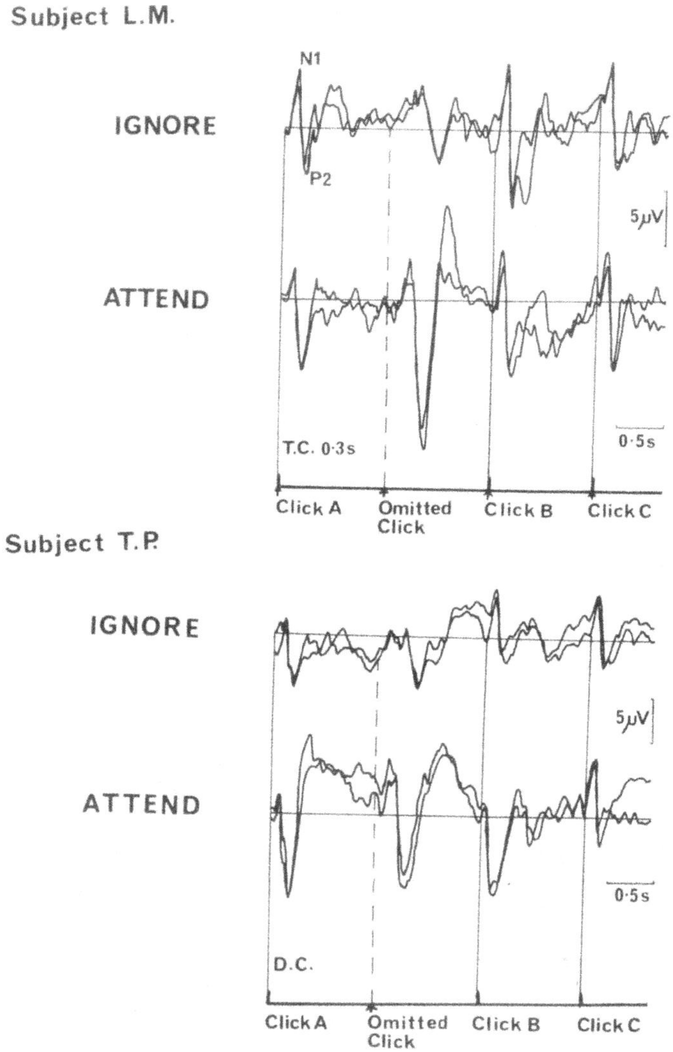

Fig. 19. Cortical potentials evoked by clicks and by omitted clicks. Clicks were presented once every 1.1 sec and occasionally one was omitted. The averaging computer was triggered by Click A immediately preceeding the omitted click and averaging was continued for four seconds. In each of the "attend" and "ignore" conditions, two separate average traces are superimposed to show the reproducibility of the results. In the upper set of traces averaging was done over 64 epochs from AC recordings whereas in the lower traces averaging was done over 32 epochs from DC recordings. All recordings were from vertex to mastoid electrodes, vertex negativity being represented by an upward deflection. (PICTON *et al.*, 1974b)

This extensive literature suggests that P_3 is associated with making a certain type of perceptual decision (HILLYARD, 1969; SMITH *et al.*, 1970; PICTON *et al.*, 1974b) — namely, the recognition of a specific target signal to which a particular cognitive or motor response is required. The temporal relation of P_3 to this decision has been assessed by several approaches. Longer P_3 latencies accompany those perceptual decisions that entail longer reaction times (RTs), such as "mismatch" as opposed to "match" decisions (POSNER *et al.*, 1973) and more difficult visual discriminations (DONCHIN, personal communication). Moreover, variability in RT has been reasonably well correlated with variability of P_3 latency during intensity discrimination (RITTER *et al.*, 1972) and omitted stimulus (PICTON *et al.*, 1974b) tasks. As shown in Fig. 20, however, the motor response typically precedes (or coincides) with the peak of the P_3 wave. This relationship is difficult to evaluate precisely, because recording the P_3 concurrently with the motor reaction contaminates the P_3 component with the pre- and post-motor potentials; on the other hand determining P_3 and RT latencies on separate trials (as in Fig. 20) leaves some doubt about the inter-trial consistency of the decision times. Allowing for such errors, it seems reasonable

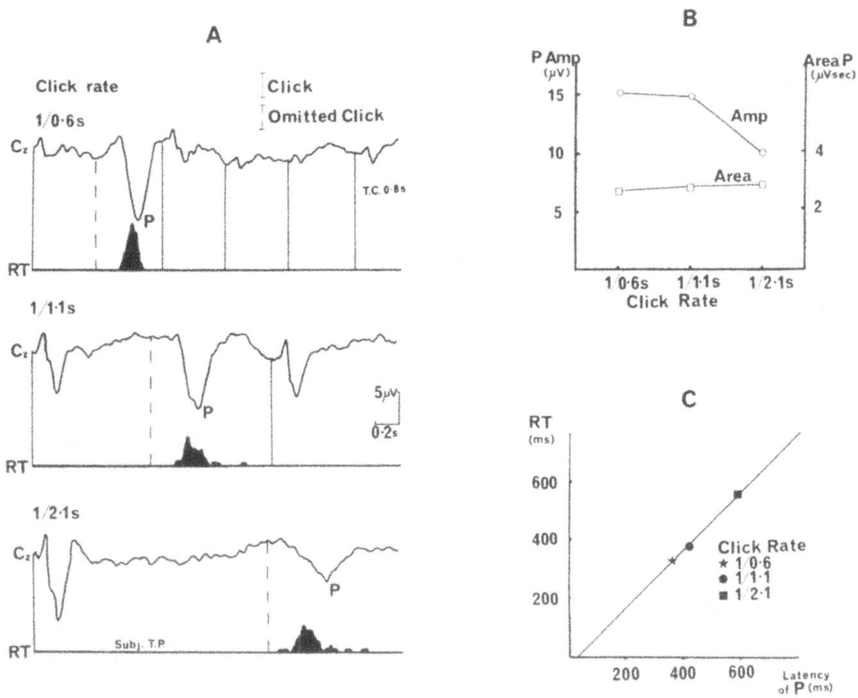

Fig. 20a—c. Latency of the late positive wave and reaction times. (a) Responses evoked by counting the omitted clicks at three different rates of click presentation. Each trace represents the average of 100 epochs. The lower tracing at each time interval represents the reaction time histogram for the same subject responding as quickly as possible to the missing click in a separate session. (b) Area and amplitude of the positive wave of the omitted stimulus response plotted against interclick interval. Combined results of three subjects. (c) Modal reaction time plotted against peak latency of the positive wave. Combined results of three subjects. (Picton et al., 1974b)

to conclude, however, that perceptual decision or recognition precedes the major portion of the P_3 wave but may coincide approximately with its onset (Ritter *et al.*, 1972). The earlier portions of the "decision complex" which precede P_3, however, (*e.g.* a negative wave at about 200 msec; Fig. 19) could represent the actual neural activity leading up to the decision.

The P_3 has been related to various characteristics of the motor response in situations where an immediate reaction is called for upon detecting a target stimulus. Wilkinson and Morlock (1967) first showed that P_3 waves were larger in response to tones requiring a motor response than to counted tones. Karlin *et al.* (1971) demonstrated that P_3 grew larger as a function of response speed in a discriminative RT task, but was largest of all following the "no-go" signals. In an elegantly designed choice RT experiment, Karlin and Martz (1972) have further shown that the magnitude of the P_3 depends upon the prior likelihood of making a given response independently from the stimulus probability factor. Donchin *et al.* (1973), however, have reported somewhat conflicting results in another choice RT task: they found that P_3 had the same amplitude when the stimulus-response was known in advance as when it was unpredictable. One problem in evaluating these results, however, is the possible contamination of the P_3 by concurrent motor potentials and by the positive "return to baseline" of the prior CNV. It is difficult to separate out positive shifts related to the perceptual decision from those strictly determined by the motor response generating mechanisms.

A final class of stimuli which elicit large P_3 waves are those which provide feedback information to a subject on whether his previous guess, response, or perceptual judgment was right or wrong. The amplitude of the P_3 waves is larger when the feedback is more improbable and unexpected (Teuting *et al.*, 1970), when it conveys more useful information (Picton and Low, 1971), and when it pronounces the subject "wrong" as opposed to "right" (Squires *et al.*, 1973a). Some of the properties of the feedback P_3 are illustrated in Fig. 21. When tone pips were simply counted, a small P_3 occurred. When the same tone conveyed feedback information, a large P_3 developed, which was larger and more delayed for the incorrect feedback. One possible explanation for these effects is that post-stimulus processing is more complex following feedback than counting and more complex still after wrong than after correct feedback, since, after wrong feedback, perceptual strategies must then be re-examined and refined. The P_3 accordingly may represent the activation of the appropriate cognitive contingencies following the recognition of a significant stimulus.

From these findings it can be concluded that the P_3 wave is associated in some way with perceptual decisions and their cognitive or motor sequelae. An alternate suggestion made by Karlin (1970) is that the P_3 reflects a non-selective "reactive change of state" (*e.g.* a termination of readiness) which follows the perceptual (cognitive) analysis of the signal. One mechanism by which this might occur is if the P_3 is largely constituted by the positive, post-decision "discharge" of the prior CNV. There appears to be little correspondence between the amplitude of the prior CNV and the subsequent P_3 (Donald and Goff, 1971; Hillyard *et al.*, 1971; Teuting and Sutton, 1972). Furthermore, the two phenomena have different scalp distributions in at least some instances, as shown in

Fig. 14, where prior to an auditory discrimination the CNV maximum is more frontal than the P_3 maximum, which is centro-parietal. Nonetheless, it is clear that, in the majority of experiments, the P_3 positivity overlaps with and is in part confounded by the descending limb of the CNV. Apart from the CNV-discharge question, the non-specific "reactive change" hypothesis experiences difficulty in accounting for why wrong feedback should elicit a larger P_3 than correct feedback, and, in the threshold signal detection task why there is little or no P_3 following a correct decision of signal absence (HILLYARD *et al.*, 1971; SQUIRES *et al.*, 1973b). The presence of P_3 on HITs but not on correct rejections supports the proposition that P_3 depends upon the matching of sensory input

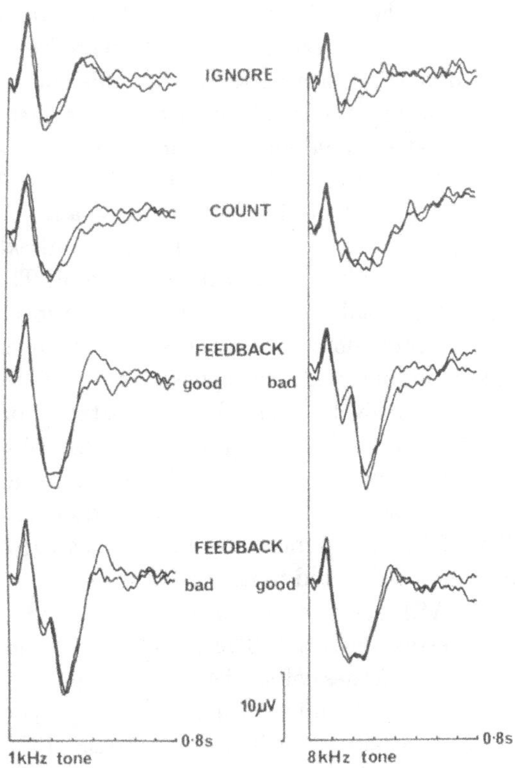

Fig. 21. Perceptual decisions and their sequelae. In this experiment an initial pair of tonepips followed by a response light preceded a final 800 msec toneburst of either 1kHz or 8kHz. In the first condition the subject read a book and ignored all stimuli. In the second condition the subject ignored the initial stimuli but counted the number of final tonebursts at each frequency — the 1kHz toneburst being twice as frequent as the 8kHz. In the last two conditions the subject performed a difficult frequency discrimination between the initial two tonepips and the final toneburst served as a feedback signal. The subject performed with an accuracy of 60—70%. The meaning of the toneburst was switched for the last condition in order to control for any stimulus dependent effects. Counting the tonebrusts caused a small late positive wave to appear in the evoked potential, especially for the less frequent signal. When the toneburst had feedback significance, however, there was a large late positive wave, the morphology of which was more related to the meaning than to the acoustic nature of the stimulus

to a "template" for the target signal, a template that is established as part of a "response set" mode of selective attention; the occurrence of the selected target stimulus leads to a decision of recognition and a triggering of the cognitive and/or motor response contingencies that were incorporated into the response set. The P_3 wave appears, therefore, to serve as a physiological index of the operation of such a response set mechanism.

C. Conclusion: Physiological Mechanisms of Attention

The most popular physiological theory of attention in recent years has been based upon a hypothetical efferent or descending inhibition of sensory transmission at peripheral levels of the auditory system (Hernandez-Peon, 1966); unattended sensory channels were presumed to be blocked from further analysis. Early experiments in animals purporting to support this concept, however, were flawed by lack of acoustic input control; with adequate methological controls there was no evidence of attentional effects upon the early analysis of auditory input (Worden, 1966; Wickelgren, 1968b). The stability of the early components of the auditory evoked potential in both animals and man would seem to indicate that auditory information is analyzed in the lemniscal auditory system in much the same way whether it is being attended or not. There certainly does exist a peripheral filtering of auditory information in the form of orienting movements to make the receptor more or less accessible, but once information has entered the nervous system, our evidence suggests that there is no further attentional filtering at brainstem levels. The relative constancy of this preliminary analysis of auditory information may form the neural basis of the primary buffer store or "echoic" memory (Neisser, 1967). Such a memory maintains a rapidly decaying record of all auditory input, whether attended or not, thereby insuring the ready availability of the last phrase or sentence of an ignored conversation if attention is by some means directed to it.

In man, the earliest AEP component shown to be altered by selective attention is the $N1$ of the vertex potential. The elicitation of the vertex potential reportedly depends on the intactness of the lemniscal input to the cortex (Jerger *et al.*, 1969; Williamson *et al.*, 1970) but also has certain properties of a modality non-specific reticular system (Goff, 1969; Fruhstorfer, 1971). It may be speculated then that the amplitude of the vertex potential reflects the degree of further processing of inputs from those selected auditory input channels that were admitted to this partially non-specific system for analysis as to content and significance under the control of a stimulus set mechanism of attention.

When a specific target signal is anticipated and its appropriate motor or cognitive response readied, a "response set" is said to exist. In metaphorical terms "templates" for possible target signals are "primed", so that those signals are recognized with a lower threshold. Such a process seems to be associated with a CNV and it is possible that the distribution of this cortical negativity reflects, in some degree, the neuronal representation of target stimulus engrams. The occurrence of such an anticipated stimulus seems to be the main requirement for eliciting the P_3 component. It is not clear whether the P_3 is a sign of the perceptual recognition (template match) or its sequelae, but it does seem to provide an accurate index of the confident recognition of a target signal for which a response set has been established.

Acknowledgement

This research was supported by NASA Grant No. 05-099-198, NIH Grant No. USPHS NS 10482-01, the Medical Research Council of Canada, and the Sloan Foundation.

References

ARDUINI, A.: Enduring potential changes evoked in the cerebral cortex by stimulation of brain stem reticular formation and thalamus. In: Jasper, H. H., Proctor, L. D., Knighton, R. S., Noshay, W. C., COSTELLO, R. J. (Eds.): Reticular formation of the brain. Boston: Little, Brown, and Company 1958.

BARLOW, J. S.: Some observations on the electrophysiology of timing in the nervous system. Electroenceph. clin. Neurophysiol. **31**, 345 (1969).

BELL, C., SIERRA, G., BUENDIA, N., SEGUNDO, J. P.: Sensory properties of neurons in the mesencephalic reticular formation. J. Neurophysiol. **27**, 961—987 (1964).

BENNET, T. H., GOTTFRIED, J.: Hippocampal theta activity and response inhibition. Electroenceph. clin. Neurophysiol. **29**, 196—200 (1970).

BICKFORD, R. G.: Physiological and clinical studies of microflexes. Electroenceph. clin. Neurophysiol. Supp. **31**, 93—108 (1972).

BIGNALL, K. E., IMBERT, M.: Polysensory and cortico-cortical projections to frontal lobe of squirrel and rhesus monkeys. Electroenceph. clin. Neurophysiol. **26**, 206—216 (1969).

BORDA, R. P.: The effect of altered drive states on the contingent negative variation (CNV) in rhesus monkeys. Electroenceph. clin. Neurophysiol. **29**, 173—180 (1970).

BORSANYI, S. J., BLANCHARD, C. L.: Auditory evoked brain responses in man. Arch. Otolaryng. **80**, 149—154 (1964).

BROADBENT, D. E.: Perception and communication. London: Pergamon Press 1958.

BROADBENT, D. E.: Decision and stress. London: Academic Press 1971.

BUCHWALD, J. S., HUMPHREY, G. L.: Response plasticity in cochlear nucleus of decerebrate cats during acoustic habituation procedures. J. Neurophysiol. **35**, 864—878 (1972a).

BUCHWALD, J. S., HUMPHREY, G. L.: An analysis of habituation in the specific sensory systems. In: STELLAR, E., SPRAGUE, J. (Eds.): Progress in Physiological Psychology Volume V. New York: Academic Press 1972b.

BUNO, W., VELLUTI, R., HANDLER, P., GARCIA-AUSTT, E.: Neural control of cochlear input in the wakeful free guinea pig. Physiol. Behav. **1**, 23—35 (1966).

BUTLER, R. A.: Effect of changes in stimulus frequency and intensity on habituation of the human vertex potential. J. acoust. Soc. Amer. **44**, 945—950 (1968).

BUTLER, R. A.: The influence of spatial separation of sound sources on the auditory evoked response. Neuropsychologia **10**, 219—225 (1972a).

BUTLER, R. A.: Frequency specificity of the auditory evoked response to simultaneously and successively presented stimuli. Electroenceph. clin. Neurophysiol. **33**, 277—282 (1972b).

BUTLER, R. A.: The auditory evoked response to stimuli producing periodicity pitch. Psychophysiology **9**, 233—237 (1972c).

CANT, B. R., BICKFORD, R. G.: The effect of motivation on the contingent negative variation (CNV). Electroenceph. clin. Neurophysiol. **23**, 594 (1967).

CAPPS, M. J., ADES, H. W.: Auditory frequency discrimination after transection of the olivocochlear bundle in squirrel monkeys. Exp. Neurol. **21**, 147—158 (1968).

CAPPS, M. J., STOCKWELL, C. W.: Lesions in the midbrain reticular formation and the startle response in rats. Physiol. Behav. **3**, 661—665 (1969).

CAREW, T. J., CASTELLUCCI, V. F., KANDEL, E. R.: An analysis of dishabituation and sensitization of the gill-withdrawal reflex in Aplysia. Int. J. Neurosci. **2**, 79—98 (1971).

Caspers, H.: Relations of steady potential shifts in the cortex to the wakefulness-sleep spectrum. In: Brazier, M.A.B. (Ed.): Brain Function Vol. 1. Los Angeles: Univ. of California Press 1963.

Castellucci, V., Pinsker, H., Kupfermann, I., Kandel, E.: Neuronal mechanisms of habituation and dishabituation of the gill withdrawal reflex in Aplysia. Science **167**, 1745—1748 (1970).

Celesia, G.G., Puletti, F.: Auditory input to the human cortex during states of drowsiness and surgical anesthesia. Electroenceph. clin. Neurophysiol. **31**, 603—609 (1971).

Cherry, E.C.: Some experiments on the recognition of speech, with one and with two ears. J. acoust. Soc. Amer. **25**, 975—979 (1953).

Clynes, M.: Dynamics of vertex evoked potentials: the R-M brain function. In: Donchin, E., Lindsley, D.B. (Eds.): Average evoked potentials-methods, results, and evaluations, pp. 363—374 Washington, D. C.: NASA 1969.

Coats, A., Dickey, J.: Nonsurgical recordings of human auditory nerve action potential and cochlear microphonic. Ann. Otol. **79**, 844—852 (1970).

Cody, D.T.R., Bickford, R.G.: Averaged evoked myogenic responses in normal man. Laryngoscope **74**, 400—416 (1969).

Cohen, J.: Very slow potentials relating to expectancy: the CNV. In: Donchin, E. and Lindsley, D.B. (Eds.): Average evoked potentials. Washington, D. C.: NASA 1969.

Cohen, J.: The contingent negative variation (CNV) and visual recognition. Electroenceph. clin. Neurophysiol. Suppl. (In press, 1973).

Cohen, J., Walter, W.G.: The interaction of responses in the brain to semantic stimuli. Psychophysiology **2**, 187—196 (1966).

Cook, J.D., Ellinwood, E.H., Wilson, W.P.: Auditory habituation at primary cortex as a function of stimulus rate. Exp. Neurol. **21**, 167—175 (1968).

David, E., Finkenzeller, P., Kallert, S., Keidel, W.D.: Akustischen Reizen zugeordnete Gleichspannungsänderungen am intakten Schädel des Menschen. Pflügers Arch. **309**, 362—367 (1969).

Davis, H.: Enhancement of evoked cortical potentials in humans related to a task requiring a decision. Science **145**, 182—183 (1964).

Davis, H., Zerlin, S.: Acoustic relations of the human vertex potential. J. acoust. Soc. Amer. **39**, 109—116 (1966).

Davis, H., Mast, T., Yoshie, N., Zerlin, S.: The slow response of the human cortex to auditory stimuli: recovery processes. Electroenceph. clin. Neurophysiol. **21**, 105—113 (1966).

Davis, H., Osterhammel, R.A., Weir, C.C., Gjerdigen, D.B.: Slow vertex potentials: interactions among auditory, tactile, electric and visual stimuli. Electroenceph. clin. Neurophysiol. **33**, 537—545 (1972).

Davis, M., Heninger, G.R.: Comparison of response plasticity between the eyeblink and vertex potential in humans. Electroenceph. clin. Neurophysiol. **33**, 283—293 (1972).

Davis, M., Wagner, A.R.: Startle-responsiveness after habituation to different intensities of tone. Psychonom. Sci. **12**, 337—338 (1968).

Debecker, J., Desmedt, J.E.: Rate of intermodality switching disclosed by sensory evoked potentials averaged during signal detection tasks. J. Physiol. (Lond.) **185**, 52—53 (1966).

Delse, F.C., Marsh, G.R., Thompson, L.W.: CNV correlates of task difficulty and accuracy of pitch discrimination. Psychophysiology **9**, 53—62 (1972).

Desmedt, J.E.: Neurophysiological mechanisms controlling acoustic input. In: Rasmussen G.L., Windle, W. (Eds.): Neural mechanisms of the auditory and vestibular systems. Springfield: Charles C. Thomas 1960.

Desmedt, J.E.: Auditory evoked potentials from cochlea to cortex as influenced by activation of the efferent olivocochlear bundle. J. acoust. Soc. Amer. **34**, 1478—1496 (1962).

Deutsch, J.A., Deutsch, D.: Attention: some theoretical considerations. Psychol. Rev. **70**, 80—90 (1963).

Dewson, J.H.: Efferent olivocochlear bundle: some relationships to stimulus discriminations in noise. J. Neurophysiol. **31**, 122—136 (1968).

Donald, M.W., Goff, W.R.: Attention-related increases in cortical responsivity dissociated from the contingent negative variation. Science **172**, 1163—1166 (1971).

DONCHIN, E., KUBOVY, M., KUTAS, M., JOHNSON, R., HERNING, R.: Graded changes in evoked response (*P* 300) amplitude as a function of cognitive activity. Perception and Psychophysics **14**, 319—324 (1973).

DONCHIN, E., OTTO, D., GERBRANDT, L. K., PRIBRAM, K. H.: While a monkey waits: electrocortical events recorded during the fore-period of a reaction time study. Electroenceph. clin. Neurophysiol. **31**, 115—128 (1971).

DONCHIN, E., GERBRANDT, L. K., LEIFFER, L., TUCKER, L.: Is the contingent negative variation contingent on a motor response? Psychophysiology **9**, 178—188 (1972).

ELAZAR, Z., ADEY, W. R.: Spectral analysis of low frequency components in the electrical activity of the hippocampus during learning. Electroenceph. clin. Neurophysiol. **23**, 225—240 (1967).

ELUL, R.: The genesis of the EEG. Int. Rev. Neurobiol. **15**, 227—272 (1972).

FAIDHERBE, J., DELIEGE, M.: Mise en évidence d'une "variation contingente negative" dans un état de centration representative. Arch. Int. Physiol. Biochim. **76**, 363—366 (1968).

FEX, J.: Augmentation of cochlear microphonic by stimulation of efferent fibres to the cochlea. Acta oto-laryng. (Stockh.) **50**, 540—541 (1959).

FEX, J.: Auditory activity in centifugal and centipetal cochlear fibers in cat. Acta physiol. scand. Suppl. **189**, 1—68 (1962).

FEX, J.: Auditory activity in uncrossed centifugal cochlear fibres in cat. Acta physiol. scand. **64**, 43—57 (1965).

FIRTH, H.: Habituation during sleep. Psychophysiology **10**, 43—51 (1973).

FORD, J. M., ROTH, W. T., DIRKS, S. J., KOPELL, B. S.: Evoked potential correlates of signal recognition between and within modalities. Science **181**, 465—467 (1973).

FRENCH, J. D., VERZEANO, M., MAGOUN, H. W.: An extralemniscal sensory system in the brain. Arch. Neurol. Psychiat. **69**, 505—518 (1953).

FRUHSTORFER, H.: Habituation and dishabituation of the human vertex response. Electroenceph. clin. Neurophysiol. **30**, 306—312 (1971).

FRUHSTORFER, H., BERSTROM, R. M.: Human vigilance and auditory evoked responses. Electroenceph. clin. Neurophysiol. **27**, 346—355 (1969).

FRUHSTORFER, H., SOVERI, P., JARVILEHTO, T.: Short-term habituation of the auditory evoked response in man. Electroenceph. clin. Neurophysiol. **28**, 153—161 (1970).

GALAMBOS, R.: Suppression of auditory nerve activity by stimulation of efferent fibers to cochlea. J. Neurophysiol. **19**, 424—437 (1956).

GARDINER, M. F., WALTER, D. O.: Differences between human evoked potentials elicited by the same acoustical stimuli during loudness discrimination tasks and pitch discrimination tasks. In: DONCHIN, E., LINDSLEY, D. (Eds.): Average evoked potentials-methods, results, and evaluations, pp. 335—342. Washington, D. C.: NASA, 1969.

GEISLER, C. D., FRISHKOPF, L. S., ROSENBLITH, W. A.: Extracranial responses to acoustic clicks in man. Science **128**, 1210—1211 (1958).

GERBRANDT, L. K., GOFF, W. R., SMITH, D. B.: Distribution of the human average movement potential. Electroenceph. clin. Neurophysiol. **34**, 461—474 (1973).

GERSHUNI, G. V., KOZHEVNIKOV, V. A., MARUSEVA, A. M., AVAKYAN, R. V., RADIONOVA, E. A., ALTMAN, J. A., SOROKO, V. I.: Modifications in electrical responses of the auditory system in different states of the higher nervous activity. Electroenceph. clin. Neurophysiol. Suppl. **13**, 115—124 (1960).

GILDEN, L., VAUGHAN, H. G., COSTA, L. D.: Summated human electroencephalographic potentials associated with voluntary movements. Electroenceph. clin. Neurophysiol. **20**, 433—438 (1966).

GOFF, W. R.: Evoked potential correlates of perceptual organization in man. In: EVANS, C. R., MULHOLLAND, T. B. (Eds.): Attention in neurophysiology, pp. 169—193. London: Williams Clowes and Sons (1969).

GOFF, W. R., MATSUMIYA, Y., ALLISON, T., GOFF, G. D.: Cross-modality comparisons of average evoked potentials. In: DONCHIN, E., LINDSLEY, D. B. (Eds.): Average evoked potentials-methods, results, and evaluations, pp. 95—141 Washington, D. C.: NASA (1969).

GOLDSTEIN, R., RODMAN, L. B.: Early components of average evoked responses to rapidly repeated auditory stimuli. J. Speech Res. **10**, 697—705 (1967).

GROSS, M. M., BEGLEITER, H., TOBIN, M., KISSIN, B.: Auditory evoked response comparison during counting clicks and reading. Electroenceph. clin. Neurophysiol. **18**, 451—454 (1965).

GROVES, P. M., LYNCH, G. S.: Mechanisms of habituation in the brain stem. Psych. Rev. **79**, 237—244 (1972).

GROVES, P. M., MILLER, S. W., PARKER, M. V.: Habituation and sensitization of neuronal activity in the reticular formation of the rat. Physiol. Behav. **8**, 589—593 (1972).

GROVES, P. M., THOMPSON, R. F.: Habituation: a dual-process theory. Psychol. Rev. **77**, 419—450 (1970).

GUMNIT, R.: DC potential changes from auditory cortex of cat. J. Neurophysiol. **23**, 667—675 (1960).

HALL, R. D.: Habituation of evoked potentials in the rat under conditions of behavioral control. Electroenceph. clin. Neurophysiol. **24**, 155—165 (1968).

HARDIN, W. B., CASTELLUCCI, V. F.: Analysis of somatosensory, auditory and visual averaged transcortical and scalp responses in the monkey. Electroenceph. clin. Neurophysiol. **28**, 488—498 (1970).

HARTER, M. R., SALMON, L. E.: Intra-modality selective attention and evoked cortical potentials to randomly presented patterns. Electroenceph. clin. Neurophysiol. **32**, 605—613 (1972).

HARTLEY, L. R.: The effect of stimulus relevance on the cortical evoked potentials. Quart. J. exp. Psychol. **22**, 531—546 (1970).

HAY, I. S., DAVIS, H.: Slow cortical evoked potentials: interactions of auditory, vibrotactile and shock stimuli. Audiology **10**, 9—17 (1971).

HERNANDEZ-PEON, R.: Neurophysiological correlates of habituation and other manifestations of plastic inhibition (internal inhibition). Electroenceph. clin. Neurophysiol. Suppl. **13**, 101—114 (1960).

HERNANDEZ-PEON, R.: Physiological mechanisms in attention. In: RUSSELL, R. W. (Ed.): Frontiers in physiological psychology. New York: Academic Press 1966.

HERNANDEZ-PEON, R., JOUVET, M., SCHERRER, H.: Auditory potentials at cochlear nucleus during habituation. Acta neurol. lat.-amer. **3**, 144—156 (1957).

HERNANDEZ-PEON, R., SCHERRER, H., JOUVET, M.: Modification of electrical activity in the cochlear nucleus during attention in unanaesthetised cats. Science **123**, 331—332 (1956).

HILLYARD, S. A.: The CNV and the vertex evoked potential during signal detection: a preliminary report. In: DONCHIN, E., LINDSLEY, D. B. (Eds.): Average evoked potentials-methods, results, and evaluations, pp. 349—353. Washington, D. C.: NASA (1969).

HILLYARD, S. A.: The CNV and human behavior. Electroenceph. clin. Neurophysiol. Supp. **33**, 161—171 (1973).

HILLYARD, S. A., HINK, R. F., SCHWENT, V. L., PICTON, T. W.: Electrical signs of selective attention in the human brain. Science **182**, 177—180 (1973).

HILLYARD, S. A., SQUIRES, K. C., BAUER, J. W., LINDSAY, P. H.: Evoked potential correlates of auditory signal detection. Science **172**, 1357—1360 (1971).

HIRANO, T., BEST, P., OLDS, J.: Units during habituation, discrimination learning and extinction. Electroenceph. clin. Neurophysiol. **28**, 127—135 (1970).

HOCHBERG, J.: Attention, organization and consciousness. In: MOSTOFSKY, D. I. (Ed.): Attention: Contemporary theory and analysis. New York: Appleton-Century-Crofts 1970.

HORN, G.: Neuronal mechanisms of habituation. Nature (Lond.) **215**, 707—711 (1967).

HORN, G., HILL, R. M.: Habituation of the response to sensory stimuli of neurons in the brain stem of rabbits. Nature (Lond.) **202**, 296—298 (1964).

IRVINE, D. R. F., WEBSTER, W. R.: Studies of peripheral gating in the auditory system of cats. Electroenceph. clin. Neurophysiol. **32**, 545—556 (1972).

JAMES, W.: The principles of psychology, Vol. 1. New York: Holt 1890.

JARVILEHTO, T., FRUHSTORFER, H.: Differentiation between slow cortical potentials associated with motor and mental acts in man. Exp. Brain Res. **11**, 309—317 (1970).

JASPER, H.: Nonspecific thalamo cortical relations. In: FIELD, J., MAGOUN, H. W., HALL, V. E.: Handbook of physiology, Section 1, Neurophysiology Vol. II. Washington: Amer. Physiol. Soc. 1960.

JENNESS, D.: Stimulus role and gross differences in the cortical evoked response. Physiology and Behavior **9**, 141—146 (1972).

JERGER, J. J., WEIKERS, N. J., SHARBROUGH, F. W., JERGER, S.: Bilateral lesions of the temporal lobe. A case study. Acta oto-laryng. (Stockh.) Suppl. **258**, 1—51 (1969).

JEWETT, D. L., WILLISTON, J. S.: Auditory-evoked far fields averaged from the scalp of humans. Brain **94**, 681—696 (1971).

KANDEL, E. R., TAUC, L.: Heterosynaptic facilitation in neurones of the abdominal ganglion of Aplysia depilans. J. Physiol. (Lond.) **181**, 1—27 (1965).

KARLIN, L.: Cognition, preparation and sensory-evoked potentials. Psychol. Bull. **73**, 122—136 (1970).

KARLIN, L., MARTZ, M., BRAUTH, S., MORDKOFF, A.: Auditory evoked potentials, motor potentials, and reaction time. Electroenceph. clin. Neurophysiol. **31**, 129—136 (1971).

KARLIN, L., MARTZ, M. J.: Response probability and sensory evoked potentials. In: KORNBLUM, S. (Ed.): Attention and performance. IV. New York: Academic Press 1973.

KEATING, L. W., RUHM, H. B.: Some observations of the effects of attention to stimuli on the amplitude of the acoustically evoked response. Audiology **10**, 177—184 (1971).

KEIDEL, W. D.: What do we know about the human cortical evoked potential after all? Arch. klin. exp. Ohr.-Nas.- u. Kehlk.-Heilk. **198**, 9—37 (1971).

KIANG, N. Y. S.: A survey of recent developments in the study of auditory physiology. Ann. Otol. Rhin. Laryng. **77**, 656—674 (1968).

KIMBLE, D. P.: Possible inhibitory functions of the hippocampus. Neuropsychologia **7**, 235—244 (1967).

KLINKE, R., BOERGER, G., GRUBER, J.: Studies on the functional significance of efferent innervation in the auditory system: afferent neuronal activity as influenced in contralaterally applied sound. Pflügers Arch. **306**, 165—175 (1969).

KLINKE, R., FRUHSTORFER, H., FINKENZELLER, P.: Evoked responses as a function of external and stored information. Electroenceph. clin. Neurophysiol. **25**, 119—122 (1968).

KNOTT, J. R., IRWIN, D. A.: Anxiety, stress and the contingent negative variation. Electroenceph. clin. Neurophysiol. **24**, 188 (1967).

KNOTT, J. R., PETERS, J. F.: Sex, stress and the interstimulus interval. Electroenceph. clin. Neurophysiol. Suppl. (In press, 1973).

KÖHLER, W., WEGENER, J.: Currents of the human auditory cortex. J. Cell Comp. Physiol. **45**, Suppl. 1, 25—54 (1955).

KONORSKI, J.: Integrative activity of the brain: an interdisciplinary approach. Chicago: University of Chicago Press 1967.

KOOI, K. A., TIPTON, A. C., MARSHALL, R. E.: Polarities and field configurations of the vertex components of the human auditory evoked response: a reinterpretation. Electroenceph. clin. Neurophysiol. **31**, 166—169 (1971).

KORNHUBER, H. H., DEECKE, L.: Hirnpotentialänderungen bei Wilkürbewegungen und passiven Bewegungen des Menschen: Bereitschaftspotential und reafferente Potentiale. Pflügers Arch. **284**, 1—17 (1965).

KUPFERMANN, I., CASTELLUCCI, V., PINSKER, H., KANDEL, E.: Neuronal correlates of habituation and dishabituation of the gill withdrawal reflex in Aplysia. Science **167**, 1743—1745 (1970).

LEV, A., SOHMER, H.: Sources of averaged neural responses recorded in animal and human subjects during cochlear audiometry (electrocochleogram). Arch. klin. exp. Ohr.-Nas.- Kehlk. Heilk. **201**, 79—90 (1972).

LIBERMAN, A. M., COOPER, F. S., SHANKWEILER, D. P., STUDDERT-KENNEDY, M.: Perception of the speech code. Psych. Rev. **74**, 431—461 (1963).

LICKEY, M. E., FOX, S. S.: Localization and habituation of sensory evoked DC response in cat cortex. Exp. Neurol. **15**, 437—454 (1966).

LISSAK, K., GRASTYAN, E.: The changes of hippocampal electrical activity during conditioning. Electroenceph. clin. Neurophysiol. Suppl. **13**, 271—279 (1960).

LIVINGSTON, R. B.: Central control of receptors and sensory transmission systems. In: FIELD, J., MAGOUN, H. W., HALL, V. (Eds.): Handbook of physiology, Section 1: Neurophysiology Volume 1. Washington, D.C.: American Physiological Society 1959.

LOPES DA SILVA, F. H., KAMP, A.: Hippocampal theta frequency shifts and operant behavior. Electroenceph. clin. Neurophysiol. **26**, 133—143 (1969).

LOW, M. D., BORDA, R. P., KELLAWAY, P.: "Contingent negative variation" in rhesus monkeys: an EEG sign of a specific mental process. Percept. Motor Skills. **22**, 443—446 (1966).

LOW, M. D., COATS, A. C., RETTIG, G. M., MCSHERRY, J. W.: Anxiety, attentiveness-alertness: a phenomenological study of the CNV. Neuropsychologia **5**, 379—384 (1967).

LOW, M. D., SWIFT, S. J.: The contingent negative variation and the "resting" DC potential of the human brain: effects of situational anxiety. Neuropsychologia **9**, 203—208 (1971).

LURIA, A. R., HOMSKAYA, E. D.: Frontal lobes and the regulation of arousal processes. In: MOSTOFSKY, D. I. (Ed.): Attention: contemporary theory and analysis. New York: Appleton-Century-Crofts 1970.

LYNN, R.: Attention, arousal and the orientation reaction. London: Pergamon 1966.

MACKAY, D. M.: Perception and brain function. In: SCHMITT, F. O. (Ed.): The neurosciences second study program. New York: Rockefeller 1970.

MARSH, J. T., MCCARTHY, D. A., SHEATZ, G., GALAMBOS, R.: Habituation and evoked auditory potentials. Electroenceph. clin. Neurophysiol. **13**, 224—234 (1961).

MARSH, J. T., WORDEN, F. G.: Auditory potentials during acoustic habituation: cochlear nucleus, cerebellum, and auditory cortex. Electroenceph. clin. Neurophysiol. **17**, 685—692 (1964).

MAST, T. E.: Short latency human evoked responses to clicks. J. appl. Physiol. **20**, 725—730 (1965).

MATSUMIYA, Y., TAGLIASCO, V., LOMBROSO, C. T., GOODGLASS, H.: Auditory evoked response: meaningfulness of stimuli and interhemispheric asymmetry. Science **175**, 790—792 (1972).

MCADAM, D. W., RUBIN, E. H.: Readiness potential, vertex positive wave, contingent negative variation and accuracy of perception. Electroenceph. clin. Neurophysiol. **30**, 511—517 (1971).

MCADAM, D. W., SEALES, D. M.: Bereitschaftspotential enhancement with increased level of motivation. Electroenceph. clin. Neurophysiol. **27**, 73—75 (1969).

MCADAM, D. W., WHITAKER, H. A.: Language production: electrocephalographic localization in the normal human brain. Science **172**, 499—502 (1971).

MILLER, G. A., GALANTER, E., PRIBRAM, K. H.: Plans and the structure of behavior. New York: Holt, Rinehart, and Winston 1960.

MILNER, B. A.: Evaluation of auditory function by computer techniques. Int. Audiology **8**, 361—370 (1969).

MORRELL, L. K., SALAMY J. G.: Hemispherie asymmetry of electrocortical responses to speech stimuli. Science **174**, 164—166 (1971).

MORUZZI, G.: The sleep-waking cycle. Ergeb. Physiol. **64**, 1—165 (1972).

NAATANEN, R.: Selective attention and evoked potentials. Ann. Finn. Acad. Sci. **151**, 1—226 (1967).

NEISSER, U.: Cognitive psychology. New York: Appleton-Century-Crofts 1967.

NELSON, D. A., LASSMAN, F. M.: Effects of intersignal interval on the human auditory evoked response. J. acoust. Soc. Amer. **44**, 1529—1532 (1968).

NIEDER, P., NIEDER, I.: Antimasking effect of crossed olivocochlear bundle stimulation with loud clicks in guinea-pig. Exp. Neurol. **28**, 179—188 (1970).

OHMAN, A., LADER, M.: Selective attention and "habituation" of the auditory averaged evoked response in humans. Physiol. Behaviour **8**, 79—85 (1972).

PAUL, D., SUTTON, S.: Evoked potential correlates of response criterion in auditory signal detection. Science **177**, 362—364 (1972).

PAVLOV, I. P.: Conditioned reflexes. Oxford University Press 1927.

PFALZ, R. K. J.: Centrifugal inhibition of afferent secondary neurons in the cochlear nucleus by sound. J. acoust. Soc. Amer. **34**, 1472—1477 (1962).

PICTON, T. W., HILLYARD, S. A., GALAMBOS, R., SCHIFF, M.: Human auditory attention: a central or peripheral process? Science **173**, 351—353 (1971).

PICTON, T. W., LOW, M. D.: The CNV and semantic content of stimuli in the experimental paradigm: effects of feedback. Electroenceph. clin. Neurophysiol. **31**, 451—456 (1971).

PICTON, T. W., HILLYARD, S. A., KRAUSZ, H. I., GALAMBOS, R.: Human auditory evoked potentials. Part I: Evaluation of components. Electroenceph. clin. Neurophysiol. **36**, 179—190 (1974a).

PICTON, T. W., HILLYARD, S. A.: Human auditory evoked potentials. Part II: Effects of attention. Electroenceph. clin. Neurophysiol. **36**, 191—199 (1974).

PICTON, T. W., HILLYARD, S. A., GALAMBOS, R.: Evoked responses to omitted stimuli. In: LIVANOV, M. N. (Ed.): Major problems of brain electrophysiology. USSR Academy of Science pp. 302—311 (1974b).

PORTMANN, M., ARAN, J. M.: Electrocochleography. Laryngoscope **81**, 899—910 (1971).

POSNER, M. I., KLEIN, R., SUMMERS, J., BUGGIE, S.: On the selection of signals. Memory and Cognition 1, 2—12 (1973).

PULETTI, F., CELESIA, G. G.: Functional properties of the primary cortical auditory area in man. J. Neurosurg. **32**, 244—247 (1970).

RAPIN, I.: Evoked responses to clicks in a group of children with communication discorders. Ann. N. Y. Acad. Sci. **112**, 182—203 (1964).

RAPIN, I., SCHIMMEL, H., TOURK, L. M., KRASNEGOR, N. A., POLLACK: Evoked responses to clicks and tones of varying intensity in waking adults. Electroenceph. clin. Neurophysiol. **21**, 335—344 (1966).

REBERT, C. S.: Cortical and subcortical slow potentials in the monkey's brain during a preparatory interval. Electroenceph. clin. Neurophysiol. **33**, 389—402 (1972).

REDDING, E. K.: Modification of sensory cortical evoked potentials by hippocampal stimulation. Electroenceph. clin. Neurophysiol. **22**, 74—83 (1967).

RITTER, W., SIMSON, R., VAUGHAN, H. G.: Association cortex potentials and reaction time in auditory discrimination. Electroenceph. clin. Neurophysiol. **33**, 547—556 (1972).

RITTER, W., VAUGHAN, H. G.: Averaged evoked responses in vigilance and discrimination: a reassessment. Science **164**, 326—328 (1969).

RITTER, W., VAUGHAN, H. G., COSTA, L. D.: Orienting and habituation to auditory stimuli: a study of short term changes in averaged evoked responses. Electroenceph. clin. Neurophysiol. **25**, 550—556 (1968).

ROESER, R. J., PRICE, L. L.: Effects of habituation on the auditory evoked response. J. Aud. Res. **9**, 306—313 (1969).

ROSE, D. E., MALONE, J. C.: Some aspects of the acoustically evoked response to the cessation of stimulus. J. Aud. Res. **5**, 27—40 (1965).

ROSE, D. E., RUHM, H. B.: Some characteristics of the peak latency and amplitude of the acoustically evoked response. J. Speech Res. **9**, 412—422 (1966).

ROTH, W. T.: Auditory evoked responses to unpredictable stimuli. Psychophysiology **10**, 125—138 (1973).

ROTH, W. T., KOPELL, B. S.: The auditory evoked response to repeated stimuli during a vigilance task. Psychophysiology **6**, 301—309 (1969).

ROTHMAN, H., DAVIS, H., HAY, I. S.: Slow evoked cortical potentials and temporal features of stimulation. Electroenceph. clin. Neurophysiol. **29**, 225—232 (1970).

RUHM, H. B., WALKER, E., FLANIGAN, H.: Acoustically-evoked potentials in man: mediation of early components. Laryngoscope **77**, 806—822 (1967).

SATTERFIELD, J. H.: Evoked cortical response enhancement and attention in man: a study of responses to auditory and shock stimuli. Electroenceph. clin. Neurophysiol. **19**, 470—475 (1965).

SEGUNDO, J. P., BELL, C. C.: Habituation of single nerve cells in the vertebrate nervous system. In: HORN, G., HINDE, R. A. (Eds.): Short-term changes in neural activity and behaviour. Cambridge University Press 1970.

SELFRIDGE, O. G.: Pandemonium: a paradigm for learning. In: The mechanisation of thought processes. London: H.M. Stationery Office 1959.

SHARPLESS, S. K.: Reorganization of function in the nervous system — use and disuse. Ann. Rev. Physiol. **26**, 357—388 (1964).

SHARPLESS, S. K., JASPER, H.: Habituation of the arousal reaction. Brain **79**, 655—682 (1956).

SHEATZ, G. C., CHAPMAN, R. M.: Task relevance and auditory evoked response. Electroenceph. clin. Neurophysiol. **26**, 468—475 (1969).

SHELBURNE, S.A.: Visual evoked responses to word and nonsense stimuli. Electroenceph. clin. Neurophysiol. **32**, 17—25 (1972).

SHERRINGTON, C.S.: The integrative action of the nervous system. New Haven: Yale University Press 1906.

SMITH, D.B.D., DONCHIN, E., COHEN, L., STARR, A.: Auditory average evoked potentials in man during binaural listening. Electroenceph. clin. Neurophysiol. **28**, 146—152 (1970).

SOHMER, H., FEINMESSER, M.: Cochlear action potentials recorded from the external ear in man. Ann. Otol. **76**, 427—436 (1967).

SOKOLOV, E.N.: Neuronal models and the orienting reflex. In: BRAZIER, M.A.B. (Ed.): The central nervous system and behavior, third conference. New York: Josiah Macy Foundation 1960.

SOKOLOV, E.N.: Perception and the conditioned reflex. New York: Pergamon Press 1963a.

SOKOLOV, E.N.: Higher nervous functions: the orienting reflex. Ann. Rev. Physiol. **25**, 545—580 (1963b).

SPONG, P., HAIDER, M., LINDSLEY, D.B.: Selective attentiveness and cortical evoked responses to visual and auditory stimuli. Science **148**, 395—397 (1965).

SQUIRES, K.C., HILLYARD, S.A., LINDSAY, P.H.: Cortical potentials evoked by confirming and disconfirming feedback following an auditory discrimination. Perception and Psychophysics **13**, 25—31 (1973a).

SQUIRES, K.C., HILLYARD, S.A., LINDSAY, P.H.: Vertex potentials evoked during auditory signal detection: relation to decision criteria. Perception and Psychophysics **14**, 265—272 (1973b).

STARZL, T.E., TAYLOR, C.W., MAGOUN, H.W.: Collateral afferent excitation of reticular formation of brainstem. J. Neurophysiol. **14**, 479—496 (1951).

SUTTON, S., BRAREN, M., ZUBIN, J.: Evoked potential correlates of stimulus uncertainty. Science **150**, 1187—1188 (1965).

SUTTON, S., BRAREN, M., ZUBIN, J., JOHN, E.R.: Information delivery and the sensory evoked potential. Science **155**, 1436—1439 (1967).

SYNDULKO, K.: Cortical slow potential shifts in humans during sensory and motor tasks. Doctoral dissertation, UCLA (1972).

TECCE, J.J.: Contingent negative variation (CNV) and psychological processes in man. Psychol. Bull. **77**, 73—108 (1972).

TEUTING, P., SUTTON, S.: The relationship between prestimulus negative shifts and poststimulus components of the average evoked potential. In: KORNBLUM, S. (Ed.): Attention and performance. IV. New York: Academic Press 1972.

TEUTING, P., SUTTON, S., ZUBIN, J.: Quantitative evoked potential correlates of the probability of events. Psychophysiol. **7**, 385—394 (1970).

THOMPSON, R.F., SPENCER, W.A.: Habituation: a model phenomenon for the study of neuronal substrates of behavior. Psychol. Rev. **73**, 16—43 (1966).

TRAHIOTIS, C., ELLIOT, D.N.: Behavioral investigation of some possible effects of sectioning the crossed olivocochlear bundle. J. acoust. Soc. Amer. **47**, 592—596 (1970).

TREISMAN, A.M.: Selective attention in man. Brit. Med. Bull. **20**, 12—16 (1964).

TREISMAN, A.M.: Strategies and models of selective attention. Psych. Rev. **76**, 282—299 (1969).

TREISMAN, A.M., GEFFIN, G.: Selective attention: perception or response? Quart. J. exp. Psych. **19**, 1—17 (1967).

VANDERWOLF, C.H.: Limbic-diencephalic mechanisms of voluntary movement. Psych. Rev. **78**, 83—113 (1971).

VAUGHAN, H.G., RITTER, W.: The sources of auditory evoked responses recorded from the human head. Electroenceph. clin. Neurophysiol. **28**, 360—367 (1970).

VINOGRADOVA, O.S.: Registration of information and the limbic system. In: HORN, G., HINDE, R.A. (Eds.): Short-term changes in neural activity and behaviour. Cambridge University Press 1970.

WALTER, W.G.: The convergence and interaction of visual, auditory and tactile responses in human nonspecific cortex. Ann. N. Y. Acad. Sci. **112**, 320—361 (1964a).

WALTER, W.G.: Slow potential waves in the human brain associated with expectancy, attention and decision. Arch. Psychiat. Nervenkrank. **206**, 309—322 (1964b).

WALTER, W. G.: Brain responses to semantic stimuli. J. Psychosom. Res. **9**, 51—61 (1965).

WALTER, W. G., COOPER, R., ALDRIDGE, V. J., MCCALLUM, W. C., WINTER, A. L.: Contingent negative variation: an electric sign of sensorimotor association and expectancy in the human brain. Nature (Lond.) **203**, 380—384 (1964).

WEBER, B. A.: Habituation and dishabituation of the averaged auditory evoked response. J. Speech Hear. Res. **13**, 387—394 (1970).

WEBSTER, W. R.: The effects of repetitive stimulation on auditory evoked potentials. Electroenceph. clin. Neurophysiol. **30**, 318—330 (1971).

WEBSTER, W. R., AITKIN, L. M.: Evoked potential and single unit studies of neural mechanisms underlying the effects of repetitive stimulation in the auditory pathway. Electroenceph. clin. Neurophysiol. **31**, 581—592 (1971).

WEINBERG, H.: The contingent negative variation: its relation to feedback and expectant attention. Neuropsychologia **10**, 299—306 (1972).

WEINBERG, H., WALTER, W. G., CROW, H. J.: Intracerebral events in humans related to real and imaginary stimuli. Electroenceph. clin. Neurophysiol. **29**, 1—9 (1970).

WEINBERGER, N. M., GOODMAN, D. A., KITZES, L. M.: Is behavioral habituation a function of peripheral auditory system blockade? Comm. Behav. Biol. 3A, 111—116 (1969).

WEITZMAN, E. D., KREMEN, H.: Auditory evoked responses during different stages of sleep in man. Electroenceph. clin. Neurophysiol. **18**, 65—70 (1965).

WICKELGREN, W. O.: Effect of state of arousal on click-evoked responses in cats. J. Neurophysiol. **31**, 757—768 (1968a).

WICKELGREN, W. O.: Effects of walking and flash stimulation on click evoked responses in cats. J. Neurophysiol. **31**, 769—776 (1968b).

WICKELGREN, W. O.: Effects of acoustic habituation on click evoked responses in cats. J. Neurophysiol. **31**, 777—784 (1968c).

WIEDERHOLD, M. L.: Variations in the effects of electrical stimulation of the crossed olivocochlear bundle on cat single auditory-nerve-fiber responses to tone bursts. J. acoust. Soc. Amer. **48**, 966—977 (1970).

WILKINSON, R. T., HAINES, E.: Evoked response correlates of expectancy during vigilance. In: SANDERS, A. F. (Ed.): Attention and Performance. III. Amsterdam: North-Holland Publ. Comp. pp. 402—413 (1970).

WILKINSON, R. T., LEE, M. V.: Auditory evoked potentials and selective attention. Electroenceph. clin. Neurophysiol. **33**, 411—418 (1972).

WILKINSON, R. T., MORLOCK, H. C.: Auditory evoked response and reaction time. Electroenceph. clin. Neurophysiol. **23**, 50—56 (1967).

WILLIAMS, H. L., TEPAS, D. I., MORLOCK, H. C.: Evoked responses to clicks and electroencephalographic stages of sleep in man. Science **138**, 685—686 (1962).

WILLIAMSON, P. D., GOFF, W. R., ALLISON, T.: Somatosensory evoked responses in patients with unilateral cerebral lesions. Electroenceph. clin. Neurophysiol. **28**, 566—575 (1970).

WOOD, C. C., GOFF, W. R., DAY, R. S.: Auditory evoked potentials during speech perception. Science **173**, 1248—1251 (1971).

WORDEN, F. G.: Attention and auditory electrophysiology. In: STELLAR, E., SPRAGUE, J. M. (Eds.): Progress in physiological psychology, Vol. 1. New York: Academic Press 1966.

WORDEN, F. G.: Auditory habituation. In: Peeke and Herz. Habituation: behavioral studies and electrophysiological substrates. New York: Academic Press 1973.

YOSHIE, N.: Auditory nerve action potential responses to clicks in man. Laryngoscope **78**, 198—215 (1968).

YOSHIE, N., OHASHI, T.: Clinical use of cochlear nerve action potential responses in man for differential diagnosis of hearing losses. Acta oto-laryngol. Suppl. **252**, 71—87 (1969).

Chapter 9

Mathematical Models of the Mechanics of the Inner Ear

C. DANIEL GEISLER, Madison, Wisconsin (USA)

With 6 Figures

Contents

I. Introduction

This chapter is a description of the mathematical models of the mechanical functioning of the inner ear that have been developed since BÉKÉSY's observations first became widely known. Theories of hearing developed prior to that time are interesting from an historical point of view, but they lack the modern insights that BÉKÉSY provided. They will, therefore, not be discussed here. The interested reader is referred to the comprehensive review of the older theories written by WEVER (1949).

The scope of this review is further limited to mathematical models and will not attempt to describe the mechanical models of the inner ear that have been developed. This omission does not imply that the mechanical models are unimportant simulations. On the contrary, the mechanical models, especially the many ingenious ones developed by BÉKÉSY, have provided much valuable insight into the workings of the cochlea and should be carefully studied by anyone interested in cochlear function. However, since full descriptions and summaries of the principle mechanical models are already easily accessible (BÉKÉSY, 1960, 1970; TONNDORF, 1970a and b), they will not be repeated here.

The chapter will be divided into two main sections, corresponding to the two different types of models that have been developed. One type, termed here the physical model, starts with observed anatomical and physical properties of inner ear structures and builds from there, using basic physical laws to describe the interactions of the various parts. The result, if successful, is a model whose output mimicks the behavior of the inner ear and whose individual sections are analogous to or isomorphic with the specific physiological structures involved. By contrast, the other type of model, often termed the computational model, represents the mechanical function of the inner ear solely in terms of the relationship between its input and its output. If successful, it will compute motion of the basilar membrane for a particular stapes input to some specified degree of accuracy. The various sections of a computational model have, however, no necessary connection with various parts of the inner ear.

II. Physical Models

A. Derivation of Basic Equations

The physical models of the cochlea which have been developed are based on the equations of acoustic wave motion valid for small motions. To derive these equations, we proceed as outlined in BIRD *et al.* (1960) and start with a fluid which, in the absence of sound, has a uniform density ϱ and uniform pressure p. Effects of fluid viscosity, unless otherwise noted, are assumed to be negligible as are the effects of thermal conductivity.

The first equation needed describes the conservation of matter. To develop this equation, consider the stationary volume element $\Delta x \Delta y \Delta z$ shown in Fig. 1. The rate of mass flowing into the volume through the face lying perpendicular to the x-axis at x is $\Delta y \Delta z\ (\varrho\, u_x)|_x$, where u_x is fluid velocity in the x-direction. The rate of mass flowing out through the face lying parallel to the first at $x + \Delta x$ is $\Delta y \Delta z\ (\varrho\, u_x)|_{x+\Delta x}$. We can write analogous expressions for the other pairs of faces. The conservation of mass in the volume element requires that the rate of mass accumulation within the volume element must be equal to the net rate of mass flowing into the volume. Therefore,

$$\begin{aligned} \Delta x\, \Delta y\, \Delta z \frac{\partial \varrho}{\partial t} = {} & \Delta y\, \Delta z\, [(\varrho u_x)|_x - (\varrho u_x)|_{x+\Delta x}] \\ & + \Delta x\, \Delta z\, [(\varrho u_y)|_y - (\varrho u_y)|_{y+\Delta y}] \\ & + \Delta x\, \Delta y\, [(\varrho u_z)|_z - (\varrho u_z)|_{z+\Delta z}]. \end{aligned} \tag{1}$$

Dividing both sides of the equation by the volume of the element and taking the limit as each of the element's dimensions approaches zero, we have,

$$\frac{\partial \varrho}{\partial t} = -\left[\frac{\partial}{\partial x}(\varrho u_x) + \frac{\partial}{\partial y}(\varrho u_y) + \frac{\partial}{\partial z}(\varrho u_z)\right]. \tag{2}$$

This equation, known as the *equation of continuity*, can be simplified somewhat for our purposes. Each term on the right hand side can be differentiated by the chain rule, giving pairs of terms:

$$\frac{\partial}{\partial x}(\varrho u_x) = u_x \frac{\partial \varrho}{\partial x} + \varrho \frac{\partial u_x}{\partial x}. \tag{3}$$

Notice that, in Eq. (3), $u_x (\partial \varrho / \partial x)$ consists of the product of two terms that are both assumed to be small, while $\varrho (\partial u_x / \partial x)$ has only one small term. We will therefore discard $u_x (\partial \varrho / \partial x)$ from Eq. (3). We will also make use of the usual approximation that any change in density will be proportional to pressure change and that the proportionality constant is equal to $\varrho \varkappa$ where $\varkappa$ is adiabatic compressibility. Utilizing this approximation and neglecting terms with second-order smallness, Eq. (2) becomes

$$\varkappa \frac{\partial p}{\partial t} = -\left(\frac{\partial u_x}{\partial x} + \frac{\partial u_y}{\partial y} + \frac{\partial u_z}{\partial z}\right) \tag{4}$$

which is the form of the equation of continuity that we will use.

The second equation needed can be derived using Newton's second law of motion. Consider again the volume element of Fig. 1. If we assume the fluid has

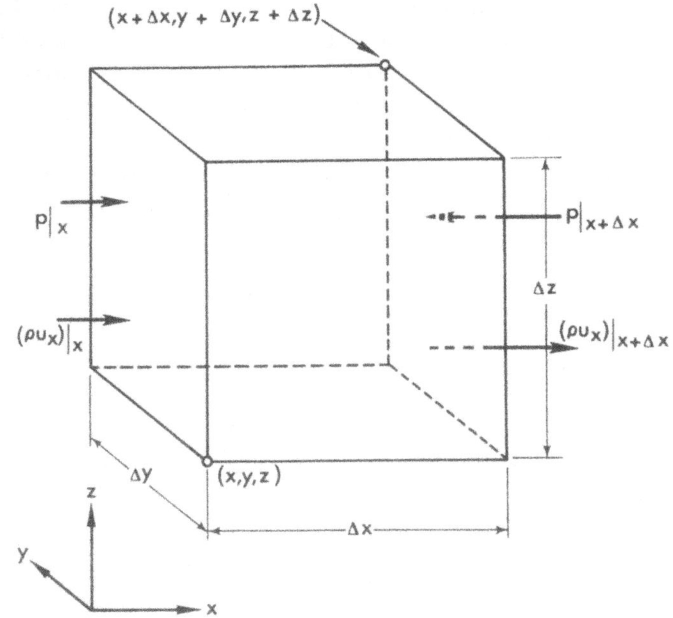

Fig. 1. Volume element $\Delta x\, \Delta y\, \Delta z$ fixed in space with arrows indicating pressures and fluid flows

negligible viscosity, the force on the face lying perpendicular to the x-axis at x is $\Delta y \Delta z p|_x$ and the force on the parallel face lying at $x + \Delta x$ is $\Delta y \Delta z\, p|_{x+\Delta x}$. The net force on the fluid in the volume element in the x-direction must equal the time rate of change of its x-momentum,

$$\Delta y\, \Delta z p|_x - \Delta y\, \Delta z p|_{x+\Delta x} = \Delta x\, \Delta y\, \Delta z \frac{d}{dt}\, (\varrho u_x). \tag{5}$$

Dividing through by $\Delta x \Delta y \Delta z$ and taking the limit as the volume goes to zero, we have, again ignoring second-order terms,

$$\frac{\partial p}{\partial x} = -\varrho \frac{\partial u_x}{\partial t}\,. \tag{6}$$

Similar equations exist for the other two coordinates. If we differentiate Eq. (4) by t and Eq. (6) and the two analogous equations in the y and z coordinates by x, y, and z, respectively, we can eliminate the velocity terms. The result is the familiar wave equation

$$\frac{\partial^2 p}{\partial x^2} + \frac{\partial^2 p}{\partial y^2} + \frac{\partial^2 p}{\partial z^2} = \frac{1}{c^2} \frac{\partial^2 p}{\partial t^2} \tag{7}$$

where $c^2 = (\varkappa\varrho)^{-1}$. For sinusoidal pressures, Eq. (7) becomes

$$\frac{\partial^2 p}{\partial x^2} + \frac{\partial^2 p}{\partial y^2} + \frac{\partial^2 p}{\partial z^2} + \left(\frac{\omega}{c}\right)^2 p = 0 \tag{8}$$

where ω is radian frequency. With Eq. (8), we are now in a position to begin our analysis of cochlea function.

The equations we have developed must be solved subject to the constraints (boundary conditions) put on them by the structure of the cochlea. The description of the cochlea used to determine these boundary conditions cannot be too detailed or else solution of the equations will become prohibitively difficult. Hence, the description of the cochlea generally used to determine the boundary conditions is as simple as possible. It ignores the curvature of the cochlea and represents it as composed of two straight channels, as seen in Fig. 2. A thin

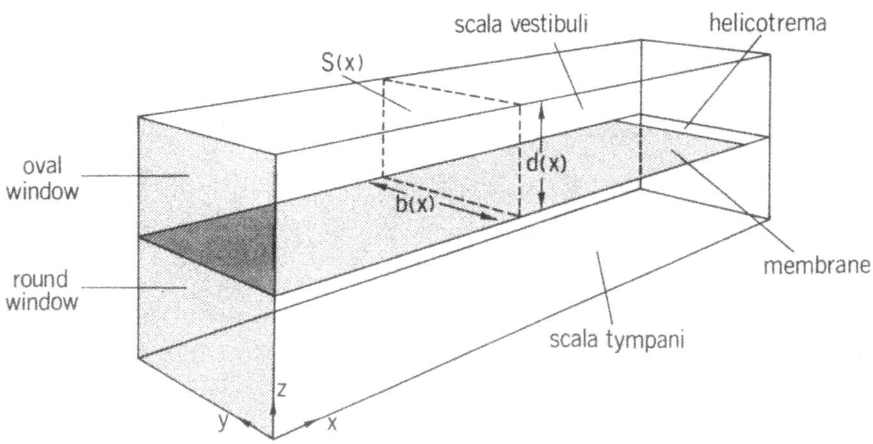

Fig. 2. Model of the inner ear

membrane represents the entire basilar partition and separates the two channels, which communicate at the apical end through the helicotrema. The oval window and round window seal the basal ends of their respective channels. The width of the membrane, the acoustic impedance of the membrane, and the cross sectional areas of the scalae are all taken to be functions of the longitudinal dimension x. Unfortunately, this variation of the model parameters with longitudinal distance and the presence of two communicating channels creates a formidable problem, and a complete solution for this representation has not yet been found. However, a number of different researchers have successfully tried various approximations and further simplifications of the model.

B. Single Uniform Duct

Before considering these various solutions of the cochlea model let us solve Eq. (8) in a related but much simpler system: the inside of a single uniform rectangular duct which has three rigid walls and one wall with a uniform finite acoustic impedance. The complete description of acoustic wave propagation in this system has been obtained (MORSE and INGARD, 1968), and will prove instructive for us. Let us set the x-axis parallel to the axis of the duct and let the duct extend from $x = 0$ to $x \to \infty$. For sinusoidal excitation at $x = 0$, the solution of Eq. (8) will be in the form of a pressure wave traveling in the x-direction and will therefore contain the term $e^{j(\omega t - k_x x)}$ where k_x, called the wave number, is a complex number. The pressure must then be of the form

$$p = \psi\,(x, y, z)\,e^{j(\omega t - k_x x)}. \tag{9}$$

Due to the fact that the properties of the duct walls are uniform in the x-direction, and hence that the boundary conditions are the same at every point along the x-axis we can show that the term ψ is not a function of x. It follows that

$$p = \psi(y, z)\,e^{j(\omega t - k_x x)} \tag{10}$$

where the exponential term determines the form of the traveling wave. A substitution into Eq. (10) shows that the real part of k_x will determine the phase velocity of the wave while the imaginary part will determine the attenuation of amplitude with distance. The transverse term ψ determines the form of the pressure distribution across the duct. When we substitute Eq. (10) into Eq. (8), we find that ψ must satisfy.

$$\frac{\partial^2 \psi}{\partial x^2} + \frac{\partial^2 \psi}{\partial y^2} + \zeta^2 \psi = 0,\ \zeta^2 = \left(\frac{\omega}{c}\right)^2 - k_x^2. \tag{11}$$

Equation (11) must hold true at all points in the duct, in particular at the boundaries. The constraints imposed by these boundaries are such that a solution of Eq. (11) does not exist for every value of the constant ζ, but only for a certain set of discrete values. These values are called characteristic values or eigenvalues. The corresponding solutions are called characteristic functions or eigenfunctions; the characteristic function corresponding to a particular value ζ_n will be called $\psi_n(y,z)$. ψ_n is not only a solution of Eq. (11), but we can show that it is also orthogonal to any other characteristic function. Hence, the complete solution for Eq. (11) is a sum of all of the characteristic functions. That is,

$$p = \sum_n A_n \psi_n (y,z) e^{j(\omega t - k_n x)} \tag{12}$$

where the A_n are constants to be specified by the input source. It remains for us to find the characteristic values and the associated characteristic functions.

To specify the characteristic functions, we must consider the boundary conditions prescribed by the duct walls. For this purpose it is convenient to set the duct at $x = 0$ with the x-axis lying along a corner of the duct, away from the soft wall, as shown in the lower duct of Fig. 2. The duct is assumed to have breadth b in the y-direction and depth d in the z-direction. For the rigid wall at $z = 0$, u_z, the fluid velocity perpendicular to the surface, must be zero. Hence, according to the z-coordinate version of Eq. (6),

$$\frac{\partial p}{\partial z} = 0, \text{ at } z = 0. \tag{13}$$

By the same reasoning

$$\frac{\partial p}{\partial y} = 0, \text{ at } y = 0, \; y = b. \tag{14}$$

For the wall at $z = d$, we specify that it is locally reactive (that is, the motion of one portion of the wall is dependent only on the acoustic pressure incident on that portion and independent of the motion of any other part of the wall). We describe this local reaction by assigning a specific acoustic impedance, defined as $Z = p/u_z$, to each point on the wall. Therefore, the boundary condition to be satisfied everywhere on the reactive wall is,

$$\frac{\partial \psi}{\partial z} = -\frac{j\varrho\omega}{Z}\psi, \text{ at } z = d. \tag{15}$$

Together, Eqs. (13) — (15) form the boundary conditions imposed by the duct walls.

The characteristic function that satisfies all of the duct boundary conditions simultaneously is

$$\psi_n = \cos\frac{\pi q z}{d} \cos\frac{\pi m y}{b} \tag{16}$$

where m and q are constants. Direct substitution into Eqs. (13) and (14) shows that m can be any positive integer, while Eq. (15) requires that

$$\pi q \tan(\pi q) = j\varrho\omega Y d \tag{17}$$

where specific acoustic admittance Y is the reciprocal of the specific acoustic impedance Z. When $\varrho\omega Y d$ is small compared to unity, an approximate solution for Eq. (17) can be obtained. In this case, we approximate the tangent term, which must also be small, by its argument and solve the resulting equation directly to yield

$$\begin{aligned} q &\cong (j\varrho\omega Y d/\pi^2)^{1/2}, \; r = 0 \\ q &\cong r + \frac{j\varrho\omega Y d}{\pi^2 r}, \; r > 0 \end{aligned} \tag{18}$$

where r can be any positive integer. Therefore each characteristic function and its corresponding mode of propagation is specified by a pair of integers, m and r.

We find the wave number of each characteristic function, upon substituting Eq. (16) into Eq. (11), to be

$$k_x^2 = \left(\frac{\omega}{c}\right)^2 - \left(\frac{\pi m}{b}\right)^2 - \left(\frac{\pi q}{d}\right)^2. \tag{19}$$

In the particular case where the free-fluid wavelength λ is considerably larger than either of the transverse dimensions, k_x obviously has a large imaginary part for all modes other than the fundamental mode ($m = r = 0$). Hence in this case, all higher modes are sharply attenuated and true propagation is possible only for the fundamental mode. Furthermore, since q has a very small magnitude in this case, the transverse term ψ_0 is practically a constant throughout the whole cross-section. In other words, for a duct having one wall of large but finite acoustic impedance and having transverse dimensions much smaller than a wavelength, the only wave which propagates for any appreciable distance is virtually a plane wave.

When $\varrho\omega Y d$ is not small compared to unity, we must solve Eq. (17) numerically. It is clear from an examination of that equation that in this case q can be quite large in magnitude, even for the principal wave. It follows from Eq. (16) that the principal wave will be far from a plane wave, no matter what the relation of the free-field wavelength to the duct dimensions.

C. A Two-Dimensional Model

Returning now to the cochlear model with its varying parameters, the most complete treatment of the problem has been that of Ranke (1950), the first of the modern auditory theorists, who obtained a two-dimensional solution. Starting with Eq. (8), Ranke further simplified the equation by making two additional assumptions. First, he assumed that the pressure was uniform in the y-dimension. Second, he assumed that the free-fluid velocity of sound c was essentially infinite. These two assumptions have the effect of reducing Eq. (8) to

$$\frac{\partial^2 p}{\partial x^2} + \frac{\partial^2 p}{\partial z^2} = 0 \tag{20}$$

which is the Laplace equation.

To establish the necessary boundary conditions, Ranke specified that the membrane was locally reactive, the local membrane velocity being equal to the difference in the pressure across the membrane, divided by the membrane's acoustic impedance. He further assumed that the wall of each duct opposite from the membrane was so far away that no reflections from it reach the membrane. The problem was therefore reduced to considering wave travel in a divided two-dimensional duct, the center wall having a finite acoustic impedance that varies with longitudinal distance, and the other two walls being far removed.

From this start, Ranke solved directly the differential equation representing the membrane boundary conditions. He obtained traveling wave solutions for the pressure difference and membrane displacement which have a number of interesting properties, among which is an ability of the latter to match closely some of BÉKÉSY's amplitude displacement curves for the basilar membrane. Moreover, the position of the amplitude maximum showed a shift towards the stapes as membrane damping was increased, an effect of recent interest (RHODE, 1971). Unfortunately, the solutions also exhibit very disturbing properties. These can perhaps best be illustrated by applying RANKE's method to a single infinitely long duct with three rigid walls and one of uniform finite impedance. We can show that the solution obtained for this case is

$$p = jA\varrho\omega e^{-j\varrho\omega Yz} e^{j\omega t - \varrho\omega Yx} \tag{21}$$

where A is a constant determined by the amplitude of the pressure at the origin. Notice that, except for the single constant A, the solution is totally determined. It follows that the solution cannot be fitted to an arbitary input waveform, such as constant pressure amplitude, applied along the line $z = 0$. Moreover, the wave number of Eq. 21 is $-j\varrho\omega Y$, which does not contain any factor corresponding to duct depth d. The significance of this absence of d can be illustrated by considering a duct in which the only propagating mode is the first one (cf. Eq. 12). The wave number of this propagating mode does contain d (Eq. 19) and thus differs fundamentally from that of Eq. 21. Hence it must be concluded that the RANKE assumption of a very distant wall is not valid in the case of a duct in which only a single mode propagates. These restrictions on the uniform duct solution imply that the RANKE solution for the cochlear model is not valid for those regions in which a z-axis boundary condition must be matched or in which a plane-wave approximation is justified. Thus, although the RANKE solution may be valid in certain regions, particulary near the point of maximum sensitivity where the plane-wave approximation appears unrealistic (see below), it does not give a solution that holds over the entire extent of the cochlear model. Consequently, we shall not pursue the RANKE model any further.

D. One-Dimensional Models

The problem must be further simplified by reducing it to a single dimension. Let us assume that the pressure in either scala is independent of y and z, and consequently that the pressure waves are planar or uniform in the transverse plane. Even for ducts as small as the cochlear scalae, we recall that this assumption is not necessarily valid and must be justified later on.

With the assumption of planar waves, we may rewrite one of the basic equations in a more convenient form. Let us return to Fig. 2 and consider a thin slice of the scala vestibuli at point x, having longitudinal thickness Δx. Since the pressure is constant across the scala, the point velocities are in the x-direction and are constant across the scala [see Eq. (6)]. Let us consider the conservation of mass for this slice. Following the reasoning that led to Eq. (1) we have

$$S_v \Delta x \frac{\partial\varrho}{\partial t} = (S_v \varrho u_v)|_x - (S_v \varrho\, u_v)|_{x+\Delta x} - b\Delta\, x\varrho v \tag{22}$$

where S_v is cross-sectional area of the scala vestibuli, u_v is velocity of fluid in scala vestibuli in the x-direction, and v is the velocity of the membrane in the direction from scala vestibuli to scala tympani. The last term in Eq. (22) describes the rate of fluid flow out of the scala boundaries at any moment due to the velocity of the membrane. Taking the limit and making the same assumptions regarding ϱ that were used in the derivation of Eq. (4), we have

$$\frac{\partial}{\partial x}(S_v u_v) = -\frac{S_v}{\varrho c^2}\frac{\partial p_v}{\partial t} - v\,b. \tag{23}$$

A similar equation can be derived for the scala tympani

$$\frac{\partial}{\partial x}(S_t u_t) = -\frac{S_t}{\varrho c^2}\frac{\partial p_t}{\partial t} + v\,b. \tag{24}$$

Two other equations are needed in addition to Eqs. (23) and (24). One of these is the force equation, which we can show is identical to Eq. (6), and the other describes the properties of the membrane. The usual description of the membrane used is that of a local reactance Z which can be described by the equation (ZWISLOCKI, 1948)

$$p_v - p_t = Zv. \tag{25}$$

The equations we must solve have now all been derived [Eqs. (6), (23) — (25)], but they can be simplified somewhat by the introduction of new variables. Following PETERSON and BOGERT (1950) we introduce

$$\begin{aligned} p_+ &= \tfrac{1}{2}(p_v + p_t) \qquad & p_- &= \tfrac{1}{2}(p_v - p_t) \\ u_+ &= \tfrac{1}{2}(u_v + u_t) \qquad & u_- &= \tfrac{1}{2}(u_v - u_t) \end{aligned} \tag{26}$$

where p_+ is average pressure and p_- is proportional to the pressure difference across the membrane. At this stage, let us also make the convenient assumption that the scalae have the same cross-sectional area, S, at any longitudinal point x. Further, let us confine our attention to sinusoidal stimulation and write each variable in its complex form (e. g., $p_v = P_v e^{j\omega t}$). When the indicated equations are combined and the new variables inserted, two new equations emerge:

$$\frac{1}{S}\frac{\partial}{\partial x}\left(S\frac{\partial P_+}{\partial x}\right) + \left(\frac{\omega}{c}\right)^2 P_+ = 0, \tag{27}$$

$$\frac{1}{S}\frac{\partial}{\partial x}\left(S\frac{\partial P_-}{\partial x}\right) + \frac{\omega^2}{c^2}\left(1 - \frac{j\,2\,\varrho\,Y b\,c^2}{\omega S}\right) P_- = 0. \tag{28}$$

We must solve Eqs. (27) and (28) simultaneously to obtain the various pressures, and then combine them with Eq. (25) to find membrane displacement.

1. Solution for Average Pressure, $p_+(x)$

The equation for average pressure, Eq. (27) has been solved by PETERSON and BOGERT (1950). They found the closed-form solution to be

$$p_+(x) = \{A J_0[\omega/c(5.8 - x)] + B N_0[\omega/c(5.8 - x)]\} e^{j\omega t} \tag{29}$$

where J_0 and N_0 are zero-order Bessel functions of the first and second kind, respectively, and A and B are unknown constants that we must now evaluate.

To determine the amplitude of the average pressure, boundary conditions must be specified at the oval window, at the round window, and at the helicotrema. In the initial work on this problem, PETERSON and BOGERT (1950) assumed that these boundary conditions were: 1) zero pressure at the round window; 2) a known pressure applied just inside the oval window [*i. e.*, $p_v(0) = P_0 e^{j\omega t}$;]; 3) zero pressure difference between the scalae at the helicotrema; and 4) continuity of fluid flow at the helicotrema. The solution for $p_+(x)$ obtained using these boundary conditions is

$$p_+(x) = \frac{P_0}{2}\left\{\frac{N_1(2.3\,\omega/c)\,J_0[(\omega/c)\,(5.8-x)] - J_1(2.3\,\omega/c)\,N_0[(\omega/c)\,(5.8-x)]}{N_1(2.3\,\omega/c)\,J_0(5.8\,\omega/c) - J_1(2.3\,\omega/c)\,N_0(5.8\,\omega/c)}\right\} e^{j\omega t}. \tag{30}$$

Evaluation of Eq. (30) indicates that it is very close to $P_0/2$ at all values of x for frequencies below 3 kHz. For higher frequencies, the function grows rapidly and becomes unbounded just above 10 kHz. The magnitude of $p_-(x)$ at the stapes end, a quantity also found from these boundary conditions, is equal to $P_0/2$ for all frequencies. Notice that we have obtained the $p_+(x)$ solution completely independently of $p_-(x)$. Moreover, we can show that the $p_-(x)$ solution is independent of $p_+(x)$. This independence of solutions is due to the particular choice of boundary conditions: they provide no coupling between the two pressures and so allow each to be determined separately.

The first boundary condition used by PETERSON and BOGERT (1950) is that pressure just inside the round window is equal to zero. This condition is equivalent to assuming that the round-window membrane is absent, for it specifies that the displacement of fluid at the round window causes no restoring force to be exerted on the fluid. When intact, the round-window membrane does in fact exert force on the fluid in the manner of an elastic membrane, at least for low frequencies (BÉKÉSY, 1960, p. 435). Accordingly, GEISLER and HUBBARD (1972) obtained a solution for $p_+(x)$ that includes the effect of the round-window membrane. Starting with Eq. (27), they simplified it first by eliminating the x-dependence of the cross-sectional area, S. With this simplification, which we can show has relatively little effect on the solution for frequencies below 10 kHz, S cancels out in Eq. (27), which then becomes the familiar one-dimensional wave equation. The solution for sinusoidal excitation is

$$p_+(x) = Ae^{j\omega(t-x/c)} + Be^{j\omega(t+x/c)} \tag{31}$$

where A and B are complex constants that must be evaluated.

Using the last three of the PETERSON and BOGERT (1950) boundary conditions, and representing the round-window membrane as a spring of specific acoustic stiffness K, GEISLER and HUBBARD (1972) found the solution to be

$$p_+(x) = \frac{P_0\{\varrho\,\omega^2 c + Kc[P'_-(0)/P_-(0)]\}\,[e^{j\omega(t-x/c)} + e^{-2j\omega l/c}e^{j\omega(t+x/c)}]}{(1+e^{-2j\omega l/c})\,\{2\varrho\,\omega^2 c + Kc[P'_-(0)/P_-(0)] + K\omega\tan(\omega l/c)\}} \tag{32}$$

where $P'_-(0)$ is the spatial derivative of $P_-(x)$ at $x = 0$, and l is the length of the cochlea at the helicotrema. Notice that the average pressure $p_+(x)$ is no longer independent of the pressure difference $p_-(x)$. The round-window membrane now serves as a coupling between these two pressures. Notice also that $p_+(x)$ in Eq. (32) is composed of two traveling waves, one going in each direction. In fact, we can easily show by factoring Eq. (32) that $p_+(x)$ is a standing wave.

Many workers (see below) have obtained solutions of $p_-(x)$ for sinusoidal excitation. For the moment, let us assume that one of these $p_-(x)$ solutions is available and hence Eq. (32) can be evaluated. Pressure along any particular scala is then obtained by adding or subtracting $p_+(x)$ and $p_-(x)$ [see Eq. (26)]. We see that the pressure at any point in either scalae is composed of two types of pressure waves. One, the $p_+(x)$ wave, is a standing wave. The other, the $p_-(x)$ wave has been shown by many workers to be a traveling wave that has a position-dependent propagation velocity. The relative amplitudes of the two pressure waves are a function of frequency and longitudinal position.

Using a spring representation of the round-window membrane also dictates the value of the $p_-(x)$ wave at the stapes end of the cochlea. GEISLER and HUBBARD (1972) found it to be

$$p_-(0) = \frac{P_0[\varrho\omega^2 c + K\omega\tan(\omega l/c)]e^{j\omega t}}{2\varrho\omega^2 c + Kc[P'_-(0)/P_-(0)] + K\omega\tan(\omega l/c)} \tag{33}$$

An evalution of Eq. (33), using values of the term $P'_-(0)/P_-(0)$ obtained from the BOGERT (1951) solution of the $p_-(x)$ wave, indicates that the assumption of fluid incompressibility (equivalent to letting $c\to\infty$) causes negligible error for frequencies below approximately 7 kHz for the human cochlea. For shorter cochleas, proportionately higher frequencies may be used without considering fluid compressibility. The evaluation of Eq. (33) also shows that the amplitude of $p_-(0)$ is approximately proportional to $\omega^{3/2}$ at very low frequencies, if reflections from the helicotrema are ignored. At these frequencies, less and less of the pressure applied at the oval window is transmitted to the pressure difference wave.

2. Solutions for Pressure Difference, $p_-(x)$

The equation describing pressure difference, Eq. (28), must now be considered. Unfortunately, this equation has no exact solution, and various simplifications and approximations have had to be employed in order to obtain solutions. The principle approximation methods and their solutions will be presented in this section. One word of caution: many of these solutions for $p_-(x)$ were originally presented as being the only significant parts of the total solution. Equation (26) shows that such a presentation is valid only if the amplitude of $p_+(x)$ is constant throughout the cochlea. We have already shown that $p_+(x)$ behaves in this fashion only for the special case of an absent round-window membrane and only then for frequencies below 3 kHz.

a) The WKBJ Approximation. RANKE (1950), attempted to solve Eq. (28) by means of the short-wavelength or so-called WKBJ approximation (MORSE and FESHBACH, 1953). Using scalae of equal and constant areas and an incompressible fluid, he obtained the approximate solution

$$p_-(x) = P_0 e^{j(\omega t - k_x x)} \tag{34}$$

where $k_x^2 = -(j2\varrho\omega Yb/S)$. RANKE recognized that Eq. (34) is a good approximation only when the plane-wave approximation is valid. Moreover, he determined, by means of a criterion closely related to the one we discussed with regard to Eq. (17), that the plane-wave approximation is clearly valid only for certain regions of the cochlea. RANKE failed to realize, however, that the WKBJ approximation itself is valid only when k_x varies slowly over a wavelength: that is, when $k_x \gg [\partial k_x/\partial x]^{1/2}$. Unfortunately, this inequality does not hold for cochlear models at frequencies of interest. For example, when k_x is evaluated at the stapes end using representative values of Y (BOGERT, 1951), the inequality is satisfied only for frequencies much greater than 20 kHz. The variation of Y with longitudinal distance is just too pronounced for the approximation to be used at any frequencies but those with extremely short wavelengths. Since the frequencies for which the WKBJ approximation is valid are above the range of human hearing, this model cannot be considered to yield the general solution of Eq. (28), even in the regions where the plane-wave approximation is valid.

b) The Peterson-Bogert Solution. PETERSON and BOGERT (1950) obtained one of the first solutions of Eq. (28), and their results are quite instructive. Before describing these results, however, let us first consider some of the details of their method. Examination of Eq. (28) shows that cross-sectional area, membrane breadth, and membrane impedance must be specified as functions of distance before the equation can be solved. Two of these variables, the area of the scalae and the membrane breadth, have been accurately measured and there is little ambiguity concerning them. By contrast, the acoustic impedance of the basilar membrane has not been accurately specified and different workers have adopted very different functions to represent it. PETERSON and BOGERT (1950) assumed, as do most others, that the membrane impedance is described by

$$Z = \frac{k}{j\omega} + r + j\omega m \tag{35}$$

where $k(x)$, $r(x)$, and $m(x)$ are functions of x but not of frequency, and correspond to stiffness, resistance, and mass, respectively. The stiffness function was obtained from the experiments of BÉKÉSY in which he pressed hairs down onto the basilar membrane (1960, p. 467). The force exerted by the hair divided by the membrane's indentation is a measure of stiffness. Such data are difficult to translate into acoustic impedances, for the effective area over which the force was spread is not clear. The stiffness function that PETERSON and BOGERT deduced from these data is an exponential function of distance that is three orders of magnitude stiffer at the basal end than at the apical end. The mass was assumed to be that of the entire scala media and was estimated on anatomical grounds to be constant along the membrane. Membrane resistance was assumed to be negligible and was dropped from Eq. (35).

The solution of Eq. (28) obtained by PETERSON and BOGERT (1950), using numerical integration, is a traveling pressure wave which decreases monotonically in amplitude for increasing x. Membrane displacement, which is obtained from $p_-(x)$ using Eq. (25), is also a traveling wave. For any particular frequency, the displacement amplitude increases monotonically for increasing x, becoming infinite at a certain point. Beyond this point, the displacement amplitude drops extremely rapidly, becoming negligibly small within 2 or 3 mm. This behavior, while complicated, can be explained with reference to Eq. (35). At small values of x, the stiffness term dominates the membrane impedance and causes the traveling wave type of response. The exponentially decreasing magnitude of the stiffness causes the increasing magnitude of the displacement. At one point along the membrane, the stiffness drops to a value such that

$$\omega = (k/m)^{1/2} \tag{36}$$

and the impedance becomes zero (we recall that $r(x)$ was neglected in this solution). The membrane displacement accordingly becomes infinite. Beyond the resonant point, the stiffness drops still further, and the mass term comes to dominate the impedance. Since an impedance composed principally of mass does not allow true wave propagation, the displacement amplitude is rapidly attenuated.

The membrane displacements obtained from the PETERSON-BOGERT solution are similar in some respects to BÉKÉSY's (1960) observations. Traveling waves which have a displacement peak at one particular point along the membrane occur in both sets of data. Moreover, for both sets the location of this displacement peak is a function of frequency: the higher the frequency, the closer to the stapes is the resonant point. Quantitatively, however, numerical discrepancies exist between the model's output and the experimental data. The chief discrepancy, aside from the infinite peak displacement, concerns the range of frequencies which have resonant points on the membrane. BÉKÉSY's data (1960, p. 442) indicate, with some extrapolation, that frequencies ranging from approximately 30 Hz to 30 kHz cause displacement peaks. By contrast, the model allows true displacement peaks to occur over a considerably more restricteded frequency range, from approximately 500 Hz to 20 kHz. The more restricted frequency range of the model is related to Eq. (36). According to that equation, the range of frequencies for which a resonant point can occur on the membrane is limited to the square root of the range of the term k/m (SIEBERT, 1970). Since that term varies by three orders of magnitude in the PETERSON-BOGERT model, a frequency range of only $1^1/_2$ orders of magnitude results.

c) The Zwislocki Solution. For our present understanding of the pressure difference, $p_-(x)$, we are deeply indebted to ZWISLOCKI, the pioneer who first derived and solved an equation similar to Eq. (28). Indeed, his basic equation is actually somewhat more complicated than Eq. (28), because he included in his development the effects of the viscosity of the perilymph. ZWISLOCKI's solution (1948, 1965) was thus the first one to be achieved. It is presented here, out of historical order, to suit the organizational framework of this chapter.

The uniqueness of ZWISLOCKI's solution (1948) is determined by his choice of parameter values. He obtained the membrane stiffness function from BÉKÉSY's measurements (1960, p. 476) of the static displacement of the basilar membrane under a pressure difference of 1 cm of water (10^3 dynes/cm^2). While these measurements yield membrane stiffness directly, they were obtained at such high pressure levels that they must remain suspect. Fitting an analytical expression to the experimental points, ZWISLOCKI obtained an exponential stiffness function that is approximately two orders of magnitude stiffer at the basal end than at the apical end. He assumed a membrane resistance function that increased slowly along the membrane. This resistance has the general effect of reducing the magnitude of the membrane displacement peak and of shifting it towards the stapes. The membrane mass function was estimated from anatomical data and increased slowly with x. The magnitude of the mass function was considerably smaller than that assumed by PETERSON and BOGERT (1950). In fact, for the stiffness and resistance functions chosen by ZWISLOCKI, the membrane mass played almost no role at all. The pressure difference was so small at the resonant point that membrane displacement from there to the helicotrema was essentially non-existent. Consequently $m(x)$ was dropped from Eq. (35).

The complete solution for $p_-(x)$ obtained by ZWISLOCKI (1965) is in terms of Bessel functions. He calculated the membrane velocity from $p_-(x)$ using Eq. (25), and found it, with suitable approximations, to be

$$v(x) = A\, e^{\left(x - \frac{r Q \omega^2}{2 k_0} e^{2.5 x} - \frac{Q r_f}{2 \varrho} e^{x}\right)} e^{j\omega(t - Q e^{x})} \tag{37}$$

where k_0 is membrane stiffness at the basal end, r is membrane resistance, Q is a constant composed of parameter values, r_f is effective viscosity resistance, and A is a function of frequency and the input pressure source. The effect of the viscosity resistance was small at all but the lowest frequencies.

The displacement of the basilar membrane calculated from Eq. (37) agrees both qualitatively and quantitatively with BÉKÉSY's data on sinusoidal basilar membrane displacement in many respects. The shapes of the displacement curves are very similar for both sets of data and the phase velocities of the displacement waves are approximately the same in each case. Moreover, the frequencies which caused membrane displacement peaks cover about the same range in ZWISLOCKI's solution and in the experimental data. This last effect is possible, even though the stiffness function varies by only two orders of magnitude, because the ZWISLOCKI solution does not involve membrane resonances.

Recent data obtained on the motion of a single point of the basilar membrane by means of the Mössbauer technique (JOHNSTONE *et al.*, 1970; RHODE, 1971) allow a further comparison of experimental findings with Eq. (37). The experimental data of particular interest are given by RHODE (1971) in a form that is essentially the ratio of basilar membrane displacement to stapes displacement. The magnitude of this displacement ratio was observed experimentally to increase by 6 dB/octave for low frequencies. As the frequency which produced the maximum magnitude of the displacement ratio (the "best frequency") was approached, the ratio increased somewhat faster. For frequencies above the best frequency, the magnitude of the ratio decreased at approximately —100 dB/octave. The phase of the basilar membrane relative to the stapes was also observed. At very low frequencies there was a phase difference of 90°. For higher frequencies, the phase of the basilar membrane lagged further and further behind the stapes, decreasing at a faster rate as the best frequency was approached.

A careful examination of Eq. (37) shows that it does not describe the latest experimental data. First, the phase velocity, which we can calculate from the last exponential term of Eq. (37), is independent of frequency. By contrast, experimental phase velocities were found to be frequency sensitive as the best frequency was approached. Second, the membrane displacement amplitude in Eq. (37) does not describe the experimental displacement curves. Comparable amplitude displacement curves for an earlier and slightly different version of Eq. (37) (ZWISLOCKI, 1948), show drop-offs above the best frequencies of not much greater than —24 dB/octave. This value is much lower than the recently observed figure. Even manipulating the parameter values of Eq. (37) does not increase the value of amplitude drop-off appreciably. In short, the ZWISLOCKI solution describes a membrane displacement pattern that is considerably different from those that RHODE observed.

d) The Bogert Solution. BOGERT (1951) used the basic formulation and parameter functions of PETERSON and BOGERT (1950), except that he retained membrane resistance in Eq. (35). To obtain a solution, he turned to electrical analog techniques. First, he developed an electrical circuit which has equations analogous to Eqs. (25), (28), and (35) for a small section of the cochlea. He then joined together 175 of these electrical circuits to form a sectional electrical analog of the hydrodynamic equations. A short-circuit termination at the apical end of the network represented the boundary conditions at the helicotrema. The input to the network was a voltage applied at the basal end representing $p_-(0)$.

The properties of the solution obtained by BOGERT have many similarities to the experimental results both of BÉKÉSY and of RHODE (1971) and we will consider them in some detail. Due to the limited amount of data published on the performance of the original network, data obtained from a recent hybrid-computer simulation of the model (HUBBARD and GEISLER, 1972) will also be included.

The amplitude of the pressure wave $p_-(x)$ along the membrane is shown in Fig. 3 for several different frequencies. The lower the frequency, the less each section of the analog attenuates the pressure and the further the pressure wave propagates. At 315 Hz, the wave propagates to the apical termination and is reflected from it. Non-zero apical terminations representing various non-zero acoustic impedances of the helicotrema, originally suggested by FLETCHER (1951), reduce these reflections but do not eliminate them at all frequencies.

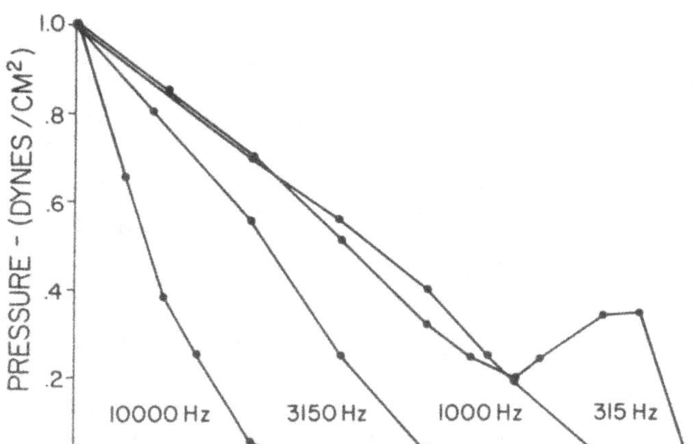

Fig. 3. Magnitude of pressure difference, $|p_-(x)|$, as a function of distance along the basilar membrane for several different frequencies. Redrawn from BOGERT (1951)

The amplitude of the membrane displacement along the membrane is shown in Fig. 4 for four different frequencies. The shapes of these displacement curves are similar to those observed in human cochleas by BÉKÉSY (1960, p. 448). However the range of frequencies which produce displacement peaks is still limited to approximately $1^1/_2$ orders of magnitude. The introduction of membrane resistance has reduced the magnitude of the response peaks and shifted each of them approximately 2 mm towards the stapes, but the resistance did not increase the frequency range.

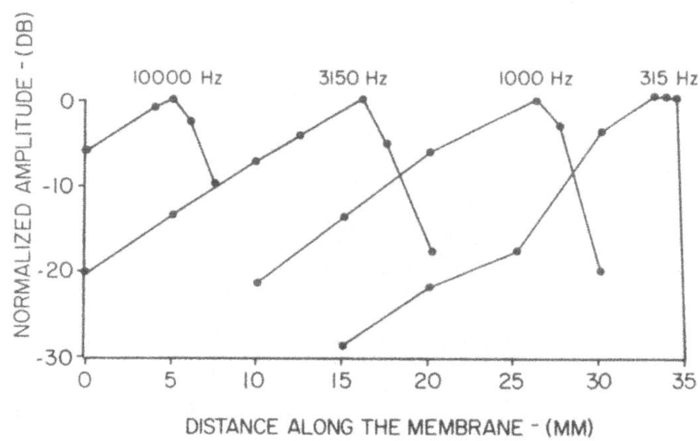

Fig. 4. Basilar-membrane displacement amplitude as a function of distance along the membrane for several frequencies. For clarity, each curve was normalized to a peak value of zero dB. Redrawn from BOGERT (1951)

Further measurements of the BOGERT analog's output have been made. Similarly to BÉKÉSY's observations, the phase of the analog's membrane displacement relative to the stapes displacement decreases monotonically with distance from the stapes. Maximum values as high as — 400° were reached. Various other comparisons between the output of the analog and BÉKÉSY's observations have been made by ZWISLOCKI (1953). Generally speaking, these comparisons indicate that the analog's output is qualitatively similar to the basilar membrane's motion observed by BÉKÉSY but that quantitative discrepancies exist.

BÉKÉSY also obtained strong evidence, both from psychoacoustic experiments (1960, p. 128) and from observations on mechanical models (1960, p. 511 ff.), that the direction of wave propagation along the cochlear partition is from base to apex, regardless of the site of stimulation. In the case where excitation is applied at the apex, therefore, waves would propagate towards the source, not away from it as is usually observed. This "paradoxical" direction of travel can also be generated in many different one-dimensional cochlear models, including the BOGERT model. Specifically, SIEBERT (1971) has shown that a general one-dimensional model, if suitably stimulated either at the apex or along the channels, will yield membrane vibration patterns that are identical to those generated by stapes stimulation, provided only that the ratio of the channel areas is the same throughout the model. SIEBERT's results, derived for incompressible fluids, can be readily extended to include those models, such as BOGERT's, which include fluid compressibility in their formulation.

To compare the model's output with the RHODE data, we must calculate the ratio of membrane displacement to stapes displacement. The membrane displacement is directly available from the analog, and the stapes displacement can be calculated from the $p_-(x)$ and $p_+(x)$ solutions. Figure 5 shows the ratio of these displacement amplitudes. The height of the peaks and the slopes on the low frequency sides of the peaks are similar to the experimental data. Moreover the curves in Fig. 5 drop off sharply past the peak (— 46 dB/octave). However, the slope does not increase appreciably as the best frequency is approached from the low frequency side, and the drop-off is not nearly as steep as the experimental curves. A reduction in membrane resistance reduces the magnitude of both of these discrepancies.

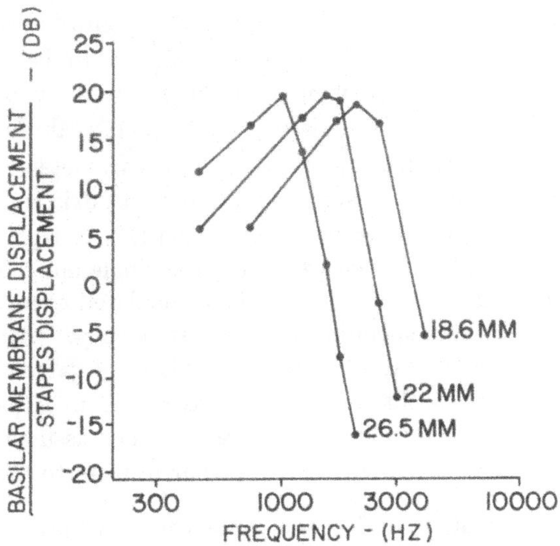

Fig. 5. The amplitude ratio of the basilar membrane displacement to the stapes displacement as a function of frequency for several positions on the basilar membrane. From HUBBARD and GEISLER (1972), with permission of the Journal of Acoustical Society of America

Figure 6 shows the phase data obtained from the model. At low frequencies the curves approach + 90°, a property shared with RHODE's experimental phase data. The general shape of the curves in Fig. 6 is also similar to the experimental

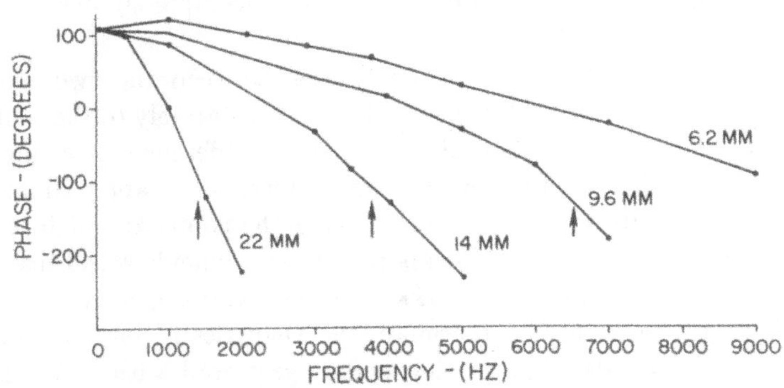

Fig. 6. Phase of the basilar-membrane displacement as a function of frequency for several membrane positions. Arrows indicate the approximate best frequency at the indicated position. Phase referenced to the stapes displacement. From HUBBARD and GEISLER (1972), with permission of the Journal of Acoustical Society of America

phase data, showing an increase in slope as best frequency is approached. The numerical agreement between the two sets of phase data, however, is poor. The maximum phase lags observed on the model were less than 400°, while experimental phase lags as great as 1600° were measured.

In his work, RHODE also showed nonlinear effects on membrane displacement as intensity was increased. Similar phenomena have been produced in the model by inserting into it a nonlinear form of the membrane resistance, $r(x)$. In both cases, increasing input pressure caused the displacement peak to become relatively smaller and more rounded, and to occur at a slightly lower frequency.

The BOGERT (1951) formulation has thus proven to be a relatively good qualitative model of the basilar membrane as observed by both BÉKÉSY and RHODE. There are, however, some major quantitative weaknesses in the model.

We should point out that the present range of parameter values has thrown doubt on one of the model's basic assumptions: the existence of only planar pressure waves. We observed in conjunction with Eq. (17) that $\varrho\omega Yd$ must be small compared to unity for planar waves to exist in a single uniform duct. However, we find that $\varrho\omega Yd$ is greater than unity when calculated at any point along the cochlear model at the corresponding resonant frequency, when Y is largest in magnitude. In accord with RANKE's warnings this large value casts considerable suspicion on the assumption that only planar waves exist in all parts of the model. Fortunately, it will be shown below that we need not assume the existence of planar waves in order to arrive at models similar in form to the BOGERT model.

e) The Fletcher Solution. Using the same basic cochlear model as BOGERT, FLETCHER (1951) arrived at a different solution that is interesting in its own right. The differences between the two solutions are basically due to the different functions chosen to represent the membrane impedance. From the BÉKÉSY probe-hair data, FLETCHER derived a different exponential stiffness function, one that is five orders of magnitude larger at the basal end than at the apical end. The mass function, which includes only the basilar membrane and the fluid near the membrane, is smaller than BOGERT's and increases with x. The damping level is essentially unchanged. FLETCHER also simplified Eq. (28) somewhat by showing that, for the impedance levels used, fluid incompressibility ($c \to \infty$) could be assumed with negligible error at all frequencies.

As might be expected from the similarities between the two models, the solutions obtained by FLETCHER are very similar qualitatively to those of BOGERT (Figs. 3 and 4). There is one notable quantitative difference. The range of frequencies which produce displacement peaks extends over approximately three orders of magnitude, from 50 Hz to 25 kHz. Thus the points at which the model's membrane has its displacement peaks approximately coincide with those observed by BÉKÉSY. Also in keeping with BÉKÉSY's observations, no large reflections from the helicotrema occur. Furthermore, the velocities of propagation for low frequency stimuli calculated from the model agree well with those calculated from BÉKÉSY's experimental data (ZWISLOCKI, 1953). Thus, there is good quantitative agreement between much of BÉKÉSY's experimental data and FLETCHER's solution. This agreement lends support to the particular values of parameters chosen. However, the stiffness function, with its change of almost five orders of magnitude over the cochlear length, seems unrealistic in view of BÉKÉSY's measurements of static membrane stiffness.

f) The Oetinger-Hauser Solution. The most complete one-dimensional model of the cochlea yet developed is that of OETINGER and HAUSER (1961). Unlike the other formulations which assume planar pressure waves in the scalae, their formulation takes account of fluid displacement in the transverse plane.

The initial basic assumptions of this solution are very similar to those made by RANKE (1950) for the two-dimensional model. Pressure in the y-direction (Fig. 2) is assumed uniform and the fluid is assumed to be incompressible. Hence Eq. (20) is one of the starting equations for OETINGER and HAUSER. They took the equation of motion for the x-coordinate as equal to Eq. (6) with a term added to account for the viscosity of the perilymph. They also took a similar equation of motion for the z-coordinate. Finally, they assumed the velocity of the membrane at any longitudinal point to be due to the difference between the pressures on either surface of the membrane divided by the local acoustic impedance $Z(x)$. For a coordinate system where the membrane lies at $z = d$ (Fig. 2), this assumption implies that

$$p_v(x, d) - p_t(x, d) = Zv \tag{38}$$

where v is membrane velocity [*cf.* Eq. (25)].

The reduction of the two-dimensional model just described to a one-dimensional representation hinges on the observation that the deflection of the basilar membrane is of primary interest. It follows from Eq. (38), therefore, that pressures need not be specified throughout the ducts but only at the membrane surface. If we average several variables across the depths of the scalae and make certain simplifying assumptions regarding the flow of fluid in the z-direction, we obtain the desired one-dimensional equations. For the scala vestibuli, we have

$$\frac{d\bar{u}_v}{dx} = -\frac{v}{d} \tag{39}$$

$$(r_0 + j\omega\varrho)\,\bar{u}_v + \frac{d}{dx}\left[p_v(x, d) + \frac{(r_0 + j\omega\varrho)d}{3}\,v\right] = 0 \tag{40}$$

where $\bar{u}_v$ is the average x-velocity across the scala in the plane x, and r_0 is a viscosity term. We obtain a similar set of equations for scala tympani. An examination of Eqs. (39) and (40) shows that, with the exception of the viscosity terms and of the last term in Eq. (40), they are identical in form to Eqs. (6) and (23). The last term in Eq. (40), therefore, is the term which approximates the effect of the fluid velocity in the z-direction. The similarity of Eqs. (39) and (40) to Eqs. (6) and (23) is very reassuring. The assumption of fluid motion in the transverse plane, at least for the assumptions of this model, does not affect the form of the equations derived assuming planar waves. Only the identity of some of the variables is changed and a single, rather simple term is added.

The final equations derived by OETINGER and HAUSER are actually a little more complicated than Eqs. (39) and (40), because they were also able to represent the fact that the basilar membrane extends only part way across the breadth of the cochlear duct. The solution to these final equations was accomplished by means of an electrical analog. This analog is unlike previous ones (*e. g.*, BOGERT,

1951) in that it represents the pressure in each scala individually, not just the pressure difference between scalae. The electrical analog, which also includes impedances to represent the window membranes, is thus somewhat more complicated than the previous ones. However, this type of representation, also adopted by SIEBERT (1971), has the considerable advantage that it gives a complete solution for the pressures, not just the $p_-(x)$ portion. The stiffness function of the membrane in the OETINGER-HAUSER model was derived from BÉKÉSY's pressure-difference measurements and decreases by approximately three orders of magnitude from base to apex. The mass of the membrane, taken from ZWISLOCKI's formulation (1948), increases by a factor of approximately 10 over the length of the cochlea. The term representing the effect of fluid velocity in the transverse plane appears as a mass term added to the static mass of the membrane.

The output of the OETINGER-HAUSER model is very similar to BÉKÉSY's data in many regards, although the approximate range of frequencies producing membrane displacement peaks in the model is only two orders of magnitude. However, the velocity of propagation of pulses and the decay behavior of the model after the termination of sinusoidal excitation are very similar to BÉKÉSY's observations. The shape of the displacement amplitude curve obtained for a particular frequency as a function af distance along the analog is however considerably broader than the comparable curves obtained by BÉKÉSY (1960, p. 448). Thus even this model cannot be considered a flawless replica of the inner ear.

g) Other Solutions. Various other workers have utilized the general one-dimensional representation of the inner ear to obtain solutions of Eq. (28) (BAUCH, 1956; WANSDRONK, 1961; CALDWELL *et al.*, 1962; KLATT and PETERSON, 1966; STEWART, 1972). Each of these representations used somewhat different functions to represent the membrane impedances, and each representation was realized by an electrical analog or a digital-computer program. Generally speaking the results obtained from these analogs are similar to comparable data obtained from one or the other of the models described above.

The possibility that truly resonant oscillations, instead of traveling waves, occur in the inner ear has recently been reintroduced by HUXLEY (1969). For his study, he used a model similar to RANKE's one-dimensional model (1950), but with elastic coupling added between adjacent parts of the cochlea. HUXLEY suggested that with certain types of elastic coupling a truly resonant behavior, with all parts moving sinusoidally in phase, is obtained. However, because of the short-wavelength approximation used to construct it, this model is properly limited to consideration of very high frequencies only and does not yield a general solution.

Several other resonant-oscillation types of models have been proposed for the inner ear. GOLD (1948) proposed a model that incorporates a feedback mechanism to obtain low damping levels. TIEDEMANN (1970) has proposed a resonance model where small sections of the tectorial membrane act as the resonant elements. LIEBERSTEIN (1971) suggested that small segments of the basilar membrane could be modeled by segments of a uniformly loaded annular plate clamped on both boundaries. All of these models are subject to the generals hortcomings of all resonant-oscillation models: their output does not match the available experimental data which indicate traveling-wave modes of vibration.

INSELBERG and FOERSTER (1970) have proposed still another mechanism of cochlear mechanics. They depict the basilar membrane as a beam hinged at either end and driven at the basal end with an angular displacement source. The output of the INSELBERG-FOERSTER model is vigorous over its entire length for sinusoidal excitation at any frequency and thus bears little relation to experimentally observed membrane displacements.

E. Summary

From an overall standpoint, the physical models of the inner ear must be judged very promising. Most of the models are able to display traveling wave phenomena that are qualitatively of the sort that BÉKÉSY observed. Moreover, virtually every set of measurements that BÉKÉSY has reported (1960) on the displacement of the human basilar membrane has been matched closely, in a quantitative sense, by at least one of the models. It has also been demonstrated that at least one of the models, the BOGERT simulation, exhibits behavior qualitatively similar to that recently observed in experimental animals by RHODE (1971). Unfortunately, no one model has yet been shown to exhibit with good quantitative accuracy all of the experimentally demonstrated characteristics of the inner ear.

The acceptance of the physical models of the inner ear is not universal. In a recent article, NAFTALIN (1968) raised objections to these models on several different grounds, chief among which is the extremely small displacements which are predicted by the models for threshold stimulation. The recent demonstration of nonlinear mechanical behavior in the inner ear by RHODE (1971) indicates that such extrapolations to threshold levels must be made with caution. However, if even the lowest-intensity results obtained by RHODE are linearly extrapolated to threshold intensity levels, membrane displacements no larger than 0.06Å are indicated. The possibility that biological tissues can vibrate coherently over such small distances is considered impossible by NAFTALIN, who states that threshold displacements on the order of molecular dimensions (1Å) are the smallest that can be expected in the organ of Corti. These considerations indicate that the excitation of the inner ear at threshold levels is neither well understood nor adequately modeled.

III. Computational Models

The computational models of the inner ear's mechanics form a small but very useful class of models. We recall that these formulations make no attempt to derive cochlear displacements from hydrodynamic considerations. They represent the mechanical function of the inner ear solely in terms of the relationship between its input, the stapes displacement, and its output, the displacement of a point on the basilar membrane. Such models are a very convenient and flexible way of summarizing existing physiological data. Moreover, if the model is linear, it can be used to predict responses to stimuli other than those used to formulate the model. Computational models have also been used to suggest errors in experimental measurements.

A. The Flanagan Models

Trying to match response data that BÉKÉSY obtained from the inner ear with sinusoidal excitation, FLANAGAN (1960) developed the first computational models of the inner ear. Each of these models, three in number, is an analytical function that exhibits terminal characteristics that match the physiological data reasonably well. The function which provided the best fit at a particular point x is

$$F_1(j\omega) = Y(j\omega)/X(j\omega) = c_1\,\beta^{4.83}\left(\frac{\varepsilon + j\,\omega}{\beta + j\,\omega}\right)\left[\frac{1}{(j\,\omega + \alpha)^2 + \beta^2}\right]^2 e^{-j\frac{3\pi\omega}{4\beta}} \tag{41}$$

where $X(j\omega)$ and $Y(j\omega)$ are the complex amplitudes of the stapes displacement and of the membrane-point displacement, respectively; $\beta = 2\alpha$ is approximately the best frequency of the cochlear point; and c_1 and ε are constants.

Even with this function, however, a totally accurate fit between the physiological data and the model's output was not achieved. For example, if ε in Eq. (41) is set to zero, its amplitude response is almost a perfect fit to some of BÉKÉSY's experimental amplitude data. However, a phase response different by 90° from the experimental phase response results at low frequencies. Other discrepancies, all of them relatively small, marred the performance of the other two models.

Bothered by the apparent imperfections of the first three models, FLANAGAN and BIRD (1962) developed another model which is a so-called minimum-phase function in series with a phase-shift network. They were able to show that this type of model, a very general one that includes all realizable discrete-element models, is not able to mimic the phase responses observed in the inner ear by BÉKÉSY: a phase discrepancy of 90° still persists at low frequencies. Either the inner ear cannot be represented with this form of model or the experimental phase and amplitude measurements were somewhat in error. Support for the latter alternative has recently been obtained by RHODE (1971), who observed that the basilar membrane was 90° out of phase with the stapes at low frequencies. On the other hand, the nonlinear aspects of the membrane displacement also described by RHODE (1971) cannot be duplicated by any such linear system.

B. The Siebert Model

A different computational model of the inner ear was developed by SIEBERT (1962), who desired a simpler form that could be easily manipulated. His equation, for frequencies of interest is

$$F(\omega, x) = 1.46\left(\frac{\omega/2\pi}{10^{5-x}}\right) e^{\left[-2\left(\frac{\omega/2\pi}{10^{5-x}} - 1\right)^2 - \left(\frac{\omega/2\pi}{10^{5-x}} - 1\right)\right]} e^{-j\left(\pi + \frac{2\omega/3}{10^{5-x}}\right)} \tag{42}$$

where $F(\omega, x)$ is the complex amplitude of the volume displacement of the membrane at point x relative to the volume displacement of the stapes. Equation (42), which is applicable to any point along the cochlea at any frequency, has interesting properties. For example, if ω is allowed to vary for fixed x, and the amplitude of the resulting function is plotted on logarithmic frequency coordinates, the shape of the curve is independent of x. The same is true for the curve of phase as a function of frequency. That is, the frequency curves obtained for different points along the membrane have exactly the same shape. Notice that the phase of Eq. (42) decreases exponently with distance. Such a phase function, as pointed out by NIEDER (1971), has a distinctive property: the pattern of zero-crossings along the membrane at any one moment is independent of frequency. Only the location of the first zero-crossing is determined by the frequency.

The shape of the amplitude curves generated by Eq. (42) is, aside from being a little too rounded at the peak, quite similar to the shapes of the comparable curves from BÉKÉSY's physiological data (1960, p. 454) except at low frequencies. It follows that relative invariance of shape is also a property of BÉKÉSY's amplitude curves. Agreement between the theoretical and experimental phase curves was not as good. As we can see from Eq. (42), its phase approaches —180° for low frequencies, while BÉKÉSY's comparable phase curves approach zero.

Along with Eq. (42), SIEBERT (1962) also developed an elegant technique for comparing different types of amplitude and phase measurements. We remember that in some of BÉKÉSY's experiments, frequency was varied for a fixed observation point. In other experiments, measurements were made along the membrane at a fixed frequency. Using the new technique, SIEBERT was able to demonstrate that these various sets of BÉKÉSY's data were in general remarkably consistent with each other. However, one set of these measurements, made at fixed frequencies (BÉKÉSY, 1960, p. 448), was not reconcilable with the others.

C. Other Models

Several other workers have developed computational models of the inner ear that are not as complete as the ones presented above. The model of SAKAI and OGUSHI (1968), for example, incorporates only the amplitude of the membrane deflection. Their representation of the deflection is similar in form to the amplitude portion of Eq. (37). NIEDER (1971), on the other hand, has proposed a model of cochlear action that is based exclusively on the phase characteristics of the traveling waves. A propagation delay that increases exponentially with distance is the specific representation used in his model. Although both of these other models show interesting effects, their usefulness is severely limited by the incompleteness of their formulations.

Acknowledgement

This work was supported in part by National Institutes of Health Program Project Grant NS-06225.

Note added in proof: Since the completion of this chapter, giant strides have been made in mathematical modeling of the cochlea. First, a complete solution for the two-dimensional equation (Eq. 20) with realistic boundary conditions was obtained, a solution valid for the entire cochlear duct [LESSER, M. B., BERKLEY,

D. A.: Fluid mechanics of the cochlea. Part 1. J. Fluid Mech. *51*, 497–512 (1972)]. SIEBERT has beautifully shown [RANKE revisited – a simple short-wave cochlear model. J. acoust. Soc. Amer., **56**, 594–600 (1974)] that both the plane-wave approximation and RANKE's two-dimensional approach are but limiting cases of this complete solution. Second, solutions to even more elaborate physical models including all three dimensions have been obtained by LIEN [A mathematical model of the mechanics of the cochlea. Monograph **212**, Biomedical Computer Laboratory, Washington University, St. Louis (1973)] and by STEELE [Behavior of the basilar membrane with pure-tone excitation. J. acoust. Soc. Amer., **55**, 148–162 (1974)]. Also of interest are an integrable one-dimensional physical model [SCHROEDER, M. R. An integrable model for the basilar membrane. J. acoust. Soc. Amer., **53**, 429–434 (1973)] and a new computational model involving nonlinear elements [KIM, D. O., MOLNAR, C. E., PFEIFFER, R. R. A system of nonlinear differential equations modeling basilar-membrane motion. J. acoust. Soc. Amer., **54**, 1517–1529 (1973)].

References

BAUCH, H.: Die Schwingungsform der Basilarmembran bei Erregung durch Impulse und Geräusche, gemessen an einem elektrischen Modell des Innenohres. Frequenz **10**, 222–234 (1956).

BÉKÉSY, G. von: His papers have been collected in: Experiments in hearing. New York: McGraw-Hill Book Co. 1960.

BÉKÉSY, G. von: Enlarged mechanical model of the cochlea with nerve supply. In: TOBIAS, J. V. (Ed.): Foundations of modern auditory theory. New York: Academic Press 1970.

BIRD, R. B., STEWART, W. E., LIGHTFOOT, E. N.: Transport phenomena, 71 ff. New York: John Wiley and Sons 1960.

BOGERT, B. P.: Determination of the effects of dissipation in the cochlear partition by means of a network representing the basilar membrane. J. acoust. Soc. Amer. **23**, 151—154 (1951).

CALDWELL, W. F., GLAESSER, E., STEWART, J. L.: Design of an analog ear. In: Biological prototypes and synthetic systems, Vol. I. New York: Plenum Press 1962.

FLANAGAN, J. L.: Models for approximating basilar membrane displacement. Bell System Tech. J. **39**, 1163—1191 (1960).

FLANAGAN, J. L., BIRD, C. M.: Minimum phase responses for the basilar membrane. J. acoust. Soc. Amer. **34**, 114—118 (1962).

FLETCHER, H.: On the dynamics of the cochlea. J. acoust. Soc. Amer. **23**, 637—645 (1951).

GEISLER, C. D., HUBBARD, A. E.: New boundary conditions and results for the Peterson-Bogert model of the cochlea. J. acoust. Soc. Amer. **52**, 1629—1634 (1972).

GOLD, T.: Hearing. II. The physical basis of action of the cochlea. Proc. roy. Soc. B. **135**, 492—498 (1948).

HUBBARD, A. E., GEISLER, C. D.: A hybrid-computer model of the cochlear partition. J. acoust. Soc. Amer. **51**, 1895—1903 (1972).

HUXLEY, A. F.: Is resonance possible in the cochlea after all ? Nature (Lond.) **221**, 935—940 (1969).

INSELBERG, A., FOERSTER, H. von: A mathematical model of the basilar membrane. Math. Biosci. **7**, 341—363 (1970).

JOHNSTONE, B. M., TAYLOR, K. J., BOYLE, A. J.: Mechanics of the guinea pig cochlea. J. acoust. Soc. Amer. **47**, 504—509 (1970).

KLATT, D. H., PETERSON, G. E.: Reexamination of a model of the cochlea. J. acoust. Soc. Amer. **40**, 54—61 (1966).

LIEBERSTEIN, H. M.: The basilar membrane as a uniformly loaded plate clamped on two spiral boundaries in a plane or on two helical-spiral boundaries; discussion of the model. Math. Biosci. **12**, 281—291 (1971).

MORSE, P. M., FESHBACH, H.: Methods of theoretical physics, 1092 ff. New York: McGraw-Hill Book Co. 1953.

MORSE, P. M., INGARD, K. U.: Theoretical acoustics, 492 ff. New York: McGraw-Hill Book Co. 1968.

NAFTALIN, L.: Acoustic transmission and transduction in the peripheral hearing apparatus. In: BUTLER, J. A. V., NOBLE, D. (Eds.): Progress in biophysics and molecular biology, Vol. 18. New York: Pergamon Press 1968.

NIEDER, P.: Addressed exponential delay line theory of cochlear organization. Nature (Lond.) New Biol. **230**, 255—257 (1971).

OETINGER, R., HAUSER, H.: Ein elektrischer Kettenleiter zur Untersuchung der mechanischen Schwingungsvorgänge im Innenohr. Acustica **11**, 161—177 (1961). An English translation is available, at a price, from Associated Technical Services, Inc., 855 Bloomfield Ave., Glen Ridge, New Jersey, 07028, USA.

PETERSON, L. C., BOGERT, B. P.: A dynamical theory of the cochlea. J. acoust. Soc. Amer. **22**, 369—381 (1950).

RANKE, O. F.: Hydrodynamik der Schneckenflüssigkeit. Zeits. f. Biol. **103**, 409—434 (1950). An English translation is available, at a price, from the Natl. Translations Center, John Crerar Library, 35 W. 33rd St., Chicago Ill., 60616, USA.

RHODE, W. S.: Observations on the vibration of the basilar membrane in squirrel monkeys using the Mössbauer technique. J. acoust. Soc. Amer. **49**, 1218—1231 (1971).

SAKAI, H., OGUSHI, K.: Simulation of the neural response in the peripheral auditory system, NHK Laboratories Note, Tokyo, Japan **117** (1968). Copies of the article (PB 179451) are available from the Clearinghouse for Federal Scientific and Technical Information, Springfield, Va. 22151, USA.

SIEBERT, W. M.: Models for the dynamic behavior of the cochlear partition. Quart. Progr. Report, R. L. E., M. I. T. **64**, 242—258 (1962).

SIEBERT, W. M.: Personal communication (1970).

SIEBERT, W. M.: "Paradoxical" waves, bone conduction, and cochlear models. Quart. Progr. Report, R. L. E., M. I. T. **100**, 214—221 (1971).

STEWART, J. L.: A theory and physical model for cochlear mechanics. Acta oto-laryng. (Stockh.) Suppl. **294** (1972).

TIEDEMANN, H.: A new approach to theory of hearing. Acta oto-laryng. (Stockh.) Suppl. **277** (1970).

TONNDORF, J.: Cochlear mechanics and hydro-dynamics. In: TOBIAS, J. V. (Ed.): Foundations of modern auditory theory. New York: Academic Press 1970a.

TONNDORF, J.: Nonlinearities in cochlear hydrodynamics. J. acoust. Soc. Amer. **47**, 579—591 (1970b).

WANSDRONK, C.: On the mechanism of hearing. Thesis, University of Leiden (1961).

WEVER, E. G.: Theory of hearing. New York: John Wiley and Sons 1949.

ZWISLOCKI, J.: Theorie der Schneckenmechanik. Acta oto-laryng. (Stockh.) Suppl. **72**, (1948).

ZWISLOCKI, J.: Review of recent mathematical theories of cochlear dynamics. J. acoust. Soc. Amer. **25**, 743—751 (1953).

ZWISLOCKI, J.: Analysis of some auditory characteristics. In: LUCE, R. D., BUCK, R. R., GALANTER, E. (Eds.): Handbook of mathematical psychology, Vol. III. New York: John Wiley and Sons 1965.

Chapter 10

Electrical Stimulation of the Ear in Man

F. BLAIR SIMMONS, M.D.
Professor of Otolaryngology Stanford University

With 2 Figures

Contents

Probably no single topic about hearing has generated as much speculation and controversy as has electrical stimulation of the ear and of hearing. Ever since VOLTA's (1800) observation of "sounds like the boiling of soup" when he placed electrodes in his own ears, men of various persuasions have sought to use "electrical stimulation" for diagnosis or elimination of ear disease, the cure of deafness, and also occasionally to better understand hearing for its own sake. A certain confusion still exists today about what happens when an audio frequency current is applied in or near the ear, because, there is more than one form of electrical hearing. VOLTA, for example, may have truly heard the sound of "boiling soup" because of electrolysis bubbles with his DC current through saline in his ear canals. He also may have actually stimulated the auditory nerve. Instead, he may have experienced *electrophonic hearing* — a sensory phenomenon peculiar to the ear which is in fact just another pathway for acoustic stimulation of hearing. Because various electrophonic effects have many times been confused with direct stimulation of the cochlea and nerve, it is important to describe the phenomenon in some detail here.

I. Electrophonic Hearing

When an audio frequency current is passed from an electrode to the skin, the electrode tip and the opposing skin surface act as the two plates of a condenser loud speaker. The resulting acoustic vibrations are transmitted to the cochlea by both air- and bone-conduction. The loudness of the sound usually depends upon the distance between the active electrode and the ear. An electrode placed in the ear canal is most likely to be heard while stimulus currents are still too low to cause tactile sensations or other side effects. In modern times, the skin transduction mechanism was first seriously explored by KAHLER and RUF (1930) who became suspicious of such an effect when they found that sounds could be heard when the electrode was placed on distant body parts. They also reported that the sound could be heard by a second observer not included in the circuit. In the English language, the most extensive studies of skin transduction are described in a series of papers by STEVENS *et al.* (1936, 1939) and by FLOTTORP (1953).

When sine waves are used, the auditory sensations are usually tonal. The pitch is impure but usually corresponds to the second harmonic. A stronger fundamental is heard if a negative direct current (a polarizing potential) is applied simultaneously through the stimulating electrode. The lower limit of frequencies heard in this manner is approximately 150 Hz, and the upper limit probably corresponds to the subject's normal air conduction acuity — perhaps 12.000 Hz or higher on the average.

The ability to perceive electrophonic sounds depends on normal or near-normal inner ear function. Thus, an individual with a high-frequency sensorineural hearing loss will likewise be limited in hearing high frequency electrophonic sensations. A maximum loudness of about 40 dB sensation level (SL) is reported by most investigators before the pain threshold is reached. However, the range of loudness varies considerably with different techniques and with stimulus frequency.

Moving Electrode on Skin. The loudest and widest range of frequencies heard are apparently produced by FLOTTORP's "fricative effect". In this method, one very large electrode is placed on the forearm (inactive electrode) and the other (small electrode) is continuously moved over the skin (usually on the auricle) as audio frequencies are introduced. If the electrode is stationary, the sound disappears in a few seconds as the skin impedance drops. Using this system, FLOTTORP achieved thresholds between 20 and 16.000 Hz, and attained a maximum loudness of 60 dB SL at 1.000 Hz. Distortion was altered by changing the stimulus site or type of electrode. A metal electrode on dry skin over bony parts produced a larger second harmonic component, whereas wet mucous tissue (palate) produced more first harmonic.

Fixed Electrode on Skin. If an active electrode with a larger surface area (>150 sq mm) is used, sound can be heard when the active electrode remains stationary. Threshold is elevated and the maximum loudness that can be perceived is about 35—40 dB above normal threshold. Both threshold and loudness are proportional to applied voltage and to the surface area of the electrode. The skin under the electrode must be dry. The low-frequency limit of hearing is about 150 Hz. Second harmonic is more prominent below 2.000 Hz, whereas the fundamental is more pronounced above 5.000 Hz. A piece of cellophane between electrode and skin increases the low-frequency response, but at 125 Hz only a sensation of vibration centered deep within the head is perceived. The insertion of cellophane also partially stabilizes the transient character of the sensation. Without that dielectric, the auditory sensation diminishes to inaudibility in about 30—40 sec during steady-state stimulation (FLOTTORP, 1953). This second, or fixed-electrode, method of producing sounds by electromechanical transduction at a skin boundary forms the basis for many of the earlier reports of "electrical hearing" (SCHEPPEGRELL, 1898; EICHHORN, 1931; JELLINEK and SCHEIBER, 1930).

A similar range of sensations can also be produced by modulating a radio frequency carrier (40—100 kHz and higher) with audio frequencies. With this method, however, a steady state stimulus sustains a reasonably constant auditory sensation and does not disappear. Within reasonable limits, pain is not a stimulus parameter problem and speech transmission is quite intelligible. This electrophonic mode has enjoyed some of the popular enthusiasm common to the early 1930 descriptions (*Life*, September 14, 1962). Some "therapeutic" applications for treatment of sensorineural deafness which are reminiscent of the 1860's are apparently also undergoing a renaissance (MANFREDI and BOMBELLI, 1963; PUHARICH and LAWRENCE, 1969).

Electrode in External or Middle Ear. In the classical applications of this technique, the ear canal is partially filled with saline and an electrode placed in the saline (BRENNER, 1868). If an alternating current (ac) voltage is passed to the ear canal, tympanic membrane or middle ear (*via* tympanic membrane perforation), sounds are heard. The fidelity and loudness of those sounds vary considerably from one location to another and also vary according to small differences in the methods of stimulation. The majority of these sensations do not seem to differ in any important way from the description already given for effects of fixed electrodes on skin.

Historically, however, there has been much more controversy about the site of stimulus transduction than with stimulation of other body areas, presumably because of proximity to the cochlea in cases with tympanic membrane perforations where sounds were heard when electrodes are placed on the round window or promontory.

In 1940, JONES *et al.* reported on the results of stimulations in 20 ears lacking tympanic membranes. Most of the patients had undergone a radical mastoidectomy. The active electrode was a saline-soaked cotton-tipped wire, placed in the oval or round window areas:

> Nine subjects heard tones corresponding in pitch to the frequency of the applied voltage; five heard a "buzzing" noise whose character was roughly independent of the stimulating frequency; two heard both the pure tone and buzzing noise, although at different frequencies; and four heard nothing. Of these [last] four, two had large amounts of scar tissue filling the middle ear; one had no cochlea (removed by operation); and one had labyrinthitis with complete loss of hearing.

Significant additional observations on those subjects who heard pure tones included the fact that only the first harmonic was heard. Direct current polarization did not change the perception but did elevate threshold sensitivity. The responses did not obey a square law. The pitch difference limen (DL) was equivalent to the DL obtained by ordinary acoustic stimulation. Beats were heard if electrical and acoustical stimuli were presented simultaneously but at slightly different frequencies. (The appearance of beats during simultaneous acoustical and electrical stimulation also occurs with external canal stimulation, in association with either first or second harmonics, GERSUNI, 1936; CRAIK *et al.*, 1937; KELLAWAY, 1946). The range of frequencies heard as tones did not extend below 100 Hz. Very slight differences in the placement of the electrode created unpredictable and very wide variations in threshold and frequency response.

Most of these observations on tonal sensations were similar to those reported earlier by the Russian investigators (ANDREEF, 1934; GERSUNI and VOLOKHOV, 1936). These investigators also felt that the tonal sensations at frequencies above 100 Hz were electromechanically transduced but from within the cochlea and that a normal or near-normal cochlea was required for their perception.

One historically interesting difference remains in the general conclusions of the Russian and American investigators which has occasionally made parallel interpretations of their work confusing. The Russians placed the site of electromechanical transduction exclusively within the cochlea. They did not distinguish between the character of sensations produced by electrodes near the cochlear fenestrae and those produced by stimulation in the external canal (intact tympanic membrane). This might have been because the Russians observed that the auditory sensations were identical in either location. It now appears likely that identical sensations were produced because they used a saline-pool conductor at both sites; whereas JONES *et al.*, who found differences between the outer and middle ear locations, used saline in the ear canal and a saline-soaked cotton-tipped wire in the middle ear. FLOTTORP (1953) demonstrated that even this slight difference in technique would be adequate to change the harmonic content of the perceived sound. He argues convincingly that all such tonal sensations result from one of several electromechanical transducers at or near the electrode-skin or electrode-mucosa boundary.

Most evidence at this moment suggests that the cochlea is not directly involved in electrical excitation by sinusoids or other waveforms in the middle ear whose frequency is greater than about 100 Hz. The other limits imposed on electrophonic hearing are: a normal cochlea; the impedance characteristic of the electrode-skin junction; and the current density at which pain, tactile sensations, dizziness, or muscle twitching occur.

II. Auditory Nerve Excitation

Other types of electrical stimulation, especially within the middle ear, probably also have caused direct excitation of the auditory nerve in addition to electrophonic hearing. The Russian investigators were the first to describe these sensations in detail, but their reports did not always clearly distinguish between auditory nerve excitation and one of the several electrophonic effects reviewed above. ANDREEF *et al.* (1934) reported that during stimulations of persons with inner and middle ear defects, auditory sensations were produced with sine wave stimuli at frequencies between 1.5 and 14.000 Hz. In the subject with:

> ... an affected auditory organ (injury) [sensorineural hearing loss of unknown severity] ... sensations arise with frequencies of 1.5 Hz and bear the character of separate short noises. At frequencies of the order of 30—40 Hz fusion of these separate sensations into a smooth buzzing noise occurs; beginning with frequencies of from 100—200 Hz to 6.000 Hz, the character of sensations remains unchanged. On increasing the current strength it is possible to observe in some cases besides sensations of noise also tonal sensations. The pitch of the tone is constant during all the frequencies ... besides auditory sensations, the arising of cutaneous (tactile, pain, temperature) sensations are observed. Irritation of the vestibular apparatus can also take place. (STEVENS did not accept perception of such low frequencies by

sinusoidal stimulation as originating within the cochlea. He suggested that the Russians' stimulator probably produced a distorted stimulus, rich in higher-frequency harmonics, and that these harmonics were the effective stimulus. [The Russians did not use an oscilloscope to monitor their stimuli.] STEVEN's objection was probably valid.)

Proceeding on the assumption that all these stimuli actively excited the nerve, this same group performed other (more extensive) observations employing direct currents and condenser discharges, calculated chronaxy, rheobase, loudness growth, etc. They interpreted these observations to indicate that the auditory nerve was electrophysiologically similar to other peripheral sensory somatic nerves. Loudness was said to increase at a rate 45 times that for acoustical stimuli.

It will be recalled that the JONES *et al.* (1940) study included seven subjects who also heard sounds at frequencies below 250 Hz during round and oval window stimulation. At frequencies around 10 or 20 Hz the sound was intermittent, "like the chirp of a cricket". It had a rhythmical quality below about 50 Hz. Above 100 Hz the character of the noise did not change appreciably. Over the range below 250 Hz, only rather large changes in stimulus frequency could be detected, and the reported pitch change bore no relation to the direction of the frequency change. Small changes in frequency were occasionally reported as changes in loudness. Tonal stimulations in the nontest ear were not at all like those produced by the electrical stimuli. The loudness of the noise increased very rapidly as stimulus intensity increased. In one subject, a 4 dB electrical change corresponded to a 13.5 dB acoustic loudness change. The loudness of the sounds decreased very rapidly when the stimulation was continued for several seconds.

DJOURNO and EYRIES (1957a, b) and DJOURNO *et al.* (1957) reported the first attempt at stimulation of the acoustic nerve by direct application of an electrode. During reoperation of a 50-year-old man who had previously undergone bilateral surgery for cholesteatoma and was totally deaf, a single electrode was placed on the nerve and this was attached to an induction coil. The indifferent electrode and coil were implanted in the temporalis muscle. The coil was later stimulated by induction currents from a second coil placed against the overlying skin. The French investigators initially used an electrophrenic stimulator producing pulsed stimuli at a rate of 100/sec, interrupted 20 times/min. The patient described sounds like "crickets" or a "roulette wheel". Although in later experiments the pitch of various stimuli remained undistinguishable, the patient seemed able initially to perceive a change in the character of the perceptions with changes of stimulus frequency up to 1.000 Hz, described as various degrees of undertone. Above 1.000 Hz, "confusion was total". The sound was reported as "stronger" when the frequency was lower. A short time later MASPETIOL, working with DJOURNO, placed a round window electrode in a girl deaf from streptomycin treatment. The findings were similar (see ZOLLNER and KEIDEL, 1963). Long-term attempts to develop speech discrimination in these two patients failed.

SIMMONS *et al.* (1964) reported the first bipolar stimulation of the eighth nerve, through a posterior craniotomy approach in an 18-year-old patient undergoing surgery for a recurrent tumor. The findings were somewhat unexpected when considering these previous reports. The bipolar electrodes were placed about 4.5 mm apart, parallel with the long axis of the nerve. Using bipolar square-wave stimulation, rate differences were distinguishable up to 3.500/sec. Between 20/sec and about 900/sec the subject was able to distinguish rate differences quite easily, and at 850/sec a DL of about 5/sec was measured. Above about 1.000/sec, rate difference detection diminished considerably. Thresholds were quite sharp and growth of loudness was very rapid above threshold. Because of the presence of near-normal cochlear function in the stimulated ear, the possibility existed that electrophonic hearing was taking place, rather than a direct or selective stimulation of the acoustic nerve. This, however, seemed unlikely.

The most detailed description of long-term 8th nerve stimulation is a report by SIMMONS (1966). He placed six electrodes in the modiolus of a man who had a total sensorineural hearing loss and observed stimulus responses for a period of 18 months. The following paragraphs are abstracted from these observations.

Pitch Sensations: Four variables were found to cause pitch changes. A characteristic pitch was described for each of the electrodes, presumably corresponding to the nerve fibers stimulated and to the classical place theory for pitch localization on the basilar membrane. A group of *rate pitch* sensations were described which depended on stimulus repetition rate, and corresponding with classical concepts of volley or synchronous pitch coding. A *waveform pitch* dependency was observed which was related to the shape of individual stimuli (*e.g.*, sine vs rectangular pulses) and modified both characteristic and rate pitch sensations. An *intensity pitch* effect occurred wherein pitch (especially characteristic pitch) rose whenever the stimulus intensity increased. The percept arising from any repetitive stimulus was always related to a combination of these pitch effects.

Characteristic Pitch: Even a single stimulus pulse produced a pitch, and this pitch was different in each electrode. In particular, when the stimulus was a 1/sec monopolar biphasic rectangular pulse, and when this stimulus was adjusted to produce equally loud sensations in each electrode, one electrode had a considerably higher pitch than any of the others; two were equal in pitch and lower than the first; two others were slightly lower still and about equal; one consistently produced the lowest pitch. For example, a single pulse in one electrode was described as a "ping" or "tapping on the side of a glass", and another electrode was "duller", more like "tapping on a door". It was impossible to determine exactly what these pitches were, but judging from his descriptions they were high on the pitch scale, probably well above 1.000 Hz and correspond to locations in fibers from the basal turn of the modiolus. These pitch rankings amongst electrodes were generally independent of stimulus waveforms or repetition rates, even though the pitch percept itself was modified by such changes. Thus, at a rate of 300—400/sec, stimulation of one electrode produced a steady high-pitched sound "like a violin" while the next lower-rank electrode produced a lower steady sound, "more like a horn or trumpet". There was a similar pitch ranking of electrode pairs during bipolar stimulation, but in a more complex manner since the ranking of some combinations was changed by changes in the stimulating waveform.

Repetition Rate Pitch: Change in pitch with increasing stimulus rates did not seem to be an orderly perceptual continuum from low to high pitch. Stimulations at 1/sec were called "pings, dings, hammering on [sheet] metal". At 4/sec, the ringing quality disappeared. The sounds were "clicks" or simply "short sounds".

At 10/sec these "short sounds" were "faster", and occasionally buzzings. At 20/sec almost all stimuli were described as more or less continuous sounds, "whistles, telephone bells, buzzing, or burrs", depending upon the electrode stimulated, the stimulus waveform, loudness, and the context of the stimulus. In general, these sounds correspond with percepts of low frequency modulation (rate pitch) of a higher frequency signal (characteristic pitch).

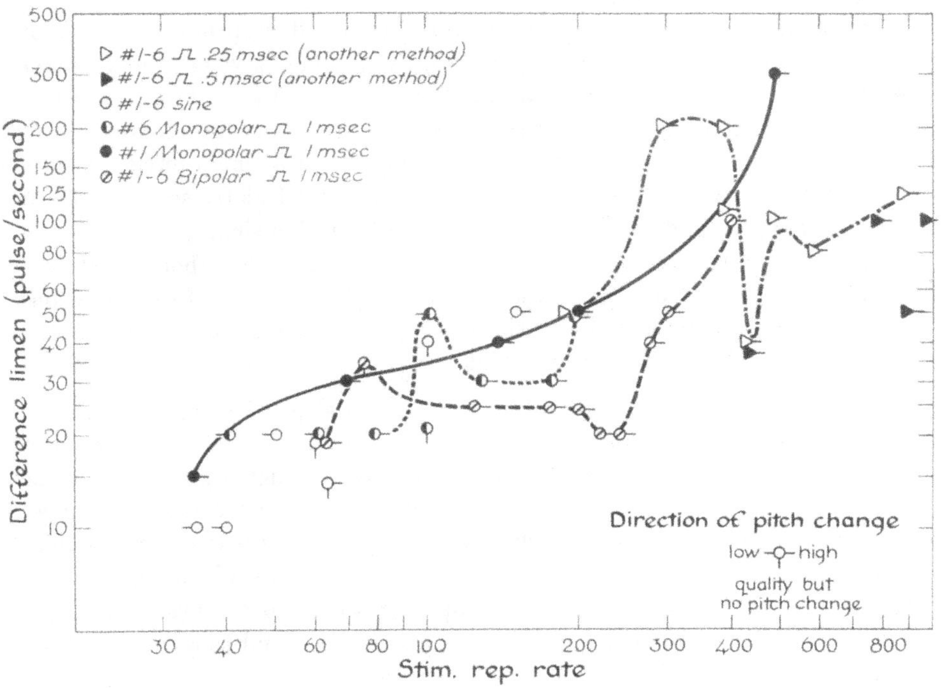

Fig. 1. Repetition rate difference limen (DL). Pitch or distinctly different sound quality DL for several different types of stimulation are plotted on the ordinate using a logarithmic scale. (Each plot point indicates the highest stimulus rate of the compared pair. Subtract the DL from this point to obtain the rate of the lower member of the pair.) The pitch usually increased with rate and this rising pitch is indicated by a right-hand orientation of the plot point symbols. A left-hand orientation indicates a drop in pitch with a rate increase, and downward or no orientation indicates a sound quality change without pitch change. All DL's for the several stimulus conditions were obtained at subjective "comfortable loudness" — about 5—10 dB above threshold — and were balanced for equal loudness. Judgments were obtained by presenting a two- or three-second stimulus at one rate followed by a one- to two-second pause, then the second stimulus rate. The subject judged the pitch of the second rate, relative to the first. At the higher frequencies, another method was also used *(open and closed triangle plot points)*. The two rate samples were alternated several times in succession, until the subject judged, "high, low, high ...", or, "all the same"

Fig. 1 shows several rate-pitch difference limens for stimulus rates greater than 20/sec. The degree of pitch change between about 20 and 90/sec was not large. In all but one electrode the pitch decreased slightly at 40/sec before gradually rising at higher stimulus rates.

Major changes in the quality of the sound occurred in the 20—90/sec stimulus range. Using rectangular pulses, 20 and 40/sec sounds were the same quality, but at 40/sec the "individual sounds are shorter and closer together". All rates below 50/sec were called "rough, rattling, or crackling". All rates above 90/sec were "smooth steady sounds". The transition between rough to steady sounds was gradual and was affected by the shape of the stimulating pulse. For example, sine waves were smooth sounds at 60/sec but 1 msec rectangles only became smooth between 80 and 90/sec.

Percepts at 100/sec included bee buzzings, auto and peep horns. Sounds at rates above 100/sec universally had a steady tonal quality whose pitch always rose with rate increases. They were described as horns, violins, and whistles whose individual characteristics changed with envelope patterns and test context. Thus a 400/sec stimulus in one test session was simply called a "high-pitched steady sound". When it was automatically switched on and off at 0.3 sec intervals it became a "ding, ding, ding of a railroad crossing [warning signal]".

The highest repetition rate pitch changes occurred at either about 4—500/sec or near 1.000/sec, depending upon the test method. The pitches of the sensations themselves were estimated to be much higher, perhaps corresponding to acoustic sensations in the 2.000 Hz range and higher.

Waveform pitch changes were related to the onset slope of a single stimulus or of repetitive trains. In general, stimuli with longer pulse durations and slow onset slopes had lower pitches. Rectangular pulses always had higher pitches than sine waves. Ramp functions were even lower-pitched if their rise times were longer than corresponding sine waves. Pitch or quality differences between rectangular and sinusoidal stimulation were present at all repetition rates. When, for example, a 200/sec sine wave was used, then abruptly changed to a 200/sec rectangle, "[The sound] went from a lower pitch to a higher pitch and they were both on together".

The description just given and others like it suggest that the *rate* of the 200 Hz sine wave first established the lower pitch. Then, when the stimulus was abruptly changed to a 200/sec rectangle, the periodicity component continued unchanged while the waveform change caused another (higher) sound to be heard at the same time. If this is correct, it fits a more general conclusion that waveform differences affected the characteristic pitch of an electrode. It must then also be concluded that characteristic pitch depended upon both the excitation of a specific group of fibers and upon the temporal dispersion of that excitation.

Threshold and Loudness: Fig. 2a shows the stimulus currents required for threshold perception during monopolar and bipolar stimulation with several waveforms. The energy requirements at threshold were not as widespread as the Fig. 2a data might suggest. When calculated in coulombs, all thresholds were between 0.1 and 8 μcoulombs/sec, but each pulse required nearly the same 0.015 μcoulombs/pulse. Ascending thresholds were worse than descending thresholds, typically by a two-fold difference in stimulus current.

Fig. 2b shows some typical loudness difference limens as stimulus voltage was increased from threshold to an intensity said to be "uncomfortably loud" by the subject. This intensity probably corresponded to an acoustic sensation level of

100 dB. The control of loudness and loudness matches were easily obtained. Most other observations were carried out between 5 and 10 dB above threshold — a range said to be comfortably loud by the subject. There was no problem with

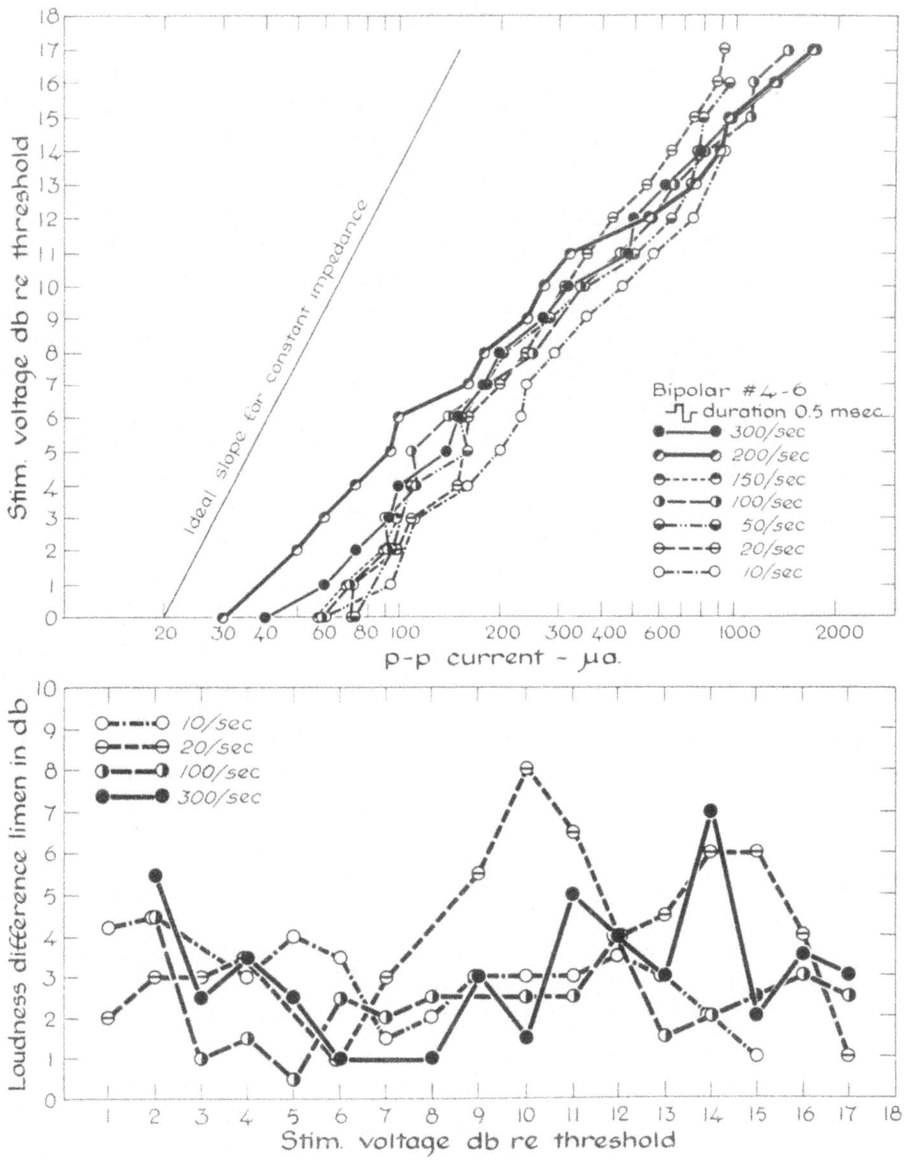

Fig. 2. Loudness and stimulus magnitude. *Top*, Peak-to-peak current flow resulting from 1 dB increments in stimulus voltage from perceptual threshold. A 0.5 msec biphasic, rectangular waveform (bipolar) at several repetition rates was used. Note that current flow was not linear and that the impedance decrease was most marked at rapid repetition rates. *Lower*, Relation of loudness difference limen (in decibels of voltage) to stimulus intensity. The data were obtained by the two-stimulus comparison method during the same series of tests. Note that the most sensitive DL's were about 5—7 dB above threshold

stimulus spread to vestibular neurons or the facial nerve. No painful sensations were reported at any time.

Threshold adaption during steady state stimulation did occur. With most waveforms and electrode combinations, the sound was heard for at least three minutes when the intensity was twice its average threshold value.

Multi-Electrode Stimulation: When more than one pair of electrodes were stimulated at the same time, or when two different waveforms were superimposed in the same electrode(s), a variety of perceptual descriptions were obtained. The subject often heard more than one sound simultaneously. At times, combination stimuli retained their individual perceptual identity. In other instances, the combination lost individual components and produced a sound which was different from that obtained by stimulating either electrode alone. Simultaneous stimulation through several electrodes did not increase threshold sensitivity. Furthermore, only on a few occasions was there any indication that stimuli, only slightly above threshold individually, interacted when introduced simultaneously. At intensities more than a few decibels above threshold, the combined-stimulation loudness was considerably less dependent on current flow than during single-channel stimulation. When contiguous tissue areas were stimulated (an assumption based upon the use of one electrode common to two bipolar pairs), the pitch usually rose and loudness changes were unpredictable. The perceptual identity of a single-channel's stimulus was most frequently retained during simultaneous multichannel stimulation if its sound seemed to be markedly different from the other sounds. The perceptual difference was related to a difference in characteristic pitch, large difference in repetition rate, and differences in waveform. A stimulus in one channel could "modulate" the perception of a steady-state stimulus in another channel (suprathreshold) without that modulating stimulus also being identified by the subject. Simultaneous stimulation of more than one electrode pair did not appreciably increase the perceptual resolution of simple pitch judgments, nor did it aid in the differentiation of rapidly changing or otherwise more complex waveforms.

Speech Stimuli: In the majority of speech-stimulation experiments, a tape-recorded radio commentary was used. With either tape or a live-sound source, the stimulus was immediately recognized without prior cues as speech, and occasionally as singing. The "voice" was almost always said to be male, changing in pitch and quality according to electrode selection, band-pass filtering, and tape speed. The following observations were consistent when an unmodified speech waveform was used:

1. The subject was unable to make out what was being said. This was a puzzle to him at first because he was quite certain that the sounds were speech. He suggested it was, in fact, a foreign language (Spanish) being spoken.

2. The talking was said to be very rapid, intense, question-asking or excited. Reducing the tape recorder speed by half sounded more normal to him; the voice was lower pitched and louder. A change in the emotional quality, toward more excitement, was also produced by increasing intensity or the high-frequency band-pass.

3. When all such parameters remained constant, and on specific questioning, he attributed *no pitch change* to the ongoing speech, only loudness changes.

(This was an important consistency with other findings. Pitch changes were not usually noticed by the subject during continuous stimulation unless the new waveform or rate was continued for 200—300 msec.)

4. Low-frequency speech transients were frequently described as brief "high pitched sounds" separate from the "voice". A band-pass filter set at 75—1.200 Hz produced a "normal voice".

5. Simultaneous presentation through two bipolar channels, using the 75 to 1.200 Hz filter, produced "a lot of short words ... da .. de .. de .. da" in an irregular rhythm.

6. Several different sounds (clicks, rattles) were also heard in addition to and at the same time as the "voice'.

The most intriguing observations were those collected when the subject generated his own stimulus by speaking into a microphone. At first, he was not actually given the microphone. It was held outside his visual field but close enough to pick up his fragmentary remarks. After a few moments, he spontaneously noticed he was "hearing himself". He said that he heard his voice clearly and understood every word. His voice sounded as if he were listening to it through a telephone. He was unable to describe the difference between hearing himself and listening to sounds produced by someone else — counting, for example, from one to ten. The only number he guessed correctly more times than not was seven — the only bisyllabic member of the set.

The speech waveform, filtered or unfiltered, was definitely not an optimal stimulus, even if the problem of controlling net current flow could have been ignored. Because of their longer periods, the lower speech frequencies sounded louder (occasionally higher pitched) than higher-frequency transients of equal amplitude. Changes in overall signal amplitude also modified the pitch.

A number of modified signals and multi-electrode stimulations were attempted without appreciable change in the above descriptions. The major non-linearity problems were, however, eliminated by using speech to drive a constant-width rectangular pulse generator which also had a 40-to-15 dB amplitude compression characteristic. Pulse repetition rate and amplitude were triggered and modulated by the corresponding parameters of the speech input signal. These speech-modulated rectangular pulses produced a "voice" and eliminated the pitch-inversion of low frequencies. With this type of pulse-modulated stimulus, electrode selection had a more marked effect on the quality of the "voice". In one pair, the stimulus produced "singing", not speech. In another, the "voice" was high-pitched; in a third it was low-pitched, even when the speed of the tape recorder was doubled.

When the subject himself spoke into the microphone, the effect upon his usually loud monotonic speech was remarkable. It slowed to about half its normal speed, became somewhat slurred, softer, and less distinct. He said he could hear and understand himself, but later remarked that this time it did not sound at all like his own voice. Again he was unable to tell us in what ways either his voice or other voices sounded "wrong". The one exception was his complaint that the word *two* (in the series one, two, three ...) always sounded like *three* whether spoken by him or another speaker.

Simmons concludes that: "It was abundantly clear that whenever a speech signal was used — as long as it was "recognized" as speech — we were dealing with a different part of the nervous system from the one which analyzed the other types of stimulations and made isolated pitch and loudness judgments, etc. We are absolutely certain, for example, from such nonspeech experiments, that pitch changes of major proportions occurred with a 10 dB change in stimulus intensity or with a rate change from 200/sec—300/sec. Yet the subject reported 'no change in pitch' with comparable parameter changes when he was hearing 'someone talking'. This difference in perceptual behavior during speech may have been due to a failure to distinguish rapidly changing rates and amplitudes. Or, it may have been that the subject was listening with emphasis on different components of a different set of perceptual criteria for abstract and for meaningful stimuli".

III. Summary

While the data available are clearly inadequate to set the limits for perceptions arising from electrical stimulation of the auditory nerve, some features are clear enough. All perceptions of stimuli are auditory, and most have pitch components which correspond with and confirm the classical "place" and "volley" theories of pitch coding. The upper limit of pitch by volley discharges is imprecisely known, but extends at least to 500/sec with poor difference limen discrimination when compared to acoustic hearing. The lower limit of this pitch — a sound with a steady quality — begins to emerge at about 50/sec. In between, pitch difference limens are poorer than those obtainable by acoustic stimuli. Loudness difference limens are also larger with electrical excitation, and the range from threshold to "very loud" is 15—25 dB, depending upon electrode location. Multiple pitch and waveform-related sensations can be produced when more than one site in the nerve is stimulated simultaneously. The over all input-output electrophysiological characteristics do not differ in any major way from those which might be expected in stimulating any modality specific peripheral nerve of similar size and proximity to its secondary sensory ganglion. Even so, the auditory nerve and central nervous system seem remarkably effective in detecting within these crude stimuli impressively small changes in temporal cues inherent in stimulus waveforms.

References

ANDREEF, A. M., GERSUNI, G. V., VOLOKHOV, A. A.: Electrical stimulation of the hearing organ. J. Physiol. USSR **17**, 546—559 (1934).

BELLUCCI, R. J., SCHNEIDER, D. E.: Some observations on ultrasonic perception in man. Ann. Otol. **71**, 719—726 (1962).

BRENNER, R.: Untersuchungen und Beobachtungen auf dem Gebiete der Electrotherapie. Leipzig: 1868 and 1869; see Erb. W.: Arch. Ophthal. Otol. **1**, 232—282 (1869).

CRAIK, K. J. W., RAWDON-SMITH, A. F., STURDY, R. S.: Note on the effect of A.C. on the human ear. Proceedings of the Physiological Society, May 1937. J. Physiol. (Lond.) **90** (1937).

DJOURNO, A., EYRIES, C.: Prothèse auditive par excitation electrique a distance du nerf sensoriel a l'aide d'un bobinage inclus a demeure. Presse Med. **35**, 14—17 (1957a); see also, same case: C.R. Soc. Biol. **151**, 423—425 (1957b); DJOURNO, A., EYRIES, C., VALLANCIEN, B.: Bull. franç. nat. Acad. Med. **141**, 481—483 (1957).

EICHHORN, G.: Das "Radiophon". Mschr. Ohrenheilk. **65**, 308—312 (1931).

FLOTTORP, G.: Effect of different types of electrodes in electrophonic hearing. J. acoust. Soc. Amer. **25**, 236—245 (1953).

GERSUNI, G. V., VOLOKHOV, A. A.: On the electrical excitability of the auditory organ: On the effect of alternating currents on the normal auditory apparatus. J. exp. Psychol. **19**, 370—382 (1936).

HAEFF, A. V., KNOX, C.: Perception of ultrasound. Science **139**, 590—592 (1963).

JELLINEK, S., SCHEIBER, T.: Eine neue Methode des Hörens. Wien. klin. Wschr. **43**, 417 (1930).

JONES, R. C., STEVENS, S. S., LURIE, M. H.: Three mechanisms of hearing by electrical stimulation. J. acoust. Soc. Amer. **12**, 281—290 (1940).

KAHLER, Z.: Versuch einer Hörverbesserung unter Benützung der Knochenleitung. Z. Hals-Nasen-Ohrenheilk. **27**, 437—443 (1930).

KELLAWAY, P.: The mechanism of the electrophonic effect. J. Neurophysiol. **9**, 23—32 (1946).

MANFREDI, A., BOMBELLI, U.: Radioacoustic treatment of deafness. Pubblicazioni Dell' Istituto Nazionale De Ottica, Serie IV, N. 408 (1963).

PUHARICH, H. K., LAWRENCE, J. L.: Hearing rehabilitation by means of transdermal electrotherapy in human hearing loss of sensorineural origin. Acta Oto-laryng. **67**, 69—83 (1969).

SCHEPPEGRELL, W.: Electricity in diseases of the nose, throat and ear. New York: G. P. Putnam's Sons 1898.

SIMMONS, F. B., MONGEON, C. S., LEWIS, W. R., HUNTINGTON, D. A.: Electrical stimulation of acoustical nerve and inferior colliculus: Results in man. Arch. Otolaryng. **79**, 559—567 (1964).

SIMMONS, F. B.: Electrical stimulation of the auditory nerve in man. Arch. Otolaryng. **84**, 2—54 (1966).

STEVENS, S. S.: On hearing by electrical stimulation. J. acoust. Soc. Amer. 8, 191—195 (1936).

STEVENS, S. S., JONES, R. C.: The mechanism of hearing by electrical stimulation. J. acoust. Soc. Amer. **10**, 261—269 (1939).

VOLTA, A.: On the electricity excited by mere contact of conducting substances of different kinds. Trans. roy. Soc. Phil. **90**, 403—431 (1800).

ZÖLLNER, F., KEIDEL, W. D.: Gehörvermittlung durch elektrische Erregung des *Nervus acusticus*. Arch. Ohr.-Nas.-Kehlkopfheilk. **181**, 216—223 (1963).

Chapter 11

Electrical Stimulation of the Auditory System in Animals

G. M. GERKEN

With 1 Figure

Contents

In recent years, increased emphasis has been placed on the nature of neural functions in the behaving animal, and electrical stimulation of the central nervous system has proved to be a technique well suited to the study of this conscious mode of brain activity. Yet electrical stimulation of the central portions of a sensory system typically produces either a behavioral response that rapidly habituates with repeated stimulus presentations, or no response at all. The use of the electrical signal as a cue for the performance of a learned behavior, however, establishes a sustained behavioral responsiveness to the electrical stimuli, which in turn permits accurate and repeatable measurement of the effectiveness of the central stimulation.

The kinds of questions that may be asked with the combined stimulation-behavioral approach can be roughly divided into two categories: those concerned with sensory quality, and those concerned with neural mechanisms and neural organization.

I. The Question of Sensory Quality

The nature of the sensory experiences that are produced in animals by peripheral stimulation must be inferred from behavioral data. The operant conditioning techniques used in *behavioral psychophysics* (see BLOUGH, 1966; STEBBINS, 1970) constitute one source of such data. Inferences may also be based on a wide range of other behavioral procedures related, for example, to generalization, masking, and orientation responses. These same behavioral methods must also be used to infer the sensory effects produced by electrical stimulation. While the behavioral methods available necessarily permit only limited inferences of sensory quality, the combination of stimulation and behavioral procedures yields results that are otherwise unobtainable.

NIEDER and NEFF (1961), for example, classically conditioned four cats to respond to sound and obtained immediate generalization to stimulation of inferior colliculus. Only one animal, however, of a group of three animals trained initially on collicular stimulation showed immmediate generalization to sound. Why generalization should appear to have a directional quality is not clear. Perhaps this effect is related to the quality of auditory sensation produced by collicular stimulation but, in addition, there is the possibility that collicular stimulation produces effects other than sensory experience. These non-auditory effects may be of critical importance in interpreting the results of this experiment.

Other investigators have employed measures of generalization or transfer as indicators of the similarity of effect produced by stimulation of various brain loci (NIELSON *et al.*, 1962; DOTY and RUTLEDGE, 1959; COLAVITA, 1970). There is little indication of generalization among a number of unrelated subcortical structures (NIELSON *et al.*, 1962; DOTY, 1969) and, hence, little indication of similarity of sensory quality among unrelated brain areas.

Generalization may occur, however, within a group of related structures. Rate of extinction, used as a measure of generalization between brain stimulation and a photic stimulus (KITAI, 1966), indicated that the effect produced by stimulation of optic chiasma was most similar to the effect produced by the photic stimulus. This was followed in decreasing order by stimulation of occipital cortex, superior colliculus, and frontal cortex. A similar experiment based on auditory system electrode placements would seem worthwhile.

Inferences of sensory quality may be based on the behaviorally measured interactions between two stimuli. In auditory masking, for example, the fact that one sound masks another indicates to a first approximation that the masking sound is the louder of the two. Several forms of interaction between auditory and electrical stimuli were demonstrated with an electrode located in the superior olivary complex (GERKEN, 1970). Detection threshold for 3 Hz, 0.3 msec electrical pulses was elevated by the presence of synchronized noise bursts. The 20 msec noise bursts were repeated throughout each experimental session and, hence, could not serve as a cue for the behavioral response. One interpretation of the elevation of electrical threshold by the noise is that the noise bursts were louder than the sensation produced by the electrical stimulation. An increase in current level was required to make the electrical pulses detectable in the presence of the noise bursts, implying that the larger current probably produced a louder sensation. This interpretation is supported by the finding that a further increase in noise intensity required a still further increase in stimulation current to maintain detectability.

In a second demonstration using briefer noise bursts, the time interval between noise and electrical pulse was varied over a 30 msec range. Detection of the electrical pulse was demonstrated to be critically dependent upon the time of occurrence of the pulse relative to the noise; thus, it was concluded that the sensation produced by the pulse was probably of brief duration. Finally, electrical detection threshold was shown to be related to the frequency spectrum of a background sound, which may indicate the presence of tonality in the sensation produced by electrical stimulation. Because of the multiple interactions between the acoustic and electrical stimuli, it may be concluded that the predominate effect of applying stimulation through this one electrode was auditory in nature. Further speculations could also be made as to the loudness, duration, and pitch of the electrically induced sensation.

Three other electrodes placed in trapezoid body, centrally in inferior colliculus, and in medial geniculate were tested in a similar fashion, but evidence of interaction between electrical and acoustic stimulation was not obtained. This apparent lack of interaction was studied in more detail for several medial geniculate placements (GERKEN, 1971 a). It was found that an interaction was clearly present at the level of medial geniculate but that it was both more complex and more subtle than the interaction obtained at the level of the superior olive. A far more extensive set of interaction data for electrodes in the various auditory nuclei might well permit rather detailed inferences concerning the nature of the auditory sensations produced by electrical stimulation of these nuclei.

Another aspect of sensory quality concerns the apparent directionality of the sensation produced by electrical stimulation. WESTER (1971) obtained orienting responses to electrical stimulation of various thalamic structures. Behavioral orientation produced by stimulation of the thalamic sensory relay nuclei rapidly habituated in contrast to the orientation produced by stimulation of the intralaminar thalamic group. WESTER interprets stimulation of relay nuclei, including medial geniculate, as producing a sensory experience that is of no intrinsic signal value, and consequently the animal soon comes to ignore the stimulation effects. Not all electrode sites produced an orientation response, but, for lateral thalamic placements, the direction of orientation was to the contralateral side. Similar results for inferior colliculus and medial geniculate placements were obtained in my laboratory (GERKEN, 1970). Cochlear nucleus placements that yielded a directional response produced orientation to the ipsilateral side (GERKEN, 1970). Of three placements in superior olivary complex, one yielded ipsilateral orientation while two produced contralateral orientation. Since higher level auditory nuclei receive both ipsilateral and contralateral projections from the cochlea, these results would seem to indicate a functional contralateral dominance at the higher levels.

The fact that orientation responses are not associated with all placements in the auditory system suggests that the directional aspect of auditory sensation, and possibly the information necessary for localization as well, is mediated by restricted portions of the auditory system. This would not, of course, imply that single units in other portions of the auditory system do not differentially respond to changes in the location of a sound source. The question is a functional one that concerns the use made by the behaving animal of the auditory neural information.

The question of sensory quality, if pushed to the extreme, is that of exactly defining the sensations produced by electrical stimulation in terms of the peripheral stimuli that yield the identical sensation. The mapping of the equivalences between the sensations produced by electrical stimulation and the sensations produced by peripheral stimuli seems at present to be an unrewarding task. Furthermore, considering the different distributions of neural activity produced by central and peripheral stimuli, it is not at all apparent that the effects of central stimulation can be completely equated to the effects of peripheral stimulation.

In any event, such a mapping would be a monumental task that can be pursued far more efficiently with human subjects.

It should be clear that animal research on the question of sensory quality has hardly begun. Yet, it is already apparent that certain aspects of auditory sensation are differentially distributed within the auditory system. The question of sensory quality is thus changed from "what does it sound like ?" to "how are sensations x, y, and z related to a given group of neurons ?" — a question which in essence concerns neural organization.

II. The Question of Neural Organization

The electrical stimulus activates hundreds or thousands of neurons; hence, the experimental results obtained must be basically coarse-grained. On the other hand, the experimental results probably reflect the predominant properties related to the region stimulated. From electrical stimulation work, we may expect an outline of auditory neural functioning, rather than a detailed listing of neuronal interrelations.

In comparison to auditory psychophysical research, electrical stimulation work is only in the beginning stages. One of the necessary first steps is to determine the lower limits of responsiveness of the various auditory loci to electrical stimuli. Specification of these sensitivities should then permit use of electrical stimulation of proper intensity, insuring the use of an adequate, but not excessive, stimulus in further studies of the auditory system.

Detection of Electrical Stimulation. Presently available data indicate that sensitivity to electrical stimulation of the subcortical auditory system is closely related to anatomic locus (GERKEN, 1970, 1971a). Behaviorally measured detection thresholds for electrode placements in cochlear nucleus ranged from 8 μA to 60 μA with a mean of approximately 22 μA. Thresholds for placements in superior olivary complex or the central nucleus of inferior colliculus ranged from 20 μA to 50 μA, while thresholds for placements in apical inferior colliculus or medial geniculate nucleus were 75 μA and above. Mean threshold for the anterior portion of medial geniculate is 90 μA, while thresholds for posterior placements in geniculate are at least twice this value (GERKEN, 1971a). The interesting question of the neural basis for these differences in threshold presents an opportunity to correlate events on the anatomic and physiologic levels with occurrences in the behavioral realm.

Measurement of detection threshold for electrical stimulation requires the use of sophisticated behavioral methodology. Operant conditioning techniques seem most powerful in this regard and a number of specific procedures have been developed for a wide range of psychophysical experiments using animal subjects (BLOUGH, 1958, 1966; STEBBINS, 1970). Operationally, auditory and electrical-stimulation thresholds can be measured using the same behavioral procedures. The useable dynamic range for electrical stimulation is frequently no more than 20 or 30 dB and, hence, is much smaller than the range for acoustic stimulation. I have found that intensity increments of less than 1 dB are appropriate for the measurement of electrical stimulation thresholds. It is of considerable importance to note that specific threshold values, such as those listed above for the several auditory nuclei, are dependent upon the particular behavioral procedures used. It is safe, however, to regard these thresholds as indicating the relative sensitivities of the auditory nuclei.

Complete specification of electrical detection thresholds requires, in addition to specification of the behavioral procedures, reference to several stimulation parameters other than pulse current and pulse duration. For a simple train of monophasic pulses, these parameters include repetition rate, polarity, waveform, and current density. For example, lower current-thresholds are typically obtained with longer pulse durations or higher repetition rates (Davis and Forbes, 1936; Doty *et al.*, 1956; Gerken, 1970).

Minimizing current threshold is not necessarily the most desirable strategy. A given current threshold may also be expressed as a coulomb threshold, for example, and the coulomb threshold can be the quantity minimized. Unfortunately, it is not clear whether current threshold, coulomb threshold, or even some other measure is most appropriate for use as the measure of the effectiveness of the electrical stimulus. It is clear, however, that application of presently available knowledge of electrodes and electrode properties can greatly benefit brain stimulation research (Greatbatch, 1967; Greatbatch *et al.*, 1969; Terasawa and Sawyer, 1969; van Heeckeren, 1969; Weinman, 1965; Weinman and Mahler, 1964; Wetzel *et al.*, 1969).

A question of special importance is whether electrical thresholds are constant over time. The data available for non-auditory cortical placements indicate that detection thresholds are stable over a period of months (Delgado, 1955; Doty and Rutledge, 1959). This does not seem to be the case for placements in brainstem and thalamus. Figure 1 shows two groups of threshold data for subcortical placements tested with the standard 0.3 msec duration, cathodal pulses presented at 3 Hz. Group 1 animals were each tested exclusively on one medial geniculate placement (Gerken, 1971a). Various parameters of stimulation were employed in addition to the standard parameters mentioned above so that the animals received extensive experience on this one electrode. Group 2 animals were multiple electrode cats and testing was rotated among electrodes (Gerken, unpublished). In an animal, for example, with two placements in medial geniculate, two placements in cochlear nucleus, and one placement each in lateral geniculate and hippocampus, a particular electrode would be tested once every sixth session. Only the standard 3 Hz stimulation was used with Group 2 animals. Final average thresholds for the data presented in Fig. 1 are shown in Table 1.

The result most apparent in Fig. 1 is that substantial decreases in threshold over test sessions were obtained for all placements. In addition, the decreases in normalized threshold follow a roughly parallel course. The similarity of Group 1 and Group 2 medial geniculate data, as well as the near equality of final medial geniculate thresholds (see Table 1), indicates that the threshold decrease was not related to the amount of testing experience on a particular electrode.

The total amount of electricity delivered through each electrode was roughly proportional to: the number of sessions in which the electrode was used, the pulse repetition rate used, and the threshold level for that electrode. The calculated total coulombs per electrode presented in Table 1 were obtained by calculating the number of coulombs presented in each threshold session and then summing over sessions. It may be seen that medial geniculate placements in Group 1 received over six times as much electricity as did medial geniculate placements in Group 2, principally because Group 1 placements were tested every session, whereas Group 2 placements were tested in rotation. Total coulomb differences among Group 2 placements reflect the differences in threshold that characterize the several brain loci, since the animals had equal experience with each electrode. Thus, no relation is apparent between threshold decrease and the number of coulombs of electricity applied through a given electrode.

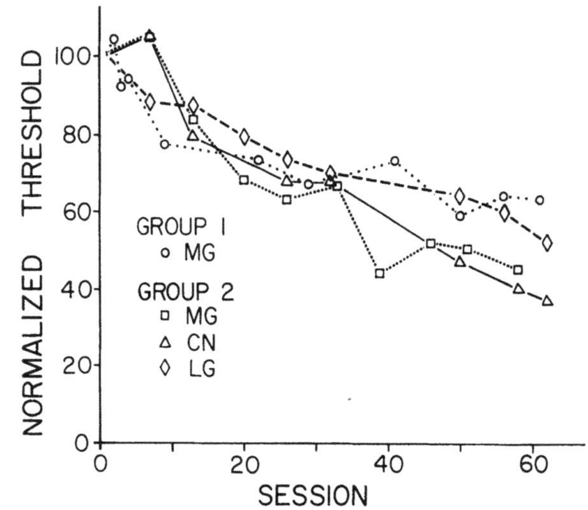

Fig. 1. Normalized electrical detection thresholds. Thresholds were normalized by taking the first detection threshold obtained for each electrode as 100%. Data for Group 1 were obtained from three medial geniculate (MG) placements in three animals. Group 2 animals had multiple electrode placements. Graphs for Group 2 animals were based on data from 5 MG electrodes, 5 cochlear nucleus (CN) electrodes, and 4 lateral geniculate (LG) electrodes. For convenience in displaying the results obtained from these multielectrode cats, session numbers for each electrode were counted from the session of the first threshold determination using that electrode. Session number, however, includes all threshold sessions, not just those using a particular electrode

Table 1. Total coulombs per electrode summed across all sessions shown in Fig. 1, and final mean thresholds

	Placement	Total coulombs per electrode	Final mean threshold, μA	Number of electrodes
Group 1	medial geniculate	1.47×10^{-3}	100.2	3
Group 2	medial geniculate	0.23×10^{-3}	103.8	5
	cochlear nucleus	0.04×10^{-3}	21.6	5
	lateral geniculate	0.18×10^{-3}	94.8	4

The general similarity of the normalized plots for cochlear nucleus and medial geniculate data indicate that threshold decrease is not related to threshold differences *per se*. In addition, comparison of auditory system placements with lateral geniculate placements indicates that threshold decrease is not peculiar to auditory brain regions. Regardless of the degree of experience with electrical stimulation, however, the sensitivity of one brain region with respect to another region tends to remain constant.

Some auditory threshold data are available that were obtained using the same behavioral procedures as were used to obtain the data of Fig. 1. Average threshold in four animals for 3 Hz presentation of a brief transient sound (GERKEN, 1971b) did not significantly change over an average interval of eleven sessions with other auditory thresholds measured in that interval. Furthermore, in three animals, average threshold for 3 Hz clicks did not significantly change over an average interval of 85 sessions with only *electrical* thresholds measured in the intervening interval. Hence auditory thresholds prove to be stable and are unaffected by extensive experience with electrical threshold measurement.

In summary, the decreasing detection thresholds illustrated in Fig. 1 do not seem to be critically related to: (i) the amount of experience on a particular electrode, (ii) the number of coulombs presented through an electrode, or (iii) the threshold level *per se*. Furthermore, significant threshold decrease as a function of number of sessions was obtained with electrical stimulation but not with acoustic stimulation. Collectively, these results would seem to rule out local effects such as anatomic changes in the region of the electrode tip, since these effects logically should be a function of some of the factors listed above. The general conclusion, therefore, is that the threshold decreases shown in Fig. 1 point to a process central to any of the electrode loci. Quite possibly, the animal is "learning" to utilize what amounts to a novel mode of sensory input. Whether, in a strict sense, these threshold changes indicate the occurrence of learning is both an important and difficult question that is, in any event, beyond answer by the presently available data.

Other Aspects of Detection. It cannot be assumed *a priori* that electrical stimulation of a sensory system, even when current is applied at elevated intensity levels, is necessarily detectable.

In an extreme case, an animal with placements in pars principalis of the right and left medial geniculate bodies never learned to perform satisfactorily when tested with electrical stimulation (GERKEN, unpublished). The animal experienced extensive training over a period of months, alerted to stimulation, and even responded many times to the stimulation, thus receiving a number of food reinforcements. Performance was never reliable enough, however, to permit measurement of electrical detection threshold. The cat readily transferred to photic stimulation and was an excellent subject when tested with acoustic stimulation.

Another animal (cat 127) showed a similar pattern of behavior in response to electrical stimulation but, with difficulty, several electrical detection thresholds were obtained (GERKEN, 1971a). Only one electrode was positioned in this animal but the electrode design was such that it could be adjusted as to depth of penetration in the brain. Following a ventral movement entirely within medial geniculate nucleus of approximately 0.8 mm, the behavior of the animal during stimulation changed markedly and further threshold testing was accomplished without difficulty. As best as could be determined, detection thresholds before movement of the electrode were approximately the same as those measured after movement of the electrode, so that the problems of detection were not related to the intensity of the stimulation.

In still another case, a lesion contralateral to a medial geniculate placement disrupted performance with electrical stimulation for 2 1/2 months while leaving responsiveness to acoustic or photic stimulation unaffected (GERKEN, 1971c). Other instances of this sort have been encountered in the past but were not extensively studied. For example, severe problems were encountered in obtaining adequate performance using stimulation of apical inferior colliculus (GERKEN, 1970). The fact that no instance of difficulty of this sort has ever been encountered using electrodes in areas with detection thresholds of less than 75 μA suggests that thresholds above this level may be indicative of the *functional* organization of the neurons stimulated. The high threshold would, thus, indicate a diffuse neural organization that was inherently difficult to activate with punctate stimulation from a single electrode. Alternately, a high detection threshold may be indicative of the presence of substantial inhibitory effects.

An area for further research has been opened by MILLER and his associates (MILLER *et al.*, 1969; MILLER and GLICKSTEIN, 1967). They demonstrated that, for electrodes in auditory and visual cortices, behavioral reaction time decreased as intensity of stimulation increased. Behavioral reaction time is also a function of the intensity of peripheral auditory or visual stimuli. Combining the two sets of results provides an objective means of equating the effects of peripheral and central stimulation.

Continued effort to elucidate neural mechanisms should ultimately result in a picture, albeit a coarse-grained picture, of the roles of the various auditory nuclei in the auditory functions of the conscious animal. A very incomplete picture of this sort can already be sketched for one auditory nucleus — inferior colliculus. The significance of the sketch lies principally in the points that differ from, or add to, the traditional picture of collicular function.

The Composite Effect of Stimulation: Inferior Colliculus. Electrical stimulation of the auditory system produces not only auditory sensations but possibly motivational, affective and motor responses as well. The production of these other responses in most instances, requires substantially more electrical energy. There is available a very limited mapping of affective and motor responses from auditory system electrode placements (GERKEN, 1970); again, much more needs to be done. Several studies have centered on various aspects of the responses mediated by inferior colliculus; these studies will be cited to illustrate the composite effect of stimulating this important auditory locus.

Stimulation of the central nucleus of the inferior colliculus is detectable and can be used as a cue for the performance of a behavioral response (COLAVITA, 1969; GERKEN, 1970; PATTERSON, 1971). There is more rapid acquisition of classical conditioning when collicular stimulation is used as the conditioning stimulus (CS) than when acoustic stimulation is used as the CS (COLAVITA, 1969; PATTERSON, 1971). If less intense collicular stimulation is used, acquisition of learning proceeds at about the same rate as for acoustic stimulation (PATTERSON, 1971). The intensity of an acoustic CS has not been observed to produce such marked changes in the rate of acquisition of learning; thus, it seems reasonable to conclude that collicular stimulation, and in particular strong collicular stimulation, produces not only an auditory sensation, but also yields another effect which acts to speed learning. This effect may be an affective response which functions as a motivational factor.

Support for the view that collicular stimulation yields motor and motivational effects may be found in the report that strong stimulation of colliculus (0.1 msec biphasic pulses of 1.4—2.4 mA presented at 10 Hz) may serve as the unconditioned stimulus (US) in classical conditioning (COLAVITA and SZELIGO, 1971). The US produced a backward movement of the head and closure of the eyelids. In this experiment, stimulation of inferior colliculus at a lesser intensity (0.15—0.5 mA) served as the CS. In two control animals, unpaired presentations of the CS and US did not yield evidence of pseudo-conditioning. In all animals, the use of bipolar stimulating electrodes eliminated the aversive effects that result from a strong flow of current through an indifferent electrode placed outside the nervous system.

In studies with chronic and acute animals, motor responses such as pinna movements, eye movements, and pupillary dilation have been obtained (SYKA and STRASCHILL, 1970; SYKA and RADIL-WEISS, 1971). Stimulation consisted of 1.0—2.0 sec trains composed of pulses 0.5 msec in duration with estimated current intensities of 75—220 μA and repetition rates of 100 Hz. Some of these motor effects are conveyed, no doubt, by the direct anatomic pathways between the inferior and superior colliculi (TARLOV and MOORE, 1966; POWELL and HATTON, 1969).

The functional relation between inferior colliculus and the reticular formation was studied further by COLAVITA (1970). Cats trained on collicular stimulation generalized to stimulation of reticular formation, although cats trained on reticular stimulation did not generalize to stimulation of colliculus. These results were interpreted as demonstrating the presence of a unidirectional functional pathway linking the auditory and reticular systems. Perhaps these findings may also be linked to the results of NIEDER and NEFF (1961) mentioned earlier in this chapter.

That a particular portion of the nervous system should mediate sensory, motor, motivational, and affective functions should not be especially surprising, since these functions are aspects of hearing and hearing-related behavior. This conclusion however, assumes that spread of stimulating current to other neural structures is not a significant factor. Basically, four types of data can be used to support this assumption: comparison of effects obtained from several electrode positions (SYKA and RADIL-WEISS, 1971; GERKEN, 1970), the sharply defined effects of electrode movement (STONEY *et al.*, 1968), unidirectional generalization (COLAVITA, 1970), and comparison of monopolar and bipolar stimulation data (WETZEL, 1970). Without discussing the matter in further detail, current spread, in general, does not appear to be a serious problem in many stimulation situations; but, in critical instances, lack of spread to adjacent neural structures must be demonstrated experimentally.

Concluding Remarks. The use of electrical stimulation to study central processing is, in many ways, analogous to discovering a hitherto unknown sensory system. As in the case of the newly discovered system, certain information is much in need, such as: definition of the adequate stimulus, anatomic delineation of the locus responsive to stimulation, development and calibration of stimulus sources, and establishment of stimulation standards. Work of this sort has been carried out in a number of laboratories but a great deal more is required for the full potentialities of the electrical stimulation method to be realized.

In a limited brain region, probably thousands of neurons are simultaneously activated by gross electrode stimulation, but punctate activation of this sort may not occur in the course of normal auditory functioning. Experimental support for this view is found in the work of CLARK (1969) which demonstrated that the neuronal firing patterns which are produced in the superior olivary complex by acoustic stimuli cannot be simulated by electrical stimulation of the auditory nerve or cochlea. I would guess that a neuronal firing pattern more closely allied to naturally occurring patterns within the auditory system may be produced by rapid, sequential stimulation of an array of electrodes using current levels near threshold. Such an array may well be used to take advantage of existing interneuronal relationships to the extent that the effects produced will be primarily a function of the stimulation sequence.

Finally, the auditory system does not stand by itself but is interrelated with numerous other brain areas, such as the claustrum, caudate nucleus, cerebellar cortex and the septal region. In recent years, these interconnections have received increased attention (GOLDEN and LUBAR, 1971; OTELIN, 1970; LAGRUTTA *et al.*, 1970; HASSMANNOVA and SPECTOR, 1967; DIAMOND *et al.*, 1969; POWELL and HOELLE, 1967; ADES, 1941). As stimulation work on the auditory system continues, it will be a task of considerable importance to evaluate the functional role in the behaving animal of these anatomic interconnections.

Acknowledgements

This work was supported in part by a grant from the National Institute of Neurological Diseases and Stroke.

References

ADES, H. W.: Connections of the medial geniculate body in the cat. Arch. Neurol. Psychiat. **45**, 138—144 (1941).

BLOUGH, D. S.: A method for obtaining psychophysical thresholds from the pigeon. J. exp. Anal. Behav. **1**, 31—43 (1958).

BLOUGH, D. S.: The study of animal sensory processes by operant methods. In: Operant behavior: areas of research and application. New York: Appleton-Century Crofts 1966.

CLARK, G. M.: Responses of cells in the superior olivary complex of the cat to electrical stimulation of the auditory nerve. Exp. Neurol. **24**, 124—136 (1969).

COLAVITA, F. B.: Electrical brain stimulation used as a CS. Commun. behav. Biol. **3**, 315—317 (1969).

COLAVITA, F.B.: The reticular formation and avoidance conditioning. Physiol. Behav. 5, 1423—1426 (1970).

COLAVITA, F.B., SZELIGO, F.: Classical conditioning with brain stimulation at one site serving as both CS and US. Physiol. Behav. **6**, 41—44 (1971).

DAVIS, H., FORBES, A.: Chronaxie. Physiol. Rev. **16**, 407—441 (1936).

DELGADO, J.M.R.: Evaluation of permanent implantation of electrodes within the brain. Electroenceph. clin. Neurophysiol. **7**, 637—644 (1955).

DIAMOND, I.T., JONES, E.G., POWELL, T.P.S.: The projection of the auditory cortex upon the diencephalon and brain stem in the cat. Brain Res. **15**, 305—340 (1969).

DOTY, R.W.: Electrical stimulation of the brain in behavioral context. Ann. Rev. Psychol. **20**, 289—320 (1969).

DOTY, R.W., RUTLEDGE, L.T.: "Generalization" between cortically and peripherally applied stimuli eliciting conditioned reflexes. J. Neurophysiol. **22**, 428—435 (1959).

DOTY, R.W., RUTLEDGE, Jr., L.T., LARSEN, R.M.: Conditioned reflexes established to electrical stimulation of cat cerebral cortex. J. Neurophysiol. **19**, 401—415 (1956).

GERKEN, G.M.: Electrical stimulation of the subcortical auditory system in behaving cat. Brain Res. **17**, 483—497 (1970).

GERKEN, G.M.: Behavioral measurement of electrical stimulation thresholds for medial geniculate nucleus. Exp. Neurol. **31**, 60—74 (1971a).

GERKEN, G.M.: Electrophysiological observations relevant to masking. Audiology **10**, 97—109 (1971b).

GERKEN, G.M.: Behaviorally measured interactions between medial geniculate nuclei. J. acoust. Soc. Amer. **50**, 118 (1971c).

GOLDEN, G.H., LUBAR, J.F.: Effect of septal and fimbrial stimulation on auditory and visual cortical evoked potentials in the cat. Exp. Neurol. **30**, 389—402 (1971).

GREATBATCH, W.: Electrochemical polarization of physiological electrodes. Med. Res. Eng. **6**, 13—17 (1967).

GREATBATCH, W., PIERSMA, B., SHANNON, F.D., CALHOON, S.W. JR.: Polarization phenomena relating to physiological electrodes. Ann. N. Y. Acad. Sci. **167**, 722—744 (1969).

HASSMANNOVA, J., SPECTOR, I.: Relations fonctionnelles entre relais acoustique (G. M.) et claustrum. J. Physiol. (Paris) **59**, 427—428 (1967).

KITAI, S.T.: Generalization between photic and electrical stimulation to the visual system. J. comp. physiol. Psychol. **61**, 319—324 (1966).

LAGRUTTA, V., AMATO, G., MILITELLO, L.: The responsiveness of acoustic area after stimulation of the caudate nucleus. Experimentia (Basel) **26**, 259—260 (1970).

MILLER, J.M., GLICKSTEIN, M.: Neural circuits involved in visuomotor reaction time in monkeys. J. Neurophysiol. **30**, 399—414 (1967).

MILLER, J.M., MOODY, D.B., STEBBINS, W.C.: Evoked potentials and auditory reaction time in monkeys. Science **163**, 592—594 (1969).

NIEDER, P.C., NEFF, W.D.: Auditory information from subcortical electrical stimulation in cats. Science **133**, 1010—1011 (1961).

NIELSON, H.C., KNIGHT, J.M., PORTER, P.B.: Subcortical conditioning, generalization, and and transfer. J. comp. physiol. Psychol. **55**, 168—173 (1962).

OTELLIN, V.A.: The auditory cortex projections to the caudate nucleus and probable role of the nucleus as an associative subcortical area. Sechenov physiol. J. U.S.S.R. **56**, 967—972 (1970).

PATTERSON, M.M.: Inferior colliculus CS intensity effect on rabbit nictitating membrane conditioning. Physiol. Behav. **6**, 273—278 (1971).

POWELL, E.W., HATTON, J.B.: Projections of the inferior colliculus in cat. J. comp. Neurol. **136**, 183—192 (1969).

POWELL, E.W., HOELLE, D.F.: Septotectal projections in the cat. Exp. Neurol. 18, 177—183 (1967).

STEBBINS, W.C. (Ed.): Animal psychophysics. New York: Appleton-Century-Crofts 1970.

STONEY, S.D., Jr., THOMPSON, W.D., ASANUMA, H.: Excitation of pyramidal tract cells by intracortinal microstimulation: effective extent of stimulating current. J. Neurophysiol. **31**, 659—669 (1968).

SYKA, J., RADIL-WEISS, T.: Electrical stimulation of the tectum in freely moving cats. Brain Res. **28**, 567—572 (1971).

SYKA, J., STRASCHILL, M.: Activation of superior colliculus neurons and motor responses after electrical stimulation of the inferior colliculus. Exp. Neurol. **28**, 384—392 (1970).

TARLOV, E. C., MOORE, R. Y.: The tecto-thalamic connection in the brain of the rabbit. J. comp. Neurol. **126**, 403—414 (1966).

TERASAWA, E., SAWYER, C. H.: Electrical and electrochemical stimulation of the hypothalamo-adenohypophysial system with stainless steel electrodes. Endocrinology **84**, 918—925 (1969).

VAN HEECKEREN, D. W., HOGAN, J. F., GLENN, W. W. L., BROOKS, M. S.: Engineering analysis of pacemaker electrodes. Ann. N. Y. Acad. Sci. **167**, 774—784 (1969).

WEINMAN, J.: Biphasic stimulation and electrical properties of metal electrodes. J. appl. Physiol. **20**, 787—790 (1965).

WEINMAN, J., MAHLER, J.: An analysis of electrical properties of metal electrodes. Med. Elect. and Biol. Eng. **2**, 299—310 (1964).

WESTER, K.: Habituation to electrical stimulation of the thalamus in unanesthetized cats. Electroenceph. clin. Neurophysiol. **30**, 52—61 (1971).

WETZEL, M. C.: Identification of self-stimulation elements for adjacent electrodes in the cat. Physiol. Behav. **5**, 899—905 (1970).

WETZEL, M. C., HOWELL, L. G., BEARIE, K. J.: Experimental performance of steel and platinum electrodes with chronic monophasic stimulation of the brain. J. Neurosurg. **31**, 658—669 (1969).

Chapter 12

Cochlear Mechanics

C. R. STEELE*, Stanford, California

With 16 Figures

Contents

Abstract

Three successively more elaborate physical models for the fluid-elastic interaction in the cochlea are analyzed by asymptotic methods, with which an *a priori* assumption of "long" or "short" wavelengths is not necessary. Appropriate stiffnesses are estimated from BÉKÉSY's static point and pressure load measurements. Most calculations are for a "two-mode" model which admits an independent motion of the arches of CORTI and the pectinate zone of the basilar membrane. The phase, location of maximum response, and arrival times correlate well with recent measurements of basilar membrane response, electrical and neural activity. The model cannot reproduce with any reasonable change in stiffness or fluid viscosity, the sharpness of decay observed at a fixed point for high frequency, nor the severe post-mortem changes in amplitude. This indicates that the organ of CORTI has a significant mechanical function not taken into consideration by the present models. The "three-mode" model, which includes the flexibility of the bony shelf tip, is briefly considered. The results indicate that for frequencies over 1 kHz no "long" wavelengths occur in the human cochlea.

Introduction

Under the heading "mechanics", we consider the behavior of the cochlear fluids and the elastic tissue of the cochlear partition, without any consideration of

* Professor of Aeronautics and Astronautics, Stanford University.

possible feedback from the electrical and chemical activity of the cochlea. Even with this restricted view, the problem is formidable and far from a satisfactory resolution. The general objective would be (1) to explain the purpose of the gross anatomical features such as the coiling, the bone construction, the fibrous arrangement of the basilar membrane and its attachment, but including the structural details of the organ of CORTI and even the cilia, and (2) to determine quantitative information on the relation between external sound excitation and the mechanical environment (stress, strain) of the receptor cells.

A historical survey of the many and varied "theories of hearing" is given by WEVER (1949), none of which anticipated the actual dynamic response of the cochlea observed in 1928 by BÉKÉSY (1960). Since it is more difficult to imagine an effective neural stimulation through traveling waves than, for instance, through local resonance, BÉKÉSY's observation was not readily accepted. No one has been able or willing to repeat BÉKÉSY's direct measurements with the light microscope. Qualitative confirmation has been obtained, however, by measurement of a radioactive source placed on the basilar membrane, JOHNSTONE and BOYLE (1967), RHODE (1971, 1973), by capacitive probe, WILSON and JOHNSTONE (1972), and by laser illumination, KOHLLÖFFEL (1973). Nevertheless, a fundamental understanding of the traveling wave phenomena is gained most easily through a mathematical treatment.

An examination of the pre-BÉKÉSY "theories" shows that, although giving a completely false general description of cochlear mechanics, each contains some truth. Furthermore, a main reason for straying so far from reality is that most of these "theories" involved not only speculation about an appropriate physical model for the cochlea, but speculation about the behavior of the model. For example the famous suggestion from HELMHOLTZ of sharply tuned, basilar membrane fibers cannot be supported by any reasonable model with the same mass density of fluid and elastic tissue. If HELMHOLTZ had performed either an experiment or mathematical analysis of his stretched string model, he would have found the broadly tuned, traveling waves. Whether the basilar membrane is equivalent to a set of transverse strings under tension, a thin membrane under some tension as in the experimental models of BÉKÉSY (1960), or an isotropic plate, is irrelevant to the qualitative features of the traveling waves. It has been clearly demonstrated by the mathematical studies, for instance, of RANKE (1950) and ZWISLOCKI (1953), summarized in DALLOS (1973), that a monotonic variation along the cochlea in effective compliance of the cochlear duct will produce traveling waves under a pure tone excitation.

The first step of a study of the mechanics is the formation of a simplified physical model, which hopefully simulates certain features of the actual cochlea. Next comes an investigation of the response of the physical model through mathematical analysis of the exact equations for the model, or through actual construction of the model and experimentation. Close agreement with the available physiological data for the cochlea indicates that the model does contain significant features of the cochlea; a lack of agreement indicates that important features have been omitted. Even in the latter situation a gain in understanding is accomplished.

A difficulty has been that the simplest physical model involves the interaction between three-dimensional fluid motion and the elastic partition, so the equations cannot be solved by usual methods. Except for RANKE (1950) all investigators have made use of the assumption of long wavelength in order to obtain a reasonably simple equation, ZWISLOCKI (1953), DALLOS (1973). Although this is referred to as the long-wave "model", it provides a limited representation of the physical model. From the many model experiments of BÉKÉSY (1960, p. 437) and from his observation of radial waves on Reissner's membrane for frequencies over 1 kHz BÉKÉSY (1960, p. 496), it can be concluded that the significant portion of the gross response of the cochlea duct is in fact short-wave. Thus, it is never clear whether disagreements between results from the long-wave model analysis and the physiological data should be attributed to inadequacies in the physical model or in the long-wave approximation.

It is shown in STEELE (1974a) that it is possible to obtain reasonably simple solutions for a cochlear model without the long-wave assumption. In the present article the approach is reviewed and extended to a more accurate physical model. In addition, the transient response to click excitation is treated.

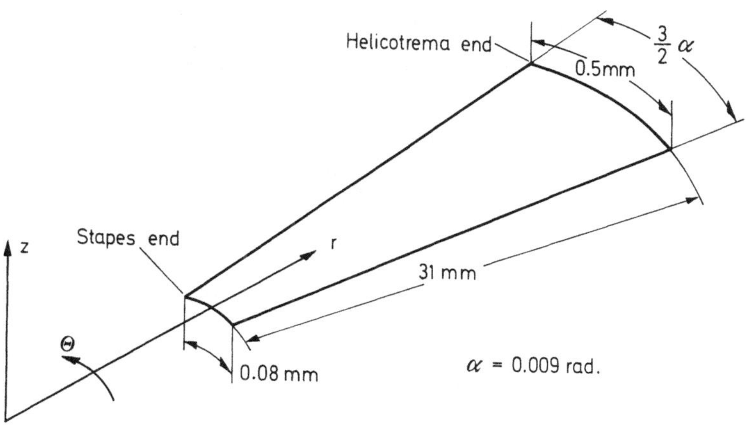

Fig. 1. Nominal human basilar membrane

The "nominal" basilar membrane is shown in Fig. 1. BÉKÉSY's static tests, on a linear scale (Fig. 2), indicate that the arches of CORTI have a substantial stiffness, while his observation of the dynamic response indicates the contrary. To resolve this, the possibility for an independent motion of the arches and the remaining portion of the basilar membrane is considered (Fig. 3). What seem to be reasonable elastic stiffnesses are deduced from BÉKÉSY's static point load and pressure tests. The displacement of the tip of the bony shelf is a third mode which is briefly considered in this investigation. Because this deformation becomes significant near the stapes, the 2-mode model has much less volume compliance in this region (Fig. 2b).

A very simple explanation of the waves in the cochlea can be obtained by considering the basilar membrane as a simply-supported, massless, tapered plate strip immersed in an infinite body of fluid. For a given frequency of pressure fluctuation, prescribed in the fluid far from the plate, the plate response is shown in Fig. 4. To the left of zero, the "transition point", where the plate is more narrow, only the *Gi* function is significant and gives the response in phase with

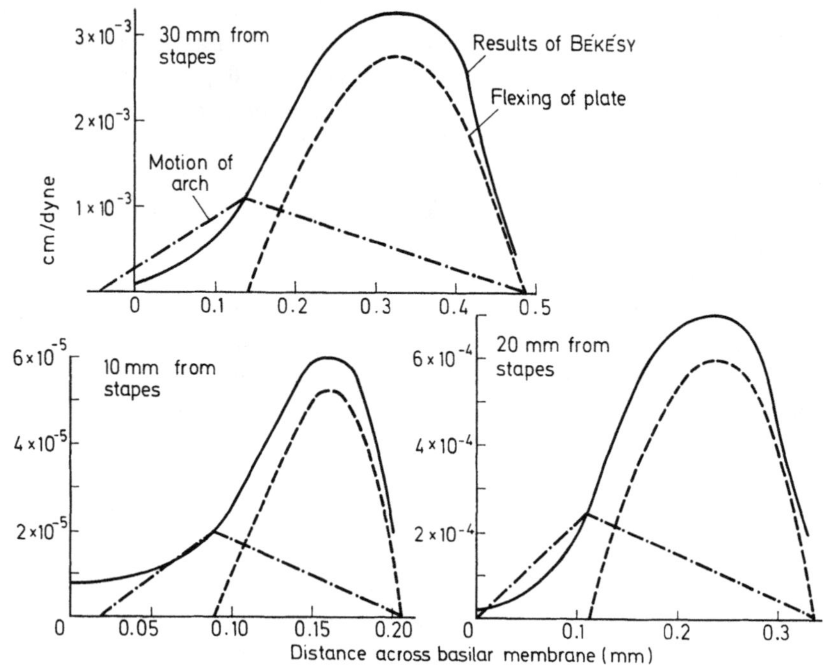

Fig. 2a

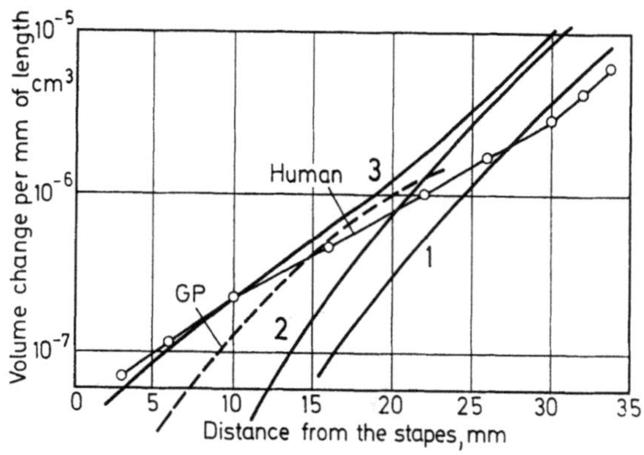

Fig. 2b

Fig. 2a. Response of basilar membrane to concentrated load (Békésy, 1960, pp. 467—468). b Volume displacement for 1 cm water pressure for cochlea (Békésy, 1960, pp. 476, 510) and for models with 1, 2, and 3 modes included

the driving pressure. To the right of the transition point, in the wider more compliant region of the plate, the out-of-phase component of the displacement, given by *Ai*, combines with the *Gi* function to produce the wave traveling away from the transition point. The amplitude of this wave decreases rapidly when the viscosity of the fluid is taken into consideration. Thus the transition point is very near the point of maximum amplitude of plate response.

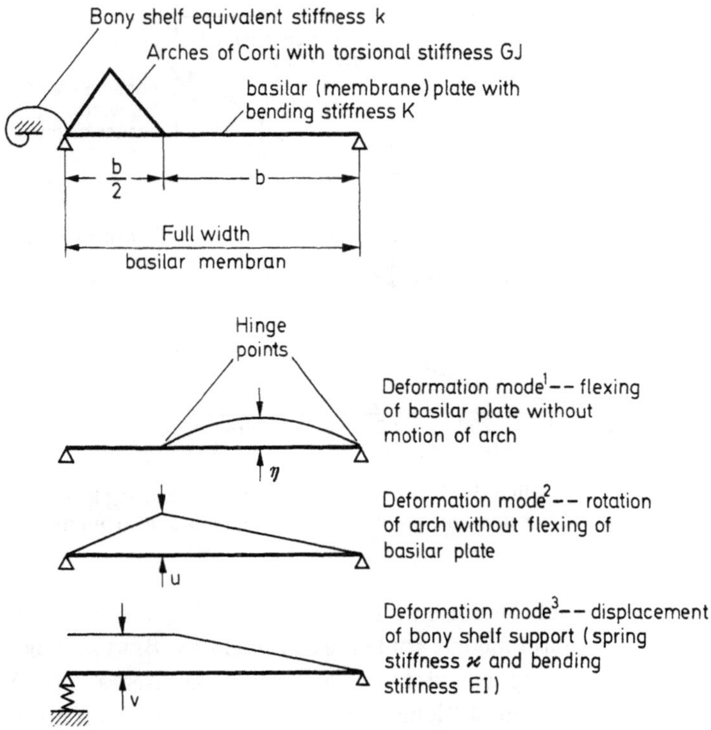

Fig. 3. Structural model for basilar membrane

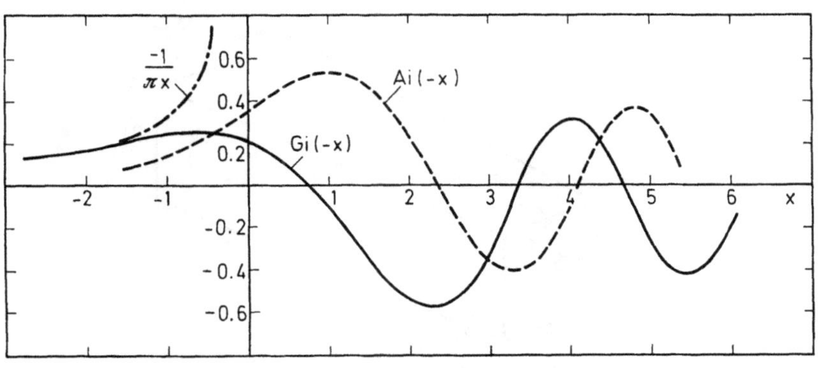

Fig. 4. Airy functions $A\,i\,(-x)$ and $G\,i\,(-x)$

The location of the transition point depends on frequency, as shown in Fig. 5, for the assumptions of perfectly flexible and perfectly rigid arches of Corti. The localization which occurs in the actual cochlea is bounded by these two extremes, except for the low frequencies for which the end effect of the helicotrema becomes significant, and for the high frequencies for which the deflection of the bony shelf becomes important. Thus, we can conclude that the motion observed by BÉKÉSY is an intrinsic characteristic of a tapered plate immersed in a fluid.

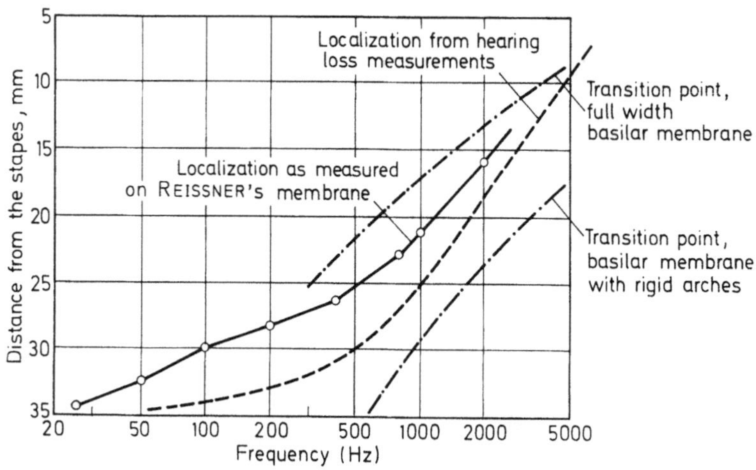

Fig. 5. Localization observed directly (BÉKÉSY, 1960, p. 442) from hearing loss (STEVENS et al., 1935), compared with transition point for basilar membrane in infinite fluid

To obtain the effect of the finite walls, the model of Fig. 6 is considered, which resembles the experimental models studied extensively by BÉKÉSY (1960) and by TONNDORF (1970). By using an extension of the "phase integral" method, with which an *a priori* assumption of "long" or "short" wavelengths is not necessary, a simple solution is obtained in terms of (1) a phase function, (2) an (inviscid) amplitude function, and (3) a damping function due to fluid viscosity.

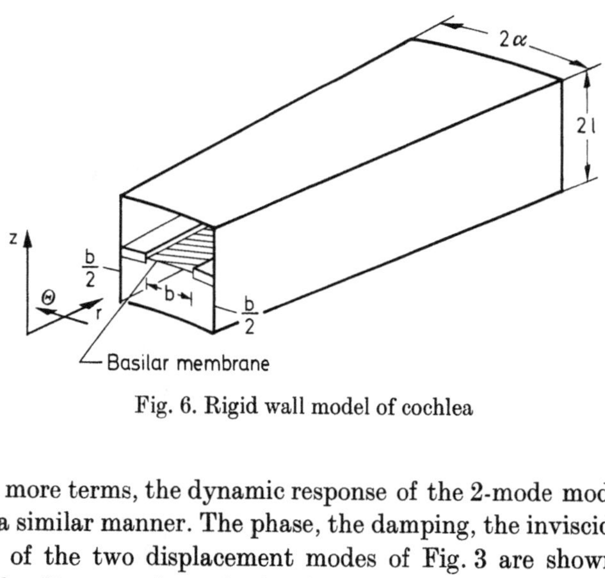

Fig. 6. Rigid wall model of cochlea

By adding more terms, the dynamic response of the 2-mode model of Fig. 7 is considered in a similar manner. The phase, the damping, the inviscid amplitude ψ, and the ratio of the two displacement modes of Fig. 3 are shown in Fig. 8 as functions of the distance along the basilar membrane, normalized with respect to the distance to the transition point (given by the lower curve of Fig. 5). Putting these together for an excitation of 1000 Hz gives the amplitude envelopes of Fig. 9. The location of the points of maximum amplitude for different frequencies is shown in Fig. 10.

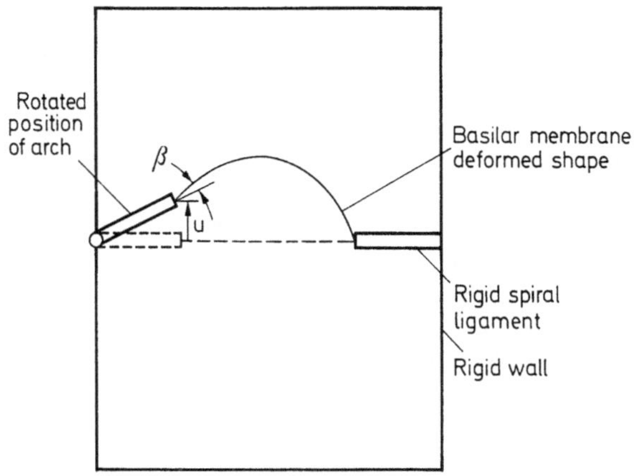

Fig. 7. Rigid wall model of cochlea with flexible arches of CORTI

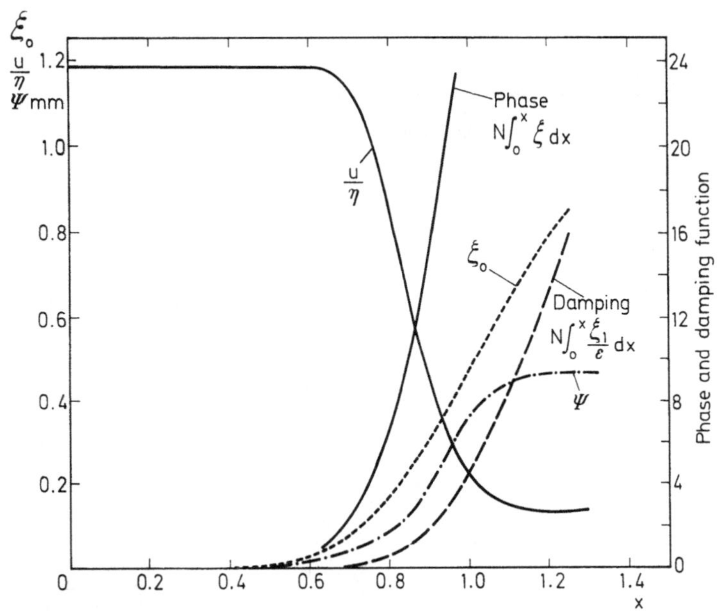

Fig. 8. Phase, amplitude, and damping functions

BÉKÉSY's curve in Fig. 10 is actually for the maximum displacement of REISSNER's membrane (BÉKÉSY, 1960, p. 441). He observed that, below 3 kHz (later revised to below 1 kHz, p. 496), the components of the organ of CORTI all have the same phase, and everyone has assumed the amplitude ratios are the same. The results for the model of Fig. 7, as well as BÉKÉSY's 1953 observation (p. 497), indicate that this assumption is unwarranted. The REISSNER and the tectorial membranes could very well have a lively motion of their own, but might be expected to follow, on the whole, the radial motion of the arches. Indeed the point of maximum arch motion of Fig. 9 comes close to the point of maximum motion observed by BÉKÉSY.

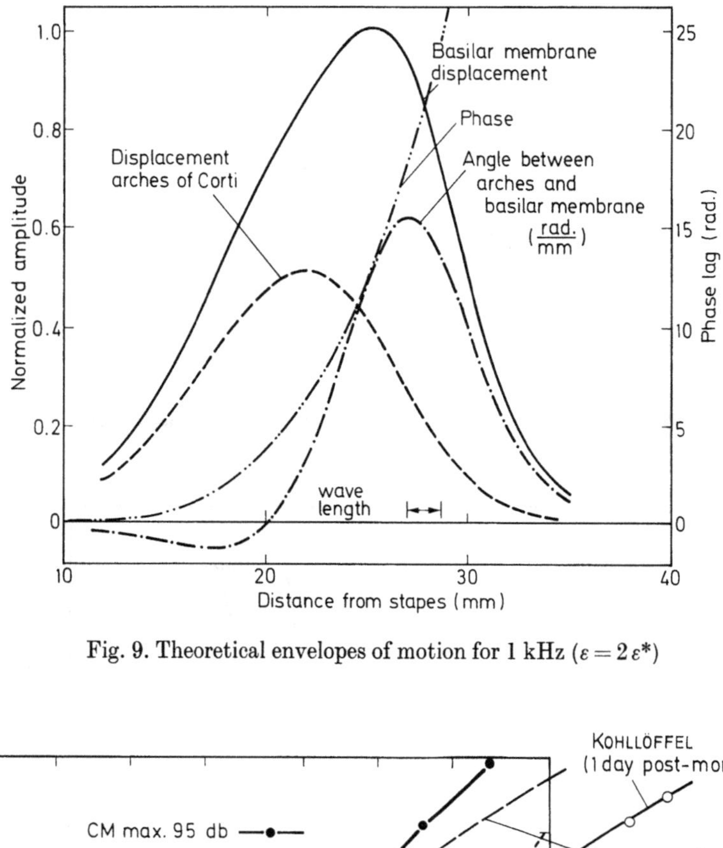

Fig. 9. Theoretical envelopes of motion for 1 kHz ($\varepsilon = 2\varepsilon^*$)

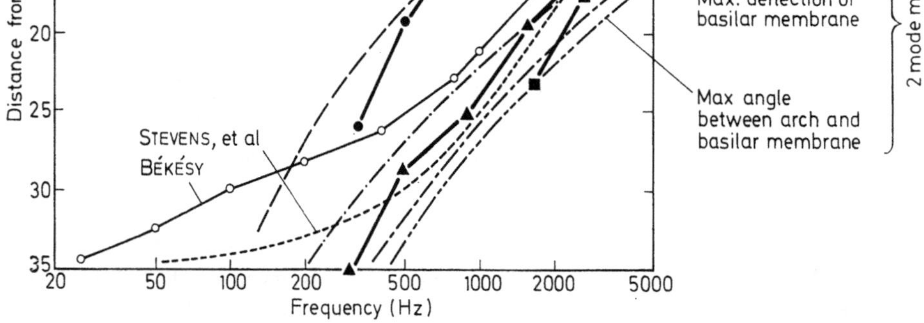

Fig. 10. Spatial localization in model for fixed frequency compared with measurements of electrical field (HONRUBIA and WARD, 1968, 1969) and basilar membrane (KOHLLÖFFEL, 1973)

Numerical results for the model response at a fixed point as the frequency is varied have not yet been calculated. However, a direct comparison can be made with the measurements of spatial distribution at a fixed frequency made by HONRUBIA and WARD (1968, 1969) and KOHLLÖFFEL (1973) in Fig. 10. The location of the maximum DC summating potential (SP) is in the region of maximum activity indicated by the model. The maximum AC cochlear microphonic (CM) is shifted some distance toward the stapes, very close to the boundary of the basal region in which, according to the model, the wavelength is "long". This supports the suggestion that considerable cancellation occurs in the microphonic signal when the wavelength is short, so that the measurement does not accurately indicate the distribution of CM generation (KOHLLÖFFEL, 1971). The measurements of maximum basilar membrane displacement obtained by KOHLLÖFFEL (1972) when rescaled in Fig. 10 are close to the model curve for maximum arch motion. His results for a point near the stapes do not show much difference in the "best frequency" of the live and one day post-mortem conditions. However, RHODE (1973) shows roughly an octave decrease during the first post-mortem hours at points with a best frequency of around 7 kHz. A one-octave shift would place KOHLLÖFFEL'S points in Fig. 10 near the model curve for maximum basilar membrane deflection.

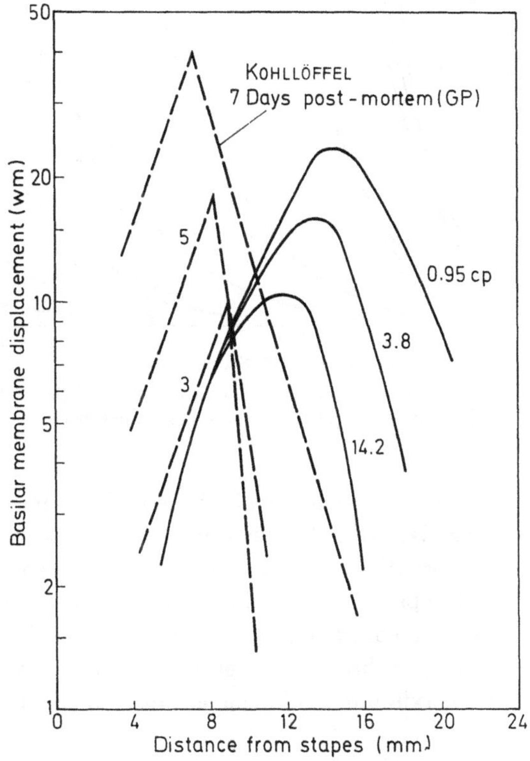

Fig. 11. Basilar membrane amplitude from 2-mode model with different values of fluid viscosity compared with observation of KOHLLÖFFEL (1973) for 8 kHz excitation. The maximums of the lowest curves for model and observation were arbitrarily placed together near an amplitude of 10

The envelopes for 8 kHz are shown in Fig. 5 for a fluid viscosity of 0.95 cp which would correspond to the measurements of endolymph and perilymph of MONEY, et al. (1966) und ZWICKER (1973), and viscosities 4 and 16 times higher. All other Figures show results for 3.8 cp, but we see that the model is fairly insensitive to changes in fluid viscosity. The results from KOHLLÖFFEL (1973) show similar slopes. However, all investigators show much sharper apical slopes for *in vivo* measurements, which cannot be obtained by any reasonable change in the model viscosity. Furthermore, as the model viscosity increases the peak magnitude decreases, so the conclusion is that the post-mortem changes are not attributable to fluid viscosity changes.

KOHLLÖFFEL (1973) and RHODE (1973) find that the post-mortem change in phase is not so pronounced. Figures 12 shows that the model results are quite close to KOHLLÖFFEL's measurements, but deviate from BÉKÉSY's low frequency

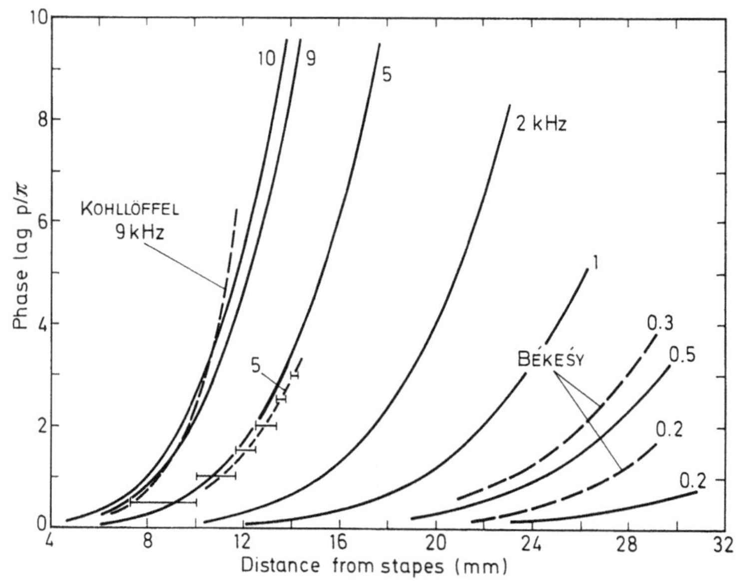

Fig. 12. Phase from 2-mode model compared with observations of BÉKÉSY (1960, p. 462) and KOHLLÖFFEL (1973) (5 days post-mortem)

results, which may be due to the end effect of the helicotrema not considered in the model. In Fig. 10 we also see a deviation in the localization indicated by the model and BÉKÉSY's observation. The two deviations tend to nullify each other in Fig. 13, which shows the phase at the point of maximum arch motion and at the point of maximum basilar membrane motion, according to the model. The indication is that REISSNER's membrane does tend to follow the model arch motion, while the phase at the maximum basilar membrane motion agrees with RHODE (1971).

The effect of the bony shelf deflection on the impedance at the stapes is shown in Fig. 14. The peculiar behavior in BÉKÉSY's experimental curve near 1 kHz corresponds to a transition from "long" to "short" wavelengths at the stapes of the model.

The transient response of the model to a "click" excitation is shown in Fig. 15. The arrival time agrees with BÉKÉSY's observation and the deduction based on CM measurements by DALLOS and CHEATHAM (1971). The most striking correlation occurs between the arrival time estimated from the phase locking of single fiber

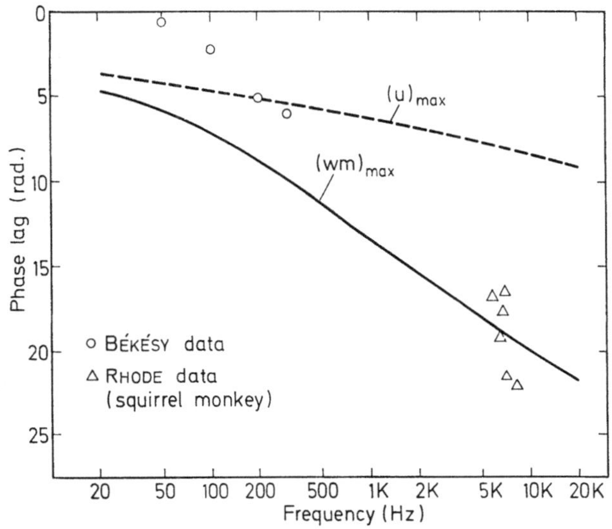

Fig. 13. Phase lag at maximum amplitude of arch and basilar membrane motion from model ($\varepsilon = 2\varepsilon^*$) compared with data from BÉKÉSY (1960, p. 462) and RHODE (1971)

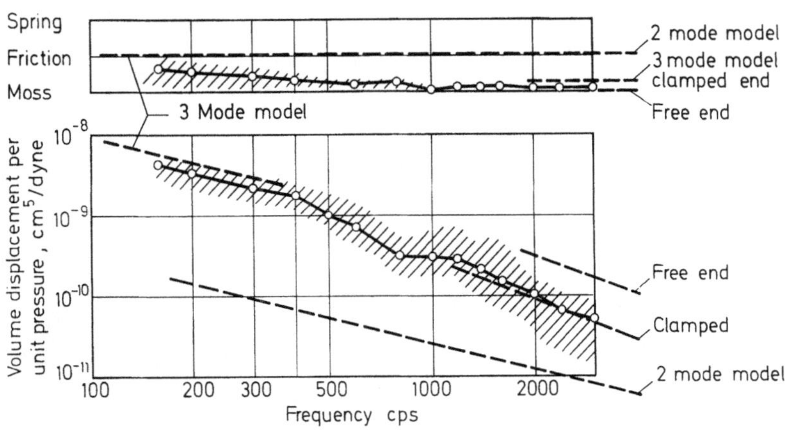

Fig. 14. Volume displacement of the cochlear fluid when the stapes and round-window membrane were removed (from BÉKÉSY, 1960, p. 435) compared with model

recordings and from the model as shown in Fig. 16. ANDERSON, et al. (1971) concluded that there was no correlation with BÉKÉSY's observations; the model results show the contrary.

For the negative aspects, we note that the model is based on BÉKÉSY's post-mortem stiffness measurements, so agreement with *in vivo* data would seem fortuitous. However, the result shown in Fig. 16 for neural activity at 90 db and the SP data in Fig. 10, show too strong a correlation to be dismissed lightly. Secondly, the model fails to show the sharpness of basilar membrane tuning

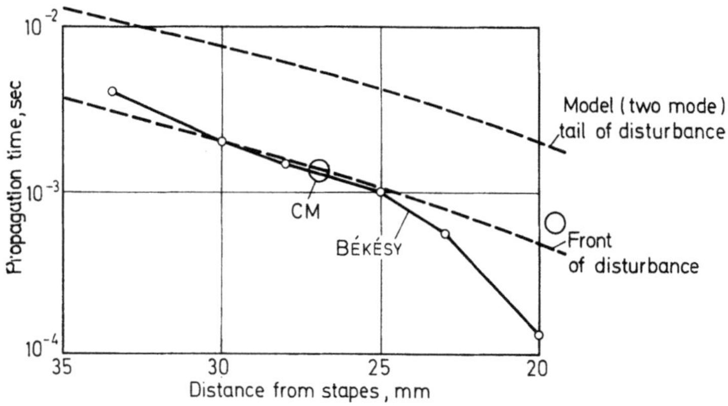

Fig. 15. Propagation of click for cochlea (Békésy, 1960, p. 458) and 2-mode model. Points are computed from CM data by Dallos and Cheatham (1971)

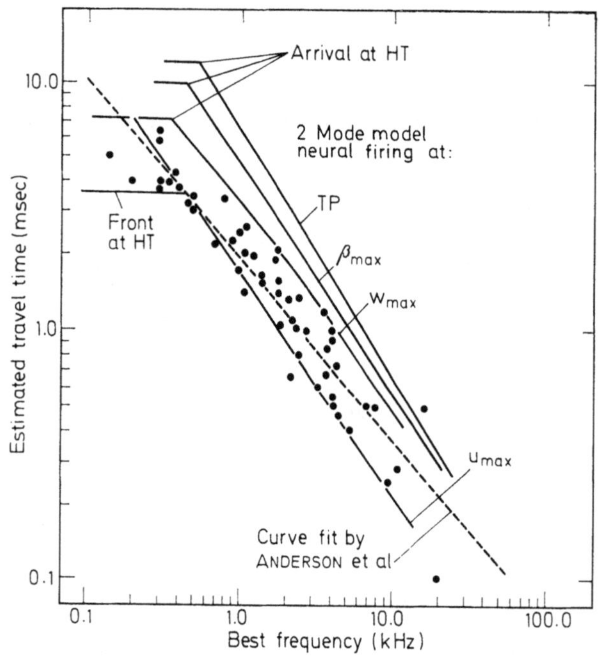

Fig. 16. Travel time estimated from nerve fiber recordings by Anderson et al. (1971) compared with 2-mode model results ($\varepsilon = 2\varepsilon^*$)

found by the direct *in vivo* measurements and cannot obtain such sharpness by any reasonable change in fluid viscosity or elastic properties. But this can be interpreted as indication that the organ of Corti, omitted from the model, does have a significant mechanical function. Such a possibility is strongly suggested by the neural tuning, which is an order of magnitude sharper than that of the basilar membrane EVANS and WILSON (1973). This has motivated the suggestion by TIDEMANN (1970) of resonating tectorial membrane fibers, as well as the speculation on subtectorial membrane fluid flow by STEELE (1973). Consideration of the elaborate structure of the organ of Corti, its systematic geometric variation shown by TIDEMANN (1970), and the highly orthotropic, visco-elastic behavior of the tectorial membrane shown by BÉKÉSY (1960, p. 490) would indicate that the mechanics of this tissue is as important as the basilar membrane mechanics. Thus we can report little progress toward the goal of obtaining the mechanical environment of the receptor cells.

For the purpose of the gross anatomical features of the cochlea, we have the definite analytical result that flexibility of the basilar membrane supporting structure causes a loss in high frequency capability. This is confirmed by the comprehensive study by FLEISCHER (1973), in which he shows that animals with high frequency capability always have a substantial bony shelf, with thick bone connections between the upper and lower surfaces, a well-developed secondary osseous spiral lamina, and solid bone cochlear walls. Except for the *Monotremata*, which have a cochlea resembling the lagena of a bird, FLEISCHER finds coiled cochleas in all classes of mammals. Thus the use of the spiny anteater to justify a straightened model of the cochlea is not proper. A preliminary effort to include curvature in a cochlear model was made by HUXLEY (1968). In STEELE (1974b), it is shown that the curvature can change the effective stiffness of Reissner's membrane by an order of magnitude. Another aspect is the shape of cross-section of the scalae which is greatly distorted in the model Fig. 6. FLEISCHER finds a variety of shapes and variations in shape which must serve a mechanical purpose.

Thus we show that a physical model of the cochlea, free from artificial parameters, can yield simple but sufficiently accurate solutions, which provide some interesting correlations with physiological data. However, the fundamental questions concerning the mechanics of the cochlea remain unanswered.

Elastic Properties

Many investigators have utilized the test data obtained by BÉKÉSY for the volume displacement of the cochlear partition due to a static pressure difference in the scala vestibuli and scala tympani. If the details of the cochlear motion are sought, it is, however, necessary to have values for the stiffnesses of the individual elements in the partition. Such values can be deduced from BÉKÉSY's remarkable test results for the deflections of the various elements under a concentrated load. The point load tests were performed at three sections of the cochlea and clearly demonstrate that it is the basilar membrane whose properties change significantly (BÉKÉSY, 1960, pp. 467–8). BÉKÉSY further demonstrated by static and dynamic tests that the basilar membrane is not under significant tension. If it is not under tension, then the resistance to deformation must come, for sufficiently small amplitudes of deformation, from the bending rigidity. Thus the basilar membrane is not a "membrane" but, in the terminology of mechanics (FLÜGGE, 1962), a plate. Furthermore, BÉKÉSY observed that the deformation pattern around the concentrated load was nearly circular, except near the stapes, so to a good approximation the basilar membrane is an isotropic, elastic plate. This is confirmed by the microstructure shown by IURATO (1962). The separation of the two layers of collagen fibers in the pectinate zone forms a "sandwich" construction which has substantially greater bending stiffness. For stretched strings there would be no mechanical advantage gained by this separation.

The nominal shape of the human basilar membrane as given by WEVER (1949) is shown in Fig. 1 and is used for all calculations. However, all results from the model, as well as data from the guinea pig, are converted to the 35 mm cochlear scale used by BÉKÉSY.

The results for the point load tests are plotted by BÉKÉSY (1960, p. 467—468) on a logarithmic scale, so that the values for the basilar membrane and the softer tissues may appear together. The point of the basilar membrane at which the maximum deflection occurs appears to be roughly in the center. However, DOTSON (1974) realized that the deviation from the center is significant. He replotted the point load response on a linear scale, in Fig. 2a, which shows clearly a sharp change in the curve at the region one-third the distance across. By no coincidence this is the region at which the outer pillar of the arch of CORTI is attached to the basilar membrane. Thus, the arches do provide a substantial stiffening.

Since the pillars of the arches are relatively stiff compared to the basilar membrane, it seems reasonable to consider the cross-section of the arch as rigid. The total displacement of the basilar membrane then consists of the modes shown in Fig. 3: the first, a plate flexing of the pectinate zone; the second, a rotation of the arch; and the third, a deflection of the support under the inner pillar of the arch. As shown by IURATO (1962), the two fiber layers of the pectinate zone come together at the foot of the outer pillars and at the spiral ligament, which seems to be nature's way of forming essentially momentfree hinge support of the lateral edges of the pectinate zone.

If the curves of Fig. 2a are split into the parts due to each of the modes of deformation, the flexing deformation is, to a good approximation, symmetric about the point between the foot of the arch and the spiral ligament, so the use of these two modes seems to be reasonable. The magnitude of the maximum flexing deformation due to the concentrated load η_P/P and the deflection due to the concentrated load at the end of the arch u_P/P from Fig. 2 are shown in Table 1. Also shown is BÉKÉSY's result for the change in cross sectional area, *i.e.* the volume displacement per unit length, of the entire cochlear duct due to a static pressure difference in the scalae (BÉKÉSY, 1960, p. 476).

The deflection η_P under a concentrated load P at the center of a long plate simply supported at the edges is (FLÜGGE, 1962, p. 39–8)

$$\frac{\eta_p}{P} = \frac{b^2}{2\pi^3 K}\left[1 + \frac{1}{3^3} + \frac{1}{5^3} + \cdots\right] \approx \frac{b^2}{2\pi^3 K} \tag{1}$$

where K depends on the YOUNG's modulus E for the material and the plate thickness h

$$K = \frac{E h^3}{9} \, .$$

Thus with Eq. (1) the values of K in Table 1 are directly calculated from the known geometry and BÉKÉSY's test results. The value of K varies nearly with the inverse of the cube of the width. It is most reasonable that E is constant, since it is a material property. Thus the point load results indicate that the pectinate zone thickness is inversely proportional to width. According to the detailed measurements of the water buffalo *(Anoa bubalis)* by TIEDEMANN (1970), the product of arcuate zone width and thickness is almost constant, with a maximum deviation of about 10%. So, for the model, the value of K given in Table 2 will be used, which fits the value in Table 1 at the midpoint and follows the b^{-3} relation. It should be noted, however, that hb = constant is not satisfied by the high-frequency echolocators, in particular *Rhinolophedea* (PYE, 1967).

Just from the geometry, it is evident that if the arches were a tube with a thin-walled, triangular cross section, continuous along the length, then the torsional stiffness GJ would be excessively large; *i.e.* the arches would be essentially rigid against any local deformation of the remaining portion of the basilar membrane. However, the arches are not continuous with the length, but are separate parallel rods joined only at the corners. Thus the torsional stiffness could have a value compatible with the plate bending of the basilar membrane. An additional resistance to the rotation of the arch would come from the attachment to the bony shelf and from the attachment of the cilia to the tectorial membrane (LIM, 1972), which is represented by the coiled spring constant k in Fig. 3. Thus the GJ is a measure of the resistance to relative rotation of two cross-sections of the arches of CORTI, while k measures the resistance to rotation of all the arches together.

The equation for the arches is

$$GJ \frac{\partial^2}{\partial r^2} u - ku = \frac{2}{b} \mathfrak{m} \tag{2}$$

where $\mathfrak{m}$ is the total moment acting on the hinge. It can be shown, by a more elaborate analysis, that the variation in the r direction can be ignored in the determination of the local values of k and GJ.

The deflection under the static point load P is

$$\frac{u_p}{P} = \frac{b^2}{8(kGJ)^{1/2}} \tag{3}$$

so the factor kGJ can be readily obtained from the data in Table 1.

The deflection decreases to 14% a distance away

$$|r - r_0| = 2\,(GJ/k)^{1/2} . \tag{4}$$

Table 1. Data from BÉKÉSY's static tests

Distance from stapes %	η_P/P mm/dyne	u_P/P mm/dyne	$\Delta A/\Delta p$ mm^4/dyne	K dyne mm
29	5.3×10^{-4}	2×10^{-4}	2.24×10^{-5}	0.55
57	6×10^{-3}	2.4×10^{-3}	7.85×10^{-5}	0.122
86	2.8×10^{-2}	1×10^{-2}	2.85×10^{-4}	0.05

Near the stapes, as seen in Fig. 2a, the deflection of the tip of the bony shelf becomes significant. This is taken into consideration by the third deformation mode shown in Fig. 3, consisting of a displacement of the arch without rotation. Since there is a resistance to displacement and bending, the behavior is that of a beam on an elastic foundation, with the equation

$$EI\frac{\partial^4 v}{\partial r^4}+\mathscr{H}v=R_e \tag{5}$$

where R_e is the distributed load. The solution for the deflection under a concentrated load P is

$$v/P=[2^{3/2}(EI)^{1/4}\mathscr{H}^{3/4}]^{-1}.$$

From Fig. 2a, at the 20 mm station, we have

$$v/P=7\times10^{-5}\ \text{mm/dyne}$$

which will be assumed to be constant along the cochlea.

For the model of Fig. 3, the volume displacement per unit length for a static pressure difference Δp is

$$\frac{\Delta A}{\Delta p}=\frac{b^2}{\mathscr{H}}+\frac{9b^4}{64k}+\frac{b^5}{120K}. \tag{6}$$

Figure 2b shows the experimental values. Without much justification, we assume that the contribution of the plate bending and arch rotation should be about the same. Thus k is chosen as shown in Table 2. The bony shelf stiffness is chosen so that Eq. (6) will match the data near the stapes

$$\mathscr{H}=910\ \text{dynes/mm}^2.$$

The Curve 1 in Fig. 2b shows the last term in Eq. (6), the Curve 2 shows the additional effect of arch rotation, and Curve 3 shows all three terms of Eq. (6).

With $\mathscr{H}$ determined, the above concentrated load result gives the bending stiffness

$$EI=8.6\times10^5\ \text{dyne mm}^2.$$

From Fig. 2, it is seen that, to an excellent approximation, the ratio of the maximum arch to maximum plate deflection under the point load is the same at each section. Thus, from Eq. (1) and Eq. (3), with the previous result that K varies with b^{-3}, the torsional stiffness GJ must vary with b^{-2}.

The decay distance for the deformation of the model due to a point load at the outer foot of the arch, from Eq. (4) shown in Table 2, does not seem to be

Table 2. Properties of model

Distance from stapes %	mm	Distance from origin r mm	Plate width b mm	$K(\sim b^{-3})$ dyne mm	$k(\sim b^{-4})$ dynes	$GJ(\sim b^{-2})$ dyne mm^2	$2(GJ/k)^{1/2}$ mm
0	0	5.9	0.053				
29	9	14.9	0.135	0.48	43.5	2	0.44
57	17.7	23.6	0.213	0.122	7	0.8	0.69
86	26.7	32.6	0.293	0.047	2	0.42	0.85
100	31.0	36.9	0.333				

contradicted by BÉKÉSY's observations. Thus, the properties in Table 2 appear to give good approximations to the properties of the human basilar membrane and arches of CORTI.

The basilar membrane in man and guinea pig are generally about the same. We note that the (rescaled) volume compliance for the guinea pig in Fig. 2b is very close to the human in the apical end, but is about one-tenth as much near the stapes. This can be attributed to the distance between the edge of the bony shelf and the foot of the inner pillar, which is negligible for the guinea pig, cat, etc., but is substantial for man (and water buffalo TIEDEMANN (1970)). In addition, the shear stiffening between the upper and lower bone plates of the shelf is noticeably weaker in man (FLEISCHER, 1973). Thus the "two-mode" model, i.e. with mode 3 in Fig. 3 neglected, for which the detailed calculations have been carried out, may simulate the guinea pig cochlea better than the human.

Infinite Fluid

One of the obstacles to an accurate analysis of cochlear activity is the necessity of handling three dimensional motion of the fluid. The model experiments by BÉKÉSY (1960, pp. 437–9) indicate that the essential features of the activity are insensitive to large variations in the size of the fluid chamber, location of the excitation of the fluid, etc. Thus, there must be a significant local intrinsic property of the structure-fluid interaction. The simplest solution for a tapered plate, in the shape of the basilar membrane in Fig. 1, simply-supported along the sides and immersed in an infinite fluid, can be obtained by using the cylindrical coordinates r, Θ, z for both plate and fluid.

Free Vibration. For an incompressible, inviscid fluid the equation for the velocity potential is

$$\Delta\Phi + \frac{\partial^2}{\partial z^2}\Phi = 0 \tag{7}$$

where Δ is the Laplacian operator for the r, Θ plane. A solution which decreases with the distance above the plate is

$$\Phi = J_N(\lambda r)\, e^{i\omega t - \lambda z} \cos N\Theta \tag{8}$$

where $\omega/2\pi$ is the frequency, λ is a constant parameter, and J_N is the BESSEL function. Thus, at the plane $z=0$, we obtain the relation between the fluid pressure above the plate p and the plate displacement w

$$p = i\varrho w\Phi = \frac{\varrho\omega^2}{\lambda} w \tag{9}$$

in which ϱ is the density. Only the sign of Eq. (9) is changed for the fluid pressure under the plate. For an elastic, homogeneous, isotropic plate of constant thickness, the equation is (FLÜGGE, 1962)

$$K\Delta\Delta w = -2p \tag{10}$$

in which the pressure loading from Eq. (9) is doubled for the fluid on both sides of the plate. Since the Laplacian operator is in the equations for both the fluid and the plate, substitution of Eq. (9) into Eq. (10) gives the relation between the constants

$$K\lambda^5 = 2\varrho\omega^2 . \tag{11}$$

Thus, for a given frequency, the value of λ can be calculated.

This solution actually gives the vibration of a complete circular plate, immersed in fluid, in a mode with nodal lines along the radial lines an angle π/N apart. Because of the asymmetry about the nodal lines, they are lines of zero displacement and bending moment. If the portion of the basilar membrane between the arches and the spiral ligament (Fig. 3) is considered to be the simply supported tapered plate in the fluid, then the taper angle is α shown in Fig. 1 and one obtains $N = 350$. Since N is so large, the asymptotic approximation (ABRAMOWITZ and STEGUN, 1966, p. 368) can be used.

$$J_N(\lambda r) = \gamma(r)\, Ai\,(-\zeta) + 0\,(N^{-1}) . \tag{12}$$

$0(N^{-1})$ denotes terms bounded by a constant, presumably near unity, divided by N, and where γ is a "smooth" function, the details of which are not particularly important. The argument of the AIRY function has the expansion near $r = N/\lambda$

$$\zeta = \lambda(2/N)^{1/3}(r - N/\lambda)\,[1 + 0\,(r - N/\lambda)] . \tag{13}$$

When the curve for the AIRY function Fig. 4 is considered, the significance of the transition point $r_t = N/\lambda$ can be appreciated. For smaller values of r, the function is exponentially small; for larger values, the function is oscillatory.

Such a "transition", or "turning" point, arises in a variety of physical problems, several of which are discussed in WILCOX (1964), and is similar to the behavior observed in the cochlea (BÉKÉSY, 1960, pp. 421–2, 461–2) and various models of the cochlea (BÉKÉSY, 1960, pp. 514–534). These all have the common properties:

1) The stiffness varies monotonically with length.
2) A local section, if isolated, would be an independent resonator.

For a given frequency of excitation, the transition point is at the section which would resonate, if isolated. Because of the coupling between sections, however, the transition point marks the boundary between the "soft" and "stiff" regions in which waves can and cannot occur. For a higher frequency of excitation, the transition point moves toward the stiffer region, thus giving the general dependence on frequency observed by BÉKÉSY and previously discussed by RANKE (1950), ZWISLOCKI (1953), and DALLOS (1973).

Since the width at the transition point, $b_t = \pi r_t/N$, we have the simple relation between frequency and the location of the transition point r_t

$$\omega^2 = \frac{K\pi^5}{2\varrho b_t^5} = \frac{KN^5}{2\varrho r_t^5} . \tag{14}$$

Figure 5 is taken from BÉKÉSY (1960, p. 442) and shows the location of the maximum basilar membrane amplitude observed by BÉKÉSY as a function of frequency. Also shown is the curve from STEVENS *et al.* (1935) relating the loss of hearing of a particular frequency to a region of damage on the guinea pig cochlea. The lower curve in Fig. 5 gives the location of the transition point from Eq. (14)

with the use of the values from Table 2, the density of water, and rescaling the distance for the 35 mm cochlea.

It appears, from Fig. 5, that the transition point might have some relation to the behavior of the actual cochlea. If the transition point for a tapered plate with the full width of the basilar membrane is computed, *i.e.* if b_t is replaced by $3b_t/2$ in Eq. (14), then the upper curve in Fig. 5 is obtained. Thus the observed data is neatly bounded by the simple model with the rigid arches, which is too stiff, and the simple model with no arches, which is too flexible. Note that, since $K \sim b^{-3}$, the variation of transition point with frequency is just $\omega \sim b_t^{-4}$.

Forced Vibration. So far only the free vibration of the plate in the fluid has been considered. The transition from a constant phase to a traveling wave along the plate strip is obtained if a uniform fluctuation in the fluid pressure at a large distance from the plate is prescribed. Without worrying over an exact solution for the forcing pressure, the behavior is shown by adding to Eq. (9) the term

$$\frac{p_0 r_0}{r} e^{i\omega t} \cos N\Theta \tag{15}$$

where $p_0 r_0$ is a constant. This is a pressure in the fluid independent of z and decreasing slowly along the plate strip. The solution can be obtained by using the HANKEL transform, with the result for the plate deflection

$$w = \eta \cos N\Theta$$

$$\eta = -p_0 r_0 e^{i\omega t} \int_0^\infty \frac{\lambda}{K\lambda^5 - 2\omega^2 \varrho} J_N(\lambda r)\, d\lambda\,. \tag{16}$$

It can be shown that, since N is large, the maximum contribution of the integrand comes from the region near the transition point of the BESSEL function, $\lambda = N/r = \pi/b$. Hence, an approximation is

$$\eta \sim -\frac{p_0 r_0}{r} e^{i\omega t} \frac{\frac{\pi}{b}}{K\left(\frac{\pi}{b}\right)^5 - 2\omega^2 \varrho}\,. \tag{17}$$

Physically, the approximation Eq. (17) corresponds to neglecting the fluid and elastic coupling along the plate strip, so the system consists of independent oscillators. Thus, for the narrow end of the tapered plate, the stiffness dominates; at the wide end, the fluid inertia dominates; and at the transition point we have resonance, *i.e.* unbounded response to the driving fluid pressure.

However, the argument giving Eq. (17) is not valid near the transition point for which the integrand of Eq. (16) is singular. Instead the approximation Eq. (12) is used and the singular term retained, so the integral is similar to

$$\int_{-\infty}^{\infty} \frac{Ai|(-y)}{y-\zeta} dy = \pi\,[Gi(-\zeta) - iAi(-\zeta)] \tag{18}$$

in which $Gi(-\zeta)$ is a particular solution of AIRY's equation discussed in ABRAMOVITZ and STEGUN (1966) and shown in Fig. 4. The improved approximation to Eq. (16) is

$$\eta = -\frac{p_0 r_0 e^{i\omega t}}{r} \frac{\frac{\pi}{b}(-\pi\zeta)}{K\left(\frac{\pi}{b}\right)^5 - 2\omega^2 \varrho} [Gi(-\zeta) - iAi(-\zeta)] \tag{19}$$

where ζ is defined by Eq. (13). This result is not singular and shows the true character of the response. In the stiff region, ζ is negative, $Gi(-\zeta)$ approaches $(-\pi\zeta)^{-1}$, while $Ai(-\zeta)$ is exponentially small; thus Eq. (19) coincides with the "uncoupled" approximation Eq. (17) with the deflection exactly in phase with the pressure. As the transition point $\zeta=0$ is approached, the out-of-phase component of the response given by the Ai function becomes significant. For the soft region of positive ζ, both Gi and Ai are oscillatory and form a wave progressing away from the transition point. The variety of models studied by BÉKÉSY with a variety of loading distributions (in particular BÉKÉSY, 1960, p. 517), all exhibit this characteristic.

The result [Eq. (19)] does have a resemblance to the behavior of the cochlea; however, much is dissimilar. This will be shown to be due to the difference in the solution of this section, which allows whatever lateral motion of the fluid required to make the solution simple, and the solution in the next section for rigid walls. Another important difference concerns the damping. When the viscosity of the fluid is included, the pole of the integrand of Eq. (16) is shifted below the real axis, and the argument of the functions in Eq. (19) become slightly complex, providing a more rapid diminishment of the wave progressing from the transition point.

Fluid compressibility can easily be included and shown, in agreement with the discussion by ZWISLOCKI (1953), to be negligible, as is also the mass of the plate.

Damping. For a real fluid, the solution of the Navier-Stokes equation (FLÜGGE, 1962) must be used. Instead of the result [Eq. (9)] which permits slipping of the fluid on the plate surface, the result for the viscous fluid which does not slip on the plate is

$$w_r = J'_N(\lambda r)\cos N\Theta\, e^{i\omega t}\left[e^{-\lambda z} - e^{-\beta z}\right]$$

$$w = J_N(\lambda r)\cos N\Theta\, e^{i\omega t}\left[e^{-\lambda z} - e^{-\beta z}\lambda/\beta\right]$$

$$\sigma_z = \frac{\varrho\omega^2}{\lambda} J_N(\lambda r)\cos N\Theta\, e^{i\omega t}\left[e^{-\lambda z} - \frac{2\lambda^2}{\lambda^2-\beta^2}\left(e^{-\lambda z} - e^{-\beta z}\right)\right] \tag{20}$$

in which σ_z is the stress normal to the plate, the parameter β is

$$\beta^2 = \lambda^2 + i\omega\varrho/\mu$$

μ is the viscosity, and w_r is the displacement of the fluid in the r-direction. At the plate, the normal stress equals the negative of the pressure. The relation between pressure and normal displacement is

$$\frac{p}{w} = -\frac{\varrho\omega^2}{\lambda}\frac{1}{1-\lambda/\beta}\,. \tag{21}$$

Even for the small dimensions of the cochlea, the ratio λ/β is less than unity, so the viscosity is significant only in a "boundary layer" near the plate. However, β is complex valued, so that the viscous correction term in Eq. (21) provides the small damping which has a considerable effect on the envelope of the basilar membrane deformation.

Expanding Eq. (21) gives

$$\frac{p}{w} = -\frac{\varrho\omega^2}{\lambda}\left[1 + \frac{1-i}{2}\varepsilon + \cdots\right] \tag{22}$$

where, since $\lambda = \pi/b_t$,

$$\varepsilon = \frac{\pi}{b_t}\left(\frac{2\mu}{\varrho\omega}\right)^{1/2}.$$

Thus, ε gives the ratio of the viscous boundary layer thickness to the plate width. Since $b_t \sim \omega^{-1/4}$, we have $\varepsilon \sim \omega^{-1/4}$. Békésy (1960, p. 407), in a series of tests, measured the viscosity of the human perilymph as 1.97 centipoise, (37° C). According to the more recent tests by Money et al. (1966) and Zwicker (1973), both endolymph and perilymph have a viscosity nearly that of water. Békésy (pers. comm. 1971) did comment that "to me the endolymph is something like the vitreous body in the eye and it has a different viscosity in its normal position than after it has been touched or displaced".

We shall now proceed with the more realistic model with rigid walls and not go through the details of showing the viscous correction to the solution [Eq. (19)].

Table 3. Values of viscosity parameter; ε^* from data of Money *et al.* (1966), and $\varepsilon = 2\varepsilon^*$ estimated from data and observation of Békésy (1960)

f Hz	b_t	ε^*	$\varepsilon = 2\varepsilon^*$
20	0.764	0.514	1.028
50	0.606	0.408	0.816
100	0.51	0.343	0.686
200	0.43	0.289	0.578
500	0.341	0.229	0.458
1000	0.287	0.193	0.386
2000	0.242	0.163	0.326
5000	0.192	0.129	0.258
10000	0.161	0.108	0.216
20000	0.136	0.0915	0.183

Rigid Wall Model

From the previous section, it is seen that the general behavior of the cochlea does have the characteristics of a transition point problem. We now consider a model which is somewhat more realistic. The basilar membrane is again considered as a tapered plate, but now attached at the edges by momentless hinges to rigid plates which are attached to the rigid tube walls as shown in Fig. 6. The plate stiffness variation given in Table 2 is used. Thus, in comparison with the actual cochlea, the model has the same basilar membrane between the arches of Corti and the spiral ligament. The arches are compressed flat and considered to be rigid of width $b/2$, while the spiral ligament is flattened and stretched a bit to the width $b/2$, and also considered to be rigid. The soft cells of the spiral organ of Corti and Reissner's membrane are ignored. Finally, the curved walls of the cochlea are straightened into the rectangular cross section of Fig. 6 of constant total height $2l$ and twice the width of the basilar membrane. The tube will be considered to be of infinite extent, thus the end conditions for the helicotrema are ignored.

The above may seem to be unreasonable idealizations. However, the important feature is that the volume of fluid is preserved. When the basilar membrane is displaced at a region far down the tube, there must be an equal volume of fluid displaced at the "stapes" and "round window" at the near end. For $l = 4$ mm, the areas of the model scalae are about the same as in the actual cochlea, except in the apical turn near the helicotrema. There, however, the cochlea is so tightly wound that any straightened model could be subject to considerable suspicion. Fortunately, the solution shows that, in agreement with the model studies (BÉKÉSY, 1960, p. 437), in the region of interest for a given frequency of excitation, it is only the fluid near the basilar membrane that is of primary importance; *i.e.* the solution is insensitive to the exact value of l and, therefore, presumably, insensitive to the exact size and shape of the cross section or to the curvature.

The attractive feature of the model in Fig. 6 is that the fluid-basilar membrane interaction can be handled easily, thus resolving the difficulty discussed by RANKE (1950). For the fluid in the "scala vestibuli" $0 \leqq z \leqq l$ the velocity potential which satisfies the condition of zero flow through the walls at $\Theta = \pm\alpha$ may be written as the Fourier series

$$\Phi = e^{i\omega t} \sum_{n=0,1,2,\dots} \Phi_n(r,z) \cos nN\Theta \tag{23}$$

where $N = \pi/\alpha = 350$. For the flexing mode of Fig. 3, the displacement on the plane $z = 0$ is

$$w = \begin{cases} \eta(r) \cos N\Theta & 0 < |\Theta| < \alpha/2 \\ 0 & \alpha/2 < |\Theta| < \alpha \,. \end{cases} \tag{24}$$

The deviation from this half-sine wave displacement of the basilar membrane can be included but at a cost of considerable clutter without much effect on the final results. In the expansion [Eq. (23)], only the first two terms are significant.

Traveling Wave Solution. One possibility is to utilize the HANKEL transformation, as used in the preceding section. It turns out, however, that an exceedingly simple solution can be obtained by directly assuming an asymptotic expansion of the solution in the form of a progressing wave

$$\eta(r) = \psi(x)\, e^{i(\omega t - N \int_0^x \xi(x)\, dx)} [1 + 0\,(N^{-1})] \tag{25}$$

in which the dimensionless coordinate is $x = r/r_t$, where r_t is defined in Eq. (14). This is the usual expansion used for waves in inhomogeneous media (HEADING, 1962), and is valid when the wavelength is sufficiently short in comparison with the distance over which the properties of the medium change significantly. Here, we have N to use as the large parameter of the expansion.

As suggested by HALLAUER (1974), the potential function [Eq. (23)] can be taken in the same form with the result

$$\Phi_n(r,z) = -\,i\omega A_n \frac{\cosh(l-z)\,\mu_n}{\mu_n \sinh l\mu_n} [1 + 0(N^{-1})] \tag{26}$$

in which

$$\mu_n = \frac{N}{r_t} [\xi^2 + n^2 x^{-2}]^{1/2} \,. \tag{27}$$

In order to satisfy the condition of zero flow through the surface $z = l$, the hyperbolic function is chosen; and, to make the displacement at $z = 0$ equal to Eq. (24) we choose

$$A_0 = \frac{1}{\pi}\eta\,,\quad A_1 = \frac{1}{2}\eta$$

$$A_n = \frac{2}{\pi}\,\frac{\cos\frac{n\pi}{2}}{1-n^2}\,\eta\,.$$

To obtain a convenient solution for the plate deformation of the basilar membrane, with the hinged edges at $\Theta = \pm\alpha/2$, it is necessary to expand the pressure in the Fourier series of terms zero at the hinges

$$p = -\varrho\omega^2 \sum_{n=1,3,5,\ldots} C_n [1 + 0(N^{-1})] \cos nN\Theta$$

the first term of which is of primary importance

$$C_1 = \sum_{n=0,1,2,\ldots} \frac{A_n}{\mu_n} \coth\mu_n l \left(\frac{4}{\pi}\,\frac{\cos\frac{n\pi}{2}}{1-n^2}\right)$$

$$= \frac{4}{\pi^2}\,\frac{\coth\mu_0 l}{\mu_0} + \frac{1}{2}\,\frac{\coth\mu_1 l}{\mu_1} + \cdots\,.$$

Phase Function. With the pressure on the plate known, the deflection can be obtained from the equation of a plate with variable stiffness (Flügge, 1962). The half sine wave variation in the deflection across the plate [Eq. (24)], with the expansion [Eq. (25)] for the deflection on the centerline and the expansion for the pressure, can all be substituted into the plate equation in the usual asymptotic procedure. The leading term gives the "eikonal" equation for the phase function ξ which in dimensionless form is

$$x^{-3}[\xi^2 + x^{-2}]^2 - \frac{1}{2}\left\{\frac{8}{\pi^2}\,\frac{\coth\mu_0 l}{\xi} + \frac{\coth\mu_1 l}{[\xi^2 + x^{-2}]^{1/2}}\right\} = 0\,. \tag{28}$$

Long and Short Wavelengths. The hyperbolic functions give the effect of the finite wall at $z = l$. The argument $\mu_1 l$ is always large in comparison with unity. Thus for an excellent approximation $\operatorname{Coth}\mu_1 l = 1$. The second argument can be written in several forms

$$\mu_0 l = \left(\frac{\pi l}{b_t}\right)\xi = \frac{l}{r_t} N\xi \tag{29}$$

Again, we have a large factor $(\pi l/b_t)$, so when ξ is not too small, both coth terms in Eq. (28) can be replaced by unity. However, ξ becomes small in the region near the stapes, making the argument [Eq. (29)] smaller than unity. Thus we have the separation

$$\operatorname{Coth}\mu_0 l \approx \begin{cases} 1 & \text{for } \mu_0 l > 1 \\ (\mu_0 l)^{-1} & \text{for } \mu_0 l < 1\,. \end{cases} \tag{30}$$

In the region $\mu_0 l > 1$, which will be shown to be the region of the maximum amplitude of basilar membrane response, the fluid motion does not extend to the wall at $z = l$, but is localized near the basilar membrane. This is, then, the "short wavelength" region. In the region $\mu_0 l < 1$, the fluid motion extends to the wall $z = l$ to such an extent that the pressure [due to the first term of Eq. (23)] acting on the plate is equal to the average pressure in the fluid cross section.

This is then the "long wavelength" region. Rather than initially postulate either a long or short wavelength theory, as discussed by ZWISLOCKI (1953), we have the region of long and short wavelength behavior coming out naturally in the solution.

For the region in which $\mu_0 l > 1$, the phase relation [Eq. (28)] is rewritten

$$x^8 = \frac{2[1+(\xi x)^2]^2}{\frac{8}{\pi^2}\frac{1}{\xi x} + [1+(\xi x)^2]^{-1/2}} \qquad [31]$$

The numerical solution for ξ as a function of x is easily obtained by assuming values of ξx and then computing x. Thus, the direct calculation of the roots of the algebraic expression [Eq. (28)] is avoided. For small values of ξx, Eq. (31) gives

$$\xi \sim \frac{4}{\pi^2} x^7 .$$

Thus the restriction that $\mu_0 l$ be larger than unity gives, for $l = 4$ mm, the long-wave boundary shown in Fig. 10. Hence the significant portion of the response is given by the "short wave" approximation [Eq. (31)], independent of the distance to the wall l. This agrees with the model studies of BÉKÉSY (1960, p. 437), which show no effect of the wall until the wall distance l is decreased to 0.3 mm.

It is of interest that the seemingly more difficult rigid wall model actually simplifies the solution. Instead of the sharply defined transition region with the infinite fluid, the rigid walls cause the transition to be spread out. The phase function $\xi(x)$ is a continuous function. Thus Eq. (25) is uniformly valid and gives a single wave propagating along the cochlea, with a wavelength which is very long in the stiff region near the stapes and becomes very short as the transition point for the plate in an infinite fluid is approached. So, instead of needing the special function of Fig. 4, the single exponential function [Eq. (25)] is adequate.

Numerical evaluation will be deferred for the next section in which the flexibility of the arches is taken into consideration. We continue here with the rather simple analytic expression that can be obtained for the damping and for the "transport" function ψ of Eq. (25).

Damping. The effect of the fluid viscosity on the pressure for a mode of vibration of the immersed plate was previously obtained [Eq. (21)]. If the viscosity correction is added to Eq. (26) in a similar way, the equation for the phase [Eq. (28)] becomes

$$x^{-3}[\xi^2 + x^{-2}]^2 - \frac{1}{2}\left\{\frac{8}{\pi^2}\frac{1}{\xi}\frac{1}{\tanh\mu_0 l - \mu_0/\beta} + \frac{1}{[\xi^2+x^{-2}]^{1/2}}\frac{1}{\tanh\mu_1 l - \mu/\beta_1}\right\} = 0. \quad (32)$$

For the region $\mu_0 l > 1$, after the expansion of the viscosity term, this becomes

$$\begin{aligned} F(\xi, x) &= x^{-3}[\xi^2 + x^{-2}]^2 - \frac{1}{2}\left\{\frac{8}{\pi^2}\frac{1}{\xi} + [\xi^2 + x^{-2}]^{-1/2}\right\} \\ &= (1-i)\frac{\varepsilon}{4}\left[\frac{8}{\pi^2}+1\right] \approx (1-i)\frac{\varepsilon}{2} . \end{aligned} \qquad (33)$$

Thus the correction is

$$\xi - \xi_0 = \frac{(1-i)\,\varepsilon}{2\frac{\partial}{\partial\xi}F(\xi_0, x)} \qquad (34)$$

where ξ_0 is the undamped result

$$F(\xi_0, x) = 0 .$$

Transport Function. The transport function can be obtained either by working out the "next-to-lowest" ordered terms resulting from the substitution of the expansions into the equations, or can be obtained much more easily by considering the average rate of work performed at each cross section of the tube.

$$W = \frac{\omega}{2\pi} \int_0^{2\pi/\omega} \left\{ - \int_{-l}^{l} \int_{-\alpha}^{\alpha} p \dot{w}_r \, r \, d\theta \, dz + \int_{-\alpha/2}^{\alpha/2} \left[M \frac{\partial \dot{w}}{\partial r} - Q \dot{w} \right] r \, d\theta \right\} dt \qquad (35)$$

in which M is the moment and Q the transverse shear acting on the plate edge. Carrying out the calculation gives

$$W = \left(\frac{\omega^3 \varrho}{4\pi^3} b_t^3 \right) \psi^2 \left(x \frac{\partial F}{\partial \xi} \right).$$

For zero damping W must be constant for every cross section, so

$$\psi = C \left[x \frac{\partial}{\partial \xi} F\,(\xi, x) \right]^{-1/2} \qquad (36)$$

where C is a constant. The modification due to viscosity [Eq. (34)] has a significant effect in the exponent of Eq. (25), since it provides the real damping term, but does not have much effect on Eq. (36).

Thus, the solution is easily calculated—the phase function from Eq. (31), the damping from Eq. (34), and the transport function from Eq. (36). The results look quite similar to the observations by Békésy, but then, so do the analytic results of Ranke (1950), Zwislocki (1953), and others. Despite the advantage of the present solution in being free from parameters chosen to fit Békésy's observations of the *dynamic* response, there is still nothing that adds insight into the basic question. How can a response due to a pure tone, involving about a third of the basilar membrane in significant motion, possibly cause a very localized neural excitation necessary for a "place" theory of hearing? In the following section, the one-step more elaborate model is considered. A new aspect of the basilar membrane response is revealed, which could be a significant step closer to the answer.

Flexible Arches of Corti

The arches of Corti undergo less deflection, in comparison with the basilar membrane, according to the static point load tests of Békésy shown in Fig. 2a. In the dynamic response, the conclusion (Békésy, 1960, p. 496) is that the load on the membrane due to the pillar of the arch is small in comparison with the fluid loading, since no change in the curvature of the basilar membrane was observed at the foot of the pillar. Thus the observation of the dynamic response seems a bit in conflict with the static tests. In this section, the model in Fig. 7 is considered in which the two independent modes of motion, shown in Fig. 3, are allowed.

The analysis requires only a modification of that of the preceding section. Because of the asymmetry in the fluid caused by the arch rotation, the sine series must be added to Eq. (23)

$$e^{i\omega t} \sum_{n=1,2,\ldots} \frac{\Phi_{2n-1}}{2}(r, z) \sin\left(\frac{2n-1}{2} N \Theta \right) \qquad (37)$$

and the displacement of the surface $z=0$, instead of Eq. (24) becomes

$$w=\begin{cases}\eta(r)\cos N\Theta+u(r)\left(\frac{\Theta}{\alpha}+\frac{1}{2}\right), & \text{for } |\Theta|<\frac{\alpha}{2}\\ 2u(r)\left(1-\frac{\Theta}{\alpha}\right), & \text{for } \frac{\alpha}{2}<\Theta<\alpha\\ 0 & \text{for } -\alpha<\Theta<-\frac{\alpha}{2}\end{cases} \tag{38}$$

in which u is the amplitude of displacement at the foot of the arch, and η is the maximum displacement in flexing, as shown in Fig. 3. The same traveling wave solution [Eq. (25)] is sought, for which the new Φ functions are of the same form as Eq. (26). To satisfy the displacement on the $z=0$ plane, the coefficients must be

$$\begin{aligned}A_0&=\frac{1}{\pi}\left(\eta+\frac{3\pi}{8}u\right)\\ A_{1/2}&=\frac{8}{\pi^2}(2^{1/2}-1)u\\ A_1&=\frac{1}{2}\left(\eta+\frac{4}{\pi^2}u\right).\end{aligned} \tag{39}$$

The plate equation then provides the phase equation, which is the same as Eq. (32) but with the effect of the arch rotation appearing as the addition factor

$$\begin{aligned}x^{-3}[\xi^2+x^{-2}]^2-\frac{1}{2}\left[\left(1+\frac{3\pi}{8}\frac{u}{\eta}\right)\frac{8}{\pi^2}\frac{\coth(Nl\xi/r_t)}{\xi}\right.\\ \left.+\left(1+\frac{4}{\pi^2}\frac{u}{\eta}\right)(\xi^2+x^{-2})^{-1/2}\right]=0\end{aligned} \tag{40}$$

in which $\coth\mu_1 l$ is replaced by unity.

To obtain the relation between the two deformation modes, Eq. (2) for the motion of the arches must be used. For a momentless hinge at the connection between the arch and flexible plate in Fig. 4, the reaction at the hinge is

$$R=\int_{-\alpha/2}^{\alpha/2}\left(\frac{1}{2}+\frac{r\Theta}{b}\right)prd\Theta$$

so the moment acting on the arch is

$$\mathfrak{m}=-\frac{b}{2}R-\int_{\alpha/2}^{\alpha}r(\alpha-\Theta)\,prd\Theta\,.$$

Since the pressure above the plate is

$$p=\varrho\omega^2[B_0+B_1\cos N\Theta+B_{1/2}\sin N\Theta/2]$$

in which

$$B_n=\mu_n^{-1}A_n\coth\mu_n l$$

the integrations give

$$\mathfrak{m}=-b^2\omega^2\varrho\left[\frac{3}{8}B_0+\frac{1}{\pi^2}B_1+\frac{4(2^{1/2}-1)}{\pi^2}B_{1/2}\right] \tag{41}$$

which must be doubled to account for the pressure from the fluid below the plate.

Using the values of Table 2, Eq. (2) gives the relation

$$\left[-(5x\xi)^2-1\right]u=-4x^7\frac{N}{r_t}\left\{\frac{3}{8}B_0+\frac{1}{\pi^2}B_1+\frac{4(2^{1/2}-1)}{\pi^2}B_{1/2}\right\} \tag{42}$$

Expanding the B_n terms in Eq. (42) gives the relation between the two modes of deformation, which can be substituted into Eq. (40), yielding a rather difficult algebraic expression to solve for ξ as a function of x. However, if we define a quantity

$$v=x^8\left[(1+\xi^2x^2)^{-1/2}+\frac{8}{\pi^2}\frac{\coth\mu_0 l}{x\xi}\right] \tag{43}$$

then the first approximations are

$$\frac{u}{\eta}\approx\frac{\frac{3\pi}{16}v}{1+(5x\xi)^2-\frac{9\pi^2}{128}v} \tag{44}$$

$$v\approx\frac{2(1+x^2\xi^2)^2[1+(5x\xi)^2]}{1+(5x\xi)^2+\frac{9\pi^2}{64}(1+x^2\xi^2)^2} \tag{45}$$

which are used for a quickly convergent iterative procedure for the calculation of the phase function.

Transport Function. To the expression [Eq. (35)] giving the average work per unit time performed on a cross section of the tube, the work due to the torsion acting on the arches must be added

$$\frac{\omega}{2\pi}\int_0^{\frac{2\pi}{\omega}}\mathfrak{m}\frac{2}{b}\dot{u}\,dt\,. \tag{46}$$

In addition, the asymmetric terms of the fluid motion come into the first integral of Eq. (35). The result is not so easily compressed to a simple form, as in Eq. (36), but is

$$C^2=W\left(\frac{4\pi^3}{\omega^3\varrho\,b_t^3}\right)=x\psi^2\left\{4x^{-3}(\xi^2+x^{-2})+\left(\frac{16}{\pi^2}\frac{GJ}{bK}\right)x^{-5}\left(\frac{u}{\eta}\right)^2+\frac{1}{2\xi^2}\left[8\left(\frac{2\mu_0 l+\sinh 2\mu_0 l}{2\sinh^2\mu_0 l}\right)\left(\frac{A_0}{\eta}\right)^2+\frac{4(\xi x)^3}{(1+\xi^2x^2)^{3/2}}\left(\frac{A_1}{\eta}\right)^2+\frac{16(\xi x)^3}{(1+4\xi^2x^2)^{3/2}}\left(\frac{A_{1/2}}{\eta}\right)^2\right]\right\}. \tag{47}$$

The coefficient of the term from the torsion of the arches is

$$\frac{16}{\pi^2}\frac{GJ}{bK}=50$$

which dominates the first term, which gives the work in bending the basilar membrane, until the transition point is approached.

Damping. Fortunately, the result [Eq. (45)] remains a good approximation for $x\leq 1$ even when the phase function has a small imaginary part.

Expanding

$$\xi = \xi_0 + \xi^1 + \cdots$$

where ξ_0 is the undamped phase function, we obtain from Eq. (45)

$$v = v_0 [1 - x^2 \xi_0 \xi_1 D] \tag{48}$$

where

$$D = \frac{4}{1 + x^2 \xi^2} + \frac{50}{1 + (5x\xi)^2} - \frac{50 + \frac{9\pi^2}{16}(1 + x^2 \xi^2)}{1 + (5x\xi)^2 + \frac{9\pi^2}{64}(1 + x^2 \xi^2)^2}$$

From a similar expansion for Eq. (43), the result is obtained

$$\xi_1 = (1 - i)\,\varepsilon \frac{\xi_0^2 \left(\frac{8}{\pi^2} + 1\right) \frac{1}{2}}{\frac{8}{\pi^2} + \xi_0^3 x^3 \left(1 + x^2 \xi_0^2\right)^{-3/2} + v_0 \xi_0^3 x^{-5} D} \,. \tag{49}$$

Results

An integration of $\xi(x)$ which is computed from Eqs. (43), (44) yields the phase

$$\mathscr{P} = -N \int_0^x \xi(x)\, dx \,. \tag{50}$$

For small values of the phase, the wavelength is "long". However, for small ξ, Eq. (45) gives

$$v = \frac{2}{1 + (9\pi^2/64)} = 0.837$$

while Eq. (43) gives

$$\frac{x^7 \coth \mu_0 l}{\xi} \approx \frac{v \pi^2}{8} = 1.03 \,. \tag{51}$$

So, for very small values of ξ we have

$$\mu_0 l = \frac{\pi l \xi}{b_t} \approx \left(\frac{\pi l}{b_t} x^7\right)^{1/2} \tag{52}$$

so the phase is

$$\mathscr{P} \approx -N \frac{2}{9} \left(\frac{b_t}{\pi l}\right)^{1/2} x^{9/2} \tag{53}$$

which varies linearly with a change in driving frequency.

The approximation [Eq. (52)] can be used to obtain the overall impedance of the fluid in the model. The average pressure $\bar{p}$ and the average velocity $\bar{w}_r$ are related by the "long wave" equation (ZWISLOCKI, 1953).

$$\frac{\partial \bar{p}}{\partial r} = -\varrho \frac{\partial^2}{\partial t^2} \bar{w}_r \,. \tag{54}$$

For the traveling wave, this gives

$$-\frac{i N \xi}{r_t} \bar{p} = \omega^2 \varrho \bar{w}_r [1 + 0(N^{-1})] \,.$$

Therefore, the volume displacement of fluid at the end of the tube, the stapes, divided by the pressure difference in the two scalae at that end is

$$\frac{A_{ST}\,\overline{w}_r}{2\,\overline{p}} = -\,i\left(\frac{A_{ST}}{2\omega^2\,\varphi\,l}\right)\mu_0\,l = -\,i\left(\frac{10}{\pi^2}\times 10^{-9}\,\frac{\text{cm}^5}{\text{dyne}}\right)\left(\frac{1\text{ kHz}}{f}\right)^2\mu_0\,l \quad (55)$$

in which the average human stapes area 3.2 mm² is used. Eq. (52) gives the result

$$\frac{A_{ST}\,\overline{w}_r}{2\,\overline{p}} = -\,i\left(2.5\times 10^{-11}\,\frac{\text{cm}^5}{\text{dyne}}\right)\left(\frac{10^3\text{Hz}}{f}\right)$$

which is shown on Fig. 14 with the experimental results of Békésy (1960, p. 435). This shows the 2-mode model in its worst light, since the deflection of the bony shelf is quite significant near the stapes. Even so, the trend is correct and the amplitude is only 20 dB off.

We consider now the solution in the short-wave region. The various parts of the solution are plotted as functions of x, the normalized distance along the basilar membrane, in Fig. 8. This shows the rapid increase in phase as the transition point is approached. Also shown in Fig. 8 is the ratio u/η of the two modes of Fig. 3. As the transition point is approached, the motion of the arches becomes small in comparison with the flexing of the basilar membrane. The damping function also increases rapidly as the transition point is approached.

The amplitude of the wave [Eq. (25)] involves both the transport function ψ and the damping function

$$|\,\eta\,| = \psi(x)\,e^{-N\int_0^x \xi_1 dx}\,. \quad (56)$$

Thus, the frequency enters through the value of ε [see Eq. (49)] from Table 3. The maximum amplitude of basilar membrane deflection for the two modes of Fig. 3, which is not necessarily at the midpoint, is given by

$$wm = u\,[1-\pi^{-1}\cos^{-1}(u/\pi\,\eta)] + \eta\,[1-(u/\pi\,\eta)^2]^{1/2}\,. \quad (57)$$

The response exactly at the midpoint was also considered and found to be not much different. Using the viscosity $\varepsilon = 2\varepsilon^*$ in Table 3, with Eq. (56) and the values in Fig. 8, gives the curve labeled $(wm)_{\max}$ in Fig. 13. This passes through Rhode's points but not through Békésy's. If the curve for the maximum arch motion is plotted on Fig. 13, it does indeed pass through Békésy's points for 200 and 300 Hz. The lower frequency points are off because an end condition for the helicotrema is not considered in the model.

One striking feature of Fig. 8 is that u/η, the ratio of the arch displacement to basilar membrane flexing displacement, is essentially constant for most of the region of significant deformation. The observation (Békésy, 1960, p. 497) indicates no discontinuity in the curvature of the basilar membrane at the foot of the arch of Corti. If the angle β, between the model arch and membrane, Fig. 7 is computed

$$\beta = \frac{\pi}{b}\left(\eta - \frac{3}{\pi}\,u\right)$$

we have the result that the relative stiffnesses of arch and membrane are such that β is almost zero in the region where u/η is constant. Thus the model indicates almost no discontinuity in the basilar membrane slope over a substantial region. On Fig. 9 is shown the envelope for the arch displacement, the maximum basilar membrane displacement across the section, and the angle β. Just past the point of maximum arch motion, the angle β becomes very significant.

The consequence is a simple explanation of the transition from a radial (Θ-direction in Fig. 1) to a longitudinal (r-direction in Fig. 1) vibration of the top surface of the organ of CORTI observed by BÉKÉSY (1960, p. 497). The rotation of the arch, with a small amplitude of plate flexing, causes the radial motion of the recticular membrane and the soft cells attached. Further along the cochlea the arch motion is small in comparison with the flexing mode, and the wavelength is shorter, causing a substantial longitudinal motion of the fluid in our model, and, presumably, in the organ of CORTI in the actual cochlea, following the discussion by BÉKÉSY (1960, p. 498). Thus the model of Fig. 7, with the stiffness of Table 2 based only on BÉKÉSY's static tests, does produce a dynamic response to a pure tone in excellent agreement with the details of BÉKÉSY's observations.

This angle β has a somewhat more peaked envelope than either displacement. The location for the maximum as a function of frequency is shown in Figs. 10, which is close to the curve for the hearing loss due to local damage. The wavelength of the motion near the maximum of β is shown in Fig. 9. Thus the half wave is about 0.5 mm. Figures 11 and 12 show additional results. So it seems likely that a further consideration of more details of the motion with a more elaborate model will lead to yet more interesting results. After all, the organ of CORTI is quite an elaborate structure, only crudely represented even by the present model.

Flexible Bony Shelf

The solution of the preceding section shows that, even with the complicated motion of the basilar membrane, it is only the first term B_0 of the FOURIER series expansion for the pressure that is significant in the region between the transition point (lower curve in Fig. 5) and the stapes. With only the leading terms retained, the equations for the three modes of basilar membrane deformation (Fig. 3) for the progressing wave Eq. (25) give the relations

$$K\left(\mu_0^2 + \left(\frac{\pi}{b}\right)^2\right)^2 \eta = \frac{8}{\pi} B_0$$

$$(k + GJ\,\mu_0^2)\, u = \frac{3}{4} B_0\, b^3$$

$$(\mathscr{H} + EI\,\mu_0^4)\, v = 2\, B_0\, b$$

where B_0 is the pressure due to the average displacement

$$B_0 = \frac{\varrho\,\omega^2}{\mu_0} \coth \mu_0 l \left[\frac{1}{\pi}\eta + \frac{3}{8}u + \frac{1}{2}v\right].$$

Combining the four relations yields the simplified equation for μ_0, which is the derivative of the phase function ($\mu_0 = N\xi/r_t$).

$$\frac{\mu_0 b}{\varrho\omega^2}\tanh\mu_0 l = \frac{b^2}{\mathscr{K}+EI\mu_0{}^4} + \frac{9}{64}\frac{b^4}{k+GJ\mu_0{}^2} + \frac{8}{\pi^2}\frac{b}{K\left(\left(\frac{\pi}{b}\right)^2+\mu_0{}^2\right)^2}\,. \qquad (58)$$

Note that when the wavelength is very long, μ_0 is small, so the bending effects $EI\mu_0^4$, $GJ\mu_0^2$, and $K\mu_0^4$ are all negligible, and the right-hand-side is exactly the volume compliance Eq. (6).

Thus at the stapes, for long wavelengths Eq. (58) gives

$$\mu_0 l \approx (\varrho\,\omega^2 bl/\mathscr{K})^{1/2}$$

$$= 0.956\,(f/1\text{ kHz})\,.$$

Using this in Eq. (55) gives the upper dashed curve in Fig. 14, reasonably close to the data from Békésy for the low frequencies. Now, for frequencies greater than 1 kHz, we have the result that $\mu_0 l$ is greater than unity, so the wavelength is "short", even at the stapes! Then the EI term dominates and Eq. (58) gives the approximation

$$\mu_0^5 \approx \frac{b\,\varrho\,\omega^2}{EI}$$

so that

$$\mu_0 l = 0.76\ (f/1\text{ kHz})^{2/5}.$$

Since the bending of the support is significant, it is necessary to use the complete solution

$$v = e^{i\omega t}[e^{-iz} - D_1 e^{-ie^{-i\varphi z}} + D_2 e^{ie^{i\varphi z}}]$$

in which $z = \mu_0(r - r_{ST})$ and the complex root $(1)^{1/5}$ is $e^{i\varphi}$ where $\varphi = 2\pi/5$. The constants D_1 and D_2 are determined from the constraint condition at the stapes. Thus, these correction factors for Eq. (55) are obtained

$$-\,i\,0.36\;e^{i\pi/6.5}\ \text{(clamped)}$$

$$-\,i\,0.6\;\;e^{i\pi/6.5}\ \text{(hinged)}$$

$$-\,i\,1.4\;\;e^{i\pi/41}\ \text{(free)}\,.$$

As shown in Fig. 14, the amplitude for the most reasonable clamped condition is in the middle of Békésy's data, while the phase is not far off. The amplitude for the free end condition is somewhat high, as might be expected.

Thus the conclusion is obtained that the peculiar shape of Békésy's data in Fig. 14 near 1 kHz shows the transition from long to short waves at the stapes. Therefore, for the frequencies over 1 kHz there are no long waves in the cochlea. This agrees with the observation by Békésy (1960, p. 496) that waves travel in the radial direction on Reissner's membrane for the higher frequencies.

It can be shown that this third mode has little effect on the region of maximum excitation for the middle and low frequencies; *i.e.*, Fig. 9 should be unchanged, and it is expected that the reason for the complete loss of hearing at 20 kHz can be answered after the detailed numerical calculation is performed.

Transient Waves

For an arbitrary transient excitation of the stapes, the Laplace transformation may be used with the result

$$\eta = \int g(\omega)\, e^{i(\omega t - \int \mu_0 dr)} \psi [1 + 0(N^{-1})]\, d\omega \tag{59}$$

which may be thought of as a sum of stationary waves of the form of Eq. (25). The function $g(\omega)$ depends on the excitation. The large parameter N now makes it possible to use the "saddle point" or "stationary phase" method to evaluate this integral. Indeed, the main contribution, for fixed r and t, comes near the saddle point, at which

$$t = \frac{\partial}{\partial \omega} \int_{r_{ST}}^{r} \mu_0\, dr = t(r, \omega)\,. \tag{60}$$

For another interpretation, this equation provides, for a fixed frequency, the arrival time t at the station r of the energy associated with that frequency. For a sudden disturbance at the stapes, *i.e.*, a "click", the waves from all frequencies will be of roughly equal importance in Eq. (59), and all will start at the stapes $r = r_{ST}$ at time $t = 0$ in Eq. (60).

DOTSON (1974) has considered these waves in detail for the one-mode model. He has shown that the curves Eq. (60) for all frequencies are contained between two envelopes, without consideration of the damping due to the fluid viscosity. One envelope gives the curve for the arrival of the "front" of the transient disturbance due to the click; the other envelope gives the "tail" of the disturbance.

The curve for the pulse front is easily obtained for either the one- or two-mode models, since it is formed by the low frequency waves. Thus, Eq. (52) can be used in Eq. (60), with the simple result

$$t = (3.67 \times 10^{-3}\,\text{sec})\,(r/36.9\,\text{mm})^{9/2}\,. \tag{61}$$

This is plotted in Fig. 15; the agreement with the experimental values obtained by BÉKÉSY is remarkable, except at the 20 mm section. A preliminary study of the more complicated 3-mode model indicates that this discrepancy indeed may be due to the flexibility of the bony shelf.

In the region where $\mu_0 l > 1$, the transition point may be used to simplify Eq. (60). Again using $x = r/r_t$, where the transition point r_t varies with $\omega^{-1/4}$, we have

$$\frac{\partial}{\partial\omega} = \frac{\partial x}{\partial\omega}\frac{d}{dx} = \frac{x}{4\omega}\frac{d}{dx}\,.$$

Thus, writing Eq. (60) in the form

$$t = \frac{\partial}{\partial\omega} N \int_{x_{ST}}^{x} \xi(x)\, dx$$

one obtains easily

$$t = \frac{N}{4\omega} x\, \xi(x)\,. \tag{62}$$

Therefore the curve $\xi_0(x)$ of Fig. 8 gives directly a good approximation for the energy propagation.

The equation for the envelope is obtained by taking the derivative of Eq. (62) with respect to the parameter ω. After eliminating ω, the result is

$$x\frac{d\xi}{dx} = 3\,\xi\,.$$

This is satisfied at the point $x = 1.067$, at which $x\xi = 0.622$. This is the point at which the propagation curve for a single frequency Eq. (62) touches the envelope of the curves from all frequencies due to the click. Since we may write

$$\omega = \omega_H\,(36.9\,\mathrm{mm}/r)^4\,x^4$$

where the frequency with the transition point at the helicotrema (Fig. 5a) is

$$\omega_H = 550\ \mathrm{Hz}$$

the equation for the envelope is

$$\begin{aligned} t &= \frac{N}{4\omega_H}\,\frac{\xi_0}{x^3}\,(r/36.9\ \mathrm{mm})^4 \\ &= (12.1\times 10^{-3}\ \mathrm{sec})\,(r/36.9\,\mathrm{mm})^4\,. \end{aligned} \tag{63}$$

This curve is shown in Fig. 15 as the tail of the disturbance.

More than just the disturbance due to a click, Fig. 15 shows the propagation of the transient effect at the start of a pure tone signal. Thus, at the station 25 mm from the stapes, the first signal arrives at 1 msec, but, at 4 msec, the tail of the transient noise passes and the steady-state (stationary) condition is reached. Despite this, some 10 msec of a 1 kHz tone signal is required in order to determine the pitch. The interpretation is clear. All or most of the transient noise must reach the helicotrema, according to this model at 12 msec, where it is dissipated through the viscous orifice flow through the helicotrema, before the pitch of a tone signal can be determined.

At the end of a pure tone signal, exactly the same transient waves are generated, requiring 12 msec to reach the helicotrema. Remember that all of this analysis for Fig. 15 is *independent* of the fluid viscosity along the cochlea. Thus the fundamental paradox of the Helmholtz resonance theory, in which the damping of the resonators must be small to give quick response and sharp frequency discrimination but must be large to prevent prolonged ringing after the end of a tone, is completely avoided. For this reason the usual calculation (Dallos, 1973, p. 153) of the "resistive component of basilar membrane impedence" from Békésy's data for the transient response measured at a point on the basilar membrane is completely incorrect. The tapered membrane transports all transient effects to the helicotrema, with or without viscosity of the fluid or internal damping of the organ of Corti.

Anderson et al. (1971) present data for VIII nerve activity in the spider monkey. The average phase difference between stimulus and firings of a single fiber is shown to vary linearly with frequency. According to the simple wave equation with a constant velocity of propagation, the travel time from the point of stimulation to the point of observation is given by the slope of the phase difference — frequency curve. The results of such a calculation for 80 nerve fibers are shown in Fig. 16.

In the present investigation, it is shown that the cochlea is by no means representable by a simple wave equation. It is remarkable, however, that the calculation of ANDERSON et al. is correct. The phase curve of Fig. 8, after conversion to a frequency scale (i.e., x^4), is almost linear in the region of maximum response. The result Eq. (60), which is reduced to Eq. (2), is exactly the derivative of phase with respect to frequence. To compare with the model behavior, the time required for the propagation of energy of a constant frequency stimulus from the stapes to the transition point on the basilar membrane for that frequency, is obtained by setting x equal to unity in Eq. (62), which gives the curve TP in Fig. 16. The points of maximum arch, basilar membrane, and angle displacement occur at values of x which change slightly with frequency. The corresponding energy travel times are shown in Fig. 16.

The bounding of the neural data points, which are for 90 db intensity, and the SP points for 95 db, shown in Fig. 10, between the curves for maximum arch and maximum basilar membrane motion does not seem coincidental. The limited data given by ANDERSON et al., for lower intensities indicates an increase in the arrival time, closer to the $\beta_{\max}$ curve, just as does the SP measurement at 65 db in Fig. 10. Further discussion is given in STEELE (1973).

Acknowledgements

I thank EARL SCHUBERT for his encouragement of this work, portions of which were supported by a contract between the Physiological Psychology Branch of the Office of Naval Research and Stanford University School of Medicine, and by the Biomedicine Institute, University of Zürich.

References

ABRAMOWITZ, M., STEGUN, L. A. (Eds.): Handbook of mathematical functions. National Bureau of Standards, Appl. Math. Series 55 (1966).

ANDERSON, D. J., ROSE, J. E., HIND, J. E., BRUGGE, J. F.: Temporal position of discharges in single auditory nerve fibers within the cycle of a sine-wave stimulus: frequency and intensity effects. J. acoust. Soc. Amer. **49**, 1131—1139 (1971).

BÉKÉSY, G. VON: Experiments in hearing. New York: McGraw-Hill 1960.

BÉKÉSY, G. VON: Traveling waves as frequency analysers in the cochlea. Nature (Lond.) **225**, 1207–1209 (1970).

DALLOS, P.: The Auditory Periphery. New York: Academic Press 1973.

DALLOS, P., CHEATHAM, M. A.: Travel time in the cochlea and its determination from cochlear microphonic data. J. acoust. Soc. Amer. **49**, 1140—1143 (1971).

DOTSON, R.: Cochlear model with transient excitation. Ph. D. Dissertation, Stanford University 1974.

EVANS, E. F., WILSON, J. P.: The frequency selectivity of the cochlea. In: MOLLER, A. R.: Basic Mechanisms in Hearing. New York: Academic Press 1973.

FLEISCHER, G.: Studien am Skelett des Gehörorgans der Säugetiere, einschließlich des Menschen. Säugetierkundl. Mitt. **2**, **3**, 131—239 (1973).

FLÜGGE, W. (Ed.): Handbook of engineering mechanics. New York: McGraw-Hill 1962.

HALLAUER, W. L., JR.: Nonlinear behavior of the inner ear. Ph. D. Dissertation, Stanford University 1974.

HEADING, J.: An introduction to phase integral methods. New York: John Wiley 1962.

HONRUBIA, V., WARD, P. H.: Longitudinal distribution of the cochlear microphonics inside the cochlear duct (guinea pig). J. acoust. Soc. Amer. **44**, 951—958 (1968).

HONRUBIA, V., WARD, P. H.: Properties of the summating potential of the guinea pig's cochlea. J. acoust. Soc. Amer. **45**, 1443—1450 (1969).

HUXLEY, A. F.: Is resonance possible in the cochlea after all? Nature (Lond.) **221**, 935–940 (1968).

IURATO, S.: Functional implications of the nature and submicroscopic structure of the tectorial and basilar membranes. J. acoust. Soc. Amer., **34**, 1386—1395 (1962).

JOHNSTONE, B. M., BOYLE, A. J. F.: Basilar membrane vibrations examined with the Mössbauer technique. Science **158**, 389—390 (1967).

KOHLLÖFFEL, L. U. E.: Studies of the distribution of cochlear potentials along the basilar membrane. Acta oto-laryng. (Stockh.) Suppl. No. 288 (1971).

KOHLLÖFFEL, L. U. E.: A study of basilar membrane vibrations II .The vibratory amplitude and phase pattern along the basilar membrane (postmortem). Acustica **27**, 66—81 (1972).

KOHLLÖFFEL, L. U. E.: Observations of the mechanical disturbances along the basilar membrane with laser illumination. In: MOLLER, A. R. (Ed.): Basic Mechanisms in Hearing, pp. 95—118. New York: Academic Press 1973.

LIM, D. J.: Fine morphology of the tectorial membrane. Arch. Otolaryng. **96**, 199—215 (1972).

MONEY, K. E., SOKOLOFF, M., WEAVER, R. S.: Specific gravity and viscosity of endolymph and perilymph. (Third Symposium on the Role of the Vestibular Organs in Space Exploration). Washington, D.C.: NASA Special Publication 152, U.S. Gov't. Printing Office (1966).

PYE, J. D.: Hearing in bats. In: DE REUCK, A. V. S., KNIGHT, J. (Eds.): Hearing mechanisms in vertebrates. London: J. & A. Churchill 1967.

RANKE, O. F.: Theory of operation of the cochlea: a contribution to the hydrodynamics of the cochlea. J. Acoust. Soc. Amer. **22**, 772–777 (1950).

RHODE, W. S.: Observation of the vibration of the basilar membrane in squirrel monkeys using the Mössbauer effect. J. acoust. Soc. Amer. **49**, 1218–1231 (1971).

RHODE, W. S.: An investigation of post-morten cochlear mechanics using the Mössbauer effect. In: MOLLER, A. R. (Ed.): Basic Mechanisms in Hearing. New York: Academic Press 1973.

STEELE, C. R.: A possibility for subtectorial membrane fluid flow. In: MOLLER, A. R. (Ed.): Basic Mechanisms in Hearing. New York: Academic Press 1973.

STEELE, C. R.: Behaviour of the basilar membrane with pure tone excitation. J. acoust. Soc. Amer. **55**, 148—162 (1974a).

STEELE, C. R.: Stiffness of Reissner's membrane. J. acoust. Soc. Amer., **55**, 1252—1257 (1974b).

STEVENS, S. S., DAVIS, H., LURIE, M. H.: The localization of pitch perception on the basilar membrane. J. gen. Psychol. **13**, 297–315 (1935).

TIDEMANN, H.: A new approach to the theory of hearing. Acta oto-laryng. (Stockh.) Suppl. 277 (1970).

TONNDORF, J.: Cochlear mechanics and hydrodynamics. In: TOBIAS, J. V. (Ed.): Foundations of Modern Auditory Theory, Vol. I. New York: Academic Press 1970.

WEVER, E. G.: Theory of hearing. New York: John Wiley 1949.

Wilcox, C.H. (Ed.): Asymptotic solutions of differential equations and their applications. New York: John Wiley 1964.

Wilson, J.P., Johnstone, J.R.: Capacitive probe measures of basilar membrane vibration. Symposium on Hearing Theory 1972, IPO Endhoven, Holland, pp. 172—181 (1972).

Zwicker, E.: Wissenschaftlicher Jahresbericht, Institut für Elektroakustik, TH München (1973).

Zwislocki, J.: Review of recent mathematical theories of cochlear dynamics. J. Acoust. Soc. Amer. **25**, 743–751 (1953).

Chapter 13

On the "Residue" and Auditory Pitch Perception *

E. de Boer, Amsterdam, Netherlands

With 40 Figures

Contents

* To J. F. Schouten who "placed" his mark on a "period".

A. Trigger (Introductory Remarks)

The present chapter on *the residue phenomenon* is set up in an unorthodox way. Instead of giving a cursory review it presents the historical development in great detail. It is more a textbook on the psychophysics of pitch than a review of recent research. There are several reasons for this, as listed below:

a) Very few scientists, even those working on pitch perception, are aware of all the intricacies involved.

b) Textbooks on psychophysics or physiology of hearing in general are either outdated – the development has been very fast the last five years – or not authorative on this subject.

c) The older literature on the residue is inaccessible; as a consequence, an overview is difficult to obtain.

d) The publications include many subtleties in psychophysical experiments or advanced mathematical details of signal generation which make them difficult to understand for physiologists, etc.

e) There exist many misconceptions about the relevance of certain physiological experiments for pitch perception (and vice versa).

f) The problem of the residue is of prime importance for speech as well as for music, but a comprehensive account of the subject does not exist.

g) In some instances psychophysical or physiological studies are reported that seem to indicate that the "residue" is about to be discovered again. Such situations may be prevented by the existence of a general text.

These reasons led the present author to compile a description of the development of residue theory within a unifying framework. The account is constructed with a minimum of reference to the mathematical description of signals; as a consequence, there are only a few formulas, and those included, are very simple. In this way it is intended to reach the largest possible number of potential readers.

The treatise is rather lengthy, and the description is concentrated on only a few of the great many possible topics. The length is dictated by the wish to be instructive and clear. The choice as to which topics should be treated at length, which ones mentioned only in passing, and which ones should be skipped entirely, was difficult. The ultimate choice has been made with the greatest possible caution and after much deliberation. The strongest emphasis was put on the development of concepts; hence, many details of a procedural or methodological nature are completely left out of the discussion. There will be several subjects that seem to be "forgotten" entirely; the choice of subjects treated remains entirely the author's responsibility. The opinions ventured represent the author's own (1975) convictions. They are believed to represent also the communis opinio of the most noted scientists, but exceptions are possible, of course. The author would like to know whether his approach has been successful, in other words, whether his work can be understood by physiologists, psychologists and other scientists, and he welcomes feedback from the readers.

Many discussions with other scientists have contributed to a clear delineation of the most important ideas. Ample opportunity for discussion was provided by the conferences listed in Section I. 3. The author is especially grateful for the opportunity provided by Bell Telephone Laboratories for extensive discussions with the groups of scientists involved in speech analysis and synthesis and in hearing research. These discussions have contributed greatly to the form of the present treatise.

The general outline of the chapter is as follows. The "residue story" is described in seven sub-chapters. The intention was that every one of these can be read and understood more or less independently of the others. That is the reason why many repetitions can be found in the text. Part B contains a general introduction to methodology and terminology of psychophysical research. A short outline of FOURIER analysis is included. The earliest history on pitch research provided the path leading to the "place theory". The period encompassing the second part of the 19th century and the first few decades of the 20th century is described in Part C. The "residue theory" was conceived and described around 1940 by the Dutch scientist SCHOUTEN. Part D contains a comprehensive description of SCHOUTEN's experiments and the conception of the residue theory. That theory stressed the importance of waveform aspects of the signals employed, in particular, the periodicity. Many studies were devoted to the study of "periodicity pitch", as it was called, and Part E of the chapter describes the most important ones. The description is centered around the study of the pitch of inharmonic signals, and it appeared that a generalization of the definition of "residue" was needed to encompass all findings.

A new twist was given to the study of pitch perception when it was discovered that the main contributions to the pitch arise from low-numbered harmonics – in the original conception the main contribution was thought to arise from the unresolved high-numbered harmonics. This finding and its subsequent elaboration entailed a gradual shift of emphasis from waveform to spectrum aspects of the signals employed, and it took some time before this was established. The period in which these studies were performed is described in Part F. The relation between residue signals consisting of unresolved, closely spaced, components and those consisting of resolved, widely spaced, components remained somewhat unclear. The existence of aural combination tones (particular forms of products of nonlinear distortion) proved to be the factor that resolved this matter. Part G of the chapter gives a more detailed description of nonlinear distortion in general, and the properties of aural combination tones in particular. The newer residue theories are described in Part H; residue pitch is presently recognized to be almost entirely determined by the spectral content of the sound stimulus. This part describes the crucial experiments underlying this notion, several theories based upon it, and a few related phenomena. Some general reflections and warnings about mis-interpretations are described in the concluding Part I. The end of the story may read exactly like the begin: is it "place", or "period"? The meaning of these terms has changed completely, however.

A few words of explanation are in order on physiological aspects of the residue phenomenon. In the course of the present treatise it becomes clear why it is not likely that we will discover any clear-cut physiological mechanism responsible for the formation of residue pitch. Hence there is very little opportunity to describe physiological aspects of the residue phenomenon. An exception is formed by the topic of auditory nonlinearity (Part G).

The temporal features of stimuli appear to have only little to do with pitch. These features do play a part in perception: they are certainly related to the perception of "flutter", "rattle", "roughness", and the like. There will be physiological correlates to these phenomena, no doubt. It was decided, however, to leave these physiological aspects out of the discussion entirely since the main emphasis was to be put upon pitch phenomena.

B. Impulses of Interest (Outline of Problems, Fourier Theory)

1. Introduction

The "residue" in hearing theory is a concept that is intimately connected with the perception of *pitch*. Pitch – or as it can be called, in a slightly different context: tone height – is an attribute of sound that has been recognized as something special since the earliest documented times. Pitch plays a very important part in music and many observations and theories have been focused on this attribute during the long history of music. Scientific study of it (in the modern sense) was only possible after the development of acoustic instruments that permitted the generation of tones and signals with well-determined physical properties. Nevertheless, a most important and crucial question on pitch could already be formulated – and partly answered – on the basis of experiments with what we consider as the most primitive acoustic instrument possible, the siren. That is the question as to what physical parameter of the acoustic signal determines the pitch of the perceived sound; we will see in the sequel how this problem was attacked with unequalled ingenuity in a period where virtually no quantitative experiment could be performed.

We are not yet in a position to give a definition of what is the "residue" in hearing. However, the uninitiated reader may be satisfied at this stage by the following annotations. *Tones* are sounds that generally have a clearly determined musical pitch. Physically, tones can be regarded as combinations of a number of sinusoidal vibrations, all with different frequencies. These constituent vibrations are called *components*. Most of the tones used in music consist of combinations of sinusoidal vibrations of which the frequencies form an arithmetical sequence (*e.g.* 250, 500, 750, 1000, 1250, ... Hz). The pitch of such tones is usually associated with the lowest of these components. However, when the lowest component happens to be very weak or inaudible, the tone still has the same pitch (as if the lowest component were present). This pitch is produced by the cooperation of components of higher frequencies. Such a combined action of components which gives rise to a percept with a clear musical pitch is called a *residue*. The concept will be explained in detail later on. The most remarkable property for the moment is that a residue can have a pitch.

The study of the relation between physical properties of signals and attributes of perception belongs to the realm of *psychophysics*. In the context of a Handbook on Sensory Physiology it is necessary to devote some space to the nature of this field of scientific study in general. One principal problem in this field is the quantification of a sensation. In general, sensations cannot be measured in a numerical sense; this problem can, however, often be circumvented by the use of special techniques, such as the measurement of just noticeable differences in perception. By measuring the physical counterpart of a just noticeable change in a signal the main point of what a sensation really is, by-passed, and the limit of perceptual analysis is measured instead. By this means, it remains possible to study the properties of the analyzing mechanism without actually specifying the output. In several other branches of psychophysics, it is attempted to quantify attributes of sensations more directly; the logical consistency of experimental results is then the guideline along which the relevance of certain signal parameters is confirmed. In the field of audition this applies, *e. g.*, to the measurement of loudness.

To come back to the pitch problem: pitch is, in a sense, a directly measurable attribute because there already exists a musical scale which uniquely assigns a number (*e. g.* a frequency value) to a pitch. Conversely, we may state that this pitch scale derives its structure from the properties of human pitch perception. Pitch can be measured directly along the musical pitch scale by persons possessing "absolute pitch". Other persons may compare pitches of two sounds and so arrive at a numerical value for the pitch of a sound; this procedure is even possible with unmusical persons. In these respects, pitch has many of the properties of a "Gestalt".

In the realm of the "residue" theory, where the residue pitch is a central issue, a tangible and practical definition of pitch is called for. A *pure tone, i. e.*, the tone perceived from a sinusoidal sound signal, seems to be the clearest bearer of pitch as it is devoid of a specific timbre. For this reason, the operational definition of pitch involves the comparison of the unknown sound with a pure tone and adjusting the frequency of the latter until the two are judged to have equal pitch. This definition is almost exclusively used whenever numerical measurement of pitch is desired. Most of the sounds used in residue research have a timbre that is so widely different from that of a pure tone that the observers have great difficulties with the comparison. This is partly reflected in the results of such experiments. In some studies, a complex signal with a definite pitch is used as the comparison signal. Pitch matches are then easy to make, but the disadvantage is that the comparison signal is a multi-parameter signal, and the decision to use only one parameter as the bearer of pitch is an arbitrary one which requires justification.

The basic duality of psychophysics – direct measurement *versus* comparison experiments – causes several inherent problems. This is also the case for the pitch attribute. In the present author's opinion, this accounts for many troubles that occurred in pitch research and for the grave problems of connecting results of all research projects together in a meaningful way. This is especially true since many of the signals that have been used in pitch research – and, especially, in "residue" research – are much less tonal than most of the sounds used in music. Hence, it is easy to lead an observer astray so that, in fact, he does not use his pitch sense at all. Only very few scientists have employed listeners that were sufficiently well versed in music that they could be expected to have a well-developed sense of pitch. Pitch has many attributes of a "Gestalt", and observations on pitch require a good deal of introspection. Both aspects do not lend themselves easily to positivistic scientific experimentation based on the repeatability and reproducibility of measurements. However, if one wishes to demonstrate quite general properties of the auditory system, it is necessary to prove that the phenomena observed can be measured in what are called "naive listeners" as well. It should not be done the other way around. Even worse is to do the tests exclusively with naive listeners and to base far-reaching conclusions about perception aspects on these persons' responses.

2. Fourier Analysis

It is assumed that the reader is at least vaguely acquainted with the formalism of Fourier analysis. In order to avoid misinterpretations and to provide a unified basis for forthcoming descriptions, the principles are briefly summarized in this section. In this chapter, we shall mainly consider signals, written as a function $f(t)$ of time t, that are deterministic. That means the waveform of $f(t)$ can be predicted when only part of it is known. An important sub-class of these signals are the *periodic signals*. A periodic signal $f(t)$ with period T can be written as the sum of a number of sinusoidal signals $s_i(t)$, all with different frequencies f_i (i is an integer index). Because of the periodicity the frequencies f_i have the peculiar property that they all are integral multiples of the *fundamental frequency* $f_0 = 1/T$. The waveforms of all the constituent sinusoids $s_i(t)$, when added together, form exactly the waveform $f(t)$. The following formula expresses this mathematically (Σ denoting a summation):

$$f(t) = \sum_{i=1}^{N} s_i(t) \tag{1}$$

(the index i is an integer and in this context always limited to cover a finite range, from 1 to N).

Each of the signals $s_i(t)$ is called a *component*; it is a sinusoidally varying signal and hence can be written in the form

$$s_i(t) = a_i \cos(2\pi f_i t + \varphi_i). \tag{2}$$

For a periodic signal $f(t)$ all frequencies are, as stated, integral multiples of the frequency f_0; this is most simply expressed by using the integer index i as the multiplier:

$$f_i = i \cdot f_0 \tag{3}$$

with $f_0 = 1/T$.

Components of which the frequencies are integral multiples of a frequency f_0 are called *harmonics* of f_0. The rank number of harmonics corresponds to the index i in Eq. (3). Formerly, such components were also called *overtones*, with a rank number one lower than i. For example, the second overtone is the same as the third harmonic ($i = 3$). The lowest harmonic, with i equal to 1, is commonly referred to as the *fundamental*; to avoid ambiguity we shall often refer to it as the fundamental component. The frequency f_0 is the fundamental frequency; as stated, this is the inverse of the period T. It is confusing that a series of frequencies conforming to Eq. (3) is often called a *harmonic series*. Because of the wide acceptance of this terminology, it will be difficult to insist upon one consistent description, andit will occur sometimes that different terms are used for the same idea or concept.

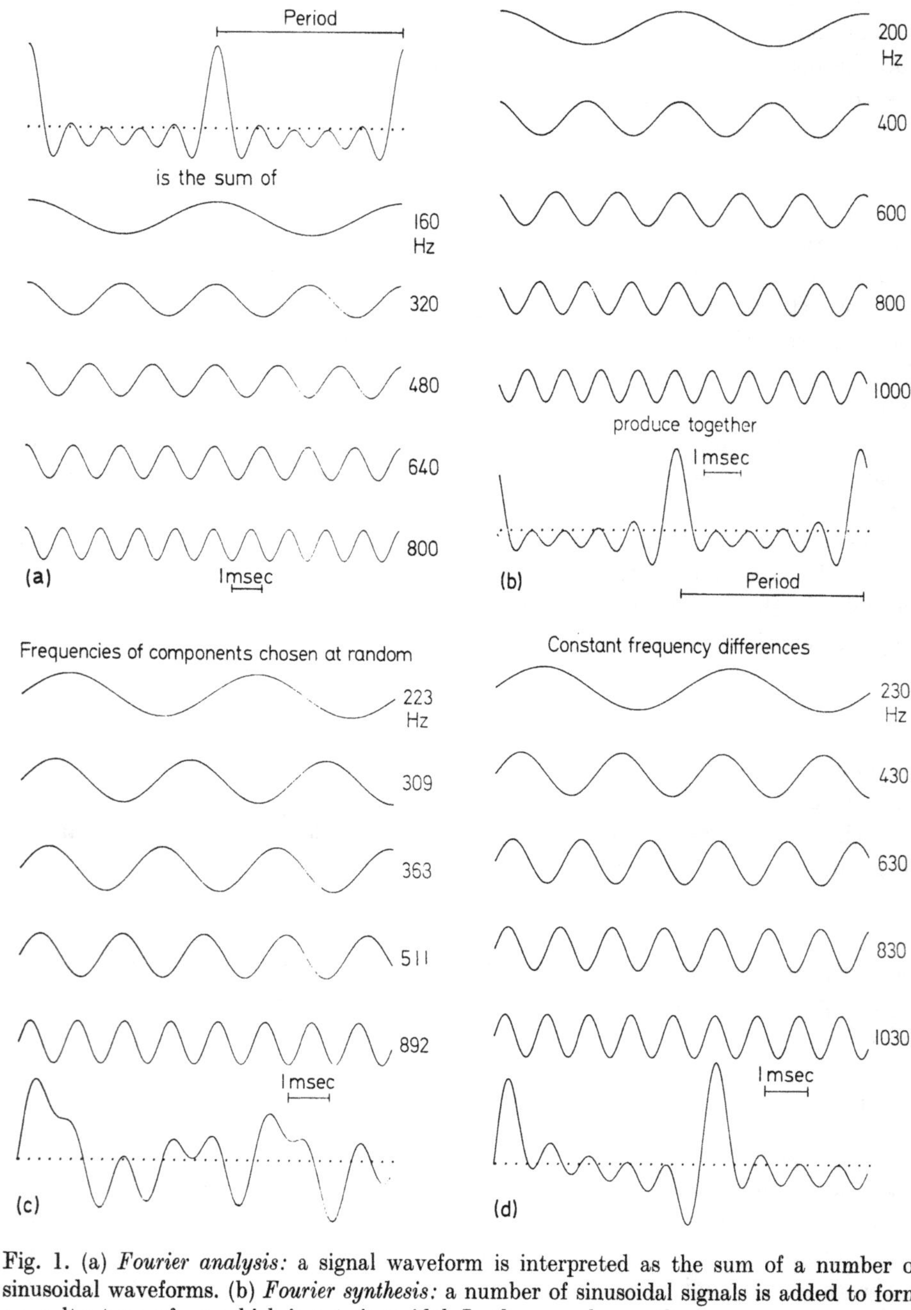

Fig. 1. (a) *Fourier analysis:* a signal waveform is interpreted as the sum of a number of sinusoidal waveforms. (b) *Fourier synthesis:* a number of sinusoidal signals is added to form a resultant waveform which is not sinusoidal. In the case shown, the component frequencies form a harmonic series; as a consequence, the resultant waveform is periodic (note that the component phases are different here). (c) *Fourier synthesis:* in this case, the component frequencies are random. (d) *Fourier synthesis:* in this case the frequencies form an arithmetical sequence

In order that relation (1) is obeyed, the amplitudes a_i and phases φ_i must have particular values for a particular signal $f(t)$. These values are found by applying the mathematical formalism of *Fourier analysis*. This process is illustrated by Fig. 1a for a periodic signal. Conversely, one may generate a particular set of sinusoidal signals $s_i(t)$, with chosen values of amplitudes and phases, and obtain the signal $f(t)$ by addition *(superposition)*. This is *Fourier synthesis*, and it will be used quite often in this chapter. See Fig. 1b.

For the waveform of the sum signal $f(t)$ the component amplitudes a_i are as important as the component phases φ_i. For auditory perception, the amplitudes are by far more important. The graph in which component amplitudes are plotted as a function of frequency is commonly referred to as the *spectrum*. Furthermore, Fourier analysis is also known as *spectral analysis*. However, it should always be remembered that, mathematically, phases are as important as amplitudes and that only certain properties of auditory analysis permit the suppression of phase data. In residue research, phase effects have played and continue to play an important part as we shall see.

For Fourier synthesis, there is no principal restriction in the choice of the component frequencies f_i. When these frequencies are not chosen to be integral multiples of a value f_0, the resulting sum signal will not be periodic, but it will still be deterministic. Such signals are usually not produced directly as specific waveforms and then analyzed, but they are produced by *synthesis* from a finite number of constituent sinusoidal components (see Fig. 1c for an illustration). In research of the residue phenomenon, the component frequencies are not random, but they are usually chosen to form an arithmetical series, *i. e.*, they have equal differences. The resulting signals, although having no simple periodicity, show a particular regularity in their waveform which has played an important part in residue theory. This will be described in the sequel. An illustration is provided by Fig. 1d.

If a part of a deterministic signal is analyzed, always the same components are found, no matter which part is taken (at least theoretically). This does not hold true for a stochastic signal like random noise. Every section of a noise signal has a different composition. For every frequency region, one can only specify the average spectral content; hence, spectral analysis of random signals can only be carried out in the "mean" sense. Moreover, the number of constituent components is not finite as in all the signals considered above, and that is the reason we cannot speak of the "amplitude of the component at a particular frequency" but are forced to use always the "average spectral content over a certain frequency region". Noise signals will only briefly be touched upon in this chapter; they are described here just for the sake of completeness.

3. Linear and Nonlinear Transformations

The theory of Fourier analysis is more than a mathematical tool. In physics, it is used a great deal to simplify the description of phenomena. This can be done wherever the system under study is a *linear* system. Put in the simplest possible terms, a linear system reacts to any disturbance in a way that is independent of the occurrence of other disturbances. This implies that when at any point the sum of two disturbances – here represented as two signals, $x_1(t)$ and $x_2(t)$ — is present, the reaction at another point is the sum $y_1(t) + y_2(t)$ of the reactions $y_1(t)$ and $y_2(t)$ brought about by each of the two x-signals separately. The notion of linearity implies also that the "output" signal (the reaction) is proportional to the "input" signal (the disturbance), *i. e.*, if $x(t)$ becomes, *e. g.*, 3 times as large, $y(t)$ will also become 3 times as large. A peculiarity of a linear system is that the reaction to a (sustained) sinusoidal signal is again a sinusoidal signal. Amplitude and phase may have been changed by the linear system, but the frequency has remained the same, of course. This property explains the utility of Fourier analysis in the domain of linear systems theory. Let us consider an input signal $x(t)$ and the resulting output signal $y(t)$, and let us decompose the former into a sum of sinusoidal signals:

$$x(t) = \sum_{i=1}^{N} {}_x s_i(t). \tag{1-a}$$

Each of the s-signals is transformed into another sinusoidal signal ${}_y s_i(t)$, in which process only the amplitude and the phase can be changed, and the output signal $y(t)$ must be the sum of these y-components:

$$\sum_{i=1}^{N} {}_y s\ (t) = y(t). \tag{1-b}$$

As a consequence, the transformation that the system performs for any input signal $x(t)$, can be described entirely by the transformations that *sinusoidal* input signals undergo. Frequency is then the only independent parameter. Hence the transformation is completely specified by the *amplitude* and *phase* characteristics describing the changes in amplitude and phase as a function of frequency.

Many transformations that take place in the peripheral auditory organs conform to the principle of linearity. For some transformations linearity fails significantly and we must then explicitly account for the *nonlinear* properties of the system. For a linear system, all Fourier components of the output signfy must already be contained in the input signal, since the system can only modial sinusoidal components, not create them. For a nonlinear system this is no longer true: a nonlinear system often reveals its nonlinearity by way of newly created sinusoidal components in the output signal. The newly created components are called *distortion products*. Moreover, in a nonlinear system, there usually is no proportionality between the amplitude of output and input signals, not even for sinusoidal signals. Nonlinear systems are extremely difficult to specify or to analyze. Let it be sufficient here to mention just the type and nature of distortion products that are relevant in the present context.

Let us start with a nonlinear system subjected to a single sinusoidal input signal $s(t)$ with frequency f_0. The output signal will not be sinusoidal, but it will have the same period as the input signal. Hence, it can be described as a sum of sinusoids like Eq. (1) and the newly created components will have frequencies that are integral multiples of f_0 [compare Eq. (3)]. In other terms, the components created are harmonics or overtones of the input signal. The amplitudes of these harmonics do not vary in direct proportion to the amplitude of the sinusoidal input signal. When the input signal is a composite signal, the situation is much more complicated. Let us consider the case where the input signal is composed of two sinusoidal signals $s_1(t)$ and $s_2(t)$, with frequencies f_1 and f_2, respectively. In this case, the frequencies are entirely arbitrary; there is no relation between them, except that f_2 is assumed to be larger than f_1. One may now expect in the output signal two series of harmonics: those of which the frequency is an integral multiple of f_1 and the same for f_2. This expectation is met indeed, but that is not all. A second group of distortion products have frequencies that are specific combinations of the frequencies f_1 and f_2. Quite appropriately, these are called *combination tones*. A few examples: the *difference tone* with frequency f_2-f_1, the *sum tone* with frequency f_1+f_2, other combination tones have frequencies like $2f_1-f_2$, $2f_2-f_1$, $3f_1-2f_2$, $2f_1+f_2$, etc. Several of these distortion products will turn out to be important for the theory of the residue phenomenon as we shall see. Moreover, combination tones have played an important part in the history of music (*cf.* PLOMP, 1965) and have been the cause of much confusion; the TARTINI pitch, for instance, may either be a simple difference tone or a higher-order combination tone.

When the input signal consists of more than two sinusoidal components, the situation becomes so complicated that it is hard to sort out everything. The principal point is that distortion products arise having frequencies which are always linear combinations of at least two of the input frequencies:

$$f_d = k_1 f_1 + k_2 f_2 + \dots .$$

In this formula, f_d is the frequency of a distortion product, and f_1, f_2 ... are the frequencies of the input signal. The coefficients $k_1, k_2, \dots$ are all (positive or negative) integral numbers. It is recalled that there is no general rule that controls the amplitude of any distortion product (*cf.* Section G. 2).

4. Pitch, Intervals, Aural Detection of Components

Long before Fourier theory was established, musicians knew that musical instruments produce multiple tones. In many musical instruments, notably bowed instruments and organ-pipe-like instruments, a tone is produced of which the waveform is periodic but definitely not sinusoidal. Such a tone can put a resonator (*e.g.* a string) into vibration whenever the resonance frequency of the resonator corresponds to one of the component frequencies of the tone. Furthermore, two tones can blend beautifully when the fundamental frequency of one corresponds to one of the component frequencies of the other. The harmonics of a tone with a fundamental frequency of about 125 Hz are shown in musical notation by Fig. 2. This figure indicates a peculiarity that has to do with the relation between the physical parameter: frequency and the subjective attribute,

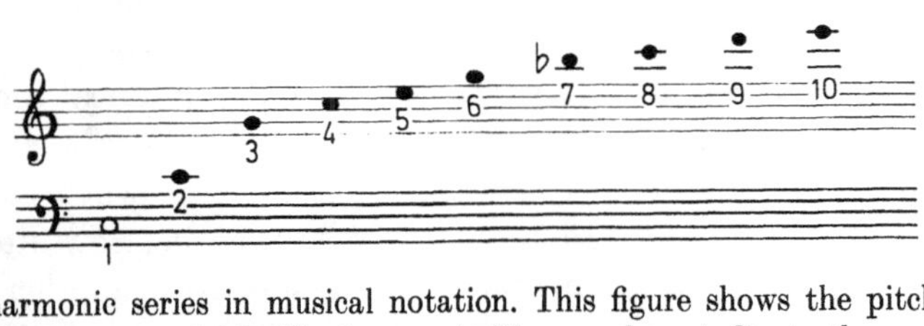

Fig. 2. The harmonic series in musical notation. This figure shows the pitches of each of the harmonics of a tone of 125 Hz (approx.). The numbers indicate the rank numbers of the harmonics

pitch. The series of frequencies f_i according to Eq. (3) form an arithmetical series, *i. e.*, their differences are constant. In musical notation, the differences are not constant: the pitch difference between the lowest two harmonics is the largest, and all subsequent pitch differences become successively smaller. The difference between the 1st and 2nd harmonics amounts to one octave, that between the 2nd and 3rd harmonic, a fifth, between the 3rd and 4th a fourth, etc. Our subjective pitch scale, in general terms, is laid out in such a way that a certain *musical interval*, *i. e.*, a difference of two pitches, corresponds to a specific *ratio of frequencies*. The ratio's 2:1, 3:2, 4:3, etc. successively become smaller, and hence the musical intervals become smaller too.

The various components of a tone can be identified (objectively) with the help of resonators. Up to a point, however, they can also be identified by the ear. That is, with a certain amount of training, a musical listener can aurally isolate the components of a complex signal. Each component is then recognized as what it actually is: a sinusoidal vibration (simple tone) that has an almost colourless tone quality. With a little bit of training, one can learn to identify at least the 1st to the 5th harmonic. Now, when one listens to a tone, two attitudes are possible. One is to listen to the sound as a whole, appreciating its pitch and perceiving the timbre as a characteristic quality of the entire sound. The other attitude is one of subjective analysis: one tries to break up the sound into constituent sounds (which happen to correspond to sinusoidal components), and the qualities of the sound as a whole are lost. In the latter case, we may allude to the situation by saying that the auditory system is attempting to carry out a Fourier analysis. That this has its limitations is self-evident. However, the possibility of this process has tremendous consequences for auditory theory.

5. Terminology

In the previous sections, several terms and their interrelations were described. There are more terms in common use which do not always conform to a strict definition. It seems appropriate, therefore, to group the terms into different categories and to try to separate them according to the categories to which they belong. The main categories will be: *descriptors of signals* in physical/mathematical terms and *descriptors of sensations*. A provisional grouping might look like Table 1. The terms are grouped according to the main category of usage. Corresponding terms in the other category are indicated within parentheses. Obvious omissions in the table can be filled in by resorting to a consistent terminology as introduced by SMOORENBURG (1970, 1972). The new term, part-tone, has been underlined in the table. Following these suggestions, we should adhere to a convention. The word *tone* and combinations of it, like simple tone and complex tone, should be used only in the perceptual sense. The corresponding physical concept should be described with the word *signal*. This will be fairly difficult since the term tone has acquired already many connotations. The reader will readily acknowledge this when he tries to re-read Section B. 4 and, noting how often the word tone is used in a dualistic sense, mentally tries to substitute another word for it. Furthermore, it is very difficult to replace the word tone whenever it is used in a musical context.

The word *partial* can be reserved exclusively for physical descriptions as soon as we can resort to a corresponding term like part-tone for its perceptual counterpart. The auditory Fourier analysis described in Section B. 4 can then be summarized by stating that a complex tone (*i. e.* a tone that is not a simple tone) can either be perceived as a tone or analyzed into part-tones. Each part-tone happens to correspond to a partial and, when attention is drawn to it, is perceived as a simple tone. Not all components can be recognized as part-tones; the remaining components form together a tone which cannot be analyzed any more. (These nonanalyzable partials constitute what has been called a "residue".)

Table 1. Terms in common use

Term, concept	Physical/mathematical meaning	Perceptual meaning
Sound	+	(+)
Tone[a]		+
Pitch		+
Musical interval	(frequency ratio)	+
Simple tone, pure tone	(sinusoidal signal)	+
Complex tone	(multi-component signal)	+
Frequency	+	
Frequency ratio	+	(interval)
Linearity	+	
Nonlinearity	+	
Distortion	+	+
Distortion product	+	+
Combination tone	(+)	+
Sinusoidal signal	+	(simple tone)
{ Frequency component	+	(part-tone)
{ Fourier component		
{ Partial	+	(part-tone)
Part-tone	(component, partial)	+
{ Harmonic	+	
{ Overtone	+	+
Fundamental frequency	+	
Fundamental (component)	+	+
Fundamental tone		+

[a] This concept is used in music in a dualistic sense.

C. Fourier's Proper "Place" (Early History, General Concepts)

1. Training to Hear Partials

In Sections B. 4 and B. 5, it has been described how the auditory system is capable of carrying out an incomplete type of Fourier analysis. The physical presence of harmonics can be proven by the use of resonators. However, as Helmholtz (1862, 1896, 1954) described, these can also be used to train an observer in auditory analysis and to make him realize that the part-tones he can hear correspond to the *partials* that can be proven to exist by physical means. The strings of a piano can be used as resonators in this type of experiment. The first test shows the presence of partials. A key is depressed which corresponds to one of the harmonics (2nd, 3rd, 4th, etc.) shown in Fig. 2. This action frees the corresponding string from its damper. While the key of, *e. g.*, the tone g_1 is depressed, the tone c is struck vigorously. When the c key is released subsequently, the tone c ceases but its 3rd harmonic g_1 is clearly heard which proves that this tone was contained in the previous sound.

By small variations of this experiment, the listener can convince himself that the partial g_1 is not only contained in the c sound, but that he can hear it in the tone c and that he can mentally isolate it. A very useful trick to train one-self to do this is to let the harmonic under question be heard previously and to direct attention to that particular pitch. With the help of a piano (or another string instrument), it is easy to hear the part-tone corresponding to the 5th or 6th harmonic. HELMHOLTZ reports that he was able to isolate aurally up to the 16th harmonic. However, he could not do this without artificial means of enhancing a partial – he used resonators in the form of hollow spheres provided with a small open tube, the Helmholtz spheres. PLOMP (1966) gives a short historical review of the attempts to determine the upper limit of aural isolation of harmonics. There is very little correspondence between the results of different experiments, mainly because of the vagueness of criteria used. By the use of very strict criteria and a very rigorous measurement procedure, PLOMP established that auditory analysis of components in a multi-component signal is well possible to the 5th harmonic, but that the power of resolution decreases quickly in the range of the 5th to the 9th harmonic. This should not rule out, however, that analysis of higher components is not possible, only that it requires a special situation. The limit found by PLOMP is related to the limit of aural resolution as it is expressed by the concept of the *critical bandwidth*. See other chapters of this volume for a description of this concept.

2. Ohm's Law

The relation between Fourier theory and auditory analysis was first formulated by OHM (1843). This was known later as *Ohm's acoustical law*. In its original version it read:

α) "... this is my formulation of the old definition of a 'tone':

a) To produce a tone of frequency m a series of periodic impressions with a period equal to $1/m$ is necessary; the form $a \cdot \sin 2\pi(mt + p)$ must be present in each period either purely or as a real component.

b) These forms must have the same value of p in successive periods.

c) The value of a must be the same in successive periods."

β) "... as the means to assess whether or not a given impression contains the form $a \cdot \sin 2\pi(mt + p)$, I use the theorem of Fourier which has become so famous because of its numerous and important applications, and which reads as follows...."

3. Acoustic Siren

It is seen that this formulation by OHM is more strict than can be substantiated by experiments, as we have seen above. We must remember, though, that the law was formulated in a time in which hardly any quantitative acoustic measurement could be carried out; a time also, in which Fourier's theorem had been formulated only two decades earlier. As Ohm put it, "... I tried to prove whether the definition of the 'tone', as it was given to us by our forbears, would contain everything necessary and sufficient to explain the newer facts or not." And he concluded, "... that right was done to the old endowned definition...."

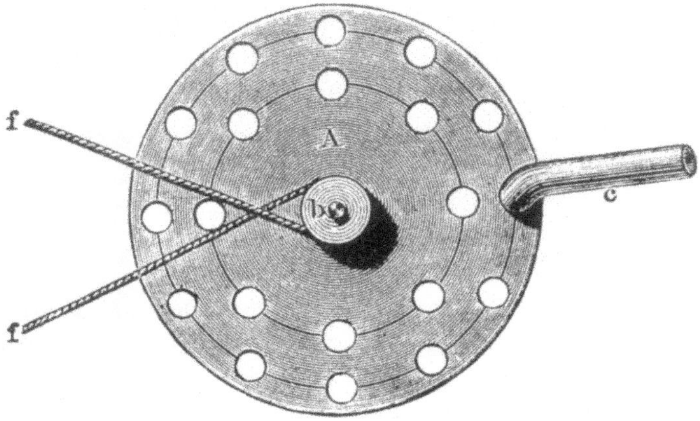

Fig. 3. The acoustical siren as used in SEEBECK's time. After HELMHOLTZ (1896)

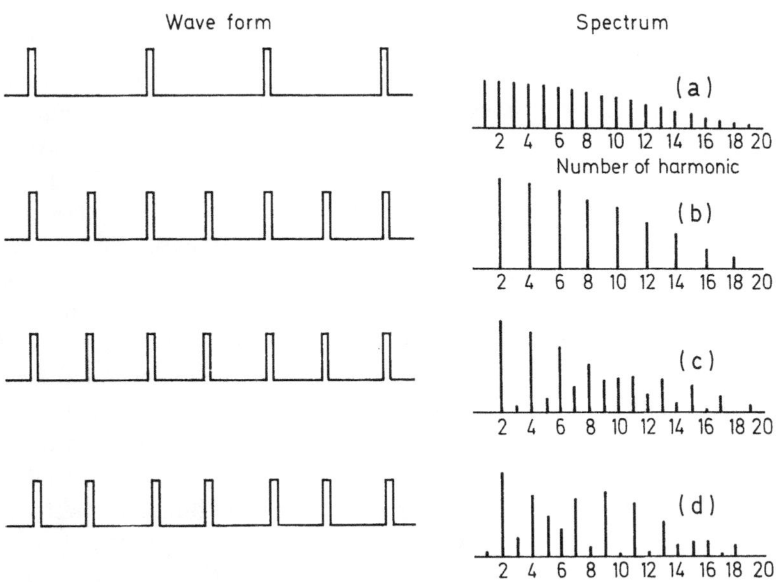

Fig. 4a—d. "Modern" interpretation of SEEBECK's principal experiment. In (a) and (b,) all pulses are equidistant. In (c) and (d), their distances alternate (see text). After SCHOUTEN (1940a)

Ohm's definition was formulated in such strict terms as a strong foothold against hypotheses put forward by Seebeck two years earlier (1841). Seebeck used an acoustic siren as sound generator. Figure 3, taken from Helmholtz' book, shows its construction. A disc A, provided with a series of holes is rotated by way of a string attachment f. Air is blown through a tube c so that a puff of air can come out whenever one of the holes is opposite the end of the tube. When the disc rotates with constant speed and the holes are equally spaced around the circumference, the resulting signal consists of a periodic series of puffs. In a stylized form, the waveform can be considered as a periodic series of rectangular pulses (see the upper trace of Fig. 4). Such a waveform has many Fourier components as the spectrum (also shown in Fig. 4) illustrates. Theoretically, the lower harmonics have almost equal amplitudes. (It goes without saying that the actual observation and analysis of acoustical waveforms could not be carried out until much later.) The corresponding part-tones can be analyzed by the ear and their loudnesses are not very different. Seebeck reported that the fundamental dominated.

4. Seebeck's Crucial Experiment

Now, Seebeck constructed a signal in which the harmonics were of highly unequal strength; he did this in two stages. His disc contained four concentric rows of holes. In the first row, the angular distance between the holes was 20°; in the second, the distance was 10°. It is clear that the tone will sound one octave higher when the tube of the siren is moved from the first to the second row. The resulting signal and its associated spectrum (highly idealized, of course) are shown in the second panel of Fig. 4. The components can again be regarded as a harmonic series but with a fundamental frequency that has become twice as high.

Seebeck's crucial experiment – the second stage – was carried out with the third and the fourth rows of holes. In these rows, the holes are not equidistant. In the third row, they are alternatingly 9.5° and 10.5° apart. The basic period of repetition thus encompasses not two but four holes, and the fundamental component is the same as for the first signal. However, since the waveform (see the third panel of Fig. 4) resembles so much that of the second row, it comes as no surprise that the second, fourth, sixth, etc. harmonics dominate and that the odd harmonics are rather weak. This is especially true for the fundamental component; the latter is so weak as to be barely visible in the figure. The fourth row of holes has distances of 9° and 11°, respectively. Waveform and spectrum, as shown by the fourth panel in the figure, should be self-evident now. The great surprise of the experiment is that the step from the second to the third row is accompanied by a change of the pitch one octave downward. If the pitch were associated exclusively with the part-tone (partial) at the fundamental frequency, it would be very weak. Seebeck concluded that the strength of (what we now call) a part-tone, is not determined by one (objective) Fourier component. Furthermore, he posed the statement that the pitch of a musical sound is not determined by the frequency of the lowest Fourier component but by the period of the signal's waveform.

It is to be noted that the change in period between the second and the third row of holes could also have been brought about by using only one row of holes and two tubes through which compressed air is blown. When the distance between the pipes is varied, all situations depicted in the figure can be obtained. Perhaps SEEBECK used this method when he discovered the effect. The principal point challenged by SEEBECK's experiments was the alleged quantitative connection between the strength of a partial and the loudness of the corresponding part-tone. When we realize how crude the experiments were in those times, we marvel at the ingenuity with which SEEBECK's attack was launched.

OHM's reply (1843) contained the aforementioned apodictical formulation of what later became known as Ohm's acoustical law, a great number of calculations proving, amongst other things, that the fundamental component must have been contained in SEEBECK's signals and no reference to any conclusive experiment that would contradict Seebeck's contentions. SEEBECK (1843) formulated his criticism a second time, devoting some attention to the effects of the width of the pulses (see Fig. 4) with respect to the period, and showing once more that in his experiments with the third and the fourth rows of holes, the subjective strength of the first and the second harmonics did not correlate with the objective strength. He concluded that each (subjective) part-tone was not simply the result of one Fourier component. He even went as far as to suggest that a number of higher harmonics might collaborate to enhance the strength of the first, or that these may produce a tone with the pitch of the fundamental (without the fundamental present). Real forebodings of the later residue theory!

5. Ohm's Reply; Helmholtz

OHM's final paper on the question was more authorative and witty than scientific. OHM admitted that he could not use his ears in experiments because "... nature had completely denied him a musical ear" (1844). He closed the argument by stating that SEEBECK's deviating observations were simply due to an auditory illusion. In his monumental book, *On the sensations of tone as a physiological basis for the theory of music*, HELMHOLTZ (1862, 1896, 1897, 1954) devoted close attention to this matter. On the basis of his arguments, he agreed with OHM, and it is most remarkable to notice that this argumentation just does *not* concern the points SEEBECK made. SEEBECK's observations led to the conclusion that some part-tones could be appreciably louder than would follow from their FOURIER counterparts. HELMHOLTZ' arguments, on the contrary, concerned mainly the reasons why part-tones could be judged to be weaker than would follow from the theory. In any event, OHM's and HELMHOLTZ' authoritative works remained the principal bases for the theory of the perception of pitch until about one century later.

One important reason for the impact of HELMHOLTZ' work was that he provided a possible physiological explanation for auditory analysis. He postulated that different parts of the organ of Corti in the cochlea are tuned to different resonance frequencies. In this way, each FOURIER component of a sound excites only a single stretch of the organ of Corti, and the nerve fibers originating from that stretch carry only information about that component. This theory also accounted in an elegant way for the fundamental law about tone quality (timbre) that HELMHOLTZ discovered. The law states that the timbre of a sound depends on the distribution of the Fourier components with respect to intensity and that timbre does not depend on the phases of the components (HELMHOLTZ was careful to leave the matter for components with a small pitch difference undecided).

The studies by VON BÉKÉSY (1960) proved that HELMHOLTZ' assertions were essentially right, with two exceptions. The first is that the apical part of the cochlea is tuned to the lower frequencies and the basal part to the higher frequencies, and not the other way around, as HELMHOLTZ supposed in his earliest works. The second point is that the mechanical damping in the cochlea is fairly high so that components will not be well resolved by the cochlear mechanism. Still later studies have shown that the situation is far better on the level of the activity of individual cochlear nerve fibers. According to the most modern findings, the frequency selectivity at this point is rather high and certainly sufficient for separating the lower harmonics (the explanation of these facts in terms of cochlear mechanics and physiology is quite another matter...). See the chapter on frequency selectivity of the cochlea by EVANS in Vol. V/2.

HELMHOLTZ also suggested a mechanism by which the impression of the fundamental pitch could possibly be enhanced. He described at great length the various types of distortion products, notably the difference tone, but he did not apply this directly to the problem brought forward by SEEBECK.

6. Fletcher, the Missing Fundamental, Distortion

From the time that vacuum tubes could be used to generate and analyze signals, research in physiological acoustics received a great boost. The problem of the pitch of complex tones received attention because of the fact that telephone exchange circuits have the property that frequencies corresponding to the fundamental of the human voice are attenuated quite heavily. Despite the absence of the fundamental (and of several of the lower components), the human voice via the telephone sounds with the natural pitch. In the time when FLETCHER wrote his first book, *Speech and Hearing* (1929), there was no doubt about this fundamental property; the phenomenon was commonly referred to as "the case of the missing fundamental". The general consensus was that aural distortion was the cause of the phenomen; the missing fundamental was restored as a distortion product. That this is quite feasible is evident when we realize that all pairs of consecutive harmonics give rise to a difference tone with the same frequency as the (objectively missing) fundamental. FLETCHER's quantitative estimates (1929, 1931) showed that this explanation could well be correct for the high levels of signal strength as used in telephone conversations. Although FLETCHER once described (1924) that the pitch of a multi-component signal without fundamental remains the same when the sound is made weaker and weaker toward the limit of audibility, no further mention is made of this property and the distortion hypothesis is considered adequate.

7. Place Theory

The "place theory" of auditory frequency analysis was established when the theory of HELMHOLTZ on resonance in the cochlea was formulated. According to the place theory, the components of a sound are directed to various locations in the cochlea, each component producing the largest vibration at the location that is tuned to its frequency. The process is referred to as; "spatial frequency analysis". In HELMHOLTZ' original conception this analysis was rather precise; each component stimulating a circumscript region of the cochlea. In later times amendments were put forward, as described above. Although we now know that at the level of responses of auditory nerve fibers, the analysis is fairly precise, this does not imply that we can explain all auditory phenomena of frequency resolution on the basis of place theory alone. In the sequel, we will have numerous opportunities to come back to the issue of the place theory; we will refine it, we will describe its limitations, etc. One point should be stressed here, however. In its purest form, the place theory assumes perfect isolation of all components in the cochlea. In this form, it is in excellent agreement with the fundamental law on timbre, as stated above. The actual analysis carried out by the cochlear mechanism will not be perfect, of course. Then, there will be components that are not analyzed perfectly in the cochlea. We may expect that the ear will not be "phase deaf" for the components that are incompletely resolved by the place mechanism in the cochlea. In this form, we may appreciate that there exists a fundamental relation between cochlear frequency analysis and phase sensitivity of the auditory system.

D. The Schouten "Period" (The Residue Theory)

1. Two Place Principles

The demonstration by VON BÉKÉSY of the spatial frequency analysis of sound in the cochlea gave rise to the formulation of the "place theory" of hearing. As a matter of fact, it is necessary to distinguish two principles in this theory. The *first* principle is that a sound of a particular frequency will be directed in the cochlea to a certain location where it will provoke the largest vibration amplitude. The location is specific for the frequency; high-frequency signals will stimulate the basal part of the cochlea, low-frequency tones, the apical part. This part of the theory is well substantiated by experiments (in point of fact, better by more modern experiments than by VON BÉKÉSY's studies which were directed at gross movement patterns). The *second* part of the place theory is founded on the possibility of the auditory analysis of part-tones corresponding to the partials of a sound signal. This principle states that stimulation of nerve fibers at a particular location gives rise to a tone sensation with a pitch corresponding to the frequency that is characteristic for that location. In short, the first place principle says: "frequency" gives "place"; the second principle says "place" gives "pitch". The second principle was tacitly assumed to be true until the Dutch scientist, SCHOUTEN, took up SEEBECK's experiments of one century earlier again and proved that the situation is really more complicated (SCHOUTEN, 1938). It is his study that led to the concise formulation of the "residue" theory (SCHOUTEN, 1940a).

2. The Optical Siren

SCHOUTEN used an optical siren to produce periodic signals of any desired waveform and to combine (superimpose) different signals. A disc with a series of narrow radial slits is rotated in front of an illuminated surface. A mask, in

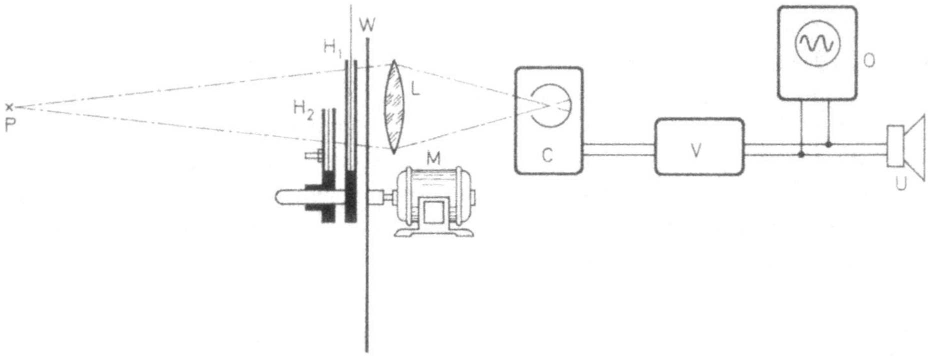

Fig. 5. Optical siren for producing synthetic sound. *P:* light source, H_1 and H_2: holders for masks, *W:* rotating disk with slits (driven by motor M), *L:* lens, *C:* photo-electric cell, V*:* amplifier, *O:* oscilloscope, *U:* loudspeaker. After SCHOUTEN (1939)

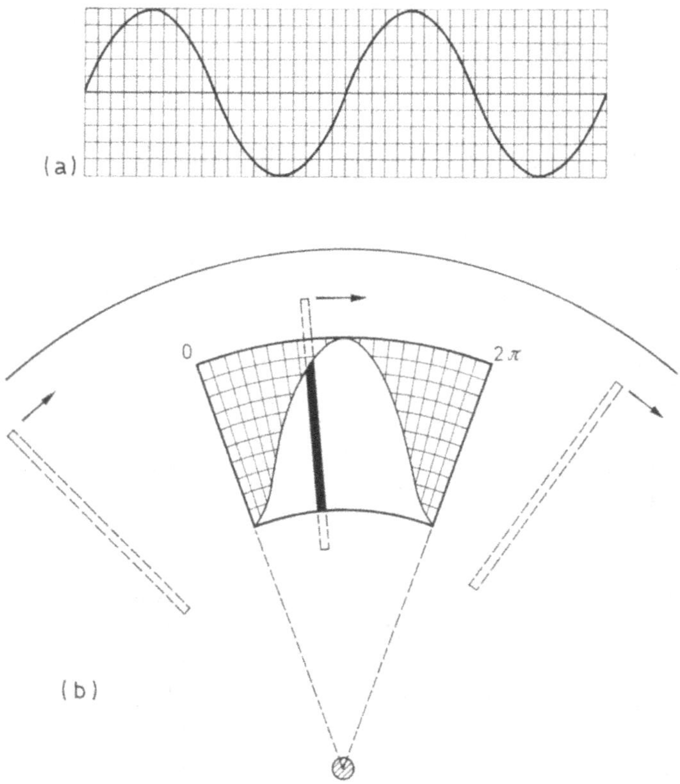

Fig. 6a and b. Sinusoidal waveform (a) transformed into a mask (b). The slits of the rotating disk are shown dotted. After SCHOUTEN (1939)

the form of a sector, is put in front of the disc so that the slits pass it successively. As a result, the amount of light transmitted varies as a function of time t, as prescribed by the form of the mask. If the slits in the disc are equidistant, the resulting light signal will be periodic. A photosensitive cell collects the transmitted light and converts it into an electric signal. In its turn, the electric signal drives a loudspeaker via an amplifier. Figure 5 shows the arrangement in detail, and Fig. 6 shows how the mask should be cut in order to obtain a sinusoidal signal.

It is fairly easy to generate a periodic series of pulses with the instrument described in Figs. 5 and 6. The frequency of repetition was 200 Hz in SCHOUTEN's experiments. The spectrum contained many harmonics of which the intensity decreased slowly with increasing index i (see Fig. 7a). The signal was presented to the ear at a sound level of about 40 dB above the threshold of audibility. The tone quality was very sharp, the pitch corresponded to the frequency of the fundamental. With the proper amount of training several of the lower part-tones can be aurally isolated. We shall refer to this sound as sound *a*.

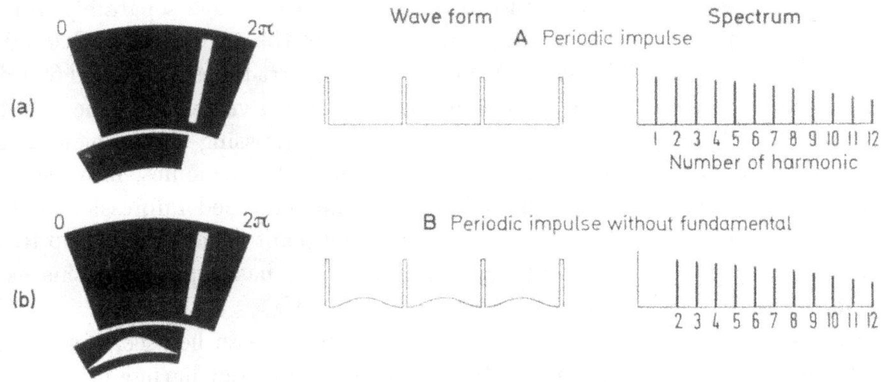

Fig. 7. (a) Periodic pulse series — waveform and spectrum. (b) Periodic pulse series with the fundamental component suppressed. The left-hand part of the figure shows the two masks used in the optical siren. After SCHOUTEN (1940a)

3. Schouten's Principal Experiment: Cancellation of the Fundamental; the Residue Hypothesis

By the addition of a second sector to the mask, the fundamental component can be removed from the signal. The added sinusoid just compensates for the corresponding component. The resulting signal and spectrum are shown by Fig. 7b. This situation is the purest form of the "case of the missing fundamental". The adjustment of amplitude and phase of the added signal is carried out with the help of a wave analyzer (an instrument which indicates the strength of the Fourier component at a specific frequency). The intensity of the fundamental component in the combined signal can thus be reduced to less than 0.5% of the original value. The sound (henceforth to be called sound *b*) looses some of its "body"; the timbre becomes somewhat sharper, but the pitch remains the same. After this, the adjustment of the compensation can be made subjectively. This proves to be fairly easy, and the part-tone, *i. e.*, the subjective component corresponding to the fundamental can be made to vanish completely. Quite contrary to expectation, the objective and the subjective settings coincide. This means that no appreciable distortion component of the fundamental frequency is formed in the ear. In other terms, the fundamental part-tone that we hear is exclusively due to the fundamental component in the sound. When the latter vanishes, so does the former, and vice versa. Schouten employed other means to verify that there was indeed no fundamental component generated in the ear, but we shall leave that aside. The surprising thing is that *the pitch ascribed to the sound b with the fundamental missing is the same as that of the original sound a.* It is definitely one octave lower than the frequency of the lowest Fourier component in sound *b*, 400 Hz. This experiment proves that the pitch of the sound is not the pitch of the lowest Fourier component present and that the fundamental is not reconstituted by nonlinear distortion.

4. New Formulation of Ohm's Law

Let us now return again to sound *a*. By concentrating the attention, the fundamental, the second and the third harmonic can be heard separately in the sound. As to actual perception, the sound consists of the pure tones of 200, 400, and 600 Hz[1] plus "something else". Sound *b* contains part-tones of 400 and 600 Hz plus "something else". In the latter case, the sound has a very sharp tone quality and this sharp tone has a pitch equal to that of the (missing!) fundamental. In the sharp tone, some part-tones, *e. g.* the 4th and 5th harmonics, may be distinguished, but the main body of it is due to the combined impression of the remaining higher-numbered components. The main point is that this sharp tone, this combined impression of unresolved components, has a pitch, in this case equivalent to the pitch of the fundamental, *i. e.* 200 Hz.

By successive removal of the next few harmonics, it can be ascertained that the sharp tone is indeed produced by the higher-numbered harmonics. Such a subjective tone is called by SCHOUTEN a "residue". Hence, *a "residue" is a subjective component of sound sensation that is the result of the combined impression of higher harmonics, namely those harmonics that cannot be resolved by the auditory organ.* In SCHOUTEN's own words (1940a), Ohm's law of subjective sound analysis may be extended as follows:

"1. The ear analyses a complex sound into a number of components each of which is separately perceptible.

2. A number of these components corresponds with the sinusoidal oscillations present in the inner-ear sound field. These components have a pure tone quality.

3. Moreover, one or more components may be perceived which do not correspond with any individual sinusoidal oscillation but which are a collective manifestation of some of those oscillations which are not or scarcely individually perceptible. Those components (residues) have an impure sharp quality."

If, in the light of this development, the difference between sounds *a* and *b* is considered again, we note that sound *a* contains *two* subjective components with the same pitch, 200 Hz. One has a pure-tone quality and is due to the presence of the (objective) fundamental component. The other, having a sharp tone quality and a rather large loudness, has a different origin, namely the mass

[1] Part-tones with pitches corresponding to 200, 400, and 600 Hz.

of unresolved components. Both subjective sound components, the fundamental part-tone and the residue, have the same pitch. In sound *b* only the residue is the bearer of the pitch – the *higher* components giving the lower *pitch*. Some part-tones may be recognized in it, with different pitches, but the pitch of the sound as a whole is determined by the residue. It should be clear from this description that proper recognition of the residue as a subjective sound component requires a good deal of abstraction and introspection. In spite of the careful and detailed description given by SCHOUTEN, the rules of the game have been followed only by very few of the later scientists working on the problem.

5. The Period as the Cue for Pitch

The next question which Schouten posed, was: what physical property of the set of higher harmonics determines the pitch of the residue? There are two obvious possibilities: all components in the sounds used have mutual frequency differences of 200 Hz, and the waveform has a repetition period of 1/200 sec. In order to solve the question, SCHOUTEN produced a signal in which these two parameters differ from one another. Consider Fig. 8a. Here a pulse series with *two* pulses per period of 1/200 sec is shown, together with its spectrum. Referred to the time interval of 1/200 sec and the fundamental frequency of 200 Hz, all components are even multiples, that is, they are integral multiples of 400 Hz. It is clear that the pitch of this sound will be 400 Hz. The second sound, Fig. 8b

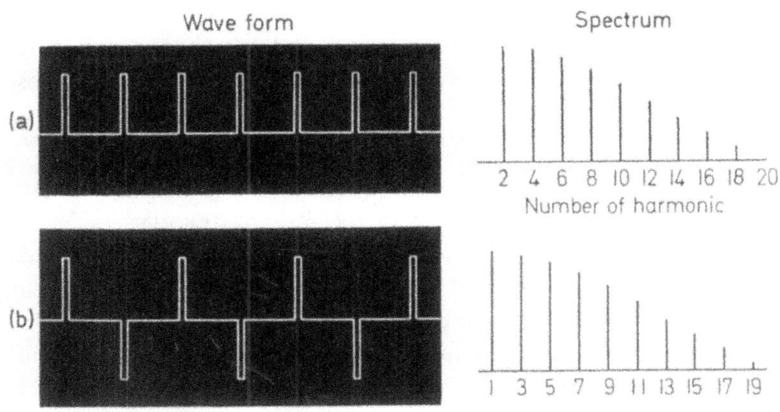

Fig. 8. (a) Periodic pulse series, fundamental frequency: 400 Hz. (b) Series of pulses with alternating signs, fundamental frequency: 200 Hz. After SCHOUTEN (1940a)

is a series of pulses with alternating signs. The components have frequencies that are odd multiples of 200 Hz, and the difference between any two successive harmonics is 400 Hz. The period of the waveform is, of course, 1/200 sec. SCHOUTEN found that the residue of this second signal, although being rather weak, had a pitch of 200 Hz. He concluded that:

"the ear thus ascribes a pitch to a residue by virtue of the periodicity of the total waveform of the harmonics which are responsible for this residue" (SCHOUTEN 1940a).

The notion of periodicity has been considerably refined by later studies and we shall come back to it later on. It has also been found that the signal of Fig. 8b is not the most suitable one for deciding on the physical parameter governing pitch, but, within the framework of an extended definition of the concept of "period", SCHOUTEN has been proved right.

6. Seebeck Revisited

The extension given by SCHOUTEN to OHM'S law is reminiscent of the extension given by SEEBECK almost one century earlier. SEEBECK (1843) wrote:

"... it follows that the tone of the siren, can at least be amplified by audible overtones. If this is the case..., then it can be supposed that it holds true for a tone that is not accompanied by harmonics, ... so that a tone with pitch m is not necessarily of the form $a \cos 2\pi(mt + \theta)$ but it may contain also terms of the form $a_s \cos 2\pi(smt + \theta_s)$ where s can be very large and a_s very small. It should not even be excluded that those latter terms, when taken together, can evoke a tone with pitch m when a term of the form $a \cos 2\pi(mt + \theta)$ is not present".

The case of the missing fundamental!

On the next page of SEEBECK's remarkable paper, we find the germs of the later residue hypothesis:

"It appears to me irrefutable that the higher terms of the cosine series control the varieties of the tone. I consider it very likely that those terms of the series which are not individually perceptible take part in this, and that these terms by their common period length evoke a specific impression on the auditory organ."

SEEBECK's experiments with the unequal pulse series (see Fig. 4) also receive a satisfactory explanation in the light of the residue hypothesis. The weakness of the fundamental component only implies that the corresponding fundamental part-tone is weak or inaudible. Of the higher harmonics, there are many that show the basic period in their combined waveform; hence, the residue will have a pitch corresponding to the frequency of the fundamental. With the optical siren, it is far easier to manipulate the parameters of the test sound and to study what happens than with the acoustical siren. SCHOUTEN reports that he repeated SEEBECK's experiments also with an acoustic siren, only to find that the effects, though present, were extremely weak and variable and that much masking noise was produced by the instrument.

7. Mechanism of Period Extraction

In a third paper, SCHOUTEN described (1940b) a possible cochlear mechanism by which the period of a complex waveform can be detected. To understand his argument, it is essential to remember that the harmonics lie the closer together (in the musical sense) the higher their index. Compare again Fig. 2. A sinusoidal signal will produce vibrations in only a limited stretch of the basilar membrane, the location being a function of the frequency. This is the first part of the place principle. The second part ("place" giving rise to "pitch") is questionable in the light of the residue theory since high components can give rise to a low pitch. We shall see presently how this part should be modified. But the first part holds true unmistakenly. Only the extent of the excited region has been left unspecified, or, what is equivalent, the width of the response curve (resonance curve) at any particular location. In view of the relation between frequency ratios and musical intervals, it is logical to assume that the width of the response curve should be expressed as a musical interval, or, in other words, as a fraction of the center frequency. HELMHOLTZ was concerned about this measure; he reasoned that the response should be less than 0.1 of its maximum value for a frequency that deviates one whole tone (two semitones) from the frequency of maximum vibration. The difference of 3 dB corresponds to 0.2 semitone in his conception (see Fig. 9). At the time of SCHOUTEN's studies several sets of data about the so-called critical bandwidth (*i. e.* the bandwidth over which the auditory system integrates sound intensity) were known but these appeared to differ widely. SCHOUTEN assumed that the frequency response characteristic at any location had a half-value width of at least a semitone. That means that the lower harmonics, being an octave, a fifth, a fourth, etc. apart, will chiefly excite narrow

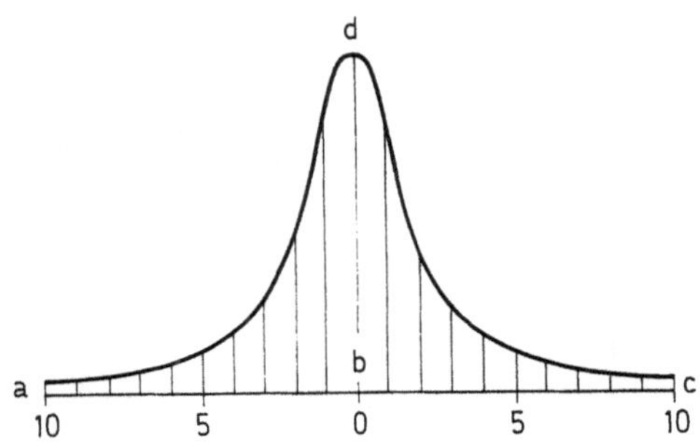

Fig. 9. Sharpness of resonance as estimated by HELMHOLTZ. Abscissa: 5 units are equivalent to a semitone. After HELMHOLTZ (1896)

stretches of receptors that are well isolated from one another by regions in which the response is comparatively small. Conversely, the receptors in those stretches will respond almost solely to isolated harmonics. Figure 10 shows the situation in SCHOUTEN's terms. Figure 11 shows the same situation in the light of more modern data on auditory frequency resolution; this figure is modified from PLOMP's doctoral dissertation (1966). Along the vertical axis, a number of response curves for selected equidistant locations along the length of the basilar membrane are plotted. The basal part of the cochlea corresponds to the top of the figure. The vertical axis is a logarithmic frequency axis so that equal musical intervals appear as equal distances along the basilar membrane. The width of the response curves appears as constant in this representation. (The response functions should be imagined to form a continuous set, only a few of them are drawn.) On the bottom of the figure, a periodic series of pulses is shown; this is the waveform with which the cochlea is supposed to be stimulated. This signal has a large number of Fourier components; for reasons of simplicity, these can all be assumed to be of equal amplitude. Their "proper" positions along the vertical axis are unequally distributed of course. In SCHOUTEN's figure, the positions for several of them are indicated. In PLOMP's figure one can use the indicated numerical values for the frequency as a guideline. The remainder of these figures shows the waveforms that can be expected at selected positions along the vertical axis. The lowest three harmonics give rise to nearly sinusoidal vibrations at the positions corresponding to their frequencies. But note, what happens to the highest harmonics! At a certain position of the basilar membrane a number of harmonics

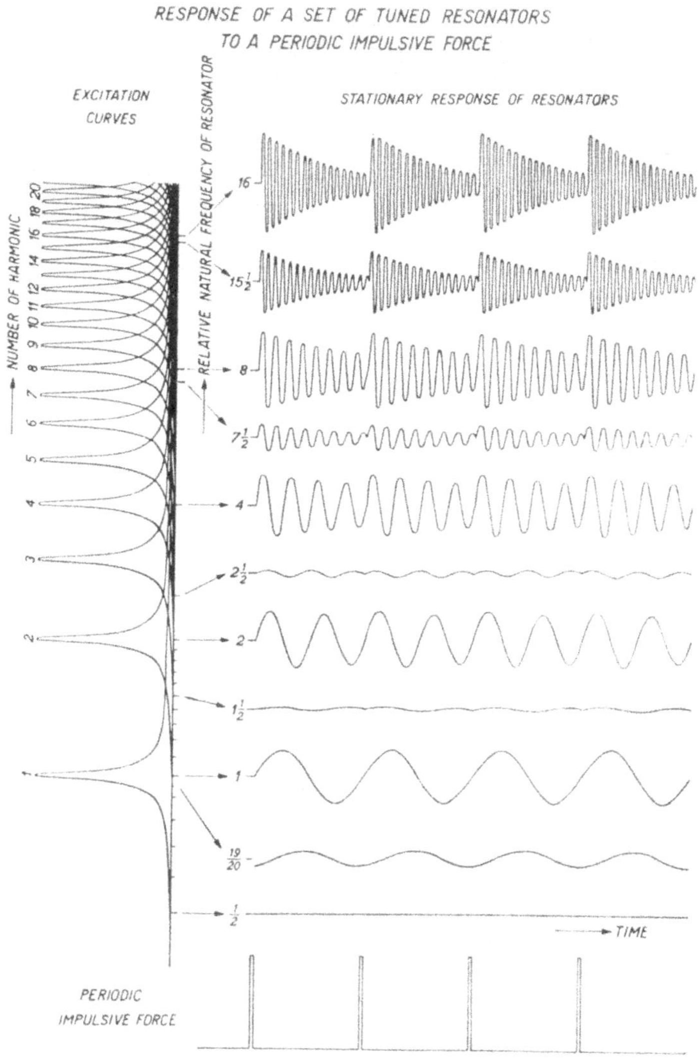

Fig. 10. Periodicity of signals and aural resolution of components: SCHOUTEN's explanation of the residue. After SCHOUTEN (1940b)

fall within the top of the response function and by interference they produce a pattern of vibration with a nonuniform amplitude. In fact, the combined excitation of such a set of higher harmonics gives rise to bursts of oscillation, and the period of these bursts is the same as the period of the pulse series that excites the cochlea. The model implied in these figures may not be quantitatively cor-

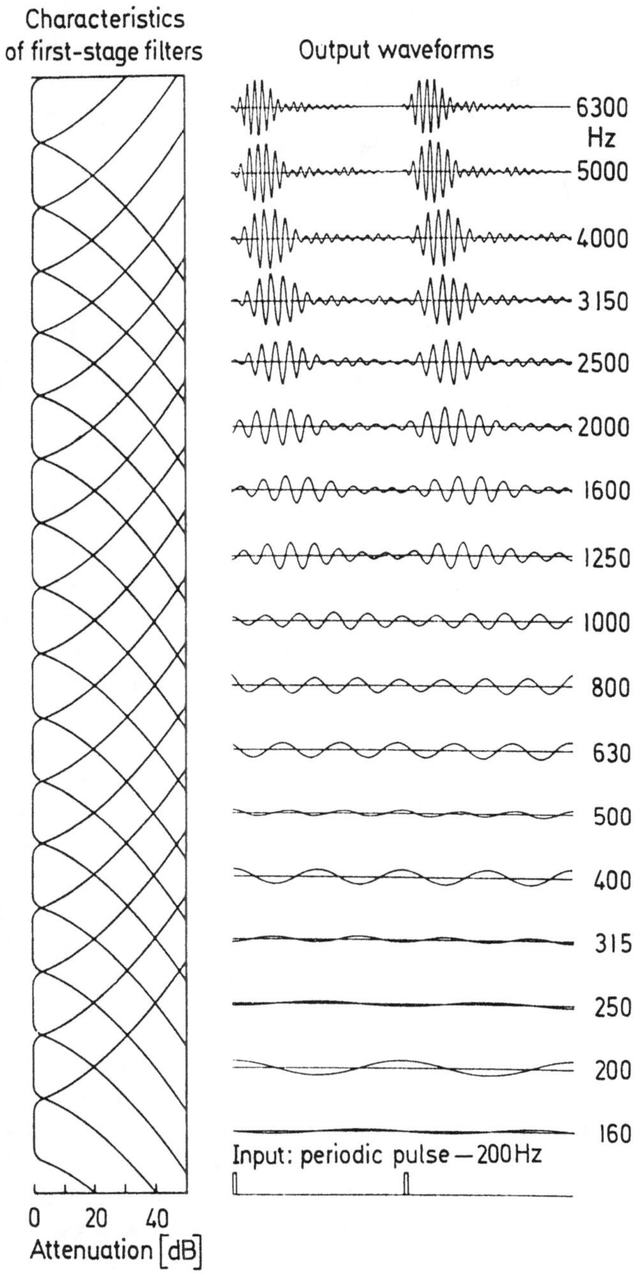

Fig. 11. Periodicity of signals and aural resolution of components: a more modern representation. After Plomp (1966)

rect, but it displays the properties to be expected from all resonating systems of analysis with a limited power of frequency resolution.

It is seen that the consideration of the first place principle, but with a limited resolving power built in, automatically leads to a response revealing the basic periodicity of the stimulus in those sections where harmonics are not resolved. That means that the second principle in the place theory should be replaced by a principle that states: when the stimulation of a particular location in the cochlea is of constant amplitude, a pitch is perceived corresponding to that location, but when the stimulation occurs in bursts, the ensuing residue has a pitch corresponding to the periodicity of the bursts, and no pitch corresponding to the stimulated location is perceived. In this theory, the nerve fibers are supposed to transmit both the quantity and the quality of the excitation of the receptors. The former is important in loudness and timbre; the latter, by virtue of the periodicity, for pitch.

8. Corollaries; Inharmonic Signals

Several phenomena acquire new perspectives in the light of the residue theory. The first is the "case of the missing fundamental" as it is encountered in the form of the telephone voice. It is clear now that the lack of the lowest harmonic, or of the lower few harmonics, will change the timbre somewhat, but there will be enough harmonics left to give a residue which lends its pitch to the sound. Whether or not the fundamental is re-instituted by nonlinear distortion is immaterial. The second point concerns the existence of more than one type of sound with the same pitch. In the signal of Fig. 7a two subjective components are present, a part-tone and a residue, both with the same pitch. In the signal of Fig. 7b, the former has disappeared, and the residue remains. The pitch is, again, 200 Hz. One can combine this second signal with a pure tone (sinusoidal signal) of *e. g.* 203 Hz; it is highly remarkable that there occur no beats (Schouten, 1940c). One hears a part-tone and a residue with slightly different pitches that coexist without causing beats. The conclusion is that beats can only occur when two signals, *e. g.*, sinusoids, stimulate one and the same receptor in the ear. Later on, we shall encounter examples of signals in which different, non-overlapping parts of the spectrum give rise to different residue pitches. The problem is, then, which of these pitches will be ascribed to the entire sound. The example cited above is the first of such signals with conflicting information (see Section F. 3).

The third phenomenon for which the residue theory contains an explanation, concerns the strike note of (carillon) bells. In general, none of the partials of a bell – and most of these are not harmonically related – corresponds to the pitch ascribed to the sound of the bell when it is struck. Furthermore, the strike note has a sharp timbre whereas each of the partials has the soft and mellow timbre characteristic for a sinusoidal signal. The hypothesis was advanced (Schouten, 1940c) that the strike note is a residue evoked by several of the partials that stand to one another in a harmonic relation. Closer inspection of the spectrum of the partials (Eigentones, as they are usually called in this case) reveals that several of these do have the required relation and that the residue pitch these partials can give corresponds to the pitch of the strike note. "Good" and "bad" bells would then be distinguished by the presence or absence of such special partials among the Eigentones.

In one of SCHOUTEN'S papers (1940c), an experiment is described that proved to be extremely important for later studies. In a purely periodic signal, the harmonics form a *harmonic series, i. e.* a series in which the frequencies are integral multiples of a fundamental frequency f_0 [see Eq. (3)]. By a special procedure, borrowed from the technology of telephone carrier circuits, it is possible to modify a signal so that all harmonics are shifted by an equal amount of Δf. The frequencies

$$f_i = i \cdot f_0$$

then become

$$f_i' = if_0 + \Delta f \tag{4}$$

and they no longer form a series of successive harmonics. We shall refer to signals with this property as *inharmonic* signals. For small values of Δf, *e. g.* 40 Hz, the 200 Hz periodic pulse series retains its tonal character, but the pitch is slightly different. This shows once more that the pitch is not determined by a distortion product such as the difference tone, since the frequency difference of the components remains the same after the shift. The same procedure was applied to a musical recording. The observed relative pitch shift was about equal to the relative frequency shift that the components in the 1000–2000 Hz region undergo. This observation can be understood with the help of the concept of dominance as it was developed later by PLOMP and by RITSMA (see Section F. 3). For the moment, we may conclude that these observations on bell tones and frequency-shifted signals indicate the plasticity of our auditory system: our ear will not only accept components forming a harmonic series but it will try to form a residue pitch when the series is nearly harmonic. Just what relations among the components are needed in order to do this remains to be seen.

9. Introspection, Slow Acceptance

Acceptance of SCHOUTEN'S findings and interpretations by the scientific world was very slow, and, perhaps, it has not even been completed in the musical world now that, scientifically, things have already taken another turn. It appears that only few of the criticizers of SCHOUTEN'S hypotheses really applied the method of introspection by which the residue is defined. So it happens that HOOGLAND (1953), when trying to disprove SCHOUTEN'S theory, only succeeded in confirming the existence of aural distortion tones, in normal as well as in abnormal ears, something that nobody would have doubted at all. HOOGLAND experimented with a residue signal generated by the method of synthesis: a number of components were generated by separate tone generators. The difficulty with which this leads to perception of a residue with a clear pitch – which difficulty is no doubt due to the problem of keeping the phases of the components constant – suggests that there really are some constraints involved in the perception of residue pitch. It was extremely difficult at that time to envisage the real consequences of these problems.

E. Wave Crests (the Impact of Periodicity Pitch)

1. Outline of this Part

Perhaps one reason for the slow acceptance of Schouten's results was the need for introspection to elucidate the main aspects of the residue. There was a definite need for convincing demonstrations that could easily be turned into well-reproducible psychophysical experiments. On the other hand, a small number of studies were published that touched upon the problem of the residue pitch from various angles, and it was attempted several times to bring such widely divergent studies into a common focus. However, the number of experimental variables is quite formidable. In this part we shall first briefly describe the demonstrations of the residue effect as they were developed by Licklider. These demonstrations, as well as a few other experiments to be described, served as a basis for a novel theory on pitch perception. The theory, Licklider's duplex theory, provides for a possible neural mechanism that carries out its operations on the neural output of the cochlear analyzer and that succeeds in extracting information about the period contained in the excitation waveform. The second part of this sub-chapter will be concerned with the extensions and modifications that were given to the residue theory by the present author around 1956. The third part describes in condensed form the great interest that temporal phenomena in hearing received until the period 1960–1965 in which a change in attitude began to be noticeable.

2. Licklider's Demonstrations

Licklider's demonstrations (1954, 1955) continue to be important because they are so ingenuously concentrated on the main aspects of the problem. Moreover, they can be repeated easily with modern equipment and they are most convincing. The frequency of the test signals was not fixed but was made to vary in order to see whether the pitch of the residue is the kind of pitch of which melodies can be made. The signals presented were, alternatingly, sinusoids and periodic pulse series (with the fundamental removed but that is not necessary). Each signal lasted about 0.5 sec and was switched on and off smoothly (the latter refinement is not essential either). In each pair of signals, the frequency of the sinusoid was the same as the repetition frequency of the pulse series, and the sinusoid was the louder signal of the two. The successive pairs progressed up and down the scale in frequency as controlled by the experimenter. While the sounds were presented in this way, a low-frequency random noise signal was turned on. This noise was produced by feeding white noise through a low-pass filter that passed only the frequency components below 1000 Hz. The low-frequency noise was sufficiently strong to mask the low-frequency channels of the auditory system. As a consequence, none of the sinusoids was audible any more as soon as the noise was turned on. However, the sharp sound produced by the high harmonics of the pulse series could be heard through the noise and it retained its low pitch. After the noise was left on for several pairs, it was turned off again, and this sequence could be repeated. Without the noise, the sinusoids and the pulse series showed both the impressed pitch course, but, after the noise was turned on, the "melody", so to speak, was only audible from the pulse series and not from the tones.

This demonstration proves conclusively that the second place principle should be modified in the sense that the receptors in the ear normally occupied with high-frequency components are really able to mediate a low pitch. In other words, there is not a one-to-one correspondence between "place" and "pitch", although there is a fairly precise projection from "frequency" (in the FOURIER sense) to "place".

3. Chopped Noise — Direct Evidence of Periodicities(?)

We have observed in the preceding sections that recognition of a temporal structure like periodicity is linked with insufficient spectral resolution. In most types of signals, it is impossible to vary the temporal structure without causing a corresponding variation in the spectral composition. There is one exception: interrupted white noise. The spectrum of noise can only be defined in statistical terms (see Section B. 2), and for white noise the average noise power content (per unit interval) is the same for all frequencies. If a white noise signal is repeatedly switched on and off at a rate of, say, 100 times per second, the spectrum, when defined in this sense, will remain the same. This is because switching a signal on and off can be regarded as a multiplication with a signal alternating between 0 and 1, this procedure causes many components to be generated that were not present in the original noise signal. Each frequency is equally likely for these new components; hence, the spectral content of interrupted white noise is the same for all frequencies, just as for uninterrupted white noise.

For high switching rates, interrupted noise cannot be distinguished from continuous noise by the ear. However, when the switching rate is low, *e. g.*, once per second, we can easily hear the temporal sequence, and the theoretical spectral content will be completely irrelevant for the ear. Somewhere in between, there is a transition. This phenomenon was studied by MILLER and TAYLOR (1948). A white noise signal was switched on and off with a duty cycle of 0.5 or more. The interruption rate could be varied between 0.1 and 5000 Hz. It was attempted to determine the pitch of the interrupted noise by comparison with a pure tone. Most listeners could produce a reliable match for interruption rates up to 200 or 250 Hz. Above 300 Hz, it was impossible to match the "buzz" of the interrupted noise to a pure tone. In a second experiment, the just noticeable variations of interruption rate were determined. (Of course this was only possible below 300 Hz.) For interruption rates below 100 Hz, the values were about twice as large as the just noticeable variations of the frequency of a pure tone. This suggests that detection of the temporal structure ("intermittency") is a major factor in the frequency discrimination of very low tones. It was not mentioned in the paper of MILLER and TAYLOR whether the "pitch" ascribed to interrupted noise is tonal enough so that "melodies" can be built from it. In the experience of the present author, the pitch is much less clear than the pitch of a residue, and not musical (DE BOER, 1956a).

4. Licklider's Autocorrelation Theory

Although auditory theories of the type of "telephone theories" had almost ceased to exist after VON BÉKÉSY's findings about the frequency-to-place transformations in the cochlea, they received some support after cochlear responses at the neural level could be studied. It soon became known that the fibers of the auditory nerve were able to follow to some extent the temporal pattern of the sound stimulus. The question is, of course, whether this frequency following plays a role in pitch perception. In his book, *Theory of Hearing*, WEVER (1949) strongly supports the hypothesis that it does. He assumed, on good grounds, that various neurons connected with a given location could follow a stimulus beyond the upper limit by frequency division. The firings of the neurons then rotate, as it were, between the members of the group of neurons; this is the famous "volley principle". At high frequencies, the volley principle may fail, whereas the place principle may fail at low frequencies. WEVER advanced the theory that both place and frequency determine pitch, the former being dominant at high frequencies and the latter at low frequencies. It is to be noted that this holds only for (sinusoidal) components and for the pitch of part-tones; the complexities of residue-like signals, as they are hypothized by SCHOUTEN, are left out. A similar attitude, the space time-pattern theory of hearing, was expressed by FLETCHER in his second book (1953), but it should be remembered that FLETCHER favoured the distortion hypothesis as the explanation of the phenomenon of the missing fundamental.

A theory directly aimed at *periodicity pitch* (under which term the residue pitch concept became known by English and American authors) was formulated by LICKLIDER (1951). It is specifically concerned with the mechanism necessary for extracting information about the period from the excitation. The first point of importance in this theory is to realize that the vibration at each location of the cochlea contains information about the frequency content of the stimulus as well as about the way the stimulus varies with time. When components are not resolved, the temporal pattern reveals the basic periodicity of the sound stimulus as Figs. 10 and 11 show. Neurons connected to this location will carry the same two types of information: by virtue of their point of origin about spectral content and by virtue of their frequency-following properties about the temporal pattern. The representation in neural terms is necessarily less accurate but that is not important at the moment.

In the theory, a network of neurons is assumed to be connected to each location of the cochlea. Figure 12 shows this network in a diagrammatical form. The principal element is a chain of delay elements (neurons) B_i; each one relays

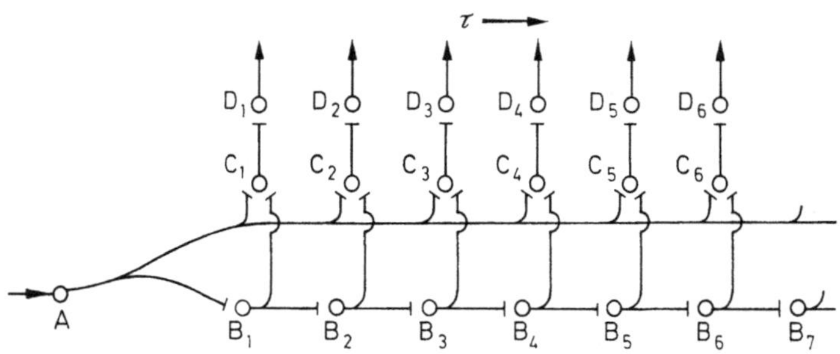

Fig. 12. Hypothetical network (neural autocorrelator), capable of measuring periodicity. See text. After LICKLIDER (1951)

the excitation at the input A after a certain delay. Each of the delay stages is connected to a "coincidence neuron" C_i which gives off an output pulse whenever it is excited nearly simultaneously at both its inputs. Consider first what happens if the system is excited by a stimulus without a definite time pattern. The delayed versions of the stimulus appearing at the neurons B_i have nothing specific in common with the original signal that is transmitted to all the coincidence neurons C_i. Hence, there will be no special pattern set up in the output neurons D_i.

Things are entirely different, however, when the excitation function is periodic. At one of the delaying stations, the output signal, being delayed by one period, is almost identical to the undelayed signal. As a consequence, the corresponding coincidence neuron is stimulated by two nearly identical input signals and that is the situation most apt to produce output pulses in this neuron. Somewhat further along the delay chain of neurons, the same situation arises; here, the delay amounts to two periods. At other places along the chain, there is no specific output. It is clear that a periodic signal evokes responses at particular locations along the neural network. In this way, the period of the stimulation is translated into the location (or, rather, locations) of the responding neurons; periodicity is encoded into a specific response pattern among the neurons.

In LICKLIDER's paper, it was shown that the analysis performed by this type of network is a form of what is mathematically known as *autocorrelation analysis*. As a matter of fact, the analysis is incomplete (a so-called running autocorrelation analysis) just as is required for the analysis of signals that can rapidly change their character.

The dimension along the delay chain may be labelled with the parameter τ. A similar arrangement is assumed to be connected to each point of the cochlea (see Fig. 13). Along the length of the cochlea, denoted by the dimension x, a limited-resolution spectral analysis is carried out. The resulting neural information can, thus, be labelled with two parameters, x and τ. Pure tones and pulse series each give rise to specific patterns of neural activity in these two dimensions.

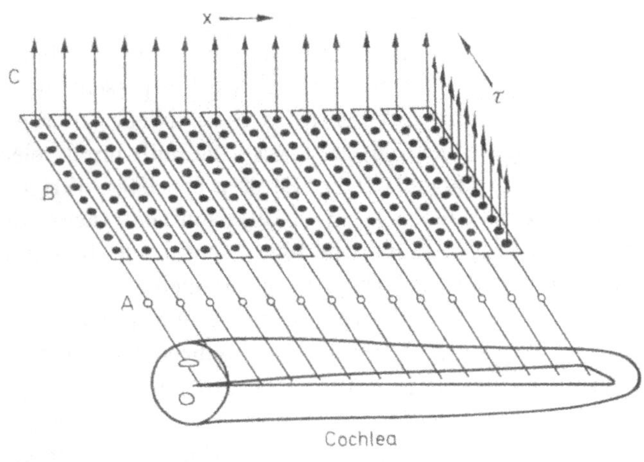

Fig. 13. Illustrating the duplex theory of hearing. After LICKLIDER (1951)

In both, the periodicity reveals itself as a succession of maxima along the τ-dimension; this may be responsible for the perceived pitch. From this two-dimensional representation, the theory derives its name, duplex theory of hearing. A related theory, in the form of a mathematical formalism, has been published by GOLDSTEIN (1957).

A later paper by LICKLIDER (1955) contains two extensions to the theory, the first of which is of considerable interest in neurophysiology. The pattern of activity, as it is analyzed by the set of networks described above, must transfer its information to higher centers in the auditory pathway of the brain. The projection may be unstructured at first, a random each-to-everyone projection. It may become structured through its own operation. The rule of modification may be that a functional connection is strengthened when it is often used and that connections which are not exercized will be weakened. When such a "plastic" system continues to operate with stimulations containing periodic signals, such as human vowels, the gradual reorganization may lead to projection of periodic points along the τ-dimension to a common point in an upper stratum of the brain. The main impetus for such a reorganization is the repeated occurrence of periodic sounds of low frequency or, rather, the occurrence of high-frequency signals with periodic envelopes. The principal result of such a process would be that periodicities detected by an autocorrelation-type of analysis could be brought into one sphere with the ordered series of excitations produced by cochlear analysis of sinusoidal signals. Pitch is not the only attribute to which such a process might apply; timbre may be another one. This would explain why listeners when presented with residue-like signals, especially those with only few Fourier components, have difficulty in separating pitch from timbre.

The second extension of the Duplex theory, which makes it into a Triplex theory, takes binaural phenomena into account. There are several types of pitch that can manifest themselves only by binaural presentation (in fact, by dichotic presentation), *i. e.*, different signals are led to the two ears. We will come to speak about these in a later section (Section H. 9).

5. Seebeck Re-Revisited

At a time that the residue theory was already more than ten years old and it continued to be challenged from several sides, the present author attempted to pinpoint once more the requirements for the existence of the phenomenon. Instead of an optical siren, like SCHOUTEN used, he built purely electronic equipment for the generation of signals. The first step consisted of rigourous application of SCHOUTEN's recipe: introspective realization that there are two possible bearers of pitch in a complex signal, the fundamental part-tone and the residue. This was considerably facilitated when the fundamental component was added in counter-phase to a periodic pulse series, just as in SCHOUTEN's central experiment. A repetition frequency of 200 Hz was confirmed to be optimal for such experiments. When the residue is easily recognized, repetition of SEEBECK's fundamental experiment (see Fig. 4b–d) once more confirms the independence of a residue and a part-tone. The experiment is performed by the addition of two periodic pulse series of 200 Hz with a variable delay between them. When pulses of one series fit exactly midway between those of the other, the pitch is the octave, 400 Hz, of the basic frequency. When they are slightly off-centre, the residue pitch jumps to 200 Hz, but the corresponding part-tone is inaudible. The lowest part-tone in the sound is still 400 Hz. An even more striking effect, which was tried but could not be demonstrated so easily in SEEBECK's days, is produced when three pulse series are combined. When all pulses are first equidistant and then one of the three series is shifted in timing, the pitch jumps down a duodecime or a twelfth (an octave plus a fifth). Other experiments were carried out with pulse series filtered by band-pass filters so as to attempt to "grow the residue as a culture". Because these experiments are also performed by other authors who appear to have exploited them more completely, they will not be described here (see Section E. 12).

6. De Boer's Experiments on Inharmonic Signals

The principal experiments of DE BOER (1956a, b) are extensions of SCHOUTEN'S endeavours with inharmonic tones described at the end of Section D. 8. The test signals were produced with a *modulator*, an electronic circuit that produces at its output a signal $z(t)$ which is the product of the two signals $x_1(t)$ and $x_2(t)$ at the two inputs:

$$z(t) = x_1(t) \cdot x_2(t). \tag{5}$$

This modulation process can also be considered in the frequency domain. Suppose that $x_1(t)$ contains a Fourier component of frequency f_1 and $x_2(t)$ a component of frequency f_2. Then the output, $z(t)$, will contain two Fourier components with frequencies $f_1 + f_2$ and $f_1 - f_2$, respectively. The modulator is a nonlinear circuit with the peculiarity that only the sum and difference frequencies are produced; the original components have disappeared completely. In DE BOER's experiments, the signal $x_1(t)$ was a sinusoidal signal, commonly referred to as the carrier signal. In accordance with later usage, the *carrier frequency* will be designated by the letter f. The second signal, $x_2(t)$, commonly called the modulation signal, was made to contain three components, with frequencies g, $2g$, and $3g$, respectively. This signal was derived from a pulse series with repetition frequency g by sharp low-pass filtering. Figure 14 gives a diagram of the setup; the figure indicates the nature as well as the spectral content of the various signals. When the modulation signal contains only the components g, $2g$, and $3g$, the output signal of the modulator contains the frequencies:

$$f - 3g,\ f - 2g,\ f - g,\ f + g,\ f + 2g,\ f + 3g. \tag{6}$$

Via a separate pathway, a fraction of the carrier signal (frequency: f) is added so that a full arithmetical series of frequencies arises. The series is harmonic only when f happens to be an integral multiple of g; in the other case, the series is characterized as an arithmetical series, *i. e.*, a series with constant frequency differences [cf. Eq. (4)]. In most of the experiments, f was sufficiently high so that the lowest Fourier component according to the series (6) had a positive frequency.

Let us start by assuming $f = 2000$ (Hz) and $g = 200$ (Hz). The resulting components then form a harmonic series:

$$1400, 1600, 1800, 2000, 2200, 2400, 2600 \text{ Hz}.$$

Needless to say that the waveform is periodic. This output signal is presented to the ear of the listener via earphones. The signal constitutes a pure form of the residue; it is well-nigh impossible to distinguish aurally any of the constituent components. The residue has a clear pitch that is readily shown to be equivalent to 200 Hz, the fundamental frequency belonging to the series of component fre-

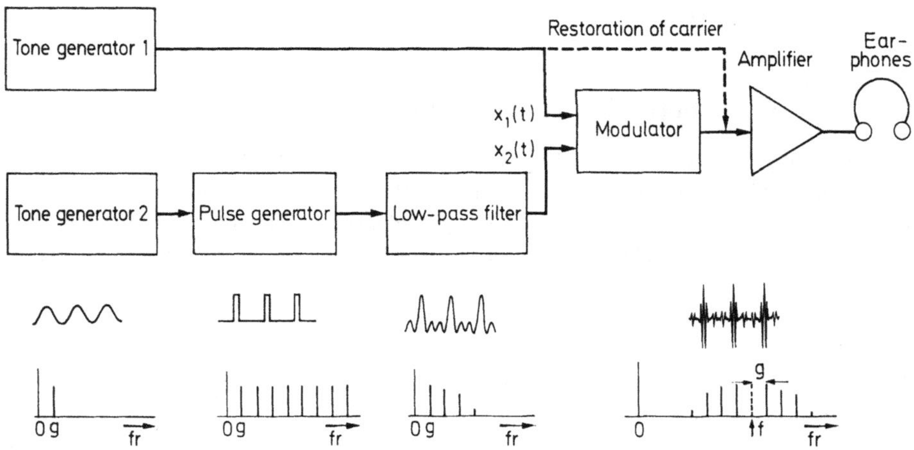

Fig. 14. Block diagram of DE BOER's signal generator. Waveforms and spectra of the signals at various points of the setup are illustrated. The spectral component shown by a dotted line is the carrier component (which is not passed by the modulator)

quencies. When instead of 2000 Hz, another integral multiple, *e. g.*, 2200 Hz, is chosen for f, the signal will again be periodic and the frequencies will again be a harmonic series, this time from 1600 to 2800 Hz. The signal again gives a residue pitch of 200 Hz, and the two signals sound much alike.

When, in going from 2000 to 2200 Hz, the carrier frequency passes intermediate values, the situation described by Eq. (4) arises. It is surprising that the sound does not reveal the prevailing inharmonicity at all; the residue does not sound much different. Only the pitch differs from 200 Hz. Consider the case $f = 2030$ Hz; the component frequencies will be (g is still 200 Hz):

$$1430, 1630, 1830, 2030, 2230, 2430, 2630 \text{ Hz}. \tag{7}$$

These frequencies do not have a common divisor in the neighbourhood of 200 Hz. Nevertheless, the residue is tonal and the pitch corresponds to approx. 205 Hz. When the carrier frequency goes upward from 2000 Hz, the pitch goes up too, a little more than proportionally since, *e. g.*, 205 Hz is higher than 203 Hz (one tenth of 2030 Hz). Similarly, when the carrier frequency goes down from 2000 Hz, the pitch goes down too. The same will hold true when the carrier frequency is decreased from 2200 Hz; the pitch will go down from 200 Hz. Some kind of paradox is indicated since a continuous variation of f from 2000 to 2200 Hz should lead to the same pitch again. Figure 15 shows the results of pitch matches as a function of the ratio f/g in this range. The matches were obtained not with a sinusoidal comparison tone but with a purely periodic residue signal of about the same (though harmonic) spectral composition. These measurements confirm that the pitch around a harmonic situation varies somewhat more than proportionally with the carrier frequency.

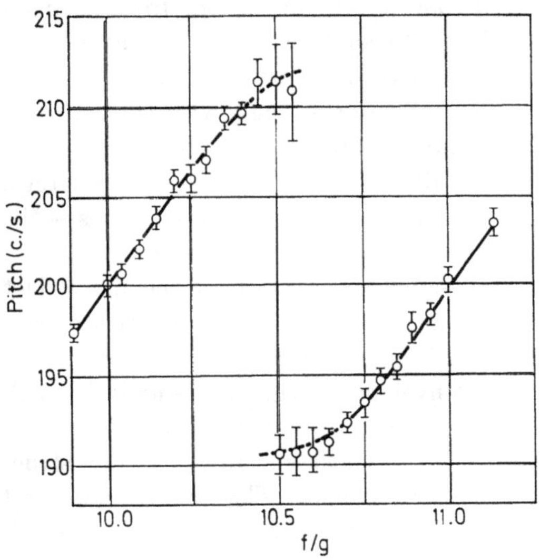

Fig. 15. Pitch of inharmonic signals as measured by DE BOER (1956b)

There are two pitch courses visible in the figure, and, somewhere in the centre of the interval, the attention of the listener seems to switch over from one to the other pitch. Clearly pitch is ambiguous in this region, and the mind can be focused on any one of the two possibilities. Both these pitches, however, are near 200 Hz. The point half-way between the harmonic situations is characterized by a peculiarity both in the waveform and in the spectrum. For instance, if $f/g = 10^1/_2$, the component frequencies are:

$$1500, 1700, 1900, 2100, 2300, 2500, 2700 \text{ Hz} \tag{8}$$

and these are all odd multiples of 100 Hz. It comes as no surprise that the waveform will be *anti*-symmetrical with a period of 1/100 sec. In other words, after 1/100 sec, modulation signal and carrier are in the same relative phase again. It is remarkable that, contrary to expectations, a pitch of 100 Hz is *not* heard. There are two possible pitches and both are near to 200 Hz. This observation constitutes the only substantial deviation from Schouten's results. Note, however, that SCHOUTEN utilized a signal with a full range of components and DE BOER a "cultured" signal containing only a few components.

7. First and Second Effect, the Pseudo-Period

The phenomena described in the previous section were investigated over the pitch range of 100 to 400 Hz. Provided the carrier frequency f is not too high with respect to the modulation frequency g, the pitch shifts can be easily observed. In all cases, the pitch varies a little more than proportionally with f and the amount of this deviation is large when the ratio f/g is low. The deviation does not tend to disappear when f/g increases up to a value of 10. Beyond that value the quality of the pitch diminishes rapidly. This suggests that it is appropriate to consider the actual pitch as being in essence proportional to f – the "first" effect of pitch – and to consider the deviations from proportionality as a perturbation – later called the "second" effect. The existence of the second effect implies that the pitch should go down when f is kept constant and g increases. This experiment is somewhat more difficult with the setup of Fig. 14, but the results confirm this expectation (de Boer 1956a, b). Since the second effect has been a major tool in novel developments in this field by later authors – notably the recognition of the importance of combination tones – the actual measurement results will be left out of the present discussion.

We now turn to a possible explanation of the first effect. In the light of Schouten's periodicity theory, it is logical to consider the waveform. Figure 16a shows the waveform in the harmonic case; this waveform is purely periodic. The dotted lines indicate the "envelope", imaginary boundaries within which all oscillations are confined. The envelope originates from the modulation signal $x_2(t)$ fed into the modulator. In this harmonic case, the fine structure repeats itself exactly in every lobe of the envelope. The arrows indicate the period of the waveform; this is, of course, equal to the period of the envelope. In Fig. 16b, the situation is drawn for an inharmonic signal obtained by the same procedure but with the carrier frequency shifted away from the harmonic position (Figure 1d shows another illustration of an inharmonic signal.) The envelope has remained the same, but the fine structure is not the same in successive lobes of the envelope. However, it is easy to mark a "pseudo-period" as the time distance over which the waveform repeats itself in an approximate way. This is indicated by the arrow in Fig. 16b. If the auditory analyzer measures the period in the case of a periodic signal, it is not far-fetched to hypothize that it will sort out the pseudo-period in an inharmonic signal. In the case drawn, the period as well as the pseudo-period encompasses ten oscillations of the carrier frequency. Hence, this concept causes the pitch to vary as a sub-multiple of the carrier frequency; this hypothesis is sufficient to explain the "first" pitch effect. The proportionality can be expressed by the following formula:

$$p = \frac{f_0}{\mathrm{n}}. \tag{9}$$

Here, f_0 is the central frequency (the carrier frequency of the complex signal); p is the inverse of the pseudo-period; and n is an integer number, namely, the rank order of the central component. The pseudo-period theory predicts that the measured pitch is equal to p. In the following discussion, this formula will repeatedly be referred to; the meaning of p can then be described as: the frequency equivalent to pitch.

The third part of Fig. 16 shows the situation in the odd-harmonic case. Here, the carrier frequency is midway between two harmonic positions; the waveform is *anti*-symmetrical in the sense that the phase of the fine structure alternates in successive lobes of the envelope. The true period is 1/100 sec, but the signal has *two* possible pseudo-periods as indicated by the horizontal arrows. It is readily understood why the pitch should be ambiguous at and around this situation. Even these pitches are preferred by the auditory system over the pitch (100 Hz) corresponding to the true period of this signal (presumably only for a narrow-band signal).

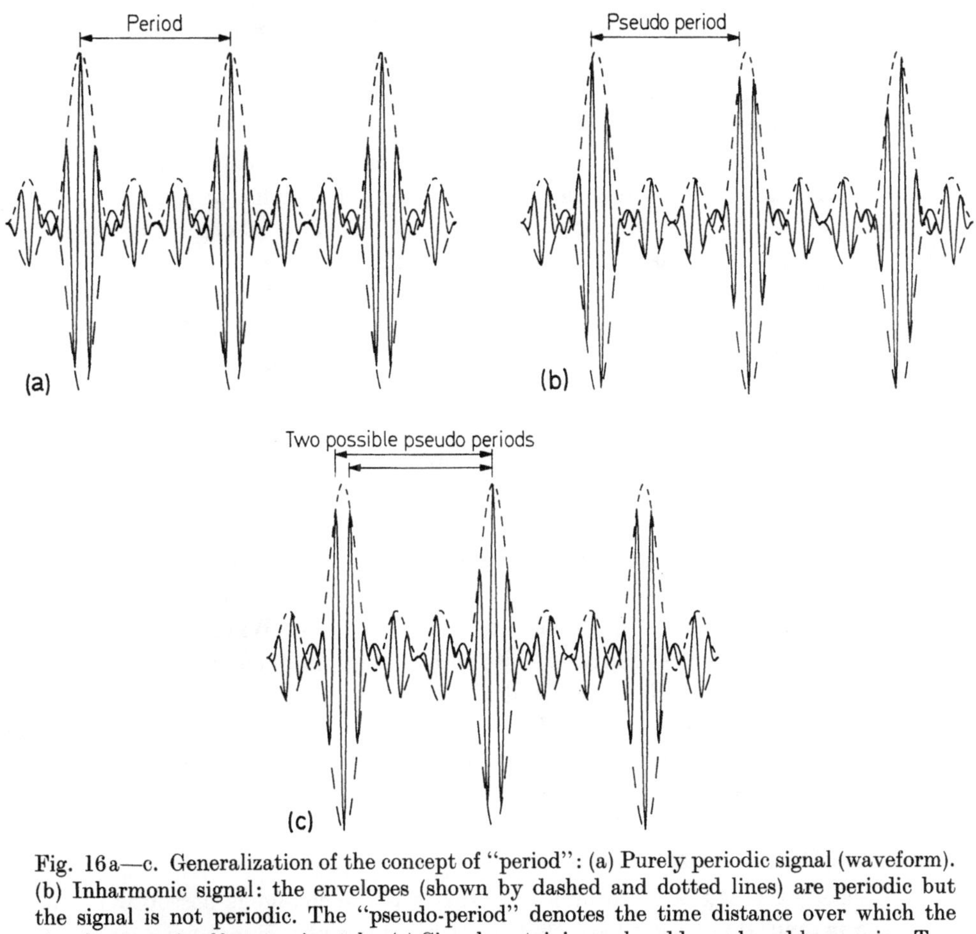

Fig. 16a—c. Generalization of the concept of "period": (a) Purely periodic signal (waveform). (b) Inharmonic signal: the envelopes (shown by dashed and dotted lines) are periodic but the signal is not periodic. The "pseudo-period" denotes the time distance over which the signal repeats itself approximately. (c) Signal containing only odd-numbered harmonics. Two pseudo-periods are possible

8. De Boer's Phase Rule

The fact that a slightly inharmonic signal sounds almost as tonal as a harmonic one is somewhat surprising. If the carrier frequency is very near to a harmonic position, the fine structure of the waveform drifts slowly through the lobes of the envelope (*cf.* Fig. 16b). We do not perceive a change of timbre related to this drifting. Hence, for these signals the timbre of the sound does not depend upon the phase of the fine structure with respect to the envelope. The invariance of timbre for this type of phase change is described by DE BOER's phase rule (1956a, 1961): *The phases φ_i of the components of a sound can be altered by an amount $\Delta\varphi$ that is a linear function of frequency:*

$$\left.\begin{aligned} \varphi_i &\to \varphi_i + \varphi_0 + c \cdot f_i \\ \Delta\varphi &= \varphi_0 + c \cdot f_i \end{aligned}\right\}^2 \tag{10}$$

without causing a change of timbre. [For the meaning of the symbol φ_i we refer to Eq. (2)].

The constant phase change φ_0 represents a phase change such as is caused by a very slight inharmonicity. For instance, a 1 Hz deviation of the carrier frequency causes φ_0 to vary so slowly as to complete one cycle per second. The phase changes described by the term φ_0 leave the envelope invariant and cannot be detected by the ear. The term $c \cdot f_i$, proportional to frequency, simply represents a shift of the origin of the time axis which is obviously imperceptible.

All other phase changes may lead to an observable change of timbre. Phase changes not obeying (10) can, for instance, be effected by changing the phase relations among the components of the modulating signal $x_2(t)$, see Eq. (5). Or else, the carrier component (shown dotted in Fig. 15) can be reintroduced in a different phase. Such phase changes do not affect pitch (in general) but they do affect timbre. By the term, "phase effects", is usually meant the dependence of timbre upon the phases of the components; hence, phase effects can only be demonstrated by introducing phase changes that do *not* obey DE BOER's phase rule.

Whether such phase changes are accompanied by detectable changes of timbre depends on two factors. The first factor has to do with the relative frequency separation of the components. When the components of the signal are spaced wide apart, each component stimulates more or less an isolated region of the cochlea. For signals with such a spectrum, no phase effects are audible; this case is described by HELMHOLTZ' fundamental law of timbre. When, on the other hand, the components are relatively close to one another, their patterns of excitation in the cochlea overlap a great deal. A change of phase, then, leads to a change of composite waveform and this may lead to a change of timbre. It appears that there is a close relation between perceptibility of phase changes and aural resolution of components. This relation was recognized much earlier (MATHES and MILLER, 1947), and the argument has been investigated repeatedly (see, *e. g.* LICKLIDER, 1955; GOLDSTEIN, 1967a).

The second factor that determines whether a phase change is perceptible concerns the magnitude of the phase change. If we think of a signal with narrowly spaced components, the phase change should cause a waveform variation exceeding a certain minimum variation in order to be perceptible. This waveform variation should pertain to a spectral width of approx. one critical band; hence, it would be logical to expect that the threshold for just noticeable phase changes can be expressed in terms of the phase deviations relative to a linear phase function [*cf.* Relation (10)] per critical band. As far as the author is aware, this line of reasoning has not been pursued systematically (probably because the

[2] $\to$ Means: is replaced by. $\Delta\varphi$ indicates a change of phase.

influence of sound intensity is so large). Phase effects of the nature considered here have continued to play an important part in residue theory, but other factors than those described above have been found to be important as well. However, the phase rule (10) has proven again to describe the phase changes for which the auditory system is "phase deaf". We shall come back to this point in Section H. 12.

9. The Pseudo-Fundamental Theory

The connection between perception of the residue and insufficient aural resolution of components was explicitly contained in SCHOUTEN's original definition. In this light, it is highly remarkable that DE BOER found that a residue pitch could be perceived quite well under conditions where the components are almost completely resolved. Such a residue shows clear changes of pitch when the signal is made inharmonic. Moreover, the pitch variations are larger than those expressed by Eq. (9), testifying to the fact that the "second effect" is quite large.

This result makes it impossible to advocate the pseudo-period theory as the *sole* explanation for pitch shifts due to inharmonicity. As an alternative, DE BOER proposed a theory operating on the frequencies of the individual (probably resolved) components. According to this theory, the auditory system tries to find a harmonic series of frequencies that corresponds in the best possible way with the frequencies of the components presented. For instance, the series of frequencies (7) can be approximated best by a harmonic series with 203 Hz as the fundamental frequency; the lowest components are just a bit too low and the highest components too high but on the average the deviations are minimal. The best-fitting fundamental frequency can be called the "pseudo-fundamental".

A more detailed formulation of this theory (DE BOER 1956a) shows that in first approximation the pseudo-fundamental is equal to an integral submultiple of the carrier frequency. Hence, the first effect of pitch shifts is again described by Eq. (9), the integer n being interpreted as the rank number of the carrier component. Actual pitch shifts are larger, of course, and the pseudo-fundamental theory has an inherent possibility to account for this fact. The determination of the best-fitting pseudo-fundamental must be made on the basis of some sort of criterion as to what is the "best" fit. In this process, the various components can be given different weights. For instance, the lower components can be considered as more important than the higher ones. In an inharmonic signal, the relative shift of the lower components is larger than that of the higher ones, and the resulting relative shift of the pseudo-fundamental will be larger when the lower components are given a larger weight. It will be seen that later developments in residue theory have utilized the same consideration. At the present stage of the description, we are not yet in a position to judge or appreciate these developments; the reader must abide his time: at least one major wave in scientific thinking is yet to come...

10. Two Types of Residue

According to DE BOER's findings, there are *two* types of residue. The first arises when components are relatively close together and cannot be resolved aurally. The pitch is probably derived from the waveform; the "pseudo-period" serves as the first-order determinant of the pitch for inharmonic signals. This type of residue is strongly phase sensitive – this term to be interpreted in the sense as described in the second part of Section E. 8. The second type of residue arises when the components are spaced relatively widely. This residue shows no phase effects, and the components are probably nearly completely resolved. The "pseudo-fundamental" can be proposed as a first approximation for the pitch of inharmonic residues of this type.

The two types of residue were named by DE BOER "intermittent" and "continuous" residue, respectively. These names are appropriate in an experimental setting in which phase effects are deliberately and continuously introduced: the intermittent residue then shows alternating periods of prominence and absence corresponding to the sharpness of timbre, and the continuous residue does not show any change with time. For the present, other names are to be preferred, names that have no connection with a particular experimental paradigm. We suggest short terms like *narrow* and *wide* residue; what is meant to express here is that the spectral components have narrow and wide spacings, respectively. These terms cannot easily be misinterpreted.

It might be objected that the word "residue" is a misnomer for the case of the wide residue since this is not the result of incomplete aural analysis. The term, "residue", is well known nowadays and there is no reason to abandon it now. Let us, therefore, continue to use this term, but let us use it in a wider sense. *The term "residue" is a universal descriptor for the joint perception of a number of components.* Whether the components are resolved or not, they give birth to a special percept by way of their combined action.

The two types of residue invoke different explanations of the observed pitch shifts due to inharmonicity. For a narrow complex, *i. e.* a signal yielding a narrow residue, the pseudo-period theory describes the pitch shifts in first approximation. For a wide complex, the pseudo-fundamental theory provides a more plausible explanation. There remain some difficulties in the explanation of the "second" effect. The pseudo-fundamental theory seems a bit more flexible, but we will see in the sequel that the pseudo-period theory must be amended also, and it finally receives about the same degree of flexibility as the pseudo-fundamental theory.

11. Multiple Modes of Pitch Perception

The present part of this chapter, in accordance with the title, wave crests, is mainly concerned with period-type aspects involved in residue perception. Hence, we continue with a short description of developments in the study of temporal phenomena, more specifically, the part played by the temporal order of pulses within one period. The experiments by the Bell group (FLANAGAN and GUTTMAN, 1960a, b; GUTTMAN and FLANAGAN, 1964) show that the question of periodicity perception is really somewhat more complex than previous work would suggest. Typical time sequences within one period are shown by Fig. 17. In the experiment, sequences of one type were matched with sequences of another type. When the repetition period of any of these signals is extremely low, *e. g.*, one second, one will hear one click per second for signal Number 1 but two clicks per second for signal Number 2, etc. When the repetition rate approaches 100 Hz (*i. e.* the period is repeated 100 times per second), the signals will be matched on the basis of their periodicity. This can be explained as the result of a pitch match, either of the fundamental's pitch or of the residue. For a signal like Number 4, the two modes differ by a factor of 4: for very low repetition rates, the signal is matched to a signal Number 1 with a repetition rate four times as high, whereas, at intermediate rates the best match is obtained when the rates are equal. There is a third mode, especially evident when the signals presented are devoid of their lower-order components. The match then occurs on the basis of the lowest component present; this mode is only evident for repetition rates above 500 Hz, hence, above the region which is important for periodicity pitch. An effort is made to correlate the findings with mechanistic events in the cochlea as reproduced by an analog model of the basilar membrane. All three "pitch modes" were found to be manifested in the mechanical operation of the cochlea. However, we think some caution is necessary. If we wish to explain the findings in terms of period detection, we do well to define exactly what we mean by period, and we must invoke specific assumptions as to what the auditory system will accept as a "periodic repetition" when in fact the repetition is only approximate (compare, *e. g.*, Signals 1 and 2).

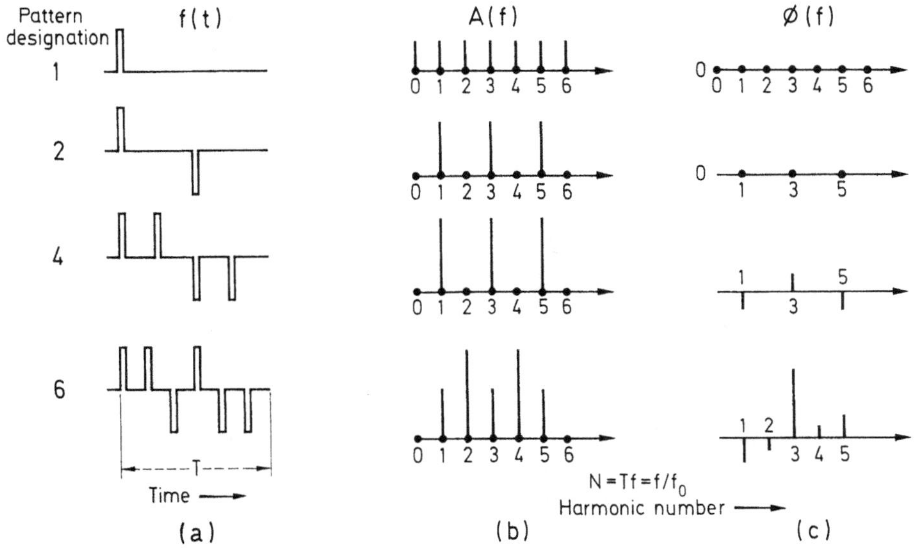

Fig. 17a—c. Waveform and spectrum of the signals used by FLANAGAN and GUTTMAN (1960a). (a) Waveforms $f(t)$ of the four signals used; T indicates the period of repetition. (b) Spectral amplitude $A(f)$ of the signals. (c) The phases $\Phi(f)$ of the spectral components, shown in a relative sense

12. Small's Work, Time Separation Pitch

That there are more subtleties involved in the perception of periodic multiple-pulse series is shown by the work of SMALL and collaborators. A signal most apt to give rise to periodicity pitch was produced by interrupting a pure tone, the carrier, repeatedly with a modulator. Typical signals were a carrier of 1000 Hz interrupted 100 times per second and a carrier of 5000 Hz interrupted 100 times per second. These signals are referred to as signals 1000/100 and 5000/100, respectively. The spectrum of such a signal is centered around the carrier frequency; to keep the spectral width down, each signal was filtered after the modulator by a band-pass filter centered around the carrier frequency. The pitch of the signal was determined by comparison with a pure tone. In contradistinction to usual methods, the matches were also carried out with a fixed tone of 100 Hz and a modulation rate which could be varied by the listener. The experiments confirmed that a low pitch of about 100 Hz is the main aspect of the signal; a match to a frequency in the region of the most prominent spectral components either could not be made or could be made with difficulty by the listeners (SMALL, 1955).

The most conspicuous finding is reported for a type of signal in which two of these pulse series are combined. Both series have nearly the same repetition frequency, *e. g.*, 100 Hz. At a certain moment, the sum of the two signals is a double pulse series as is schematically indicated by Fig. 18. (In this figure the pulses are drawn as rectangular, but, in fact, they are small sections of an oscillating waveform.) As time progresses, the pulses of one series drift with respect to those of the other series, to complete one period in something like 5 sec. THURLOW and SMALL (1955) reported that in this type of signal one can hear a pitch that is associated with this course of the time separation τ. When τ is very

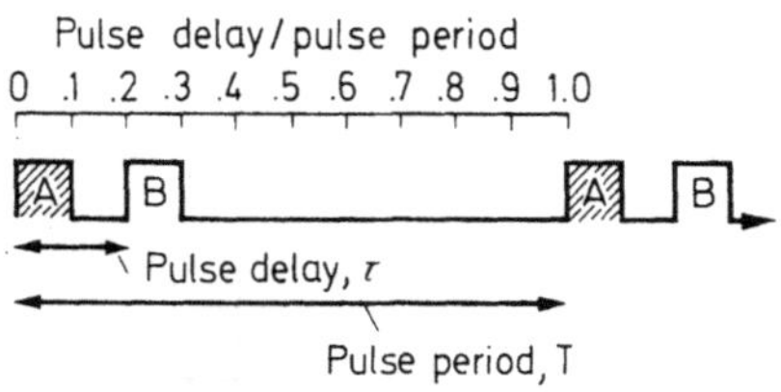

Fig. 18. Signal to demonstrate the "sweep pitch" (time-separation pitch). After SMALL and MCCLELLAN (1963)

small, this pitch is high. When τ gradually increases, the pitch drops downward. From the point that τ passes the center of the period, the pitch goes up again. The lowest pitch corresponds, of course, to the octave of the basic repetition frequency, in this case, to 200 Hz. The highest pitch was difficult to judge; in the 5000/100 condition it was considered to be higher than 1000 Hz. The effect was the most noticeable when the bandwidth of the spectrum was rather wide, a reason for experimenting with unfiltered pulse series later. In view of the experimental paradigm, this pitch was named the "sweep pitch". Since it appears to be closely associated with the separation in time between pulses, the later adopted term, "Time Separation Pitch (TSP), is a better one. It is to be noted that this type of pitch can best be heard in a situation just as the one described: a signal consisting of two pulse series with slightly different repetition frequencies. It is then recognized because of its sweeping character.

In a later study (SMALL and MCCLELLAN, 1963), it was experimentally confirmed that time separation pitch corresponds to the frequency $1/\tau$. In this study, the value of τ was constant in one experimental run. To concentrate the attention of the listener upon time separation pitch, one amongst three signals could be chosen: a single pulse series, the double pulse series, and a pure tone. The results were remarkably accurate; the largest deviations were 20 cents (*i. e.* 0.2 of a semitone; 100 cents is equivalent to one semitone). Some incidental deviations occurred but few of these were investigated further. In these experiments, the basic repetition frequencies were 25, 100, and 400 Hz, and the pulses were approximately rectangular. The relative pulse delay τ/T (see the figure) could be varied between 0.1 and 0.5. The resulting pitch had a range between 50 and 4000 Hz.

The results of SMALL and MCCLELLAN are considered to confirm that the major cue for pitch determination consists in the timing aspects of the waveform. There is no mention made as to whether a melody can be made out of time separation pitches. The study of pitch perceptions related to time separations has in later times been taken up again under the heading, repetition pitch (BILSEN, 1966; see Section F. 8). The case described in the present section appears to be just an example of the great variety of signals for which some hidden type of repetition is heard as a pitch. A more general case is a noise signal to which a delayed version of the same noise signal is added; such a signal also acquires a pitch inversely proportional to the delay time. Since the philosophy of this type of experiment involves concepts which yet have to be developed, we must defer the description of this work until later.

13. Averaging of Pseudo-Periods and Pseudo-Fundamentals

From the findings described in the preceding sections, it is evident that even the most straightforward period theory runs into difficulties when confronted with experimental findings. The situation becomes quite complicated when we realize that the actual excitation at a particular location in the cochlea has the character of a band-filtered form of the stimulus. The time separations, which are so clear from the waveform of the sound stimulus as presented to the ear, are not nearly as evident from bandpass-filtered waveforms. Moreover, it is not certain that the time distance between peaks in the waveform of filtered signals is equal to the corresponding distance in the unfiltered waveform. Consider, for example, a wide-band inharmonic signal. For the waveform of the actual stimulus, the pseudo-period can readily be determined (see Fig. 16b). If we consider, however, a location on the basilar membrane tuned to a frequency in the lower part of the signal's spectrum, we observe a pseudo-period that deviates more from the period $1/g$. We may refer to Eq. (9) but note that the integer constant n is now equal to the rank order of the strongest component passed by the filter. For a wide-band inharmonic signal, there will exist an ensemble of pseudo-period values corresponding to different cochlea locations; these pseudo-periods will all be different. Consequently, when we hear but a single pitch, the pseudo-period values must be weighed and averaged in some way by the auditory system. The situation is still more complicated since the pseudo-period will not always be an integral submultiple of the local carrier. This is the result of phase modulation exhibited by the filtered signal. In fact, this process has been studied by FISCHLER as a possible means to explain the second effect (FISCHLER, 1967). We may conclude that although a residue theory on the basis of temporal phenomena may be attractive at first sight, the actual situation is by no means simple. Due appreciation of the ensemble of pseudo-periods, as described above, makes the pseudo-period theory considerably more flexible. In the process of averaging all pseudo-periods, we may consider giving different weights to different frequency regions. It is then easy to explain the existence of the "second" effect just as with the pseudo-fundamental theory. However, the magnitude of the second effect still presents difficulties.

14. Pitch Ambiguity; the Relation between Phase Effects and Aural Resolution

The studies reported in the period 1950–1960 have clearly shown the basic dilemma in residue theory. Most of the experimental findings fit well within the framework of a theory based on periodicity concepts. In this respect, the research reported in the preceding sections is a straightforward extension of SCHOUTEN's work. Two points are of special interest in this connection and are worthy of mention in a summary. The first point is that the auditory system appears to be able to utilize temporal information of greater subtlety than that contained in basic periodicity. The "sweep-note" effect discovered by THURLOW and SMALL proves that detailed repetitions contained in the signal's waveform can provide a cue for pitch. Later, the pitch associated with time separation was called, time-separation pitch; this name appropriately describes the most probable cue.

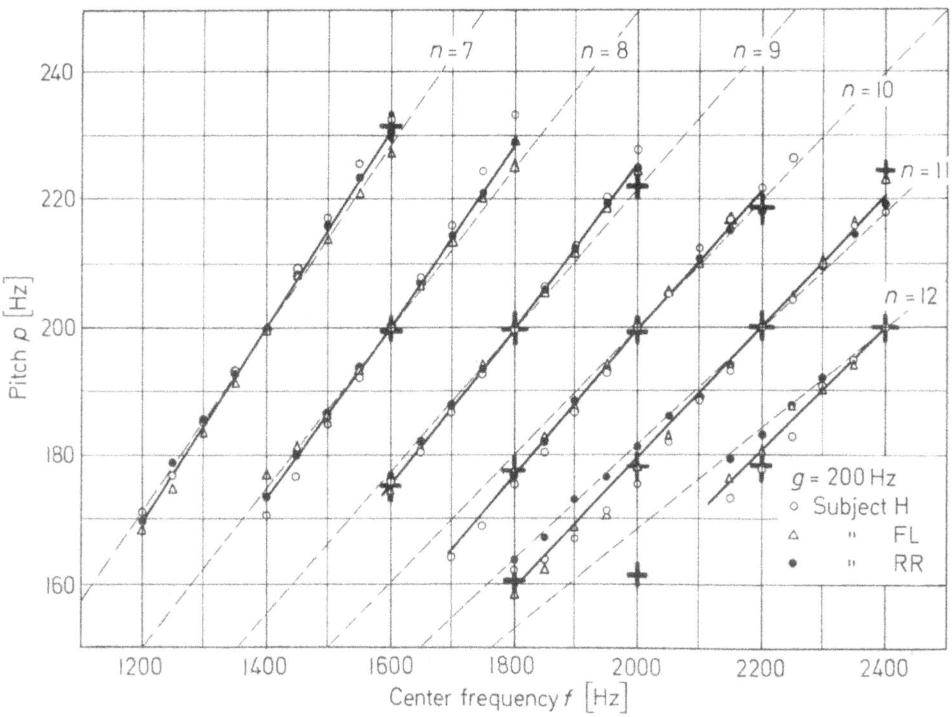

Fig. 19. Pitch measurements for three-component signals. Difference of component frequencies: 200 Hz. After SCHOUTEN *et al.* (1962)

The second point about temporal cues in a signal's waveform concerns ambiguity. In DE BOER's experiments on inharmonic signals, the situation midway between two consecutive harmonic situations led to two possible pitches. In terms of the signal waveform involved, this ambiguity is readily explained (see Fig. 16c). Which of the two possible pitches will be perceived depends on the state of attention, the signals heard previously, and so on. SCHOUTEN *et al.* (1962) repeated the experiments on inharmonic signals with complexes consisting of 3 components instead of 5 or 7. Their findings confirmed the existence of the "first" and "second" effects, but, moreover, they extended the concept of ambiguity of pitch. Figure 19 shows the results, pitch (p) as a function of the central frequency (f) of the complex. We observe that the lines connecting the data points can be extended over a wider range than is possible for DE BOER's results (Fig. 15). At any particular value of f, three or more pitches are possible. This does not necessarily imply that all of these pitches are equally prominent, of course.

We may note in passing that, apart from the second effect, the lines in Fig. 19 can be labelled on the basis of different values of n in Eq. (9). The existence of more than one pitch value then implies that the auditory system may utilize different values of n. The experimental procedure (a gradual increase of f, for instance) forces the subject to stick to a particular value of n but eventually his attention goes astray and he may pick up another pitch, corresponding to a different value of n.

We arrive at the remarkable conclusion that even in a purely harmonic complex a number of discrete pitches are acceptable to the subject. This finding was confirmed by a special experiment in which the listeners were instructed to try to find all possible pitches in a harmonic complex. The crosses in Fig. 19 show the results of this procedure; each cross stands for the centre of a cluster of data points.

Not all experimental results fit well within the framework of a "periodicity" theory. The experiments described in Section E. 11 clearly indicate that the auditory system possesses capabilities to adjust itself differently to the same situation. The clearest example is the finding of the existence of the "wide" residue, a residue formed out of a series of components that are probably almost completely resolved by the ear. This residue has all the properties of the "narrow" residue, except that it does not show phase effects. In particular, it is (at least) equally tonal. A pure temporal theory runs into difficulties when it is applied to a signal with widely spaced components. The pseudo-fundamental theory seems more fruitful in this case. It should be noted that the pseudo-fundamental theory can be regarded as an extension of the "old" place theory: the pseudo-fundamental frequency is determined on the basis of the frequencies of the components but it can equally well be based upon the "places" at which the components produce the largest excitations in the cochlea.

The last subject which should be mentioned in this summary concerns phase effects. It is well to remember at this stage the following properties of the residue:

a) The timbre of the residue is not affected by a phase change conforming to relation (10).

b) Equivalently, even the slightest amount of inharmonicity of the signal [of the type corresponding to Relation (10)] is inaudible.

c) Phase changes that do not agree with Relation (10) may cause changes of timbre; whether they do, depends greatly on the relative frequency spacing of the components. In this sense, phase effects are usually considered indicators of insufficient frequency resolution of signal components.

F. The Next "Cycle": Forebodings of a New Way of Thinking

1. Introduction

The period from 1960 to 1970 has witnessed a change in attitude toward the residue theory because a few new concepts have been formulated. Again, it has taken a long time before the findings were generally interpreted in what appeared to be scientifically the most advanced way. In the present part of this chapter, we shall describe this development. As has been explained in the introduction, there will be no room for an elaborate description of all of these newer studies; the relevant literature is easily accessible. We shall instead concentrate upon the conceptual development. Let it be repeated that the emphasis placed upon the various aspects of the work is the result of personal opinions of the present reviewer. Admittedly, other interpretations are possible; the one expressed here ties in with the newest developments and agrees with present views of most other experts in the field.

The major argument is concerned with the fact that there exists more than one type of residue. Furthermore, these residues are not equivalent to one another. Since one type of residue may be considered as "inferior" to another one, a relation like Eq. (9) for pitch shifts due to inharmonicity acquires a new perspective. In particular, the value of n in this equation need not be the rank number of the central component. It may be adjusted to be relevant to the more dominant part of the residue signal, as we shall see. In any event, the explanation of various properties of the residue has acquired a new dimension. The increased complexity of the matter has not lessened the trouble necessary for theoretical explanation of the experimental findings. For the moment, it seems better to stick to rather formal types of theorizing. Later developments may perhaps provide new insight that will serve to make simple what seemed quite complicated at first.

2. The Existence Region of the Residue (Ritsma)

It was Ritsma, one of Schouten's pupils, who made the first important contribution in this era (1962). He was intrigued by Hoogland's (1953) failure to detect a low-frequency pitch when the signal presented consisted of a number of components that were relatively close to one another ($f = 3000$, $g = 100$, for instance) and less than 60 dB SPL in level. Ritsma guessed that such sound complexes would indeed give a residue but one which is essentially without pitch. Consequently, he set out to explore the tonality of residue sounds for widely divergent values of the central frequency f and the component spacing g. He produced his 3-component signals with the modulation method (see Section D. 6 for an explanation). When the carrier frequency is f and the modulation frequency g, the resulting components will have the frequencies $f-g$ and $f+g$. A third component (carrier) with frequency f is added. In all signals f and g are harmonically related. One further experimental variable, m, is introduced by

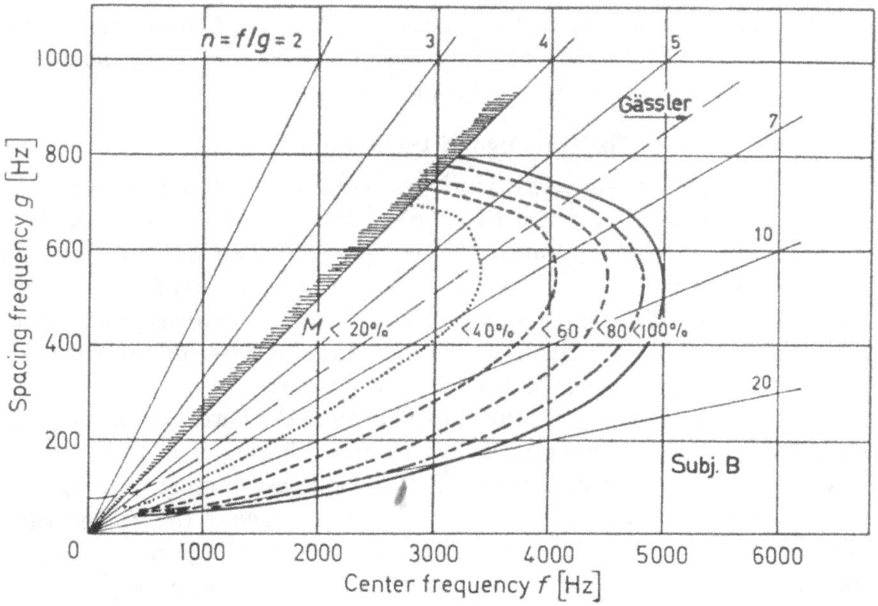

Fig. 20. Existence region for three-component residue signals. M is the modulation depth (called m in the text). The line marked "Gässler" indicates the critical bandwidth. After Ritsma (1962)

making the former two components variable in strength with respect to the latter. The amplitudes of these so-called sidebands are $^1/_2\, m$ as against unity for the carrier component. The constant m, the "modulation index", could be varied between 0.2 and a little over 1.0 (see Ritsma's paper for further details). In one experimental run, one of the parameters f, g, or m was varied while the others were kept constant.

Subjects were instructed to determine the limiting values for the variable parameter so as to find the boundary of the region of parameter values that leads to a *tonal* pitch. To aid in the judgement of tonality, a comparison signal was provided with a fixed modulation index m of 1.00, the same value of g and a considerably lower value of f. A typical result is shown in Fig. 20. The line $f/g = 4$ is a natural boundary because the value of 3 would lead to a signal of which the lowest component is just an octave above the residue pitch, a situation which would be too confusing for the listener.

Consider now the line for $m = 1.00$. This delineates the largest area in which residue signals of this type can be perceived as having a definite pitch, *the existence region of the tonal residue*. One of the most noteworthy features of this region is that it shows no evidence of being linked to the limits of auditory frequency analysis. The line which depicts the width of the critical band (*cf.* Zwicker *et al.*,

1957) corresponds to $f/g = 6$; this line (marked "Gässler" in Fig. 20) does not lie near the boundary of the existence region of the three-component residue. On the contrary, it runs right through it.

We may realize, however, that the resolution of components lying outside each other's critical bands is far from complete. A period-extracting procedure may then very well be postulated as an universal mechanism. RITSMA's (1962) paper gives further details about this mechanism; this development from earlier models of this kind (LICKLIDER, 1951) was made possible by the advances in our knowledge of the auditory system in the preceding period.

3. The Principle of Dominance I

The experiments that have led to the second important step were simultaneously, and apparently independently, carried out by RITSMA (1967) and PLOMP (1967a). In fact, the experiments were carried out in two different countries (USA and the Netherlands), and the manuscripts were received by the editor within one month. We shall describe mostly RITSMA's experiments. PLOMP's method was essentially similar and led to the same results. PLOMP's paper is, furthermore, recommended for its historical introduction.

In RITSMA's (as well as in PLOMP's) experiments, the lower components were derived from a repetitive pulse series by low-pass filtering. The higher components were derived from another pulse series by high-pass filtering. The repetition frequencies of the two pulse series were not the same. One of the residue signals (A) consisted of the lower harmonics with fundamental frequency f_0, up to a cut-off frequency f_c; the components above f_c were harmonics belonging to a fundamental frequency $f_0 + \Delta f$ (see Fig. 21). In the comparison signal (B), the

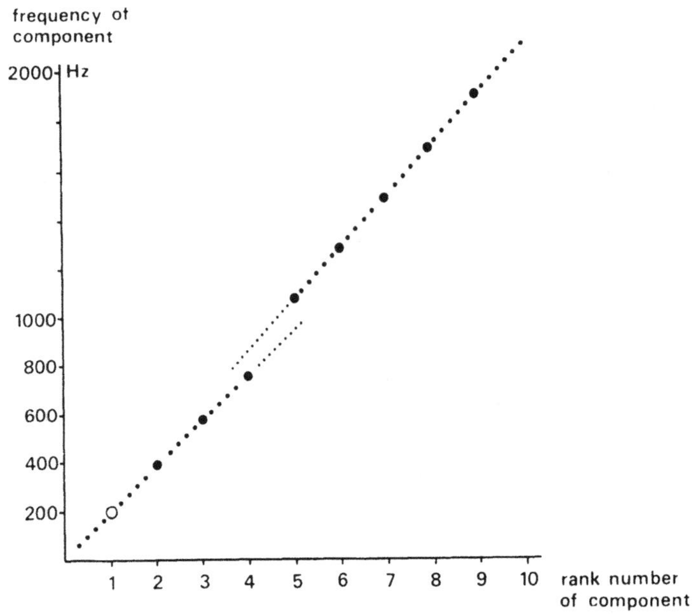

Fig. 21. Components of signal containing two conflicting types of information for pitch. The slopes of the dotted lines indicate the frequencies f_0 and $f_0 + \Delta f$. Only the A-signal is shown. The fundamental of the lower band is indicated by an open circle. Note that both dotted lines meet at the origin

roles of f_0 and $f_0 + \Delta f$ were interchanged; the subjects were to judge which of the tones had the higher pitch. The relative difference $\Delta f/f_0$ was 3 or 6%. For low values of f_c, Signal A was always judged to be higher in pitch; for high values of f_c Signal B had a higher pitch. The cross-over point depended somewhat upon the listener. For $f_0 = 100$, it was in the range 400–700 Hz; for $f_0 = 200$, it was

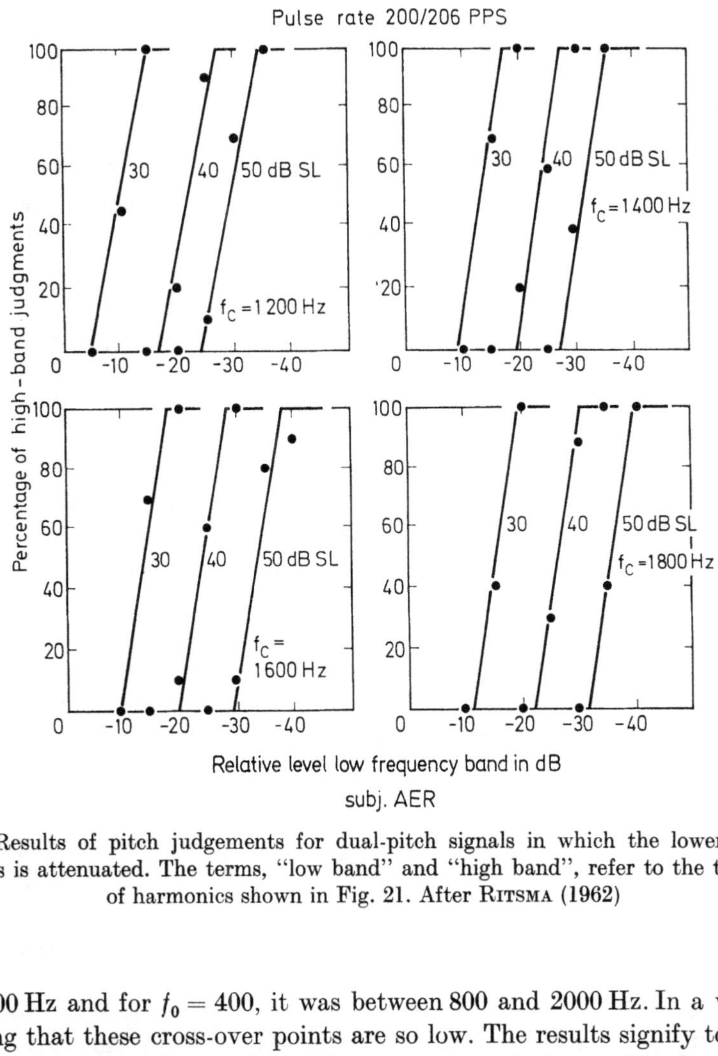

Fig. 22. Results of pitch judgements for dual-pitch signals in which the lower group of harmonics is attenuated. The terms, "low band" and "high band", refer to the two groups of harmonics shown in Fig. 21. After Ritsma (1962)

800–1400 Hz and for $f_0 = 400$, it was between 800 and 2000 Hz. In a way, it is surprising that these cross-over points are so low. The results signify to the fact that even a foursome harmonics of frequency f_0 against a multitude of components (all components above the fourth) with a fundamental of $f_0 + \Delta f$ force the total sound to have a pitch corresponding to f_0. The lower components are clearly *dominant*. Even though they are much less numerous, they outweigh the higher components.

To bring out this fact still further, Ritsma attempted to determine how strong these lower components should be to exercise this dominance. In his second experiment, f_c was fixed, and the lower components were attenuated by a variable amount. Again, the signals were presented in a two-alternative forced-choice test, and the subjects were required to judge which signal was higher in pitch. Some typical results, judgement percentage as a function of the attenuation level of the lower components, are presented in Fig. 22. It is this figure that gives the clearest demonstration of the principle of dominance: the lower components assume dominance within a level range of 5–10 dB. The threshold depends on the overall sound level in such a way that it seems that the lower components assume dominance once they surpass a certain threshold level, approximately 10 dB SL.

4. The Principle of Dominance II

In the third series of experiments, Ritsma attempted to reduce the number of components in the dominant part of the residue still further. The low-frequency part of the signal was filtered in such a way that only 2 or 3 components were left; all others were attenuated so much as to be inaudible. The lowest fundamental frequency was 200 Hz in this series. Again, there was a sharp transition in judgements when the level of this low-frequency part was varied. The general conclusion of this experiment is that at least two of the three components 600, 800, and 1000 Hz have to be present to exercise their dominance. The dominance becomes manifest as soon as these components are more than 10 dB above the subjective threshold.

Before we try to draw general conclusions, some minor points should be mentioned. Some listeners reported an ambiguity of pitch when the cut-off frequency f_c of the filters was in the dominant region. They reported no beats; apparently two neighbouring pitches can be present in a sound and this does not necessarily lead to beats. A second point is that in both Ritsma's and Plomp's basic experiments the fundamental was present as one of the components. The results of the experiments indicate that the residue formed by higher components, all except the first, is dominant. In other words, the fundamental is *not* dominant, a point which is repeatedly stressed by Plomp.

5. Some Reflections, the Second Effect

In the following sections, we shall encounter more examples of the principle of dominance. But before we describe further experiments, it is good to reflect on some previous findings and the possible connection with dominance. One of the most puzzling aspects has been the so-called "second effect" (see Section E.7). It is relatively easy to understand that the pitch of an inharmonic signal would be proportional to the frequency of the central component. That the relative pitch deviations actually are larger than the relative variations of the central component points to a more complex mechanism. In Section E. 13, it was pointed out that for an inharmonic signal the various pseudo-periods that can be associated with different locations in the cochlea are all different. Hence, if pitch is determined by the pseudo-period, it surely is an average of these pseudo-periods that should be considered. Conversely, if we want to assume a mechanism analogous to finding the pseudo-fundamental, it is again an average measure of this kind that should be envisaged. The averaging is performed over the domain of component frequencies, and soon it has been realized that the lower frequency regions carry the larger weight in the averaging process. There appear now to be *two* reasons for this. The first is related to the fact that our auditory frequency scale is a logarithmic one; in other words, the lower harmonics are wider apart, in a musical sense, than the higher ones. This differential weighing has been pointed out as a possible contribuant from the beginning period of the study of inharmonic signals on. In general, this type of weighing has been found insufficient.

RITSMA's and PLOMP's findings have contributed a second reason: the lower components are dominant with respect to pitch, and, hence, they should carry a far larger weight. The distribution of weights is very uneven indeed. The best agreement between experiment and theory can be obtained only by giving the lower components an overwhelmingly larger weight. Thus, WALLISER (1968, 1969a) could report that the pitch of the inharmonic residue is given by the frequency of the *lowest* component in the complex divided by its rank number. In other terms, the "centre of gravity" of the complex lies at the lowest component.

6. The Residue in a New Definition, Resolution of Components

The discovery of the principle of dominance has a profound effect on our thinking. If we recall that the residue was originally defined as the joint perception of the unresolved components, we are surprised to find that the dominant part of a residue signal resides in the region of lower components. Clearly, the sound that we perceive associated with the lower components has all the aspects of the residue. Hence, the definition should be modified so as to incorporate specifically this dominant part of the spectrum where components can be resolved almost perfectly by a trained ear. The new, less restrictive, definition reads:

A residue is the joint perception of a number of consecutive components.

It then becomes paramount to study the question as to which components in a residue signal can be resolved by the ear and which cannot. The dividing line between frequency resolution and spectral integration is provided by the "critical bandwidth". Abundant references can be found throughout the literature (for a short survey see DE BOER and BOUWMEESTER, 1974). For the frequencies of interest, the width of the critical band is approx. 16% of the frequency. This is represented, *e.g.*, by the line $f/g = 1/0.16$ in Fig. 20 (marked "Gässler").

Specific experiments on aural resolution in residue signals have been carried out by PLOMP (1964). The results of these experiments indicate the extent to which a component can be aurally separated from the complex. We shall describe only one of the experiments. A listener can choose, by way of a switch, to listen to a periodic residue signal or a pure tone. Actually, he has two possible pure tones at his disposal, one of which coinciding with one of the harmonics of the periodic signal and the other lying midway between two consecutive harmonics. The situation is symbolized in Fig. 23. The listener's task is to select from the two pure tones the one he considers to correspond to one of the audible harmonics of the periodic signal.

The experiment is conducted with the familiar two-alternative forced choice method. When the comparison tones are in the extreme high part of the spectrum, the probability of a correct answer is 0.50. Of course, the lower components can be detected with a probability of 1.0. Results were, in short, that the percentage of correct responses dropped from 100 to 50 in the range of n = 4 to n = 9.

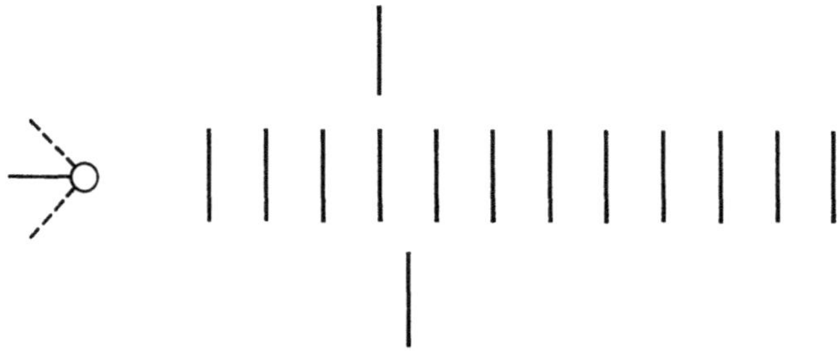

Fig. 23. The three signals from which the subject can choose in PLOMP's (1964) experiments on aural resolution. The lines indicate frequencies of components. The circle symbolizes the selection switch. After PLOMP (1964)

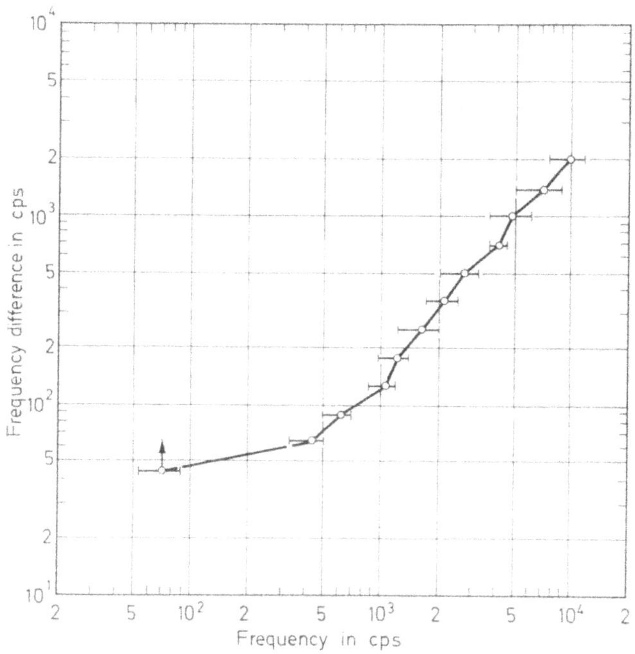

Fig. 24. Frequency difference between harmonics required to hear the part-tones separately. The course of the measured thresholds as a function of frequency corresponds closely to that of the critical bandwidth. After PLOMP (1964)

The results were essentially similar for inharmonic signals. The frequency difference of components that can be aurally resolved depends upon the central frequency in a way that is closely similar to the characteristics of the critical bandwidth. The relation is depicted in Fig. 24.

The results of PLOMP's study once more underline the fact that the dominant region of a residue signal is a region in which single components can be picked out of the signal with nearly perfect certainty. It should be noted, however, that this does not imply that the determination of the pitch of the residue cannot possibly be performed on a temporal basis. That a component can be aurally separated does not mean that components do not interact in the ear. The arguments provided by studies like this are only suggestive; for the dominant part of the residue, it is likely that interaction of components is minimal.

7. Audibility of High Partials

Although the higher components of a periodic pulse signal cannot be distinguished from one another, this does not mean that they cannot be detected under any circumstance. With a special procedure, even extremely high harmonics can be made audible. This effect has been studied by DUIFHUIS (1970, 1971). A brief description of the experiments follows. The basic signal is a periodic pulse series with fundamental frequency f_0. The repetition frequency f_0 was rather low, 25–100 Hz. A sinusoid of (exactly) the frequency $n \cdot f_0$ is generated separately and added to the pulse series. The phase of this extra component is fixed in such a way that the n-th harmonic in the sum signal can be present at any desired intensity and with positive as well as negative polarity.

The threshold of detection for the reconstituted n-th component can be determined as a function of its polarity. For values of n below 10, the threshold is the same for both polarities, as expected. For extremely high values, above 28, polarity has a profound effect. The result is that, when the n-th harmonic is added with the amplitude it normally has in the periodic pulse series, it cannot be detected. The *absence* of this harmonic can be detected very well. Similarly, the n-th harmonic can be detected when it has twice its normal amplitude. In the region with n between 10 and 28, a gradual transition appears between the two types of behaviour.

In DUIFHUIS' paper, a possible interpretation of the results for high n values is given. Consider the response of a high-frequency band-pass filter (tuned to the n-th harmonic) to a periodic pulse series, *e.g.*, from Fig. 11. The response to each pulse is extremely short. If we subtract the n-th component from the signal, it shows up in the response as a sinusoid filling up most of the period between the pulses. It can now be understood why we are able to hear the n-th component as a pure tone when it is actually absent in the spectrum. Furthermore, this explains why the complex sounds exactly the same when the n-th component is present with double its normal amplitude and when the n-th component is completely absent.

In the second paper (DUIFHUIS, 1971), the full consequences of the idea suggested earlier were pursued. Consider again the response of a high-frequency band-pass filter tuned to the n-th harmonic, and let the stimulus be a not-modified series of pulses. The response of the filter comes in bursts synchronous with the pulses. Between the pulses, there is little excitation, and it is likely that an extremely short tone burst can be detected when it is presented at just the right instant between the pulses. The threshold will be higher when the tone burst coincides with the peak of the filtered signal. This reasoning is borne out by the results of measurements. The short tone bursts were made to contain approximately 8 complete sinusoidal oscillations; the harmonic numbers used were 20,

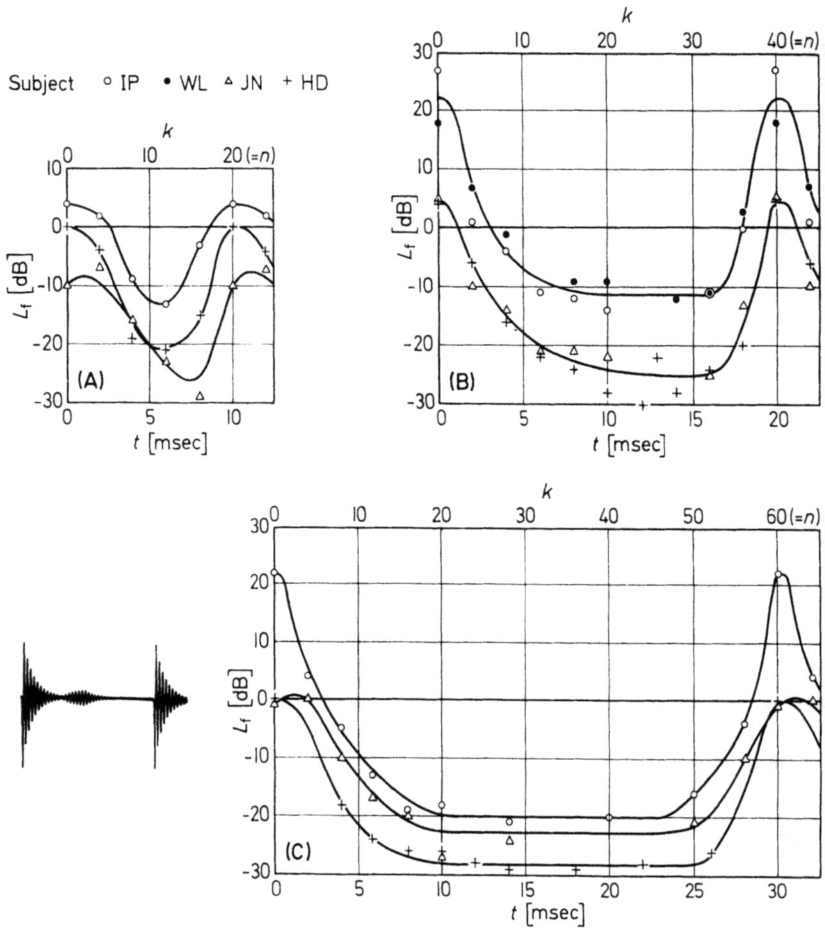

Fig. 25. Threshold of a tone pulse as a function of its temporal position in the period of a periodic pulse series. The tone frequency is 2 kHz; in A, B, and C the repetition frequencies are 100, 50, and $33^1/_3$ Hz (hence the harmonic numbers are 20, 40, and 60, respectively). The inset shows schematically how we conceive of the response of the "auditory filter" tuned to 2 kHz to the stimulus. After DUIFHUIS (1970)

40, 60, and 80. The threshold (not the threshold of audibility but the lowest level at which the added component could be recognized as a pure tone) was studied as a function of the delay t, between the pulse and the centre of the tone bursts. The results are presented as a function of the dimensionless variable k, defined as $k = nt/T$ where T is the time between successive pulses. Figure 25 shows the results for three different values of T and a fixed value of 2 kHz for the frequency of the n-th component. This figure shows that the threshold declines smoothly when the tone burst is moved away from the pulse. The course of this decline reflects the decay of activity of the auditory filter at this frequency after it has been excited by a pulse. DUIFHUIS was able to estimate the value of 10 as the best fitting value of the so-called "quality factor" of the pertinent resonant circuit. This value agrees well with similar values determined from responses of auditory nerve fibers (KIANG *et al.*, 1965). Corresponding values obtained from psychophysical measurements of masking patterns indicate similar or somewhat higher values.

8. Repetition Pitch

We conclude this part with the description of auditory phenomena that are not readily explained by either a temporal or a spectral analysis. "Time-separation pitch" (see Section E. 12) as studied by SMALL and associates seems at first sight a purely temporal phenomenon: pitch is closely associated with time separation. This simple-minded notion is reinforced when we realize that this pitch remains clear when the repetition rate of the pulse pairs is made very low or when the pulse pairs (always with the same interval) appear at a random rate (MCCLELLAN and SMALL, 1967). However, the pitch deviates when the second pulse of each pair is inverted (FOURCIN, 1965). As will be seen later, one possible explanation of this effect includes spectral filtering and the manifestation of a region of spectral dominance.

In the present section, we shall describe an effect that likewise suggests a purely temporal type of auditory processing but that turns out later to be more complex in nature. The effect is called "repetition pitch" (BILSEN, 1966) and we shall consider here only the monaural case. To the ear of the listener is presented the sum of two signals, a white-noise signal $n(t)$ and the identical white-noise signal delayed by a time τ. The waveform is then

$$x(t) = n(t) + pn(t - \tau), \tag{11}$$

where $p = +1$. This signal acquires a peculiar timbre due to the presence of the echo but by varying the delay τ it readily becomes apparent that there is a pitch associated with it. It comes as no surprise that the pitch corresponds to the frequency $1/\tau$ just as for time-separation pitch. The name "repetition pitch" (RP) seems quite appropriate since the phenomenon is manifest only when the delayed signal is highly correlated with the first signal. When the polarity factor p is made -1, the echo has the opposite polarity. There results a definite shift of the pitch of a little over two semitones (*cf.* FOURCIN, 1965). BILSEN (1966) made careful measurements of these pitch shifts, and he found that there were two pitches possible. These corresponded to the frequencies $1.14/\tau$ and $0.87/\tau$, respectively. Essentially the same values were obtained when the identical procedure was repeated but with randomly presented pulse pairs (Time Separation Pitch). Under the conditions tested, the accuracy of pitch matches appeared to be somewhat better for time-separation pitch than for repetition pitch.

The $p = -1$ condition is obtained by inverting the delayed version of the original input signal $n(t)$; or, in other words, shifting the phases of all components of the delayed signal over 180 degrees. A situation "halfway" between $p = +1$ and $p = -1$ can be obtained by shifting the phases of all components of the delayed input signal over 90° before adding the echo to the input. This case cannot be described by a specific value for p in Eq. (11) since the waveform of the "echo" is now quite different from that of the original signal $n(t)$. In fact, waveforms like these can only be obtained with sophisticated signal processing methods. The procedure resulted in pitch shifts about halfway between those discussed above. The pitch for the 90° condition was approximately $1.08/\tau$; this holds for both repetition pitch (RP) and time-separation pitch (TSP). Note that such a result cannot be accounted for by a simple temporal processing mechanism, a point to which we will return later.

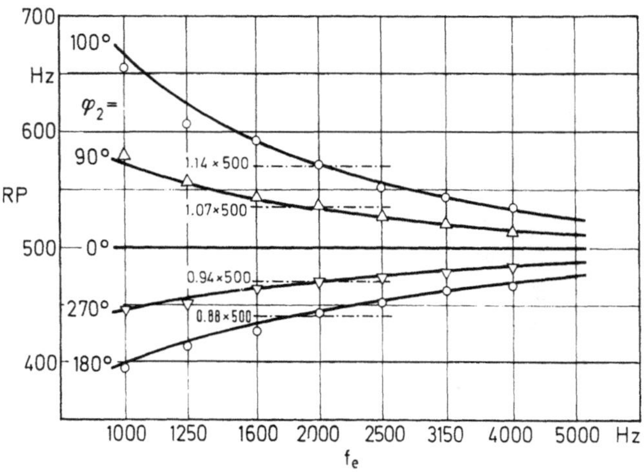

Fig. 26. The pitch of repetition pitch (RP) for four experimental conditions. Signals are filtered to a 1/3-octave bandwidth. Time delay τ: 2 msec. Abscissa: centre frequency of the filter. Central line: p = +1. Circles: p = —1 (two pitches). Triangles: echo phase shifted over +90° or —90°. Solid lines: computed according to $RP = 1/(\tau \pm 1/2f_0)$ for p = — 1 and $RP = 1/(\tau \pm 1/4f_0)$ for the ±90° conditions. Dashed lines: unfiltered signal with p = —1. After BILSEN and RITSMA (1969/1970)

In a later series of experiments, BILSEN and RITSMA determined the pitches for filtered signals. In view of the intimate relation between RP and TSP, they performed their experiments only with one type of signal, a series of pulse pairs with time interval τ. The (average) repetition rate was 20 times per second; the pulse pairs could be presented periodically or with random inter-pair intervals. The signal was filtered by a third-octave band-pass filter before being led to the ear. Figure 26 shows a representative result, the measured pitch for four conditions of the "echo" as a function of the central frequency of the band-pass filter. A theoretical estimate of expected pitch shifts can be obtained as follows. The response of the third octave filter with central frequency f_0 to the first pulse is a short-duration oscillation with frequency f_0 (the filter "rings" because it has relatively low damping). The response to the second pulse is similar but it differs in details depending upon the phase shift that the second pulse has undergone. For the case $p = +1$ the distance between the most prominent peaks will be an integral number of periods $T_0 = 1/f_0$. This distance will be close to τ, of course. For $p = -1$, the distance will be an odd number of half periods. This leads to the prediction that for the $p = -1$ condition the pitch will be $1/(\tau \pm 1/2f_0)$. A similar prediction can be made for the 90° and 270° conditions. These theoretical functions are drawn as solid lines in Fig. 26. It is seen that the measured points are all quite close to these lines.

The same reasoning can be applied backwards for the case in which the signal is not filtered. The measured pitch shifts then correspond to the pitch shifts for a value of f_0 which is about 4 times $1/\tau$. See the dashed lines in the figure. This can be formulated in terms of a dominant region; for wide-band RP signals, the pitch shifts are determined from the frequency region that is centered at 4 times $1/\tau$. The authors conclude that it is not possible to explain the properties of RP solely in the temporal domain. Neither is it possible to find a explanation in the spectral domain. We shall come back to this point later (Section H. 14). Only a combined approach, in which a temporal analysis is carried out from the signal as it appears filtered in the dominant frequency region, is fruitful. It remains puzzling that the auditory system does not employ a fixed dominance region but seems to adjust it on the basis of the time difference τ between signal and echo.

G. The Missing Link (Towards a Unified Framework)

1. Nonlinear Processes, Combination Tones

Several of the studies described in the preceding sections have put more emphasis on the spectral properties of residue signals than on the periodicity. This trend was initiated by the work on dominance (Section F. 4ff.) and it has been substantiated by later studies. In view of this aspect, it is necessary to give additional details about the internal representation of the spectrum. Two aspects of this have already been described, aural resolution (or critical-band filtering) and specific temporal effects induced by isolated high-frequency components. There is one aspect in which the internal representation of the spectrum differs from the objective spectrum, even when these two points are taken into account. Under special circumstances, our auditory system generates distortion products that contribute significantly to our perception. The presentation of a residue signal consisting of just a few components makes this effect especially noticeable. That is the reason why we have to be more specific about auditory nonlinearity than we were in Section B. 3.

The process of nonlinear distortion is usually studied in the case of a simple nonlinear transfer system. Consider a system in which an input signal $x(t)$ is transformed into an output signal $y(t)$ in such a way that each value of $y(t)$ is just a function of the value of $x(t)$ at the same instant of time:

$$y(t) = F\{x(t)\}. \tag{12}$$

Such a system is an instantaneous nonlinear transform system, often referred to as "memoryless". If the function F(a) which is the descriptive function of this system, were linear in a, no new Fourier components would be generated. Suppose now that $F(a)$ is a quadratic function of a, then the effect of Eq. (12) would be that each signal would appear to be multiplied by itself. Compare Eq. (5) of Section E. 6 when $x_1(t)$ and $x_2(t)$ refer to the same sinusoidal signal $x(t)$. Two new components will arise, one with the frequency 0 (which is immaterial in this context) and one with the double frequency. Hence, such a nonlinearity produces the second harmonic of a sinusoidal input signal. If the input signal $x(t)$ contains two components with frequencies f_1 and f_2, the output will consist of these harmonics and two further components having frequencies equal to $f_2 - f_1$ and

$f_2 + f_1$. Such a purely quadratic distortion is rarely encountered, however. It would be more appropriate to consider $F(a)$ as mixed:

$$F(a) = c_1 a + c_2 a^2. \tag{13}$$

Such a system transmits the original frequencies f_1 and f_2, and it generates distortion products with frequencies $2f_1$, $2f_2$, $f_2 - f_1$, and $f_2 + f_1$. A more complicated nonlinear system is described by

$$F(a) = c_1 a + c_2 a^2 + c_3 a^3. \tag{14}$$

The third-order term produces the following distortion products for a two-component stimulus:

a) the third harmonics of each component, frequencies $3f_1$ and $3f_2$,

b) third-order combination tones, frequencies $2f_1 \pm f_2$ and $2f_2 \pm f_1$.

Of these, the $2f_1 - f_2$ term turns out to be extremely important. Higher-order terms in a series like:

$$F(a) = c_1 a + c_2 a^2 + c_3 a^3 + c_4 a^4 + c_5 a^5 + \dots \tag{15}$$

produce higher-order harmonics of each input component and combination tones of corresponding complexity [see Eq. (6) of Section B. 3].

Let us consider now a residue signal consisting of a small number of consecutive harmonics of a fundamental frequency f_0. The lowest possible number of components is two, so let the frequencies be:

$$\begin{aligned} f_1 &= n f_0 \\ f_2 &= (n+1) f_0 \quad (n \text{ integer}). \end{aligned} \tag{16}$$

The third-order difference tones now have the frequencies:

$$\begin{aligned} 2f_1 - f_2 &= (n-1) f_0 \\ 2f_2 - f_1 &= (n+2) f_0. \end{aligned} \tag{17}$$

These are just the neighbouring components in the full harmonic series. If these combination tones are audible, it may well be that they play a role in residue perception.

2. Amplitude Functions

Before turning to experiments on the detectability of combination tones, we have to discuss one more topic of interest, the amplitude behaviour. We saw that each term of the series (15) gives rise to distortion components with frequencies $k_1 f_1 \pm k_2 f_2$, where $k_1 + k_2$ is equal to the order m of that term[3]. The creation of such components can be proven mathematically by substituting a two-component signal:

$$x(t) = A_1 \cos 2\pi f_1 t + A_2 \cos 2\pi f_2 t \tag{18}$$

into the corresponding term of (15). The reduction of the trigonometric formulae then shows one other important fact. The amplitude A of the distortion component with frequency $k_1 f_1 \pm k_2 f_2$, generated by the m-th term in the series (15),

[3] k_1 and k_2 are restricted to be positive numbers in this section.

depends in the following way upon the amplitudes A_1 and A_2 of the input components:

$$A_d = \text{const.}\ A_1^{k1} \cdot A_2^{k2} \tag{19}$$

with $k_1 + k_2 = m$. Hence, the third order-combination tone with frequency $2f_1 - f_2$ should have an amplitude proportional to the square of A_1 and to the first power of A_2. Note that this special amplitude dependence is dictated by the use of a power term in Eq. (15). Note also that the amplitude dependence will be different when more than one term in the series (15) contributes to a particular distortion product.

That the individual exponents of the factors in (19) are just k_1 and k_2 is difficult to see without mathematics. That the sum of the exponents should be equal to the degree m of the corresponding term is easily seen as follows. Consider the case where we first stimulate the system with a certain signal with amplitude A_0 (*e. g.*, $A_1 = A_2 = A_0$, but such a restriction is not necessary) and that we observe the combination tones generated by the term of the m-th degree. When the system is stimulated next with the same waveform but with the amplitude kA_0, this term will produce the same combination tones but the amplitude will be multiplied by k^m. Hence, the sum of the exponents in (19) must be equal to m, the degree of the term that produces the combination tones under study.

3. The Difference Tone ($f_2 - f_1$)

With this somewhat more detailed knowledge about distortion products, we turn to experimental evidence about the audibility of harmonics and combination tones. When one moderately loud purely sinusoidal signal is presented to the ear, the second harmonic can easily be distinguished; it sounds an octave higher than the primary tone. With various methods, the effective strength of the second harmonic can be measured as a function of the intensity of the primary tone. In general, the effective strength of the second harmonic behaves as the theory predicts: this distortion product can be described as if it were generated by the second term of the series (15). The primary tone has to be rather strong; when it is below 50 dB, no second harmonic is heard. Once the second harmonic is audible, it tends to have an effective intensity that rises as the square of the intensity of the primary tone. Or, in terms of decibel levels, for each 10 dB increase in level of the primary tone, the second harmonic increases by the double amount, 20 dB. Very little is known about the third aural harmonic; it probably is not significant.

There is a rich variety of distortion products when a signal is presented that contains two sinusoidal components. Let us call the frequencies of the two primary components f_1 and f_2, as before. Of these frequencies, f_1 is the lower. A quadratic term in the series (15) would produce (apart from the second harmonics of the two components) two combination tones, the so-called *difference tone* with frequency $f_2 - f_1$ and the *sum tone* with frequency $f_1 + f_2$. The difference tone has had a long history in music (*cf.* PLOMP, 1965). Scientific investigation has shown that its behaviour can be described very well by the quadratic term in (15). In particular, the effective strength of the difference tone behaves as the square of the amplitude of the components, as the theory predicts (ZWICKER,

1955). In the days of HELMHOLTZ, the source for the underlying type of non-linearity was sought in the middle ear. More recent experiments indicate that the frequency ratio f_2/f_1 has a larger influence on the difference tone than is compatible with a middle-ear origin (PLOMP, 1965; HALL, 1972a). It is possible that both the middle and the inner ear contribute to the production of the difference tone. The sum tone is audible only under special circumstances; in most cases, it is masked by the primary components (masking extends more toward the higher than toward the lower frequencies) and the second harmonics of the two primary components. Hence, it is not known whether the strength of the sum tone is compatible with that of the difference tone as the theory requires.

4. The Cubic Difference Tone ($2f_1 - f_2$)

The cubic difference tone (CDT) with frequency $2f_1 - f_2$ is unusual in all respects. A distortion product with this frequency would be generated by the term of the third order in (15). As is pointed out in Section G. 1, the CDT could contribute to residue perception if it were audible. Many studies have been devoted to the properties of this particular combination tone, and it has turned out that this distortion product has bridged the gap between older theories of the residue and the newer developments that have been hinted at in Section G. 1. As a consequence, we shall devote special attention to the properties of the CDT.

First, a few words about measurement techniques. The primary signal consists of two (sinusoidal) components with frequencies f_1 and $f_2 (f_2 > f_1)$. When a distortion tone is audible because it is generated in the ear, it is generally quite difficult to estimate its loudness; the primary tones produce too much interference. The strength of the distortion product is, therefore, determined by an indirect method. The signal presented to the ear is made to contain an additional

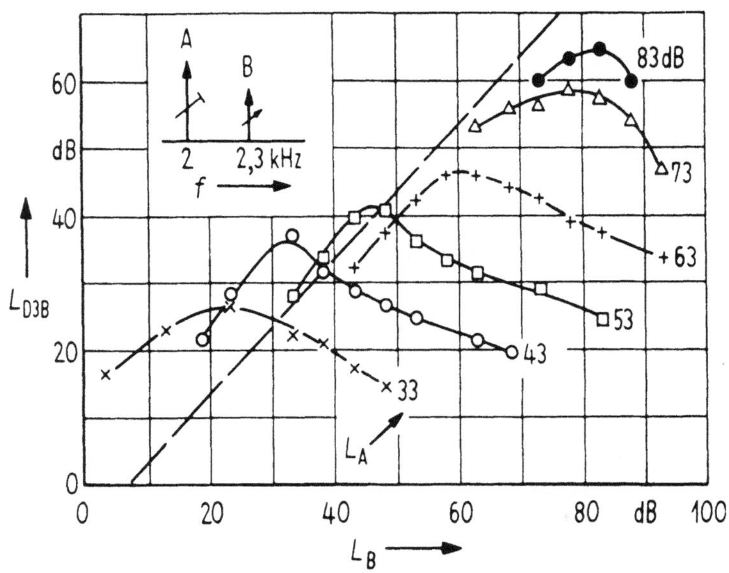

Fig. 27. Level of the cubic difference tone (CDT) as a function of the level of the higher component. Frequencies of the primary components: 2 and 2.3 kHz. The parameter is the level of the lower component. After ZWICKER (1968)

component with (exactly) the frequency $2f_1 - f_2$ of which amplitude and phase can be adjusted. The additional tone is called, cancellation tone, and the experiment is aimed at compensation of the aural distortion product by the cancellation tone. In the experiment, amplitude and phase of the cancellation tone are adjusted in such a way that the distortion product becomes completely inaudible. The adjustment is carried out by the subject himself.

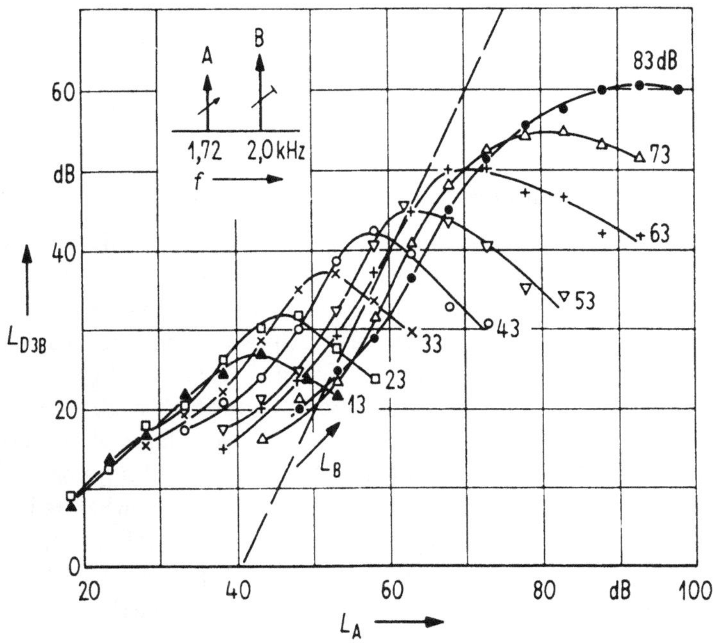

Fig. 28. Level of the cubic difference tone (CDT) as a function of the level of the lower component. Frequencies of the primary components: 1.72 and 2.0 kHz. The parameter is the level of the higher component. After ZWICKER (1968)

For the moment, we shall be concerned primarily with the amplitude of the CDT. ZWICKER, in 1955, was the first to report the unusual amplitude behaviour of the CDT with frequency $2f_1 - f_2$. Figures 27 and 28 taken from a later paper by ZWICKER (1968), serve to illustrate the findings. For Fig. 27, two tones, labelled A and B, were presented. The lower one had a fixed amplitude; the higher one was varied in level as the experimental variable. Theoretically, the level of the CDT should be varying precisely as much as the level of the higher primary tone in this situation (see the dashed line in the figure). It is seen that only the extreme left-hand parts of the experimental amplitude functions agree with theory. The main parts of the functions are quite different. In Fig. 28, the upper component is held at a fixed level and the lower one is varied. For this situation, the theory predicts a quadratic behaviour; the level of the CDT should vary over 20 dB for each 10 dB of variation of the lower-tone level (see the dashed line). It is seen that only a very small part of the curves has this theoretical slope. And, again, the main part is quite different.

One other feature of these findings is remarkable. The combination tone is audible when the components are rather weak. This is completely unlike the properties of, *e. g.*, the difference tone described above and is in complete disagreement with theory. When both primary components are varied in level simultaneously, the CDT should theoretically vary three times as much (30 dB for every 10 dB). The facts are quite different. For levels up to 60 dB, the CDT level varies at the same rate as the primary components. Hence, in this range, the *relative* CDT level is almost constant. Or, in other words, the percentage of distortion is almost constant. For primary-tone levels above 60 dB, the CDT level does not grow as much; it seems to saturate and reaches a maximum of 50 dB for primary levels of 100 dB. In this range, the percentage of distortion decreases with increasing level.

5. Essential Nonlinearity, Goldstein's Work

These findings indicate that the distortion underlying the CDT is not limited to high intensities as is the case for harmonic distortion and production of the difference tone. On the contrary, the distortion is manifest over almost the entire range of intensities. For low intensities, the distortion tone level may lie 15–20 dB below the level of the primary tones; this holds true almost down to threshold. Hence, even for very low levels the distortion is not at all negligible. Figure 29 illustrates the relative level of the CDT (relative to the level of the primaries). This figure is taken from a comprehensive paper on auditory nonlinearity by GOLDSTEIN (1967b). The cancellation-tone method was somewhat refined by an expedient intended to help the subject decide when the CDT disappeared completely. The stimulus, consisting already of three components (the two primary tones and the cancellation tone) was made to include a fourth tone. This tone,

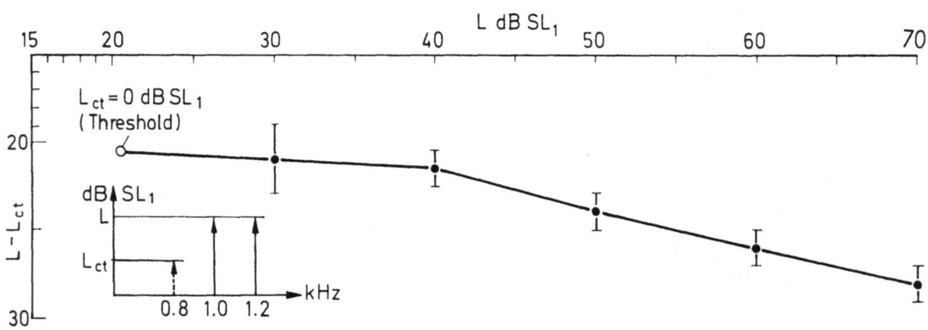

Fig. 29. Relative level of the CDT as a function of the level of the primary components. The inset shows the stimulus configuration in spectral terms (subject: JLG). After GOLDSTEIN (1967b)

termed probe tone, had a frequency differing a few Hz from that of the cancellation tone and was presented at a rather low intensity. As long as the compensation of the aural CDT by the cancellation tone is not perfect, the probe tone produces beats and these can serve to facilitate the adjustment for perfect compensation.

Figure 29 shows GOLDSTEIN's measurements of the relative CDT level as a function of the sensation level of the two primary tones. For low levels, the relative CDT level is almost constant which means that the relative amount of distortion is almost constant. For higher levels, the CDT level tends to saturate with the result that the relative CDT level begins to decrease.

Theoretically, the relative amount of distortion should always increase with increasing level. Hence, it is clear that the type of distortion that underlies the production of the CDT is completely unlike any mechanism that leads to a series development as (15). The nonlinearity that is responsible for CDT production has been termed an "essential nonlinearity" by GOLDSTEIN (1967 b), and later authors have continued to use this term (see, *e. g.*, SMOORENBURG, 1972 b). The theoretical aspects of essential nonlinearities have not been studied exhaustively although a few scattered results which are pertinent to the problem at hand are available (SCHROEDER, 1975; DE BOER, 1975; DUIFHUIS, 1975).

Two other aspects of the CDT findings are of interest. The first is that the CDT level is strongly dependent upon the frequency separation of the two primary tones. The CDT is strongest when the two tones are very near to one another, *e. g.*, when $f_2/f_1 = 1.1$. The CDT becomes much weaker when the tones are separated. The limiting point is a frequency ratio f_2/f_1 of 1.2–1.3 for sound levels of 40 dB; the CDT becomes rapidly weaker when the frequency ratio is increased. When we realize that cochlear mechanics causes each component to excite only a limited part of the organ of Corti, this strong frequency dependence is suggestive of a cochlear interaction process as the origin of the CDT. Moreover, no frequency selectivity of comparable sharpness is found in the middle ear. The problem of aural distortion, thus, appears to be very important for the study of cochlear physiology, a point to which we shall return later.

Up to this point, no mention has been made of the phase data that are produced by the experiments discussed. For difference tones and aural harmonics, the phase of the cancellation tone necessary to achieve compensation is almost independent of level. The phase data for the CDT, however, are strongly level dependent, especially in the region of low intensities. This property makes it difficult to give a description in general terms. A complicating factor is that recent studies have borne out that, in special situations, the level dependence of the CDT is not always as smooth as shown in Figs. 27 and 28. Any irregularity in the amplitude values is accompanied by irregularities in the phase. Representative papers have been written by HELLE (1969, 1970) and HALL (1972 a, b); SMOORENBURG (1972 a, b) has encountered the same phenomenon. The relevance of the CDT phase data for revealing the properties of aural frequency resolution has been discussed by SCHROEDER (1969).

The cubic difference tone (CDT) with frequency $2f_1 - f_2$ is not the only combination tone with the remarkable amplitude behaviour described above. There are combination tones with frequencies

$$f^{(k)} = f_1 - \mathrm{k}(f_2 - f_1) \quad (\mathrm{k} = 1, 2, 3 \ldots) \tag{20}$$

that have similar properties. The case k = 1 corresponds to the CDT. For k = 2, we encounter a combination tone of the fifth order; for k = 3, of the seventh, etc. Note that all these combination tones, whenever they would be audible, can act as extensions of the spectrum of a residue signal [compare Eq. (16) and (17)]. More will be said about these higher-order combination tones later.

Finally, we must mention the fact that most studies have concentrated on combination tones that lie below the frequency region of the primary tones. In contrast to the CDT with frequency $2f_1 - f_2$, the CDT with frequency $2f_2 - f_1$ lies above the primary tones. This CDT is somewhat elusive; although it tends to be masked by the primary tones, this is by no means certain, yet its existence has not been described.

For the sake of completeness, we note that some confusion has arisen concerning the basic properties of the difference tone with frequency $f_2 - f_1$. Depending upon the detection criterion used, the difference tone can show the same type of amplitude behaviour as the CDT (see, *e.g.*, HALL, 1972b). The reasons why different experiments can yield such widely divergent results are not clear at the moment.

6. Residue and Combination Tones — Smoorenburg

After this excursion to the domain of aural distortion, we return to the perception of the residue. Successive parts of the present chapter have been concerned with residue signals with an ever decreasing number of components. SCHOUTEN used stimuli with a large, indefinite number of components. DE BOER reduced the number to 7 and 5; RITSMA (in his principal experiments) to 3. SMOORENBURG (1970) took the next step; he studied the perception of signals with only *two* frequency components (the ultimate step of the perception of single-component signals related to residue phenomena has also been taken; we shall come to speak about this in the concluding section). In his first experiment, SMOORENBURG used 42 test subjects; they were required to judge which of two signals had the higher pitch. One of the signals had components of 1800 and 2000 Hz, the other of 1750 and 2000 Hz. The former signal thus had a fundamental frequency of 200,

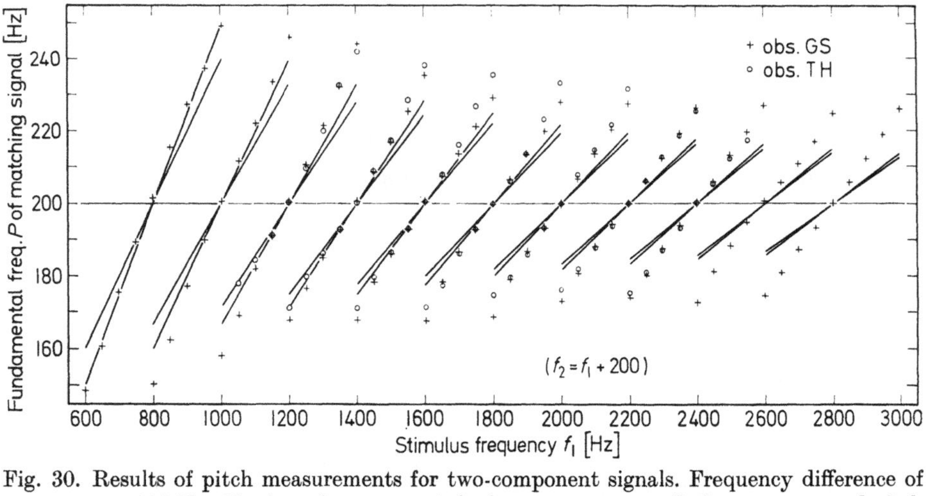

Fig. 30. Results of pitch measurements for two-component signals. Frequency difference of components: 200 Hz. Abscissa: frequency of the lower component. Ordinate: measured pitch value. The thin lines correspond to pitch shifts according to Eq. (9). After SMOORENBURG (1970)

the latter of 250 Hz. If a listener perceives a residue pitch, he will judge the second signal as having the higher pitch. If the listener's first impression of pitch is mediated by the components (in his perception, the part-tones; see the discussion on terminology in Section B. 5), his judgement will be the opposite one. From the results it appears that one of the two possible criteria is used consistently by each subject; there seems to be no rivalry between the two ways of judging the pitch. In about half of the subjects, the primary pitch impression was based on the complex tone being perceived as a whole and not on the part-tones.

Two of the subjects of the latter group participated in an extensive study of the pitch of two-tone complexes. The two components were produced by two tone generators; the components were kept 200 Hz apart; for this value of the frequency difference a residue pitch is audible when the stimulus frequencies are varied over a wide range. Another two-component signal was used as the comparison signal. This second signal was always harmonic; it was generated with special electronic equipment. To avoid the possibility that pitch matches were inadvertently based on part-tones, the ratio n of the lower component (frequency f_1) to the frequency difference was chosen so as to be different from n of the test signal. It is to be noted that the residue pitch for these two-component signals is quite weak, especially when $f_1/200$ is high. Nevertheless, reliable pitch matches were obtained for values of $f_1/200$ well over 10 (compare this with the limit of 20 reported by Ritsma in 1962 for three-component signals).

Figure 30 shows the results of the pitch measurements for the two observers. The abscissa is the frequency f_1 of the lower component; the frequency of the second component is 200 Hz higher. The ordinate is the "pitch" of the comparison signal, *i. e.*, the fundamental frequency of the comparison signal. When the test signal is harmonic, the pitch is observed to be equivalent to 200 Hz. For inharmonic signals, the pitch goes up and down around this value just as for signals with more than two components (compare Fig. 30 with Figs. 15 and 19). The full-drawn lines in Fig. 30 indicate the pitch course in the sense of the "first effect of pitch" (Section E. 7) computed according to Eq. (9) with n equal to $f_1/200$ and $f_2/200$, respectively. Remember that $f_2 - f_1 = 200$ (Hz) throughout these measurements. It is observed that the actually observed pitch shifts of inharmonic signals are larger, in other words, that the "second effect" is quite substantial.

The result is surprising. If we recall that in the pseudo-fundamental theory (see Section E. 9) the second effect can be explained by weighing the lower component more heavily than the higher one, we realize that for a two-component signal there would be very little space for a second effect. The same holds true when different pseudo-periods, measured at different locations of the basilar membrane, are considered (see Section E. 13). The largest pitch shift is obtained when the constant n in Eq. (9) is taken equal to $f_1/200$. However, the actual pitch shifts are much larger. Or, stated in a different way, the centre of gravity (*cf.* Section F. 5) lies completely outside the complex!

This point raises the question, do combination tones play a part in pitch perception? Combination tones with frequencies as given by Eq. (20) with low integral values of k would extend the given spectrum at the low-frequency side with equidistant components. If the two primary frequencies are shifted upwards over Δf Hz, all combination tones shift by the same amount. Hence, if these combination tones are audible, the aural spectrum is much richer in components than the objective one. This idea was investigated by SMOORENBURG in great detail and with several methods. Only part of this work will be described here: the remainder can be found in SMOORENBURG's papers (1970, 1972a, b).

7. Existence Region for Combination Tones

The first question is: under what conditions are the combination tones audible? This question was answered by a systematic search directed at the *existence region* for combination tones. First, f_2 was chosen twice the value of f_1, and then f_2 was gradually lowered in frequency while f_1 was kept constant. The subjects were instructed to notice the appearance of successive combination tones. The appearance of a new combination tone was noticed easily; recognition is facilitated because the pitch of the combination tone changes in the direction opposite to that of f_2. By comparison with a sinusoidal signal, the pitch of the combination tone was determined and this immediately yielded the appropriate value of k [see Eq. (20)]. In this way, the audibility of combination tones of different order (3, 5, 7..., corresponding to k = 1, 2, 3...) was determined for all possible combinations of f_1 and f_2. Figure 31 shows the results, interpolated for the situation where $f_2 - f_1 = 200$ (Hz). The result is expressed in the form of a variable λ, which is to be interpreted as follows. At a specific combination of f_1 and f_2 the

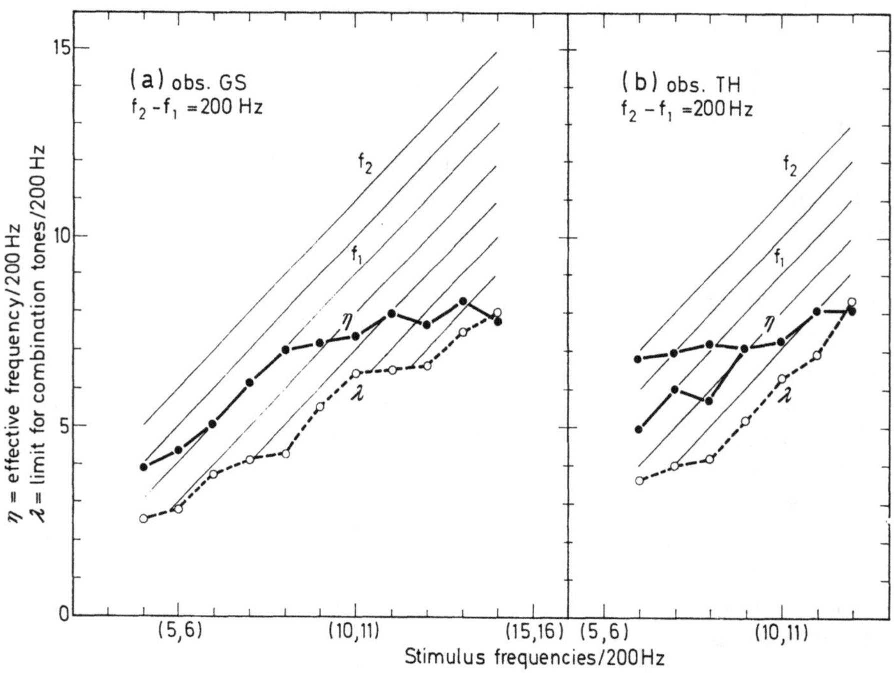

Fig. 31. Lower limit λ of the existence region of combination tones. Effective rank number η corresponding to measured pitch shifts for inharmonic two-component signals. Both functions are plotted against frequency (shown in a relative sense). The solid lines indicate the components of the "internal spectrum". Modified from SMOORENBURG (1970)

frequency f_λ of the lowest audible combination tone is measured. This frequency, divided by the difference $f_2 - f_1$ (200 Hz for this figure), yields λ. Hence, λ can also be regarded as the rank number of the lowest audible combination tone when all components are considered as harmonics (note that this interpretation holds only when the complex is harmonic). That λ turns out to be non-integral is the result of averaging over a number of experiments.

The upper two straight lines in Fig. 31 denote the primary components themselves (note that the abscissa is labelled in a relative sense). To improve clarity, several other lines have been drawn, each corresponding to one combination tone. These lines are all parallel and terminate on the function depicting λ. The figure, thus, gives an accurate account of the richness of the spectrum as it is perceived by the ear.

The second function depicted in Fig. 31 results from the pitch matches shown by Fig. 30. For inharmonic signals, the pitch deviates more from 200 Hz than is accounted for by Eq. (9). Let us rewrite this equation for deviations of pitch Δp rather than the pitch itself, and let us introduce an arbitrary constant η instead of n:

$$\Delta p = \frac{\Delta f}{\eta}\cdot \tag{21}$$

Here, Δp is the difference of the pitch with respect to the nearest harmonic situation, and Δf is the deviation of f_1 and f_2 from the nearest harmonic values. The constant η can be interpreted as the rank number of the harmonic that acts as the centre of gravity of the complex. However, it is no longer restricted to be an integral number. If the aural spectrum would consist of the two primary components only, η could only lie between n and n + 1 when n is the rank number of the lower component. The results of the pitch matches indicate that this does not hold true. In terms of Eq. (21), η should be lower than n to account for the data. From each pitch match, the equivalent value of η can be computed and the average values of η so obtained are included in Fig. 31. If we interpret η as the rank number associated with the centre of gravity of the aural spectrum, we see from the figure that η always lies *inside* the existence region of the combination tones. This lends considerable support to the assumption that the combination tones act as extensions to the spectrum and are involved in the determination of residue pitch.

Several additional arguments in favour of this hypothesis can be formulated. At the outset of Section G. 6, it was mentioned that there are essentially two categories of listeners. There proved to be a significant correlation with the existence region: the lower limit λ of the existence region for combination tones was lower for those subjects that judged pitch on the basis of the complex perceived as a whole, and it was higher for those subjects that judged pitch on the basis of individual part-tones. In further experiments, the effective width of the existence region for combination tones was experimentally manipulated. The existence region becomes smaller when the signals are weaker, and one may expect a larger value of λ as well as η. Similar effects are expected when the frequency region below the two primary tones is masked by a band-limited noise signal. Both expectations were confirmed by experiments.

From this work, we can conclude that we now have a fair understanding of the large pitch shifts found in experiments with inharmonic signals consisting of a very low number of components. If the primary components have low rank numbers, the effective rank number η will tend to refer to the fourth harmonic because of the principle of dominance. If the stimulus frequencies are all above the dominant region, the pitch will be determined by the lowest components perceived by the ear. In most cases, the effective rank number η then points to the region where combination tones have considerably enriched the spectrum.

For the highest complexes for which a pitch determination was reported to be possible, the effective value of η was limited to about 8. This suggests that generation of residue pitch by two-component signals requires at least one part-tone (combination tones included) that corresponds to a frequency not exceeding the eighth harmonic. In the series of experiments reported, this limiting situation occurred for $n = 14$. Note that in PLOMP's experiment (1964) all harmonics up to the ninth were found to be at least partly analyzable (see Section F. 6). The experiments reported in this section cannot yield a decision between the two alternatives for the residue pitch mechanism, temporal versus spectral processing. The results do lend more support to the theory involving spectral pattern recognition. Combination tones behave like tones that are physically present in the ear (see the next section). Thus, a pitch mechanism based upon the spectrum may be simply extended to include combination tones. An appropriate non-symmetrical weighing of the components will lead to predicted pitch values that agree with experimental ones. At the point where the analyzability of components fails completely, about the ninth to tenth harmonic, the pitch mechanism fails as well.

A simple spectral pattern recognition theory cannot account for all experimental results. For instance, RITSMA reported that for a three-component signal, pitch matches could be made for signals with harmonic numbers up to 20. Even when combination tones are included, such signals have only components with harmonic numbers of 14 and higher. And even the lowest components of such a complex cannot be analyzed by the ear at all. Most likely the mechanism of pitch determination is a combination of two processes, one based on temporal and the other on spectral cues. Reference may be made to the work by WALLISER (1969b) in which it is suggested that a first estimate is based on temporal properties and that the final pitch value is selected as the submultiple of the frequency of the lowest component that is closest to the first estimate. In any event, the results of the experiments reported by SMOORENBURG suggest strongly that detection of the residue pitch requires at least spectral information and confirm that combination tones considerably enrich the aural spectrum.

8. Physiological Considerations

The experiments described above have contributed enormously to our knowledge of the properties of residue pitch. It has not yet been possible to decide upon the most probable underlying mechanism of pitch determination. In any event, a process of pattern recognition of partly resolved spectral components is almost certainly involved. If that is true, a search for the physiological counterpart of the residue pitch mechanism will be extremely difficult if not impossible at this moment. It does not seem likely that we know enough about the physiological processing of signals to be able to pinpoint any physiological mechanism as being the residue pitch processor. Furthermore, we must consider all physiological evidence with extreme caution. From time to time, there appear reports about neurons in the auditory pathway that have properties closely associated with the envelope of auditory waveforms. Although temporal processing may play a part, the ultimate determination of residue pitch seems more likely to be based on spectral cues. Hence, the temporal mechanisms discovered may be involved in residue processing but almost certainly they are *not* related to the ultimate pitch processor. This is one of the reasons why the present author has considered it necessary to describe residue theory at such a length and to discuss so many auxiliary phenomena so deeply. For a complicated, and possibly multi-stage process like the one under discussion, it seems unlikely that the neurophysiological counterpart will be discovered soon; neurophysiologists should be aware of this situation. The author hopes that neurophysiologists do find the required background in the present text and invites readers to communicate their opinions, criticisms and questions to him.

The situation is entirely different for auxiliary phenomena like the production of harmonics and combination tones. Distortion products in electro-physiological potentials have received considerable attention (*e. g.*, WEVER and LAWRENCE, 1954; DALLOS, 1969; TONNDORF, 1958). There is every reason to believe that the cause for the perceptual appearance of distortion products is located in the cochlea, and, hence, the physiological findings are highly relevant. Let us concentrate on the CDT which is the most interesting distortion component in the present context.

The CDT is also the component about which the largest amount of physiological knowledge has been gathered, but not conclusive evidence as we shall see presently. Distortion products are prominent in the cochlear microphonic potential (CM). Harmonics and difference tones as well as higher-order distortion products are readily detected with specialized electronic equipment. A systematic study of the properties of the CDT (DALLOS, 1969) has yielded the result that the CDT in the CM follows the theoretical description rather accurately. No evidence about an essential nonlinearity was found. In this respect, the physiological findings are quite contrary to the psychophysical results as described above. This discrepancy has led DALLOS to conclude that the microphonic potential, although undoubtedly due to important physiological events in the cochlea, is an epiphenomenon that does not reveal the presence of all audible components.

DALLOS' results are somewhat remarkable since there are many reasons why the cause of CDT production is to be sought either in the mechanics of the cochlea or in the sensori-neural transduction process, and it seems strange that the distortion does not reflect back on the CM. Let us now consider cochlear mechanics and the generation of action potentials in single fibers of the auditory nerve in somewhat more detail. The most direct evidence that cochlear movements are nonlinear has been obtained by RHODE (1971). He measured the response of a particular spot on the basilar membrane as a function of frequency. The experiments were performed in squirrel monkeys and detection of the minute movements of the basilar membrane was possible by the use of an advanced measurement method borrowed from nuclear physics. The location chosen for observation showed a clear and pronounced resonance at a frequency near 7 kHz but only for weak sound stimuli. For sound signals of over 70 dBL, the resonance was observed to be damped, and at 90 dBL, the peak demonstrating the resonance had almost disappeared. Unfortunately, Rhode could not perform measurements at sound levels below 70 dB; hence, we have no direct evidence on mechanical nonlinearity at extremely low levels. The observations suggest, however, that the mechanical nonlinearity operates only at high levels, and that it dampens the resonance progressively when the stimulus level exceeds 70 dB.

The type of nonlinearity observed by Rhode is of the right type to yield a CDT, and, as such, it has been used as a basis for models of cochlear mechanics (Kim and Pfeiffer, 1973; Hall, 1974). The models constructed do show production of a CDT (and higher-order combination tones) but only for moderately loud to loud stimuli. Insofar as explanation of CDT behaviour at these higher levels is concerned, such models are quite powerful (*cf.* Schroeder, 1975). If our inference from Rhode's data is correct, cochlear mechanics on the level of basilar-membrane movement does not contain essential nonlinearities. Hence, the origin for the observed CDT at low sound levels is probably not located in cochlear mechanics.

9. Single-Fiber Responses

Let us now turn to the responses of single fibers of the auditory nerve. Here, we find neurophysiological counterparts of several psychophysical phenomena, notably frequency selectivity and masking (see the authorative review by Evans and Wilson, 1973). The sharpness of frequency selectivity is much higher than the sharpness reported for cochlear mechanics by von Békésy (1960). Although it is well recognized now that von Békésy's experiments were performed at such high levels that nonlinear distortion must have swamped out almost all resonance, and that more modern methods have yielded considerably sharper resonance curves, there is still no agreement about the question whether mechanical selectivity is sufficient to explain neural selectivity. The most widely held opinion is that the selectivity displayed by responses of single fibers is substantially sharper than the selectivity of mechanical response curves. However, it could be that mechanical sharpness is greater than measurements have hitherto revealed it to be.

If we adhere to the most common opinion, we must allow frequency selectivity to be achieved in two stages, the first by way of hydrodynamical transformations in the cochlea and the second via the mechano-neural transduction mechanism. The two stages are referred to as the *first* and the *second filter*, respectively. Although the existence of a second filter is usually assumed, there is no evidence at all as to its nature (several theoretical possibilities are currently being worked out (see, *e. g.*, Steele, 1973; Helle, 1974; Zwicker, 1974; Duifhuis, 1975). Furthermore, the part played by outer hair cells versus inner hair cells in the cochlea, insofar as achieving the ultimate frequency selectivity is concerned, is not clear at all (*cf.* Ryan and Dallos, 1975).

Responses of auditory-nerve fibers reveal many nonlinearities (*cf.* Pfeiffer and Kim, 1973). For the purpose of the present review, it is most important to note that the firings of an auditory-nerve fiber may be linked to the CDT. This property has been studied by GOLDSTEIN and KIANG (1968). They found that responses of a nerve fiber, when the sound consists of two components with frequencies f_1 and f_2, can show synchrony to the compound waveform but to the CDT with frequency $2f_1 - f_2$ as well. Synchrony is to be interpreted in a probabilistic sense: firings do not occur in every cycle of the waveform, but the probability of firing goes up and down just like the waveform. Hence, if the firings are observed on a time scale that is synchronous with periods of the CDT, it is noted that the firing probability may have a tendency to show the same period as the CDT. About the proper interpretation of these results, some discussion arose, but the net result was that we may safely assume that auditory-nerve fibers respond to a CDT as if this distortion product is physically present in the cochlea (GOLDSTEIN, 1970). This property tallies with the conclusion from psychophysical experiments: aural combination tones act as if they were part of the sound stimulus.

In this way we are led back to the problem, where in the chain from cochlear movement pattern to excitation of a nerve fiber are combination tones generated by a mechanism displaying all the properties of an essential nonlinearity? Rather than answering this question directly, we turn once more to psychophysical evidence and ask whether we can distinguish several stages in the production of the CDT. The answer to this question is affirmative. The subjective strength of the CDT is strongly dependent upon the frequency ratio f_2/f_1 (see Section G. 5). This suggests that the stimulus undergoes a certain amount of filtering before the site of the nonlinearity is reached. Secondly, the CDT behaves as a normal spectral component; hence, it should undergo a filtering process before the locus of its detection (nerve fibers tuned to its frequency) is reached. There appear to be two filters involved in the processing of the CDT, and the nonlinearity can be viewed as sandwiched in between. How far these filters coincide with the two filters involved in straight frequency selectivity is not known. Moreover, it may well be that the two filters involved in this concept of CDT production are partially coincident.

It may be concluded that, from psychophysical as well as neurophysiological evidence, we have obtained a fair idea about the mechanisms involved in CDT production. As to the exact site of production, we have as yet no idea (see, however, the literature cited above). And, about the nature of the nonlinearity, we know little more than that it appears to be an essential nonlinearity. Chances are likely that the same nonlinearity is responsible for other manifestations of nonlinearity in the cochlea (SMOORENBURG, 1972b; DE BOER, 1975), notably two-tone suppression (SACHS and KIANG, 1968).

H. Return to Place (?) (Increasing Importance of Spectral Concepts)

1. Doubts About Relevance of Periodicity

Are we right in concluding that "residue pitch" is growing away from "periodicity pitch"? On the basis of the foregoing, it certainly would seem so. Originally, the residue was considered as intimately connected with periodicity, but, as research progressed, more and more emphasis was put on spectral resolution rather than on interference of unresolved components. Doubts about the necessity of purely temporal processing arose from various sides. WHITFIELD (1970) reported that extensive neurophysiological research had failed to uncover a mechanism capable of measuring relatively long (several milliseconds) time intervals to a 1% accuracy. This does not prove that such a mechanism does not exist, of course, but the argument is very suggestive. In a completely different context, SIEBERT (1970) showed that the representation of nervous activity in the auditory nerve is accurate enough to account for human frequency discrimination, and that temporal information is not needed by the central nervous system. Again, not a conclusive proof, but an important piece of knowledge.

Let us recall, at this moment, which psychophysical experiment was the most important one that served to stress spectral aspects relative to temporal phenomena. That experiment was the finding of the dominant spectral region for residue pitch. In the dominant region, the components of the signal are well resolved by the auditory system, and it appears unlikely that the dominant residue is mediated by the remaining weak interactions between adjacent components. It is easier to believe that, in this case, pitch is mediated by a mechanism that tries to detect the pseudo-fundamental, a mechanism that can be described as an extension of the place theory.

Let us look now at the evidence from the other side. One of the main arguments in favour of temporal processing has been the existence of phase effects (see Section E. 8). The timbre of a sound was found to depend on the phase relation between components only when the components were close to one another in frequency. Since, in that case, adjacent components interfere because of insufficient resolution, the idea of waveform processing is immediately strengthened. For sound complexes showing clear phase effects, it would be unreasonable to assume that the residue pitch is mediated by the frequencies of the only marginally resolved components.

What part have combination tones played in the problem of theories on temporal versus spectral processing? Since combination tones are audible only when the (relative) frequency spacing is small, they seem to have strengthened the position of the temporal theory. Combination tones might even be important for phase effects (just how much, will be seen later). May we conclude that we would have been much more inclined earlier to accept an extended place theory for pitch, if there were no combination tones? The experiments to be reported in the next sections suggest an affirmative answer to this question.

2. Houtsma and Goldstein's Experiments

An essential basis for practising the art of music is the human auditory system's ability to perceive melody. On listening to a sequence of musical sounds, one can generally retrieve the series of "notes" played regardless of the spectrum generated by the particular musical instrument. Melodies can be recognized even when the sound signals are passed through a bandpass filter which only passes a small number of spectral components. Hence melody appears invariant over a large class of spectral transformations. HOUTSMA and GOLDSTEIN (1971, 1972) reported a series of psychophysical experiments that were designed within a musical framework to explore how the auditory system retrieves pitch from a sequence of periodic sound signals. These experiments have had a profound influence on contemporary theories about residue pitch – so much, in fact, that an almost complete reversal of opinion has taken place.

The experiments differed in several respects from all earlier ones. First, instead of single sounds, a simple musical message consisting of a series of sounds was used as the material. Second, the experimental subjects had an extensive musical

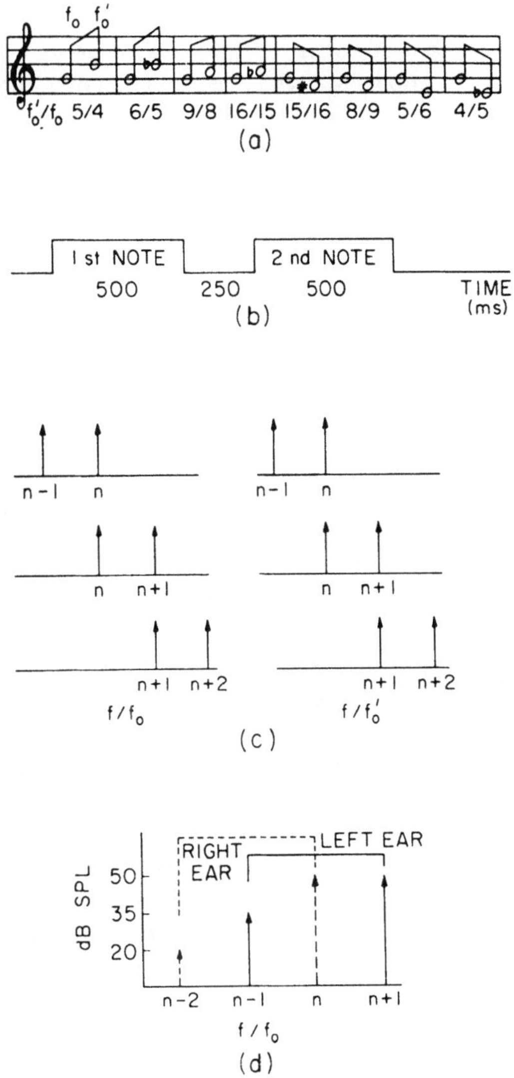

Fig. 32a—d. Experiments on recognition of musical intervals: (a) Musical intervals to be identified. (b) Timing of the stimulus tones. (c) The three possible two-component stimuli for each of the two tones; for each tone, a random choice was made among the three possible stimuli. (d) Stimulus presentation for the dichotic experiments, with the addition of simulated combination tones (see Section H. 3). After HOUTSMA and GOLDSTEIN (1972)

background. In order to test whether the experiments truly reflected the musical behaviour of melody perception, several control tests were carried out. In these control tests, the musical messages consisted of sequences of four "notes", each being a two-tone complex with two successive harmonics as components. The fundamental frequencies were in the range 200–400 Hz. The lower component was chosen randomly as the 3rd, 4th, or 5th harmonic. The subjects were required to identify the series of notes. Since all of the 10 subjects were familiar with musical dictation, an almost perfect pitch score could be expected and was, in fact, achieved. This shows that even for the unfamiliar two-tone stimulus, the subject's response reflects his natural musical skill and that very little or no special training was required for this type of task.

The main experiments were carried out with sequences of two signals. Each signal consisted of two components which were successive harmonics; for each signal, the number of the lower harmonic was chosen randomly from three successive integers, $n-1$, n, $n+1$. The parameter, n, was one of the independent parameters in the experiments. The fundamental frequencies f_0 and f'_0 of the two signals formed a musical interval: it was the subject's task to identify this interval.

The repertoire of intervals is depicted in Fig. 32a.

For reasons of convenience, all intervals are shown as starting with the same note. In the experiments, the fundamental frequency f_0 of the first signal was the second independent variable; in each series of experimental runs f_0 was the same, and, in successive runs, n was incremented by one. The intervals were presented in random order, of course. Nearly perfect scores of identification were usually achieved in the first run of a series. Increments were added to n until response dropped to chance level (12.5% correct, corresponding to one out of eight intervals guessed correctly). Section b of Fig. 32 gives details of the timing of the stimuli; Section c shows the three possibilities for the spectrum of each of the two signals. Section d will be referred to below.

Some representative results are shown by Fig. 33a. All these experiments were performed with monotic presentation[4]. The figure shows the contours for equal performance (P_c is the percentage of intervals correctly identified) in the $f_0 - \bar{n}$ plane. In Fig. 33a the ordinate $\bar{n}$ refers to an average of (integral) values of n. The results show clearly that the best performance is achieved with the lowest harmonic numbers. In other words, the larger the spacing between harmonics (on a logarithmic frequency scale), the better the performance. This is in general agreement with the principle of dominance, and it suggests once more that the two harmonics employed in this experiment are processed through separate channels of the auditory system to obtain successful identification.

3. Dichotic Pitch Recognition

The hypothesis about separate channels was tested in a second experiment employing probably the most extreme channel separation one can think of,

[4] Dichotic: Two-ear presentation; different signals are fed to the two ears. Monotic: One-ear presentation, or two-ear presentation with the same signal being fed to the two ears.

namely separate ears. The experimental paradigm was the same as in the monotic experiment, except that the components of each signal were presented dichotically, one to each ear. Figure 33 b shows results for dichotic presentation. Comparison with Fig. 33 a proves that each subject's performance is slightly below

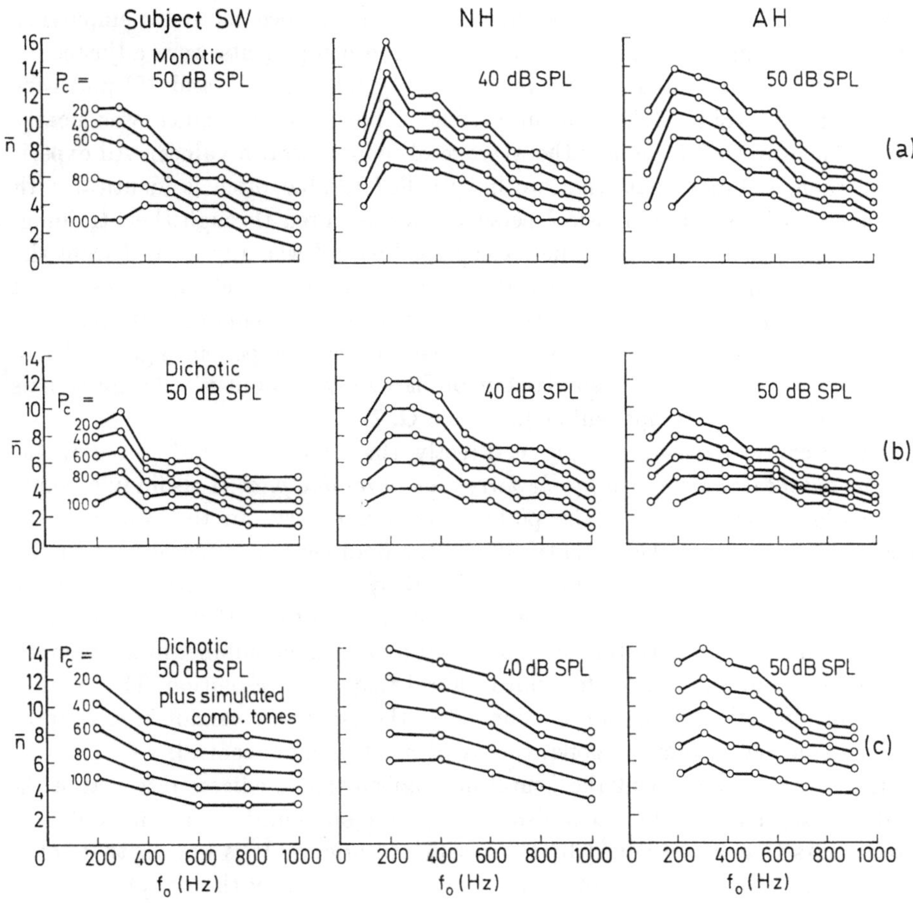

Fig. 33a—c. Equal-performance contours for identification of musical intervals. (a) Monotic presentation at 50 (40) dB SL. (b) Dichotic presentation (one component fed to each ear). (c) Dichotic presentation, with two simulated combination tones added. After HOUTSMA and GOLDSTEIN (1972)

that obtained under monotic presentation[4]. This finding considerably strengthens the hypothesis that a central mechanism integrates and processes information from both cochleas. Note that, in the dichotic case, the information from each cochlea involves only one component.

In an additional experiment, the influence of aural combination tones, which is undeniably present in the monotic case, was simulated for dichotic presentation. Two additional components were generated and distributed over the ears as is indicated by Fig. 32d. It may be expected that the total spectrum perceived in the dichotic case is now similar to that for the monotic case. As is shown by Fig. 33c, performance contours undergo an upward shift of n of approximately 2, compared to those of Fig. 33b, and there appears to be very little difference in performance between monotic and dichotic presentation of the signals. This is strong evidence that such differences in performance as occur between monotic and dichotic stimulus conditions can be attributed to aural combination tones.

Musical relevance of the experiments was tested once more by employing inharmonic stimuli. When the frequencies of the components were adjusted to produce the correct pitch despite inharmonicity (*cf.* Figs. 15 and 19) and care was taken to avoid pitch ambiguities, the subjects' performance was nearly perfect for $\bar{n}$ up to 6 ($\bar{n}$ is now the average of non-integral n-values). All experiments, then, indicate that what we have called residue pitch is identical with the concept of pitch that musical persons have acquired through their training. In the experiments described, the concept of "pitch" was approached from the side of musical intervals. Conversely, the concept of residue pitch may be extended safely toward musical intervals. The results of the experiments indicate that this holds true only for low values of n, at least for two-component signals. There are reasons to believe that a similar but probably higher limit is valid for signals with more than two components (*cf.* Section G. 7).

The dichotic experiments prove directly that *a fundamental period in the cochlear output is not required for the perception of residue pitch*. This finding points to a definite inadequacy of the period-detection theory. In the words of the authors (Houtsma and Goldstein, 1972): the findings "... suggest that fundamentals of complex-tone stimuli are retrieved by means of a central mechanism which operates on those stimulus tones or combination tones that can be resolved in the cochlea". That performance is bounded by harmonic number in the monotic case might be attributed to the limit of aural frequency resolution. That performance for dichotic stimulation is bounded in the same way cannot be accounted for by frequency resolution alone; the cause must be more central.

Little can be said about the neural mechanism that mediates retrieval of the fundamental. The central mechanism will operate on neural signals derived from components that are resolved by the peripheral organs. It is known that information about the frequency of components is preserved by the peripheral organ in two ways: "place" of activated nerve fibers and, at least for low frequencies, partial synchrony between firings of a nerve fiber and waveform of the stimulus. Either of these two cues could provide the required information for the central mechanism, and it will be quite difficult to decide between these alternatives on the basis of psychophysical experiments alone.

4. Conclusions — Wightman's Theory

The experiments by Houtsma and Goldstein have given considerable strength to the opinion that the final processor that determines pitch for a complex stimulus operates on the *spectrum* of the signal rather than on the *waveform*. There is only one aspect of the residue that seems not to agree with this opinion, namely, the existence of phase effects (see *e.g.* Section E. 14). However, it should be remembered that phase changes between components do indeed produce changes in the timbre of the sound but that the pitch remains unaffected. The arguments can be found in WIGHTMAN's first 1973 paper (1973a). Hence, it is probable that the pitch extraction mechanism operates independently of the timbre mediating mechanism, and, if that is true, the pitch mechanism might well operate entirely and solely upon spectral cues. Accordingly, two theories have been formulated that describe such a mechanism in abstract terms. We shall not endeavour to describe the theories in detail. Readers in possession of the necessary mathematical background knowledge can consult the pertinent references (WIGHTMAN, 1973b; GOLDSTEIN, 1973). The following descriptions attempt to make the ideas clear to readers who are well oriented in physiology or psychology but who are not willing to follow every step in all its abstract or formalistic detail.

In this section and in the next, we shall describe the basic ideas contained in WIGHTMAN's (1973b) pattern-transformation theory for residue pitch. We shall follow this author closely in the outline of some basic steps in a process of pattern recognition. Consider the following analogy between a visual and an auditory pattern-recognition problem. The letter "A", as it is printed here, has some particular property in common with the same letter printed elsewhere. That property allows us to identify it as an "A" despite the fact that the physical features of all A's are different. Recognition may now be described as a *sequence of transformations*; in each transformation, some of the most detailed information is lost while some specific information is preserved. After the final transformation, all information about the differences between various A's is lost and only the information relevant to the recognition of a letter remains. This is enough to enable the task of *recognition* to be performed.

In neurophysiological terms, the transformations involved are transformations of patterns of neural activity. For the pitch problem, the first transformation is carried out by the peripheral sensory system. The nervous system is assumed to carry out a transformation of the peripheral pattern of neural activity into another pattern in such a way that all stimuli with the same pitch have a similar representation. The pattern-transformation theory proposes specific forms for the transformations involved. In each of the stages, it is important to list what kind of information is preserved and what is lost. Let us take the first transformation, the transformation of the acoustical stimulus into what is termed the "Peripheral (neural) Activity Pattern" (PAP). Note that the latter pattern is not necessarily to be identified with the pattern of neural activity in the auditory nerve(s) since the experiments described in the previous sections strongly indicate that information coming from the two ears is processed jointly.

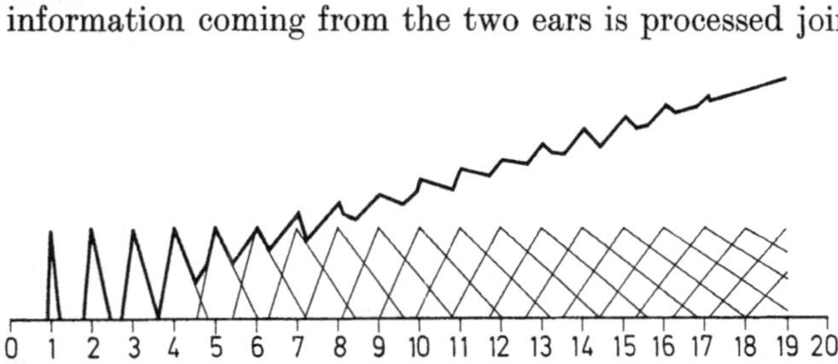

Fig. 34. The peripheral activity pattern (schematic) for a periodic pulse series. Abscissa: frequency — or location in the cochlea labelled by rank number of component. Ordinate: neural activity. Thin lines: contributions by individual components. Thick line: total activity

The first transformation (Stage I) is assumed to be a frequency analysis process with limited resolution. In many respects, it is similar to the signal transformation carried out by the cochlea, but, in the theory, only the major features are needed. The output of this stage, the PAP, is a pattern of neural activity that represents the spectral contents of the stimulus in a crude way. In factual terms, the output is a function ("amount of neural activity", for instance, the mean rate of firing) that depends on location (representing, in a way, the "place" in the cochlea). The analysis performed in this transformation is, as said, limited in resolving power just as the cochlea does not produce a single locus of neural activity for each sinusoidal component of the sound stimulus. The limit of resolution agrees in general terms with the critical band; the bandwidth is assumed to be proportional to frequency. Details about this limit are not important here, but the idea of explicitly including a limited power of resolution in this transformation is one of the main features of the theory.

As a consequence of this restriction, the representation of a multi-component stimulus is substantially smeared out; only the lower components will stand out as more or less isolated patches of neural activity (the locus of largest activity corresponding to frequency) and the higher components, *e. g.*, those with a rank number of 10 and higher, are fused. See Fig. 34 for a stylized representation of the PAP. In the transformation of Stage I, all information about phase is lost, and so is the information about the waveform formed by the fused components.

5. Wightman's Theory, Continued

The second transformation (Stage II) is intended to bring out the main features of the PAP in terms of its oscillatory properties. If the stimulus were a periodic pulse series, having a large number of equidistant components, the PAP will clearly indicate the first 10, or so, of these components. This occurs in the form of regular undulations as in Fig. 34. When the stimulus is a different signal, Stage II tries to bring out a similar feature. Hence, it is not surprising that Stage II is formally assumed to operate like a Fourier analyzer. If a more or less regular undulation is present in the PAP, the Stage II transformation brings out its "frequency". Actually, the latter parameter is a temporal parameter since a periodic repetition in the original signal is the feature that causes an oscillation in the PAP. Because of the two transformations involved, this parameter is not the same as the time t; hence, we shall designate it by a different symbol, namely τ. Summarizing, then, the output of the second stage is a function (again probably an amount of neural activity) dependent upon τ. Whenever a specific form of undulation or oscillation is present in the PAP, Stage II shows that activity is larger for a certain value of τ.

The third stage of the proposed model identifies the maximum in the transformed version of the PAP, and pitch is assumed to be directly associated with the value of τ for which the maximum occurs. As an extra feature, the magnitude of the maximum gives an indication of the subjective strength, or the "clearness", of pitch, a feature that no other theory possesses. In WIGHTMAN's paper, the predictions of the model are compared with the results from several experiments on residue pitch. In many cases, a satisfactory agreement is found, somewhat surprising in view of the extreme simplifications that have been built in to make the model manageable in computational terms.

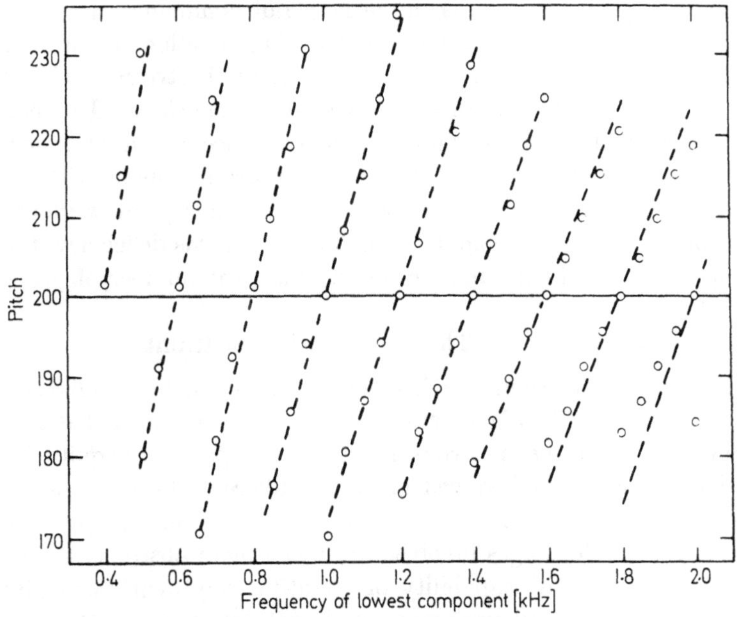

Fig. 35. Comparison between theory (circles) and experiment (dashed lines) on the pitch of inharmonic signals. After WIGHTMAN (1973b)

For example, the model rather accurately predicts the pitch shifts for inharmonic signals. Data are taken from PATTERSON's (1973) measurements, and the comparison between theory and experiment is shown by Fig. 35. Contrary to common usage, the circles in this figure are predictions from the theory and the dashed lines indicate the trend of the experimental results. Due to the fact that limited aural resolution is built in, and that, therefore, the lower components are more prominent in the PAP, the first as well as the second effect of pitch are represented accurately. An exception is formed by the region of higher frequencies where the theory predicts smaller pitch shifts than the measured ones. Two modifications appear necessary. The first is the addition of combination tones to the PAP. The second modification is that these combination tones should be represented with an intensity nearly that (within a few decibels) of the stimulus components. The latter modification implies some kind of amplitude-compression scheme. It should be stressed that these points constitute only refinements; the basic theory successfully predicts much of the experimental data.

WIGHTMAN's model predicts more than just pitch *value*; it also gives estimates of pitch *strength*. It appears that the theory is rather insensitive to changes of parameters in the Stage I transformation as regards pitch values. With the exception of the point discussed in the preceding paragraph, the parameters of the model can, thus, not easily be fixed by comparing theory and experiment for pitch values. The predictions for pitch strength, however, are strongly dependent upon the parameters inserted in the model. There are as yet too few experimental results on this issue, but the theory in its present form agrees with the tendencies reported in the literature.

One aspect of pitch strength is the principle of dominance. The theory predicts that pitch strength is a smoothly declining function of harmonic rank number. The upper limits are in good agreement with Ritsma's (1962) values for the existence region for the three-component residue signal. The model fails, however, to account for the lower limit of the existence region, and, hence, does not predict that the 3rd, 4th, and 5th harmonics are dominant with respect to pitch. It appears difficult to improve the theory on this point without making the model considerably more complicated. Apart from this deficiency, the theory ties together in a meaningful and elegant way a great number of properties of residue pitch.

6. Goldstein's Theory — Basic Constraints

A second theory on residue pitch has been published by Goldstein (1973). In one sense, it is related to Wightman's theory: it is assumed that *all* cues for pitch are obtained from the spectrum. In all other respects, it is quite dissimilar; in particular, the concepts involved are quite different. Furthermore, the concepts used in Goldstein's theory do not allow a simple interpretation in terms of neural activities. The stages involved are much more abstract; the beauty of the theory lies more in its capability of quantitatively synthesizing inferences from all available sets of relevant psychophysical data than on the possibilities for experimental verification of its essential features.

Basically, the central processor is viewed as a recognizer of spectral patterns that are supplied by the peripheral frequency analyzers. The *peripheral analyzer* extracts from a complex stimulus all the components that differ from their neighbours by more than some resolution limit. It then produces *only* information about the frequency of each component to the central processor. The following constraints are involved in the analysis stage:

a) only aurally *resolved* components contribute,

b) the *phase* relations are irrelevant,

c) only the *presence* of a component is reported – the amplitude is irrelevant (within limits),

d) the information about component frequency is basically *inaccurate*, a non-negligible variability is involved.

The *central processor* accomplishes recognition by selecting out of its repertoire of stored patterns the one that is best matched to the information received. The matching is done on the basis of maximum likelihood estimation. The stored patterns with which the matching is carried out have one constraint:

e) it is assumed that the information received corresponds to stimuli in which the components are *successive harmonics*.

The points listed under a) through e) above, are the fundamental restrictions under which the proposed mechanism is assumed to operate. Goldstein's paper describes these points in detail, providing all the relevant justification for each one of them. We suffice by mentioning a few basic relations. Assumptions a) and b) appear reasonable in view of the growing role of spectral concepts in residue theory that we have witnessed. Assumption c) was already necessary in WIGHTMAN'S theory and can be traced back to SMOORENBURG'S work. Assumption d) is based on the motivation that frequency information about resolved components is conveyed to the central nervous system by noisy neural channels.

The last Assumption (e) is the one involving successive harmonics. One argument is contained in DE BOER'S observation that a signal consisting of odd harmonics of 100 Hz does not convey a residue pitch of 100 Hz but yields two possible pitches in the 200 Hz region (see Section E. 6 and Fig. 15). Hence, it is better to assume that the central processor operates on the principle that successive harmonics are present than that a periodic stimulus is present. It is to be noted that the central processor has no information about which rank number is to be associated with each component. The estimation of the best-fitting series of (successive) rank numbers is an essential part of the pitch recognition procedure, and it directly accounts for ambiguities in pitch as they are often observed (see Section E. 14).

The only free parameter in the theory is the one describing variability (fundamental inaccuracy) associated with frequency information. This parameter is assumed to be a function only of frequency. It proved possible to derive a functional form for this parameter (labelled σ) that is sufficient to produce good agreement between theory and experiment. The experimental data were taken from HOUTSMA and GOLDSTEIN'S work on recognition of musical intervals (1971, 1972). The best estimates for the standard deviation $\sigma(f)$ that is associated with the measurement of a component frequency f are depicted in Fig. 36. With the appropriate parameter values inserted, the theory can predict performance in the musical interval experiment in great detail, as Fig. 37 shows. Experimental data are averaged over various stimulus conditions (compare Fig. 33a). Because of its strictly statistical structure, the theory is capable of predicting contours of equal performance, and the agreement with experimental results is observed to be quite good.

Unlike WIGHTMAN'S theory, the present theory predicts several details of the existence region for residues as well as of the region of dominance. In this way, it accounts for RITSMA'S (1967) as well as PLOMP'S (1967) data, albeit that there are indications that the highest components should be given a smaller weight in some way or other. [Note: this is difficult in view of Assumption (c)]. In particular, the theory accounts for the fact that the lowest components – including the fundamental – do not belong to the dominant region. One reason for this effect is seen in Fig. 36; for low frequencies, the standard deviation σ increases when frequency decreases.

A separate check on the derived values of the measurement uncertainty σ is possible on the basis of measurements of frequency discrimination of residues. RITSMA (1963) tried to measure the fundamental accuracy of pitch matches by comparing two residues with one another. To avoid matches based on perception of part-tones, the two signals to be compared comprised disjoint frequency regions; the test stimulus consisted, *e. g.*, of harmonics 6–8, and the standard stimulus of harmonics 9–11. Goldstein shows that his theory is in excellent agreement with these data. Incidentally, the accuracy with which residue pitches are determined is decidedly inferior to that with which the pitch of pure tones can be determined. Hence, the variance $\sigma(f)$ describing the precision with which

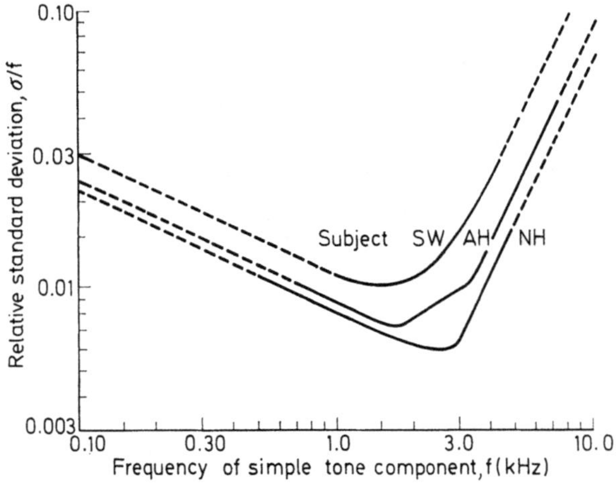

Fig. 36. Relative standard deviations characterizing the precision with which frequency in formation from aurally resolved components is conveyed to the central pitch processor. After Goldstein (1973)

frequency information is conveyed to the central processor, has a considerably larger value than the variance corresponding to pure-tone frequency discrimination. The conclusion that the accuracy of representation of components is inferior to that of isolated pure tones is also possible outside the framework of Goldstein's theory; as yet there seems to be no reasonable explanation for this property.

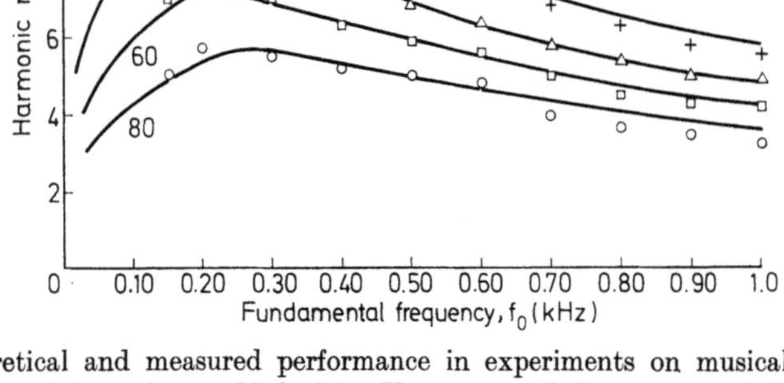

Fig. 37. Theoretical and measured performance in experiments on musical intelligibility. Data are averaged from data published by Houtsma and Goldstein (1972). After Goldstein (1973)

7. Goldstein's Theory — Verification

A major point concerns, of course, the pitch shift associated with inharmonicity of the sound stimulus. GOLDSTEIN'S theory predicts, in an approximate form, that the effective rank number η describing the pitch shifts is the average of the rank numbers of the lowest and the highest component:

$$\eta = \frac{n_{low} + n_{high}}{2} . \tag{22}$$

For the meaning of η, we refer to Eq. (21) and the discussion in Section G. 7. If we include combination tones, the predicted values of η in Fig. 31 would lie midway the curve for λ (the lower limit for combination tones) and the line representing f_2, the highest component (higher combination tones being ignored). Up to $n = 10$, the agreement is quite remarkable; it is recalled that n is the rank number of the lower one of the primary components.

Above $n = 10$ there are deviations; to account for these, it is necessary to add the rule that only components that are more than 10% remote from one another contribute information to the central processor. It is exactly at this point that the limit of peripheral aural resolution creeps in. In this connection, it is interesting to note that the frequency inaccuracy implied in σ reflects a different dependence on f than the limit of aural resolution as represented by, *e. g.*, the critical band. In particular, σ is observed to increase sharply above 3000 Hz, a fact which is not paralleled by critical-band behaviour.

The role of combination tones is unseparable from the concept of inharmonicity pitch shifts. A rather lengthy part of GOLDSTEIN'S paper is devoted to the confounding role of the combination tones. During the history of the residue theory, there were several instances in which experimental evidence indicated primary involvement of the spectrum rather than the waveform. The first of these findings was DE BOER'S description of the "wide residue" (Sections E. 9 and E. 10). The second was the discovery of the principle of dominance (see Sections F. 2 and F. 3). The third point to be mentioned in this connection is the frequent underestimation of pitch shifts due to inharmonicity. But it appears that the contributions of combination tones, associated with narrow spacing of components as they are, have over-emphasized the possible role of interaction between components. Once the confounding role of the combination tones was recognized, many properties of the residue appeared as less puzzling. One point stressed in GOLDSTEIN'S paper is that combination tones must be resolved by the auditory system in order to be effective in pitch determination. It is suggested that combination tones would also be responsible for at least some of the effects associated with narrow-band sound complexes. As stated earlier, we shall come back to this subject later (Section H. 11).

8. General Conclusions

GOLDSTEIN'S theory describes a unifying logic that underlies the residue phenomenon and, thereby, defines a problem for physiology to solve. The frequency of the constituent harmonics is communicated to the central processor in a noisy way, and the question is left open whether the signals are coded by their place or their temporal course. Present physiological knowledge is insufficient to answer the question.

The theory starts from the assumption that the properties of residue pitch cannot be accounted for by peripheral events localized within a small region of frequencies; the pitch processor synthesizes information from wide frequency regions as well as from both ears. In this respect, the theory is much more than a consistent framework describing the formation of a pseudo-fundamental frequency. When aural frequency analysis fails because of insufficient resolution, residue pitch ceases to exist. However, more often residue pitch ceases to exist because of too much ambiguity. Hence, the peripheral analysis of the stimulus into its constituent components is a necessary but not a sufficient step in the creation of residue pitch. The emphasis of the pitch-determining mechanism is displaced from a peripheral to a central site. It is then logical to see the mechanism of pitch extraction equipped with properties typical for a neural network; despite the noisy way in which information is received, a remarkable consistency of the result of the processing is evident. Yet the pitch extraction mechanism has an innate tendency to arrive at ambiguous pitch values; a fact that is corroborated by many experimental findings. In GOLDSTEIN's theory this tendency can be traced to the problem of determining the proper value of n. WIGHTMAN's theory has the same tendency, but here it is more difficult to pinpoint the underlying cause. With these somewhat more general remarks, we close the discussion on unifying theories of residue pitch.

9. Dichotic Pitch Phenomena — Dichotic Repetition Pitch

Long before the period we are describing here, several dichotic pitch phenomena were known. To elicit these effects, two signals are presented to the two ears that are the same in many respects but differ in one. For the HUGGINS pitch, for example, two white-noise signals are used that differ only in the interaural phase relation over a narrow range of frequencies (CRAMER and HUGGINS, 1958). A faint pitch is heard corresponding to the frequency region for which the signal is truly dichotic, *i. e.*, for which the two signals at the two ears are different. Another manifestation of dichotic pitch perception is described by FOURCIN (1970). Repeated attempts were made to explain these phenomena but they remained puzzling. A relation with lateralization seemed evident and has even led to definite studies of this relation even for monaural residue phenomena (NORDMARK, 1963). More recently, this type of study has been taken up again (possibly prompted by the success of HOUTSMA and GOLDSTEIN's work on dichotic interval recognition) and it appears that the results now allow for a more consistent interpretation. We shall describe some experiments on "Dichotic Repetition Pitch" as reported by BILSEN and GOLDSTEIN (1974) and point out in due course the relation with, *e. g.*, the FOURCIN pitch.

We recall that "repetition pitch" (RP) is produced when to a noise signal $n(t)$ the same signal, but delayed in time, is added. Monaural repetition pitch (MRP) is described in Section F. 8, and Eq. (11) describes the stimulus used. Monaural repetition pitch can be heard when the time delay τ is between 1 and

10 msec. A much fainter but distinct pitch can be heard when the original noise signal $n(t)$ is led to one ear and the delayed version $n(t-\tau)$ of the same noise signal to the other. The pitch heard is called "dichotic repetition pitch" (DRP). Unlike MRP, DRP exists only when the time delay exceeds 3 msec. (Note that the time delays associated with lateralization are smaller than 1 msec.)

The pitch of DRP was measured by matching it with an MRP stimulus; this procedure proved possible over the range of τ indicated above. Furthermore, it proved possible to determine DRP with tests involving musical intervals. It is not surprising to find that DRP corresponds to the frequency $1/\tau$.

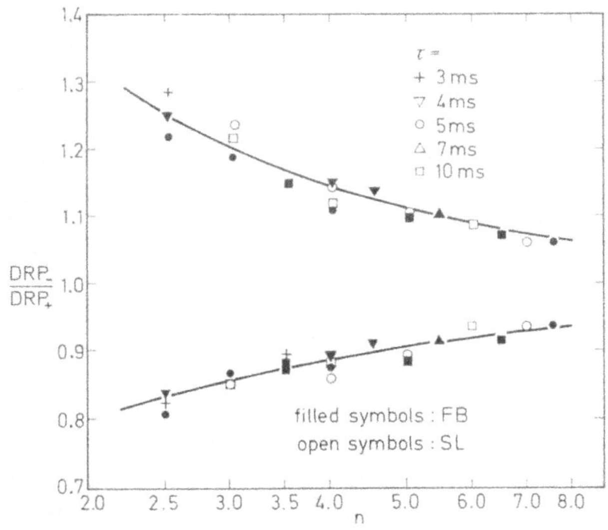

Fig. 38. Relation between DRP_- and DRP_+ for band-pass filtered signals. The thick lines are computed from $DRP_-/DRP_+ = \tau/(\tau \pm 1/2f_0)$, where f_0 is the centre frequency of the filter. Note that the abscissa is labelled as $n = f_0 \cdot \tau$. After BILSEN and GOLDSTEIN (1974)

Just as for MRP, further experiments were carried out on the effect produced by inverting the delayed noise signal $n(t-\tau)$ before it is presented to the ear. Let us designate dichotic repetition pitch by DRP_+ when the two signals are presented with the same polarity, and by DRP_- when the delayed version is inverted. It was found that DRP_- deviates significantly from DRP_+. In general, two DRP_- pitches can be perceived, one a little higher, the other a little lower than $1/\tau$. For wide-band signals, the best agreement was obtained when, for DRP_-, the actual time delay τ (in msec) was increased or decreased by 0.8 msec; the measured pitches corresponded well with $1/(\tau+0.8)$ and $1/(\tau-0.8)$. Note that this result holds for DRP only; for MRP it is different (see Section F. 8).

The wide-band signals employed covered the frequency region up to 2 kHz. Experiments with the same paradigm but executed with narrow-band signals (bandwidth: one third of an octave) yielded pitch deviations that were a distinct function of the central frequency f_0. In Fig. 38, the results are plotted. The ordinate shows the relation between DRP_- and DRP_+ values; the abscissa is labelled as n, the equivalent rank number associated with f_0 (actually, n is calculated from $n = f_0 \cdot \tau$). The two sets of data correspond to the two possible pitches. If we compare this figure with Fig. 26, we see a very close correspondence. For the narrow-band DRP_ pitches, the same formula is proposed as for MRP with negative p; the pitch corresponds to $1/(\tau \pm 1/2f_0)$. This relation is presented in the figure in the form of two solid lines, the experimental data points are observed to be described rather accurately by this formula.

Returning once more to wide-band signals, the results of the experiments indicate that there is a single frequency region of dominance; the value of 0.8 msec is equivalent to half a period of a centre frequency of 625 Hz. This dominant region appears to be effective for all values of τ employed. It is recalled that in the monaural case the dominant region appears to adjust itself to the value of τ used in the experiment (Section F. 8).

10. Relation with "BMLD" and the "EC" Theory

It is clear that the DRP phenomenon cannot be explained by simply assuming that the two spectral representations produced by the two peripheral hearing organs are added. There must be involved some subtle form of interaction. Binaural interactions are well-known phenomena in view of directional hearing, lateralization, etc. Regrettably, there is not one type of binaural interaction that is capable of tying together all experimental evidence of this nature. Perhaps the auditory phenomenon that is closest to DRP is the so-called Binaural Masking-Level Difference (BMLD). Space does not permit a full description, so only a few basic remarks will be presented, sufficient to convey the gist of the ideas involved. Suppose a tone is presented at such a level that it is just masked by a (wide-band) noise signal. If tone and masking signals are presented identically at the two ears, there will be no advantage over the monaural situation; in this case, the binaural masked threshold is the same as in the monaural condition. Now, let the polarity of the tone signal as it is presented to one of the ears be inverted. The tone at the other ear remains the same, and the noise is presented to the two ears with identical waveforms, as before. The surprising fact is that the masked threshold can be considerably lower in this situation.

This "release from masking" (as it is sometimes called) can be explained if we assume that somewhere in the nervous system an operation is performed which is equivalent to a subtraction of the two waveforms of the two stimuli. Even when such a subtraction would be imperfect, contaminated by neural noise, for instance, the tone would stand out in the resulting signal with respect to the noise. This idea has been worked out in great detail by DURLACH (1972). The subtraction stage was characterized as the process of "cancellation". To account for all experimental results on BMLD's, it was necessary to assume that the subtraction process did not involve the signals as they are presented at the ears, nor the signals as they might be processed by the peripheral organs. In DURLACH's theory, another idea is incorporated; before being subject to the subtraction process, the signals originating from the two ears are made alike as much as possible. That is, they are made to have the same average amplitude, and, furthermore, they are assumed to be shifted in time so as to make them as similar as possible. This part of the mechanism is referred to as the "equalization process".

The basic ideas involved in this EC-theory (Equalization and Cancellation) are taken over by BILSEN and GOLDSTEIN to the domain of dichotic repetition pitch. In order to achieve a resulting signal that displays the characteristics of an MRP signal, addition is postulated instead of subtraction. In this way, the properties of DRP are brought back to those of MRP. In line with recent developments, the explanation of the properties of pitch is sought entirely in the spectral domain. In other words, the proposed addition process is invoked only to obtain a resulting signal with the spectral properties required for an MRP.

The theory also offers a qualitative description for the FOURCIN pitch. In FOURCIN's experiments, two independent signal pairs, each of the type described above, were used. The first pair consists of the noise signal $n_1(t)$ and its delayed version $n_1(t - \tau_1)$. The second pair consists of another noise signal $n_2(t)$ and the same noise, delayed over a different time interval τ_2, to be written $n_2(t - \tau_2)$. The signals presented at the ears consist of various combinations of these four signals. It appears reasonable to assume that the "equalization stage" is presented with partly conflicting cues, and it thus sets a different standard for each condition. By the use of this expedient, many aspects of FOURCIN's work receive an explanation. The FOURCIN pitch then appears as an extension of the dichotic repetition pitch, and the latter appears as the more fundamental phenomenon.

A monaural version of the FOURCIN pitch experiments has been studied by ROSENBERG (1975). The sum of three signals was presented to the ear: a noise signal $n(t)$, a delayed version of it $n(t - \tau_1)$ and a second delayed version $n(t - \tau_2)$. Among the several pitches audible there was one corresponding to $\tau_1 - \tau_2$. If the resulting signal is inspected on its temporal properties, *e. g.*, in terms of its autocorrelation function (*cf.* Section E. 4 where an operational neural model is described capable of carrying out the analysis), this result is easy to understand. In terms of the recognition of the shape of the spectrum, the location of peaks and valleys, etc., the existence of this pitch is more difficult to visualize. We mention this experiment mainly because of its connection to the FOURCIN pitch phenomenon; the consequences of ROSENBERG's experiment have not yet been worked out in detail.

11. The Internal Spectrum

We now come to the latest types of evidence that are relevant to the problem of spectral versus temporal processing. One of the major arguments in favour of a theory of temporal processing of residue signals has always been based on the existence of *phase effects* (see, *e. g.*, Sections E. 8 and E. 14). Figure 16 shows several typical waveforms of three-component residue signals. The waveforms are characterized by prominent envelopes (indicated by the dotted lines). Any change of the phase relation of the components that leaves the waveshape of the envelope the same does not lead to an audible change of timbre. All phase changes obeying DE BOER's phase rule (1956a, 1961) belong to this class [see the description in Section E. 8 and Relation (10)]. Any *other* type of phase change may be perceptible, especially when the spacing of components is relatively narrow. Such phase changes affect the prominence of peaks in the waveform of the envelope; in the framework of a temporal residue theory, this would lead to changes in the synchronization of nerve firings and, ultimately, to changes in prominence of the residue. If, in line with the recent trends as described in the preceding sections, we are led to believe that all residue processing is based upon spectral amplitudes, the phase effects remain a puzzle. There are strong indications that phase effects are intimately connected with combination tones. Evidence for this notion is presented in the following paragraphs.

First, it should be made clear that the "spectrum", upon which the central residue processor is assumed to operate, contains the combination tones in exactly the same form as the acoustic components. In a series of tests, it was shown by BUUNEN *et al.* (1974) that a combination tone and an objective acoustic component of exactly the same frequency follow the normal rules of addition when they are combined. The second point demonstrated in BUUNEN'S paper is that the residue is the most prominent for that phase relation of the components for which the strength of the (third-order) combination tone is highest.

A third piece of what may be termed circumstantial evidence is the proof that a combination tone that is coincident in frequency with one acoustic component shows exactly the same phase change as that component for all phase changes obeying DE BOER'S phase rule. This proof is described in the same paper. We present the proof here in a simplified form. Consider a three-component signal, the upper two component frequencies being called f_1 and f_2. The third-order combination tone with frequency $2f_1 - f_2$ is coincident with the lowest acoustical component. If all acoustical components are given the same phase change φ_0 [*cf.* Relation (10) in Section E. 8], the combination tone acquires a phase change of $2\varphi_0 - \varphi_0$ and this is equal to φ_0, the phase change of the lowest acoustic component. A phase change proportional to frequency is equivalent to a shift in the origin of the time axis, and, therefore, cannot affect any combination tone in another way than an acoustic component. This completes the proof that the combination tone with frequency $2f_1 - f_2$ acquires exactly the same phase change as the objective component of the same frequency. It is thus seen that the phase rule not only describes situations leaving the envelope of the waveform invariant but also the situations leaving the relation between combination tones and objective components invariant.

From these studies, it can be concluded that the "internal spectrum" is composed of both objective components and combination tones without distinction between these two. For phase changes of the objective signal that conform to the linear phase rule (10), the internal spectrum remains the same no matter whether combination tones contribute or not. The residue is the most prominent when the internal spectrum shows the largest component amplitudes.

12. Phase Effects — Buunen's Work

We now turn to the phase changes that do not obey the linear-phase rule (10). The associated changes in timbre are most easily noticed when the components of a three-component signal are not locked to one another but are produced by free-running oscillators. We can represent that signal in the following way: assume first that the frequencies are exactly equidistant and replace one of the components by one with a slightly different frequency. BUUNEN and BILSEN (1974) describe several experiments executed with this type of signal of which we will present the one that is the most relevant at this stage. The original frequencies are labelled $f_c - \Delta f$, f_c, and $f_c + \Delta f$. (The symbol f_c is equivalent to the carrier frequency f of Section E. 6ff., F. 2, etc. and Δf is equivalent to g.) The components with frequencies $f_c - \Delta f$ and $f_c + \Delta f$ are presented directly to the ear, but f_c is replaced by f'_c deviating a few Hz from f_c. If $\Delta f/f_c$ is sufficiently small (*e. g.* < 0.15), beats are heard that are easily associated with the varying phase relation between the f'_c-component and the other components. Note that the phase of the central component differs from the average phase of the two outer components and that, consequently, the phase variations do not conform to (10).

A component is added to the signal with a frequency of $2f'_c - (f_c + \Delta f)$, exactly the same frequency as the aural cubic difference tone (CDT). Amplitude and phase of this component can be adjusted by the listener just as in a cancellation experiment (see Section G. 4). If the phase effects would result from variations of the signal's envelope, no setting of amplitude and phase of the added component would result in their disappearance. BUUNEN and BILSEN report that their listeners were able to adjust the cancellation tone so that the beats disappeared. Unfortunately, they give no details as to whether the setting corresponds to that in which the combination tone is fully cancelled. In an informal experiment, the present author was able to corroborate their finding. At a particular setting of amplitude and phase of the cancellation tone, the timbre beats of the residue disappear, only a very faint beat associated with the lowest part-tone remains. The setting necessary to achieve this is very close to that for cancellation of the CDT.

The implication of these findings is clear: phase effects are strongly related to combination tones. We may extrapolate from these findings the following. Changes in the timbre of the residue are related to changes in the internal spectrum composed as it is of acoustical components and combination tones. Any phase change that leaves the internal spectrum the same does not affect the residue timbre. Any phase change that causes one or more of the internal components to change its amplitude may produce an audible change of the residue timbre. The prominence of residue pitch is a monotonic function of the strength of those components of the internal spectrum that are dominant with respect to pitch. It should be noted that these remarks are extrapolations which may not be justified in the most general situation, *e. g.*, the effect produced by changes in the phase of only one component amidst a great many components. It can be expected that such a situation is a most difficult and complicated one from the experimental point of view since several combination tones contribute to the internal spectrum.

13. Binaural Diplacusis and the Residue (van den Brink)

The importance of aural isolation of partials is confirmed by a series of experiments by VAN DEN BRINK (1970, 1975a, b). Binaural diplacusis is used as a tool to measure details about the way the pitch of the residue is derived from the pitches of the (resolved) partials. When a pure tone is presented alternatingly to the left and to the right ear, the pitch may not seem the same. The pitch difference "between the ears" can be measured by presenting tones with different frequencies alternatingly to the two ears and having the observer adjust the frequency of the tone at one ear so as to achieve equality of pitch. The pitch differences measured in this way show an irregular pattern when viewed as a function of frequency; this pattern may show day-to-day variations but over a period of several hours it is fairly stable. *Binaural diplacusis* is the term denoting the phenomenon that the same tone may have a different pitch at the two ears; the magnitude of this effect can be expressed as the (relative) shift of frequency that is necessary to compensate for the difference in pitch.

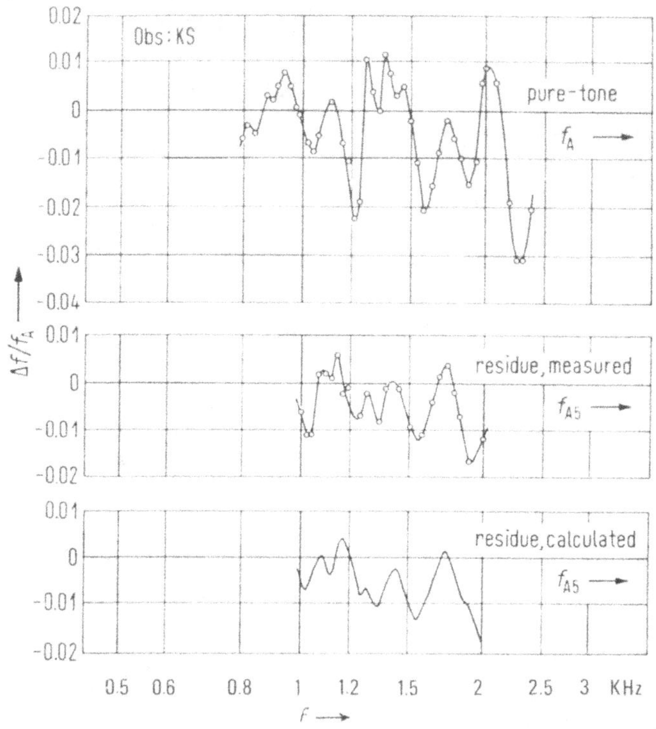

Fig. 39. Measured diplacusis for pure tones and residue signals (upper and centre panels). The lower panel shows the theoretical prediction (see text). The abscissa is the frequency f of the pure tone or the 5th harmonic. After VAN DEN BRINK (1975a)

What is described here for pure tones holds true also for residue signals; binaural diplacusis for residue pitch can be measured by essentially the same method. In all cases, a great measurement accuracy is needed, of the order of 0.1%. In VAN DEN BRINK's experiments, the residue signals consisted of the 4th, 5th, and 6th harmonics. Signal A (fundamental frequency f_A) presented to the left ear was alternated with Signal B (frequency f_B) presented to the right ear. The subjects were instructed to vary f_B until the pitches of the sounds at the two ears were the same. Care was exercised to ensure that the pitch matches were indeed based upon judgements of residue pitches and not on the comparison of aurally isolated partials (part-tones). The magnitude of diplacusis can be plotted as the ratio $(f_B - f_A)/f_A$ necessary to achieve equality of pitch; the central panel of Fig. 39 shows some representative results. The abscissa (f) is the frequency of the central component, in this case five times the fundamental f_A. The upper panel of the figure shows diplacusis values for pure tones; the abscissa is now the frequency of these tones. Evidently, there is some similarity between these two sets of data for one observer.

From the pure-tone diplacusis values, a prediction can be made about the diplacusis of the residue. For any of the residue signals employed, the diplacusis values can be determined for each of the components; averaging of these values yields the data plotted in the lower panel of the figure. It is surprising how well this prediction agrees with experimental results for residues (central panel). The pitch of the residue apparently correlates well with the (average of the) pitches that each of the components would have if it were presented in isolation. *It is the "pitch information" of the part-tones rather than the "frequency information" of the components that determines the pitch of a residue.* If we translate the pitch information contributed by each component into the "place" in the cochlea corresponding to maximal excitation, we arrive at an extended place theory, just as DE BOER implied in his pseudo-fundamental theory (Section E. 9) or as it is crystallized in WIGHTMAN'S and GOLDSTEIN'S theories. Compare also WALLISER'S results (1968). This conclusion holds true only under the conditions described: signals containing components near the region of spectral dominance. With higher rank numbers of the components, there will be a larger overlap of the excitation patterns in the cochlea and a non-negligible contribution of combination tones; indeed it was observed that the agreement between theory and experiment deteriorates drastically for rank numbers beyond 8. This point will not be pursued in the present review. The main results of the study were corroborated by several experiments in which the pitch-frequency relations of one of the ears were manipulated. The application of low-pass noise or the execution of the test where one ear is under the condition of auditory fatigue are examples of the methods used in additional experiments. In all cases, the basic findings could be confirmed.

One of VAN DEN BRINK'S experiments (1975b) is interesting also because of the pitch percepts involved. Signal A consisted of the 4th, 5th, and 6th harmonics (of frequency f_A), all presented to the left ear. Signal B consisted of the same harmonics (of a different frequency, f_B) but these were divided between the ears; the 4th and 6th harmonics were presented to the left ear while the 5th harmonic was presented to the right ear. Here, we have the peculiar situation that the components at the left ear have a fundamental one octave above f_B. Yet the residue pitch corresponds to f_B provided the sound is not too loud. Another surprising fact is that this residue is localized near the left ear. The pitch perceived on the left jumps by one octave when the right-ear signal is switched off. A pure-tone sensation corresponding to the single component at the right ear is perceived at that side. During the pitch matches it proved quite easy to concentrate upon the residues perceived on the left side and to disregard the pure-tone percept on the other side.

In the light of HOUTSMA and GOLDSTEIN's work, these observations are not too surprising. They suggest that the information coming from the two ears interacts to determine residue pitch, and the same pitch is then associated with the side receiving the most complex information. The experiments described here were intended to serve quite another purpose, namely, to determine accurately how much the pitch information of one single component contributes to the pitch of the residue. It could be concluded that the weights of the three components are about equal in this process. This holds for signals consisting of the 4th, 5th, and 6th components. For other rank numbers, the results are not conclusive.

14. Spectral Aspects of Time Separation Pitch and Monaural Repetition Pitch

The main tendency of the studies reported in the preceding sections is that information about pitch is mainly conveyed by spectral information and not by temporal information. So we must have another look at those experiments that once seemed to confirm that pitch is strongly related to periodicity. Let us reconsider, therefore, the interpretations of time-separation pitch. (Section E. 12) and repetition pitch (Section F. 8). There is no doubt that the simplest explanation of the presence of pitch can be based on temporal aspects of the signals. The signals involved have the peculiarity that the waveforms are almost identical to time-shifted versions of themselves, and it is not too far-fetched to conclude that a neuron arrangement like the one of Fig. 12 would bring out this property easily. An interpretation in spectral terms is slightly more difficult. Since the spectral description of a noise signal is more involved than that of a deterministic signal, we shall consider the case of a double-pulse series like that depicted in Fig. 18. This signal leads to perception of time-separation pitch (TSP).

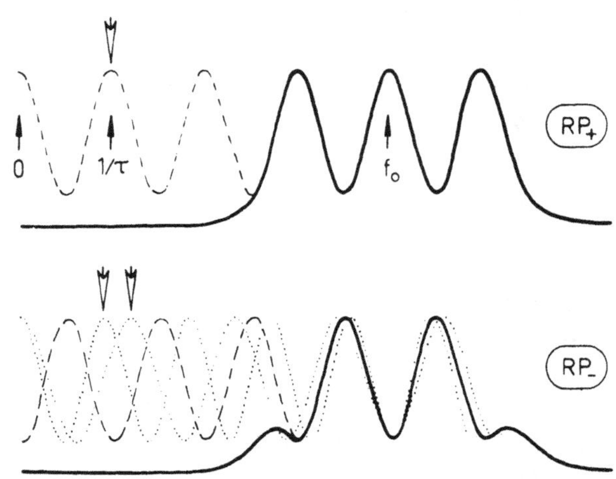

Fig. 40. Illustrating the matching procedure carried out by the central pitch processor. The thick lines indicate the spectrum of the (filtered) stimulus. The dashed line is the spectrum of the same stimulus but unfiltered. The dotted lines show the spectrum that the central processor tries to match to the actual spectrum. The two panels pertain to two possible repetition pitch (RP) conditions, RP_- and RP_+. In the latter case two different matches are possible arrow. After BILSEN and GOLDSTEIN (1974)

One periodic series of pulses has a spectrum consisting of many components (see, *e. g.* Fig. 4a). The presence of the "echo" causes undulations in the spectrum. In particular, the components with frequencies at or near odd multiples of $1/2\tau$ (τ is the delay time) will be reduced drastically. The spectrum will show peaks between these points, at integral multiples of $1/\tau$; *i. e.*, at even multiples of $1/2\tau$. When the polarity of the "echo" is inverted, the spectral magnitude will be reduced at even multiples of $1/2\tau$, including the frequency zero. (The same type of spectral modification occurs when an echo is added to a noise signal; note that in this case the spectrum must be interpreted in the statistical sense.) In terms of the newer residue theories, we must assume that the general shape of the spectrum is recognized by the central processor and that the successive peaks are interpreted as successive "harmonics" of a common "fundamental frequency". The latter frequency is the pitch of the corresponding residue.

Now, if the signal presented is band-limited, *i. e.*, restricted in its frequency range, the task for the central pitch processor is much more difficult. An idea of how the interpretation in terms of "successive harmonics" is achieved is presented in Fig. 40, taken from Bilsen and Goldstein's (1974) paper. The two cases illustrated pertain to "echo's" of positive and negative polarities, respectively. For reasons of clarity, the spectra are not shown as groups of lines (each line corresponding to an integral multiple of the fundamental frequency) but as continuous functions. In this respect, the same figure describes also the average spectrum of the signals used for repetition pitch (This explains why the two panels are labelled by RP_+ and RP_-.)

For the upper panel (positive polarity of the echo), a satisfactory match is achieved between the actual spectrum and a hypothetical one (dashed line) containing lobes at integral multiples of $1/\tau$. This makes it plausible that the pitch will correspond to $1/\tau$ despite the fact that the spectrum is incomplete. For the lower panel, the actual spectrum is a part of a spectrum that has zero amplitude at a frequency of zero and that has maxima at odd multiples of $1/2\tau$ (see the dashed line). The spectrum is interpreted by the central processor as a "regular" spectrum (one that has a maximum also at the frequency zero); this is indicated by the figure. Actually, there are two possible matches – in terms of other theories: there are two possible pseudo-fundamentals. Both matching spectra are shown as thin dotted lines.

The principal point illustrated by this figure is that the determination of a pitch value is achieved by a process of pattern recognition. Compare Wightman's theory in this respect; in the present case, the central processor tries to find the best index (pseudo-fundamental) to describe the observed undulations in the spectrum. If we assume that the accuracy of the matching procedure is determined by the critical band on the one hand, and the irrelevance of the lower spectral lobes on the other hand, we can easily understand why for a wide-band signal the region of spectral dominance seems to adjust itself in accordance with the value of τ (*cf.* Section F. 8). In all conditions, the third to fifth peaks in the spectrum will be the most important ones for the determination of pitch, and, as a result, the frequency region of these peaks acts as the dominant region.

I. "Time-Out" (General Reflections)

1. The Importance of "Set"

Must we say goodbye to the "residue"? We might be inclined to say: yes. In the course of this treatise, we witnessed the gradual change of meaning of the term "residue", a change that finally led to a new and less restrictive definition (see *e. g.* Section E. 10). At the same time the musical aspects of "residue pitch" grew more and more important. Was the residue originally thought to be one bearer of pitch, later it appeared that the residue formed by a few of the lower components is dominant even with respect to the fundamental. What has remained is the notion that the percept of the residue can only be brought about by a particular form of collaboration of components, and, in this form, the residue is dominant even with respect to the fundamental. Allusions to phenomena like the "pitchiness" of chopped noise belong to the past; a much more refined correlation between spectral components is necessary to invoke a pitch percept in the musical sense. Instead of chopped noise, we nowadays discuss phenomena like repetition pitch and combination tones.

What is also new is the ambiguity involved in residue pitch. This was recognized rather hesitantly at first (Section E. 6); later, it was considered an essential feature of the mechanism (Section E. 14). How essential it is did not become completely clear before the work on two-tone complexes and musical intervals (Section H. 2). In last instance, even the harmonic number n of the lower partial appeared to be essentially ambiguous (Section H. 6). The ambiguity involves one other concept that is, in the opinion of the present reviewer, of the greatest importance. Every psychophysical result is the product of the specific methodology involved and the "set" or "state of conditioning" of the subject. When we listen to a sound, we do not perceive this or that aspect of the sound all the time; what we perceive depends completely on our training. Let us recall, for instance, the introspection involved in the recognition of the residue in SCHOUTEN's terms (Section D. 9), the "classical" counterpart of the "instruction phase" involved in present-day psychophysics. In this connection, we recall also that there are two groups of listeners as regards their primary reaction to two-tone signals (Section G. 6). But we must appreciate as well that a particular listener involved in a particular task produces a result that is highly dependent upon his training, motivation, ability, etc. Hence, the fact that the result of a particular experiment turns out to be extremely clear-cut does not necessarily imply that every naive listener is able to perceive the signals in the same way. It is not too difficult to associate a (residue) pitch with a two-tone complex presented monaurally. But to do the same with a two-tone complex presented dichotically is quite another matter. A similar difference obtains for repetition pitch: every naive listener can immediately perceive monaural repetition pitch but the dichotic phenomenon (Section H. 9) is so much weaker that many listeners experience extreme difficulties with it. Yet, in both cases, we see that psychophysical tests (admittedly executed under ideal circumstances) indicate a performance that is nearly the same for dichotic and monotic conditions.

We may conclude that we must be extremely cautious in our conclusions. The "normal" mechanism for extracting pitch is not "connected" to the two ears as it appears to be functioning in HOUTSMA and GOLDSTEIN'S dichotic experiments (Section H. 3). But by proper training and instruction, the mechanism can switch from the monaural to the binaural mode and it seems to operate with the same perfection and with the same limitations. It is then logical to endow the underlying mechanism with a set of constraints that operate in the same way under both types of conditions. However, there is no direct evidence that this is fully justified – it remains a theory.

We may carry this scrutiny over to the domain of dichotic repetition pitch, and, in that case, the conclusion may be slightly different. In order to explain dichotic repetition pitch (Section H. 4), it is necessary to postulate some interaural interaction that is partly based on waveform aspects. The idea is borrowed from work on binaural masking level differences (BMLD's), and it serves its purpose well. But we do not necessarily have to conclude that a similar mechanism is operative under "daily listening conditions". Moreover, there is no indication as to whether or not the subjective "strength" of dichotic repetition pitch is comparable to that of BMLD phenomena, and we have no inkling as to whether or not the same amount of additional training is needed to perceive it. The negative results of HOUTSMA and GOLDSTEIN'S experiments (1971) on the perceptibility of dichotic phase effects only augment our doubts. This is one of the fundamental problems in the interpretation of advanced psychophysical experiments; comparison of different experiments must proceed with the greatest possible caution. The present reviewer hopes that the reader will interpret with the same caution all that has been written in this chapter on the residue phenomenon.

2. Guide to Related Literature

In collecting and selecting the material for this chapter, many subjects were left out of the discussion entirely. As is pointed out in the introduction, the selection process was a careful and deliberate one. Apologies are due to numerous authors that have contributed to residue research but do not find their work cited appropriately. No attempt will be made to fill that gap, or to be complete in that respect, but some indications are in order as to where to find other pertinent material in the literature. This may guide the cautious and interested reader to domains of pitch phenomena that have not been treated in the present text.

Residue pitch is an important aspect of speech perception. Yet it has proved extremely difficult to incorporate it in the analysis and synthesis of speech. Many different types of "pitch extractors" have been proposed but none of these was entirely satisfactory. We mention only two possibilities for a pitch extractor. The "cepstrum" technique (NOLL, 1964) is, in a way, analogous to WIGHTMAN'S pattern-transformation theory (Sections H. 4 and H. 5) but without the limited frequency resolution of this theory. SCHROEDER (1968) proposed two pitch extractors that symbolize the two fundamental aspects upon which the present chapter is concentrated; one extractor operates on regularity in the temporal, the other on regularity in the spectral domain. The latter type of pitch extractor can be connected with GOLDSTEIN'S theory (Section H. 6) and could be modified easily to mimic almost all aspects of our perception of intonation in speech. Many other pitch extractors work on the principle of reconstituting the fundamental by non-linear distortion; as we have seen, these procedures have no connection with pitch perception.

Pitch in music has important uses in the formation of melodies and of harmonies (chords). Studies on the relation between musical scales and fundamental properties of the auditory system can be found in TERHARDT's work (1972a, b, 1974a). Musical intervals exist in two forms, successive and simultaneous. The concepts of consonance and dissonance are crucial for simultaneously presented tones. The relation between consonance and frequency analysis in hearing was studied by PLOMP and LEVELT (1965). Unfortunately, this work was not continued with residue signals; hence, the conclusions are partly the result of extrapolation and relate more to the physics of signals than to the logic of perception. More modern views on, *e.g.*, beats of mistuned consonances (PLOMP, 1967a) invoke the involvement of combination tones (HALL, 1972b). At present, much work is concentrated on dynamic aspects of pitch successions; the opinions seem not to be crystallized enough to cite one authorative review.

In its original conception, the term "residue" was conceived to encompass phenomena associated with the perception of unresolved components, hence, with the perception of temporal phenomena. This aspect of the residue has received less and less emphasis, at least in studies where especially the musical pitch aspects have been pursued. This does not imply, of course, that the perception of temporal properties of signals has been neglected. On the contrary, several schools of research have concentrated on this subject. The entire range of possibilities between tonal residues (distinguished by a clear pitch) and a-tonal residues (distinguished by a rattle-like quality) has been explored by RITSMA and HOEKSTRA (1974). The perception of roughness has been studied very thoroughly by TERHARDT (1968, 1974b), who was amongst the first authors to question the alleged relationship between pitch perception and unresolved components (1970, 1972).

A completely novel way of studying psychophysical phenomena has been introduced by HOUTGAST (1972, 1973). Normally, thresholds are determined as the limits for detecting the presence of a signal. In the pulsation threshold method, the signal under study alternates with another one (encompassing the same frequency region). Under appropriate conditions, an auditory illusion is created; the listener does not perceive the alternations but hears the test signal as a continuous signal. By varying the stimulus conditions the limit of continuity is determined; this is called the "pulsation threshold". This new method has opened up a vast area of applications; the first of these have already been quite successful, a definite confirmation of the fact that a phenomenon like lateral suppression exists also for auditory perception (HOUTGAST, 1972). The consequences of this type of work may reach very far, indeed; at present, they cannot even be assessed in a very approximate way.

3. Conferences

Many European scientists have contributed to residue research. They have had the opportunity to discuss their work in a truly international setting in three important conferences. The first two of these meetings took place in the Netherlands; the third, in Germany. It is interesting to note the shifts in emphasis from the published proceedings of these conferences (PLOMP and SMOORENBURG, 1970; LOPES CARDOZO, 1972; ZWICKER and TERHARDT, 1974). At the time of the first conference (in Driebergen, 1969), emphasis was still on the periodicity aspects of residue signals. This applies to the psychophysical as well as to the physiological research reported. Opinions that tended to disagree with the current view were ventured rather casually and with great reserve, yet they caused a great deal of discussion. The second conference was held in 1972 at the IPO in Eindhoven (SCHOUTEN's institute). At that time, the major part of the switch from periodicity aspects to spectral pattern recognition had already taken place. In the present author's recollection, several of the discussants seemed almost too eager in accepting the newer theories and denouncing the older ones. The balance between enthousiasm and sound criticism was reached somewhat later; the proceedings of the third conference (held in Tutzing, 1974) indicate a major shift of focus. It is no longer general pitch theory that holds the main part of attention. It was recognized that the neural mechanisms underlying the extraction of pitch information are too complex to allow for a fruitful study. Consequently, most of the papers describe research directed at more fundamental aspects of the mechanism of the cochlea, and very few papers have a direct bearing on pitch perception.

At present, there seem to be more puzzling problems concerning basic cochlear operation – problems about mechanics, sharpening, nonlinearity, to name but a few – than in pitch. However, *do we have to solve all these problems completely before we can tackle other questions*? Questions such as: in what form is information about the frequency of partials transferred to the central nervous system? Is it by way of "phase" or by "periodicity" (in the sense of partial synchrony between the stimulus waveform and the firings of auditory nerve fibers)? And: why is information about partials substantially less accurate than that for isolated pure tones?

4. Place and Period Coding in Nerve Fibers

Because of his personal interests, the present author cannot refrain from making some comments on these fundamental issues. The concept of "place" has received a different meaning nowadays. When a pure tone is presented to the ear, the activity (average firing rate) is maximal in a confined group of auditory nerve fibers. This group is characterized by rather sharp boundaries but not by a well localized or very pronounced maximum. Every nerve fiber carries information about the spectral content of the stimulus in a specific frequency region; this is the "principle of specific coding" (DE BOER, 1973). The information, when considered in terms of rate of firing, is not too precise, so that "place" information is not very specific. However, a nerve fiber also carries information in its pattern of firing. In fact, the firings are partly synchronous with a (band-pass) filtered form of the stimulus, the type of filtering being specific to the nerve fiber. If the ear is stimulated by a complex signal consisting of a number of components, many nerve fibers will be excited by more than one component. Still, for many fibers one component will be dominant over the others, and the nerve fiber's firings will be predominantly synchronous with that particular component (ROSE *et al.*, 1969; HIND *et al.*, 1967; DE BOER, 1973). This is what we mean by stating that information about components of a stimulus is also carried in terms of temporal aspects of nerve firings.

One of the major questions at issue during the 1969 Driebergen conference was whether the central nervous system possesses the means of extracting periodicity information from nervous activity patterns contributed by many nerve fibers. Recent research has suggested very strongly that this question is irrelevant insofar as the cues for residue pitch are concerned. Hence, a more modern question would be whether or not *the central nervous system utilizes temporal information from neural firing patterns for the isolation of partials.* This question cannot be fully answered now. But it is difficult to understand auditory analysis of highly specialized signals such as, *e. g.*, the ones used by DUIFHUIS (Section F. 7) on the basis of a "pure" place theory, with neural firing rate as the only variable.

It should be emphasized that it is not implied that the pitch of a partial is measured on the basis of the periodicity of nerve firings. The arguments presented above only concern the *isolation* of a partial, *i. e.*, the tying together of the information conveyed by the nerve fibers from a region in which one partial dominates. In the light of these elaborations, the author expresses the desire that, in the near future, research will be devoted to the processing of periodicity and regularity of firing patterns by the central nervous system. Such a study would be essential in a quest for revealing the mechanisms involved in the isolation of partials.

5. The One-Tone Residue

Returning once more to the subject of residue pitch, we have witnessed a continuous reduction of the number of components. Remarkably enough, the musical quality of the signals used has increased. It has been pointed out in Section I. 1 how cautious we must be in the interpretation of this statement; the listener must be brought into a certain "state" of competence and attention in order to perform the required task. The most extreme form of this effect is encountered in the case of the "one-component residue" (HOUTGAST, 1974). The experiment can only be carried out in a situation of low signal-to-noise ratio; *i. e.*, the signals are presented at levels slightly above the threshold (the threshold may be elevated by a continuously presented wide-band noise signal). The stimuli are two-tone complexes consisting of successive harmonics just as in SMOORENBURG's and in HOUTSMA and GOLDSTEIN's work. By way of a task of pitch comparisons, the subject is brought into a state in which he has to utilize his "central pitch processor". In the course of the experiment, one of the stimuli is sometimes replaced by a single component (one harmonic). The subject appears not to notice this, and his scores, when evaluated for those more or less isolated instances, are in line with his other scores. Apparently, the central pitch processor has substituted a subharmonic of the single harmonic just as it has tried to determine common subharmonic frequencies for all the two-component signals.

This experiment demonstrates in an extreme form how much a pattern-transformation process can be fooled before it ceases to operate. When one of the single-component stimuli is presented in isolation, there is no listener who would ascribe a pitch to it corresponding to a subharmonic, *i. e.*, an integral submultiple of the frequency. Yet, in the paradigm of HOUTGAST's experiment, these instances are bound to occur. Should we conclude that the listener is subject to illusions? Certainly not, or else we should conclude that all residue pitch perception phenomena are illusions. The experiment only demonstrates the distinction between *performance* in a task and *perception* in an introspective sense. Quite a few authors, when writing about the residue (in the classical sense, associated with periodicity pitch) failed to include the notions about introspection that were so clearly described and emphasized by SCHOUTEN. Modern authors should try to avoid a related pitfall; there is no one-to-one relation between perception and the outcome of a particular experiment.

HOUTGAST's experiment serves another function; it points once more to the modern-day dilemma described in the previous section. Is the pitch of the subharmonic recognized on the basis of the temporal pattern of nervous activity? Or on the basis of "place", *i. e.*, the locus of maximal activity? These are the same fundamental questions as before but their meaning has become quite different.

Formerly, these questions had to do with the periodicity of the sound and its processing. In this sense the situation is clear:

Is there a "place" for "periodicity"? The answer is: no.

Are we in a "period" of "place"? Answer: it seems so.

At present, the same questions can be asked about recognition and isolation of part-tones:

Is there a "place" for "periodicity"? The answer is: probably.

Are we in a "period" of "place"? Answer: not necessarily.

"Place" seems necessary in the present "period". But it may not be sufficient; partials may be processed by temporal mechanisms. We do not know for certain.

Period.

References

BÉKÉSY, G. VON: Experiments in hearing. New York: McGraw-Hill Co. 1960.

BILSEN, F. A.: Repetition pitch: Monaural interaction of a sound with the repetition of the same, but phase shifted, sound. Acustica **17**, 295—300 (1966).

BILSEN, F. A., GOLDSTEIN, J. L.: Pitch of dichotically delayed noise and its possible spectral basis. J. acoust. Soc. Amer. **55**, 292—296 (1974).

BILSEN, F. A., RITSMA, R. J.: Repetition pitch and its implication for hearing theory. Acustica **22**, 63—73 (1969, 1970).

BOER, E. DE: On the "residue" in hearing. Academic thesis, Amsterdam 1956a.

BOER, E. DE: Pitch of inharmonic signals. Nature (Lond.) **178**, 535—536 (1956b).

BOER, E. DE: A note on phase distortion and hearing. Acustica **11**, 182—184 (1961).

BOER, E. DE: On the principle of specific coding. J. Dynamic Systems, Measurement, and Control (Trans ASME) **95**-G, 265—273 (1973).

BOER, E. DE: Spectral transformations by essential nonlinearities. Internal memorandum Bell Telephone Laboratories (1975).

BOER, E. DE, BOUWMEESTER, J.: Critical bands and sensorineural hearing loss. Audiology (Basel) **13**, 236—259 (1974).

BRINK, G. VAN DEN: Experiments on binaural diplacusis and tone perception. In: PLOMP, R., SMOORENBURG, G. F. (Eds.): Frequency analysis and periodicity detection in hearing. Leiden, Netherlands: Sijthoff 1970.

BRINK, G. VAN DEN: The relation between binaural diplacusis for pure tones and for complex sounds under normal conditions and with induced monaural pitch shift. Acustica **32**, 159—165 (1975a).

BRINK, G. VAN DEN: Monaural frequency-pitch relations as the origin of binaural diplacusis for pure tones and residue sounds. Acustica **32**, 166—174 (1975b).

BUUNEN, T. J. F., BILSEN, F. A.: Subjective phase effects and combination tones. In: ZWICKER, E., TERHARDT, E. (Eds.): Facts and models in hearing. Berlin-Heidelberg-New York: Springer 1974.

BUUNEN, T. J. F., FESTEN, J. M., BILSEN, F. A., BRINK, G. VAN DEN: Phase effects in a three-component signal. J. acoust. Soc. Amer. **55**, 297—303 (1974).

CARDOZO, B. L.: Proceedings IPO conference on hearing theory. Eindhoven, Netherland: IPO 1972.

CRAMER, E. M., HUGGINS, W. H.: Creation of pitch through binaural interaction. J. acoust. Soc. Amer. **30**, 413—417 (1958).

DE BOER, E.: See under B.

DALLOS, P.: Combination tone $2f_1—f_2$ in microphonic potentials. J. acoust. Soc. Amer. **46**, 1437—1444 (1969).

DUIFHUIS, H.: Audibility of high harmonics in a periodic pulse. J. acoust. Soc. Amer. **48**, 888—893 (1970).

DUIFHUIS, H.: Audibility of high harmonics in a periodic pulse. II. Time effect. J. acoust. Soc. Amer. **49**, 1155—1162 (1971).

DUIFHUIS, H.: Cochlear nonlinearity and second filter; possible mechanism and implications. Submitted for publication, J. acoust. Soc. Amer. (1975).

DURLACH, N. I.: Binaural signal detection: equalization and cancellation theory. In: TOBIAS, J. V. (Ed.): Foundations of modern auditory theory. New York-London: Academic Press 1972.

EVANS, E. F., WILSON, J. P.: The frequency selectivity of the cochlea. In: MØLLER, A. A. (Ed.): Basic mechanisms in hearing. New York-London: Academic Press 1973.

FISCHLER, H.: Model of the "secondary" residue effect in the perception of complex tones. J. acoust. Soc. Amer. **42**, 759—764 (1967).

FLANAGAN, J. L., GUTTMAN, N.: On the pitch of periodic pulses. J. acoust. Soc. Amer. **32**, 1308—1319 (1960a).

FLANAGAN, J. L., GUTTMAN, N.: Pitch of periodic pulses without fundamental component. J. acoust. Soc. Amer. **32**, 1319—1328 (1960b).

FLETCHER, H.: The physical criterion for determining the pitch of a musical tone. Phys. Rev. **23**, 427—437 (1924).

FLETCHER, H.: Speech and Hearing. London: McMillan 1929.

FLETCHER, H.: Auditory patterns. Rev. Mod. Phys. **3**, 258—278 (1931).

FLETCHER, H.: Speech and hearing in communication. New York: Van Nostrand 1953.

FOURCIN, A. J.: The pitch of noise with periodic spectral peaks. In: Proceedings 5th International Congress on Acoustics, Liège, Vol. Ia, B 52 (1965).

FOURCIN, A. J.: Central pitch and auditory lateralization. In: PLOMP, R., SMOORENBURG, G. F. (Eds.): Frequency analysis and periodicity detection in hearing. Leiden, Netherland: Sijthoff 1970.

GOLDSTEIN, J. L.: Auditory spectral filtering and monaural phase perception. J. acoust. Soc. Amer. **41**, 458—479 (1967a).

GOLDSTEIN, J. L.: Auditory nonlinearity. J. acoust. Soc. Amer. **41**, 676—689 (1967b).

GOLDSTEIN, J. L.: Aural combination tones. In: PLOMP, R., SMOORENBURG, G. F. (Eds.): Frequency analysis and periodicity detection in hearing. Leiden, Netherland: Sijthoff 1970.

GOLDSTEIN, J. L.: An optimum processor theory for the central formation of the pitch of complex tones. J. acoust. Soc. Amer. **54**, 1496—1516 (1973).

GOLDSTEIN, J. L., KIANG, N. Y.-S.: Neural correlates of the aural combination tone $2f_1—f_2$. Proc. IEEE **56**, 981—992 (1968).

GOLDSTEIN, M. H. JR.: Neurophysiological representation of complex auditory stimuli. MIT-RLE, Technical Report **323** (1957).

GUTTMAN, N., FLANAGAN, J. L.: Pitch of high-pass-filtered pulse trains. J. acoust. Soc. Amer. **36**, 757—765 (1964).

HALL, J. L.: Auditory distortion products f_2-f_1 and $2f_1-f_2$. J. acoust. Soc. Amer. **51**, 1863—1871 (1972a).

HALL, J. L.: Monaural phase effect: cancellation and reinforcement of distortion products f_2-f_1 and $2f_1-f_2$. J. acoust. Soc. Amer. **51**, 1872—1881 (1972b).

HALL, J. L.: Two-tone distortion products in a nonlinear model of the basilar membrane. J. acoust. Soc. Amer. **56**, 1818—1828 (1974).

HELLE, R.: Amplitude und Phase des im Gehör gebildeten Differenztones dritter Ordnung. Acustica **22**, 74—87 (1969, 1970).

HELLE, R.: Selektivitätssteigerung in einem hydromechanischen Innenohrmodell mit Basilar- und Deckmembran. Acustica **30**, 301—312 (1974).

HELMHOLTZ, H. VON: Die Lehre von den Tonempfindungen als physiologische Grundlage für die Theorie der Musik. Braunschweig: Vieweg 1862. Fifth edition 1896. On the sensations of tone as a physiological basis for the theory of music. First English edition 1897. Paperback edition. New York: Dover 1954.

HIND, J. E., ANDERSON, D. J., BRUGGE, J. F., ROSE, J. E.: Coding of information pertaining to paired low-frequency tones in single auditory nerve fibers of the squirrel monkey. J. Neurophysiol. **30**, 794—816 (1967).

HOOGLAND, G. A.: The missing fundamental. A place theory of frequency analysis in hearing. Academic thesis, Utrecht (1953).

HOUTGAST, T.: Psychophysical evidence for lateral inhibition in hearing. J. acoust. Soc. Amer. **51**, 1885—1894 (1972).

HOUTGAST, T.: Psychophysical experiments on "tuning curves" and "two-tone inhibition". Acustica **29**, 168—179 (1973).

HOUTGAST, T.: Personal demonstrations (1974).

HOUTSMA, A. J. M., GOLDSTEIN, J. L.: Perception of musical intervals: evidence for the central origin of the pitch of complex tones. MIT-RLE, Technical Report **484** (1971).

HOUTSMA, A. J. M., GOLDSTEIN, J. L.: The central origin of the pitch of complex tones: evidence from musical interval recognition. J. acoust. Soc. Amer. **51**, 520—529 (1972).

KIANG, N. Y.-S., WATANABE, T., THOMAS, E. D., CLARK, L. F.: Discharge patterns of single fibers in the cat's auditory nerve. Cambridge, Mass.: MIT-Press (1965).

KIM, D. O., MOLNAR, C. E., PFEIFFER, R. R.: A system of nonlinear differential equations modeling basilar-membrane motion. J. acoust. Soc. Amer. **54**, 1517—1529 (1973).

LICKLIDER, J. C. R.: A duplex theory of pitch perception. Experientia (Basel) **7/4**, 128—134 (1951).

LICKLIDER, J. C. R.: "Periodicity pitch" and "place pitch". J. acoust. Soc. Amer. **26**, 945 (A) (1954).

LICKLIDER, J. C. R.: Auditory frequency analysis. In: Proceedings Third London Symposium on Information Theory 1955.

LOPES CARDOZO, B.: See under C.

MATHES, R. C., MILLER, R. L.: Phase effects in monaural perception. J. acoust. Soc. Amer. **19**, 780—797 (1947).

MCCLELLAN, M. E., SMALL, A. M., Jr.: Pitch perception of pulse pairs with random repetition rate. J. acoust. Soc. Amer. **41**, 690—699 (1967).

MILLER, G. A., TAYLOR, W. G.: The perception of repeated bursts of noise. J. acoust. Soc. Amer. **20**, 171—180 (1948).

NOLL, A. M.: Short-time spectrum and "cepstrum" techniques for vocal-pitch detection. J. acoust. Soc. Amer. **36**, 296—302 (1964).

NORDMARK, J.: Some analogies between pitch and lateralization phenomena. J. acoust. Soc. Amer. **35**, 1544—1547 (1963).

OHM, G. S.: Über die Definition des Tones, nebst daran geknüpfter Theorie der Sirene und ähnlicher tonbildender Vorrichtungen. Ann. Phys. Chem. **59**, 513—565 (1843).

OHM, G. S.: Noch ein Paar Worte über die Definition des Tones. Ann. Phys. Chem. **62**, 1—18 (1844).

PATTERSON, R. D.: The effects of relative phase and number of components on residue pitch. J. acoust. Soc. Amer. **53**, 1565—1572 (1973).

PFEIFFER, R. R., KIM, D. O.: Considerations of nonlinear response properties of single cochlear nerve fibers. In: MØLLER, A. A. (Ed.): Basic mechanisms in hearing. New York-London: Academic Press 1973.

PLOMP, R.: The ear as a frequency analyzer. J. acoust. Soc. Amer. **36**, 1628—1636 (1964).

PLOMP, R.: Detectability threshold for combination tones. J. acoust. Soc. Amer. **37**, 1110—1123 (1965).

PLOMP, R.: Experiments on tone perception. Academic thesis, Utrecht (1966).

PLOMP, R.: Beats of mistuned consonances. J. acoust. Soc. Amer. **42**, 462—474 (1967a).

PLOMP, R.: Pitch of complex tones. J. acoust. Soc. Amer. **41**, 1526—1533 (1967b).

PLOMP, R., LEVELT, W. J. M.: Tonal consonance and critical bandwidth. J. acoust. Soc. Amer. **38**, 548—560 (1965).

PLOMP, R., SMOORENBURG, G. F.: Frequency analysis and periodicity detection in hearing. Leiden, Netherland: Sijthoff 1970.

RHODE, W. S.: Observations of the vibration of the basilar membrane in squirrel monkeys using the Mössbauer technique. J. acoust. Soc. Amer. **49**, 1218—1231 (1971).

RITSMA, R. J.: Existence region of the tonal residue. I. J. acoust. Soc. Amer. **34**, 1224—1229 (1962).

RITSMA, R. J.: On pitch discrimination of residue tones. Intern. Audiol. **2**, 34—37 (1963).

RITSMA, R. J.: Frequencies dominant in the perception of the pitch of complex sounds. J. acoust. Soc. Amer. **42**, 191—198 (1967).

RITSMA, R. J., HOEKSTRA, A.: Frequency selectivity and the tonal residue. In: ZWICKER, E., TERHARDT, E. (Eds.): Facts and models in hearing. Berlin-Heidelberg-New York: Springer 1974.

ROSE, J. E., BRUGGE, J. F., ANDERSON, D. J., HIND, J. E.: Some possible neural correlates of combination tones. J. Neurophysiol. **32**, 402—423 (1969).

ROSENBERG, A. E.: Personal communication (1975).

RYAN, A., DALLOS, P.: Effect of absence of cochlear outer hair cells on behavioural auditory threshold. Nature (Lond.) **253**, 44—46 (1975).

SACHS, M. B., KIANG, N. Y.-S.: Two-tone inhibition in auditory-nerve fibers. J. acoust. Soc. Amer. **43**, 1120—1128 (1968).

SCHOUTEN, J. F.: The perception of subjective tones. Proceedings Kon. Acad. Wetensch. (Neth.) **41**, 1086—1094 (1938).

SCHOUTEN, J. F.: Synthetic sound. Philips Tech. Rev. **4**, 153—180 (1939).

SCHOUTEN, J. F.: The residue, a new component in subjective sound analysis. Proc. Kon. Acad. Wetensch. (Neth.) **43**, 356—365 (1940a).

SCHOUTEN, J. F.: The residue and the mechanism of hearing. Proc. Kon. Acad. Wetensch. (Neth.) **43**, 991—999 (1940b).

SCHOUTEN, J. F.: De toonhoogtegewaarwording. Philips Technisch Tijdschr. **5**, 298—306 (1940c).

SCHOUTEN, J. F., RITSMA, R. J., CARDOZO, B. L.: Pitch of the residue. J. acoust. Soc. Amer. **34**, 1418—1424 (1962).

SCHROEDER, M. R.: "Period histogram and product spectrum", new methods for fundamental-frequency measurement. J. acoust. Soc. Amer. **43**, 829—834 (1968).

SCHROEDER, M. R.: Relation between critical bands in hearing and the phase characteristic of cubic difference tones. J. acoust. Soc. Amer. **46**, 1488—1491 (1969).

SCHROEDER, M. R.: The amplitude behavior of the cubic difference tone. J. acoust. Soc. Amer. **58**, 728—732 (1975).

SEEBECK, A.: Beobachtungen über einige Bedingungen der Entstehung von Tönen. Ann. Phys. Chem. **53**, 417—436 (1841).

SEEBECK, A.: Ueber die Sirene. Ann. Phys. Chem. **60**, 449—481 (1843).

SIEBERT, W. M.: Frequency discrimination in the auditory system: place or periodicity mechanisms? Proc. IEEE **58**, 723—730 (1970).

SMALL, A. M., Jr.: Some parameters influencing the pitch of amplitude modulated signals. J. acoust. Soc. Amer. **27**, 751—760 (1955).

SMALL, A. M., JR., MCCLELLAN, M. E.: Pitch associated with time delay between two pulse trains. J. acoust. Soc. Amer. **35**, 1246—1255 (1963).

Smoorenburg, G. F.: Pitch perception of two-frequency stimuli. J. acoust. Soc. Amer. **48**, 924—942 (1970).

Smoorenburg, G. F.: Audibility region of combination tones. J. acoust. Soc. Amer. **52**, 603—614 (1972a).

Smoorenburg, G. F.: Combination tones and their origin. J. acoust. Soc. Amer. **52**, 615—632 (1972b).

Steele, C. R.: A possibility for sub-tectorial membrane fluid motion. In: Møller, A. A. (Ed.): Basic mechanisms in hearing. New York-London: Academic Press 1973.

Terhardt, E.: Über die durch amplitudenmodulierte Sinustöne hervorgerufene Hörempfindung. Acustica **20**, 210—214 (1968).

Terhardt, E.: Frequency analysis and periodicity detection in the sensations of roughness and periodicity pitch. In: Plomp, R., Smoorenburg, G. F. (Eds.): Frequency analysis and periodicity detection in hearing. Leiden, Netherland: Sijthoff 1970.

Terhardt, E.: Zur Tonhöhenwahrnehmung von Klängen. I. Psychoakustische Grundlagen. Acustica **26**, 173—186 (1972a).

Terhardt, E.: Zur Tonhöhenwahrnehmung von Klängen. II. Ein Funktionsschema. Acustica **26**, 187—199 (1972b).

Terhardt, E.: Pitch, consonance, and harmony. J. acoust. Soc. Amer. **55**, 1061—1069 (1974a).

Terhardt, E.: On the perception of periodic sound fluctuations (roughness). Acustica **30**, 201—213 (1974b).

Thurlow, W. R., Small, A. M., Jr.: Pitch perception for certain periodic auditory stimuli. J. acoust. Soc. Amer. **27**, 132—137 (1955).

Tonndorf, J.: Localization of aural harmonics along the basilar membrane of guinea pigs. J. acoust. Soc. Amer. **30**, 938—943 (1958).

Van den Brink, G.: See under B.

Walliser, K.: Zusammenwirken von Hüllkurvenperiode und Tonheit bei der Bildung der Periodentonhöhe. Academic thesis, Stuttgart 1968.

Walliser, K.: Zusammenhänge zwischen dem Schallreiz und der Periodenhöhe. Acustica **21**, 319—329 (1969a).

Walliser, K.: Über ein Funktionsschema für die Bildung der Periodentonhöhe aus dem Schallreiz. Kybernetik **6**, 65—72 (1969b).

Wever, E. G.: Theory of hearing. New York: Wiley 1949.

Wever, E. G., Lawrence, M.: Physiological acoustics. Princeton: University Press 1954.

Whitfield, I. C.: Central nervous processing in relation to spatio-temporal discrimination of auditory patterns. In: Plomp, R., Smoorenburg, G. F. (Eds.): Frequency analysis and periodicity detection in hearing. Leiden, Netherland: Sijthoff 1970.

Wightman, F. L.: Pitch and stimulus fine structure. J. acoust. Soc. Amer. **54**, 397—406 (1973a).

Wightman, F. L.: The pattern-transformation model of pitch. J. acoust. Soc. Amer. **54**, 407—416 (1973b).

Zwicker, E.: Der ungewöhnliche Amplitudengang der nichtlinearen Verzerrungen des Ohres. Acustica **5**, 67—74 (1955).

Zwicker, E.: Der kubische Differenzton und die Erregung des Gehörs. Acustica **20**, 206—209 (1968).

Zwicker, E.: Ein hydromechanisches Ausschnittmodell des Innenohres zur Erforschung des adequaten Reizes der Sinneszellen. Acustica **30**, 313—319 (1974).

Zwicker, E., Flottorp, G., Stevens, S. S.: Critical bandwidth in loudness summation. J. acoust. Soc. Amer. **29**, 548—557 (1957).

Zwicker, E., Terhardt, E.: Facts and models in hearing. Berlin-Heidelberg-New York: Springer 1974.

Chapter 14

Infrasound

H. E. von Gierke and D. E. Parker
Yellow Springs and Oxford, Ohio (USA)

With 16 Figures

Contents

I. Introduction

Human beings ordinarily detect only a small portion of the sound energy to which they are exposed. Indeed, sound is usually defined in terms of the limited range of frequencies to which the human ear readily responds — the "audiofrequency" range. However, sound energy at frequencies below this audiofrequency range can elicit both auditory and nonauditory responses from human beings. It is energy in this infrasound range that is the focus of the present chapter. This chapter deals with air-transmitted infrasound only; structure-borne infrasound, usually described as vibration, is not included.

Although infrasound is generated by many sources both within the body and in the external environment, recent development of artificial sources that generate high levels of this energy has necessitated a detailed examination of the effects of infrasound on human beings. The initial results from various laboratories appear to present a consistent picture. While it would be unreasonable to suggest that the findings concerning infrasound have reached a maximum, suggested by von Békésy (1974, Vol. V/1, Chapter 1) as the best time to write a handbook, the recent results dispel many of the errors and misconceptions that have been rife in the infrasound literature.

Exposure to infrasound elicits a variety of auditory and nonauditory responses. At threshold, the observer initially becomes aware of an intermittent chugging or motorboating sound. As stimulus intensity is increased, observers consistently report a sensation of pressure build-up in the middle ear. The pressure sensation appears related to tympanic membrane retraction and vascular infusion into the blood vessels of the tympanic membrane. The observers may also detect vibration of hair or clothing as well as a modulation of vocal signals at these infrasound levels. Further increases in intensity may result in pain, damage to middle ear structures, and temporary or permanent hearing loss.

The substantive material to be considered in this chapter is organized into seven main sections. Section II briefly reviews environmental and physiological infrasound sources as well as laboratory simulators. Some of the difficulties in measuring infrasound are also considered. Section III includes a discussion of the biomechanical principles of infrasound reception and a brief examination of external, middle, and inner ear responses. Direct auditory responses to infrasound (thresholds, loudness, and masking) are summarized in Section IV; damage to the ear associated with high intensity infrasound stimulation is also considered. Section V deals with the changes in audiofrequency sound reception due to the simultaneous presence of infrasound and/or static pressure. The effect of modulating an audiofrequency sound at an infrasound frequency is discussed briefly. Indirect auditory responses to infrasound are presented in Section VI. Included in this section are those responses which are mediated by the cochlea but which are not themselves primarily auditory. Indirect auditory responses can be physiological, such as cardiovascular and endocrine changes, or behavioral, such as disturbances of complex task performance and annoyance. By stimulating structures other than the cochlea, infrasound can elicit nonauditory responses; vestibular and respiratory nonauditory responses to infrasound are summarized in Section VII. The infrasound effects similar to those produced by structure-borne vibration are also examined in Section VII. Finally, proposed exposure limits for infrasound are presented in Section VIII.

The information considered in this chapter provides support for three basic points concerning infrasound. First, contrary to the statements contained in most treatments of hearing and a definition of the term itself, infrasound can produce auditory responses in human observers. Confusion might be reduced if we replaced the word "infrasound" with the phrase "low frequency sound". Second, the dangers of infrasound suggested by some scientists (GAVREAU *et al.*, 1966; GREEN and DUNN, 1968; BRYAN and TEMPEST, 1972) and in the popular press have been exaggerated. While very high levels of infrasound may produce damage or disturbance, the levels encountered in nearly all environments are not dangerous. Third, both auditory and nonauditory responses to infrasound are clarified by biomechanical analysis. Of particular interest is the suggestion that the auditory sensations evoked by infrasound can be understood by analyzing the distortion products of middle ear nonlinearities.

II. Infrasound Sources

A. Environmental and Physiological Sources

Infrasound is usually defined as airborne sound energy at frequencies below 16—20 Hz. While there seems to be a general consensus concerning the upper limit of the infrasound spectrum, there is less agreement regarding the lower frequency cutoff. Many investigators would place the low frequency infrasound limit at 0.1 Hz; other investigators suggest that the infrasound spectrum should extend to static pressure (PIMONOW, 1974). In this chapter, we generally consider 0.1 Hz as the lower limit for biologically significant infrasound effects, although static pressure, along with other forms of stimulation that share properties with infrasound, is discussed in Section V. However, the traumatic effects of large overpressures (blast waves) on the ear are not included (see HIRSCH, 1968).

The infrasound to which human beings are exposed during everyday activities derives from widely diverse natural and artificial sources. Natural infrasound sources include earthquakes and volcanic eruptions, water turbulence such as ocean waves and waterfalls, air turbulence, and thunder. Because of their long wavelength, infrasound disturbances can be propagated over great distances; STEPHENS (1971a) has suggested that the loss of energy from a 0.1 Hz wave traveling around the earth may be as little as 5%. Even though the atmospheric environment may seem silent to the human observer, pressure changes in the infrasound frequency range are continuously present. Pressure fluctuations in the range of 10^{-3} to 5 N/m^2 that can be correlated at observation points located several km apart have been labeled microbaroms. These microbaroms are distinguished from the large random pressure fluctuations, which may be as high as 50 N/m^2, that accompany winds of 30 km/h. Several observations of infrasound produced by natural events are included in Table 1.

Environmental infrasound that derives from man-made indoor and outdoor sources, such as transportation, industrial processes, and the operation of machinery, has received little attention until recently. The infrasound levels produced by large aerospace systems such as large rocket boosters and jet engines for supersonic transport-type aircraft primarily focused practical attention on this area (MOHR *et al.*, 1965; COLE *et al.*, 1966). As with audiofrequency sound surveys, environmental infrasound levels reported in the literature vary widely. In some

Table 1. Environmental infrasound and low frequency sound

Source of sound	Peak frequency (Hz)	Peak intensity dB SPL	Spectrum character	Ref.
Low freq. wind excited noise in a 16 story building during a storm (on 16th floor)	< 1	118	sharp	Brüel and Olesen (1973)
Low freq. wind excited noise in a 14 story building in stormy weather (on 13th floor)	< 1	120	sharp	Brüel and Olesen (1973)
Atmospheric pressure fluctuations	< 1	100	—	Nixon and Johnson (1973)
General pattern of noise from earth-quakes and explosions	10	86	rounded	Stephens (1971a)
Tuyère furnace, on the charging platform	25	123	—	Leventhall (1974)
Shaker tables in a foundry knock-out plant	25	120	—	Leventhall (1974)
Factory compressor noise	25	114	rounded	Leventhall (1974)
Noise near a blast furnace	7	115	sharp	Leventhall (1974)
Noise in boiler house of apartment block	41	89	sharp	Leventhall (1974)
Hand-held pile-driver at 20 yards	30	82	flat	Stephens (1971a)
Ventilation system noise				
factory	20	86	sharp	Leventhall (1974)
laboratory	33	91	sharp	Leventhall (1974)
office	30	78	sharp	Leventhall (1974)
Farm tractor noise	2, 4, and 30	80	flat	Stephens (1971a)
Noise in diesel train	2—32	100	flat	Leventhall (1974)
Noise in train on London subway	20	90	flat	Stephens (1971a)
Noises on a ship				
engine room (400 ton car ferry)	15	133	sharp	Leventhall (1974)
control room (cross-channel passenger vessel)	8	103	sharp	Leventhall (1974)
first class lounge (cross-channel passenger vessel)	32	110	sharp	Leventhall (1974)
Aircraft noise				
BAC 1—11 on take off	6 and 30	75	flat	Stephens (1971)
Riding in an aircraft	<10	120	—	Tempest (1971)
Helicopter noise				
inside a 2-seater	15	118	sharp	Leventhall (1974)
inside a 5-seater	28	120	sharp	Leventhall (1974)
Inside a space capsule	1—20	145	—	Tempest (1971)
Large rockets	1—20	150	—	Tempest (1971)
Inside a submarine	5—20	140	—	Tempest (1971)
Car noise				
saloon car traveling at 100 km/h with the quarter-light windows open	2	115	rounded	Leventhall (1974)
Saloon car traveling at 100 km/h with the rear window open	16	112	sharp	Leventhall (1974)

Table 1. (continued)

Source of sound	Peak frequency (Hz)	Peak intensity dB SPL	Spectrum character	Ref.
Car noise (cont'd)				
Volvo station car, one side window halfway open, 100—110 km/h	< 1	117	sharp	Brüel and Olesen (1973)
Fiat 500 with the sun roof removed	< 1	107	sharp	Brüel and Olesen (1973)
One-litre saloon car with the windows closed				
70 mph	1—5	103	flat	Tempest (1971)
60 mph	2	102	sharp	Tempest (1971)
40 mph	2	98	sharp	Tempest (1971)
One-litre saloon car with the driver's window open, 60 mph	2	115	sharp	Bryan and Tempest (1972)
Noise within a taxi cab				
windows closed	3 and 13	95	flat	Stephens (1971a)
windows open	28	92	flat	Stephens (1971a)
Running	2—4	90	—	Nixon and Johnson (1973)
Swimming	0.3—0.7	140	—	Nixon and Johnson (1973)
Physiological noise level with enclosed ear	16—20	75	rounded	Shaw (1974) Vol. V/1, Chapter 14

instances, differences in reported infrasound levels can be attributed to different recording procedures. Apparatus for recording infrasound and some of the difficulties in performing these measurements have been discussed by Brüel and Olesen (1973), Leventhall and Hood (1971), and Stephens (1971b). Differences in recording conditions also account for variation in reported environmental infrasound levels; this is particularly true for reports on infrasound generated in transportation.

Infrasound levels recorded inside automobiles vary as a function of several factors including vehicle speed, vehicle size, road conditions, windows open or closed, and so on. Figure 1 illustrates differences in the spectral distribution of infrasound pressures recorded inside automobiles under varying conditions. With windows open at high velocity (100 km/h), sound pressure levels between 110 and 120 dB (re 20 μ N/m^2) in the 2—20 Hz frequency range have been observed. At lower vehicle velocities and with the windows closed, infrasound levels drop to 90—100 dB.

Ships generate infrasound with peaks corresponding to the firing rate of the diesel engines. Sound pressure levels of 130—135 dB have been recorded in the engine room of a small car ferry; at other locations on various ships infrasound levels are in the 100—110 dB range.

Infrasound levels in regular (100 km/h) trains correspond with the levels seen in cars. Recently developed high speed trains generate acoustical environments which differ significantly from those encountered with regular trains. Fox and Vardy (1973) have calculated pressure variations up to 160 dB at the head of a

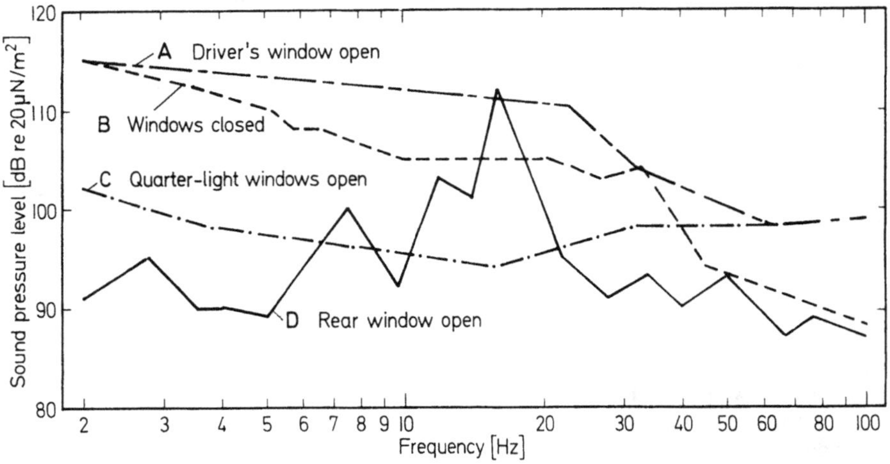

Fig. 1. Low frequency noise levels inside sedans traveling at 100 km/h under varying conditions of window closure. Data from Bryan and Tempest (1972) and Leventhall (1974)

train traveling through a parallel sided tunnel at 180 km/h. Oscillation of this pressure as a result of reflection from the far portal may have a frequency of 0.25 Hz, depending upon tunnel length. Observations on infrasound levels generated in transportation as well as by other artificial sources are included in Table 1.

Infrasound is also produced by the natural functioning of physiological systems within the body or by the activities pursued by human beings. Walking, jogging, or swimming should produce pressure changes at the tympanic membrane that are identical to the infrasound generated by a specific source. Nixon and Johnson (1973) calculated that jogging in a manner which causes the head to vary 15 cm in altitude should produce a pressure variation of about 90 dB at the basic frequency of the vertical oscillation (2—4 Hz). Swimming in a manner such that the ear oscillates between the air and a submerged depth of 7.5 cm produces pressure fluctuation equivalent to 141 dB (0.3—0.7 Hz). Infrasound due to physiological noise from circulation and muscle activity in the occluded external auditory meatus is in the order of 75 dB at 16—20 Hz (Shaw, 1974, Vol. V/1, Chapter 14); the infrasound due to physiological activity must be assumed to rise further at lower frequencies, at least down to the fundamental pulse frequency. These noise levels were measured under quiet listening conditions; infrasound levels from other activities such as chewing are not known but might well be higher.

The intensity of environmental infrasound, particularly that produced in the natural environment or by an individual's normal activities, is of interest because it may suggest minimum damage tolerance levels. It seems unlikely that physiological structures would survive phylogenic development unless those structures could withstand without impairment exposure to the stimulation ordinarily present in an organism's environment.

B. Laboratory Simulation

Artificial production of infrasound for laboratory investigation has employed a variety of sources ranging from simple manometers and pistonphones to whole-body enclosures. Several investigators have noted the importance of accurate analysis of the acoustical energy generated by these infrasound sources. One aspect of this analysis problem involves measurement of the infrasound signal components. The signal transducer and associated electronic analyzer should have a DC capability to insure detection of the entire signal. Further, the signals should be analyzed with narrow band filters (maximum of 5%) or on a "per cycle" basis. Also, the investigator must specify the audiofrequency components of the signal generated by the infrasound source. Harmonics produced by the infrasound source that are in the audiofrequency range may be easily detectable by the observer in an experiment.

Two related questions are central in evaluating the results of experiments that employ infrasound stimulation. First, does the infrasound source produce a pure signal, *i.e.*, to what extent are higher harmonic distortion products present in the signal? Second, does the investigator offer an adequate analysis of the total acoustical signal, particularly with respect to the higher harmonics? The problem of higher harmonics can be illustrated by referring to Fig. 4, which presents hearing thresholds as a function of frequency. At 10 Hz the threshold for detection is approximately 120 dB. Harmonic distortion products must be less than 80 dB at 20 Hz and less than 40 dB at 100 Hz in order to remain inaudible. It is very difficult to produce infrasound signals of high intensity that are sufficiently pure (higher harmonic distortion products might be introduced due to the nonlinearity of the air at high intensities even for purely sinusoidal piston motion). In the absence of detailed consideration of this problem by a particular investigator, it is difficult to be sure that the results attributed to infrasound are not in fact produced by audiofrequency distortion products.

Characteristics of several infrasound generation systems are summarized in Table 2.

III. Reception of Infrasound Energy

A. Body Surface

Because infrasound wavelengths ($\lambda = 34$ m at 10 Hz) are much larger than body dimensions, the body is ordinarily immersed in a conphase pressure or velocity field during infrasound exposure; *i.e.*, the excitation is the same all over the body surface. Since the basic physical properties of body tissue are those of a viscoelastic fluid (von Gierke *et al.*, 1952) much less compressible than air, the pressure effects on tissue as such and therefore on the total body are minimal. Acoustically speaking, due to the large mismatch of the acoustic impedance of air to the acoustic impedance of tissue practically all mechanical energy is reflected at the body surface and the energy entering the body as part of the compression wave is negligible. This situation would change if only part of the body surface

Table 2. Performance of representative infrasound sources used in research

Facility	Generator	Operation	Performance	Ref.
Thermophone	Loudspeaker coupled via manometer to ear	Beating of two AC inside thermophone capsule; frequency response down to 1 Hz	154—174 dB	von Békésy (1936)
Pistonphone mercury manometer	Motor driven pistonphone; manual control manometer	Alternating pressures up to 50 Hz	165 dB alternating pressure; 180 dB static pressure	von Gierke *et al.* (1953)
Whole-body enclosures; and free field: jet engine; high pressure air source; low frequency test chamber	Hydraulic loud-speakers; high velocity air flow; low frequency siren	Normal operating modes for various devices and facilities	Discrete tones and bands of noise at levels of 150—154 dB	Mohr *et al.* (1965)
Pistonphones	Coupled to ear via closed tube	Motor driven alternating pressures	165 dB + alternating pressure	Nixon (1974)
Whole body pressure chamber 9 × 1.2 × 1.8 m	Four .38 m diam. loud-speakers: 300 W amplifier	Operates as a Helmholtz resonator tunable over range of 3—18 Hz	145 dB for single frequency; 126 dB for noise band	Leventhall and Hood (1971)
Monaural/binaural head-phones from 0.3 m diameter loudspeakers	Earmuffs; drivers worked into volume of 1 l	Response flat up to 200 Hz	Maximum SPL is 150 dB at 1 Hz	Yeowart (1971)
Whole body 1200 l cabinet	Six 0.46 m diameter loud-speakers on sides of chamber	Electrodynamic	Maximum SPL is 140 dB	Yeowart (1971)
Whole body chamber 1557 l	Hydraulic driven 1.8 m diam piston and .46 m diam piston	Alternating pressures, 0.5—30 Hz	1.8 m piston: 172 dB (0.5—10 Hz) falling to 158 dB at 30 Hz .46 m piston: 144 dB (1—10 Hz) falling to 135 dB at 20 Hz	Johnson (1974)
Whole body chamber	Hydraulic driven piston	7.5 Hz	130 dB	Borredon and Nathié (1974)

were exposed to infrasonic pressures or forces. In this case – as is easily demonstrated by a small piston indenting a small surface area overlying soft tissue — the tissue is not purely compressed but escapes at a right angle to the applied force: transverse shear waves are set up in the body tissue which could not have developed in the case of the omnidirectional immersion of the body in an infrasound field. The smaller the body area exposed to infrasound pressures, the higher percentage of the impinging energy is absorbed at the body surface and enters the body (von Gierke *et al.*, 1952). This type of excitation with pressure or force acting on restricted body areas, such as one side of the torso, the buttocks area or the grip area of the hand, is practically equivalent to structure-borne vibration exposure as it is studied in vibration research with infrasonic frequencies. In these cases, the infrasound results predominantly in shear waves inside the tissue with considerably larger energy transfer to the body and relatively large vibration amplitudes and tissue stresses between body segments and organs. The mechanical impedance of a small surface area of the body or of the whole body of a seated man exposed to unidirectional forces is therefore completely different from the impedance of a whole man exposed to omnidirectional pressure, even if the infrasonic frequency is the same in both cases. Based on these differences in mechanical energy transfer and mechanical excitation, the injury problems and the physiological and psychological effects are completely different. Most normally occurring infrasound environments do not produce appreciable vibration levels in tissue, comparable to the vibration levels excited by structure-borne vibration.

Exceptions to the foregoing exist wherever the human body encloses an air volume as an integral part of the body structure. In the case of the ear, such configuration evolved with the sole purpose to increase mechanical energy absorption over the small, protected surface area of the tympanic membrane and to match the inner ear impedance to the impedance of the air surrounding the body. Again, the important tissue displacements in the inner ear are reached not by tissue compression but by shear loading (von Gierke, 1958). In this way the ear absorbs more than 90% of the acoustical energy, whereas the other body areas absorb much less than 10% or even 1%. In the case of the lungs, the pressure across the chest wall is equalized at low frequencies by air passing through the trachea; only at higher frequencies is the impedance of the airways sufficiently high that the lungs act like an enclosed air volume, which is compressed by the pressure on the chest wall. Maximum wall vibrations and energy transmission to the lungs occur at the resonance frequency of the lung volume plus chest wall system (40—60 Hz in man). At the low frequencies (< 1 Hz) the lung volume connected through the open airways to the outside has another resonance as a Helmholtz resonator but this is a resonance of the air flowing in and out through the airway and not primarily a vibration of body parts. However, high flow rates and pressure changes in the enclosed volume can produce subjective sensations and physiological effects (see Section VII. C). Similar considerations apply to the sinus cavities.

With respect to the transmission of infrasound energy to the whole body or the respiratory system, it is important to keep in mind that the considerations presented depend on the ratio sound wavelength to body dimensions. For animals smaller than man, equivalent infrasound whole body effects will appear at correspondingly higher frequencies. The chest resonance appears between 40 and 60 Hz in man, around 500 Hz in the rabbit, and 1100 Hz in the mouse (VON GIERKE, 1968).

In the following, our discussion focuses on the ear; the special cases of infrasound stimulation of the vestibular system (via the middle ear) and the respiratory apparatus are considered in Section VII.

There is relatively little specific information concerning the biomechanical effects of infrasound on the ear. However, extrapolation of existing data on the ear's audiofrequency response to the infrasound region appears appropriate in many instances.

B. External Ear

Properties of the external ear are detailed by SHAW (1974) in Vol. V/1, Chapter 14. In addition to protecting the tympanic membrane, the external ear aids detection of the direction of a sound source and adds considerable acoustic gain at higher frequencies.

Due to the long wavelength of the infrasound stimuli relative to the length of the external auditory meatus (2.3—2.7 cm), there is practically no change in sound pressure between the free field and the tympanic membrane for these stimuli. Figures 5, 9, and 10 in SHAW's Chapter 14illustrate that the acoustic gain attributable to the external ear approaches zero at frequencies below 1 kHz. For the same reason, interaural phase differences approach zero for infrasound stimuli (Fig. 4, SHAW, Vol. V/1, Chapter 14) and sound pressure levels at the tympanic membrane do not vary as a function of the azimuth angle of incident infrasound (Fig. 5, SHAW, Vol. V/1, Chapter 14).

In order to account for differences between minimum audible field (MAF) and minimum audible pressure (MAP), several investigators have examined physiological noise levels in the enclosed ear. The MAF-MAP difference increases with decreasing frequency, amounting to as much as 10 dB at 100 Hz. Physiological noise levels in the external auditory meatus range between 70 and 75 dB at 16—20 Hz following supra-aural enclosure and must be expected to increase further for lower frequencies (Fig. 22, SHAW, Vol. V/1, Chapter 14). One might speculate that the evolutionary restriction of the ear's sensitivity in the low audiofrequency and infrasound range was determined by the necessity to attenuate response to physiological noise.

C. Middle Ear

The middle ear serves as an impedance matching transformer, providing efficient transfer of sound energy from air to the cochlear fluids. Information regarding the response of the middle ear to infrasound has been obtained by examination of pressure changes in the perilymph and can be extrapolated from direct observations of the motion of the ossicular chain.

KOBRAK (1948) calculated the linear displacement of the umbo from measurements of tympanic membrane angular rotation induced by static pressure changes in the external auditory meatus using human cadavers. These measurements, which are illustrated in Fig. 2, indicate that the umbo's response was approximately linear for negative pressures but became increasingly nonlinear at higher levels of positive pressure. The outward excursion of the umbo was greater than the inward excursion at corresponding levels of negative and positive pressure. The implications of Kobrak's observations are twofold: First, harmonic distortion

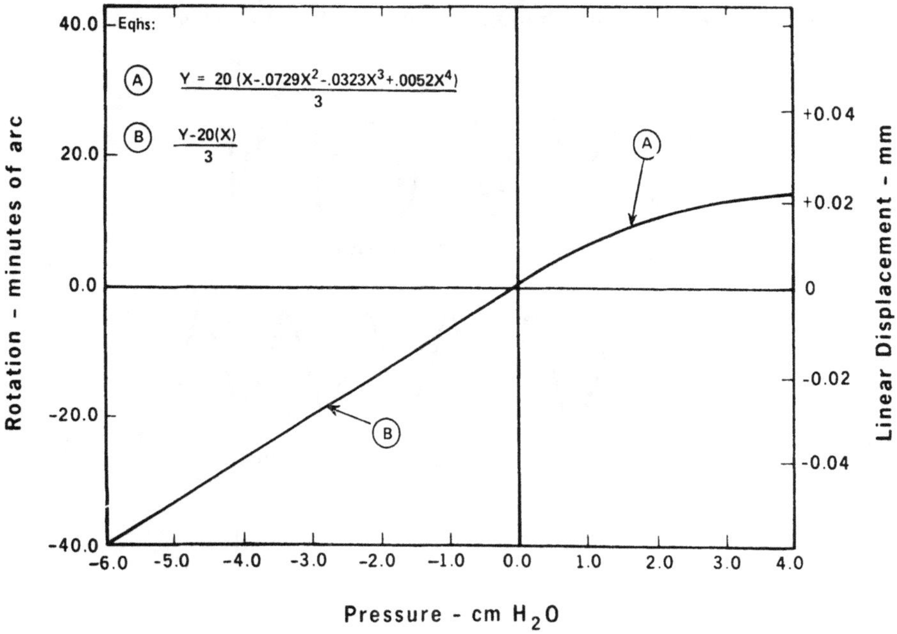

Fig. 2. Tympanic membrane angular rotation (left ordinate) and calculated linear displacement of umbo (right ordinate) as a function of static pressure [recorded from a human cadaver by KOBRAK (1948)]. Nonlinear middle ear response to increased pressure is described by Eq. (A); linear response to decreased pressure is described by Eq. (B). From JOHNSON and VON GIERKE (1974)

is introduced by the middle ear when stimulus intensities exceed 110—120 dB; the importance of this distortion for perception of infrasound is considered in Section IV. Second, static pressure changes exceeding 0.5—1.0 cm H_2O change the transmission characteristics for simultaneously presented alternating pressure; this is discussed in Section V.

GUINAN and PEAKE (1967) observed the vibration amplitude of the cat's stapes at frequencies down to 20 Hz. Their observations indicate that the peak-to-peak amplitude of the stapes and the phase angle between the stimulus and the stapes motion remain essentially constant at frequencies below 400 Hz [see Fig. 4, MØLLER (1974), Vol. V/1, Chapter 15].

Observations of perilymph pressure changes produced by infrasound stimulation support the view that the middle ear introduces nonlinear distortion at high infrasound stimulus intensities. Figure 3 illustrates perilymph pressure changes (top line in each pair of traces) evoked by infrasound stimulation at 5.7 Hz. For A) the stimulus intensity was 150 dB, and for B) the stimulus intensity was 112 dB. These pressure recordings were obtained from the superior semicircular canal in a guinea pig (PARKER, 1976). Similar data have been published for audiofrequency stimulation (see WEVER and LAWRENCE, 1954, p. 167).

D. Inner Ear

The auditory analyzer located in the cochlea performs a sophisticated transformation on incoming signals: pressure by time stimuli are transformed into displacement by distance along the basilar membrane by time responses. This transformation is discussed by Eldredge (1974) in Vol. V/1, Chapter 17.

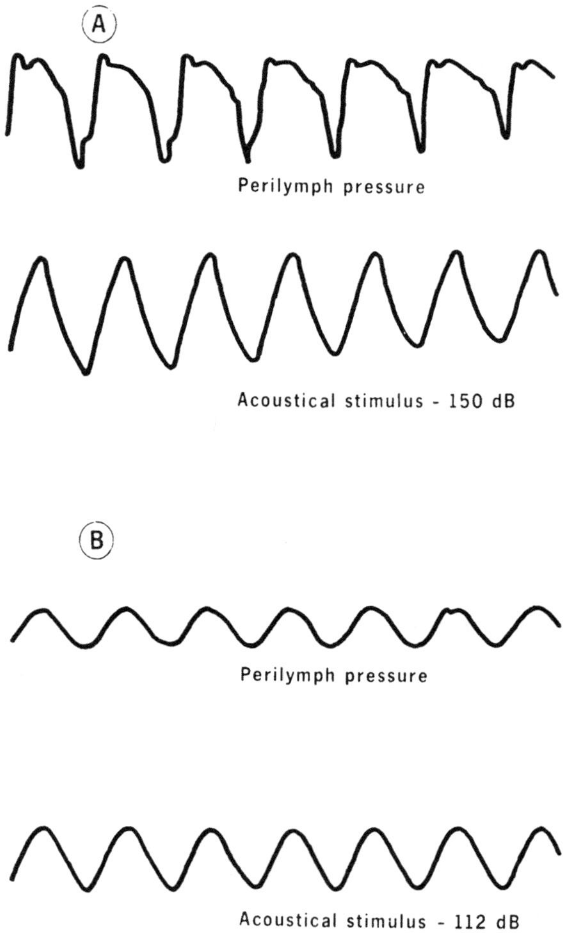

Fig. 3 A and B. Perilymph pressure changes in superior semicircular canal (top traces) during infrasound stimulation (bottom traces) at 5.7 Hz. Stimulus intensities: (A) 150 dB; (B) 112 dB. From Parker (1976)

Von Békésy (1943) described the relative amplitude of vibrations along the basilar membrane as a function of the frequency of the stimulus. For frequencies of 50 Hz and above the basilar membrane displacement shows a clear peak (maximum). For 30 Hz and below von Békésy described a gradual increase in the basilar membrane displacement all the way to the apex; no point of maximum displacement was observed (Fig. 2, Eldredge, Vol. V/1, Chapter 17). As discussed by Dallos (1973), the cochlea can be modeled as a high-pass acoustic filter. The helicotrema and the cochlear partition form a parallel acoustic circuit, and the acoustic shunt represented by the helicotrema becomes increasingly effective at lower stimulus frequencies. The importance of these observations for our purposes it that stimuli in the infrasound frequency range apparently have no "place" on the basilar membrane.

There is a clear relationship between the patterns of basilar membrane displacement observed by VON BÉKÉSY and the "tuning curves" of single neurons in the eighth nerve. Although neurons with best frequencies as low as 100 Hz have been observed (KIANG, 1965), clearly the sharpness of the tuning curve ("Q") decreases with decreasing frequency [see EVANS (1975), Vol. V/2, Chapter 1].

It is possible for the neurons of the auditory system to encode the periodicity of infrasound stimuli. However, the observations that infrasound stimuli are perceptually different from audiofrequency stimuli and that infrasound detection can probably be accounted for by considering distortion products (Section IV) mitigate against a frequency theory (WEVER, 1949) for infrasound representation, and by extension, for any auditory signals.

IV. Direct Auditory Response to Infrasound

Exposure to infrasound elicits a variety of sensations ranging from an apparent "gentle massage" of the tympanic membrane through pressure build-up to pain. In contrast to statements prevalent in the literature, infrasound stimulation can also produce a clear auditory sensation that is frequently described as a chugging or motorboating sound. The first part of this section describes the auditory perceptual effects associated with infrasound stimulation, including thresholds, loudness, and masking. In the second part, indicators of damage including tissue destruction and threshold shifts are considered.

A. Perception

1. Thresholds

Figure 4 summarizes the results of several experiments concerning thresholds for detection of low audiofrequency sound and infrasound. The detection threshold rises sharply from about 90 dB at 20 Hz to 130—140 dB at 1 Hz. Agreement among different investigators is quite good. Hearing thresholds for narrow bands of noise are included in Fig. 4. While there are no differences between narrow band noise and pure tones in the audiofrequency range, noise thresholds are lower than pure tone thresholds by about 4 dB for frequencies below 16 Hz. This difference can be attributed to distortion products produced by the peak components of the noise signals.

The hypothesis that the audibility of infrasound is primarily the result of harmonic distortion products generated in the audiofrequency range has been suggested by JOHNSON and VON GIERKE (1974). This distortion product hypothesis was initially proposed because observers indicate that tonal quality is lost at frequencies below 19 Hz (GUTTMAN and JULESZ, 1963) and because of the difference in thresholds for pure tones and noise. The source of the distortion products is the nonlinearity of the middle ear. Kobrak (1948) measured the middle ear nonlinearity of a human cadaver; these measurements and a mathematical description of the curve are illustrated in Fig. 2. The effect of the nonlinear distortion observed by Kobrak on pure tones of various intensities was calculated and the

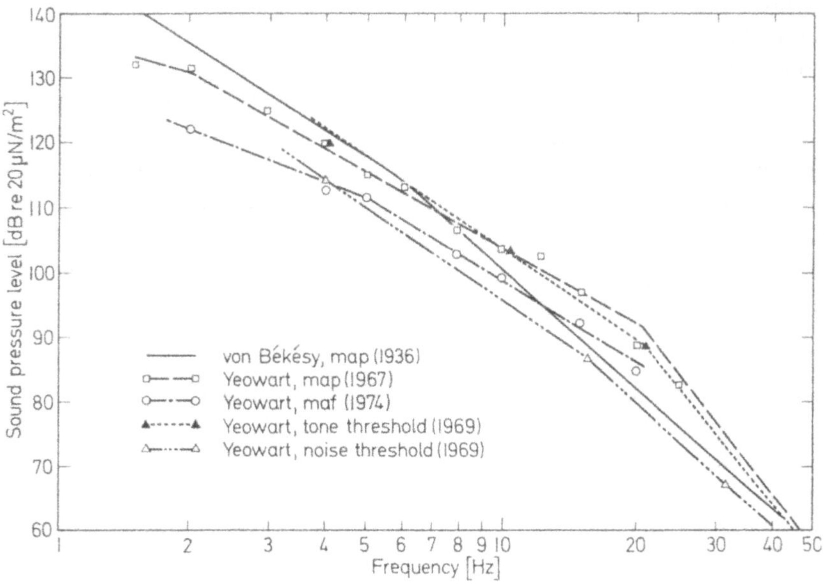

Fig. 4. Infrasound and low frequency sound detection thresholds

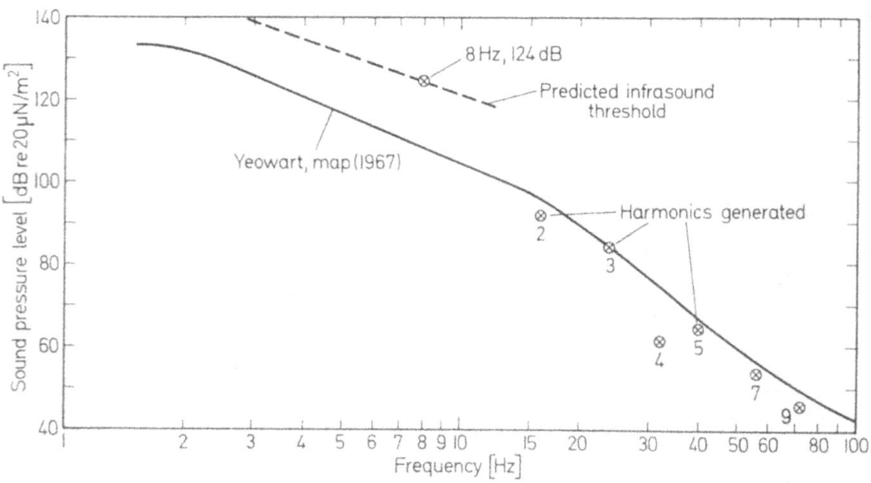

Fig. 5. Threshold for audibility of infrasound (dashed line) due to middle ear nonlinear distortion calculated from equations of Fig. 2. Solid line represents experimentally obtained threshold function. The middle ear's response to an 8 Hz 124 dB tone yields several higher harmonic distortion products that fall on the low audiofrequency threshold function; therefore, the 8 Hz infrasound should be audible due to distortion generated in the audiofrequency range. From Johnson and von Gierke (1974)

Fourier coefficients of the harmonics generated by this distortion were determined. An example of the procedure employed by JOHNSON and VON GIERKE is presented in Fig. 5. The third harmonic (24 Hz) of an 8 Hz, 124 dB pure tone was calculated to have a sound pressure level of 83 dB. The intensity of the 24 Hz harmonic falls on the threshold curve; therefore, the distortion produced by the middle ear at 24 Hz should cause the 8 Hz, 124 dB tone to be audible. In a similar manner other harmonic intensities were calculated and the results plotted in Fig. 5. Several of these harmonics are close to the detection threshold; this could account for the report that the 8 Hz stimulus sounds more like a rumble than a pure tone. The dashed line in Fig. 5 illustrates the threshold for audibility of pure tones in the range of 2–12 Hz on the basis of middle ear distortion. This predicted threshold lies 10—15 dB above the observed threshold curve. The discrepancy between observed infrasound thresholds and those predicted on the basis of nonlinear distortion might be accounted for by considering other sources of distortion in the ear, by modifying the equation for middle ear nonlinearity slightly, or by assuming a slightly lower audiofrequency threshold detection curve (*e.g.*, SIVIAN and WHITE, 1933). On the other hand, the predicted audibility threshold due to the harmonic distortions is based on pure tone thresholds for individual frequencies and not on the simultaneous presence of a whole harmonic spectrum in a fixed phase relation. The latter, resulting in a modulated sound pattern, might be responsible for the lower observed threshold. In an experimental test of their hypothesis, JOHNSON and VON GIERKE demonstrated that the threshold for detection of infrasound pure tones was elevated when the pure tone was presented simultaneously with masking noise in the low audiofrequency range.

The hypothesis and observations described by JOHNSON and VON GIERKE focus attention on one of the fundamental problems of performing research on infrasound, *i.e.*, the generation of distortion-free stimuli. If the distortion product hypothesis is correct, failure on the part of an experimenter to eliminate stimulus distortion could invalidate the obtained data. Comments from YEOWART (1974) indicate that stimulus distortion produces strong effects. In one of his experiments, YEOWART noted that the observer was reliably detecting infrasound tones at lower levels than had been obtained previously. Upon investigation YEOWART found that the observer's earcup was not seated properly and that air was escaping at one point. The air leak produced a slight hissing sound which apparently contributed to the observer's detection capability.

2. Loudness

Two related problems concerning the loudness of infrasound stimuli are considered in this section. First, equal loudness contours are examined. Second, observations on the growth of perceived loudness as a function of increased intensity of the physical stimulus are considered.

Observations on the loudness of infrasound stimuli are limited; apparently the only systematic observations available have been performed by WHITTLE *et al.* (1972). Two aspects of loudness were addressed by WHITTLE and his colleagues: loudness matching across frequencies and the form of the loudness function at a single frequency.

Table 3 summarizes the results of equal loudness matches for frequencies of 50, 25, 12.5, 6.3, and 3.15 Hz. In all cases the original reference stimulus was at 50 Hz. Loudness matches were usually obtained for tones differing by one octave although checks were made by making comparisons across a range up to three octaves. The intensity of the 50 Hz tone was set at one of three levels: 60, 73, and 86 dB. The

Table 3. Sound pressure levels for equal loudness (dB re 20μ N/m²) (Whittle *et al.*, 1972)

Frequency of tone (Hz)	SPL and standard error		
	"Low"	"Medium"	"High"
50	60.0[a]	73.0[a]	86.0[a]
25	78.0 (1.2)	87.7 (1.2)	97.8 (1.2)
12.5	97.7 (1.2)	104.7 (1.3)	112.6 (1.1)
6.3	110.9 (0.6)	118.0 (0.5)	125.6 (0.6)
3.15	126.5 (0.4)	132.9 (0.2)	137.6 (0.2)

[a] Reference levels.

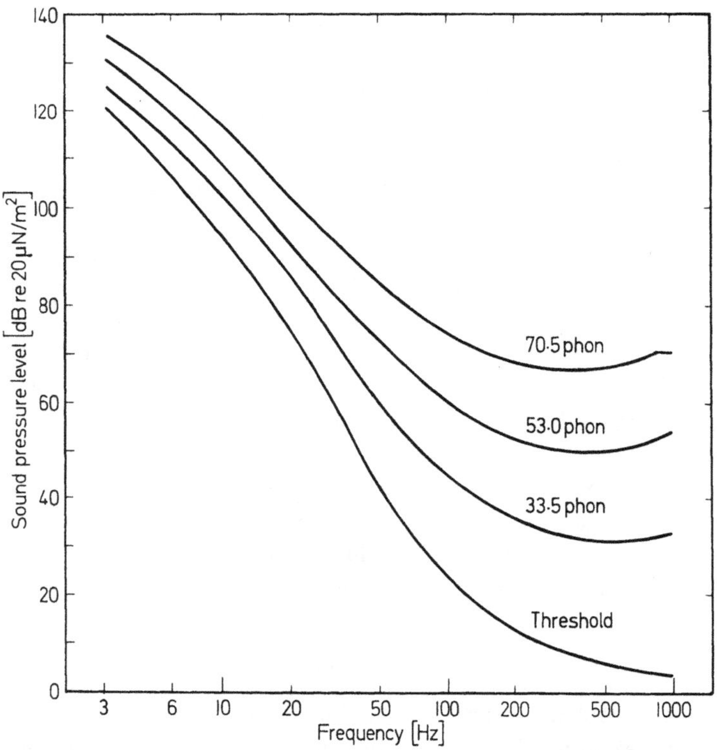

Fig. 6. Equal loudness and threshold contours. Contours above 20 Hz based on ISO R226; contours below 20 Hz based on observations of Whittle *et al.* (1972)

data in the table indicate the stimulus intensities at the other frequencies required to produce sound subjectively as loud as the three levels of the 50 Hz tone. Figure 6 illustrates the ISO equal loudness contours with extensions into the infrasound frequency range based on the observations by Whittle *et al.*

Determination of the loudness functions employed a magnitude estimation procedure. The results of the magnitude estimation observations at frequencies of 50, 25, 12.5, 6.3, and 3.15 Hz are presented in Fig. 7. Differences among the loudness functions can be most readily summarized by considering the changes in the value of n in the equation

$$S = k(I^n - I_0^n) ,$$

where S indicates perceived loudness, I is the intensity of the tonal stimulus, I_0 signifies the least intense stimulus that can be detected because of noise, k is a constant that varies as a function of the modulus, and n is the exponent chracteristic of a particular stimulus. Table 4 presents the exponents derived from the curves illustrated in Fig. 7.

The relative positions of the curves for the different frequencies on the y-axis were determined using the data obtained in the "high intensity" equal loudness contour study. The fact that the "medium intensity" equal loudness points fall in the appropriate places lends an encouraging consistency to the data.

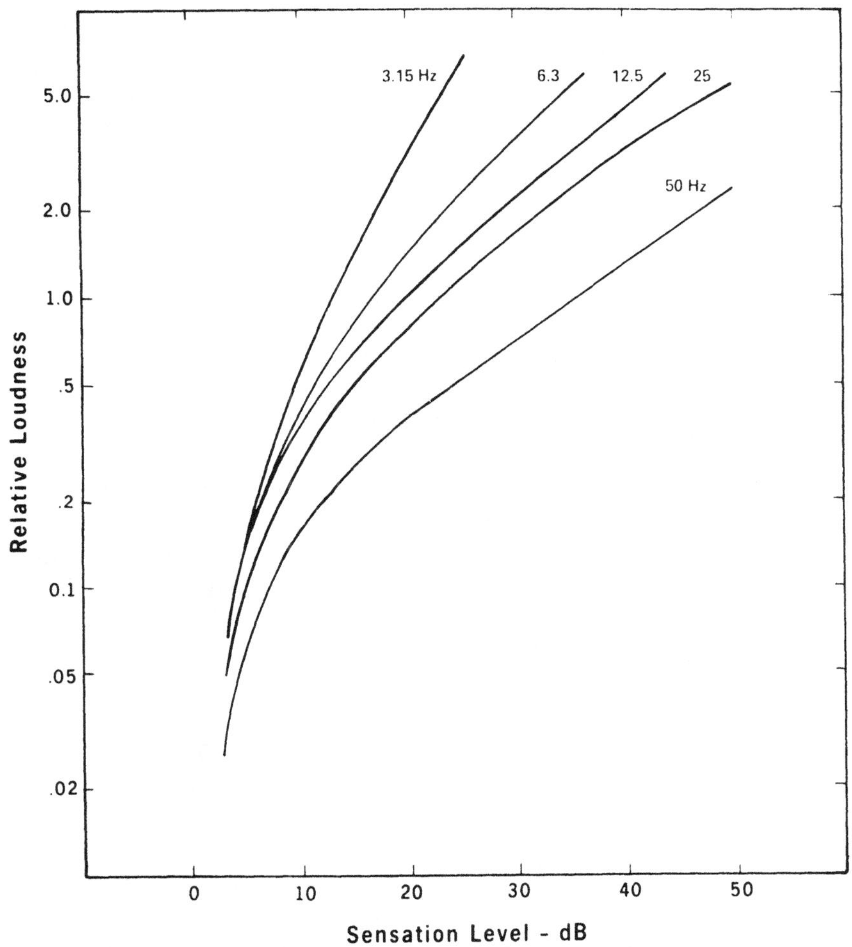

Fig. 7. Relative perceived loudness as a function of stimulus intensity. Sensation level = 10 log I/I_0. The parameter is stimulus frequency. Data obtained by Whittle *et al.* (1972) with a magnitude estimation procedure

3. Masking

To the extent that middle ear nonlinearities result in higher harmonic distortion products during high intensity infrasound exposure, it is reasonable to expect that masking of audiofrequency signals would result from infrasound stimulation.

Table 4. Loudness exponents derived from magnitude estimations (Whittle *et al.*, 1972)

Frequency (Hz)	n
3.15	0.66
6.3	0.34
12.5	0.23
25	0.22
50	0.21

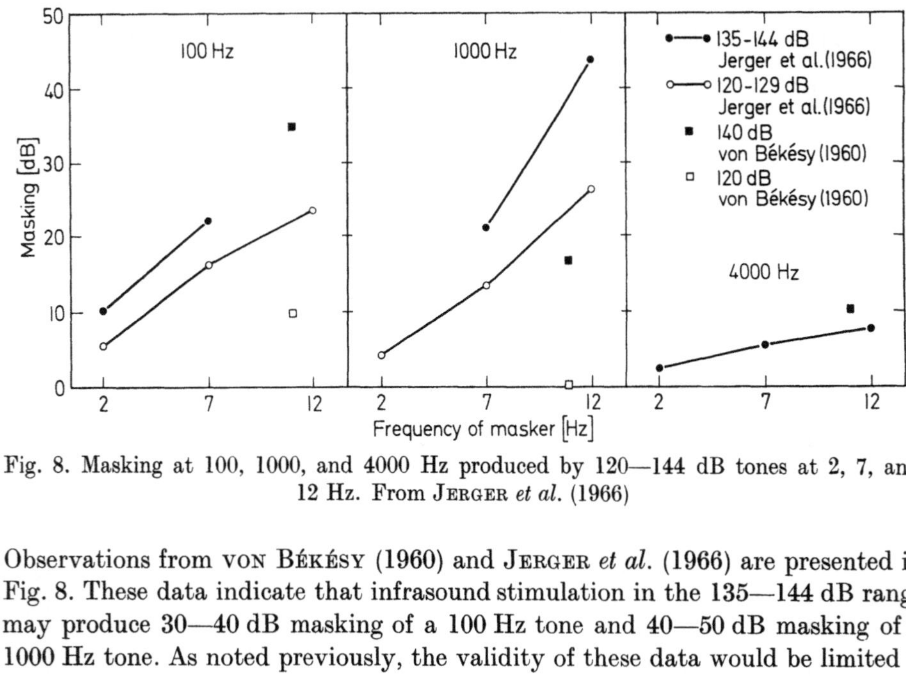

Fig. 8. Masking at 100, 1000, and 4000 Hz produced by 120—144 dB tones at 2, 7, and 12 Hz. From Jerger *et al.* (1966)

Observations from von Békésy (1960) and Jerger *et al.* (1966) are presented in Fig. 8. These data indicate that infrasound stimulation in the 135—144 dB range may produce 30—40 dB masking of a 100 Hz tone and 40—50 dB masking of a 1000 Hz tone. As noted previously, the validity of these data would be limited if distortion were introduced by the stimulus apparatus as well as by the middle ear. Jerger *et al.* suggest that the discrepancies between their observations and those of von Békésy might be accounted for by differences in the listening conditions of the two experiments; however, because the stimulus was not completely analyzed by Jerger and his colleagues, the possibility that the differences in the results are attributable to stimulus distortion cannot be ruled out.

B. Overstimulation

1. Tissue Damage

Determination of the levels of mechanical stimulation, including infrasound, that produce damage to the auditory system or otherwise impair the performance of human beings has been one of the tasks pursued in our laboratory. As indicated in Fig. 7, the growth of loudness, indicated by the value of the exponent n, is more rapid for infrasound than for audiofrequency sound. Consequently, the difference between stimulus intensities that can just be detected and stimulus intensities that may result in permanent tissue damage should be smaller in the case of infrasound than for normal audiofrequency sound. Because of the small range of intensity difference between detection and damage, infrasound can be potentially more dangerous to an individual than audiofrequency sound (as has been proposed by several investigators, although not necessarily for the reasons that they suggest).

Tympanic membrane injury may occur as a result of intense acoustic exposures which drive the middle ear system beyond the mechanical limits of its normal modes of operation and which may exceed the rupture strength of the membrane itself. Severe middle ear damage is usually accompanied by some inner ear damage as well. Drum membrane ruptures usually heal with little residual effect on hearing; however, ossicular chain and inner ear effects may be much more persistent. The threshold for human tympanic membrane rupture occurs at average static pressure changes of around 4.15×10^4 to 5.53×10^4 N/m^2. Since peak pressures for tympanic membrane rupture must be expected to decrease from the value for static pressure with increasing frequency, the rupture pressure for infrasound will undoubtedly be higher than the rupture pressure for audiofrequency sound. The few accidental data points available for audiofrequency sound point to pressures well over 160 dB. Pressures of this magnitude rarely occur as stationary phenomena, but so far have been of interest only in connection with the low frequency components of the overpressures from explosions and gun blasts (HIRSCH, 1968).

Observations on damage to the auditory apparatus following intense infrasound exposure have been limited to gross inspection of the tympanic membrane and middle ear. Guinea pigs, chinchillas, dogs, and monkeys as well as human beings have been examined. Moderate levels of exposure (130—140 dB) result in tympanic membrane retraction and dilation of the tympanic membrane blood vessels. Tympanic membrane retraction probably results from a rectifier action of the Eustachian tube: the volume of air flowing from the nasopharynx to the middle ear during the rarefaction phase of the stimulus is less than the volume of air flowing from the middle ear to the nasopharynx during the condensation phase. This tympanic membrane retraction is probably the cause of the feeling of pressure build-up that the observers report.

Experimental animals have been exposed to the highest levels of infrasound available in our laboratory (172 dB at frequencies of 2—8 Hz). The animals were either placed inside the pressure chamber (whole-body exposures) or stimulated monaurally through a tube and earcup. Exposure durations varied from 5—32 min. Tympanic membrane retraction and vascular infusion similar to that noted previously with the human beings were observed. Subsequent dissection revealed bleeding in the middle ear in the chinchilla; however, this bleeding was not seen in dogs and monkeys (JOHNSON, 1973).

2. Pain

Pain in the ear is easily recognized by individuals and is related to displacement of an otherwise normal middle ear system beyond its mechanical limits of normal operation. Aural pain is not directly related to sensitivity, as evidenced by the fact that normal and hard-of-hearing persons have the same average aural pain thresholds. Likewise, it is neither associated with nor a warning for sensorineural hearing loss, which can become very severe without any experience of pain. Pain may be experienced during infrasound exposure at levels that pose no risk to hearing function.

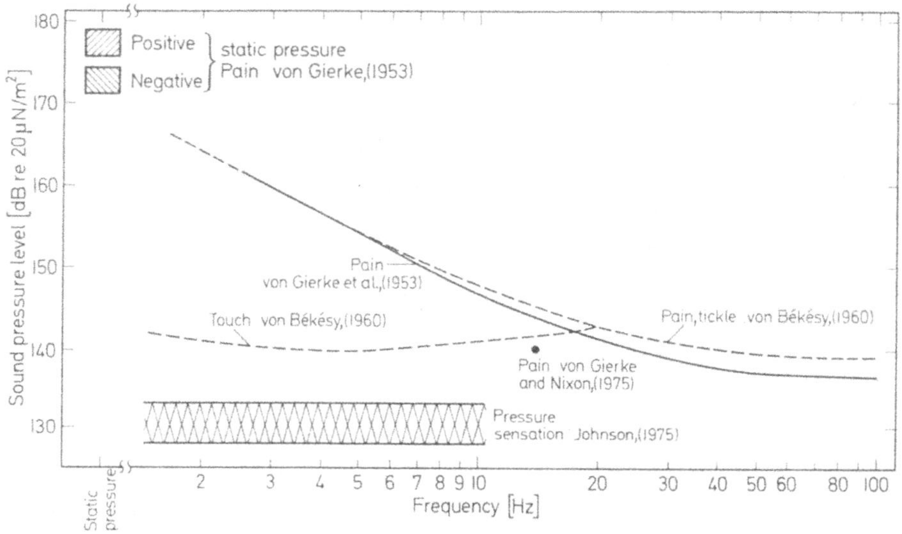

Fig. 9. Pain, touch, tickle, and middle ear pressure build-up thresholds for static pressure, infrasound, and low audiofrequency sound

Thresholds for aural pain are summarized in Fig. 9. The data from von Békésy (1936, 1960) and von Gierke *et al.* (1953) are highly consistent. The single data point in the figure represents a condition where one observer reported pain during a pistonphone exposure of about 140 dB at 14 Hz; in this instance the pain disappeared after a few minutes and did not return during a subsequent 30 min exposure at the same level (von Gierke and Nixon, 1975). The pain threshold appears to be about 140 dB around 20 Hz, rapidly increasing to about 162 dB at 2 Hz. Pain produced by static pressure on the ear, either positive or negative, appears between 175 dB and 180 dB. Any form of aural pain during infrasound exposure must be considered an indicator that the tolerance limits of the mechanical elements of the auditory system have been reached and the exposure should be terminated and avoided in the future.

3. Temporary Threshold Shift

Temporary threshold shift (TTS) has been widely used as an indicator of potential noise-induced permanent threshold shift (NIPTS), although the correlation between TTS and NIPTS is imperfect.

Table 5. Threshold shifts following infrasound stimulation

Exposure	Hearing response	Recovery	Ref.
Submarine diesel room 10—20 Hz, no level given	Depression of upper limits of hearing as measured by number of seconds a tuning fork was heard—no conversion to MAP	Recovery in a few hrs outside diesel room	TONNDORF (1950)
Discrete tones; narrow band noise in 10—20 Hz region; 150—154 dB exposures of about 2 min	No change in hearing sensitivity reported by *S*s; no TTS measured about one hr post exposure	—	MOHR *et al.* (1965)
Successive 3 min whole-body exposures, 7—12 Hz; 119—144 dB	TTS in 3000—6000 Hz range for 11 of 21 *S*s (TTS of 10—22 dB)	Recovery within hrs	ALFORD *et al.* (1966)
Pistonphone coupled to ear via earmuff. 18 Hz at 135 dB. Series of 6.5 min exposures rapid in succession	Average TTS of 0—15 dB after 30 min exposures	Recovery within 30 min	NIXON and JOHNSON (1973)
Pistonphone coupled to ear via earmuff. 14 Hz at 140 dB. Six individual exposures of 5, 10, 15, 20, 25, and 30 min	Three experienced *S*s—no TTS in 1 *S*; slight TTS in 1 *S*; 20—25 dB TTS in 1 *S*	Recovery within 30 min	NIXON and JOHNSON (1973)
Ear only: pressure chamber coupled to ear via tuned hose and muff:			
171 dB (1—10 Hz) 26 sec, 1 *S*	No TTS		
168 dB (7 Hz) 1 min, 1 *S*	No TTS		
155 dB (7 Hz) 5 min, 2 *S*s	No TTS		
140 dB (4, 7, 12 Hz) 30 min, 1 *S*	14—17 dB TTS	Recovery within 30 min	NIXON and JOHNSON (1973)
140 dB (4, 7, 12 Hz) 5 min, 8 *S*s	8 dB TTS for 1 *S*		
135 dB (6, 1.6, 2.9 Hz) 5 min, 12 *S*s	No TTS		
126 dB (6, 1.6, 2.9 Hz) 16 min, 11 *S*s	No TTS		
Whole body: all exposures with 2 *S*s:			
8 min at 8 Hz at SPLs of 120, 126, 132, 138 dB	No TTS		
8 min at 1, 2, 4, 6, 8, 10 Hz at 144 dB	No TTS	—	NIXON and JOHNSON (1973)
8 min at 12, 16, 20 Hz at 135—142 dB	No TTS		

In one of the early reports, Tonndorf (1950) described the effects of infrasound in the diesel engine rooms of submarines on the hearing of crew members. Elevation of hearing thresholds was demonstrated by the decreased time periods during which the sound from a tuning fork was audible. Recovery occurred after various time periods outside the engine room.

Mohr *et al.* (1965) exposed observers to infrasonic signals, both pure tones and noise bands, for 2 min or less at levels up to 150–154 dB. Audiometry was not performed immediately following the exposures; however, measures taken about 1 h later showed no TTS. In Mohr's study the exposure signal was experienced only once, while on-board submarine exposures were experienced daily.

Alford *et al.* (1966) exposed 21 males to repeated 3 min signals of from 2–12 Hz at levels of 119 dB to 144 dB. TTS of 10 dB or more in the range of 3000–8000 Hz was found in 11 of the 21 observers after exposures of 137—141 dB. All TTS values were small, ranging from 10–22 dB. The authors indicate that the 7–12 Hz exposures at high levels did produce considerable energy in the audiofrequency range (100—4000 Hz). Unfortunately, spectra of the various exposure signals are not included in the report. It seems likely that at least some of the measured TTS may have been caused by the audiofrequency components of the fatiguing stimuli.

A number of studies of TTS and infrasound have been conducted in our laboratory using a pistonphone and a large pressure chamber as signal generators. With a pistonphone coupled tightly to the ear via an earmuff, Nixon and Johnson (1973) investigated effects on hearing thresholds of 14 Hz at 140 dB and 18 Hz at 135 dB for 30 min exposure durations. Some observers experienced no changes in hearing for standard audiometric test frequencies due to the exposures, while others showed various amounts of TTS, with one observer showing a maximum 20 dB change at one test frequency in one ear.

In another series of investigations, Nixon and Johnson measured the effects of short duration auditory exposures of 135—171 dB at 0.5–12 Hz and whole-body exposures of 135–144 dB at 1–20 Hz. The pressure chamber described in Table 2, which provided whole-body exposures to infrasound at levels as high as 172 dB, was used to generate the stimuli. Exposure durations varied from 26 sec of 1–10 Hz at 171 dB to 30 min of 4, 7, and 12 Hz at 140 dB. The various exposure parameters, effects on hearing (if any), and recovery are itemized in Table 5.

V. Effects of Infrasound on Audiofrequency Sound Reception

When infrasound or static pressure, which can be considered as very low frequency infrasound, act on the auditory system in the presence of audiofrequency sound, several interaction phenomena occur. Most of these phenomena can be understood as a consequence of the nonlinear transmission characteristic of the ear (Fig. 2). Although a uniform quantitative theoretical treatment of all these effects has not yet been attempted and the experimental data might not yet be complete enough to do this, most of the observations can be qualitatively explained on the basis of these nonlinear effects. The observations are: (a) static pressure across the tympanic membrane changes the auditory acuity for audiofrequency sound, (b) infrasound modulates the reception of speech signals, (c) impulse noise with an infrasound component is associated with a lower risk of hearing loss than the same audiofrequency impulse noise without the infrasound component, and (d) audiofrequency sound modulated with infrasound can result in vestibular manifestations similar to those produced by infrasound by itself (Section VII. A). Phenomena a—c can be explained by the fact that the relatively large middle ear displacements caused by the static pressure or infrasound shift the operating point on the transmission characteristic, reducing and/or modulating the gain of the middle ear transmission. Phenomenon d has been hypothesized (PARKER and VON GIERKE, 1971) to be the result of the demodulation properties of the nonlinear middle ear transmission. The modulated audiofrequency sound of high intensity would therefore result in static pressure changes or infrasound at the output of the middle ear transformer and would evoke vestibular effects in a manner similar to primary static pressure and infrasound stimuli. The auditory phenomena and observations of combined infrasound and audiofrequency sound exposures (a—c), which do not yet conclusively support the hypothetical framework proposed, are discussed in the remainder of this section. The nonauditory, vestibular effects are reviewed in Section VII. A.

A. Static Pressure

MØLLER (1974, Vol. V/1, Chapter 15) reviewed the effects of static air pressure on the transmission properties of the middle ear. Several investigators have examined the effects of static pressure on detection thresholds for human observers to audiofrequency sound. The results of these studies indicate a decrease in the sensitivity of the ear which is most marked at low frequencies. These threshold changes result primarily from changes in the transmission characteristics of the middle ear (Fig. 2). VON BÉKÉSY (1960) and MØLLER (Fig. 18, Vol. V/1, Chapter 15) have demonstrated that a pressure difference of 10 cm H_2O across the tympanic membrane results in a 10—20 dB decrease in transmission at low frequencies (250—1000 Hz). These observations support the suggestion that in complex acoustical environments the infrasound components may actually afford an observer some degree of protection against damage from the audiofrequency sound components.

B. Effects of Infrasound on Speech Reception

The effects of low audiofrequency sound and infrasound on speech perception have been examined by PICKETT (1959) and by VON GIERKE and NIXON (1975). In Pickett's study, a low frequency noise spectrum was produced that was approximately parallel to the speech spectrum. Overall noise levels were set at 85, 105, and 115 dB, and the low noise frequencies were removed by a set of filters that provided high-pass cutoff frequencies of 20, 75, 150, 300, and 600 Hz. The effects of these various noise stimuli on intelligibility of PB words were examined; the results are summarized in Fig. 10. These data indicate that noise components as low as 20 Hz significantly influence speech intelligibility. Pickett suggested that these effects must be accounted for by a spread of masking above 300 Hz because removal of speech signal frequencies below 300 Hz had no influence on intelligibility.

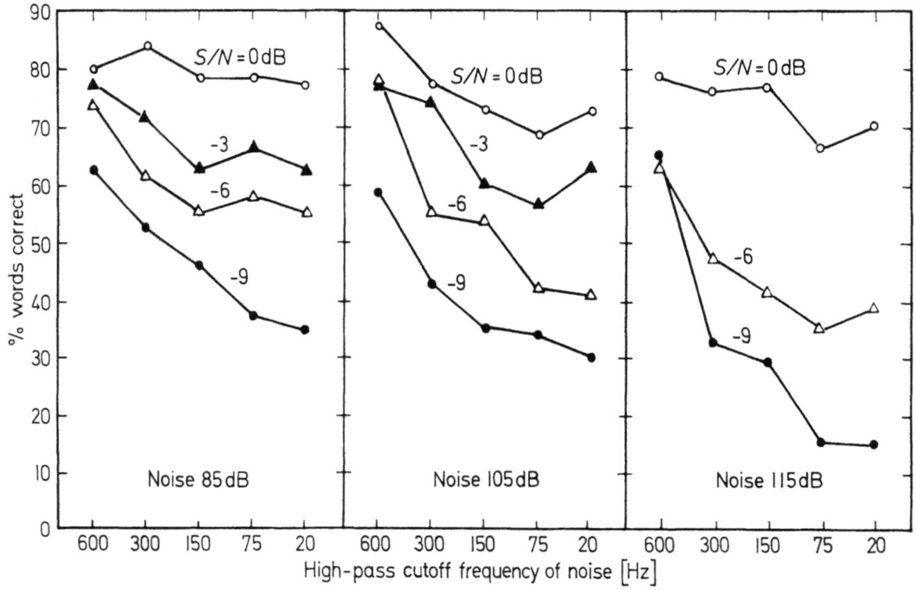

Fig. 10. Effects on speech intelligibility of low frequency noise. Ordinate indicates percentage of PB words correctly detected. Abscissa indicates the high-pass cutoff frequency of a filter which acted on a low frequency noise source; decreasing cutoff values are associated with increased levels of low frequency noise. The parameter in each panel (S/N) is the speech to noise ratio. From Pickett (1959)

Von Gierke and Nixon (1975) reported that observers had little difficulty in understanding speech in a face-to-face situation during whole body infrasound exposures at intensities up to 150 dB in spite of clear infrasound modulation of the speech signal. On the other hand, some observers reported minor difficulties in understanding speech presented through headphones during whole-body infrasound exposure. These observations have not been pursued to determine whether the reduced intelligibility is due to effects of the infrasound on the earphone, the auditory apparatus, or a combination of these two factors. However, it is obvious that infrasound should produce loudness modulations of the speech sounds at twice the frequency of the infrasound due to nonlinear middle ear transmission (Fig. 2) and the demonstrated change in auditory acuity with static pressure.

C. Impulse Noise

On the basis of their energy density spectra, the impulsive noise from sonic bangs and air bag restraint devices contain infrasound components. Nixon (1974) has recently reviewed the effects of impulse noise, particularly on the auditory system.

Sonic bangs, generated by aircraft in supersonic flight, have been alleged to adversely affect human hearing. The sonic bang is an impulsive sound with peak acoustical energy in the infrasound region. The energy density spectra of idealized sonic bangs of different durations are shown in Fig. 11. The maximum energy, with a roll-off of 6 dB/octave, is found at about 20 Hz for a fighter-type aircraft ($T = 0.04$ sec) and drops to below 2 Hz for supersonic transport-type aircraft ($T = 0.4$ sec).

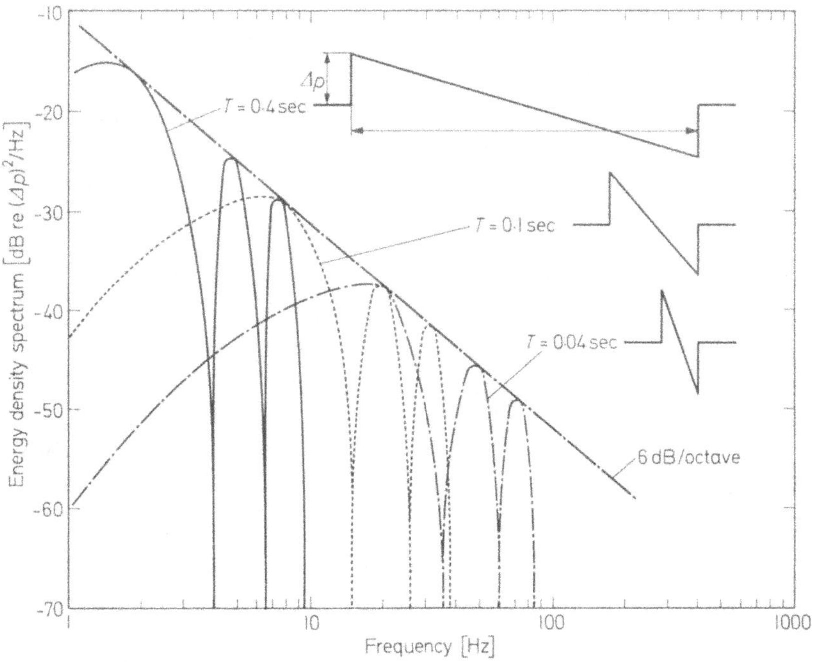

Fig. 11. Energy density spectra calculated for idealized sonic bangs of different durations. From NIXON *et al.* (1968)

Sonic bangs experienced in the community range from about 25—96 N/m² on the average. Field investigations and experience with exposure of humans to sonic bangs as intense as 6.91×10^3 N/m² have revealed no adverse effects on hearing. During a study at White Sands, New Mexico, USA, on structural response to sonic bang, personnel experienced about 30 sonic bangs daily over two 30 day periods separated by one month. Sonic bangs were increased in intensity from about 2.4×10^2 N/m² early in the program to 1.34×10^3 N/m² late in the study. Audiometric data collected at frequent intervals showed no changes in hearing due to the intense exposures. At Tonopah, Nevada individuals experienced sonic bangs on the ground at levels of 2.40×10^3 to 6.91×10^3 N/m² with no adverse effects on hearing (NIXON *et al.*, 1968). On the basis of these as well as other data on sonic bang exposures of human beings, it may be concluded that the intense infrasound present in high level sonic bangs does not constitute a problem for the human auditory system.

A new concept in automobile personal restraint safety devices is the "air bag system". This system involves the use of large hollow cushions which are concealed collapsed in the dashboards of automobiles and which, when the car encounters a forward crash, rapidly fill with gas and occupy the space between the dashboard of the car and its occupants to cushion the forward impact of the latter. The extremely rapid deployment of these prototype systems is accompanied by an intense impulsive noise which is experienced by the occupants. For purposes of our discussion, the frequency content of the air bag inflation noise can be generally described by the idealized spectra of Fig. 11, showing maximum energy at the lowest infrasound frequencies. Some high level, low audiofrequency energy present in the air bag noise is not shown.

In one study, 91 observers experienced the air bag noise inside a test automobile at a median peak pressure level of 168 dB (NIXON, 1969). Analysis of the air bag noise indicated the presence of acoustical energy in the low audiofrequency regions. About 50% of the observers experienced some TTS with about 95% of these recovering to pre-exposure threshold on the same day. About 5% required a little longer to recover, and one observer showed a slight shift at one frequency for several months.

In another study, the air bag impulse noise was separated into its component parts, a low frequency pressure pulse associated with displacement of the internal volume of the automobile by the inflating bag and a high frequency noise burst associated with activation of the system, gas flow turbulence, bag unfolding, and

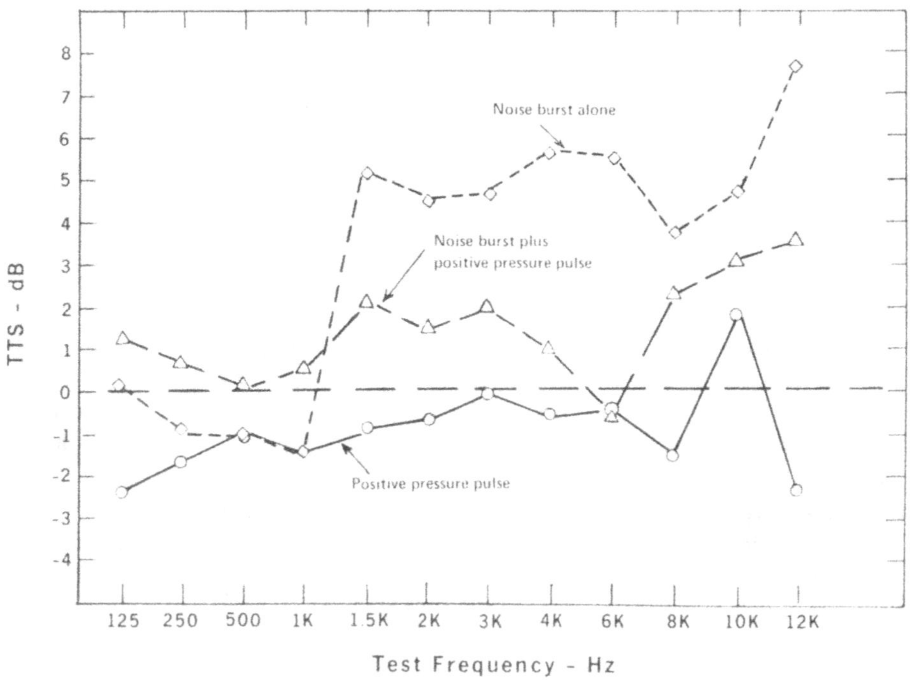

Fig. 12. TTS produced by simulated air bag noise components (audiofrequency noise burst and pressure pulse) presented individually or in combination. From SOMMER and NIXON (1974)

the like (SOMMER and NIXON, 1974). Volunteers experienced each of three noise exposures: the low frequency pressure pulse, the high frequency noise burst, and the composite air bag noise (both components simultaneously). The results, shown in Fig. 12, indicate that maximum TTS was caused by the noise burst, no TTS was caused by the pressure pulse, and for the total signal the noise burst effects were reduced by the pressure pulse resulting in less TTS than for the noise burst alone.

Although the sonic bang and the air bag inflation noise may not satisfy the "definition" of infrasound, the very intense infrasound components certainly qualify them for consideration. There is no clear-cut evidence that the infrasound in either of these signals in any way adversely affects the ear. On the other hand, it is suggested that the infrasound components may act to ameliorate undesirable effects of higher frequency energy. Certainly, there is clear evidence that loading the middle ear system with static pressure or very slow pressure changes (VON GIERKE *et al.*, 1953; VON GIERKE and WARREN, 1953) does reduce transmission of acoustic energy to the inner ear and may be considered protective. Whether or not intense infrasound might serve to reduce the adverse effects of intense audio-frequency energy on the ear is a worthy subject for further investigation.

VI. Indirect Auditory Response to Infrasound

In addition to the direct auditory effects discussed in Section IV, a variety of indirect physiological and behavioral effects, which generally have been observed during audiofrequency sound exposure, have been sought and/or studied in response to infrasound. These effects include changes in autonomic nervous system/endocrine system activity, disturbance of sleep, disturbance of complex task performance, and annoyance.

Several investigators have examined peripheral physiological responses associated with infrasound exposure. BORREDON and NATHIÉ (1974) exposed observers to infrasound of 7.5 Hz at a level of 130 dB. Measurement of systolic and diastolic blood pressure as well as heart rate was undertaken during periods of quiet, infrasound exposure (up to 50 min duration), and broad band audiofrequency noise. Responses to infrasound were minimal and reached statistical significance only in the case of diastolic blood pressure. FECCI *et al.* (1971) reported small cardiovascular and respiratory changes for workers in a nuclear research facility where the ventilating system produced infrasound in the 70–80 dB range. However, the adequacy of the control group and the consequent attribution of the effects observed to infrasound *per se* in the study by FECCI *et al.* is questionable. ALFORD *et al.* (1966) were unable to detect changes in EKG attributable to infrasound stimulation at intensities up to 144 dB. BONDAREV *et al.* (1970) investigated the effects of 10–20 Hz infrasound at 80–84 dB on pituitary-adrenal axis activity in rats. The effects associated with infrasound were negligible, although the combination of infrasound with vibration resulted in marked changes. The study by BONDAREV and his colleagues illustrates a basic difficulty in interpreting many of the anecdotal reports of infrasound effects in real-life situations. Because infrasound is combined with other stimuli in everyday situations, it is difficult to know what proportion of the response observed, if any, should be attributed to the infrasound component of the total stimulus environment. Since the effects of infrasound have been relatively unknown, it seems that people have leapt to the conclusion that the effects observed were the result of the infrasound. This conclusion has probably been unwarranted in most cases.

In contrast to the problem of sleep disruption encountered with intense audiofrequency sound exposure, there have been isolated reports that infrasound induces fatigue and drowsiness (GAVREAU, 1966; LEVENTHALL, 1974). However, there are no systematic investigations of the effects of infrasound on sleep. [JOHNSON (1973), did note that one dog apparently fell asleep during exposure to a peak stimulus intensity of 172 dB at 1 Hz over a period of 1.5 h.]

The conditions under which noise exposure may result in disturbance of complex task performance have been extensively investigated (see PARKER and VON GIERKE, 1974). LEVENTHALL (1974) found statistically significant performance decrements for a reaction time task and a complex tracking task during noise exposures of 115–120 dB in the 3–15 Hz frequency range. It is possible that Leventhall's observations may have resulted from loss of attention rather than some effect of the infrasound stimulus; this interpretation is supported by the observation that performance improvements, attributed to "arousal", were observed at higher stimulus intensity levels. In contrast to the report by LEVENTHALL, VON GIERKE, and NIXON (1975) reported no disturbance of visual acuity or a finger dexterity task during short term exposure to tones of 3–7 Hz at 152 dB. Exposure to approximately equivalent levels of stimulation at 43–73 Hz, however, did produce significant visual decrements by both subjective and objective measures. Similarly, ALFORD *et al.* (1966) were unable to detect decrements in reaction time or in performance of a reasoning task during exposure to infrasound at levels up to 144 dB. The experiments reported by VON GIERKE and NIXON and ALFORD *et al.* do not support the hypothesis that infrasound, even at very intense levels, is detrimental to human performance.

The final topic to be considered in this section is annoyance. Annoyance can be considered displeasure or resentment reported by individuals in response to noise exposure and may result in action by those individuals to eliminate the noise source. Annoyance is a complex response which frequently reflects implications that a particular noise has for an individual, as well as physical characteristics of the noise itself (see CONNOR and RUDMOSE, Vol. V/3, Chapter 7). Some people report annoyance as soon as they are able to detect a particular noise; however, in most instances the threshold for annoyance is greater than the threshold for detection. Certainly the lower limit for annoyance should be the infrasound threshold function described in Fig. 13 (Curve C). Any argument for much lower levels is difficult to support in view of the natural physiological infrasound levels in the ear. In the United States an Ldn of 55 has been suggested as an annoyance threshold for sound in the audiofrequency range; this level is approximately equal to the 45 phon curve which can be estimated from the data of WHITTLE *et al.* (1972) and which is plotted in Fig. 13 (Curve B_2). Because of the rapid growth of loudness in the infrasound frequency range (Fig. 7 and Table 4), the 45 phon level is close to the threshold for detection. At infrasound frequencies below 5 Hz indirect and nonauditory effects may determine annoyance. These effects would include detection of structural vibration and perceived middle ear pressure; Curve B_1 is a conservative threshold for these effects (JOHNSON, 1975). The 120 dB level has been employed for short-term community exposure at the Cape Canaveral rocket launch site; ten years of observation suggest the validity and/or preventive character of this level (VON GIERKE, 1974).

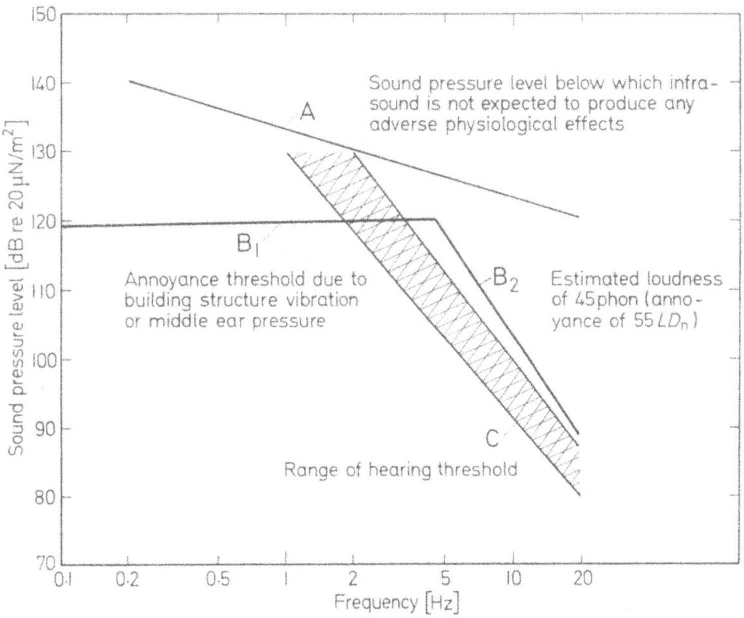

Fig. 13. Estimated infrasound annoyance thresholds. Curve B_2 is the level of infrasound which should produce 55 Ldn . Curve B_1 indicates a conservative estimate of annoyance due to nonauditory effects. Curve C is the range of hearing thresholds under various stimulus conditions for tones and noise. Curve A is the estimated threshold for damage. From JOHNSON (1975)

VII. Nonauditory Responses to Infrasound

Infrasound of high intensity can affect several mechanoreceptors in addition to those of the cochlea. As noted in Section III, because of the impedance mismatch between body tissues and air, most infrasound energy is reflected at the interface between body surfaces and the surrounding air. This section focuses on two major physiological systems that may be affected by infrasound stimulation, the vestibular system and the respiratory system, and discusses infrasound and related vibration effects.

A. Vestibular Stimulation

Among the most disturbing effects occasionally attributed to infrasound are disorientation and vertigo, supposedly mediated through vestibular receptors. Consequently, several experiments have been undertaken to explore possible vestibular activation by infrasound.

Given the cochlea's exquisite sensitivity to acoustical stimulation, the vestibular system's relative insensitivity to sound is perhaps surprising. The vestibular system is quite insensitive to pressure stimulation while retaining very high sensitivity to small displacements produced by linear and angular acceleration of the skull.

Static pressure in the external auditory meatus may produce nystagmus and other vestibular reflexes in experimental animals as well as vertigo and disorientation in human beings. Employing guinea pigs, Parker *et al.* (1968) and Reschke *et al.* (1970) demonstrated nystagmus and counterrolling in guinea pigs following static pressure increments of 13—20 cm H_2O. Direct recording of vestibular ganglion cell activity supports the view that these responses resulted from vestibular activation (Parker and von Gierke, 1971).

Investigation of the effects of static pressure on human beings has received a major impetus from reports of disorientation and vertigo by undersea divers. Kennedy (1972) has compiled an annotated bibliography of studies in this area. Ingelstedt *et al.* (1974) demonstrated vertigo and nystagmus in 5 of 79 otologically healthy observers who were exposed to pressure changes of $\pm$ 45 cm H_2O. Incidence of vertigo was correlated with an unusually high forcing pressure (level of pressure necessary to force the Eustachian tubes open) in one ear.

A considerable amount of information has been collected concerning the response of the vestibular system to acoustical energy (see Parker, 1976). With our co-workers we have added to this effort in recent years. At this point we have examined both physiological and biophysical responses to infrasound in human beings, monkeys, and guinea pigs. Our main measures of physiological response have been the reflexive eye movements, including counterrolling and nystagmus, evoked by vestibular stimulation.

Parker (1976) described a series of experiments in which restrained, awake guinea pigs and monkeys were exposed to intense infrasound (172 dB at 1, 2, and 4 Hz; 169 dB at 10 Hz; 162 dB at 20 Hz; and 158 dB at 30 Hz) that was generated by the dynamic pressure chamber described by Johnson (1974). Whole-body exposures were performed with the experimental animals located inside the dynamic pressure chamber. Two whole-body exposures of guinea pigs were performed after the external auditory meatus on one side had been sealed with bone wax. When the animals were located outside the chamber, infrasound was presented to one ear through a hollow earbar that was sealed in the external auditory meatus and connected to the dynamic pressure chamber with plastic tubing. Responses from 5 guinea pigs and 4 monkeys were examined.

Consistent, repeatable eye movements of the types which are ordinarily associated with vestibular stimulation (nystagmus and counterrolling) were *not* observed in response to infrasound. Two of the guinea pigs exhibited a few nystagmus beats during stimulation, but these observations were not repeatable. One of these animals also exhibited a very small oscillatory eye movement which was apparently in phase with the stimulus, but the response was too small to record with electrophysiological techniques. None of the monkeys demonstrated any evidence of vestibular-induced eye movements.

The failure to observe physiological vestibular responses to infrasound was surprising in view of an earlier study (PARKER *et al.*, 1968) in which we demonstrated nystagmus to pressure oscillations of 166 dB at about 1 Hz. In the earlier study, however, the pressure oscillation was generated by an animal respirator, and the oscillations were between ambient pressure (0 cm H_2O) and +50 cm H_2O rather than being symmetrical around ambient pressure. Therefore, the response in the earlier study can be attributed to static pressure, which has been demonstrated to elicit nystagmus in the guinea pig (PARKER and RESCHKE, 1972).

In the studies with human beings, visual nystagmus and postural equilibrium were employed as measures of vestibular activation by infrasound stimulation. Visual nystagmus was monitored with recording electrodes, and postural equilibrium was determined with a rail task (GRAYBIEL and FREGLEY, 1963). Infrasound was coupled from the dynamic pressure chamber via a large diameter flexible hose to short secondary hoses at the earmuff devices which enclosed the ears. Adjustment of the length of the coupling hose and of the secondary hoses allowed presentation to one or both ears and of phase differences in the signals to the two ears.

Visual nystagmus was studied on volunteers who experienced infrasound monaurally, bilaterally in-phase, and bilaterally 180° out-of-phase at levels of 142–155 dB. The results may be summarized by the statement that visual nystagmus was not observed for any of the conditions investigated.

Postural equilibrium, as indicated by ability to stand on narrow rails, was evaluated for infrasound exposures at levels ranging from 110–140 dB. Exposure conditions were the same as those employed in the study on visual nystagmus. Statistical analysis of the data obtained in this experiment revealed no effects of infrasound on postural equilibrium for the conditions evaluated. While infrasound stimulation failed to elicit vestibular responses, audiofrequency stimulation employing the same methodology yielded clear effects beginning at exposure levels of 105 dB (HARRIS and SOMMER, 1968).

In a recent non-systematic observation, two investigators exposed themselves to infrasound at intensities up to 172 dB and frequencies of 2–8 Hz for periods up to 25 sec. The investigators were unable to detect disorientation or nystagmus at these exposure levels (JOHNSON, personal communication).

The results of our investigations correlate with those of ALFORD *et al.* (1966), who reported that only 1 of 21 observers exhibited transient, mild vertigo during exposure to 140 dB infrasound at 12 Hz. In contrast to the results from our laboratory and those described by ALFORD *et al.* (1966), EVANS (1971), and EVANS and TEMPEST (1972) have reported that infrasound at 7 Hz applied for approximately 1 min can elicit nystagmus at intensities as low as 125 dB. Reconciliation of the discrepant observations concerning the effects of infrasound on the vestibular system is difficult without more complete information than we have available; however, the Evans and Tempest reports leave open two areas for examination. First, it is possible that the nystagmus was produced by audiofrequency sound which was a distortion product of the infrasound signal. Several observations place the threshold for nystagmus response to audiofrequency sound in the 130-dB range.

Second, in the absence of adequate controls, including "blind" evaluation of the data, the evaluator's prior information may intrude excessively on his evaluation of the ambiguous nystagmus records.

Because of its potential similarity to infrasound and because it approximates some forms of environmental noise, the effects of interrupted audiofrequency sound on the vestibular system have been pursued in our laboratory.

Experiments on the effects of interrupted audiofrequency sound employing experimental animals are incomplete. Initial results indicate that transient eye movements in phase with stimulus bursts can be observed in guinea pigs and monkeys stimulated by transient tone bursts of 130–140 dB and 500–1000 Hz at repetition rates of 1–5/sec. Eye movements have not been consistently observed in human beings; however, human observers report transient tilting or displacement of the visual field correlated with intermittent tone bursts in the 115–125 dB intensity range (Reschke *et al.*, 1975). Harris (1972) reported that observers exhibited significantly lower scores on an equilibrium test when they were exposed to intermittent audiofrequency stimulation at 95 and 105 dB than when the stimulation was continuous.

The apparent discrepancy between vestibular effects evoked by infrasound and vestibular effects produced by intermittent audiofrequency stimulation might again be explained by considering the distortion mechanism in the middle ear discussed in Section V (Parker and von Gierke, 1971). Audiofrequency sound either modulated with infrasound or interrupted must result in a rectified component at the output of the middle ear which would manifest itself as true infrasound or changing static pressure at the input to the inner ear. It might therefore be more effective with respect to vestibular stimulation than primary infrasound or static pressure stimuli at the tympanic membrane, which would be considerably attenuated by the middle ear. Further experimental data to clarify these mechanisms are required.

B. Infrasound and Body Vibrations

Von Gierke (1974) and Jansen (1974) have reviewed relationships between infrasound and vibration. In determining these relationships, the most important factor to consider is the interaction of infrasound energy with the body; this interaction is discussed in Section III.A. Practically all effects of mechanical energy, vibration and sound, are caused by displacement of tissue. Displacement of tissue primarily occurs if some air is displaced or some air is compressed. Other tissue displacements and tissue compressions can occur, but they are negligible at these low frequencies compared to the motions facilitated by air enclosures. Therefore, motions at low frequencies are directed toward the enclosed air spaces because that is where the body surface is soft (*i.e.*, exhibits a low impedance). Vibration exposure of the whole body (at infrasound frequencies) when the body is sitting on a vibrating platform produces body deformations which are generally similar to but differ in detail from those produced by airborne infrasound. In this case, the inertial forces act on the masses in the body, primarily on the abdominal mass, which moves in and out of the abdominal cavity and rib cage and thereby compresses air in the lungs. No matter if the body is exposed to longitudinal vibration or transverse vibration (front to back), the main subsystem responding to the stimulation is the abdominal mass and it vibrates, compressing the air in the lungs. Therefore, for practical purposes all the organs in the abdominal cavity vibrate in phase. This produces what is generally called the main body resonance or the fundamental natural frequency of the human body or of the abdominal system.

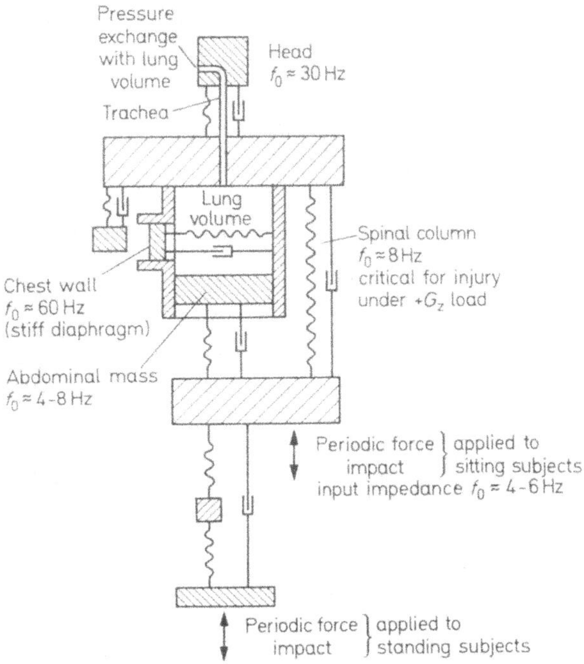

Fig. 14. Lumped parameter biodynamic model of human thorax-abdomen system. From VON GIERKE (1964)

Figure 14 demonstrates a model for the human body which was developed based on the findings of vibration and sound studies. It is helpful in understanding, calculating, and explaining the various low frequency resonances of the human body as well as their location and interaction (VON GIERKE, 1964). If one exposes this whole system to low frequency sound or infrasound, then the pressure acts on the abdomen and pushes the diaphragm upwards and acts simultaneously on the chest walls and causes chest wall motion; at the same time the pressure acts on the air going into the mouth, through the trachea and communicating with the air volume in the lungs. Since the pressure acts at these three areas (abdomen, chest, mouth) simultaneously, the system is much stiffer to the pressure exposures than it is to linear vibration exposure through the buttocks. That is why the resonance of the chest to sound occurs in the 40–60 Hz range, whereas abdominal/chest resonance under vibration occurs in the 4–8 Hz range. Unfortunately, this important difference in the response of the body to omnidirectional infrasound compared to unidirectional vibration has been overlooked in many discussions; the thorax-abdomen resonance for infrasound is at almost 10 times higher frequencies than for unidirectional vibration.

All of the masses, elasticities, and dampings indicated in Fig. 14 are quantitatively known; the impedances of the various surfaces are also known; therefore, the response of the model to various pressure excitations can be determined. From human blast accidents, the compression and extension of lung volume required to produce various degrees of lung injury can be estimated. [A considerable amount of information is available on the response of humans or animals exposed to explosion waves – see BOWEN *et al.* (1968)]. Based on these data one can estimate under what infrasound vibration of the chest the same lung damage would occur as occurs in a one time compression or extension of the thorax under explosion waves. There is a definite relation between what occurs in explosion waves and what might occur at extremely high intensities – although never observed in practice – in infrasound fields.

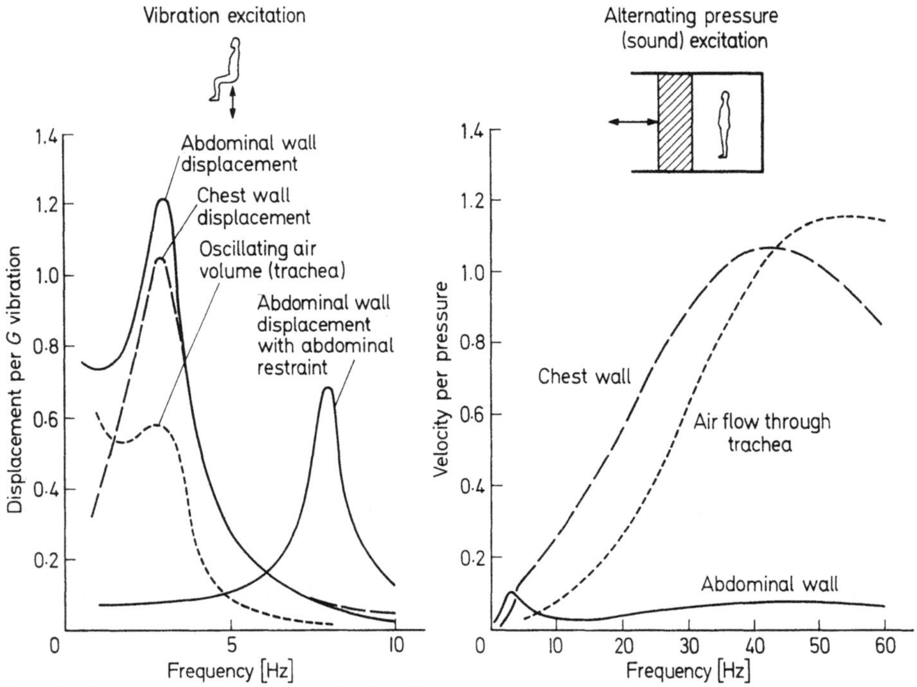

Fig. 15. Response of model described in Fig. 14 to linear translation (left) and whole-body sound exposure (right)

Figure 15 presents the results of calculations for the model of Fig. 14 and illustrates the differences in resonance frequencies which occur in human beings submitted to vibrations and to infrasound. The model is rextremely useful in studying any potential modification of the system. For example, it has been proposed many times that personnel exposed to low frequency vibration or sound fields should wear abdominal belts to suppress abdominal vibration. The model can give us a quantitative indication of the consequences of such action and tells us – as illustrated for one example in Fig. 15 – that suppressing one specific resonance can result in a potentially more dangerous resonance in a higher frequency range.

Up to the present time practically all controlled infrasound experiments have been performed in pressure chambers, where the sound fields are stationary and no propagation effects occur. If possible, these experiments should be conducted not only in pressure chambers but also in standing wave tubes, where the effects of the phase of the sound wave could be examined (*e.g.*, at points where velocity effects are maximum and pressure effects are minimum). However, based on knowledge from the biological effects of blast waves, one would expect that for human beings the pressure effects are the more severe ones. The velocity effects of blast waves do not produce directly severe effects or long term damage, although they can result, due to nonlinearity, in a unilateral pressure on the body. Observers can detect these effects (like being "hit" from one side by the sonic bang wave). In a high amplitude blast wave the velocity effects can be indirect; they can push the whole body in one direction and damage the observer by throwing him to the ground. In general, it appears on the basis of these data that with respect to infrasound the pressure is the most significant quantity which should be studied.

C. Respiratory Response

The possibility that infrasound might produce respiratory effects was deduced from the observations by MOHR *et al.* (1965) of coughing and choking during siren exposures at 150–154 dB in the 50–100 Hz frequency range. Initial observations of anesthetized animals in the dynamic pressure chamber revealed a dramatic decrease or even cessation of respiration. JOHNSON (1974) performed a series of systematic observations on this respiration reduction phenomenon using anesthetized dogs. An impedance respirometer and visual observation were used to monitor the dogs' breathing. Thresholds for respiratory decline or cessation were in the 165–166 dB range. At stimulus frequencies below 1 Hz the chest wall appeared stationary, while at higher frequencies (1–8 Hz) the chest wall appeared to move in phase with the infrasound stimulus. JOHNSON developed a model to account for this phenomenon. Assuming that the lungs can be treated as a rigid bottle open at the bottle neck, the following equation describes the airflow into the bottle:

$$V_m = (2.67 \times \mathrm{FRC} \times 10^{SPL-194/20} - V_D)\, 60\mathrm{f}\,,$$

where V_m is the effective volume of air reaching the alveoli per min, FRC is the functional residual capacity, SPL is sound pressure level re 20 μ N/m^2, V_D is dead space, and f is frequency in Hz. Assuming an FRC of 300 ml and a V_D of 30 ml, an exposure of 172.5 dB at 1 Hz will result in a V_m of 2340 ml/min. This is well within the range of 1500–3000 ml/min ordinarily required for resting dogs and could account for cessation of breathing.

The respiratory phenomena associated with intense infrasound exposure apparently lead to infrasound modulation of speech produced in the sound field which is similar to the modulation of speech produced by a talker experiencing whole body vibration. The latter has been studied extensively (NIXON, 1962; NIXON and SOMMER, 1963). This effect on the speech generation mechanism is in addition to the modulation of the hearing acuity by infrasound on the reception side (Section V.B).

VIII. Proposed Exposure Limits

Tolerance levels for exposure of human beings to infrasound have been considered by NIXON and JOHNSON (1973) and by VON GIERKE and NIXON (1975). Limit levels for infrasound exposure may be prescribed on the basis of experience with auditory and whole-body responses. Our discussion has revealed that human performance and vestibular function were not influenced by short time exposures at levels as high as 140–155 dB. Under some stimulus conditions auditory and respiratory effects were observed. The auditory system appears to be more sensitive to possible adverse effects of infrasound than the other systems evaluated, except for possible whole body responses at intense short duration exposure levels. Consequently, to define limit levels primarily in terms of the auditory system responses should also provide protection for the other, less susceptible, systems and functions. The tentative exposure limits were derived with respect to safety and interference with and preservation of general bodily functions. Subjective annoyance and/or comfort were not part of the considerations.

Tentative limit noise levels which may be considered as acceptable for 8-min exposures are 150 dB at 1–7 Hz, 145 dB at 8–11 Hz, and 140 dB at 12–20 Hz. These levels apply to discrete frequencies or octave bands centered about the stated frequencies. Maximum exposure duration is 8 min with 16 hrs rest between exposures. The use of good insert earplugs may increase the permissible levels by 5 dB for the same exposure times by reducing the aural contribution to the overall response. Earplugs are strongly recommended for all intense infrasound exposures to minimize subjective sensations; however, the use of earmuffs should be avoided. While good earmuff protectors may provide about 10 dB attenuation between 20 and 100 Hz, protection from infrasound stimuli appears to be negligible; in some instances the noise levels under the muff appear to increase (NIXON *et al.*, 1967). Levels above 150 dB should be avoided even with maximum hearing protection until additional technical data are accumulated.

If one were required to specify safe criteria for long duration exposures to infrasound, some extrapolation would be called for in the absence of complete data. The proposed 24 hrs exposure limits presented in Fig. 16 represent such an estimate. The data described earlier indicate essentially no effects at 20 Hz for exposures of 8 min at levels up to 141 dB. Using the equal energy rule of 3 dB per doubling or halving of time and some rounding, and extrapolating from 8 min out to 24 hrs reduce the limit level to about 118–120 dB at 20 Hz.

Table 6. Recommended maximum permissible exposures to infrasound

Duration (hr)	Frequency (Hz) 1	5	10	20
1	145	138	135	132
8	136	129	126	123
24	131	124	121	118

For computation purposes, we adopted the method of representing exposure in terms of level and of number of cycles (frequency times time) as parameters. Accepting the set of conditions cited above as a base for acceptable exposure, the formulation becomes:

$$\text{Limit SPL} = 10 \log \frac{t}{8\ \text{min}} + \log \frac{f}{20} + 141\ .$$

Limit levels for selected frequencies of 1 – 20 Hz and exposure durations of 1 – 24 hrs are contained in Table 6. The 24 hrs duration levels are represented in Fig. 16 as the proposed infrasound limit curve between 1 Hz and 20 Hz. As shown

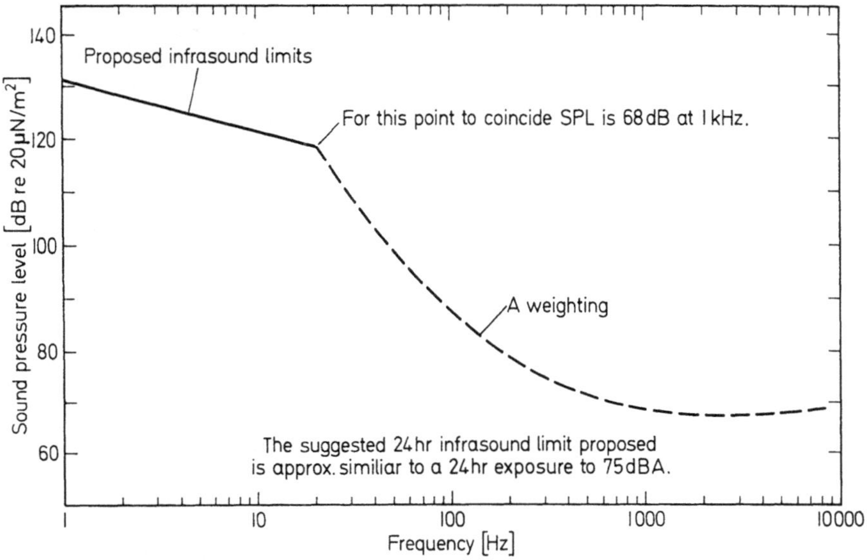

Fig. 16. Proposed 24 hrs infrasound limit (solid line) and audiofrequency 24 hrs limit of 75 dBA

in that figure, the suggested 24 hrs infrasound limit is approximately similar to a 24 hrs exposure to 75 dBA. The reader is reminded that limit values, although in line with present-day health analysis of the U.S. Environmental Protection Agency (U.S. Environmental Protection Agency, 1973, 1974), were derived by extrapolation and should be used with care.

References

Alford, B. R., Jerger, J. F., Coats, A. C., Billingham, J., French, B. O., McBrayer, R. O.: Human tolerance to low frequency sound. Amer. Acad. Ophthalm. Otolaryng. Transact. **70**, 40—47 (1966).

von Békésy, G.: Über die Hörschwelle und Fühlgrenze langsamer sinusförmiger Luftdruckschwankungen. Ann. Physik **26**, 554—566 (1936).

von Békésy, G.: Über die Resonanzkurve und die Abklingzeit der verschiedenen Stellen der Schneckentrennwand. Akust. Z. 8, 66—76 (1943). Also: On the resonance curve and the decay period at various points on the cochlear partition. J. acoust. Soc. Amer. **21**, 245—254 (1949).

von Békésy, G.: Experiments in hearing. New York: McGraw-Hill 1960.

von Békésy, G.: Introduction. In: Keidel, W. D., Neff, W. D. (Eds.): Handbook of sensory physiology, Vol. V/1, pp. 1—8. Berlin-Heidelberg-New York: Springer 1974.

Bondarev, G. I., Sinitsina, A. D., Efimov, I. N.: On the combined effect of low-frequency vibration and noise on the pituitary-adrenal cortex system. Gigiena i Sanitariya (USSR) **35**, 106—108 (1970).

Borredon, P., Nathié, J.: Effects physiologiques observés chez l'homme exposé a des niveaux infrasonores de 130 dB. In: Pimonow, L. (Ed.): Colloque international sur les infrasons, pp. 59—84. Paris: Centre National de la Recherche Scientifique 1974.

Bowen, I. G., Fletcher, E. R., Richmond, D. R., Hirsch, F. G., White, C. S.: Biophysical mechanisms and scaling procedures in assessing responses of the thorax energized by air-blast overpressures or by non-penetrating missiles. Ann. N. Y. Acad. Sci. **152**, Art. 1, 122—146 (1968).

Brüel, P. V., Olesen, H. P.: Infrasonic measurements. Internoise **73**, 599—603 (1973).

Bryan, M., Tempest, W.: Does infrasound make drivers "drunk"? New Sci. **53**, 584—587 (1972).

Cole, J. N., Mohr, G. C., Guild, E., von Gierke, H. E.: The effects of low-frequency noise on man as related to the Apollo space program, AMRL TR-66-119. Wright-Patterson Air Force Base, Ohio: Aerospace Medical Research Laboratory 1966.

Connor, W., Rudmose, W.: Community response to noise. In: Keidel, W. D., Neff, W. D. (Eds.): Handbook of Sensory Physiology, Vol. V/3. Berlin-Heidelberg-New York: Springer 1976.

Dallos, P.: The auditory periphery, p. 180. New York-London: Academic Press 1973.

Eldredge, D. H.: Inner ear — cochlear mechanics and cochlear potentials. In: Keidel, W. D., Neff, W. D. (Eds.): Handbook of sensory physiology, Vol. V/1, pp. 549—584. Berlin-Heidelberg-New York: Springer 1974.

Evans, E. F.: Central nervous system — eighth nerve and primary cochlear nucleus. In: Keidel, W. D., Neff, W. D. (Eds.): Handbook of sensory physiology, Vol. V/2, pp. 1—108. Berlin-Heidelberg-New York: Springer 1975.

Evans, M. J.: Infrasonic effects on the human organs of equilibrium. Proceedings of Fall Meeting of the British Acoustical Society paper 71—104 (1971).

Evans, M. J., Tempest, W.: Some effects of infrasonic noise in transportation. J. Sound and Vibration **22**, 19—24 (1972).

Fecci, R., Barthelemy, R., Bourgoin, J., Mathias, A., Eberle, H., Moutel, A., Jullien, G.: L'action des infra-sons sur l'organisme. Med. Lavoro **62**, 130—150 (1971).

Fox, J., Vardy, A.: The generation and alleviation of air pressure transients caused by the high speed passage of vehicles through tunnels. In: International Symposium on the Aerodynamics and Ventilation of Vehicle Tunnels. Paper G 3. Cranfield, England: BHRA Fluid Engineering 1973.

Gavreau, R., Condat, R., Saul, H.: Infra-sons: générateurs, détecteurs, propriétés physiques, effects biologiques. Acustica **17**, 860—866 (1966).

von Gierke, H. E.: Discussion of Dr. Lawrence's paper on "Process of sound conduction". Laryngoscope **68**, 347—354 (1958).

von Gierke, H. E.: Biodynamic response of the human body. Applied Mechanics Review **17**, 951—958 (1964).

von Gierke, H. E.: Response of the body to mechanical forces — an overview. Ann. N. Y. Acad. Sci. **152**, Art. 1, 172—186 (1968).

von Gierke, H. E.: Effects of infrasound on man. In: Pimonow, L. (Ed.): Colloque international sur les infra-sons, pp. 417—435. Paris: Centre National de la Recherche Scientifique 1974.

von Gierke, H. E., Davis, H., Eldredge, D. H., Hardy, J. D.: Aural pain produced by sound. Benox Report, Contract HG ori-020, Task Order 44, ONR Project Nr. 144079. Chicago: University of Chicago 1953. (DDC AD 24685, National Technical Information Service, Springfield, Va.)

von Gierke, H. E., Nixon, C. W.: Effects of intense infrasound on man. In: Tempest, W. (Ed.): Infrasound and low frequency vibration. London-New York: Academic Press 1976.

von Gierke, H. E., Oestreicher, H. L., Franke, E. K., Parrack, H. O., von Wittern, W. W.: Physics of vibrations in living tissues. J. appl. Physiol. **4**, 886—900 (1952).

von Gierke, H. E., Warren, D. R.: Protection of the ear from noise. Benox Report, Contract HG ori-020, Task Order 44, ONR Project Nr. 144079. Chicago: University of Chicago 1953. (DDC AD 24685, National Technical Information Service, Springfield, Va.)

Graybiel, A., Fregley, A. R.: A new quantitative ataxia test battery, Report No. 107. Pensacola, Florida: Naval School of Aviation Medicine 1963.

Green, J. E., Dunn, F.: Correlation of naturally occurring infrasonics and selected human behavior. J. acoust. Soc. Amer. **44**, 1456—1457 (1968).

Guinan, J. J., Jr., Peake, W. T.: Middle ear characteristics of anesthetized cats. J. acoust. Soc. Amer. **41**, 1237—1261 (1967).

GUTTMAN, N., JULESZ, B.: Lower limits of auditory periodicity analysis. J. acoust. Soc. Amer. **35**, 610 (1963).

HARRIS, C. S.: Effects of increasing intensity levels of intermittent and continuous 1000 Hz tones on human equilibrium, AMRL TR-72-11. Wright-Patterson Air Force Base, Ohio: Aerospace Medical Research Laboratory 1972.

HARRIS, C. S., SOMMER, H. C.: Human equilibrium during acoustic stimulation by discrete frequencies, AMRL TR-68-7. Wright-Patterson Air Force Base, Ohio: Aerospace Medical Research Laboratory 1968.

HIRSCH, F. G.: Effects of overpressure on the ear — a review. Ann. N. Y. Acad. Sci. **152**, Art. 1, 147—162 (1968).

INGELSTEDT, S., IVARSSON, A., TJERNSTRÖM, Ö.: Vertigo due to relative overpressure in the middle ear. Acta oto-laryng. (Stockh.) **78**, 1—14 (1974).

JANSEN, G.: Survey of research done in Germany concerning the effects of infrasound on humans. In: PIMONOW, L. (Ed.): Colloque international sur les infra-sons, pp. 85—106. Paris: Centre National de la Recherche Scientifique 1974.

JERGER, J. B., ALFORD, A., COATS, A., FRENCH, B.: Effects of very low frequency tones on auditory thresholds. J. Speech Hearing Res. **9**, 150—160 (1966).

JOHNSON, D. L.: Animal exposure to infrasound. J. acoust. Soc. Amer. (Abstr.) **53**, 293 (1973).

JOHNSON, D. L.: Various aspects of infrasound. In: PIMONOW, L. (Ed.): Colloque international sur les infra-sons, pp. 337—358. Paris: Central National de la Recherche Scientifique 1974.

JOHNSON, D. L.: Auditory and physiological effects of infrasound. Internoise **75**, 475—482 (1975).

JOHNSON, D. L., VON GIERKE, H. E.: Audibility of infrasound. J. acoust. Soc. Amer. (Abstr.) **56**, 37 (1974).

KENNEDY, R. S.: A bibliography of the role of the vestibular apparatus under water and pressure: content oriented and annotated, Report No. 1. Pensacola, Florida: Naval Medical Research Institute 1972.

KIANG, N. Y-S.: Discharge patterns of single fibers in the cat's auditory nerve, pp. 84—92. Cambridge, Mass.: The M.I.T. Press 1965.

KOBRAK, H. G.: Construction material of the sound conduction system of the human ear. J. acoust. Soc. Amer. **20**, 125—130 (1948).

LEVENTHALL, H. G.: Man-made infrasound — its occurrence and some subjective effects. In: PIMONOW, L. (Ed.): Colloque international sur les infra-sons, pp. 129—153. Paris: Centre National de la Recherche Scientifique 1974.

LEVENTHALL, H., HOOD, R.: Instrumentation for infrasound. Proc. Fall Meeting Brit. Acoust. Soc. paper 71—101 (1971).

MOHR, G. C., COLE, J., GUILD, E., VON GIERKE, H. E.: Effects of low frequency and infrasonic noise on man. Aerospace Med. **36**, 817—824 (1965).

MØLLER, A. R.: Function of the middle ear. In: KEIDEL, W. D., NEFF, W. D. (Eds.): Handbook of sensory physiology, Vol. V/1, pp. 492—517. Berlin-Heidelberg-New York: Springer 1974.

NIXON, C. W.: Influence of selected vibration upon speech. I. range of 10—50 Hz. J. Auditory Res. **2**, 247—266 (1962).

NIXON, C. W.: Human auditory response to an airbag inflation noise, PB-184-837. Washington: Department of Transportation 1969.

NIXON, C. W.: Human auditory response to intense infrasound. In: PIMONOW, L. (Ed.): Colloque international sur les infra-sons. Paris: Centre National de la Recherche Scientifique 1974.

NIXON, C. W., HILLE, H. K., KETTLER, L. K.: Attenuation characteristics of earmuffs at low audio and infrasonic frequencies, AMRL TR-67-27. Wright-Patterson Air Force Base, Ohio: Aerospace Medical Research Laboratory 1967.

NIXON, C. W., HILLE, H. K., SOMMER, H. C., GUILD, E.: Sonic booms resulting from extremely low altitude supersonic flight: measurements and observations on houses, livestock and people. AMRL TR-68-52. Wright-Patterson Air Force Base, Ohio: Aerospace Medical Research Laboratory 1968.

NIXON, C. W., JOHNSON, D. L.: Infrasound and hearing. In: WARD, W. (Ed.): Proceedings of the international congress on noise as a public health problem, pp. 329—348. Washington: U.S. Environmental Protection Agency 1973.

Nixon, C. W., Sommer, H. C.: Influence of selected vibration on speech (range of 2—20 Hz and random), AMRL TDR-63-49. Wright-Patterson Air Force Base, Ohio: Aerospace Medical Research Laboratory 1963.

Parker, D. E.: Effects of sound on the vestibular system. In: Tempest, W. (Ed.): Infrasound and low frequency vibration. London-New York: Academic Press 1976.

Parker, D. E., von Gierke, H. E.: Vestibular nerve response to pressure changes in the external auditory meatus of the guinea pig. Acta oto-laryng. (Stockh.) **71**, 456—461 (1971).

Parker, D. E., von Gierke, H. E.: Sound, vibration, and impact. In: Slonim, N. B. (Ed.): Environmental physiology, pp. 119—162. Saint Louis: C. V. Mosby 1974.

Parker, D. E., von Gierke, H. E., Reschke, M.: Studies of acoustical stimulation of the vestibular system. Aerospace Medicine **39**, 1321—1325 (1968).

Parker, D. E., Reschke, M. F.: Mechanisms of acoustical vestibular stimulation. I. Middle ear nonlinearity. Minerva Otorinolaringologica **22**, 240—249 (1972).

Pickett, J. M.: Low frequency noise and methods for calculating speech intelligibility. J. acoust. Soc. Amer. **31**, 1259—1265 (1959).

Pimonow, L.: Apercu general du domaine infra-sonore. In: Pimonow, L. (Ed.) Colloque international sur les infrasons, pp. 33—58. Paris: Centre National de la Recherche Scientifique 1974.

Reschke, M. F., Homick, J., Landreth, J.: Acoustical vestibular stimulation in man. Minerva Otorinolaringologica **24**, 253—260 (1975).

Reschke, M. F., Parker, D. E., von Gierke, H. E.: Stimulation of the vestibular apparatus in the guinea pig by static pressure changes: head and eye movements. J. acoust. Soc. Amer. **48**, 913—923 (1970).

Shaw, E. A. G.: The external ear. In: Keidel, W. D., Neff, W. D. (Eds.): Handbook of sensory physiology, Vol. V/1, pp. 455—490. Berlin-Heidelberg-New York: Springer 1974.

Sivian, L. J., White, S. D.: On minimum audible fields. J. acoust. Soc. Amer. **4**, 288—321 (1933).

Sommer, H. C., Nixon, C. W.: Primary components of simulated airbag noise and their relative effects on human hearing, AMRL TR-73-52. Wright-Patterson Air Force Base, Ohio: Aerospace Medical Research Laboratory 1973.

Stephens, R. W. B.: Infrasound. Revista de Acoustica **2**, 48—55 (1971a).

Stephens, R. W. B.: Natural sources of low frequency sound. Proceedings of Fall Meeting of the British Acoustical Society, paper 71—105 (1971b).

Tempest, W.: Low frequency noise in road vehicles. Proceedings of the Fall Meeting of the British Acoustical Society paper 71—106 (1971).

Tonndorf, J.: The influence of service on submarines on the auditory organ. In: Chapter D II, Appendix to German Aviation Medicine in World War II. Dept. of the Air Force (1950).

U.S. Environmental Protection Agency: Public health and welfare criteria for noise, 550/9-73-002. Washington, D. C.: Environmental Protection Agency 1973.

U.S. Environmental Protection Agency: Information on levels of environmental noise requisite to protect public health and welfare with an adequate margin of safety, 550-9-74-004. Washington, D. C.: Environmental Protection Agency 1974.

Wever, E. G.: Theory of hearing, p. 189. New York: J. Wiley; London: Dover Publ. 1949.

Wever, E. G., Lawrence, M.: Physiological acoustics, p. 167. Princeton, N. J.: Princeton University Press 1954.

Whittle, L. S., Collins, S. J., Robinson, D. W.: The audibility of low frequency sounds. J. Sound Vibration **21**, 431—448 (1972).

Yeowart, N. S.: Low frequency threshold effects. Proc. Fall Meeting Brit. Acoust. Soc. paper 71—103 (1971).

Yeowart, N. S.: The effect of infrasound on man. In: Pimonow, L. (Ed.): Colloque international sur les infra-sons, pp. 289—306. Paris: Centre National de la Recherche Scientifique 1974.

Yeowart, N. S., Bryan, M. E., Tempest, W.: The monaural m.a.p. threshold of hearing at frequencies from 1.5—100 c/s. J. Sound Vibration **6**, 335—342 (1967).

Yeowart, N. S., Bryan, M., Tempest, W.: Low frequency noise thresholds. J. Sound Vibration **9**, 447—453 (1969).

Yeowart, N. S., Evans, M. J.: Thresholds of audibility for very low-frequency pure tones. J. acoust. Soc. Amer. **55**, 814—818 (1974).

Chapter 15

Electrocochleography

J. J. EGGERMONT, Leiden (The Netherlands)

With 53 Figures

Contents

I. Introduction

Electrocochleography (ECoG) is the recording of stimulus-related potentials generated in the human cochlea, including the first-order neurons forming the auditory nerve. These potentials are the cochlear microphonics (CM), the summating potentials (SP), and the compound action potential (AP). The history of electrocochleography is relatively long, because only a few years after the discovery of CM in animals (WEVER and BRAY, 1930) a round-window recording of CM in man was reported (FROMM *et al.*, 1935), although the responses were so small that no cathode-ray display could be obtained. Improved recording and amplification techniques gave better CM recordings (ANDREEV *et al.*, 1938; PERLMANN and CASE, 1941; LEMPERT *et al.*, 1947, 1950). The term cochleogram was proposed by LEMPERT *et al.* (1947), who in 1950 suggested the placement of a needle electrode through the eardrum onto the promontory. Despite this suggestion, all of the early recordings were made during ear surgery. These studies represent the first era of electrocochleography.

The work was taken up ten years later by RUBEN and his co-workers, who were the first to obtain clear CM responses from the round window (RUBEN *et al.*, 1959, 1960). Progress in the recording techniques resulted in measurable click-evoked compound action potentials (RUBEN *et al.*, 1961, 1962; RUBEN and WALKER,

1963; Bordley *et al.*, 1964; Ronis, 1966), but all recordings were still made during surgery. Reviewing his work, Ruben (1967) mentioned three important topics in electrocochleography: 1. the correlation of physiological and psychoacoustic properties, 2. the investigation of certain diseases, and 3. the objective diagnosis of individual cases of deafness. This second epoch of ECoG was characterized by improved CM measurements and clear AP recordings at high click levels. It was still impossible to measure the AP near the subjective threshold of hearing and ECoG based on round-window recording remained an operating-room technique.

The ultimate step by which ECoG became a routine diagnostic procedure was taken independently by Japanese (Yoshie *et al.*, 1967) and French scientists (Portmann *et al.*, 1967). Yoshie recorded from the outer ear canal but later also used promontory recording. The Bordeaux group used solely promontory recording. The use of average response computers for routine electrocochleography has made it possible to record compound action potentials to stimuli having an intensity close to the subjective hearing threshold. So both the use of the averager and of the transtympanic or extratympanic approach have converted the method from an operating-room technique to a routine office procedure (*e.g.*, Montandon *et al.*, 1975a).

Attempts to develop a non-surgical technique for ECoG were made by Sohmer and Feinmesser, also in 1967; they recorded click-evoked potentials from the earlobe. The recorded response included the compound action potential and a series of waves having longer latencies. These long-latency responses were claimed to originate from the various brainstem nuclei and were in general larger than the compound AP from the auditory nerve. Technical improvements of the method were reported (Sohmer *et al.*, 1972; Lev and Sohmer, 1972; Sohmer and Feinmesser, 1973), and other recording sites such as the hard palate (Spreng and Keidel, 1967; Keidel, 1971) proved to be useful. In the last few years, this far-field technique of brainstem potential recording has led to a new field of electric response audiometry: brainstem audiometry (Terkildsen *et al.*, 1973; Thornton, 1975), which will not be considered in this paper.

II. Methods

A. Stimulation techniques

Sound stimuli capable of evoking compound action potentials from the auditory nerve have to be quickly changing in time since a well defined triggering of the nerve fibre activity is required. Such acoustic stimuli are. *e.g.*, clicks and short tonebursts but also amplitude- and frequency modulated continuous tones. The stimuli used may be divided into two major groups: stimuli with a broad-band spectrum and stimuli with a narrow-band spectrum.

1. Wide-band Stimuli

Wide-band stimuli such as clicks were the first stimuli used in electrocochleography. Like the electric shock used in neurophysiology, the acoustic click provides the best synchronization of the individual nerve fibre responses (Aran *et al.*, 1972;

YOSHIE, 1971). Depending on the type of transducer used and on the duration of the electric signal (usually 50–150 μsec), a click comprises a large number of frequencies, which means that the whole cochlea may be stimulated. Some authors call it advantageous that the whole cochlea can be investigated with one type of stimulus (ARAN *et al.*, 1971a), but the disadvantage of the lack of frequency specificity is felt (MONTANDON *et al.*, 1975b). Electrocochleography with clicks provides a general impression of cochlear functioning rather quickly. In cases of a flat hearing loss, one obtains an exact threshold determination and considerable information about the supraliminal behaviour of the cochlea (*e.g.* the presence of recruitment may be indicated). Most of the evidence on this point has been provided by ARAN *et al.* (1971a) and YOSHIE (1971). A somewhat more frequency-specific but still wide-band stimulus is the 2000 Hz half – sinewave used by ELBERLING and SALOMON (1971) and delivered by a specially shielded TDH-39 dynamic headphone (ELBERLING and SALOMON, 1973). At relatively moderate stimulus intensities (about 75 dB p.e. SPL), the major excitation takes place in the 1–4 kHz region (ELBERLING, 1974).

2. Narrow-Band Stimuli

The use of filtered clicks, produced by ringing a suitable band-pass filter with an electric pulse, improves the frequency selectivity in threshold determinations (ARAN *et al.*, 1971b). The filtered clicks were produced by a 100 μsec, rectangular impulse passed through an Allison-2AB band pass filter having a slope of 30 dB/octave for central-frequency filter settings from 300–9600 Hz. Some statistical evaluation was made for the wide-band click data but not for the filtered click results. It was concluded that the use of filtered clicks with central frequencies of 4800 and 9600 Hz could offer information additional to the wide-band click results and concerning the shape of the audiogram. It seems that the use of the relatively broadly tuned filter induced part of the low reliability of the data obtained, since it limits the resolution of an audiogram to about 30 dB/octave. This limitation was felt by ZERLIN and NAUNTON (1975), who proposed the use of third-octave filtered clicks with a spectrum slope of about 60 dB/octave at all frequencies. The filtered clicks typically had a rise time of about 3 periods and a decay time of more than 6 periods. These stimuli are expected to prove useful in electrocochleography.

A different approach was adopted by YOSHIE (1971) and by EGGERMONT and ODENTHAL (1974a, b, c), who used short trapezoidal tonebursts, which also give good threshold frequency specificity. In addition, the longer duration and the flat plateau of the toneburst considerably facilitates the quantification of the CM and SP. The pure tone bursts used (EGGERMONT *et al.*, 1974a) have two periods of the sinewave during the rise time and fall time and at least six periods during the plateau. This, like filtered clicks, makes the duration of the toneburst dependent on the stimulus frequency. However, the shortest rise time used was 0.33 msec and the plateau duration was never made less than 4 msec to assure reliable CM and SP measurements.

When tonebursts and filtered clicks are used, cancelling of the CM becomes important. This can be achieved for the filtered clicks by presenting the electric pulses alternately in polarity to the filter used; by adding the responses, the CM is cancelled. When tonebursts are used, two methods can be employed: rolling (random) phase stimulation (YOSHIE, 1971) or presentation of the tonebursts alternately in phase and counterphase with an electronic commutator (EGGERMONT *et al.*, 1974a). Both methods have advantages. In rolling phase stimulation, the even harmonics present in the CM at high intensity levels are also cancelled, which is not the case using alternating phase stimuli; however, the CM information is completely lost. In alternating-phase presentation, the CM can also be obtained free of AP by additionally commutating the responses recorded and averaging them separately (SPOOR, 1974).

3. Amplitude and Frequency Modulation

A type of acoustic stimulation less often used in electrocochleography is the amplitude- or frequency-modulated continuous tone. For amplitude modulation, the stimuli have the same trapezoid-shaped envelope but now added in-phase to a continuous tone of the same frequency as used for the toneburst (EGGERMONT and ODENTHAL, 1974b). The use of intensity increments which run from 1 dB to 15 dB offers a suitable means to achieve objective recording of the SISI-test or the difference limen of intensity.

In frequency-modulation (EGGERMONT and ODENTHAL, 1974b), the rise and fall times are to be interpreted as the time in which the continuous tone frequency changes to a new frequency, at which it remains for at least 4 msec or 6 periods before returning to the original frequency. These changes take place in two periods of the original sinewave. The modulation can be upwards ($+\Delta f$) or downward ($-\Delta f$) in frequency for an amount of $1-15\%$ of the original tone frequency.

4. A Fast Method for Electrocochleography

A rather ingeneous type of stimulation was designed by SPOOR (1974), who used a series of six tonebursts, each successive burst being 10 dB higher in intensity. The whole series in which during each 10 or 20 msec a new toneburst is generated is presented two times per second. The analysis interval of the averager is set at about 60 or 120 msec, and it is possible with two recording series to cover the whole intensity range of $0-100$ dB for one frequency. There is less perstimulatory adaptation, but to avoid the masking effect from the last intense stimulus of a series to the 50-dB-weaker first one of the new series, the relatively low repetition rate of 2/sec for the whole series is indicated. As a first introduction to some features of electrocochleography, the difference in recordings obtained in a normal and in a recruiting ear using this technique is shown in Fig. 1. Although the thresholds for both ears differ widely, the output of the cochlea (*i.e.*, the compound action potential amplitude) is about the same at the highest intensity used.

B. Recording Techniques

Stimulus related potentials from the cochlea and eighth nerve can be recorded from various sites around the peripheral hearing organ. The most remote places are the surface of the skull (*e.g.* the mastoid) and the earlobe, which are not especially suited for ECoG but favourable for brainstem audiometry. Recording from the external ear canal results in an augmentation of the recorded AP (about 1 μV at 90 dB SL), whereas, recording from the tympanic membrane makes the measured amplitudes about 3 μV at 90 dB SL. A further increase in potential is obtained by a promontory recording, resulting in APs of about 10 μV at 90 dB SL.

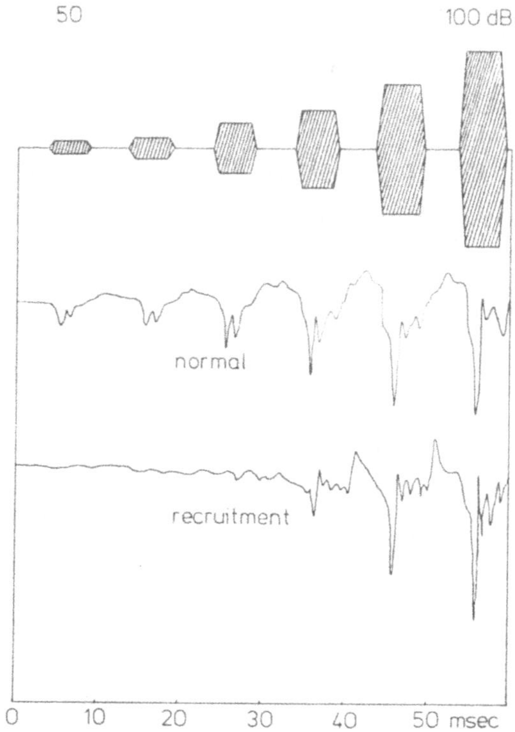

Fig. 1. Fast electrocochleography. A series of six tone bursts in which each successive burst is 10 dB higher in intensity may be used for a quick threshold estimation. The individual bursts are generated each 10 msec, the inter-series interval is chosen at about 500 msec. While each series covers an intensity range of 50 dB, two series cover the intensity region of interest for audiometry. (From ODENTHAL *et al.*, 1974)

This is the only place used when transtympanic recordings are performed. Recordings from the hard palate proved also to be of more interest for brainstem audiometry. The common placement of the electrode for a promontory recording is shown in Fig. 2, while the other recording sites are also indicated. This section will deal with the specific significance which can be obtained by either extra-tympanic, *i.e.*, ear canal or tympanic membrane recording, or by transtympanic, *i.e.*, promontory recording.

1. Extratympanic Recording

The first recording of auditory nerve potentials in man from the external ear canal were reported by YOSHIE *et al.* (1967); they used a 0.3 mm hypodermic needle, coated except at the tip, which was placed in the posterior meatal wall within a distance of about 5 mm from the annulus tympanicus. The authors state that this site is relatively close to the round-window niche. The reference electrode was placed on the earlobe. At 90 dB SL, clicks produced compound APs of about 3.5 μV in amplitude in normal ears, and about 500 responses were used for averag-

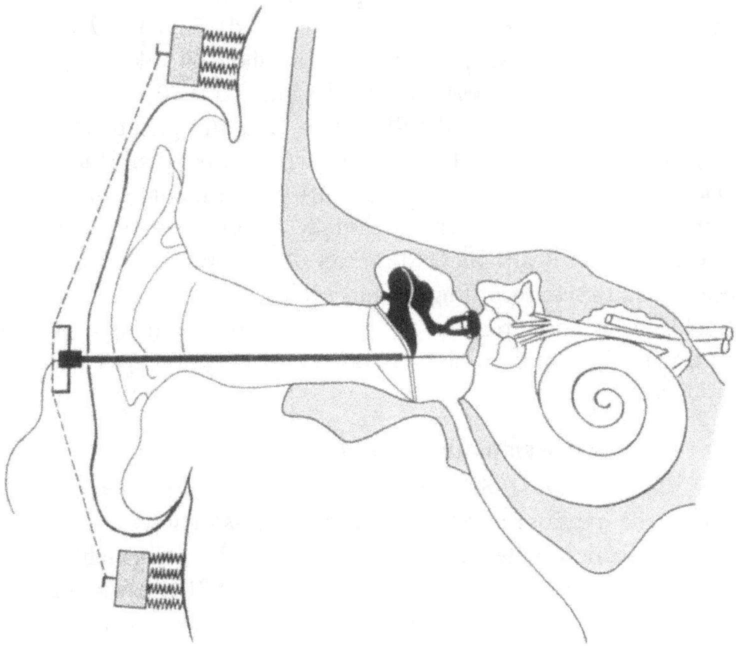

Fig. 2. Trans-tympanic electrode placement. The electrode is pierced through the eardrum and placed on the promontory; the reference electrode is a hypodermic needle placed in the earlobe. (From EGGERMONT *et al.*, 1974a)

ing. The placement of a 0.3 mm enamel insulated and nyloncoated silver wire through a 1.15 mm cannula from the planum mastoideum through the back wall of the ear canal has been advocated by SALOMON and ELBERLING (1971). The chlorided tip of the electrode was fixed under the skin about 2 mm from the limbus, and a chlorided silver needle electrode placed in the earlobe was used for reference. At about 90 dB SL, clicks produced AP-amplitudes of about 1 μV in normal ears.

A silver-foil disc (5 mm in diameter) connected to a fine nichrome or gold wire and placed on the skin of the ear canal was used as the active electrode by MONTANDON *et al.* (1975a). As a reference electrode, a silver clip was fastened at the earlobe. As in the former electrode placements, the ground electrode was on the forehead. At about 90 dB SL, clicks evoked APs of about 1–2 μV in amplitude.

Still another type of electrode was reported by COATS (1974). As an elaboration of the silverball electrode placed against the external auditory-canal skin (CULLEN *et al.*, 1972), a plastic support was designed for an insulated silver wire electrode having a silver ball contact point (0.015 in. diameter); the support held the electrode rigidly in place within 4 mm of the tympanic membrane. AP amplitudes ranged up to about 1.5 μV for stimuli of 90 dB SL. With all of these similar techniques, the active electrode is placed as near to the tympanic membrane as possible, and the reference electrode is on the earlobe. The electrode resistances are of major importance for the quality of the recorded responses. MONTANDON *et al.* (1975a) point out that electrode-electrode resistances should be less than 60 kΩ to avoid excessive noise levels, but SALOMON and ELBERLING (1971) measured electrode resistances of 2 – 6kΩ during their recordings. From a survey of the data available, it is derived that responses can be recorded down to 5 dB SL (threshold at 0.05 μV, ELBERLING and SALOMON, 1971). If the AP threshold is taken, *e.g.*, at 0.2 μV (COATS and DICKEY, 1970), one arrives at 20 dB SL, and for 0.1 μV, YOSHIE (1971) reports measurements down to 10 dB SL. These data all indicate about the same sensitivity of the measurements. It therefore, seems, quite possible to record down to the subjective threshold: however, as YOSHIE (1973) pointed out in comparing threshold estimations made with this technique to subjective ones, there can be deviations of up to 40 dB although the mean deviation is only about 15 dB. It must be recalled that these recordings in general refer to responses of subjects with nearly normal hearing, and it remains to be proven that, in ears with a considerable amount of hearing loss, the extra tympanic recording site is as reliable as the transtympanic approach.

2. Transtympanic (Promontory) Recording

Although YOSHIE *et al.* (1967) started by recording cochlear and whole-nerve potentials from the external auditory meatus, they later gave preference to the use of a transtympanic needle electrode (YOSHIE, 1971), for which an 80-micron polyurethane-coated steel wire was used. ARAN *et al.* (1971 a) used a stainless steel electrode 0.2 mm in diameter and sharpened at the tip, which type of electrode is also preferred by EGGERMONT *et al.* (1974a). The electrode is pierced through the eardrum (which requires some type of anaesthesia) and placed on the promontory between the oval and round windows. SPOOR (1974) reports an equivalent noise level (8 Hz to 10 kHz) of 6 μVpp, corresponding to an interelectrode resistance of about 3 – 5 kΩ. The compound AP amplitude at 90 dB SL click stimulation ranges up to 30 μV, which is favourable for relatively quick measurements and also facilitates recording in patients with very large hearing losses.

As to the disadvantage of perforating the eardrum, we must quote CROWLEY *et al.* (1975) who, in an elaborate survey comprising 3693 electrocochleograms from 26 clinics of which 57.1% of the ECoGs were carried out using the transtympanic approach, concluded that "the risk of persistent perforation of the tympanic membrane or of otitis media is less than 0.1%", which is interpreted as a negligible risk. As a comment to the survey, it must be said that apparently no undesirable after-effects were expected from extra tympanic electrode placement, because the questionnaire did not ask for such after-effects. However, it is conceivable that extratympanic placement of an electrode under the skin or irritation due to extensive cleaning of the external meatus in order to reduce the skin-electrode resistance, also produces after-effects (*e.g.* otitis externa).

It may be concluded that due to the placement of an electrode more near the source of the recorded potentials, especially in clinical testing of patients, the advantage of large and clear responses is of larger weight than the unease of perforating the eardrum.

3. Some Requirements for Recording Apparatus

It is advisable that the pass-band of the amplifiers used should be as large as possible. ARAN *et al.* (1971a) reported 1 Hz to 30 kHz; EGGERMONT *et al.* (1974a) used 8 Hz to 10 kHz; and ELBERLING and SALOMON (1971), 10 Hz to 5 kHz. The low cut-off frequency should be as low as possible but in accordance with the slow voltage fluctuations which are also recorded and which should be filtered out of the signal. It is the higher low-frequency settings *e.g.* 100 Hz, as used by MONTANDON *et al.* (1975a) that produce a latency change in the recorded APs and, therefore, are only tolerable for screening purposes, not for a more quantitative electrocochleographic approach. In general, the noise level of the amplifier system should be as low as possible. The 6 μVpp noise level in our equipment (SPOOR, 1974) in fact is near the upper limit for recording responses down to the subjective threshold without the necessity of averaging more than 1000 responses. The total amplification used ranges from 10000 times (ARAN *et al.*, 1971a) to even 1000000x as reported by Elberling (1971). It seems that an amplification of 20000—50000 times is the optimum value, at least for transtympanic recording. Averaging techniques are necessary for recovering the signals from the noise; the preferred analysis interval is from 10–30 msec. The stimuli should be presented at a rate of 5–10 per second, depending on the duration of the individual stimuli, to avoid diminshing of the compound AP due to adaptation (EGGERMONT and ODENTHAL, 1974a).

4. Anaesthesia and Sedation

In electrocochleography, anaesthesia or sedation are of paramount importance for the whole procedure, since restlessness of the patient during the measurements can invalidate the results of the test. The time needed for extensive electrocochleography (EGGERMONT *et al.*, 1974a) may be as much as 2 h, while a quick screening procedure using clicks may be performed in 20 min. The only pain experienced during the procedure is associated with the placement of either the extratympanic or the transtympanic needle electrode. A relatively long-lasting, light level of anaesthesia or sedation, has to be achieved to obtain the desired relative or absolute immobility of the patient. For the psychologically normal adult, local anaesthesia and additional sedation will meet the requirements for electrocochleography, but for children and mentally disturbed or anxious patients, general anaesthesia is necessary. The type of local anaesthesia applied is in general a 2% Xylocaine solution.

In children, a dissociative type of anaesthesia is used (*e.g.* Ketamine chloride) and is administered either intramuscularly or intravenously; this method is favoured when the recording period does not exceed about $^1/_2$ hour. For longer recording periods, an inhalation type of anaesthesia, *e.g.*, halothane, nitrous oxide and oxygen is preferable (ZVONAR *et al.*, 1974).

III. Receptor Potentials

A. Cochlear microphonics

1. Basic Information

The cochlear microphonics (CM) can be recorded from almost anywhere in the cochlea or from the cochlear surface. It has been demonstrated (TASAKI *et al.*, 1952) that responses to all frequencies can be derived from the first turn of the guinea pig cochlea, whereas the higher turns respond only to low frequencies. A round-window electrode seemed fully comparable with a differential recording in the first turn. The authors concluded that intracochlear differential electrode pairs sample the CM within a range of about 2 mm along the cochlear partition. The source of the CM is the hair-bearing surface of the haircells. In waltzing guinea pigs (a strain with a congenital defect of the cochlea and vestibular apparatus) having abnormal haircells, Davis *et al.* (1934) showed the absence of CM in a round-window recording. Therefore, the CM may provide some information about the validity of the cochlear haircells.

Von Békésy (1960) found the CM in the normal cochlea proportional to the displacement of the basilar membrane. Experiments in Kanamycin-intoxicated guinea pigs (Dallos *et al.*, 1972a) showed that the CM generated by the inner haircells, which appeared to be at least morphologically normal, is about 30–40 dB less sensitive than that generated by the outer haircells. This restricts the use of the CM as an indicator for outer-haircell validity only.

One of the problems encountered with promontory or round-window recording and even with differential recording of the CM is that the recorded signal is not representative for the output waveform of a given individual haircell (Whitfield and Ross, 1965). According to Kohllöffel (1971), a weighted average over the individual haircells is recorded. The weighting function incorporates the phase differences and electrotonic attenuation (6 dB/mm) along the cochlear partition. It is thus clear that the gross responses obtained from the promontory will always be diffuse; this plus the fact that only information about the basal turn is obtained indicates the difficulties encountered when conclusions have to be drawn from CM recordings in electrocochleography.

Most of the investigators in electrocochleography were only concerned in how to cancel the disturbing CM in the recordings. This is achieved by stimulating alternately with condensation or rarefaction clicks or by using tonebursts with rolling phase. After some precautions, however, it is also possible to record the CM free from intermingled AP and SP; one procedure to accomplish this is described by Spoor (1974) and is illustrated in Fig. 3.

2. Clinical Use

The clinical use of the cochlear microphonics is limited. The first quantitative data concerning the CM were reported by Yoshie and Yamaura (1969), who recorded from the promontory as well as from the ear canal. One significant finding concerned the slope of the input-output curve: for the promontory recordings, a slope equal to unity was found; whereas, it was distinctly lower for the external meatus recording. Elberling and Salomon (1973), also recording from the external ear canal, reported a slope of 0.7 in agreement with Yoshie and Yamaura. This finding is interpreted by both groups of authors as indicating that the external meatus is more favourable for recording contributions of more apically situated haircells than is the promontory recording. The 0.1 and 0.3 μV isopotential curves recorded from the meatus were in general 20 dB less sensitive than in the corresponding promontory recordings, and in normal-hearing subjects CM could be obtained from 65–120 dB SPL. HOKE *et al.* (1972), using a combination of averaging and Fourier-analysis of the CM, claim to record down to the 1 nVeff. level, which for promontory-recordings corresponds to about 40 dB SPL. The slope of the recorded input-output curves was in general slightly less than one.

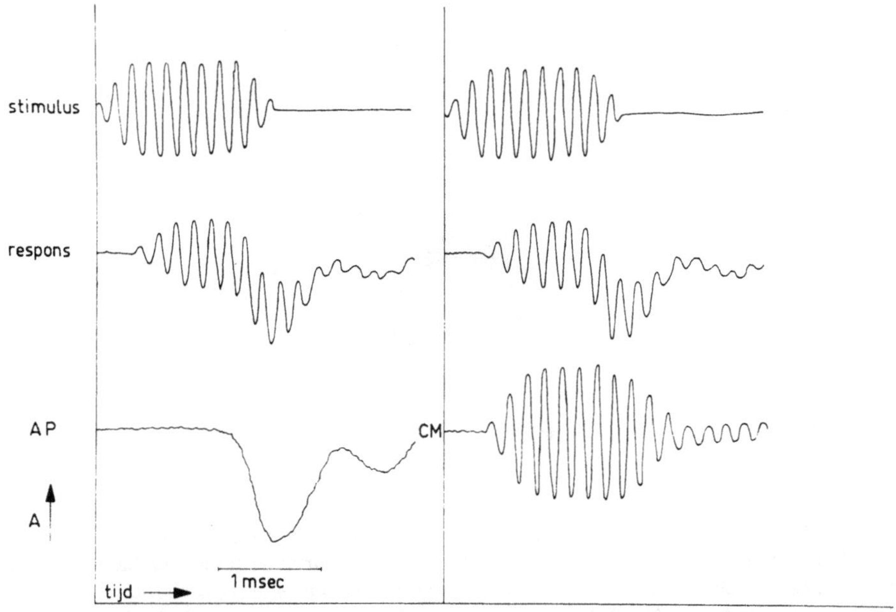

Fig. 3. Commutator action. Odd and even stimuli have opposite phase so in the corresponding responses the CM are in opposite phase. Summation leads to cancellation of the CM. The AP is cancelled simultaneously in the other channel by reversing the phase of the even responses before summation. (From EGGERMONT *et al.*, 1974a)

RUBEN (1967) compared CM output from the cochlea in ears with different types of pathology. The maximum CM-output proved not to be significantly different in conductive deafness and central deafness but was about a factor 10 lower in ears with so-called eighthnerve deafness. YOSHIE and YAMAURA (1969) observed a parallel shift of the CM input-output curve to higher intensity levels compared to normal for ears with conductive deafness. They recorded from the external meatus and also observed that the curves were somewhat steeper than those of normals, probably due to a changed electric conductance due to the presence of the middle-ear fluid. The shift of the CM curve seemed to be related to the degree of hearing loss. In sensorineural deafness, two quite distinct effects could be observed: a normal type of input-output curve in cases with a slight hearing loss and an abnormal steep curve in cases with more severe loss. In general, however, recruiting ears showed only a parallel shift compared to normal curves.

So, in general, the observations of CM lack a great amount of consistency. Although BEAGLEY (1974) finds the presence of CM and absence of AP a significant sign for a nerve deafness, the use of the CM cannot readily be quantified (ARAN, 1974). Some observations by ROSENBLITH and ROSENZWEIG (1951) must be recalled here; they recorded CM and AP at different sites of the guinea pig bulla and cochlear surface, and found at specific sites less or virtually no CM. These places can also be found on the human promontory, although only for specific frequencies of stimulation. In general, the amplitude of CM will be dependent on the recording site (Fig. 4).

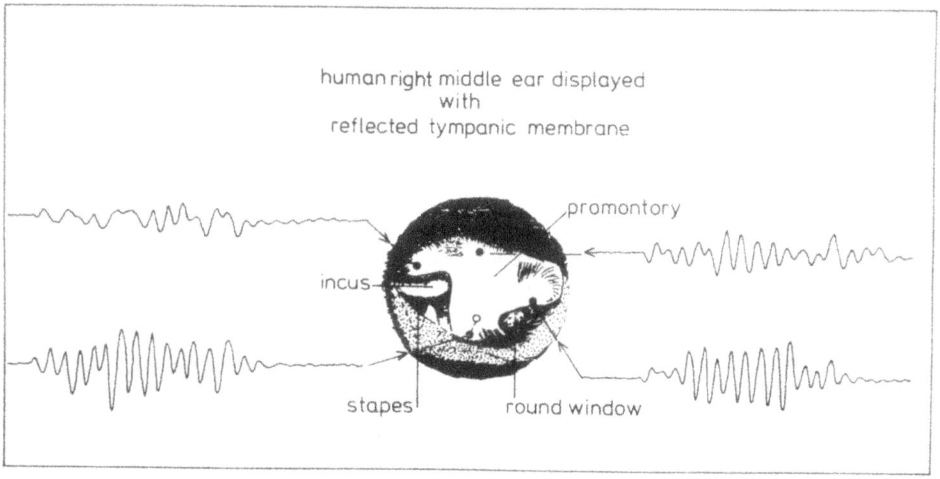

Fig. 4. Cochlear microphonic amplitude and recording site. In an ear with a large central perforation but with a normal cochlea, recordings at the four sites indicated have beenper-formed. Sites near the round window show the largest CM, while sites near the stapes show the smallest one. The AP and SP are less influenced by the recording site

One possible use of CM recordings, as indicated by ELBERLING and SALOMON (1973), is the study of the function of the middle ear (MØLLER, 1963), and for that purpose the technique of HOKE *et al.* (1972) already requiring sound measurement at the eardrum for calibration purposes, seems to be of potential value. The reliable use of promontory or external meatus recording of CM for clinical purposes of a somewhat advanced type is not seen as a promising possibility.

B. Summating potentials

1. Basic Information

A second stimulus-related haircell potential was found to be generated near the cuticular lamina of the haircells and was called the summating potential (SP). The SP appears as a DC shift of the baseline, which may be either positive or negative with respect to the scala tympanic potential (TASAKI *et al.*, 1954). For a negative summating potential (SP^-), the scala media is relatively negative with respect to the scala tympani; for a positive summating potential (SP^+), the reverse is the case.

Under various experimental conditions, *e.g.* anoxia and pressure- or electric polarization differences between the scala tympani and the scala vestibuli, a change of sign for the SP may occur. Scala media-recorded SP^- becomes more negative at increased pressure in the scala tympani. DAVIS (1960) stated that the summating potential arises as a result of a straight-forward non-linearity in the behaviour of the CM, giving rise to a DC component. However, the magnitude of the SP sometimes exceeds the peak amplitude of the CM, which led WHITFIELD and ROSS (1965) to attribute its origin to an asymmetry in the basilar membrane movement, resulting in a pressure difference between the scala tympani and the scala vestibuli during sound stimulation (*cf.* NEDZELNITSKY, 1975). This hypothesis was confirmed by DURRANT and DALLOS (1972).

When recording is not done from the scala media, the sign of the SP may lead to some misunderstanding. KUPPERMAN (1966), *e.g.*, recorded from the scala tympani relative to the neck muscles and, of course, could not relate the recorded SP sign to scala tympani polarity. He called the SP, negative, when the baseline shift was in the direction of the AP deflections; this is also a good convention when recording from the cochlear surface. An SP^+ recorded from the scala tympani corresponds, however, to an SP^- recorded from the scala media or scala vestibuli (Fig. 5). From here on the above-mentioned sign convention will be used. The SP^+ was apparently found only in stimulated parts of the cochlea (KUPPERMAN, 1966), and the SP^- in that part which was at rest. The tonotopic relationship between the SP^+ maximum at a certain frequency and the place of maximum basilar membrane displacement has been demonstrated (KUPPERMAN, 1970). The importance of the recording site for the SP was also stressed by DALLOS *et al.* (1972a). They recorded, using differential intracochlear electrodes, a differential component (DIF SP) and an overall component (AVE SP) of the cochlea. The DIF SP represents the DC-shift between scala vestibuli and scala tympani, and the AVE SP represents the DC shift of the entire cochlea relative to the neck muscle potential. The AVE SP is positive at the site of maximum stimulation and negative elsewhere in the cochlea, and therefore corresponds qualitatively with the intra-scala tympani-recorded SP.

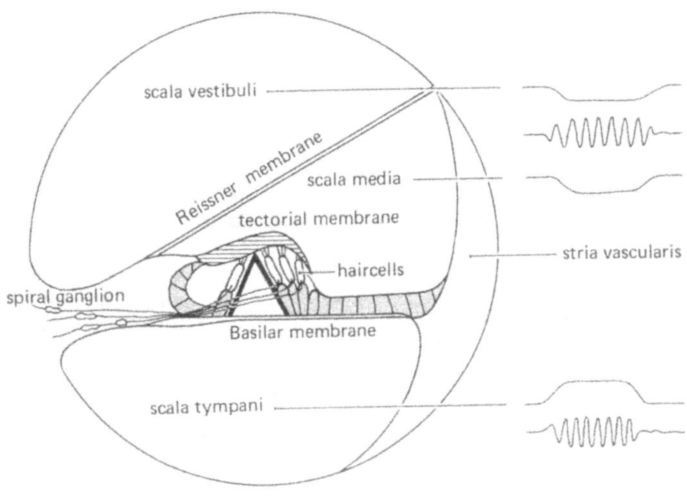

Fig. 5. Cross section of the cochlea showing the sign of the summating potential and the cochlear microphonics with respect to the intracochlear recording sites. Both the SP and the CM change sign at the cuticular laminae of the haircells. (From EGGERMONT *et al.*, 1974a)

For a round-window recording from the guinea pig, one nearly always measures a positive summating potential when stimulation occurs with high-frequency, high-intensity tonebursts. This, therefore, may be compared to the AVE SP recorded from the first turn. Recording from the cochlear surface opens the possibility that changes in the magnitude of the SP will be observed for different recording sites.

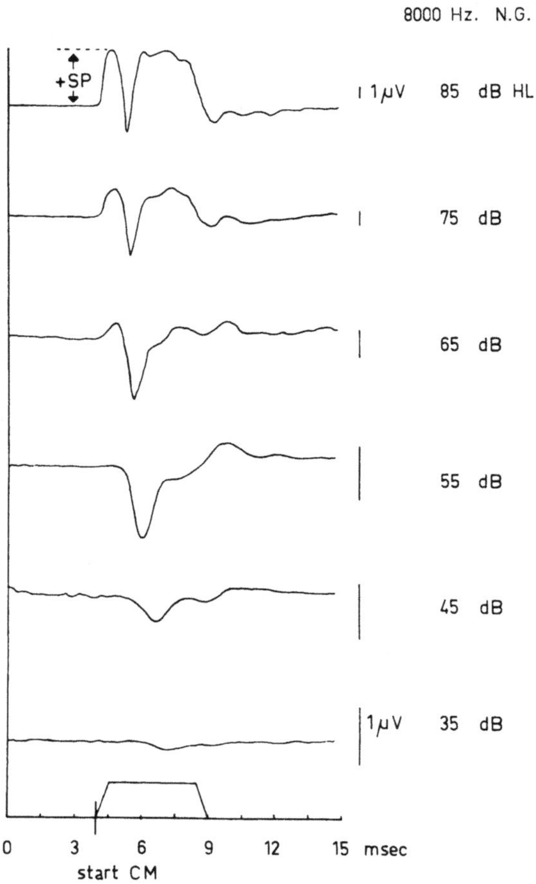

Fig. 6. The positive summating potential (SP^+) in combination with the compound AP. In some normal cochleas and, somewhat more frequently, in pathological cochleas, an SP^+ may be observed upon stimulation with high frequency tone bursts. The pattern of the SP closely resembles that of the envelope of the tone burst. The SP^+ decreases more rapidly in amplitude with intensity than does the AP. (From EGGERMONT *et al.*, 1974a)

One important thing must be noted: in recording from the round window niche or the promontory in man an SP^- is generally recorded (EGGERMONT, 1974) for all frequencies and high intensity levels. This is the opposite of what is recorded from the round window of the guinea pig, and points to a rather different electroanatomy for both cochleas.

2. Clinical Use of SP Polarity

In man, summating potentials are most easily recorded from the promontory. However, ELBERLING and SALOMON (1973) reported small but distinct SP^- for 4000 Hz toneburst stimulation in an external meatus recording. If quantitative information concerning the SP is to be obtained, a promontory recording is indicated, and tonebursts of a given minimum duration (*e.g.* 4 msec) must be used.

The SP^+, which is conveniently recorded from the guinea pig round window, can only be found occasionally when we record from the human promontory. As shown in Fig. 6, the SP^+ resembles the envelope of the toneburst and the detection threshold lies at about 55 dB HL. As already noted, an SP^- is observed far more often in promontory recording. In Fig. 7, this is shown for 8000 Hz toneburst stimulation.

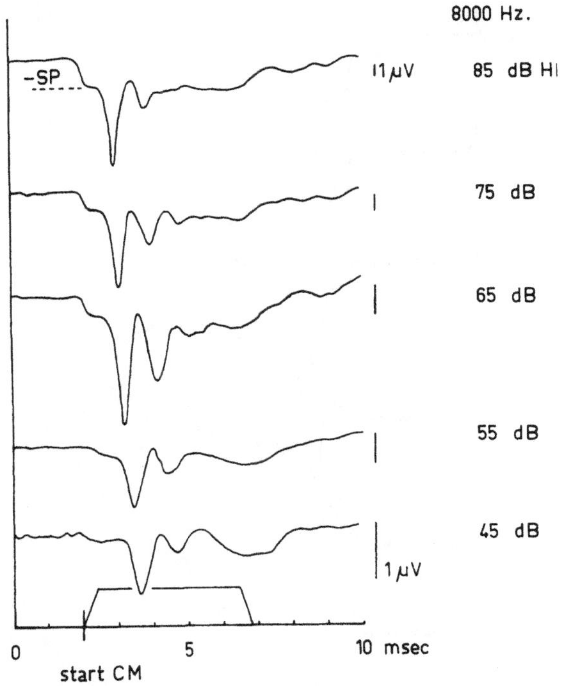

Fig. 7. The negative summating potential (SP^-). Most normal and abnormal cochleas show an SP^- at all tone burst frequencies; this is quite surprising in view of the positive sign of the summating potential recorded from the round window in the guinea pig. (From EGGERMONT *et al.*, 1974a)

Sometimes, a change of sign is observed when the frequency of the toneburst is increased at constant intensity. A sequence of this kind is shown in Fig. 8. For this ear of a patient with Menière's disease, a distinctly negative SP is observed for a stimulus of 4000 Hz at an intensity of 80 dB HL; an increase in the toneburst frequency to 4350 or 4750 Hz leads to a clear drop in the SP^- amplitude. A further increase in frequency to 5175 Hz gives a positive SP, whose magnitude increases slightly when the frequency is raised further. The same type of change is observed from the AVE SP recorded from the guinea pig's first cochlear turn (DALLOS *et al.*, 1972), where, at an intensity of 60 dB SPL, the AVE SP is typically negative for frequencies up to 3000 Hz, about zero at 6000 Hz, and positive for higher frequencies. In general, the reverse change of sign is observed for the DIF SP. It must be noted that a change from SP^+ to SP^- with increasing frequency is never found in man. The scala tympani-recorded SP from the first turn in the guinea pig usually shows the same pattern as the AVE SP, while the scala vestibuli-recorded SP has more resemblance to the DIF SP. It must, therefore, be concluded that the promontory-recorded SP generally behaves like an AVE SP, but the dominance of SP^- recordings remains puzzling.

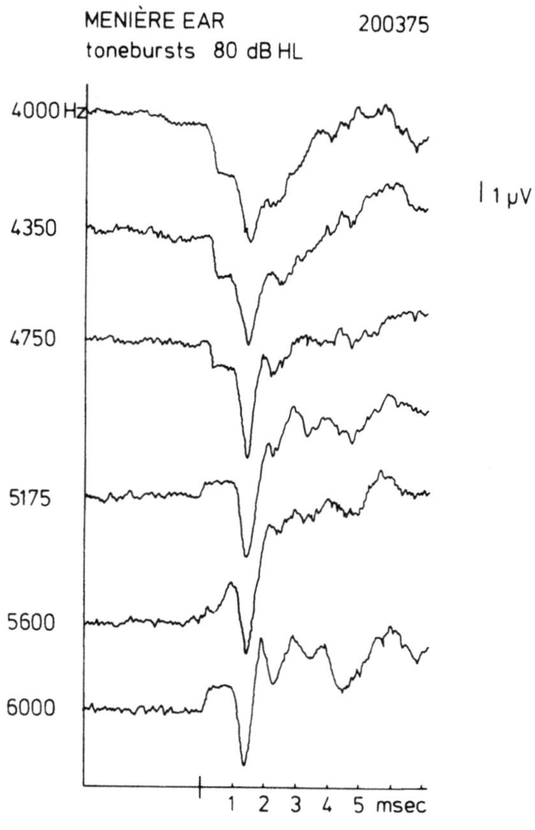

Fig. 8. Transition of negative to positive summating potential with increase in tone burst frequency. In some ears, a quite sudden change in the sign of the summating potential may be observed. In this example, a change occurs between 4750 Hz and 5175 Hz. This type of transition always occurs from SP^- to SP^+ for higher frequency and is found in Z-shaped audiograms

Of about 250 ears, all of which gave clear summating potentials at the toneburst frequencies of 2,4, and 8 kHz, only 28 ears showed a positive SP at one or more frequencies. Among these 28 ears, SP^+ was found at 8 kHz in all cases, at 4 kHz in 13 ears, and at 2 kHz in only 4. Thus, the majority of these ears showed the change of sign. In contradiction to our earlier conclusion (EGGERMONT, 1974), there seems to be a relationship between the occurrence of SP sign changes and the shape of the audiogram. In general, the audiogram shows a greater loss for the higher than for the lower frequencies, and in many cases the hearing loss increases sharply by at least 30 dB above 2000 Hz. When SP^- changed to SP^+ under increasing stimulus frequency, a few cases showed a quite typical phenomenon as can be seen in Fig. 9b. Here, the SP consists of a sharp positive peak (SP^+) followed by a smaller

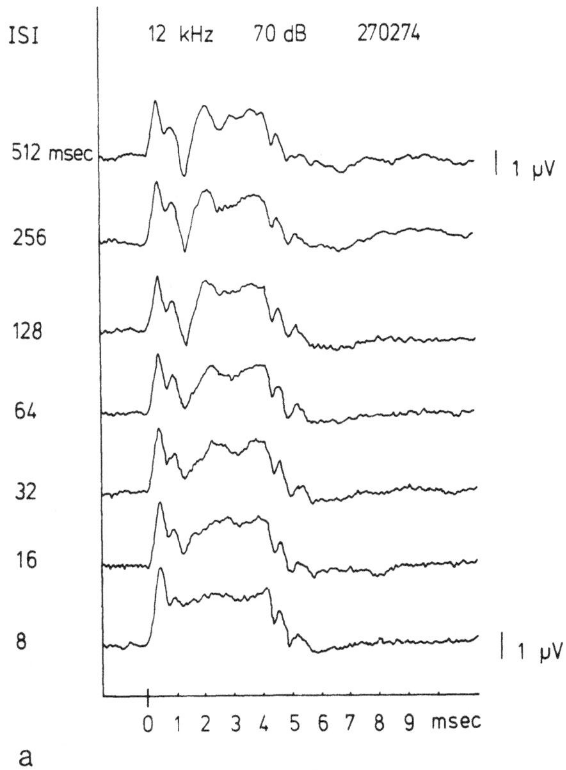

Fig. 9a

SP^- having a slightly longer latency; at lower intensities only the sharp positive peak remained. That this SP^+SP^- complex is not of neural origin is demonstrated by its persistance under lowering of the interstimulus interval, as shown in Fig. 9a. The AP disappears completely at an interstimulus interval of 8 msec, but the summating potential remains. It must be emphasized that neither the SP^+ nor the SP^- shows adaptation and that the suggestion of KUPPERMAN (1966) that the SP^- component is of neural origin does not hold, at least in this situation. The reason for this intermingled SP^+SP^- pattern may be due to the combination of the rather high stimulus frequency (12 kHz) and the more apical electrode site. The high-frequency stimulation produces SP^+ at the most basal part of the cochlea and SP^- for more apical regions, with a slight latency due to travelling-wave delay. ARAN *et al.* (1971a) tend to ascribe the occurrence of an "early positive peak" to a rather abnormal cochlear situation, but the present evidence does not permit further differential diagnosis.

3. Clinical Use of SP Amplitude

Somewhat more promising is the amplitude of the summating potential. In Fig. 10, the amplitude of the SP^- in response to 2000 Hz tonebursts is plotted as a function of stimulus intensity for 25 normal ears. A drawn line connects the calculated means. The large standard deviation is obvious. Application of this type of analysis to a group of 25 Menière ears and a smaller group of 15 ears with hearing loss due to asphyxia, noise trauma or ototoxic drugs gives mean curves like those in Fig. 11. The latter group is considered as the haircell group. It is clear that on average there will be less or no difference between the normal group and the Menière group, but the SP output is distinctly lower for the haircell-loss group.

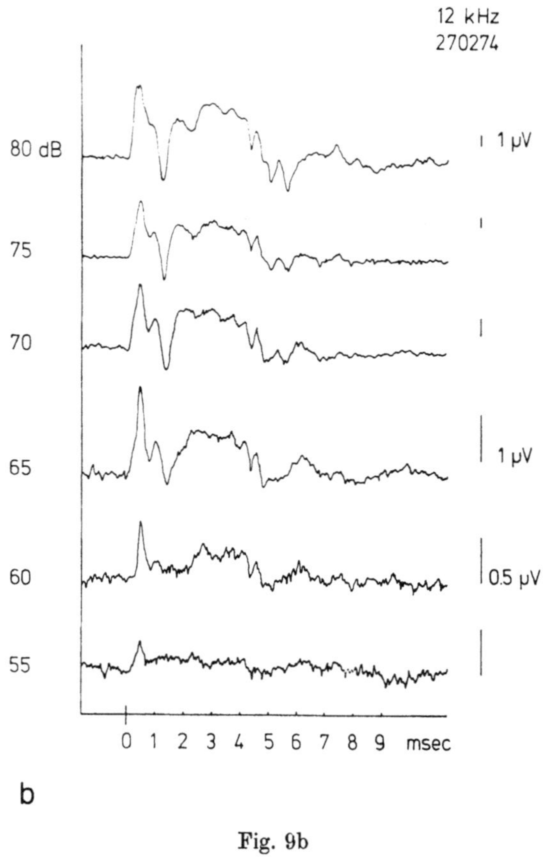

Fig. 9b

Fig. 9a, b. Combination of positive and negative summating potentials in one recording. In ears showing a transition from SP^- to SP^+ as described in Fig. 8, for very high frequencies a quite peculiar phenomenon may be observed. It appears as an SP^+ followed after some latency by a smaller SP^- thus forming an early positive peak, which is persistent to low intensity levels. A change of the repetition rate of the tone bursts shows that the combination of SP^+/SP^- does not diminish in amplitude as the AP does. Both summating potentials, therefore, are of presynaptic origin

Before making further statements, it will be appropriate to analyse the data somewhat more accurately, and, therefore, mean values and standard deviations are calculated for an intensity of 85 dB HL at three toneburst frequencies. The data for three groups, 70 Menière ears, 25 normal ears and 22 haircell loss ears are presented in Table 1.

Table 1. Summating potential amplitude distribution

	2000 Hz	4000 Hz	8000 Hz
Normal hearing	$1.5 \pm 1.4\,\mu V$	$1.8 \pm 1.8\,\mu V$	$3.0 \pm 2.6\,\mu V$
Menière ears	$3.0 \pm 2.5\,\mu V$	$1.7 \pm 1.6\,\mu V$	$1.4 \pm 1.3\,\mu V$
Haircell-loss ears	$0.2 \pm 0.2\,\mu V$	$0.25 \pm 0.20\,\mu V$	$0.45 \pm 0.35\,\mu V$

It may be observed from Table 1 that the mean values are nearly the same as the standard deviations, which points to an exponential distribution for the amplitude values of the summating potential irrespective of the state of the hearing organ. The same is found, however, for the distribution of the AP-amplitude values at 85 dB HL.

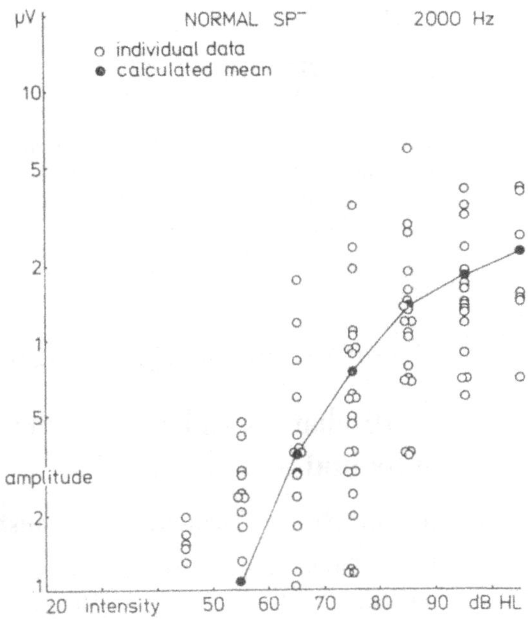

Fig. 10. Amplitude of the summating potential in normal ears. For 20 normal ears, the SP amplitude is plotted as a function of stimulus intensity for 2000 Hz tone bursts. The large dispersion in the amplitude values is obvious; the mean value tends to saturate at about $2.5\,\mu V$ for intensities above 85 dB HL. The detection threshold is around 55 dB HL. (From Eggermont, 1974)

From the data shown in Table 1, it may be concluded that although the normal ears and the Menière ears cannot be differentiated on the basis of the magnitude of the SP, the haircell-loss ears easily are. It must be kept in mind, however, that the combination of SP and AP information, especially when tonebursts of different frequencies are used, offers far more evidence for a differential diagnosis (SCHMIDT *et al.*, 1974). This conclusion will be reviewed later on in this paper.

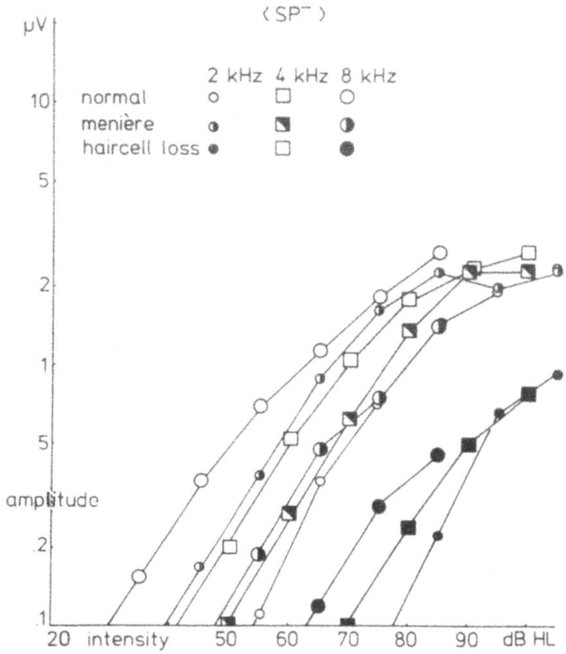

Fig. 11. Mean amplitude-intensity curves for the summating potential in normal and pathological ears at three tone burst frequencies. The amplitudes of the summating potential are significantly smaller for the ears with presumed hair-cell loss, while potentials from ears of Menière patients show the same trend as those recorded in normal ears. (From EGGERMONT, 1974)

IV. The Compound Action Potential

A. Single nerve fibre discharges and the interpretation of the compound action potential

1. Innervation and Space-Frequency Relationships

In the cat, 90–95% of the afferent nerve fibres of the auditory nerve are radial fibres innervating the inner haircells, leaving only 5–10% of spiral nerve fibres innervating the outer haircells (SPOENDLIN, 1970). In the guinea pig, these figures seem to be 85–90% and 10–15%, respectively, for radial and spiral afferent nerve fibres (MORRISON *et al.*, 1975), and there is obviously no reason to assume that the percentages will be much different in man. It follows, therefore, that the great majority of recordings of single nerve fibres are from radial nerve fibres and one must also conclude therefrom that the contributions of single nerve fibres to the compound AP will be primarily from fibres innervating the inner haircells. This will hold even at low intensity values because the sensitivity of the radial fibre inner-haircell configuration is very near the threshold of hearing (KIANG *et al.*, 1965; EVANS, 1972).

Radial nerve fibres in general innervate only one inner haircell (SPOENDLIN, 1970), and, therefore, the discharge pattern of the single nerve fibre will reflect the point response of the basilar membrane and the haircell transducer. It is known that a single fibre is most sensitive to stimulation with a particular characteristic frequency (CF). The so called tuning curve, reflecting the threshold properties of the fibre with respect to stimulus frequency, has a high-frequency slope of up to 600 dB/octave and a low-frequency slope of up to 100 dB/octave. However, for intensity values above approximately 70 dB SPL the fibre responds to nearly every frequency below the CF, and the subsequent increase of the threshold curve is only 5–10 dB/octave (KIANG and MOXON, 1974; EVANS, 1974, 1975). KIANG *et al.* (1965) have shown that the tuning curves as obtained with pure tone stimuli and tonebursts (rise-and-fall time 2.5 msec, duration 50 msec) are identical. For shorter rise times, a broadening of the tuning curve is expected, which may be relevant for electrocochleography based on tonebursts with shorter rise times.

So far, the response of one fibre to a changing stimulus has been considered. If one keeps the stimulus frequency constant, at low intensity levels only neurons having a CF close to the stimulus frequency will be excited. For increased stimulus level, some neurons with a CF below the stimulus frequency will become active and somewhat more neurons having a higher CF will respond. A plot of the CF of the activated nerve fibres *versus* the stimulus level at which they are activated (*i.e.*, the threshold level for this particular stimulus) is called the response area of the tone (KIANG and MOXON, 1974). The low CF-side (the apical side) is rather steep (about 100 dB/octave); at the high CF side (the more basal side) the curve initially is steep and at a level of about 60 dB SPL becomes relatively flat (slope about 5–10 dB/octave). It can, therefore, be stated that with increasing intensity a stimulus with a particular frequency activates a large nerve fibre population showing a nearly continuous range of threshold values. So, a compound AP to a particular toneburst will consist of contributions from a population with gradually increasing thresholds, which makes the dynamic range of the compound AP much large than for a single nerve fibre, which is at most 50 dB.

2. Responses to Clicks and the On Effect

In response to a click stimulus, a particular nerve fibre shows in the post-stimulus-time histogram (PSTH) a number of peaks spaced at regular intervals which are equal to the inverse of the CF of the fibre. The time delay between microphonics onset (as recorded from the round window) and the first peak in the PSTH was also found to be proportional to $(CF)^{-1}$ (KIANG *et al.*, 1965; EVANS, 1972). This indicates that the response latency is related to the distance between the stapes and the innervation site of the nerve fibre under study. The latency of the first peak is constant for a fairly large range of intensity values; however, at very low intensity levels the second peak may be more dominant and the first peak disappears in the spontaneous rate. For fibres with high CF's, the multiple peaks disappear from the PSTH.

In theory, as GOLDSTEIN and KIANG (1958) pointed out, the necessary well-synchronized changes in the firing rate of a simultaneously excited population of neurons, are not only the result of the abruptness of the stimulus but also reflect the timing of the unit responsiveness. This means that the population of neurons must fire synchronously with the stimulus, indicating that their latencies should be approximately the same. Under the assumption that unit responses add with equal weight at the recording electrode they arrive at:

$$A(t) = N \int_{-\infty}^{t} s(\tau) a(t-\tau)\, d\tau ,$$

in which N is the number of nerve fibres; $s(t)$ the probability density function of firing for the population, *i.e.*, the latency distribution function; $a(t)$ is the unit response as seen by a round-window electrode. In fact, if this expression is limited to the N_1-component of the AP it requires excitation in a region which is limited to the basal turn of the cochlea, especially when a click stimulus is used. The assumptions made by GOLDSTEIN and KIANG (1958) have been somewhat more elaborated by TEAS *et al.* (1962), who point out the diphasic nature of the unit response when recorded with either round-window or intracochlear electrodes. This has recently been demonstrated by KIANG *et al.* (1974), but it also became clear that the unit contributions differed in amplitude for the various fibres. Apart from the heuristic concept of the building-up of the AP by the convolution theorem, theoretical studies of the interrelation of the single nerve fibre ap and the compound AP have been made quite recently. The systematic change in travelling-wave delay (*i.e.*, the latency of single-nerve-fibre firings) as a function of the CF, has been analyzed by GOLDSTEIN *et al.* (1971). Under the assumption that the cochlea acts as a minimum-phase filter, they predict the group delay in the firing of a given nerve fibre from its tuning properties. Also, assuming linearity for the cochlear filter, DE BOER (1975) arrived at an accurate prediction of the compound AP latency as a function of intensity on the basis of the single nerve fibre properties. The so-called "reverse correlation method" (DE BOER, 1967) was used to extract the impulse response from individual neurons subjected to white noise stimulation. By a convolution of this impulse response, which can be considered the Fourier-transform of the fibres tuning curve, with any stimulus (*e.g.* a tone-burst), the output function of a large group of individual nerve fibres is obtained for that particular stimulus. The rate function of the units under study determines the response probability. A second convolution of the individual output-function with this response probability, followed by a summation over all contributing units, results in the model waveform of the compound AP, the basic assumptions being linearity, homogenity of the population, and equal contributions from each unit. In this way, however, correct preduction of the high-intensity part of the AP input-output curve could not be obtained. Therefore, either the unit contribution is subject to changes (*cf.* KIANG *et al.*, 1974) or the assumption of linearity is not valid for intensities exceeding 60 dB SPL. Recalling the shape of the tuning curve for individual neurons this last conclusion seems to be supported. It must be recalled that a correct latency prediction could be made based on a linear approximation.

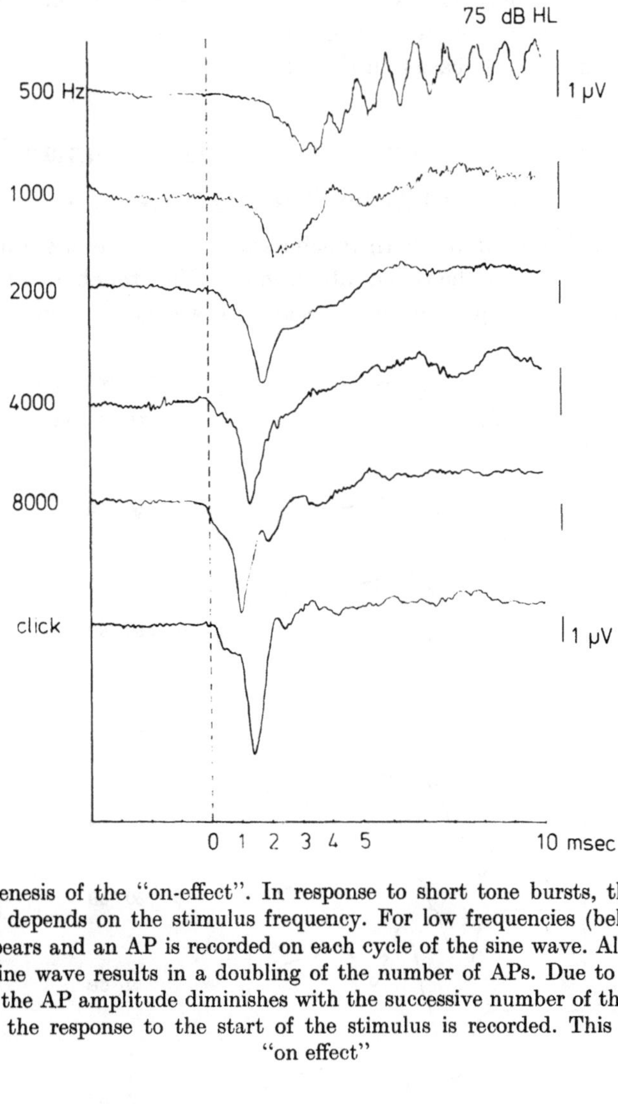

Fig. 12. The genesis of the "on-effect". In response to short tone bursts, the shape of the compound AP depends on the stimulus frequency. For low frequencies (below 2000 Hz), a phase lock appears and an AP is recorded on each cycle of the sine wave. Alternation of the phase of the sine wave results in a doubling of the number of APs. Due to adaptation and refractoriness, the AP amplitude diminishes with the successive number of the period. Above 2000 Hz, only the response to the start of the stimulus is recorded. This is the so-called "on effect"

From the above considerations, two aspects of the cochlear excitation process are revealed: 1. the mechanical (linear) filtering controlling the place of excitation of the nerve fibres and, therefore, to a large extent the latency of firing, and 2. the (non-linear) transducing stage influencing mainly the actual number of synchonized firings. The amount of synchronization of the individual firings is very important for the shape of the compound AP. For low frequency signals (500 and 1000 Hz), the AP is found at a fixed phase of the sinewave in the cochlear microphonics. When the tone frequency increases, adaptation gains progressively in importance (EGGERMONT and SPOOR, 1973), *i.e.*, APs on subsequent cycles of a low-frequency toneburst become increasingly smaller until a final value is reached. This final value depends on the tone-frequency: increasing frequency results in decreasing final values. For 1500 or 2000 Hz, the compound AP still appears during a fixed phase of the sine wave, but, due to adaptation, only the APs on the first cycles are present. For higher frequencies only one AP remains. This is called the "on-effect" (Fig 12). Measurements of the compound AP from the human promontory or the external ear canal are in most cases based on this on-effect.

B. Input-Output Relations for Normal Human Ears

1. Compound Action Potential Waveforms

When the ear is stimulated with tonebursts or clicks presented alternately in phase, certain factors must be taken into account. With tonebursts having a tone frequency high enough to prevent phase locking between the nerve fibre discharges

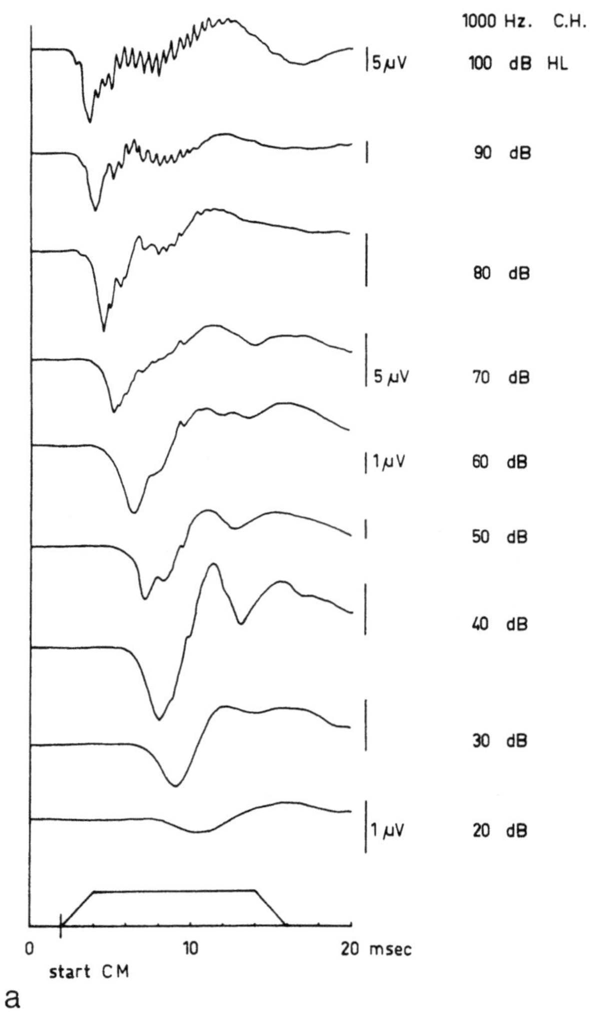

Fig 13a

and the sine wave, alternation of the phase has little or no influence on the AP-waveform. This holds for frequencies of about 3000 Hz and above. For low stimulus frequencies (500 and 1000 Hz), alternation of the stimulus phase in the toneburst to abolish the CM leads to a half-period shift of the preferred discharge phase. This in turn causes a doubling of the number of AP's with respect to the sine wave period. These closely spaced APs overlap partially, thus forming a broad average

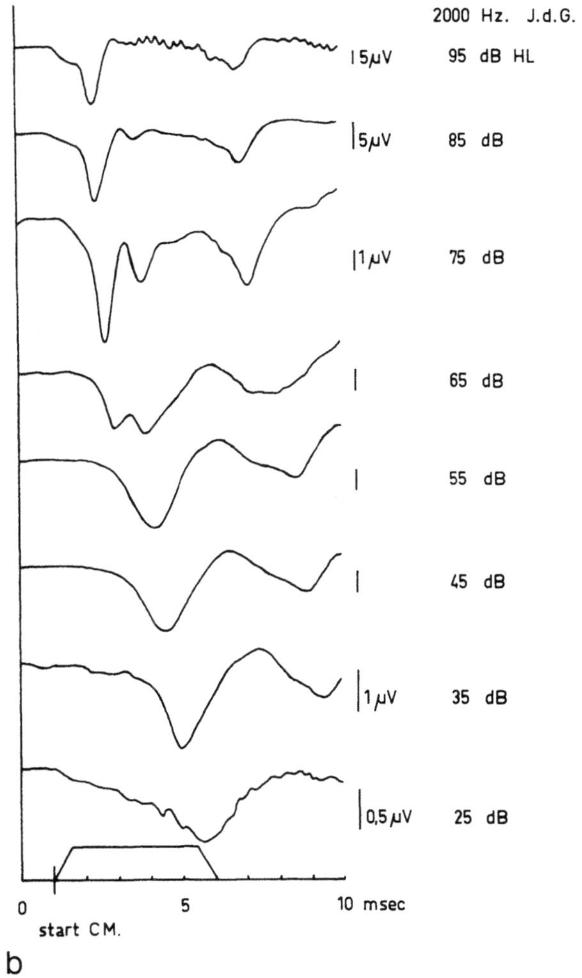

Fig. 13b

response in which only the AP tips indicate the phase lock. The AP waveforms obtained for tonebursts of 1000 and 2000 Hz are shown in Fig. 13a, b. It must be kept in mind that the toneburst duration and the rise-and-fall time depend on the stimulus frequency, and it should be noted that the analysis interval is 20 msec for 1000 Hz and 10 msec for 2000 Hz series. A series of AP responses to an acoustic click is shown in Fig. 13c.

In the 2000 Hz toneburst series, an interesting transition takes place around 65 dB HL. If the intensity of 65 dB is taken as a starting point for the analysis, it is evident that an increase in intensity leads to a relative increase of the first peak of the compound AP with respect to the second, whereas lowering the intensity favours the second peak over the first (EGGERMONT *et al.*, 1974a). A careful analysis of the same phenomenon obtained in response to a 2 kHz half-sine wave from the external ear canal was carried out by ELBERLING (1973), in consecutive 2.5 dB steps over the intensity range of 72.5–95 dB p.e. SPL. The two peaks were of about the same magnitude at 85–90 dB p.e. SPL, which corresponds to about 65–70 dB SL.

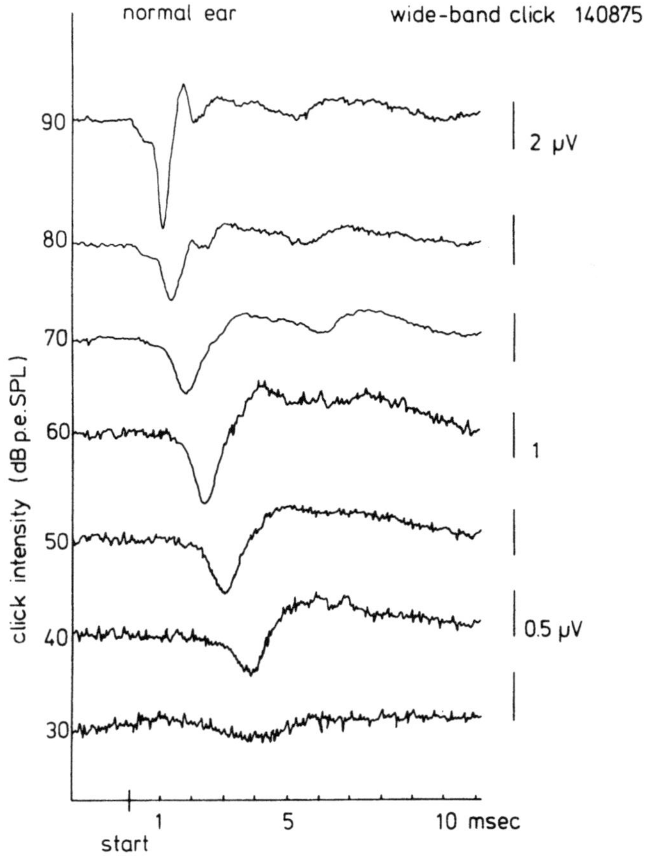

Fig. 13c

Fig. 13a, b, c. Action potential waveforms for 1000 and 2000 Hz tone bursts and for click. The tone bursts have two periods of the sine wave during rise and fall times and at least six during the plateau. For the 1000 Hz response series, the time scale is twice as large as for the other two series. The tone burst envelope is drawn under the AP traces on the same time scale. For the 1000 Hz stimuli, the phase-lock to the sine wave is noted. When the stimulus intensity decreases, the amplitude decreases and the latency increases. Note the occurrence of a double peaked AP at 2000 Hz, 65 dB HL. For the click series, the intensities are given in dB p.e. SPL; threshold for normal hearing on the average is at 20 dB p.e. SPL. (From EGGERMONT *et al.*, 1974a)

2. Amplitude-Intensity Relationships

A more accurate description of intensity-dependent phenomena can be obtained from AP-amplitude input-output curves. For a normal hearing subject, the amplitude-intensity curves are drawn for tonebursts of 2, 4, and 8 kHz and for clicks, and it may be observed that the curves become steeper the higher the toneburst frequency (Fig. 14). For the 8000 Hz series, the increase in AP-amplitude is

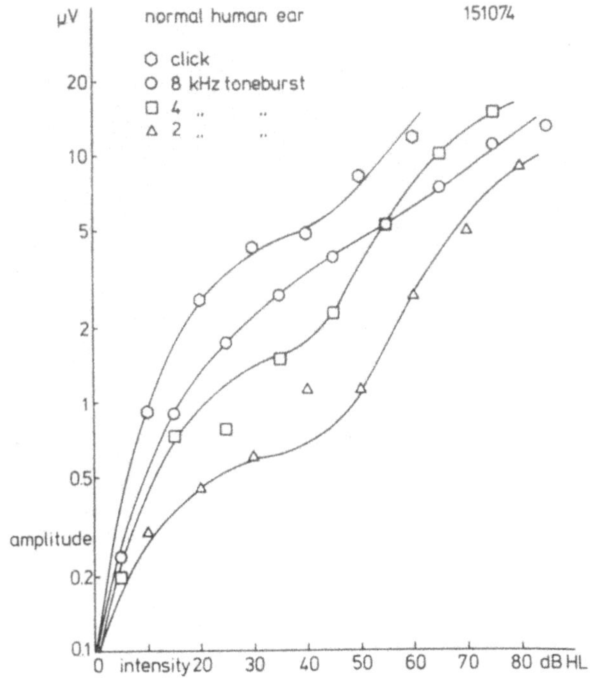

Fig. 14. Input-output curves for a normal ear at different tone burst frequencies and click. The rate of increase of the AP amplitude with intensity is largest for the click and for the higher frequencies. With the exception of the 8 kHz series, the input-output curves show some plateau around 40 dB HL (for click 0 dB HL ≃ 20 dB p.e. SPL)

gradual, but for lower frequencies and for the click stimulus, the rate of increase becomes small at intermediate intensity levels, thus forming a plateau in the input-output curve. For intensities above 50 dB HL, however, the increase rate becomes larger again. The plateau in the input-output curves is in general most obvious for the 2000 Hz toneburst stimuli; Fig. 15, shows input-output curves for six normal ears. The curve up to about 60 dB HL represents the amplitude behaviour of the second peak in the AP, while the fast rise of the curve above 60 dB HL is due to the dominance of the first peak. This is somewhat easier visualized by replotting the data on a linear amplitude scale (Fig. 15a). The amplitude-intensity curves are now subdivided clearly in a low (L-part) and a high (H-part) section (Yoshie, 1968), in which the L-part corresponds with the second peak and the H-part with the first peak. In general, amplitude-intensity curves are drawn on a linear scale, often with the largest amplitude value (*e.g.* at 90 dB SL) taken as 100% (ARAN *et al.*, 1971a; MONTANDON *et al.*, 1975a; YOSHIE, 1968); however, the major advantage of logarithmic curve plotting is that the threshold value is more accurately extrapolated from a few measuring points below 20 dB

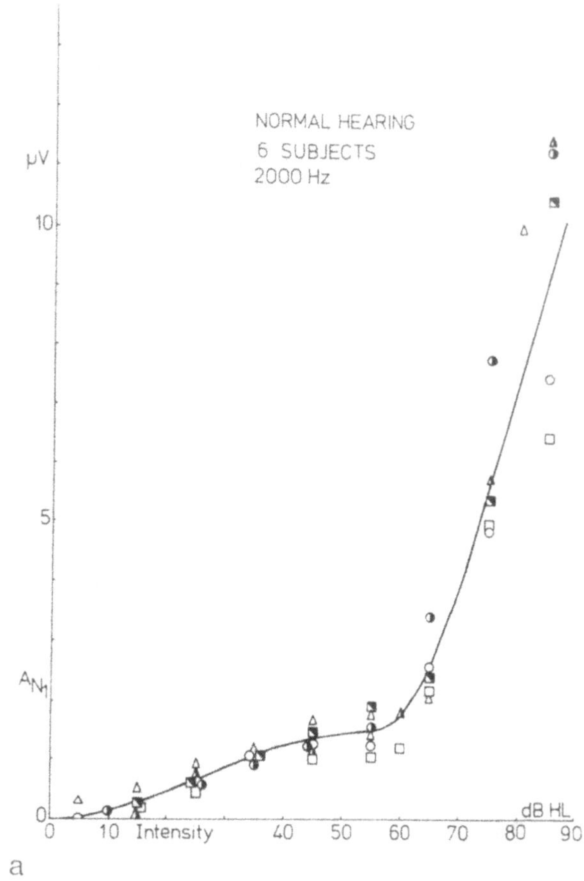

Fig. 15a

SL (EGGERMONT *et al.*, 1974a; YOSHIE, 1971). The large difference in cochlear output for normal ears is illustrated in Fig. 16 in which AP-amplitudes in response to 2000 Hz toneburst stimulation have been plotted as a function of stimulus intensity. The arithmetic mean is indicated. As for the summating potential data (*cf.* Fig. 10), the distribution of amplitude values is nearly exponential. In a statistical study, CHARLET DESAUVAGE and ARAN (1973) evaluated 61 normal ears tested with click stimulation. Normal output for a click of 85 dB SL ranged from 1.5 μV to 38.5 μV (compare to the 2–20 μV range in Fig. 16) with an average of 12.1 μV for children and 16.9 μV for adults. Average input-output curves were obtained both for the children and the adults; for the adults the curve showed a distinct plateau around 50–70 dB SL, while for the children group no plateau appears. This is probably due to differences in the external and middle ear resonances of the adult and childgroups. The resonance differences produce a shift in the maximum excitation in the cochlea.

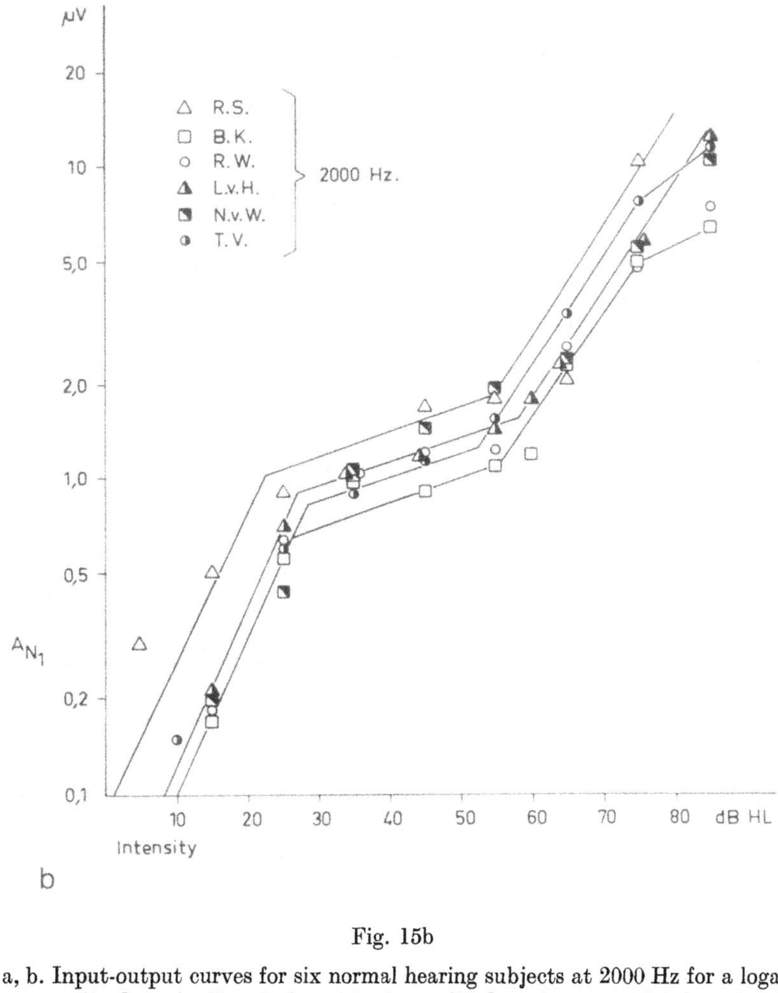

Fig. 15b

Fig. 15a, b. Input-output curves for six normal hearing subjects at 2000 Hz for a logarithmic and linear amplitude scale. For the logarithmic amplitude scale, it appears that the slope for the six curves below 1 μV is about the same. The plateau is very clear from about 25—60 dB HL. For the same data on a linear amplitude scale, the mean curve for a group of 20 normal ears is drawn in. The shallow part of the curve corresponds with the second peak in the AP (double peaked at 65 dB HL; *cf.* Fig. 13b) which dominates at low intensities. The steep part corresponds to the first peak in the AP, which increases rapidly above 65 dB HL. (From EGGERMONT *et al.*, 1974a)

3. Latency-Intensity Relationships

From the AP-responses shown in Fig. 13a, b, c, it can be observed that the AP-latency, measured from CM-onset to the largest AP-peak, increases with decreasing stimulus intensity. The occurrence of the double-peaked AP may cause a relatively large shift in the latency curve because, by convention, the largest peak is taken for the calculation of AP-latency. If the logarithm of latency is plotted as a function of the stimulus intensity for the same ear, as in Fig. 14, one obtains a nearly

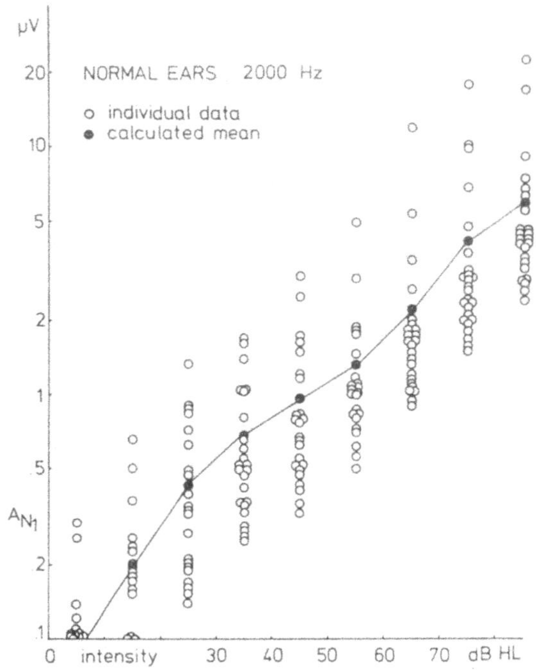

Fig. 16. Compound action potential amplitudes as a function of intensity for 20 normal ears at 2000 Hz. The dispersion observed in the amplitudes at a given stimulus intensity is less than for the SP (*cf.* Fig. 10), and the mean curve also shows the relatively flat region around 40 dB HL. (From EGGERMONT, 1974)

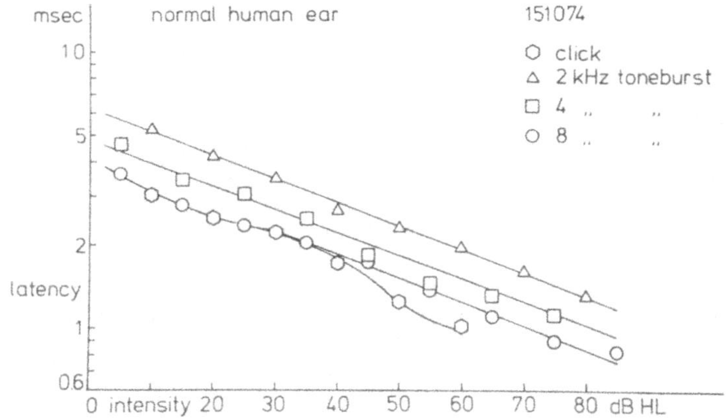

Fig. 17. Latency-intensity curves for a normal ear for different tone burst frequencies and for click. The relation between log latency and intensity for tone burst stimulation may be approximated by a straight line indicating an exponential relationship. The curve for the click shows a less simple relationship. The curves for the three tone burst frequencies are completely parallel

linear relationship in case of toneburst stimulation (Fig. 17), and the curves for the three tone frequencies are nearly parallel. For the click, a somewhat different behaviour is observed. If for a large group of normal ears the AP-latencies are

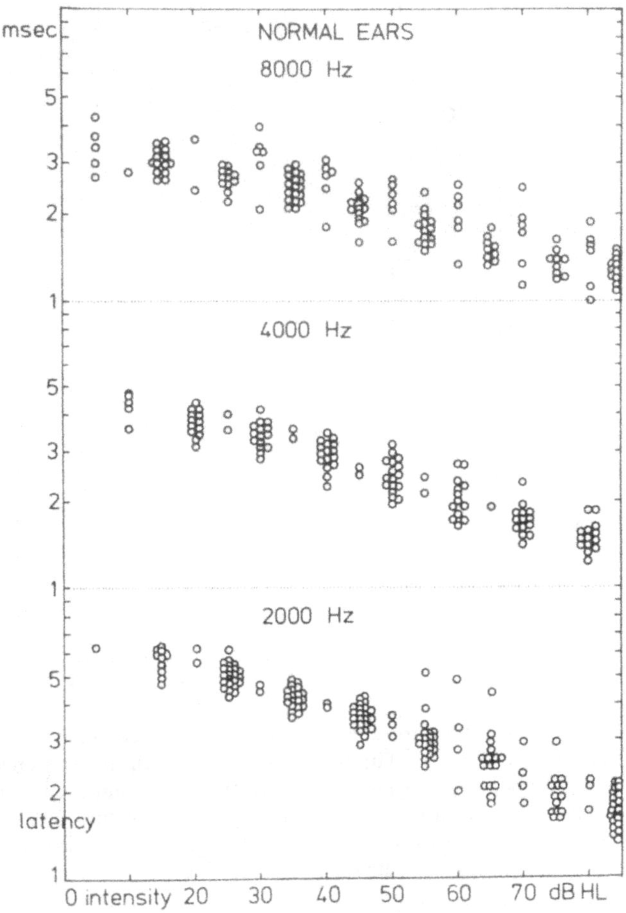

Fig. 18. Latency-intensity data for a group of normal ears at three tone burst frequencies. Latency values range from about 1 msec at 8000 Hz, 85 dB HL to about 7 msec for 2000 Hz at near threshold values. Also, for the average of a group of normal ears, the relation between latency and intensity is an exponential one. (From EGGERMONT, 1976b)

plotted as a function of intensity for three tone-frequencies (Fig. 18), it becomes clear that there will be in general such a linear relation between log latency and intensity. In nearly all papers on ECoG, latency is plotted on a linear scale (YOSHIE and OHASHI, 1969; COATS and DICKEY, 1970; ARAN *et al.*, 1971a; ELBERLING, 1973; MONTANDON *et al.*, 1975a, b), even in the report of CULLEN *et al.* (1972) despite the fact that the last noted group calculated a regression line showing an exponential dependency of latency on intensity.

If AP-latency reflects in part the travelling-wave delay up to the point of maximum contribution to the compound AP, which point changes with stimulus intensity, and if single nerve fibre discharge latency depends exponentially on the CF (GOLDSTEIN *et al.*, 1971), one would expect a linear relationship between log latency and stimulus intensity. The latency range for click is generally more

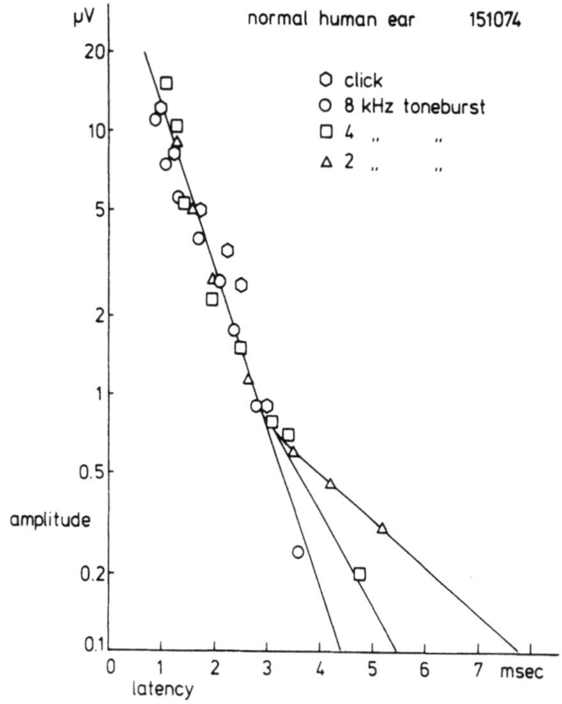

Fig. 19. Amplitude-latency functions for a normal ear for three tone burst frequencies and for click. It appears that, for a large range of amplitude-latency values, the relation is independent of the type of stimulus used. This suggests that only the site of innervation of the excited neurons is of importance. For low amplitude, *i.e.*, near threshold values, the latency is larger for lower frequencies, which points to the frequency selectivity of stimulation. (From EGGERMONT, 1976a)

restricted than for tonebursts. For a group of 61 normal ears, CHARLET DE SAUVAGE and ARAN (1973) found a mean latency at 85 dB SL of 1.5 msec (the same for adults and children) and the mean latency at threshold was 4.5 msec for children and slightly larger for adults (5 msec).

4. The Amplitude-Latency Relationship

So far, the intensity dependency of the AP-amplitude and AP-latency have been described. It is felt that a relation between AP-amplitude and latency may reflect additional properties of the compound AP (EGGERMONT *et al.*, 1974a).

A plot of log amplitude *versus* latency (Fig. 19) for the same data used in Figs. 14 and 17 shows that for a wide range of values the relationship is nearly independent of the frequency content of the stimulus. However, for low amplitude values (below about 1 μV), a separation for different stimulus frequencies is observed.

The fact that the AP amplitude seems to be uniquely related to latency for a range of about 1–10 μV suggests that synchrony of single nerve fibre firings (determining to a large extent the AP-amplitude) is related to the place of innervation of the fibres (as reflected in the latency). For clinical purposes, it proved useful to plot the amplitude and latency data both on logarithmic coordinates because in that way a linear relation could be obtained for each frequency (EGGERMONT *et al.*, 1974a), *e.g.* for 2000 Hz stimulation:

$$\log A_N = 1.2 - 2.2 \log \tau_N,$$

and the group behaviour could easily be quantified. For comparison with the results obtained in pathologic cochleas and in ears with conductive hearing loss, the regression analysis provided an adequate data reduction (ODENTHAL and EGGERMONT, 1974c). In general, a rather high correlation is found between both AP-parameters.

C. The Building-Up of the Whole-Nerve Action Potential

As we have seen, the compound AP is built up from a large number of nerve-fibre contributions, but the AP-amplitude and latency reflect only the most synchronously responding part. This part originates at different intensities (changing latency) from different parts of the cochlea. Therefore, the compound AP-waveform must be separated into contributions from relatively small parts of the cochlear partition before any further conclusions can be drawn.

1. The High-Pass Noise Masking Technique and the Derivation of Narrow-Band APs

A wide-band click stimulates, in a normal ear, almost the whole cochlear partition. If a wide-band masking noise is applied, having a level so that complete masking of the click-evoked AP can be achieved, no click-synchronous firings can be recorded from the cochlea. When this noise is passed through a high-pass filter (slope 96 dB/octave) with a cut-off frequency of, *e.g.*, 1.5 kHz, there will be no masking in the apical apart of the cochlea and click-synchronous firings from that region, *i.e.*, a compound AP, may be recorded. For a slightly lower cut-off frequency, *e.g.*, 1 kHz, a smaller region responds to the click, and a smaller AP having a longer latency is recorded. Subtraction of this latter AP from the former (larger) one results in a so-called "derived AP" (TEAS *et al.*, 1962; ELBERLING, 1974a; EGGERMONT *et al.*, 1974b). This is the click-synchronous response from a group of cochlear nerve fibres masked by the 1 kHz high-pass noise but not by the 1.5 kHz high-pass noise. This response originates from a $^1/_2$-octave (−3 dB)-wide region centered around a frequency of 900 Hz, corresponding to a length of about 3 mm along the cochlear partition approximately 25 mm from the stapes. We call this response the narrow-band AP. A complete narrow-band analysis of click stimulation is shown in Fig. 20. The response for a central frequency of 2.6 kHz, *e.g.*, is obtained by subtraction of the AP recorded in the presence of 3 kHz-high-pass noise from the AP response obtained during masking with 4 kHz high-pass noise. For higher central frequencies, the narrow-band AP latency is lower and the amplitude is higher. The responses have a disphasic shape irrespective of the narrow-band central frequency. It is clear that the N_1-peak of the unmasked click response corresponds to firings from units innervating the most basal part of the cochlea. The N_2-component, having a latency of about 4–5 msec, corresponds to contributions having central frequencies of 900 and 500 Hz. The entire frequency range in between contributes only to the positivity between N_1 and N_2 due to mutual cancellation of the narrow band contributions.

2. The Amplitude-Space Distribution for Click and Toneburst Stimulation

A plot of the narrow-band AP-amplitude (negative deflection only) as a function of the central frequency, which is equivalent to distance from the stapes (VON BÉKÉSY, 1963), shows for a click intensity of 90 dB p.e. SPL (Fig. 21) a

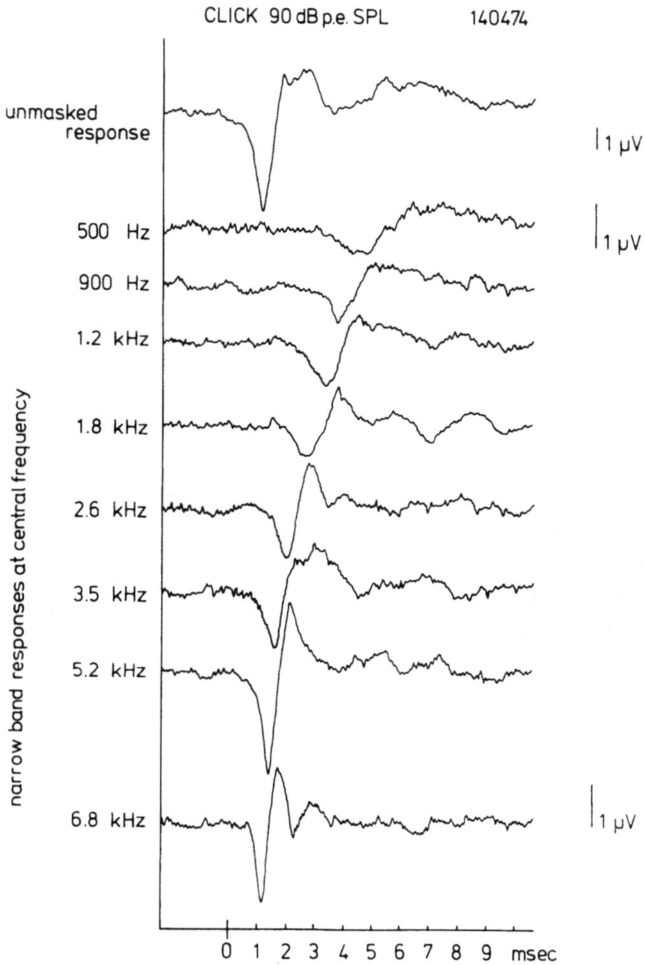

Fig. 20. Narrow-band analysis of a click evoked whole nerve action potential. Using the technique of TEAS *et al.* (1962) to derive narrow band AP responses, an analysis can be made of the composition of a whole nerve AP. The particular responses, representing synchronous firings of fibres from a $^1/_2$ octave wide region (*i.e.* about 3 mm wide) on the cochlear partition, add together to form the unmasked response. The central frequencies of the different narrow bands are indicated. Latency increases with distance from the stapes, and narrow band amplitude decreases. It is noted that the N_1 component in the click response is entirely due to contributions from fibres with high characteristic frequencies. (From EGGERMONT, 1976a)

gradual increase in amplitude for higher central frequencies. For lower click intensities, the contributions from both the high-frequency and the low-frequency side rapidly decrease, while the central region (about 3 kHz) still contributes the same. For relatively low intensities, the broad-band click spectrum and correspond-

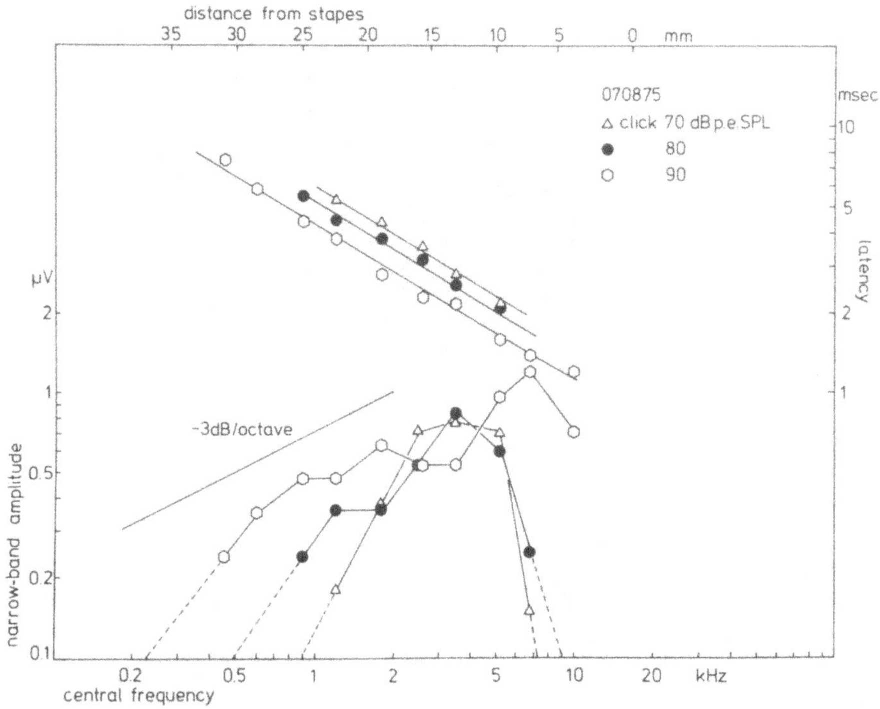

Fig. 21. Narrow band response parameters as a function of central frequency. For clicks of 70, 80, and 90 dB p.e. SPL, narrow band amplitudes are shown as a function of distance from the stapes; it is observed that for the highest intensity the amplitudes decrease by about 3 dB/octave. Lowering the click intensity results in a decrease for contributions from both the apical and basal part of the cochlea, while the central part still contributes the same. The latency data show an exponential dependency on the distance from the stapes, and a definite effect of stimulus intensity thereupon is noted

ing broad excitation area seems to be reduced to a more or less frequency-selective excitation. In this experimental situation, where the click spectrum was flat within ± 5 dB between 500 Hz and 8 kHz, the external ear canal and middle ear favour the parts in the spectrum around 2–3 kHz, where the ear has its greatest sensitivity (*cf.* ELBERLING, 1974).

The narrow-band response latencies for clicks show a linear relationship if both latency and central frequency are plotted on logarithmic coordinates. The 90 dB latency curve fits an equation

$$\tau = 1.00 \left[1 + \left(\frac{9}{\mathrm{CF}}\right)^2\right]^{1/3},$$

which is comparable to the curve fit made for the single nerve fibre discharge latency as a function of characteristic frequency (GOLDSTEIN *et al.*, 1971). For the lower intensity curves, the asymptotic latency value should be increased slightly.

If the high-pass noise masking analysis is applied to toneburst stimulation, the supraliminal frequency specificity for this type of stimulation can be derived. The narrow-band amplitude vs. central-frequency plots obtained in this situation are shown in Fig. 22a for different intensities. Compared to the click data, one observes,

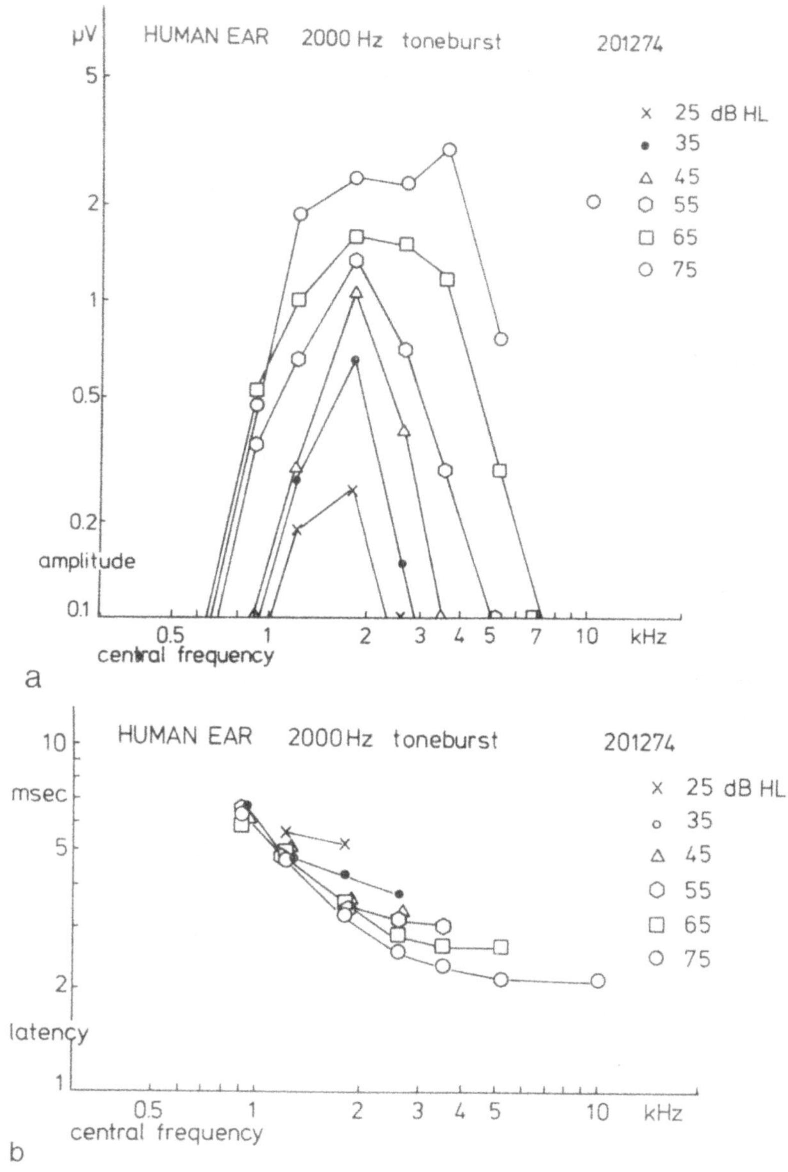

Fig. 22a, b. Narrow-band response parameters for 2 kHz tone bursts. It appears that the amplitude distribution for tone bursts is especially at the low-frequency side more restricted than observed for the click. The maximum contribution to the compound AP is at about 2 kHz, which is lower than found for the click. The latency curves show a distinctly different behaviour from what is observed for the click data. (From Eggermont, 1976a)

especially on the low frequency side, a more restricted excitation; also, the region of maximal contribution is better defined (around a central frequency of about 1.8 kHz). The narrow-band AP latencies for 2000 Hz toneburst stimulation (Fig. 22b) show a somewhat different dependency on central frequency than the narrow-band click APs. However, the slope of the linear part of the curve is the same as that for the click stimulus.

3. The Response Area for Click and Toneburst Stimulation

The response area is defined as the region in the intensity-central frequency plane bordered by the curves for which the narrow-band contributions to the compound AP have an amplitude of 0.1 μV. The derivation of the response area from the amplitude distribution is reviewed in Fig. 23, which shows the inter-

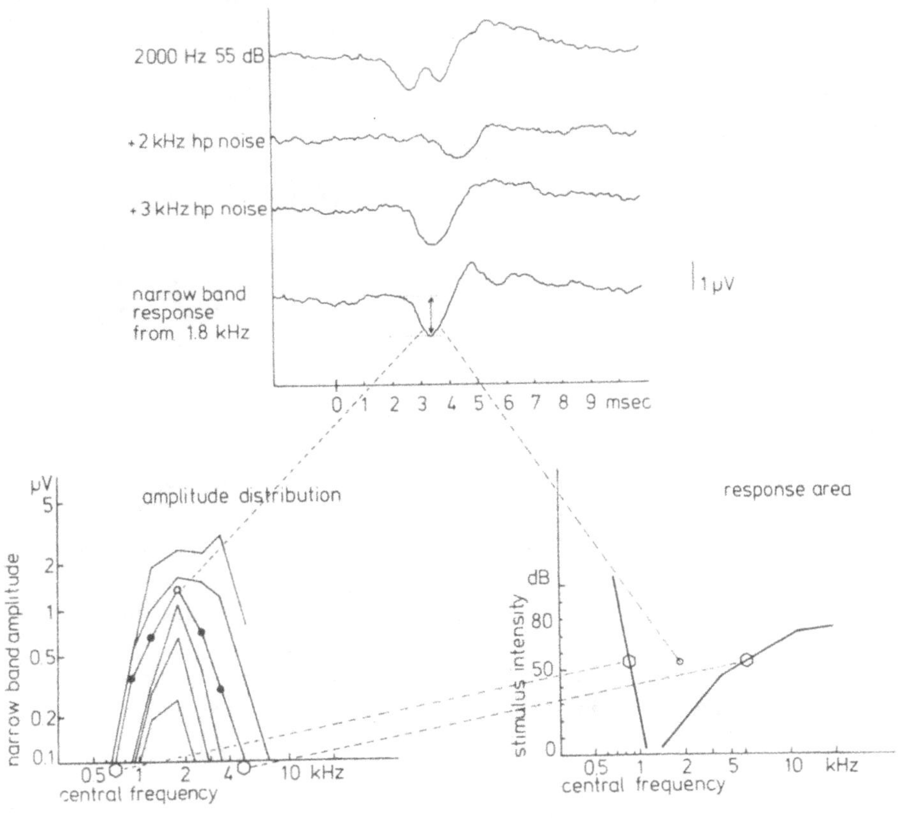

Fig. 23. The concept of the response area. The derivation of the narrow band AP for a central frequency of 1.8 kHz, obtained by subtraction of a compound AP in the presence of a 2 kHz high-pass masking noise from a response obtained in the presence of a 3 kHz high-pass masking noise is shown. The narrow band amplitudes constitute the amplitude distribution plot for different tone burst intensities. Those values for the central frequency at which the threshold for the narrow band AP is reached (0.1 μV) are used to draw the response area for a 2 kHz tone-burst. This area is formed from a narrow part for intensities below 55 dB HL and corresponding to the shallow part of the input-output curve for the whole nerve AP (*cf.* Fig. 15b) and a broad part for higher intensity levels corresponding to the steep part of the compound AP input-output curve. (From EGGERMONT, 1976b)

relations of the derivation of a narrow-band AP, the amplitude distribution and the response area. The 1.8 kHz contribution to the 2000 Hz toneburst – evoked AP is obtained by subtraction of responses recorded in the presence of 2 and 3 kHz high-pass noise. The amplitudes are plotted (*cf.* Fig. 22a) and the thresholds, for, say the 55 dB curve, are found at specific central frequencies (as indicated by the hexagonal dots); these two points form part of the response-area curve. To be more specific: at an intensity of 55 dB HL, a 2000 Hz toneburst evokes activity for an equivalent frequency range of about 900 Hz to 6 kHz. If similar analyses are made for all curves in the amplitude distribution plot, the boundary curve for the response area is obtained. It can be demonstrated that response areas for 2000 Hz tonebursts for different normal subjects are strikingly similar (EGGERMONT, 1976a). In general, the response area consists of a narrow part for intensity values below 50 dB HL, reflecting the good frequency specificity of the stimulation, especially at near-threshold values, and a broad part for intensities over 60 dB HL. From the data presented in the former section and from results obtained by ELBERLING (1974a), it can be derived that the response area for clicks will be quite different from that obtained for toneburst stimulation; the narrow-part is not present and a more symmetrical response area is obtained.

4. The Travelling-Wave Velocity in the Human Cochlea

The rapid latency increase for lower central frequencies of the narrow band is a measure for the travelling-wave delay in the human cochlea. VON BÉKÉSY (1963) explored the anatomical dimensions of the human cochlea with respect to the region of maximum displacement of the basilar membrane for different continuous tone frequencies. On the basis of these data and the latency differences (thus, neglecting the unknown values of synaptic delay) between the central frequencies, travelling-wave velocities can be calculated for each $^1/_2$-octave-wide narrow-band (Fig. 24). The mean values and standard deviations obtained are shown; the results from the narrow-band masking technique are indicated by hexagonal dots, those from masking with 1/3 octave-band reject white noise (EGGERMONT and ODENTHAL, 1974b) by open circles. The data fit well with those obtained by the high-pass noise masking technique. ELBERLING'S (1974a) results (filled circles) appear to be somewhat higher in value but show the same dependency on central frequency. Results obtained by ZERLIN (1969) based on psychoacoustic experiments also correspond well with the electrophysiologically obtained values.

Apart from a singular point around 4 kHz, which is far too high in our measurements, and the value obtained by ELBERLING (1974a) using octave-wide narrowbands, which is too low, the relation seems to be linear. A linear regression line through the displayed points is calculated for log velocity on log central frequency and has a slope of 1; the correlation coefficient is +0.91. This indicates an exponential decrease of travelling-wave velocity with distance from the stapes (EGGERMONT, 1976a).

From the data in Fig. 20, it became obvious that for higher central frequencies, *i.e.*, for more basal locations in the cochlea, the contributions to the compound AP become narrower and their amplitude increases. The narrower the AP, the better the synchrony of the individual neurons contributing to it. TEAS *et al.* (1962) have pointed out that synchrony of firing within a limited part of the cochlea, (*e.g.* a narrow-band) will be proportional to the rate of change of the basilar membrane displacement, *i.e.*, to travelling-wave velocity. If the relative width of the narrow-band APs (with respect to that obtained at a central frequency of, *e.g.*, 10 kHz) is plotted as a function of the travelling-wave velocity for the different narrow-bands,

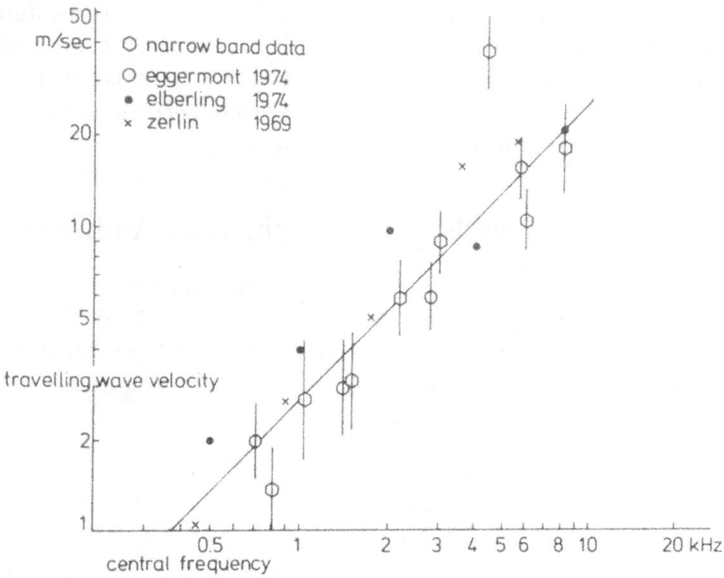

Fig. 24. The traveling wave velocity in the human cochlea. From latency differences in the different narrow band responses and the correspondence between central frequency and distance from the stapes (*cf.* Fig. 21), the traveling wave velocity may be calculated. This is done for a band-stop masking technique (O — O), high-pass noise masking techniques (○ — ○ and ● — ●), and according to a psychoacoustic method based on lateralization (× — ×). The different techniques used by either the same or different investigators result in nicely coinciding data, with the exception that in each series some irregularity is observed at about 4 kHz. (From EGGERMONT, 1976a)

the resulting curve suggests a proportionality between synchronization and the square root of the travelling-wave velocity. This may explain the dominance of basal-turn contributions to the whole-nerve AP. Using a deconvolution procedure between the recorded compound AP and a proposed unit-response waveform, ELBERLING (1975) obtained compound PST-histograms showing this relative dominance of the short latency components. Exponential transformation yielded the true excitation pattern. It is, therefore, stressed that electrocochleography performed with only one type of stimulus (*e.g.* a wide-band click) never permits evaluation of a patient's hearing in anything but a crude or predictive way. Combination with frequency-selective masking makes is more time consuming but is a far better method. The use of different frequency-specific stimuli favourably combined with frequency-selective masking, makes it possible for the investigator to surpass the range of the simple screening tests and to achieve an almost complete description of the ear under study, as will be shown in the sections that follow.

V. Threshold Electrocochleography

One of the primary features of electrocochleography is its use as a form of objective audiometry, *i.e.*, the applications yielding an audiogram or a click threshold, especially in cases where subjective audiometry is not possible. An electrocochleogram, *i.e.*, a series of thresholds for different frequencies, can only be obtained if sufficient frequency specificity of the stimulation can be obtained. This can be achieved by the use of 1/3-octave-filtered clicks (see *e.g.* ZERLIN and NAUNTON, 1975) or short tonebursts (EGGERMONT *et al.*, 1974; YOSHIE, 1973). When wide-band stimulation is used, templates or models become necessary for the estimation of the audiogram (*e.g.* ELBERLING, 1974b).

A. Click-Thresholds and the Subjective Audiogram

The first systematic study to compare click-threshold electrocochleography with behavioral audiometry appeared in 1971 (ARAN *et al.*, 1971b). The relationship between the average subjective threshold (X) for the range from 250 Hz to 8000 Hz and the electrocochleographic click threshold (Y) was calculated for 106 ears:

$$Y = 0.77\,X + 11.3\,.$$

This indicates that the click threshold will be too high for low subjective threshold values, but on the average agrees well for subjective threshold values over 80 dB.

A closer inspection of the available data shows that the agreement between subjective- and ECoG-threshold is better for 500, 1000, and 2000 Hz and to some extend also for 4000 Hz, indicating that the click threshold may be of interest to estimate the average threshold for the middle frequencies. YOSHIE (1973) for 56 ears calculated the regression lines between click threshold and pure-tone thresholds at 1000, 2000, 4000, and 8000 Hz and obtained correlation coefficients ranging from 0.45 (8000 Hz) to 0.88 (2000 Hz) and direction coefficients of the regression line from 0.40 (8000) to 0.84 (4000 Hz), with values for subjective threshold zero of +17 dB (1000 Hz) to +1 dB (2000 Hz). So YOSHIE arrived at results comparable to those of ARAN *et al.* (1971b) in showing that click thresholds are useful in evaluating the audiogram, with the exception of the higher frequencies.

Using data for 65 ears, we calculated regression lines and correlation coefficients for click threshold *versus* average threshold for 2000, 4000, and 8000 Hz and arrived at a correlation coefficient of 0.55; for click threshold versus the lowest threshold of 2000, 4000, and 8000 Hz a correlation coefficient of 0.61 was obtained and for click threshold versus 2000 Hz subjective threshold the value 0.62 was found. The slopes of the regression lines were, respectively, 0.67, 0.68, and 0.71. It seems that these findings support the conclusion that electrocochleographic click thresholds may be an indication for the audiometric threshold for the middle frequencies. This may be explained by the fact that the wide band click spectrum undergoes a transformation in outer- and middle ears which favours the part around 2000 to 3000 Hz and this frequency range becomes dominant at threshold values. A stimulus designed for optimal use of these transforming capabilities of the outer- and middle ear is the 2000 Hz half sine wave used by ELBERLING and SALOMON

(1971). In a model study, ELBERLING (1974b) proved it possible to extract the shape of the audiogram and, to a fairly good agreement, also the level thereof from the waveform and the latency behaviour of the compound AP. This may be a resolution to the difficulties encountered when using only one type of stimulation.

B. Toneburst Electrocochleogram and Subjective Audiogram

In his correlative study concerning 56 patients, YOSHIE (1973) also calculated the regression line between promontory-recorded AP thresholds (Y) for tonepips with the clinical thresholds for the frequencies 2,4, and 8 kHz (X). The pooled data resulted in

$$Y = 0.78\,X + 1.62\,,$$

with a correlation coefficient of 0.90. If the calculations were carried out for the individual frequencies, the direction coefficients ranged from 0.75 (2000 Hz) to 0.83 (4000 Hz) with correlation coefficients very near 0.90. From these data it became clear that almost all of the points in his scattergram fall within the limits, ± 15 dB, from the regression line.

In a group of 96 patients in which behavioral audiometry has been used, these thresholds (X) have been compared with electrocochleographic toneburst thresholds (Y) (SPOOR and EGGERMONT, 1976). The results are shown in Table 2.

Table 2. Comparison of ECoG thresholds and audiometric thresholds

Frequency (Hz)	Regression line	Correlation coefficient	Number of ears
500	$Y = 10.9 + 0.72X$	0.89	65
1000	$Y = 9.9 + 0.81X$	0.86	86
2000	$Y = 1.1 + 0.95X$	0.91	96
4000	$Y = 5.0 + 0.91X$	0.92	93
8000	$Y = 5.7 + 0.76X$	0.86	83

The data of Table 2 indicate that the best general fit, as for wide-band clicks, is found for the middle frequencies 1,2, and 4 kHz. However, the correlation coefficients are considerably higher for tone-burst stimuli, and the slopes of the regression lines are closer to 1. For the 500 and 8000 Hz data, the slopes of the regression line deviate considerably from 1, although the correlation coefficients remain high and are about the same as YOSHIE's (1973). An example of a scattergram for both threshold values at 2000 Hz stimulation is shown in Fig. 25a, and histograms for the threshold differences for all frequencies tested are shown in Fig. 25b.

The above studies and those of SCHMIDT *et al.* (1974) and ODENTHAL and EGGERMONT (1974a) (results incorporated in the data for Table 2) are up to now the only ones available for evaluating toneburst electrocochleography. They highly support the use of tonebursts for obtaining objective audiograms. This is further illustrated by two typical audigrams measured with both methods (Fig. 26a, b). As may be observed the results are quite convincing.

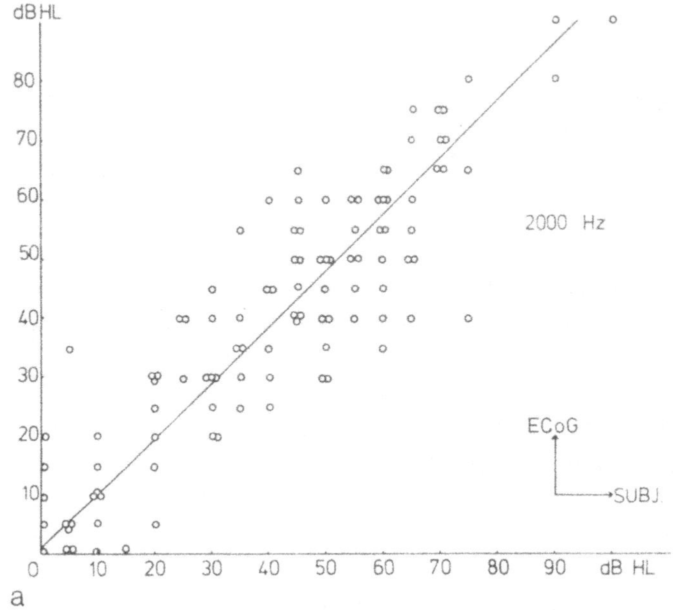

Fig. 25a

VI. Electrocochleography and Loudness Recruitment

A. The Recruitment Phenomenon

Loudness recruitment is the abnormally rapid increase in the loudness sensation with increase in intensity of an acoustic signal. The phenomenon may be quantified by using the "Alternate-Binaural-Loudness-Balance-test" if it is restricted to one ear and by the stapedius-reflex test in other cases. Although the recruitment phenomenon is well defined, considerable uncertainty and speculation concerns the underlying mechanism and therefore its value in the diagnosis of the auditory disorder. Speculations about the type of cochlear lesion responsible for the recruitment phenomenon point generally toward the loss of the outer-haircell spiral-nerve fibre population with a more or less intact inner-haircell radial nerve fibre population. The presumed less sensitive but by far larger group of radial nerve fibres retains a nearly normal cochlear function at high intensity levels although the threshold is elevated.

Based on the above hypothesis, several investigators (Yoshie and Ohashi, 1969; Portmann *et al.*, 1973; Eggermont and Odenthal, 1974a) explained their electrocochleographic findings and presented tentative criteria for recruiting ears.

Since loudness recruitment is a common phenomenon in nearly all stages of Menière's disease, the relationship between morphological loss of outer haircells and recruitment may be questioned. An alternative explanation, based on KIANG *et al.'s* (1970) findings in single nerve fibres from cochleas showing ototoxic damage,

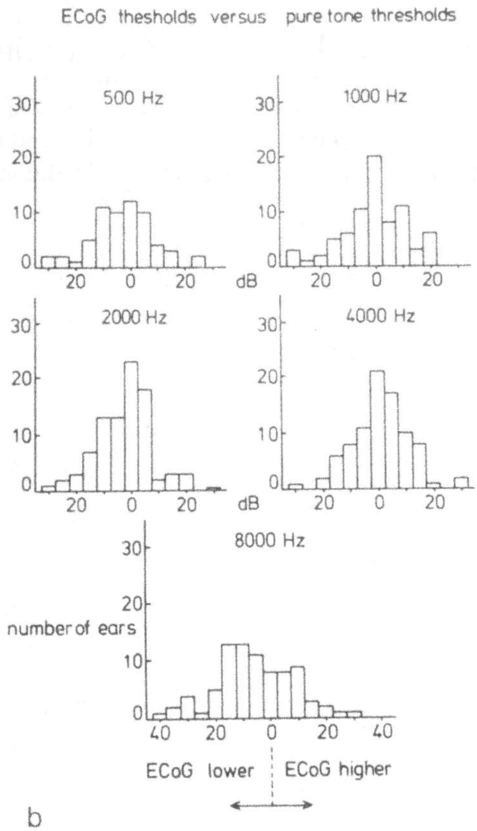

Fig. 25b

Fig. 25. Survey of threshold accuracy for tone burst electrocochleography. The scattergram (Fig. 25a) for 2000 Hz tone burst data shows that, on the average, the threshold values obtained with electrocochleography and subjective audiometry are about the same. The correlation coefficient proved to be 0.91. The histogram analysis (Fig. 25b) for the difference in threshold value obtained by the two methods shows that for 1000, 2000, and 4000 Hz this difference has a nearly normal distribution, distinctly peaked at a value of 0 dB. For both 500 Hz and 8000 Hz, the distribution is much broader. (From SPOOR and EGGERMONT, 1976)

has been proposed (EVANS, 1972; SCHMIDT *et al.*, 1974). Recruitment could be based on the conversion of normal units with narrow tuning curves into units with elevated thresholds at the characteristic frequency and broad tuning curves. EVANS (1975) concludes that due to this broadening of the tuning curves, (seen with respect to the threshold level) in some abnormal ears, a correspondingly greater proportion of the total population of neural units will be recruited with increase in stimulus level. Electrocochleographic research on the recruitment phenomenon, therefore, serves two purposes: 1. it provides evidence about the underlying mechanism(s), and 2. it yields criteria for the objective determination of recruitment. The reported findings are based on a paper by EGGERMONT (1976b) and discussed with respect to findings of YOSHIE and OHASHI (1969) and PORTMANN *et al.* (1973).

B. Input-Output Behaviour of Recruiting Ears

The waveform of the compound AP depends on the type of stimulus used as well as on the state of the ear under study. Using wide-band click stimuli, PORTMANN *et al.* (1973) defined a "recruiting response" by a diphasic waveform at all

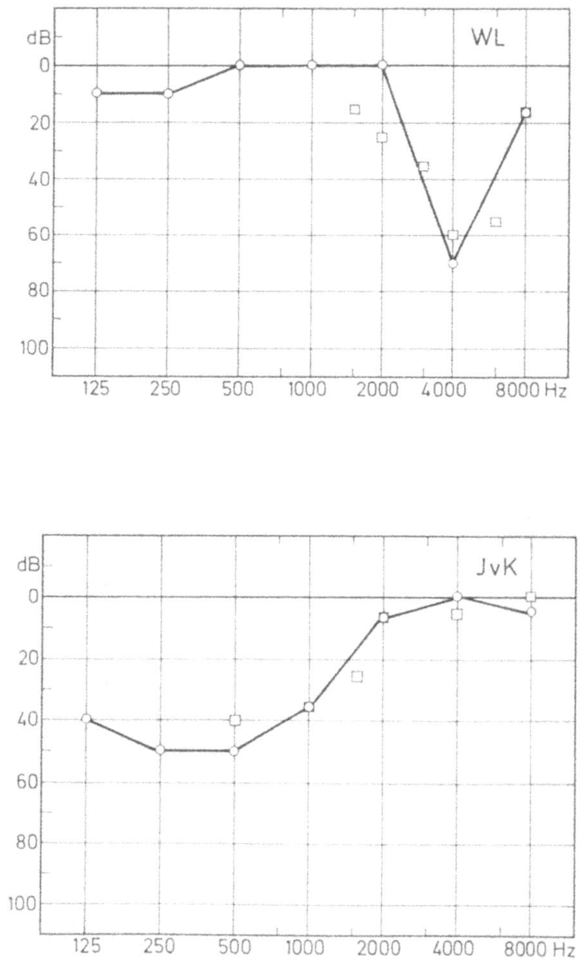

Fig. 26. Two examples of audiograms in which the electrocochleographic data and subjective data are compared show that it is quite possible to explore a sharp dip around 4 kHz or a low frequency hearing loss with an intact basal turn. The squares denote the ECoG data, and the circles the subjectively obtained threshold values. (From EGGERMONT *et al.*, 1974a)

levels, a rapid amplitude increase with intensity, without a plateau in the input-output curve, and finally a latency of less than 2 msec at the threshold. Properties assigned to responses from recruiting ears given by ODENTHAL and EGGERMONT (1974a) are not essentially different; tonebursts were used as stimuli. YOSHIE and OHASHI (1969) observed, however, an increase in latency at a given hearing level and obtained steeper input-output curves.

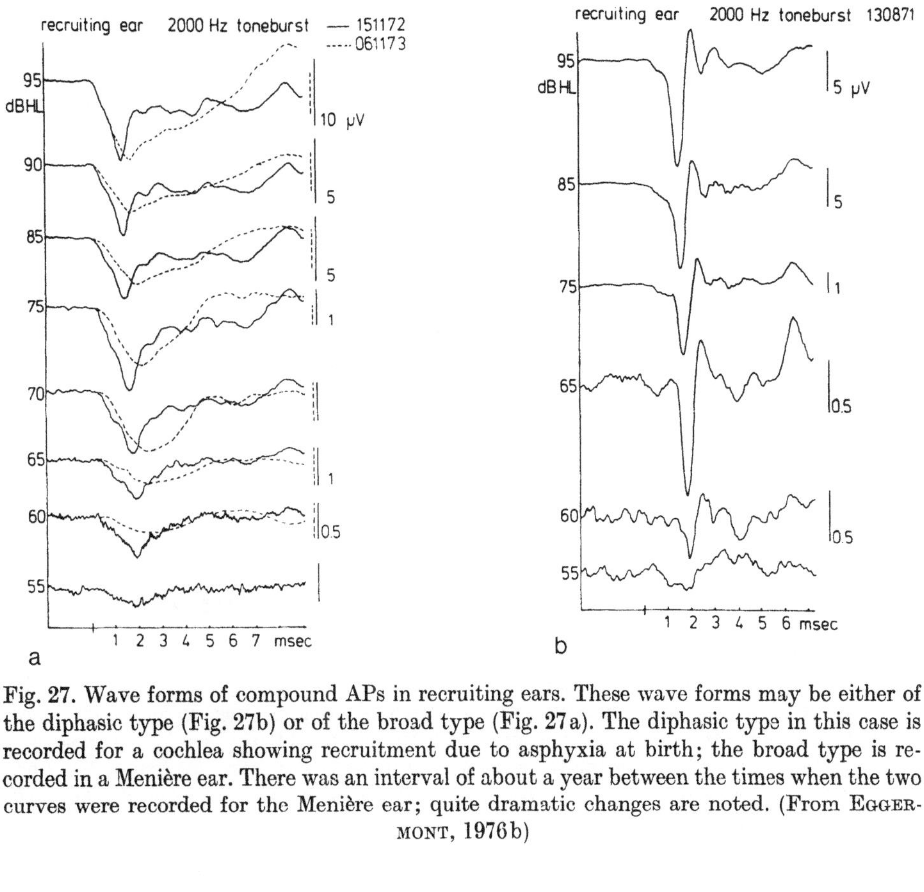

Fig. 27. Wave forms of compound APs in recruiting ears. These wave forms may be either of the diphasic type (Fig. 27b) or of the broad type (Fig. 27a). The diphasic type in this case is recorded for a cochlea showing recruitment due to asphyxia at birth; the broad type is recorded in a Menière ear. There was an interval of about a year between the times when the two curves were recorded for the Menière ear; quite dramatic changes are noted. (From EGGERMONT, 1976b)

It seems worthwhile to focus attention briefly on the three criteria mentioned above. As shown in Fig. 27b, the typical waveform obtained in a recruiting ear is clearly diphasic. The ear for which AP-waveforms are shown in Fig. 27a is also clearly recruiting as it represents a Menière patient. For both figures, responses to 2000 Hz toneburst stimulation has been used and it is found (EGGERMONT, 1976b) that the waveform of the compound AP depends more on the type of audiogram and the type of cochlear dysfunctionning than on the presence of recruitment.

The characteristic feature of the rapid increase is also reflected in the input-output curves for these ears (SCHMIDT *et al.*, 1974). A series of typical input-output curves is shown in Fig. 28 with the median curve obtained in 20 normal ears; all show the increase in steepness and the loss of the plateau. If the numerical value of the slopes (in log μV/dB) of the input-output curves for amplitude values below

1.5 μV is calculated and plotted as a function of threshold intensity for those ears, Fig. 29 is obtained. For curves obtained in 20 normal and about 80 recruiting ears in response to 2000 Hz toneburst stimulation, each ear is represented by one point. Normal cochleas are those having a threshold in this plot equal to or less than

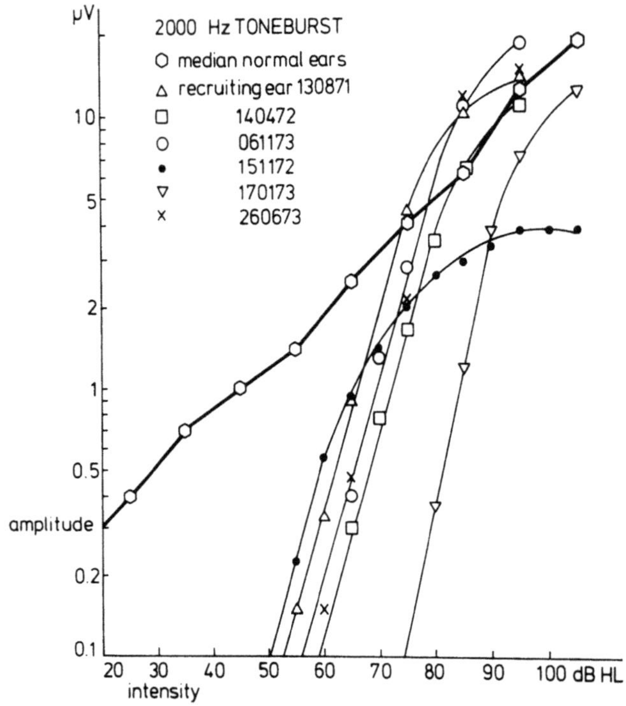

Fig. 28. Input-output curves for recruiting ears in response to 2000 Hz tone burst stimulation. For six recruiting ears, the input-output curves are drawn. The data for the three series of APs shown in the former figure are indicated by triangles (the diphasic type) and open and filled circles (the Menière ear). A common phenomenon for all curves is that the slope for amplitude values below, *e.g.*, 1.5 μV is essentially the same and much larger than that found in normal ears. The median input-output curve is based upon data for normal ears. (From EGGERMONT, 1976b)

20 dB HL. Since all other points refer to cochleas showing recruitment psychoacoustically, it becomes clear that the slope of the input-output curve is not a unique indicator for recruitment. Considering the fact that a normal ear in general will have a slope for the 2000 Hz input-output curve smaller than say 35.10^{-3} log μV/dB, one may conclude that, for the group of ears having a threshold above or equal to 40 dB HL, in about 20% of the cases the conclusion about the presence of recruitment has been wrong. The combination with data obtained at other frequencies, however, in general is more definite.

For some recruiting ears, APs with characteristic short latencies at threshold are observed. Threshold latencies are obtained by extrapolation of the regression line of log latency on log amplitude (EGGERMONT *et al.*, 1974) to the level of 0.1 μV. These values have been plotted for normal ears and recruiting cochleas as a function of threshold intensity for three toneburst frequencies (Fig. 30). The recruiting ears are separated in Menière ears and ears with presumed haircell loss due to asphyxia at birth, noise trauma, or the use of ototoxic drugs. It may be observed from the figure that the threshold latency depends to a large extent on the threshold value and, especially in the low-threshold range, also on the tone frequency.

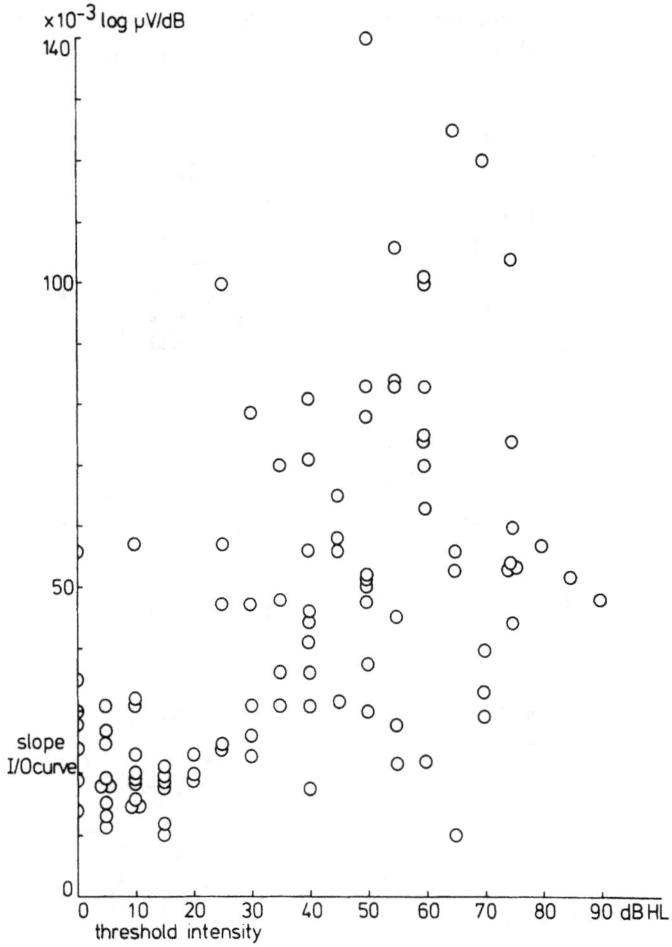

Fig. 29. Steepness of input-output curves in normal and recruiting ears for 2000 Hz tone burst stimulation. For about 20 normal ears (thresholds below 20 dB HL) and 80 recruiting ears, the numerical values of the slope of the input-output curves below the 1.5 μV level is plotted as a function of threshold intensity. It appears that on the average the slope of the input-output curve increases with increasing threshold value. It also appears that no absolute boundary for recruiting and non-recruiting ears exists. (From EGGERMONT, 1976b)

One may conclude that the criterion of latency at threshold less than 2 msec only holds for threshold values above 50 dB HL and for a small number of the data shown. In general, however, click latency is somewhat shorter than toneburst latency which may be somewhat more favourable for the fulfillment of the criterion. The point here is that if by latency at the threshold is meant the latency of a recordable AP at levels close to the threshold intensity, this may not be defined as uniquely as the extrapolated value toward the 0.1 μV amplitude level. It must be noted that the extrapolation is for a very small range only, because in general APs down to 0.15 μV amplitude are recorded.

It must be concluded therefore that the latency criterion for the presence of recruitment in fact is a threshold criterion and therefore should be used with care in the definition of recruiting responses. While the slope of the input-output curve also shows some dependency on the threshold intensity, this all taken together

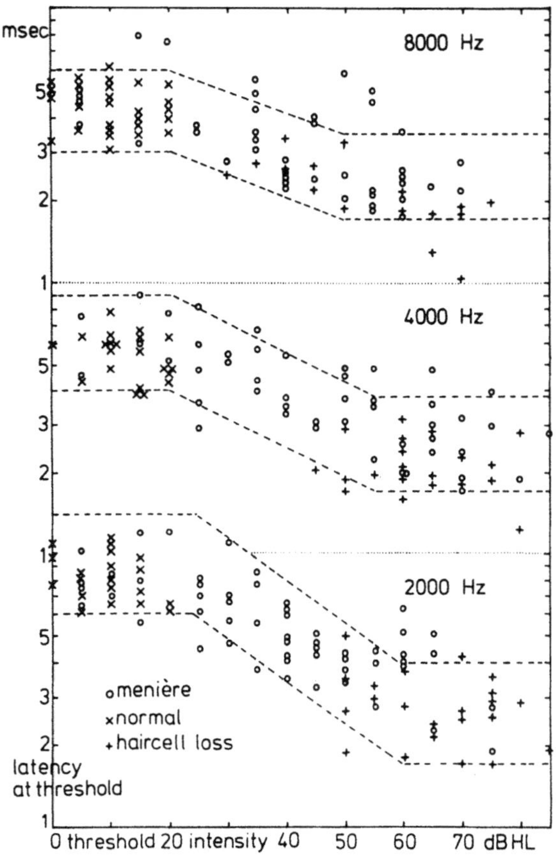

Fig. 30. Threshold latency for normal and recruiting ears for three tone burst frequencies. For threshold intensities above 60 dB HL, latencies are in general 2 to 4 msec irrespective of tone frequency. At low threshold values, however, there is a clear dependency on tone frequency: lower frequencies evoke longer threshold latencies. (From EGGERMONT, 1976b)

suggests that if one knows that an ear shows loudness recruitment, one may predict from the subjective audiogram the shape of the waveform, the slope of the input-output curve, and the latency at or near the threshold. In that case, the audiogram holds nearly unique information and the point remains to evaluate the underlying mechanism.

C. Response Areas in Recruiting Ears

From the concept of narrow-band responses (Section IV.C.), the response area is defined as that region in the intensity-central frequency plane at which supraliminal narrow-band responses can be obtained (*cf.* Fig. 23). In a normal ear, this area is narrow at low-intensity levels of the toneburst and becomes broader for high intensity stimulation. Fig. 31 shows a typical example of such a normal response area. In a way, the response area resembles a tuning curve for a single nerve fibre with a mirrored frequency scale, and it may also be obtained from single nerve fibre data (KIANG and MOXON, 1974). The finding of abnormally broad tuning curves in impaired cat-or guinea pig cochleas (KIANG *et al.*, 1970; EVANS, 1972, 1974, 1975) suggests that equivalent changes will take place with the form of the response area for tonebursts recorded in recruiting ears.

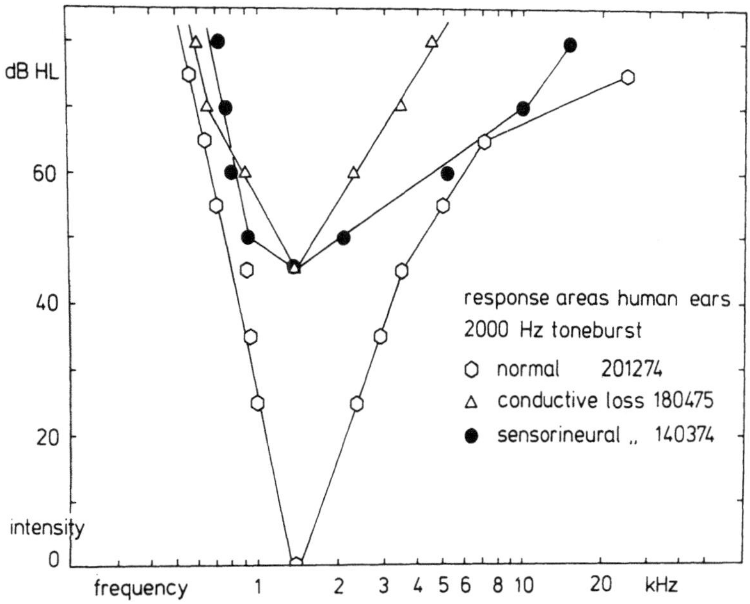

Fig. 31. Response areas for 2000 Hz tone burst stimulation in normal and pathological ears. Response areas are shown for a typical normal ear, for an ear with a pure conductive hearing loss of 45 dB HL, and for a recruiting ear. While the conduction loss curve is merely shifted upward by about 45 dB, the response area for the recruiting ear rapidly becomes as broad as the normal response curve at the same hearing level. The broad response area is thought to reflect a population of nerve fibres showing elevated thresholds at the characteristic frequency and broad tuning curves. (From EGGERMONT, 1976b)

The results obtained in two typical examples of hearing impairment are also shown in Fig. 31. Both ears had a threshold of 45 dB HL at 2000 Hz and a nearly flat audiogram. Pathology in one case was located in the middle ear and in the other in the cochlea. There is a considerable difference in the form of the response areas obtained: for the middle ear pathology, the curve is mainly shifted upwards and is only slightly broader than for normal ears; for the recruiting ear, a much broader curve is found which approaches the width of the normal response area at these hearing levels. This is what is expected from a change of a normal tuning curve into a broad one, which mechanism is held responsible for recruitment by EVANS (1974). The electrocochleogram results for ears with middle ear pathology and for recruiting ears support this new theory rather than the older two-population model. It can be shown (EGGERMONT, 1976b) that steep input-output curves are related to broad response areas, and that a relative measure of the slope of the input-output curve (*e.g.* related to a normal input-output curve in the same or the other ear) will be a valid indication for the presence of loudness recruitment.

VII. Electrocochleography in Pathological Ears

Electrocochleography can be useful in audiology applied for the differential and definitive diagnosis of hearing disorders. This means that characteristic electrocochleographic data should be compiled for each definitely known hearing impairment as well as for normal cases. These data may then characterize certain pathological conditions and subsequently serve as references for diagnosis.

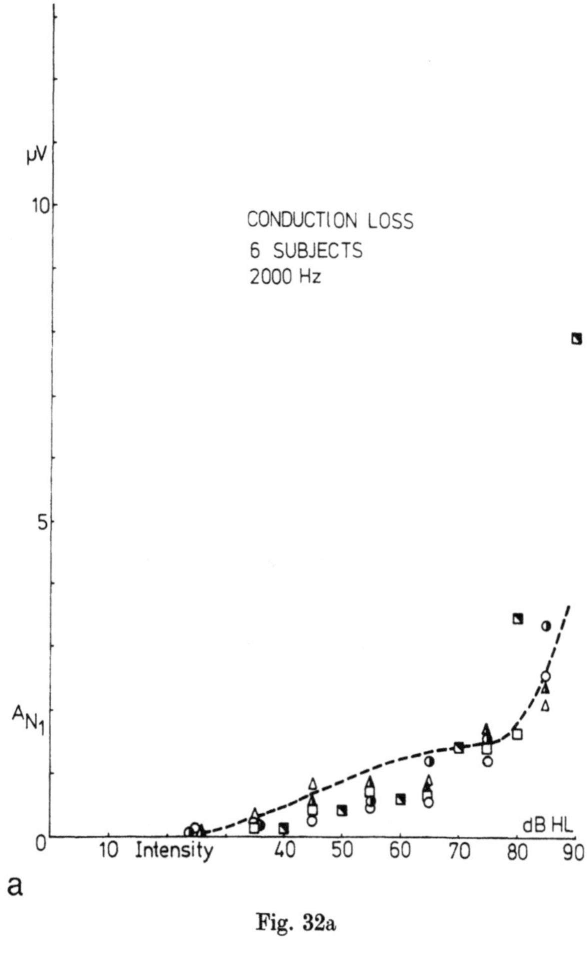

Fig. 32a

A. Findings in Conductive Hearing Loss

As may be expected from a situation with a normal cochlea but impaired middle-ear transmission, the stimulus used may be less effective than in normal ears. One observes therefore a shift to higher intensities for the amplitude input-output function, which, keeps the same shape as in normal ears (YOSHIE and OHASHI, 1969; ARAN *et al.*, 1971a; ODENTHAL and EGGERMONT, 1974a). This is illustrated by Fig. 32a, b, which show the amplitude-intensity functions for 6 ears having about the same threshold elevation due to otitis media or glue in the middle ear. On a linear scale, the average normal curve is drawn in but shifted by about

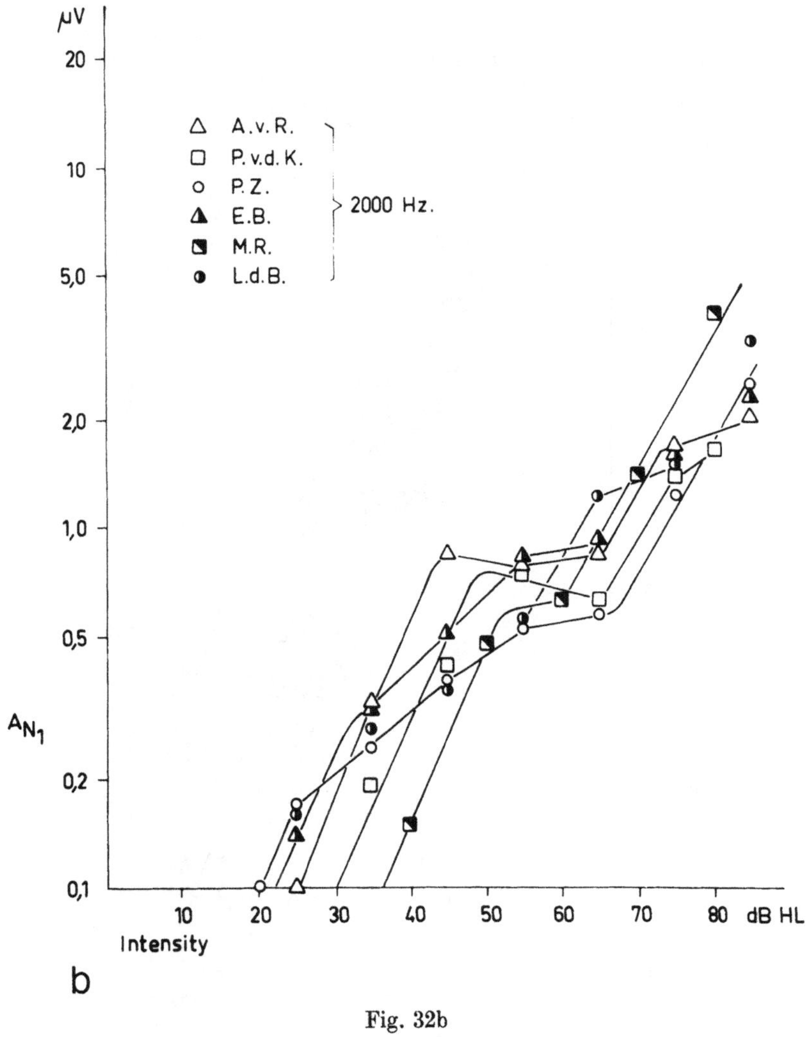

Fig. 32b

Fig. 32a, b. Input-output curves in ears showing conductive hearing loss. On a linear amplitude scale, the input-output curves have the same shape as for normal ears but are shifted to higher intensities due to the threshold elevation. This is demonstrated by the normal input-output curve which after a 25 dB shift to higher intensities corresponds well with the data. If the data are plotted on a logaritmic amplitude scale, it appears that the slope at near threshold values is about the same as in normal ears. (From EGGERMONT *et al.*, 1974a)

25 dB to the right. The curves drawn for a logaritmic amplitude scale clearly show the plateau at intermediate intensities. It must be remarked that compared to the normal input-output curves (*cf.* Fig. 15b), the intermission zone at about 50 dB HL is smaller in conductive hearing loss, at least in these examples. This means that the second steep part of the curve (for high intensities) is not shifted to the same extent as the part of the curve just above threshold. In general, this suggests a frequency-dependent hearing loss that is less for the higher frequencies.

In general, it is found that the latency-intensity function is also shifted to the right, the amount being proportional to the degree of hearing loss (YOSHIE and OHASHI, 1969). The threshold latency is in general the same as in normals (PORTMANN and NEGREVERGNE, 1973). This behaviour of the latency-intensity function

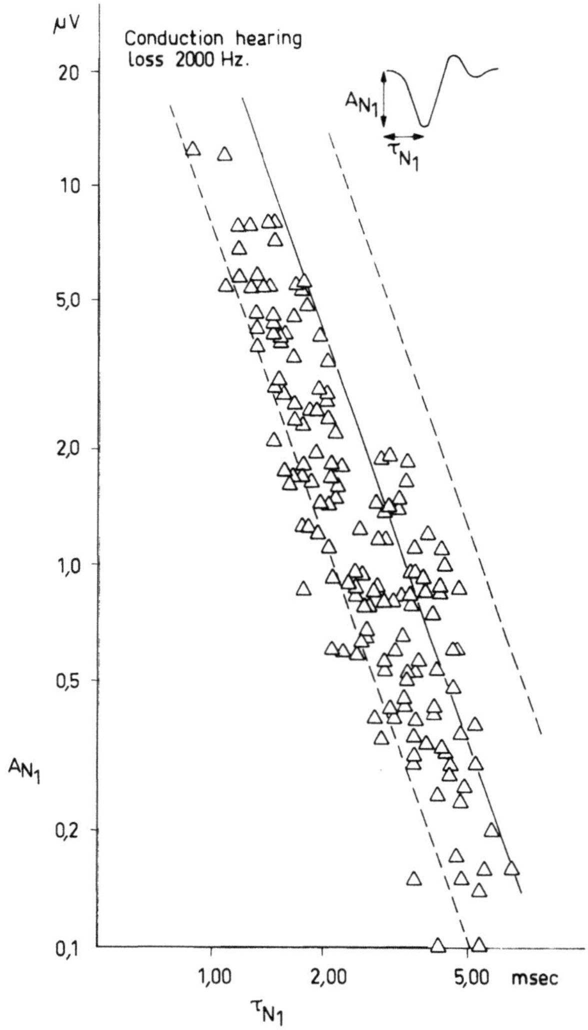

Fig. 33. Amplitude-latency scattergram for 18 glue ears for 2000 Hz tone burst stimulation. The amplitudes and latencies are both plotted on logarithmic coordinates. The regression line of log latency on log amplitude and the 2σ boundaries for the normal group are shown. The majority of the data is below the regression line, but there is no significant difference between the normal and conduction loss group. (From EGGERMONT *et al.*, 1974a)

is more consistent than the shift of an unchanged input-output curve, and, therefore, is used for separating conductive from cochlear types of hearing loss (CULLEN *et al.*, 1972). ODENTHAL and EGGERMONT (1974a) found roughly the same latency-intensity functions as in normal ears, with a tendency to longer latencies at high intensity levels. The curves could be compared to the normal ones after a shift of 20–35 dB. The characteristic jump in the latency which is found in most normal ears was not clearly present in the cases of conductive hearing loss. It must be added that conductive hearing loss due to glue in the middle ear may have altered the shunt resistances between the promontory and the external ear. In sum, one may say that it is mainly the threshold value that differs in conductive hearing loss, the shape of the compound AP and the input-output relations being normal as referred to sensation level.

If both the amplitude-intensity and latency-intensity curves have shifted to the right by the same amount, one should expect and amplitude-latency relationship that will be totally unchanged as compared to that for a normal ear. For a series of 18 ears showing conductive hearing loss, the amplitude-latency points are plotted for 2000 Hz toneburst stimulation in Fig. 33. The regression line of log latency on log amplitude and the 2σ boundaries for the normal ear group are drawn in, and, as can be seen, most of the points lie below the regression line. However, the slope of the regression line in conductive hearing loss is about the same as in normal ears (ODENTHAL and EGGERMONT, 1974a). Standard deviations and correlation coefficients also proved to be the same as in normal hearing.

B. Findings in High-Frequency Sensorineural Hearing Loss

According to results obtained with wide-band clicks, one may obtain two major types of AP waveforms in cases of sensorineural hearing loss (ARAN and NEGREVERGNE, 1973). For relatively flat cochlear hearing losses, one obtains the so-called "recruiting-responses" a series of which is shown in Fig. 27b. In cases of a restricted high-frequency loss with relatively normal hearing for low frequencies or in cases with a notch in the audiogram, a so-called dissociated response type is recorded, showing a sharp N_1-peak followed by a relatively broad second one.

In general, the input-output curves show the loss of the low-part of the curve (YOSHIE and OHASHI, 1969; PORTMANN and NEGRVERGNE, 1973; EGGERMONT and ODENTHAL, 1974a; ODENTHAL and EGGERMONT, 1974a), as illustrated by Fig. 34, which shows for a linear amplitude scale six ears with high-frequency sensorineural hearing loss and the standard normal curve. As already pointed out in the section on recruitment, the steepness of the curves is only an indication for the presence of recruitment. As MONTANDON *et al.* (1975b) have shown, input-output curves for non-recruiting high-frequency sensorineural hearing loss ears can be as steep as those for recruiting ears. The compound AP latencies in general are not changed with respect to those of normal ears at the same hearing-level, although, due to the elevated threshold, the latency at the threshold is shorter than for normal or conductive hearing loss ears (ODENTHAL and EGGERMONT, 1974a).

In ears showing rather steep audiograms, *e.g.* in cases of gentamycin intoxication, dissociated responses are recorded. At high intensity levels, a sharp N_1-peak is present which disappears quite abruptly, and the broad N_2 can be recorded down to values quite far below the threshold at that frequency. In those cases, the latency at threshold is much longer than found in normal ears (*cf.* YOSHIE and OHASHI, 1969). If the high-pass noise masking technique is used, one in general observes that these long latencies refer to contributions to the AP from the relatively unaffected part of the cochlea at, *e.g.*, 2000 Hz. This may be due to the

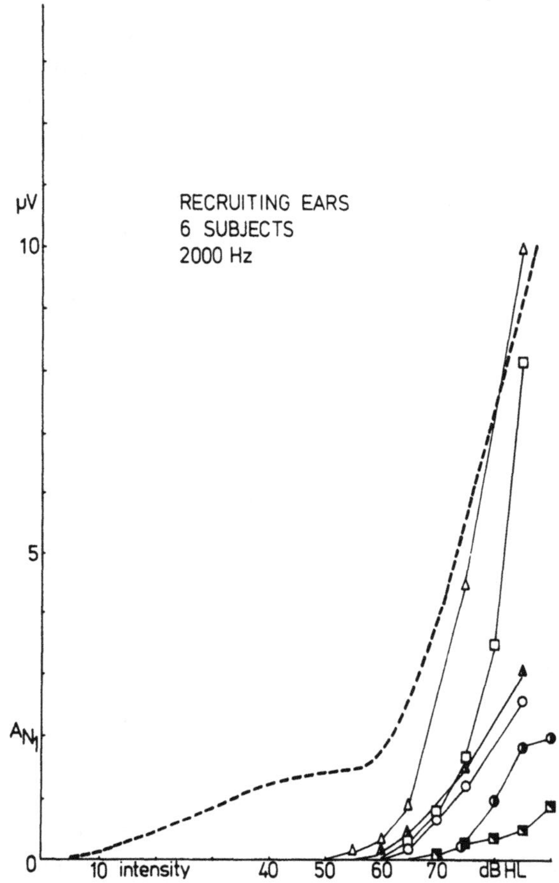

Fig. 34. Input-output for six recruiting ears at 2000 Hz tone burst stimulation. This figure shows input-output curves on a linear amplitude scale in comparison to the standard normal curve. It is observed that the flat part is nearly absent in the curves, while the output at high levels may be the same as for normal ears

shape of the toneburst spectrum showing, *e.g.*, only 50 dB suppression of the 2000 Hz component in case of 4000 Hz stimulation, and it is easily explained on the basis of the wide-band click spectrum. The dissociated AP therefore represents components from two distinctly different parts of the cochlea.

If amplitude-latency scattergrams are produced for, *e.g.*, 2000 Hz toneburst stimulation (Fig. 35), it is evident that for low amplitude values the difference between the normal area between the two dashed-lines and the points found in high-frequency sensorineural hearing loss increases with decreasing amplitude.

One finds in general a restricted range of latency values associated with a nearly normal range of amplitude values. The upper limit of the latencies recorded suggests that the effective stimulation of the 2000 Hz toneburst in these ears is restricted to somewhat more basal locations than would be expected on the basis

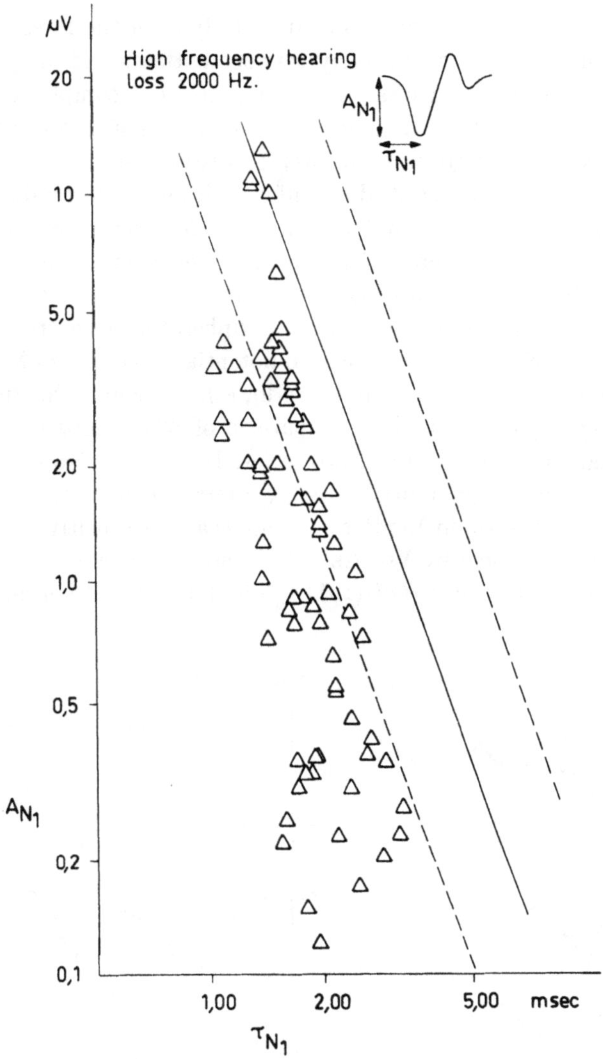

Fig. 35. Amplitude-latency scattergram for 14 ears suffering from high frequency sensorineural hearing loss. The regression line and 2σ boundaries for the normal group are indicated. At low amplitude values, the data from the impaired cochleas tend to be below the lower 2σ boundary and, therefore, are easily distinghuished from data for normal cochleas (either from normal ears or conduction loss ears). (From EGGERMONT *et al.*, 1974a)

of the toneburst spectrum (EGGERMONT, 1976a). The distinction between sensory and conductive hearing loss is usually quite clear and is made on the basis of four entities, *i.e.*, the threshold values, the slope of the input-output curves, and the parameters of the amplitude-latency curves. A problem arises, however, when a mixed hearing loss is encountered; in these situations electrocochleography performed with a well-calibrated bone-conductor (*e.g.* Yoshie, 1973) is indicated.

C. Findings in Menière's Disease

This seems a much more restricted field of study than the foregoing, but since the symptoms may differ quantitatively between patients and the pathogenesis of Menière's disease is far from clear, it is an extremely complicated field. The fluctuating hearing loss, tinnitus, and sense of fullness in the ear together with recurrent attacks of vertigo make it easy to distinguish a very large group of patients who are clinically classified as suffering from Menière's disease where no other specific causes for these complaints can be found. Electrocochleography may shed some light on these matters, at least those concerning the cochlea and auditory nerve. The ECoG thresholds are usually similar to the subjective ones, which places the origin of the hearing loss in the peripheral hearing organ.

The waveforms of the compound action potentials recorded in Menière ears are characteristic and differ widely from those in, *e.g.*, a cochlear hearing loss due to noise trauma (*cf.* Figs. 27a, b). For comparison of APs recorded in Menière ears and in a normal ear, Fig. 36 shows two series. In the Menière ear the relatively large negative summating potential strongly alters the shape of the AP (Schmidt *et al.*, 1974). The waveform in Menière's disease is a very sensitive indicator for the state of hearing as reported by Yoshie (1973) and Schmidt *et al.* (1975). For high-frequency filtered clicks, Aran *et al.* (1971a) found in a case of Lermoyez's syndrom

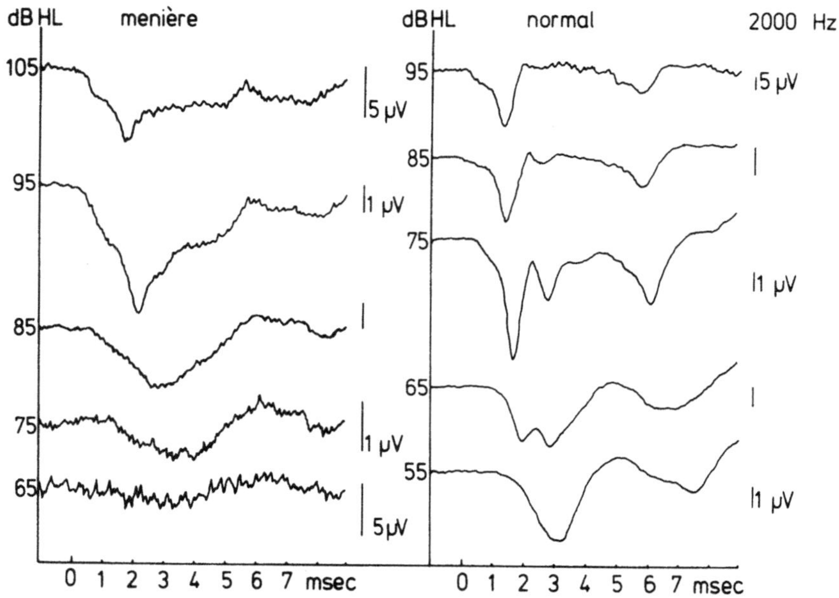

Fig. 36. Compound action potential wave forms in normal and Menière ears. For comparable 2000 Hz tone burst intensities, typical Menière AP wave forms and normal APs are shown. It appears that the pronounced negative summating potential is responsible for the broad curves obtained for Menière ears

(a variant of Menière's disease) an early positive peak, which may be an SP^{+}, and, for wide-band clicks, a negative summating potential. In general, a broad non-diphasic waveform is recorded when using click stimuli (PORTMANN and NEGREVERGNE, 1973; BRACKMANN, 1974). The results obtained so far (ODENTHAL and

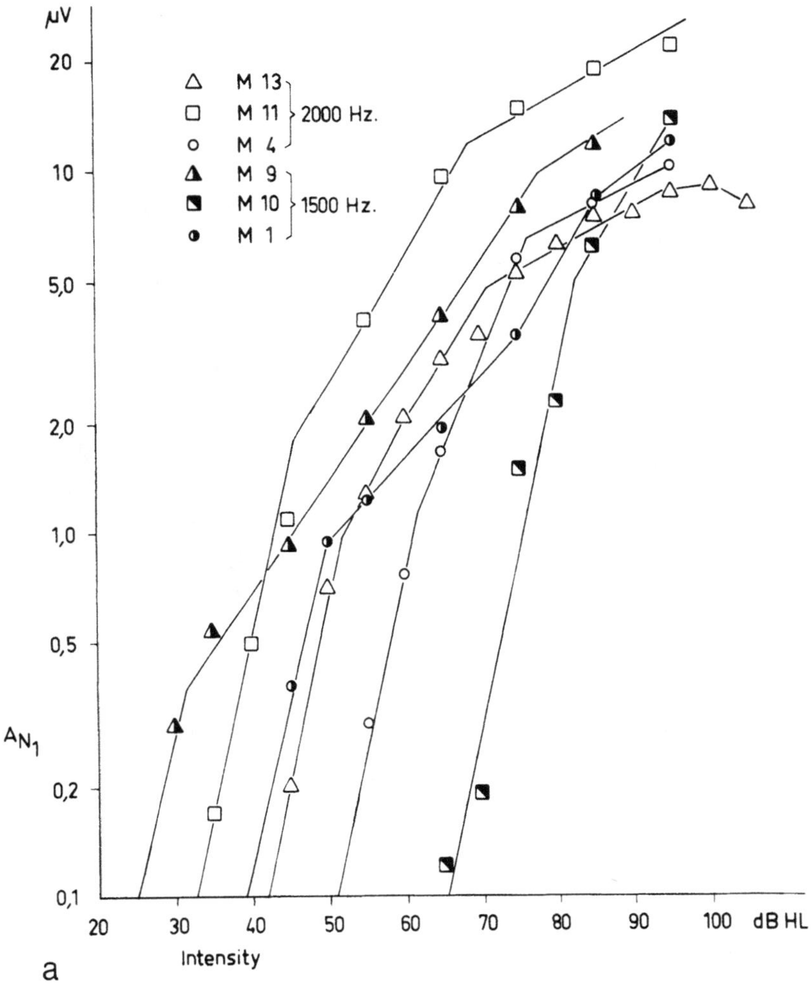

a

Fig. 37a

EGGERMONT, 1974b) point to a specific change in the SP^{-} amplitude related to the amount of hearing loss. In the fluctuant stage of hearing loss, the higher the threshold the higher the SP^{-} and vice versa. This finding may be attributed either to a mechanical displacement of the basilar membrane, which causes non-linearities in its movement as a result of the presumed endolymphatic hydrops (JOHNSTONE, 1975), or to a metabolic disturbance resulting in a larger EP, *e.g.*, due to a smaller K^{+} diffusion potential across Reisner's membrane.

In the section on summating potentials (III. A), quantitative evidence is given for the large amplitude of the SP^{-} in Menière ears. Input-output curves for the AP amplitude are usually rather steep and tend to have a saturation value which is larger than in normal ears (Fig. 37a, b); the larger saturation value may be due to the fact that normally the SP$^-$ amplitude will be incorporated to some extent in the compound AP amplitude. The latencies found in Menière ears are generally somewhat longer at a given hearing level than for normal hearing but smaller than

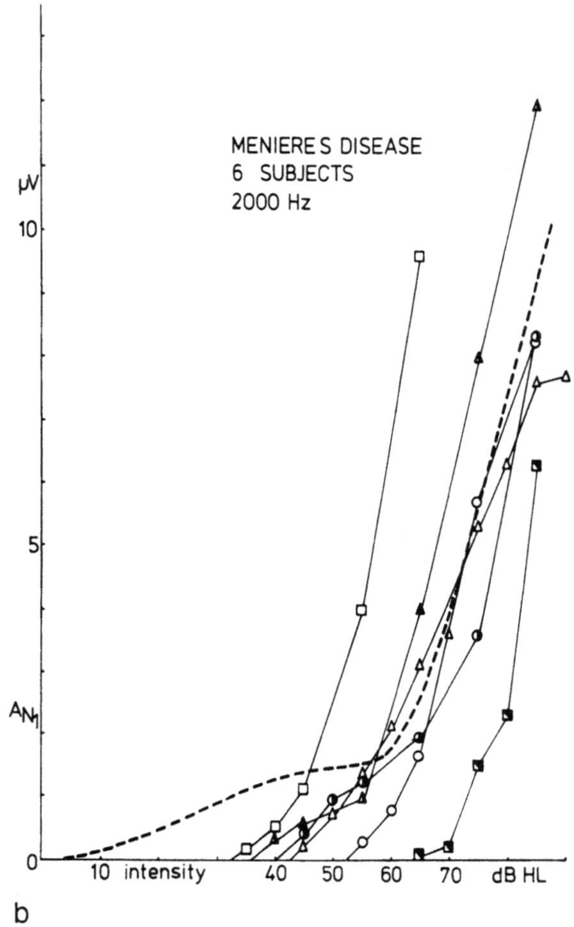

Fig. 37b

Fig. 37a, b. Input-output curves for six Menière ears. The curves plotted on a linear amplitude scale lack the shallow part found for normal cochleas; the input-output curve for a normal ear is shown. It appears that, in general, the maximum output is larger than for normal ears, a finding that may be due in part to the somewhat larger SP$^-$ which partly contributes to the compound AP amplitude. The slope of the input-output curve as seen on logarithmic coordinates appears to be greater than that for normal ears. (From EGGERMONT *et al.*, 1974a)

for normal hearing at the same sensation level. A jump in the latency-intensity curve and the corresponding transitions for the double-peaked AP are only observed in cases with small hearing losses. Surprisingly, the amplitude-latency scattergrams found in Menière ears are completely normal, especially at 2000 Hz (Fig. 38), but transitions to the type found in high-frequency sensorineural hearing loss are found for, *e.g.*, 8000 Hz. As can be seen from Fig. 38 nearly all points are within the 2σ boundaries for the group of normal ears (SCHMIDT *et al.*, 1974). Despite the fact that the latencies are somewhat shorter at the threshold relative to normal hearing, the larger compound AP amplitudes lift the points into the normal range.

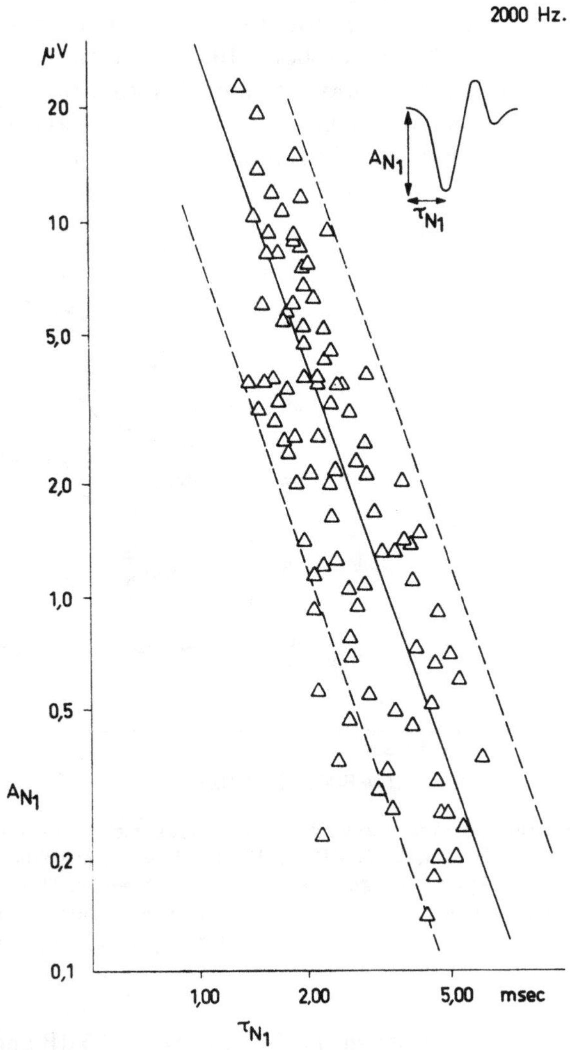

Fig. 38. Amplitude-latency scattergram for 22 Menière ears at 2000 Hz. The regression line and the 2σ boundaries for the normal group are shown. It is evident that the data for Menière ears are indistinghuishable from those of normal ears. This feature separates the Menière ears from those having high frequency sensorineural hearing loss. (From EGGERMONT *et al.*, 1974a)

This phenomenon clearly distinguishes Menière cochleas from cochleas showing haircell loss due to other causes. The relatively normal summating potentials point to nearly normal haircells and, especially, normal outer haircells. It is, therefore, suggested that the hearing loss in the initial state of the disease is due to a change in the functioning of the dendrites which reflect the changes in cochlear metabolism.

D. Findings in Acoustic Neuromas and Central Lesions

1. Acoustic Neuromas

One of the most characteristic features observed and reported for electrocochleography in acoustic neuromas is the distorted and relatively broad waveforms recorded at intermediate intensities irrespective of the type of stimulation (PORTMANN and ARAN, 1972; BRACKMANN, 1974; ODENTHAL and EGGERMONT, 1974b; BEAGLEY, 1975). Typical waveforms of this kind recorded in a patient having no hearing loss, but in whom a small acoustic neuroma was surgically confirmed, are shown in Fig. 39. APs recorded from a normal ear at the same

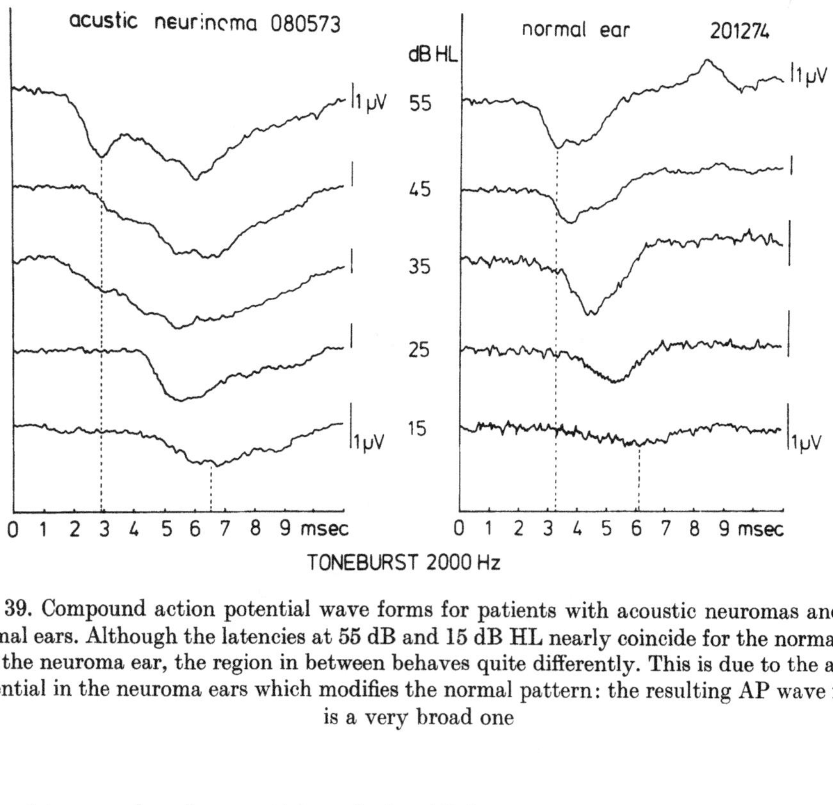

Fig. 39. Compound action potential wave forms for patients with acoustic neuromas and for normal ears. Although the latencies at 55 dB and 15 dB HL nearly coincide for the normal ear and the neuroma ear, the region in between behaves quite differently. This is due to the afterpotential in the neuroma ears which modifies the normal pattern: the resulting AP wave form is a very broad one

intensities are also shown. Although the AP latencies at 55 dB and 15 dB do not differ essentially for these series, the change in latency-intensity function is gradual in the normal ear and quite irregular in the neuroma case.

It is the above described aspect of the latency-intensity function – best observed under stimulation with 2000 Hz tonebursts and barely visible after click stimulation (ODENTHAL and EGGERMONT, 1974b) – that has been neglected in all reports but one. In a series of 91 cases of suspected acoustic neuromas, BEAGLEY (1975) predicted 88% of the surgically confirmed (49 cases) by paying most attention to the AP waveform proper. However, to understand what causes the broad AP waves and especially for the differential diagnosis between acoustic neuromas and Menière's disease, it is of the utmost importance to present the data in a more quantitative way. A study of this kind has been started by ODENTHAL and EGGERMONT (1974b). So far it covers only 14 surgically confirmed acoustic neuromas. This series comprises 6 patients with a subjectively dead ear comprising 3 cases lacking action potentials as well, 2 patients with AP thresholds of about 60 dB HL, and

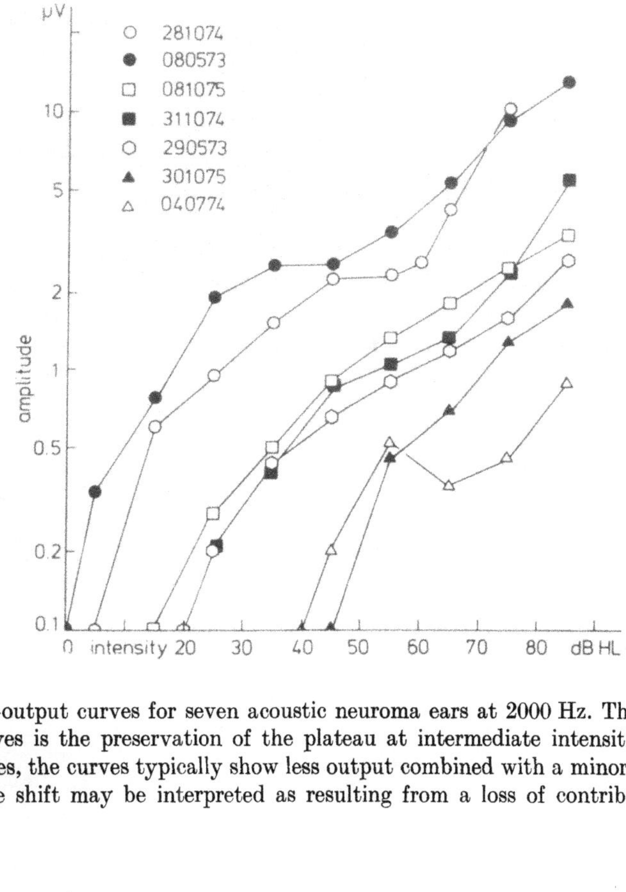

Fig. 40. Input-output curves for seven acoustic neuroma ears at 2000 Hz. The main feature of all the curves is the preservation of the plateau at intermediate intensities. For higher threshold values, the curves typically show less output combined with a minor shift to higher intensities; the shift may be interpreted as resulting from a loss of contributing neurones

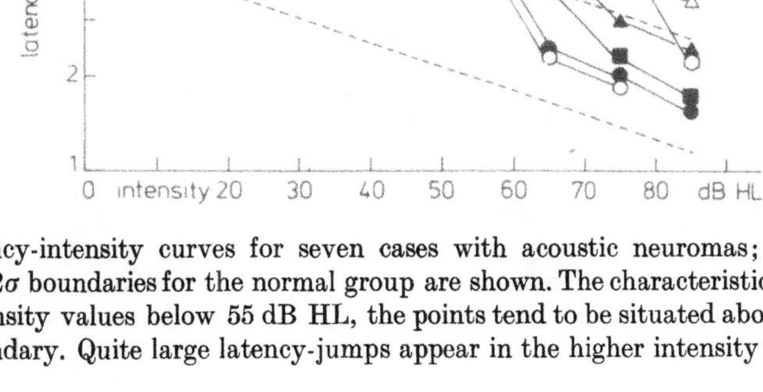

Fig. 41. Latency-intensity curves for seven cases with acoustic neuromas; stimulation at 2000 Hz. The 2σ boundaries for the normal group are shown. The characteristic for each ear is that, for intensity values below 55 dB HL, the points tend to be situated above the upper 2σ boundary. Quite large latency-jumps appear in the higher intensity range

one patient with a completely normal ECoG at all frequencies; in the remaining 8 patients, the subjective and electrocochleographic thresholds showed a good correspondence. Seven cases with less or moderate hearing loss and, with one exception, small acoustic neuromas, well be described in more detail.

The AP input-output curves for 2000 Hz toneburst stimulation are shown in Fig. 40. Two ears showed a nearly normal threshold with completely normal input-output curves, although one patient (281074) had no subjective hearing at all in that ear, from which a large extracanalicular pontine – angle neuroma was surgically removed. Three ears showed a small (15–20 dB) hearing loss and input-output curves somewhat flatter than the normal, which also may be said for the remaining two ears showing 40–45 dB hearing loss. It may be concluded that amplitude-intensity curves do not offer a consistent finding which may be used to characterize these ears, especially when there is a minor threshold elevation. However, the irregular changes in the waveform must be reflected in the latency-intensity functions (Fig. 41), which for these 7 neuromas shows a very consistent pattern for intensities below 55 dB HL. For intensities above 55 dB HL, a relatively large range of latency values is found, including transitions of about 3 msec.

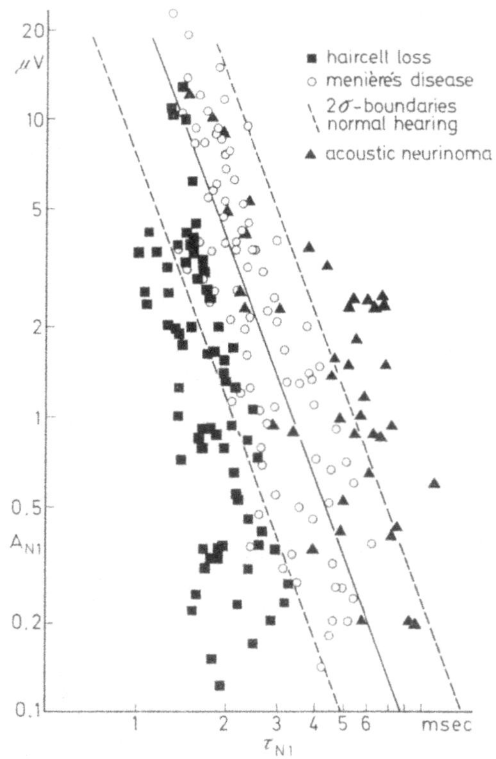

Fig. 42. Amplitude-latency scattergram for acoustic neuromas in comparison with Menière ears and hair-cell loss ears; the regression line and 2σ boundaries are shown for the normal group. The acoustic neuroma points scatter well above the normal range at intermediate amplitude values; they may be distingushed quite easily from Menière ears and even more definitely from ears with sensorineural hearing loss

For the lower intensities, the latencies are outside the 2σ boundaries of the standard normal group. These prolonged latencies may point to either a longer neural integration time or some definition-artifact in the latency. The amplitude-latency data should also reflect these changes. In order to compare with results obtained in other pathologies of the ear, Fig. 42 shows for 2000 Hz toneburst stimulation the amplitude-latency data obtained in three types of hearing pathology compared to the regression line and 2σ boundaries for the group of normal ears. The ears showing high frequency sensorineural hearing loss due to asphyxia, noise trauma, or the use of ototoxic drugs and considered as the haircell-loss group, fall below the lower 2σ boundary, but the Menière data cannot be distinguished from the normal ear range. However, the points found in acoustic neuromas are located distinctly above the upper 2σ boundary for the middle value amplitude range. It is felt that the quantification of data for this small group of acoustic neuromas may add in a significant way to the reliability of a differential diagnosis among the three types of perceptive hearing loss, namely, loss due to high frequency sensorineural hearing loss (hair-cell damage), loss due to Menière's disease, and loss due to acoustic neuroma.

2. Central Lesions

Central lesions are considered those lesions not affecting the auditory nerve, *i.e.*, located central to the cochlear nucleus. Only a few general remarks can be made with respect to the electrocochleographic findings in these cases.

A patient who was totally deaf showed two complete normal functioning cochleas (including the auditory nerve) as measured by electrocochleography. The disease apparently did not affect the cochlea or the auditory nerve and was later diagnosed as an axial ponstumor. Electrocochleograms for a patient suffering from a cerebrovascular accident with nearly complete hearing loss showed a moderate (40 dB), relatively flat, hearing loss with steep input-output curves. The patient recovered, and his hearing subjectively measured, returned to normal.

A third patient, tentatively diagnosed as having multiple sclerosis, showed fluctuations in the subjective audiogram between about 60 dB flat hearing loss and total deafness. Electrocochleography performed in both states resulted in identical recordings in agreement with a 60 dB flat hearing loss. In this case, a mixture of a stable 60 dB peripheral hearing loss and a fluctuating central component could be demonstrated. In general, therefore, no definite pattern can be assigned to this type of lesion using electrocochleography. It is felt that ECoG provides the means to differentiate between a peripheral (cochlea and auditory nerve) and a central lesion; brain-stem audiometry may provide a more detailed picture regarding the localization of the lesion.

E. Diagnosis on the Basis of Electrocochleography

The findings in normal ears and in ears with different pathologies, as reviewed in the foregoing sections, may serve as the basis for a diagnosis system that can be applied to each new ear subjected to electrocochleography. The techniques which have to be used are based on statistics and are, in fact, pattern recognition techniques. Simple patterns are more easily recognized than complex ones; this is the main reason for not making a diagnosis on the basis of the waveform of the compound AP (ODENTHAL *et al.*, 1974).

Recordings at five toneburst frequencies generally result in about 40 compound AP waveforms. As has been shown in the foregoing sections, input-output curves and amplitude-latency curves can provide sufficient information about the type of malfunction. These two curves, which are straight lines if suitable transformations are made, can be characterized by two parameters each. The part of the log AP amplitude vs intensity curve can be approximated by a straight line for amplitude values below 1.5 μV and is then characterized by the threshold value and the slope of the curve. The relation between log latency and log amplitude can also be approximated by a linear curve; this curve is characterized by the threshold latency and the slope. The four parameters so obtained can be considered the coordinates of a point in a four-dimensional space. This point characterizes the ear under study at a given frequency (HERMANS *et al.*, 1975).

For diagnosis of the hearing disorder of an individual patient, one needs reference groups of all well-known disease categories. The forming of these groups is really a difficult task. There is no problem in defining normal hearing or purely conductive hearing loss; the problems arise when one wants to form a group of ears showing haircell loss. It is presumed that high frequency hearing loss due to asphyxia at birth, noise trauma, or the use of ototoxic drugs is characterized by extensive haircell loss, so these patients may constitute a haircell loss group. As said before, even more problems emerge in forming a reference set of "true Menière" patients. Before thinking about diagnosis, however, one has to form such groups.

Each reference group is characterized at each frequency by a cloud of points in a 4-dimensional space, the more compact the cloud the more homogeneous the reference group. In general, the clouds of different reference groups will overlap partially. The position of a new point in this 4-dimensional space (a new ear to be diagnosed), therefore, can be attributed to the reference groups with some probability. The probability of belonging to each of the reference groups individually has to be calculated. From previous investigations (*e.g.* subjective audiometry), prior information concerning the type of hearing loss may be available. The presence or absence of an air-bone gap in the audiogram is prior information regarding the most likely disease categories. This prior information and the results of electrocochleography are combined to obtain a probability that the ear belongs to each of the disease categories. This is done by using Bayes Theorem (HERMANS *et al.*, 1975).

The reasons for establishing a type of diagnosis as described above are based on the hope that it will lead to a uniform procedure in decision taking on the basis of a majority of AP recordings. The paramount importance of clinically well-established reference groups is stressed because the accuracy of the procedure described above depends not only on the type of electrocochleography but also on the reliability of the reference material.

It is felt, however, that the four parameters at the five frequencies used in the diagnosis can be extended with, *e.g.*, the summating potential, and that the narrow-band AP parameters may provide additional information. With these narrow-band parameters, the final sections of this paper will deal in considerable detail.

VIII. Additional Topics in Electrocochleography

A. Adaptation and Masking

A decrease of the AP amplitude is observed when the interval between successive stimuli falls below a certain value. This is generally called adaptation, although equilibration may be a better term (Derbyshire and Davis, 1935). The characteristics of the adaptation mechanism can be studied by either repetitive stimulation or by the method of forward masking. If in forward masking experiments the interval between masker and test stimulus becomes zero, continuous masking is actually obtained, and additional mechanisms start to reduce the AP amplitude.

1. Compound Action Potentials and Repetitive Stimulation

When a train of tonebursts or clicks is presented to the ear, the resulting APs decrease in amplitude with the number of successive stimuli. In general, a stable final value is reached after the fifth stimulus; this depends on the intensity level of the stimulus and on the state of the cochlea. In a normal ear at 90 dB HL, the AP-amplitude in response to 4000 Hz tonebursts decreased slowly but continuously even after the fifth stimulus (Eggermont and Odenthal, 1974b). For a case of bilateral acoustic neuromas, an analogous effect was found at corresponding high-intensity levels (Yoshie and Ohashi, 1971). The final-value usually is quite stable (Eggermont and Odenthal, 1974a), and depends on both the stimulus intensity and the interstimulus interval (ISI). This ISI dependency is shown for six normal hearing subjects in Fig. 43 at intensities of 65 and 70 dB HL in comparison to average data from the guinea pig. The individual human data agree quite well with each other but are significantly different from those obtained in the guinea pig. Both the ISI dependency and the intensity dependency are shown in Fig. 44 for five normal human ears. A gradual decrease of the final value is found for stimulus intensities up to about 60 dB HL, after which only small changes take place. This is also observed in individual ears using tone bursts as stimuli. These findings differ from those of Stephens *et al.* (1974, 1975), who report a lowest final value for a five-click train with an ISI of 8 msec at an intensity of 80 dB SL; for intensities below or above 80 dB the final value increases again. This may be due to experimental differences of which a few will be cited. The inter-train interval used by Stephens *et al.* was 100 msec. Since in other adaptation experiments either 800 msec (Yoshie and Ohashi, 1971) or 1000 msec (Eggermont and Odenthal, 1974a, b) was used as the silent interval between the trains of stimuli, and Coats and Dickey (1972) as well as Eggermont and Odenthal (1974a, b) report full recovery of forward masking only after at least 500 msec interval, this may well influence the results.

Some further warning concerning the study of adaptation in pathological cochleas concerns the negative summating potential, which is generally included in the calculation of the compound AP amplitude, also in click stimulation. Since this SP^- is relatively large in Menière's disease, and because the SP does not show a dependency on the repetition rate of the stimuli (Eggermont, 1974), the relative diminishing of the compound AP amplitude is very minor (*cf.* Stephens *et al.*,

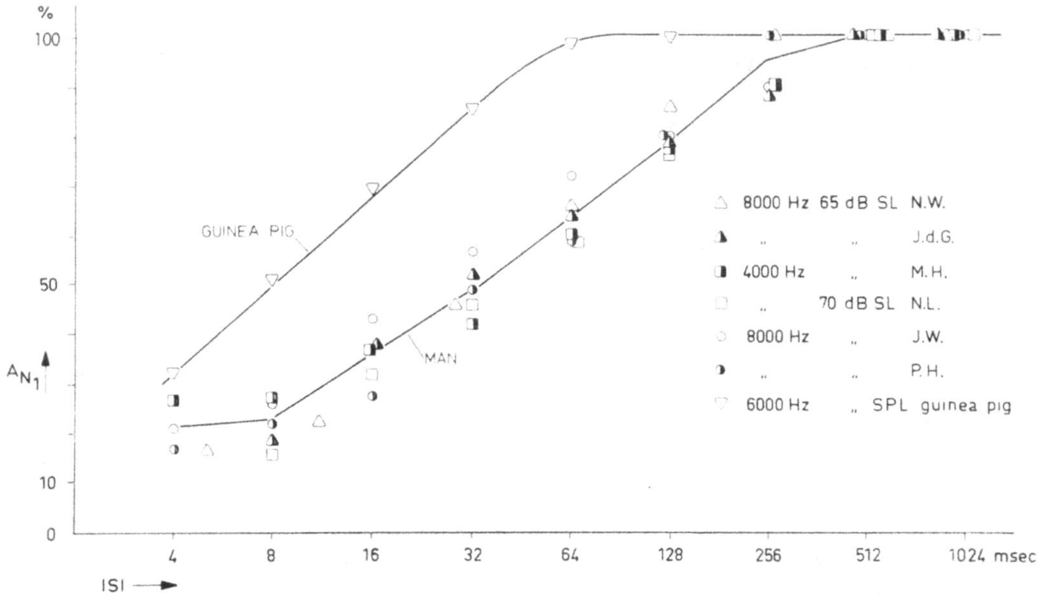

Fig. 43. Adaptation of the compound action potential. The amplitude of the compound AP depends on the interstimulus interval (ISI). For six normal human cochleas, the relative decrease in amplitude is shown; the mean curve is calculated and compared to the guinea pig curve; there is a clear difference. The 50% relative amplitude point is found at a time about four times longer in man than in the guinea pig. (From EGGERMONT and ODENTHAL, 1974a)

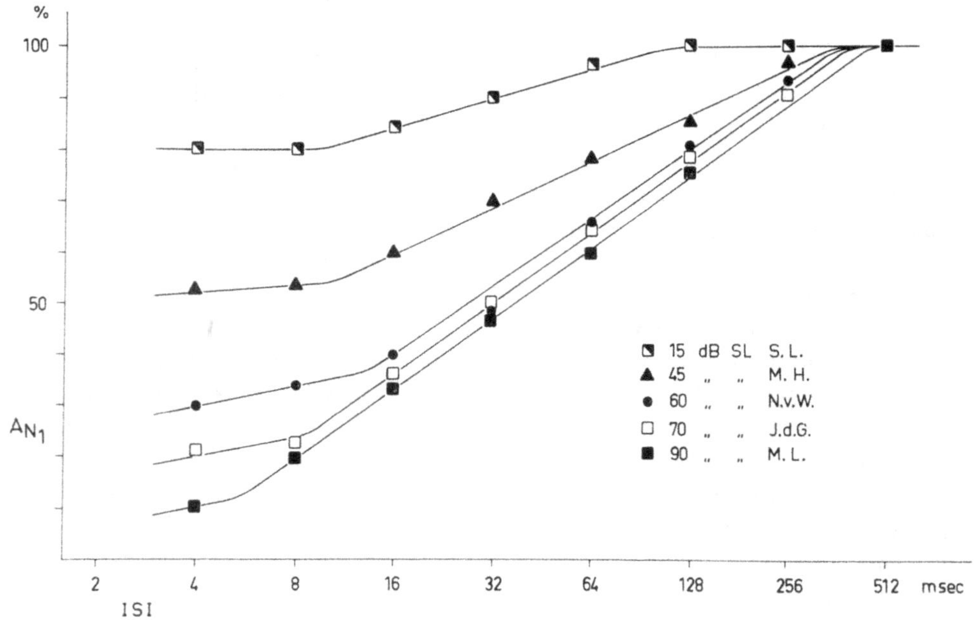

Fig. 44. Adaptation of the compound action potential amplitude for different stimulus intensities at 4000 Hz. For stimulus intensities above 60 dB HL, the adaptation curves are almost identical. Below that intensity level, considerable deviations occur in the relative amplitude behaviour. Since, for clinical electrocochleography, an ISI of 125 msec. is usually used, it is noted that for the lower intensities no adaptation occurs. (From EGGERMONT *et al.*, 1974a)

1974). The intensity dependency of adaptation of the compound AP may be in part related to the change of the excited area on the cochlear partition due to changing intensity. If adaptation is studied using a separation of the compound AP into narrow-band APs (*cf.* Section C.1) it is found that the largest adaptation is found for narrow band regions with higher central frequencies (PRIJS and EGGERMONT, to be published). Since the N_1 originates from those regions of the cochlea that are excited by the highest central frequencies and since with decreasing intensity this region shifts towards the apex of the cochlea, this may well explain the dependency on intensity. For click stimulation, the excited area differs to a large extent from that of, *e.q.*, 4000 or 8000 Hz tone bursts used in other studies.

Corresponding to the decrease in amplitude, there is a significant but generally small increase in latency that also reaches a final value after five stimuli (SPOOR and EGGERMONT, 1974). It can be shown that this latency increase is associated more with the relatively larger decrease in high-frequency contribution to the compound AP than for the narrow-bands having lower central frequency. The result is a slight shift towards the apex of the cochlea of the area contributing maximally to the N_1 amplitude, which is recorded as a slight increase in latency (up to 0.3 msec, PRIJS and EGGERMONT, to be published).

2. Forward Masking and Continuous Masking

Another method for the investigation of cochlear adaptation is forward masking, in which one studies the recovery of the compound AP to a click or short tone burst following a relatively long white noise or tonal masker. The AP amplitude and latency measured depend on both the signal-to-noise ratio and the interval between masker and toneburst. In general, it is found that after 500–1000 msec, depending on the stimulus intensity, complete recovery of the AP amplitude is obtained (COATS and DICKEY, 1972; EGGERMONT and ODENTHAL, 1974a, b) and that AP-latency is returned to normal values after 100–250 msec. These values are about 4 times as large as those found in the guinea pig (SPOOR and EGGERMONT, 1974) but also 2 to 3 times as large as found psychoacoustically in the same human subjects (COATS and DICKEY, 1972). Continuous masking experiments can be performed with wide-band masking stimuli, such as broad-band noise (EGGERMONT and ODENTHAL, 1974a, b) or high-pass filtered broad-band noise, as already discussed, or by using a tonal masker. It proved possible to measure the masking profile of a continuous 4000 Hz tone by using tone bursts of different frequencies as test stimuli (EGGERMONT and ODENTHAL, 1974c).

B. Amplitude and Frequency Modulation

Amplitude modulated continuous tones evoke compound APs whose amplitude depends on the value of the intensity increment (ΔI) of the modulation and also on the continuous tone level above which the increment is given. This is illustrated in Fig. 45. It is observed that for a normal ear the slope of the amplitude-intensity increment curve depends on the continuous tone intensity. The extrapolation to the 1 dB (ΔI) output may be of interest as a physiological correlate of the SISI test in clinical audiometry. It can be shown that a supraliminal AP is found for intensities above 55 dB HL, which is the point where the low-part and the high-part of the AP input-output curve coincide (EGGERMONT and ODENTHAL, 1974b). When the continuous tone level is set at 20 dB above the threshold, this test may serve as an objective SISI test, and some of the results thereof are compared with psychoacoustic data (SCHMIDT *et al.*, 1974). It is felt that AM stimuli may be used to validate the presumed relationship, between high SISI scores and the presence of recruitment.

Compound APs evoked by frequency modulated continuous tones depend on both the direction of the modulation and the modulation depth. The first results which were reported (EGGERMONT and ODENTHAL, 1974b) appeared to be very complex also in their intensity dependency. More consistent data can be obtained

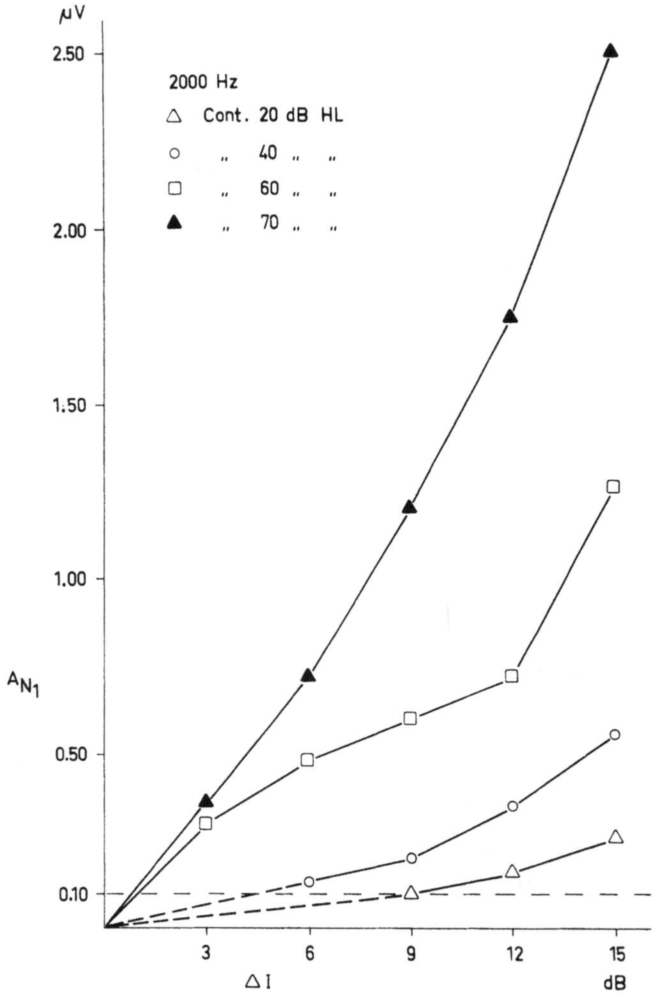

Fig. 45. The amplitude of the compound action potential in response to amplitude modulated tones as a function of the intensity increment, ΔI, for different levels of the continuous tone. The AP amplitude increases with increasing ΔI; the rate of increase depends on the continuous tone level. For a 1 dB increment, a supraliminal response (above 0.1 µV) is recorded if the continuous tone level is set at an intensity corresponding to the steep part of the input-output curve that is obtained in response to a tone burst. (From EGGERMONT *et al.*, 1974a)

by studying the AP dependency on modulation depth. Data are presented in Fig. 46 for a continuous tone of 4000 Hz of 40 dB HL, both for negative modulation ($-\Delta f$), *i.e.*, downward in frequency, and for upward modulation ($+\Delta f$). In this particular example (an early Menière patient with normal thresholds for 1000

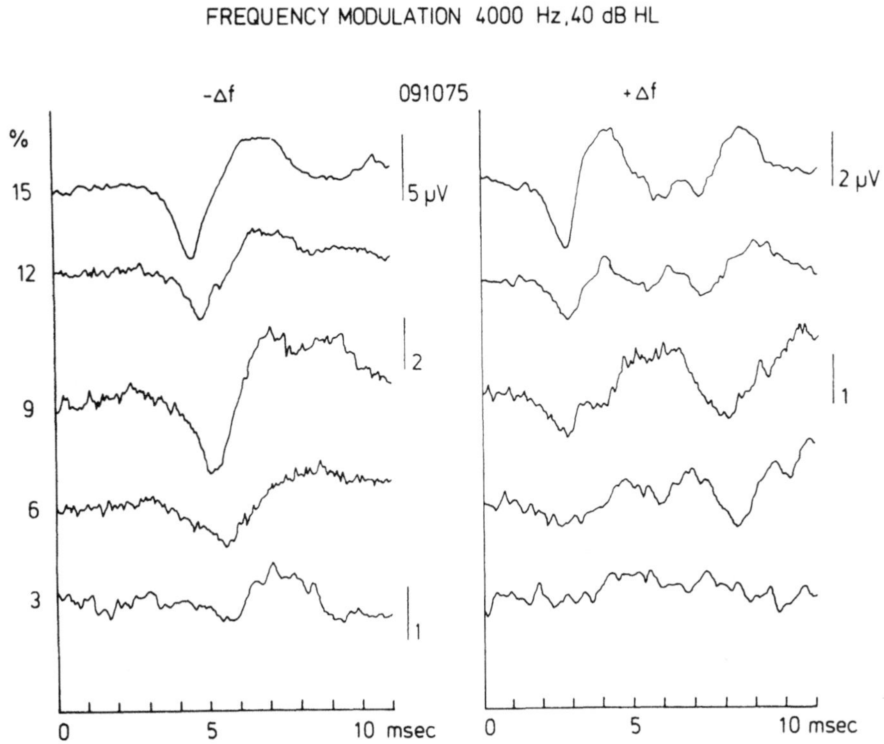

Fig. 46. Complex AP responses to upward and downward modulation in frequency for a 4000 Hz continuous tone at 40 dB HL. The amplitude depends on the depth of the modulation as well as on the direction of the modulation. Modulations downward in frequency evoke larger APs than upward modulations. The latencies also differ according to the type of modulation

to 8000 Hz), the amplitude of the responses was extremely large (up to 50 μV at 90 dB HL) which is very favourable for studying responses at low intensity values. The $-\Delta f$ series shows APs with latencies ranging from 4.5 msec to about 6 msec, for modulation depths of 15% and 3%, while the $+\Delta f$ series has considerable shorter latencies (3 to 4 msec) for the first peak. The AP amplitudes appear to be larger for the modulation downward in frequency than for the upward modulation. This seems to be related to the asymmetry in the low and high frequency slopes of the excitation profile of a continuous tone.

To investigate the frequency specificity of FM-stimuli, the high-pass noise masking technique has been applied, and the obtained narrow-band responses are shown in Fig. 47. It is observed that the main contributions to the AP arise from the 3.5 and 2.6 kHz regions, *i.e.*, below the 4 kHz tone as expected for a downward modulation. There are also contributions from the 5.2 and 6.8 kHz regions. It seems, therefore, that FM stimuli excite somewhat larger areas on the cochlear partition at a given hearing level than tonebursts. One additional feature of FM stimuli may be seen in the study of summating potentials as a function of frequency. If one adjusts the tone frequency to the edge of a region where the sign of

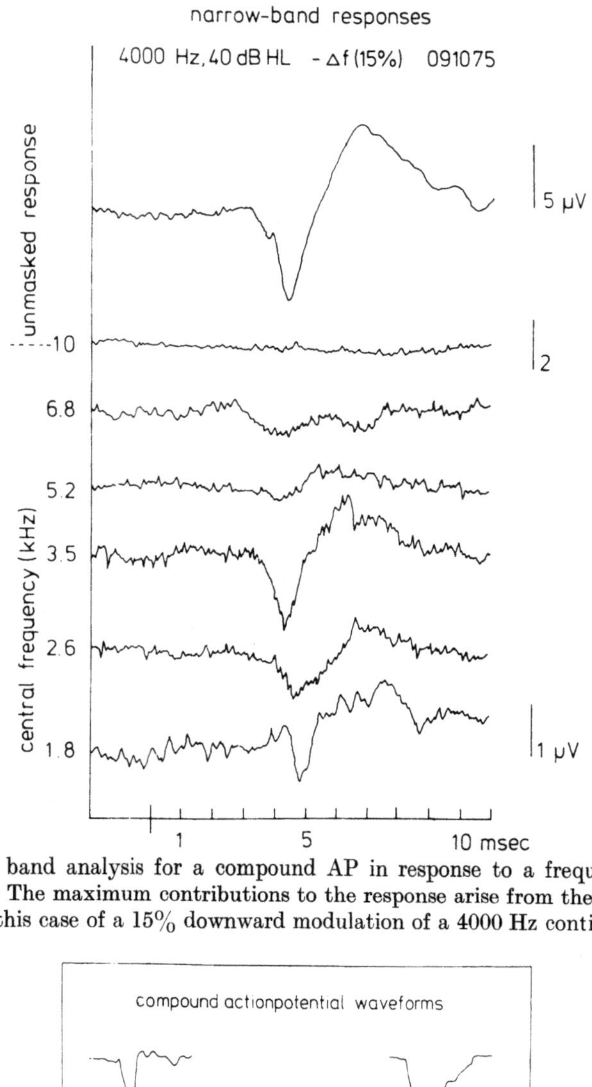

Fig. 47. Narrow band analysis for a compound AP in response to a frequency modulated continuous tone. The maximum contributions to the response arise from the 3.5 and 2.6 kHz regions in this case of a 15% downward modulation of a 4000 Hz continuous tone

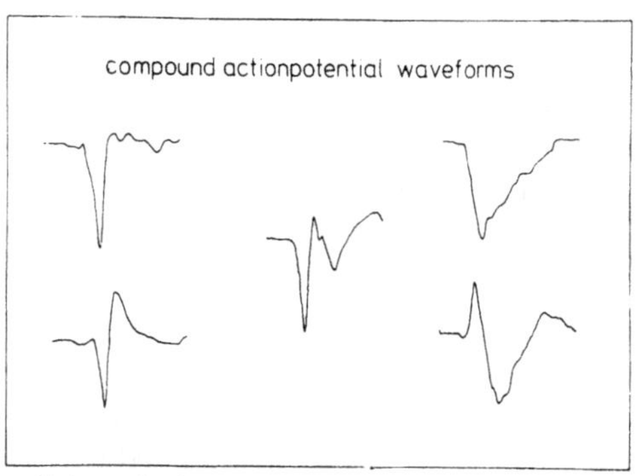

Fig. 48. Wave forms for click evoked compound action potentials. According to the Bordeaux group, one may consider five classes of compound action potentials; these are the normal type (upperleft), the recruiting type (lower left), the dissociated type (centre), the broad type (upper right) and the abnormal type (lower right). (After ARAN *et al.*, 1971a)

the SP changes, an upward ($+\Delta f$) modulation results in a large SP^+, whereas a $-\Delta f$ results in an SP^-. It seems worthwhile to elaborate some more on this type of stimulus, although at the moment no clear applications are seen.

C. The Waveform of the Compound Action Potential

Considerable attention is paid to click-evoked AP wave forms, which are an essential part of the diagnosis system advocated by the Bordeaux group (*e.g.* Aran *et al.*, 1971 a). These waveforms are differentiated into normal responses, recruiting responses, dissociated responses, broad responses, and abnormal responses (Fig. 48). The normal responses are found in normal cochleas, the recruiting and dissociated types in ears showing cochlear damage, the broad and abnormal types in, *e.g.*, Menière's disease and acoustic neuromas. These typical wave forms and their presumed reflection of the underlying disturbances in the peripheral hearing organ can be studied more thoroughly by using the narrow-band response derivation described in Section IV.C. For the normal responses, such an analysis has been shown in Fig. 20. The narrow-band contributions are essentially diphasic up to a central frequency of 6.8 kHz, at which frequency a small but distinct second negative deflection is seen. The first peak of the compound AP corresponds to synchronized firings from narrow-bands with high central frequencies; the second peak, much smaller and with a latency of 4–5 msec, is composed of narrow-band contributions from the low-frequency side. The whole cochlear region in between adds up to the small positivity between both peaks. The normal AP response to clicks is obtained by adding responses from all narrow bands along the cochlear partition; each narrow-band corresponds to about 3 mm (Fig. 21) length on the basilar membrane.

If electrocochleography is performed for an ear having a flat cochlear hearing loss, the relative dominance of the basal turn in the contributions to the click-evoked AP (*cf.* Fig. 21) will be much more pronounced, and there will be less or no contribution from regions below a central frequency of 2 kHz. This means that there will be only partial cancellation of the positivity of each narrow-band waveform at, *e.g.*, central frequencies of 3.5 kHz and 2.6 kHz, and there will be no contribution to a second negative peak with a latency around 4 to 5 msec. The result will be a pronounced diphasic AP, reflecting the diphasic nature of the narrow-band contributions. This may be an explanation for the finding of this type of "recruiting response" in patients with a flat cochlear hearing loss.

The third type of waveform – the dissociated response – is found in cochleas showing only a partial hearing loss, *e.g.*, restricted to the high frequencies or a small notch at 4 kHz. An example of a dissociated type of AP elicited by a click stimulus is shown in Fig. 49 for an intensity of 60 dB p.e. SPL corresponding to 40 dB SL. It is observed that this AP closely resembles the typical example from Fig. 48. A narrow-band analysis shows that the responses to two narrow-bands with central frequencies of 2.6 kHz and 3.5 kHz do not contribute to the compound AP. So there is a well synchronized contribution from the responses elicited in regions of the cochlea located in a basal direction from the site of damage (*i.e.*, the 5.2 and 6.8 kHz regions) and a contribution also originating in a region nearer the apex than the damaged area. The high-frequency fibre group gives rise to the sharp N_1; the low frequency fibres contribute to the second peak. The loss of the contributions from two narrow-bands results in less cancelling of the second peak than is the case in a normal ear (*cf.* Fig. 20).

The broad type of response may result from different mechanisms. It is often found in ears of Menière patients, but it is also found in cases of acoustic neuromas

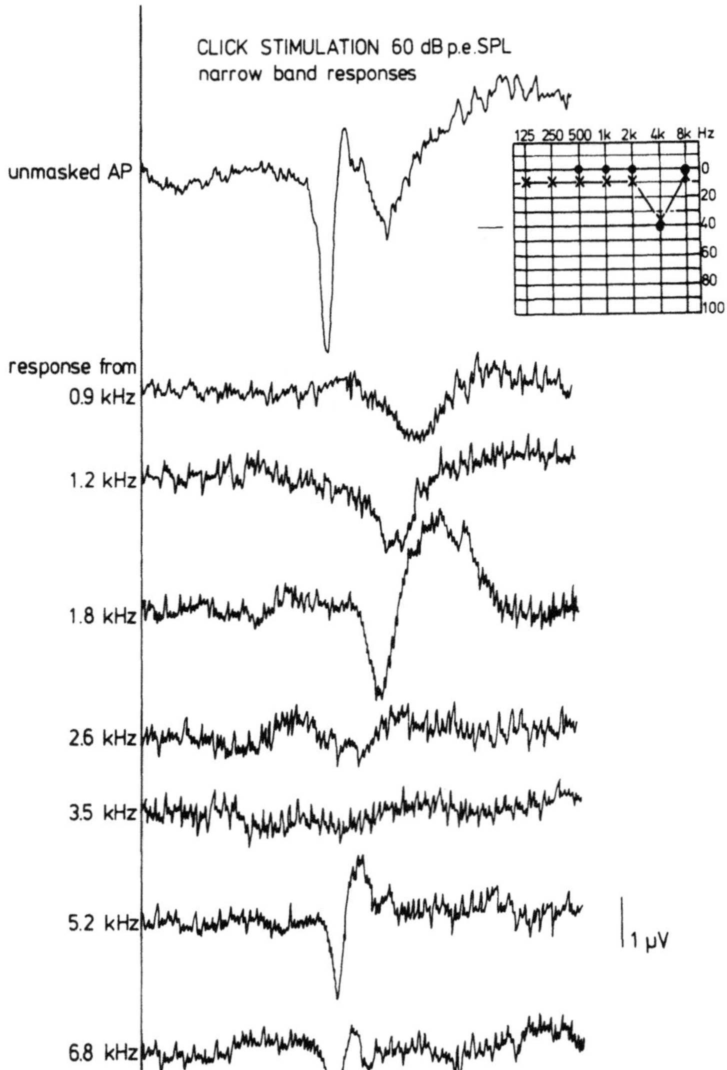

Fig. 49. Narrow-band analysis for a dissociated response. For an audiogram showing a notch at 4000 Hz, 40 dB HL, a click intensity of 40 dB SL (*i.e.* 60 dB p.e. SPL) is used. The narrow band analysis reveals that for the central frequency of 3.5 kHz no contribution to the AP is found and that the 2.6 kHz region also contributes very little. The dissociated type of response, therefore, originates from two well separated regions: one for the higher central frequencies and one for the lower

A considerable difference in the building up of such a broad waveform may exist. The first example in Fig. 50 shows four broad-type waveforms as recorded in Menière ears; the example, 180375, looks exactly like that shown in Fig. 48. It is shown that subtracting the waveform recorded for an ISI of only 4 msec, for which

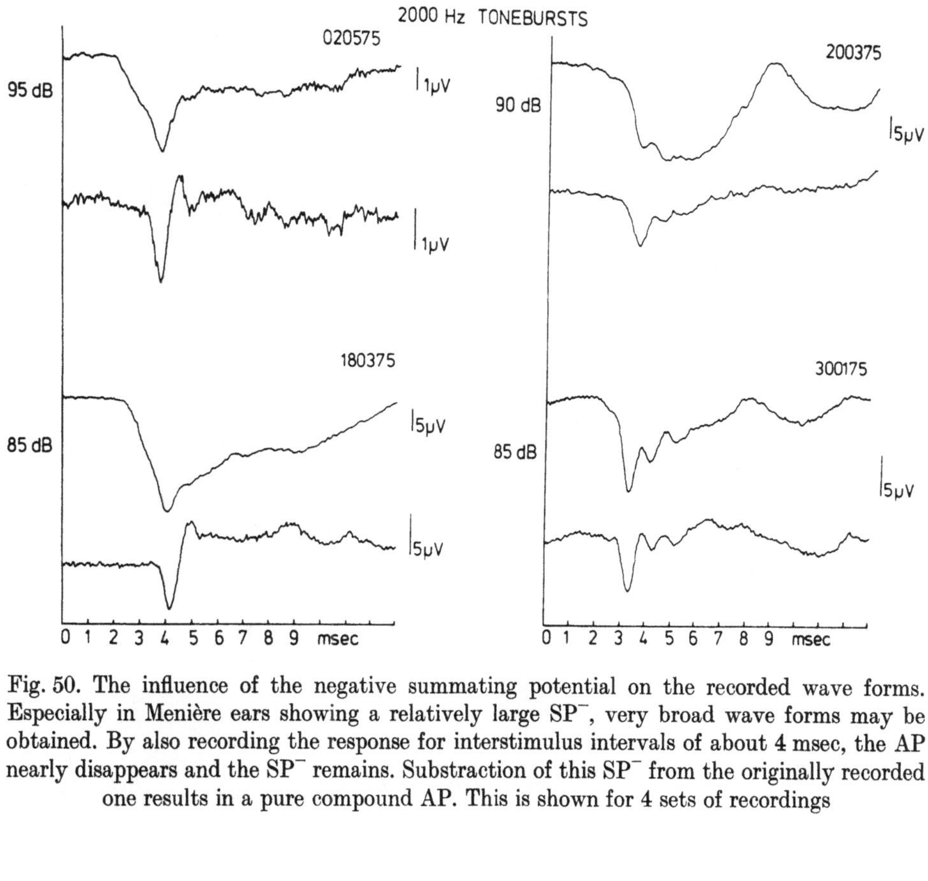

Fig. 50. The influence of the negative summating potential on the recorded wave forms. Especially in Menière ears showing a relatively large SP^-, very broad wave forms may be obtained. By also recording the response for interstimulus intervals of about 4 msec, the AP nearly disappears and the SP^- remains. Substraction of this SP^- from the originally recorded one results in a pure compound AP. This is shown for 4 sets of recordings

the compound AP nearly disappeared while the SP^- is unaffected, results in a recruiting type of response. This is also the case in the upper left example. Therefore, this broad type of response may be due to the relatively large SP^-, which is found so often in Menière ears. The same may be the case for the abnormal type of response where an early positive peak is seen. This may be explained by the mechanism illustrated in Fig. 9a, b in the section on summating potentials (III. B.).

In some cases, especially in Menière's disease, the waveform of the AP is often characterized by distinct N_1, N_2, N_3 peaks not found in normal ears. An example is presented in Fig. 51. The responses to narrow band stimuli contribute uniformly to the compound AP; some localization of the SP^- contributing regions can also be obtained (*i.e.*, 1.8–3.5 kHz regions). The low frequency contributions are only slightly diphasic, but a characteristic narrow band response for the 5.2 kHz region showing clear N_1, N_2 components is found. This is not usually observed in normal ears, in ears with hair-cell lesions (*e.g.* Fig. 49), and is reduced for stimuli with higher central frequencies (*cf.* Fig. 20). This may be the explanation for the occurrence of distinct N_1, N_2, N_3 peaks in the compound AP for Menière ears. One may also speculate that it reflects some hyperexcitability of the auditory nerve: the N_2 peak in the narrow band response may represent repeated firing of the fibres within that narrow-band.

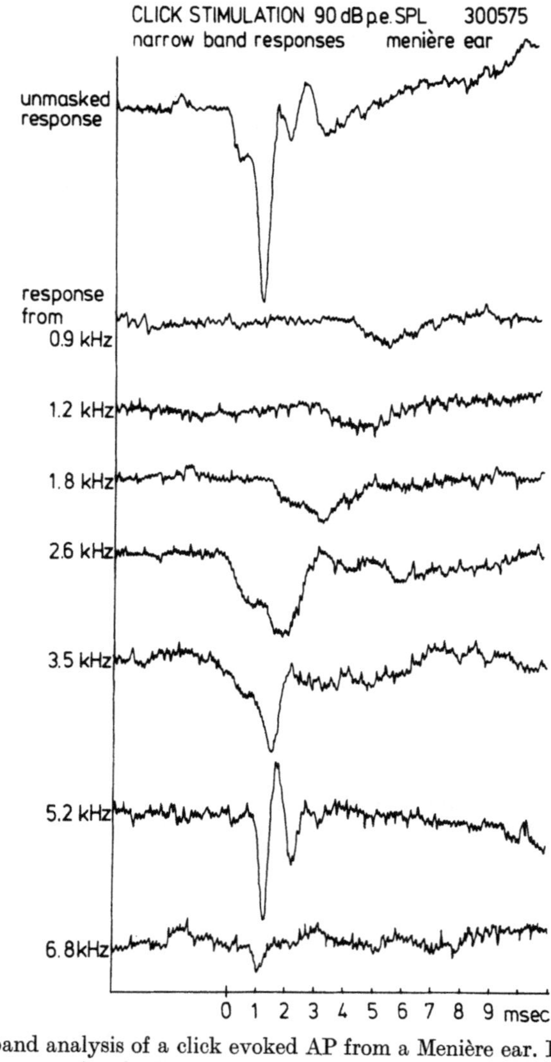

Fig. 51. Narrow band analysis of a click evoked AP from a Menière ear. Besides the presence of the SP^- in the narrow band APs, a quite typical phenomenon found in Menière ears is the triphasic narrow band response for the 5.2 kHz central frequency. This may explain the N_1, N_2, N_3 like appearance of the compound AP wave form

The broad and abnormal types of response are also found patents with acoustic neuromas. As can be observed from Fig. 52, there is only a very modest negative summating potential in the unmasked click response. Therefore, the summating potential cannot be the explanation for the occurrence of the broad response in this case. A narrow band analysis reveals that the contributions to the compound AP are no longer diphasic; they are strictly monophasic. As a result, there will no longer be any cancellation of contributions from intermediate central frequencies, and this leads to a very broad compound AP. The N_1-peak, which is still clearly present, reflects also in this case the activity of the fibres with high central frequencies (*e.g.* the **6.8** and **10 kHz** regions), the N_2 corresponds with the **3.5 kHz** region, while the end of the response corresponds with narrow-band contributions from around **500–900 Hz**. The essential difference between the broad type of

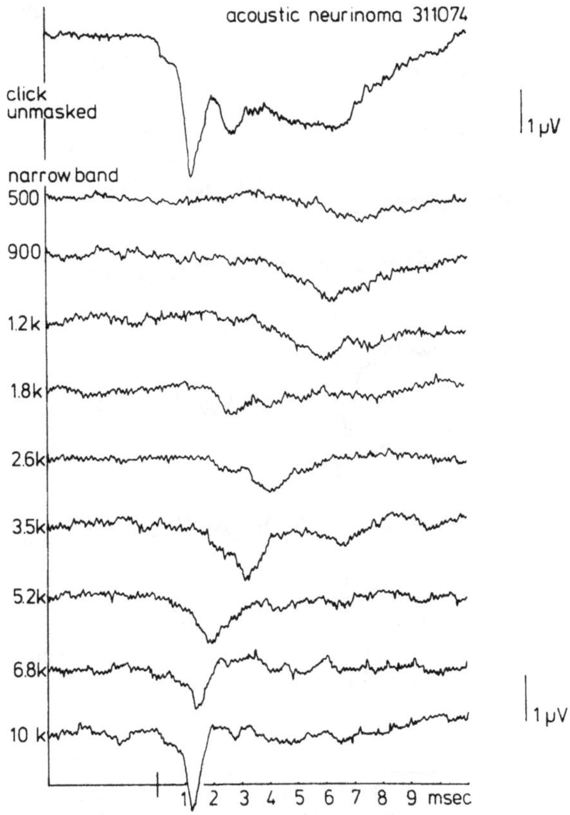

Fig. 52. Narrow band analysis of a click evoked AP in a case of an acoustic neuroma. The broad type compound AP can be built up from monophasic narrow band contributions; this does not occur for either normal ears or Menière ears

response found to Menière ears (*cf.* Fig. 50) and in cases of acoustic neuroma can only be discovered by using either the narrow-band derivation technique or by substracting the SP^- from the recordings. Since the pattern of complaints may be largely the same in Menière ears and acoustic neuromas, the use of both methods is advisable. In addition, it is also possible to distinguish between a pontine angle neuroma pressing against the pons and, *e.g.*, an axial pons tumor. In the first case, in which no hearing was present in the ear, the narrow-band waveforms (Fig. 52) differ essentially from those obtained in the second case, also without hearing. The responses (Fig. 53) are not different from those found in normal cochleas, and the conclusion that the auditory nerve was not affected by the tumor seems justified in this case. One may speculate to a large extent about the potential use of the narrow band contribution wave forms just as has been and still is done about the compound AP waveform. It is first necessary to perform an extensive survey of all types of narrow band contributions which occur and to what extent the experiment influences the results obtained. Although the narrow band contribution can be related to phenomena on the single-nerve-fibre level more easily than is the case with compound waveforms, the problem has actually only been transferred to a

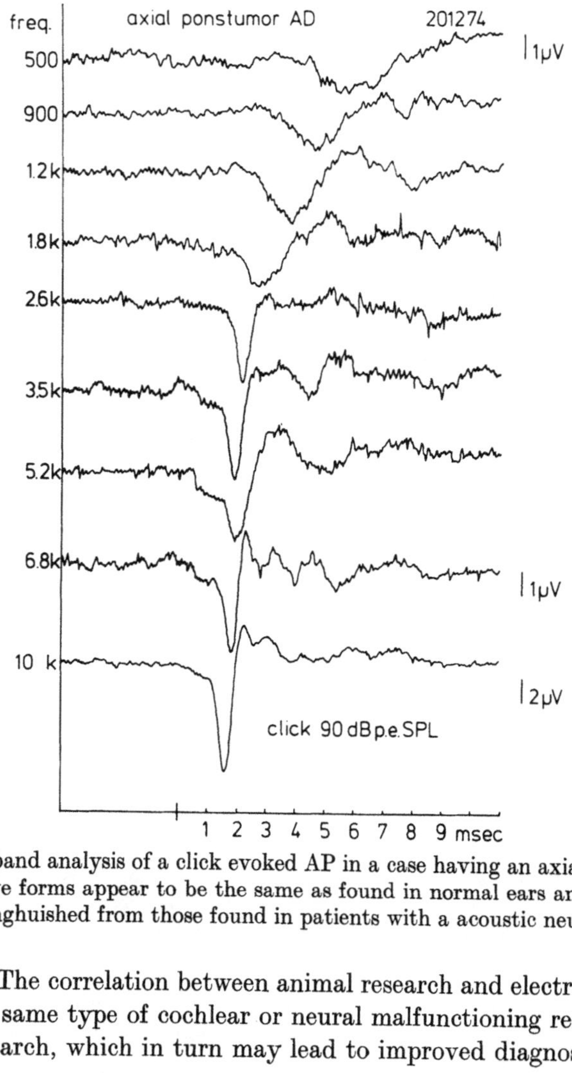

Fig. 53. Narrow-band analysis of a click evoked AP in a case having an axial ponstumor. The narrow band wave forms appear to be the same as found in normal ears and are quite easily distinghuished from those found in patients with a acoustic neuroma

different level. The correlation between animal research and electrocochleography concerning the same type of cochlear or neural malfunctioning remains the basis for further research, which in turn may lead to improved diagnosis.

Acknowledgements. The preparation of this chapter was supported in part by the Netherlands Organization for the Advancement of Pure Research (ZWO) and by the Heinsius-Houbolt Fund.

References

ANDREEV, A. M., ARAPOVA, A. A., GERSUNI, G. V.: On the cochlear potentials in man. Biul. Eksp. Biol. Med. (USSR) **6**, 495—496 (1938).

ARAN, J. M.: Value of cochlear microphonic recordings. In: RUBEN, R. J., SALOMON, G., ELBERLING, C. (Eds.): Proc. symposium on electrocochleography. 1974 (in press).

ARAN, J. M., CHARLET DE SAUVAGE, R., PELERIN, J.: Comparaison des seuils électrocochléographiques et de l'audiogramme. Etude Statistique. Rev. Laryngol. (Bordeaux) **92**, 477—491 (1971 b).

ARAN, J. M., NEGREVERGNE, M.: Clinical study of some particular pathological patterns of eight nerve responses in the human being. Audiology **12**, 488—503 (1973).

ARAN, J. M., PELERIN, J., LENOIR, J., PORTMANN, CL., DARROUZET, J.: Aspects theoretiques et pratiques des enregistrements électrocochleographiques selon la methode établie à Bordeaux. Rev. Laryngol. (Bordeaux) Suppl. **92**, 601—644 (1971a).

ARAN, J. M., PORTMANN, CL., PELERIN, J.: Electrocochléogramme chez l'adulte et chez l'enfant. Audiology **11**, 77 (1972).

BEAGLEY, H. A.: Can we use the cochlear microphonic in electrocochleography. Rev. Laryngol. (Bordeaux) **95**, 531—536 (1974).

BEAGLEY, H. A.: Electrocochleography in the diagnosis of acoustic neuroma. Symposium on electrical evoked response audiometry. Milan: Amplaid 1975.

v. BÉKÉSY, G.: Experiments in hearing. New York: McGraw-Hill 1960.

v. BÉKÉSY, G.: Hearing theories and complex sounds. J. acoust. Soc. Amer. **35**, 588—601 (1963).

DE BOER, E.: Correlation studies applied to the frequency resolution of the cochlea. J. Auditory Res. **7**, 209—217 (1967).

DE BOER, E.: Synthetic whole-nerve action potentials. J. acoust. Soc. Amer. **58**, 1030—1045 (1975).

BORDLEY, J. E., RUBEN, R. J., LIEBERMAN, A. T.: Human cochlear potentials. Laryngoscope **74**, 463—479 (1964).

BRACKMANN, D. E.: Electrocochleographic study of Menière's disease and in Acoustic neuromas. In: RUBEN, R. J., SALOMON, G., ELBERLING, C. (Eds.): Proc. symposium on electrocochleography. 1974 (in press).

COATS, A. C.: On electrocochleographic electrode design. J. acoust. Soc. Amer. **56**, 708—711 (1974).

COATS, A. C., DICKEY, J. R.: Non surgical recording of human auditory nerve action potentials and cochlear microphonics. Ann. Otol. **79**, 844—852 (1970).

COATS, A. C., DICKEY, J. R.: Post masking recovery of human click action potentials and click loudness. J. acoust. Soc. Amer. **52**, 1607—1612 (1972).

CROWLEY, D. E., DAVIS, H., BEAGLEY, H. A.: Survey of the clinical use of electrocochleography. Ann. Otol. **84**, 297—307 (1975).

CULLEN, J. K., ELLIS, M. S., BERLIN, C. I., LOUSTEAU, R. J.: Human acoustic nerve action potential recording from the tympanic membrane without anaesthesia. Acta oto-laryng. (Stockh.) **74**, 15—22 (1972).

DALLOS, P., BILLONE, M. C., DURRANT, J. D., WANG CHANG-YANG, RAYNOR, S.: Cochlear inner and outer haircells: functional differences. Science **177**, 356—358 (1972a).

DALLOS, P., SCHOENY, Z. G., CHEATHAM, M. A.: Cochlear summating potentials: Descriptive aspects. Acta oto-laryng. (Stockh.) Suppl. **302** (1972b).

DAVIS, H.: Mechanisms of excitation of auditory nerve impulses. In: RASMUSSEN, G. L., WINDLE, W. F. (Eds.): Neural mechanisms of the auditory and vestibular systems, Chap. 2. Springfield: Thomas 1960.

DAVIS, H., DERBYSHIRE, A. J., LURIE, M. H., SAUL, L. J.: The electric response of the cochlea. Amer. J. Physiol. **107**, 311—332 (1934).

DERBYSHIRE, A. J., DAVIS, H.: The action potentials of the auditory nerve. Amer. J. Physiol. **113**, 476—504 (1935).

DURRANT, J. D., DALLOS, P.: Comparison of effects of biasing the cochlear partition with electrical current and sound stimulation on the DIF SP responses. J. acoust. Soc. Amer. **53**, 325 (1973).

EGGERMONT, J. J.: Summating potentials in electrocochleography. Relation to hearing pathology. In: RUBEN, R. J., SALOMON, G., ELBERLING, C. (Eds.): Proc. symposium on electrocochleography. 1974 (in press).

EGGERMONT, J. J.: Analysis of compound action potential responses to tonebursts in the human and guinea pig cochlea. J. acoust. Soc. Amer. (To be published, 1976a.)

EGGERMONT, J. J.: Electrocochleography and recruitment. Ann. Otol. (To be published 1976b.)

EGGERMONT, J. J., ODENTHAL, D. W.: Electrophysiological investigation of the human cochlea. Audiology 13. 1—22, **1974**a

Eggermont, J. J., Odenthal, D. W.: Action potentials and summating potentials in the normal human cochlea. Acta oto-laryng. (Stockh.) Suppl. **316**, 39—61 (1974b).

Eggermont, J. J., Odenthal, D. W.: Frequency selective masking in electrocochleography. Rev. Laryngol. (Bordeaux) **95**, 489—496 (1974c).

Eggermont, J. J., Odenthal, D. W., Schmidt, P. H., Spoor, A.: Electrocochleography. Basic principles and clinical application. Acta oto-laryng. (Stockh.) Suppl. **316**, (1974a).

Eggermont, J. J., Spoor, A., Odenthal, D. W.: Frequency specificity of toneburst electrocochleography. In: Ruben, R. J., Salomon, G., Elberling, C. (Eds.): Proc. symposium on electrocochleography. 1974b (in press).

Eggermont, J. J., Spoor, A.: Cochlear adaptation in guinea pigs. A quantitative description. Audiology **12**, 193—220 (1973).

Elberling, C.: Transitions in cochlear action potentials recorded from the ear canal in man. Scand. Audiol. **2**, 151—159 (1973).

Elberling, C.: Action potentials along the cochlear partition recorded from the ear canal in man. Scand. Audiol. **3**, 13—19 (1974a).

Elberling, C.: Simulation of cochlear action potentials recorded from the ear canal in man. In: Ruben, R. J., Salomon, G., Elberling, C. (Eds.): Proc. symposium on electrocochleography. 1974b (in press).

Elberling, C.: Deconvolution of action potentials recorded from the ear canal in man. Proc. Second British Conference on Audiology. 1975, in press.

Elberling, C.: Salomon, G.: Electrical potentials from the inner ear in man, in response to transient sounds generated in a closed acoustic system. Rev. Laryngol. (Bordeaux) Suppl. **92**, 691—708 (1971).

Elberling, C., Salomon, G.: Cochlear microphonics recorded from the ear canal in man. Acta oto-laryng. (Stockh.) **75**, 489—495 (1973).

Evans, E. F.: The frequency response and other properties of single fibres in the guinea pig cochlear nerve. J. Physiol. (Lond.) **226**, 263—287 (1972).

Evans, E. F.: Auditory frequency selectivity and the cochlear nerve. In: Zwicker, E., Terhardt, E. (Eds.): Facts and models in hearing. Berlin-Heidelberg-New York: Springer 1974.

Evans, E. F.: The sharpening of cochlear frequency selectivity in the normal and abnormal cochlea. Audiology **14**, 419—442 (1975).

Fromm, B., Nylen, C. O., Zotterman, Y.: Studies in the mechanism of the Wever and Bray effect. Acta oto-laryng. (Stockh.) **22**, 477—486 (1935).

Goldstein, M., Kiang, N. Y. S.: Synchrony of neural activity in electric responses evoked by transient acoustic stimuli. J. acoust. Soc. Amer. **30**, 107—114 (1958).

Goldstein, J. L., Baer, T., Kiang, N. Y. S.: A theoretical treatment of latency, group delay and tuning characteristics for auditory nerve responses to clicks and tones. In: Sachs, M. B. (Ed.): The physiology of the auditory system. Baltimore: National Educational Consultants Inc., 1971.

Hermans, J., Eggermont, J. J., Hagedooren, J., Odenthal, D. W.: Probabilistic differential diagnosis of auditory dysfunction on the basis of electrocochleography. Meth. Inform. Med. **14**, 87—95 (1975).

Hoke, M., v. Bally, G., Landwehr, F. J.: Objektiv ermittelte Funktion des menschlichen Innenohres im gesamten Frequenzbereich mit Hilfe eines zusammengesetzten Schallsignals. Arch. klin. exp. Ohr.-Nas.-Kehlk.-Heilk. **202**, 516—521 (1972).

Jonstone, B. M.: Personal communication, 1975.

Keidel, W. D.: The use of quick correlators in electrocochleography both in oto-audiography (OAG) and in neuro-audiography (NAG). Rev. Laryng. (Bordeaux) Suppl. 709—720 (1971).

Kiang, N. Y. S.: A survey of recent developments in the study of auditory physiology. Ann. Otol. **77**, 656—675 (1968).

Kiang, N. Y. S., Moxon, E. C.: Tails of tuning curves of auditory nerve fibres. J. acoust. Soc. Amer. **55**, 620—630 (1974).

Kiang, N. Y. S., Moxon, E. C., Kahn, A. R.: The relationship of gross potentials recorded from the cochlea to single unit activity in the auditory nerve. In: Ruben, R. J., Salomon, G., Elberling, C. (Eds.): Proc. symposium on electrocochleography. 1974 (in press).

KIANG, N. Y. S., MOXON, E. C., LEVINE, R. A.: Auditory nerve activity in cats with normal and abnormal cochleas. In: WOLSTENHOLME, G. E. W., KNIGHT, J. (Eds.): Sensorineural hearing loss. London: J. & A. Churchill 1970.

KIANG, N. Y. S., WATANABE, T., THOMAS, E. C., CLARK, L. F.: Discharge patterns of single fibres in the cats auditory nerve. Cambridge, Mass.: M.I.T. Press 1965.

KOHLLÖFFEL, L. U. E.: Studies on the distribution of cochlear potentials along the basilar membrane. Acta oto-laryng. (Stockh.) Suppl. 288 (1971).

KUPPERMAN, R.: The dynamic dc potential in the cochlea of the guinea pig (summating potential). Acta oto-laryng. (Stockh.) **62**, 465—480 (1966).

KUPPERMAN, R.: The SP in connection with movements of the basilar membrane. In: PLOMP, R., SMOORENBURG, G. F. (Eds.): Frequency analysis and periodicity detection in hearing. Leiden: Sijthoff 1970.

LEMPERT, J., WEVER, E. G., LAWRENCE, M.: The cochleogram and its clinical application. Arch. Otolaryng. **45**, 61—67 (1947).

LEMPERT, J., MELTZER, P. E., WEVER, E. G., LAWRENCE, M.: The cochleogram and its clinical application: Concluding observations. Arch. Otolaryng. **51**, 307—311 (1950).

LEV, A., SOHMER, H.: Sources of averaged neural responses recorded in animal and human subjects during cochlear audiometry (electrocochleogram). Arch. klin. exp. Ohr., Nas- u. Kehlk.-Heilk. **201**, 79—90 (1972).

MONTANDON, B., MCGILL, N. D., KAHN, A. R., PEAKE, W. T., KIANG, N. Y. S.: Recording auditory nerve potentials as an office procedure. Ann. Otol. **84**, 2—10 (1975a).

MONTANDON, B., SHEPARD, N. T., MASS, E. M., PEAKE, W. T., KIANG, N. Y. S.: Auditory nerve potentials from ear canals of patients with otological problems. Ann. Otol. **84**, 164—173 (1975b).

MØLLER, A. R.: Transfer function of the middle ear. J. acoust. Soc. Amer. **35**, 1516—1534 (1963).

MORRISON, D., SCHINDLER, R. A., WERSÄLL, J.: A quantitative analysis of the afferent innervation of the organ of Corti in guinea pig. Acta oto-laryng. (Stockh.) **79**, 11—23 (1975).

NEDZELNITSKY, V.: Measurement of sound pressure in the cochleae of anaesthetized cats. In: ZWICKER, E., TERHARDT, E. (Eds.): Facts and models in hearing. Berlin-Heidelberg-New York: Springer 1975.

ODENTHAL, D. W., EGGERMONT, J. J.: Clinical electrocochleography. Acta oto-laryng. (Stockh.) Suppl. **316**, 62—74 (1974a).

ODENTHAL, D. W., EGGERMONT, J. J.: Electrocochleographic study of Menière's disease and pontine angle neurinoma. In: RUBEN, R. J., SALOMON, G., ELBERLING, C. (Eds.): Proc. symposium on electrocochleography. 1974b, in press.

ODENTHAL, D. W., EGGERMONT, J. J., HERMANS, J.: Diagnosis by electrocochleography. Rev. Laryngol. (Bordeaux) **95**, 481—488 (1974).

PERLMAN, H. B., CASE, T. J.: Electrical phenomena of the cochlea in man. Arch. Otolaryng. **34**, 710—718 (1941).

PORTMANN, M., ARAN, J. M.: Relations entre pattern cochléographique et pathologie retrolabyrinthique. Acta oto-laryng. (Stockh.) **73**, 190—196 (1972).

PORTMANN, M., ARAN, J. M., LAGOURGE, P.: Testing for "recruitment" by electrocochleography. Ann. Otol. **82**, 36—43 (1973).

PORTMANN, M., LE BERT, G., ARAN, J. M.: Potentiels cochléaires obtenus chez l'homme en dehors de toute intervention chirurgicale. Rev. Laryng. (Bordeaux) 88, 157—164 (1967).

PORTMANN, M., NEGREVERGNE, M.: Apport de l'electrocochleographie dans l'examen audiometrique de l'enfant. Rev. Laryngol. **94**, 359—379 (1973).

RONIS, B. J.: Cochlear potentials in otosclerosis. Laryngoscope **76**, 212—231 (1966).

ROSENBLITH, W. A., ROSENZWEIG, M. R.: Electrical responses to acoustic click. Influence of electrode location in cats. J. acoust. Soc. Amer. **23**, 583—588 (1951).

RUBEN, R. J.: Cochlear potentials as a diagnostic test in deafness. Sensorineural Hearing Processes and Disorders. Boston: Little-Brown 1967.

RUBEN, R. J., BORDLEY, J. E., LIEBERMAN, A. T.: Cochlear potentials in man. Laryngoscope **71**, 1141—1164 (1961).

RUBEN, R. J., KNICKERBOCKER, G. G., SEKULA, J., NAGER, G. T., BORDLEY, J. E.: Cochlear microphonics in man: A preliminary report. Laryngoscope **69**, 665—671 (1959).

RUBEN, R. J., LIEBERMAN, A. T., BORDLEY, J. E.: Some observations on cochlear potentials and nerve action potentials in children. Laryngoscope **72**, 545—554 (1962).

RUBEN, R. J., SEKULA, J., BORDLEY, J. E., KNICKERBOCKER, G. G., NAGER, T. G., FISCH, U.: Human cochlear responses to sound stimuli. Ann. Otol. **69**, 459—479 (1960).

RUBEN, R. J., WALKER, A. E.: The VIIIth nerve action potential in Menière's disease. Laryngoscope **73**, 1456—1461 (1963).

SALOMON, G., ELBERLING, C.: Cochlear nerve potentials recorded from the ear canal in man. Acta oto-laryng. (Stockh.) **71**, 319—325 (1971).

SCHMIDT, P. H., EGGERMONT, J. J., ODENTHAL, D. W.: Study of Menière's disease by electrocochleography. Acta oto-laryng. (Stockh.) Suppl. **316**, 75—84 (1974).

SCHMIDT, P. H., ODENTHAL, D. W., EGGERMONT, J. J., SPOOR, A.: Electrocochleographic study of a case of Lermoyez's syndrome. Acta oto-laryng. (Stockh.) **79**, 287—291 (1975).

SOHMER, H., FEINMESSER, M.: Cochlear action potentials recorded from the external ear in man. Ann. Otol. **76**, 427—435 (1967).

SOHMER, H., FEINMESSER, M.: Routine use of electrocochleography (cochlear audiometry) on human subjects. Audiology **12**, 167—173 (1973).

SOHMER, H., FEINMESSER, M., BAUBERGER-TELL, L., LEV, A., DAVID, S.: Routine use of cochlear audiometry in infants with uncertain diagnosis. Ann. Otol. **81**, 72—75 (1972).

SPOENDLIN, H.: Structural basis of peripheral frequency analysis. In: PLOMP, R., SMOORENBURG, G. (Eds.): Frequency analysis and periodicity detection in hearing. Leiden: Sijthoff 1970.

SPOOR, A.: Apparatus for electrocochleography. Acta oto-laryng. (Stockh.) Suppl. **316**, 25—36 (1974).

SPOOR, A., EGGERMONT, J. J.: Electrocochleography as a method for objective audiogram determination. In: HIRSH, I. J.; ELDREDGE, D. H. and SILVERMAN, S. R. (Eds): Hearing and Davis. St. Louis, Mo.: Eden Publ. Cie. 1976.

SPOOR, A., EGGERMONT, J. J., ODENTHAL, D. W.: Comparison of human and animal data concerning adaptation and masking of eight nerve compound action potential. In: RUBEN, R. J., SALOMON, G., ELBERLING, C. Proc. symposium of electrocochleography. 1974, in press.

SPRENG, M., KEIDEL, W. D.: Separierung von Cerebroaudiogram (CAG), Neuroaudiogram (NAG) und Otoaudiogram (OAG) in der objektiven Audiometrie. Arch. klin. exp. Ohr-, Nas-. u. Kehlk.-Heilk. **189**, 225—246 (1967).

STEPHENS, S. D. G., CHARLET DE SAUVAGE, R., ARAN, J. M.: Adaptation de l'electrcochleogramme: note preliminaire. Rev. Laryng. (Bordeaux) **95**, 129—138 (1974).

STEPHENS, S. D. G., CHARLET DE SAUVAGE, R., ARAN, J. M.: Gross responses from the cochlear nerve in man and in the guinea pig. Symp. Zool. Soc. Lond. **37**, 167—186 (1975).

TASAKI, I., DAVIS, H., LEGOUIX, J. P.: The space time pattern of the cochlear microphonic (guinea pig) as recorded by differential electrodes. J. acoust. Soc. Amer. **24**, 502—519 (1952).

TASAKI, I., DAVIS, H., ELDREDGE, D. H.: Exploration of cochlear potentials in guinea pig with a microelectrode. J. acoust. Soc. Amer. **26**, 765—773 (1954).

TEAS, D. C., ELDREDGE, D. H., DAVIS, H.: Cochlear responses to acoustic transients: An interpretation of whole nerve action potentials. J. acoust. Soc. Amer. **34**, 1438—1489 (1962).

TERKILDSEN, K., OSTERHAMMEL, P., HUIS IN 'T VELD, F.: Electrocochleography with a far field technique. Scand. Audiol. **2**, 141—148 (1973).

THORNTON, A. R. D.: The measurement of surface-recorded electrocochleographic responses. Scand. Audiol. **4**, 51—58 (1975).

WEVER, E. G., BRAY, C. W.: Auditory nerve impulses. Science **71**, 215 (1930).

WHITFIELD, I. C., ROSS, H. F.: Cochlear microphonic and summating potentials and the outputs of individual haircell generators. J. acoust. Soc. Amer. **38**, 126—131 (1965).

YOSHIE, N.: Auditory nerve action potential responses to clicks in man. Laryngoscope **78**, 198—215 (1968).

YOSHIE, N.: Clinical cochlear response audiometry by means of an average response computer: Non surgical technique and clinical use. Rev. Laryngol. (Bordeaux) Supp. 646—672 (1971).

YOSHIE, N.: Diagnostic significance of the electrocochleogram in clinical audiometry. Audiology **12**, 504—539 (1973).

YOSHIE, N., OHASHI, T.: Clinical use of cochlear nerve action potential responses in man for differential diagnosis of hearing loss. Acta oto-laryng. (Stockh.) Supp. **252**, 71—87 (1969).

YOSHIE, N., OHASHI, T.: Abnormal adaptation of human cochlear nerve action potential responses: Clinical observations by non-surgical recording. Rev. Laryngol. (Bordeaux) Suppl. 673—690 (1971).

YOSHIE, N., OHASHI, T., SUZUKI, T.: Non-surgical recording of auditory nerve action potentials in man. Laryngoscope **77**, 76—85 (1967).

YOSHIE, N., YAMAURA, K.: Cochlear mocrophonic responses to pure tones in man recorded by a nonsurgical method. Acta oto-laryng. (Stockh.) Suppl. **252**, 37—69 (1969).

ZERLIN, S.: Travelling wave velocity in the human cochlea. J. acoust. Soc. Amer. **46**, 1011—1015 (1969).

ZERLIN, S., NAUNTON, R. F.: Physical and auditory specifications of third octave clicks. Audiology **14**, 135—143 (1975).

ZVONAR, M., ZVONAR-KHUNDL, B., ODENTHAL, D. W.: Anaesthesia and sedation for electrocochleography. Acta oto-laryng. (Stockh.) Suppl. **316**, 37—38 (1974).

Additional Bibliography

ARAN, J. M.: The electrocochleogram: Recent results in children and in some pathological cases. Arch. klin. exp. Ohr.-, Nas.- u. Kehlk.-Heilk. **198**, 128—143 (1971).

ARAN, J. M., CHARLET DE SAUVAGE, R., BOUSSENS, J.: Comparaison des réponses normales du nerf auditif chez le cobaye, le singe et l'homme. Rev. Laryng. (Bordeaux) **95**, 31—41 (1974).

ARAN, J. M., PORTMANN, CL., DELAUNAY, J., PELERIN, J., LENOIR, J.: L'électrocochléogramme. Méthodes et premier résultats chez l'enfant. Rev. Laryng. (Bordeaux) **90**, 615—634 (1969).

BALLY, G. v., HOKE, M.: A new method for stimulus generation and signal detection in electrocochleography. Rev. Laryng (Bordeaux) **95**, 502—507 (1974).

BERLIN, C. I., CULLEN, J. K., ELLIS, M. S., LOUSTEAU, R. J., YARBROUGH, W. M., LYONS, G. D.: Clinical application of recording human VIIIth nerve action potentials from the tympanic membrane. Trans. Amer. Acad. Ophth. Otol. **78**, 401—410 (1974).

BEAGLEY, H. A.: The role of electrophysiological tests in the diagnosis of non-organic hearing loss. Audiology **12**, 470—480 (1973).

BOCHENEK, Z., FIALKOWSKA, D., BOCHENEK, W., DAWIDOWICZ, J., JASTREZEBSKI, S.: Four year experience with electric response audiometry. Audiology **13**, 403—407 (1974).

HOKE, M.: Influence of certain stimulus parameters on the compound action potential, as demonstrated at normal subjects and in some pathological cases. Rev. Laryng. (Bordeaux) **95**, 508—514 (1974).

INNITZER, J., BURIAN, K.: Vergleich der tympanale und mastoidaler Ableitung in der Elektrokochleographie. Z. Laryng. Rhinol. **54**, 268—275 (1975).

INNITZER, J.: Die Verwendung von Sinustonreizen mit langen Anstiegszeiten in der klinischen Elektrokochleographie. Z. Laryng. Rhinol. **54**, 470—476 (1975).

INNITZER, J.: Die funktionelle Überlebenszeit des Cortischen Organs beim Menschen nach Durchtrennung des N. acusticus. Z. Laryng. Rhinol. **54**, 490—497 (1975).

KHECHINASHVILI, S. N., KEVANISHVILI, Z. S.: Experiences in computor audiometry (ECoG and ERA). Audiology **13**, 391—402 (1974).

LYONS, G. D., BERLIN, C. I., LOUSTEAU, R. J., ELLIS, M. S., YARBROUGH, W. M.: Electrocochleography with retardates. Laryngoscope **84**, 990—997 (1974).

NAUNTON, R. F., ZERLIN, S.: Human whole-nerve responses to clicks of various frequency. Audiology **15**, 1—9 (1976).

PORTMANN, M., ARAN, J. M.: Electrocochleography. Laryngoscope **81**, 899—910 (1971).

PORTMANN, M., ARAN, J. M.: Electro-cochléographie sur le nourrisson et le jeune enfant. Méthode de l'audiometrie objective. Acta oto-laryng. (Stockh.) **71**, 253—261 (1971).

PORTMANN, M., PORTMANN, CL., NEGREVERGNE, M.: Four years of clinical use of electrocochleography. Rev. Laryng. (Bordeaux) **95**, 537—539 (1974).

SIMMONS, F. BLAIR.: Electrocochleography. Ann. Otol. **83**, 312—313 (1975).

SIMMONS, F. BLAIR: Human auditory nerve responses: a comparison of three commonly used recording sites. Laryngoscope **85**, 1564—1581 (1975).

TYBERGHEIN, J.: Cochleography and recruitment. Rev. Laryng. (Bordeaux) **95**, 588—514 (1974).

Chapter 16

Drug Ototoxicity

J. E. HAWKINS, JR., Ann Arbor, Michigan

With 17 Figures

Contents

I. Introduction

Ototoxicity may be defined as the tendency of certain therapeutic agents and other chemical substances to cause functional impairment and cellular degeneration of the tissues of the inner ear, and especially of the end organs and neurons of the cochlear and vestibular divisions of the VIIIth cranial nerve. Other drugs which may affect hearing or equilibrium by acting primarily on the brainstem nuclei and central pathways of the auditory or vestibular systems may be regarded as neurotoxic, but they can hardly be said to be ototoxic in the strict sense of the word.

By the latter part of the 19th century it was known that certain drugs in common use, notably quinine, the salicyclates, and oil of chenopodium, could produce vestibular disturbances, tinnitus, and temporary or even permanent impairment of hearing (SCHWABACH, 1884; NORTH, 1880). A chapter of WERNER's monograph, *Das Labyrinth* (1940) is devoted to a review of early clinical observations and animal experiments with these and other substances, including the arsenicals, ethyl and methyl alcohol, nicotine, diphtheria and staphylococcus toxins, and salts of lead and mercury. Fortunately these substances seldom pose acute threats to the integrity of the human labyrinth, although the possibility that long-term detrimental effects may be exerted by some of them, in particular the heavy metals and the components of tobacco smoke as environmental pollutants, cannot be dismissed as insignificant.

With the discovery of the antibiotic streptomycin as the first effective chemotherapeutic agent against tuberculosis came the finding that it could cause both disturbance of vestibular function and impairment of hearing (HINSHAW and FELDMAN, 1945). Other aminoglycosides subsequently introduced also proved to be effective against acid-fast or gram-negative organisms, but they often demonstrated an even greater ototoxicity than SM, especially for the cochlea. As they came to be widely used for the treatment and prophylaxis of infections, the problem of drug ototoxicity became a matter of interest and concern both for the clinician and for the investigator of inner ear mechanisms. The later introduction of the potent natriuretic agents ethacrynic acid (Edecrin®) and furosemide (frusemide, Lasix®), with a different form of ototoxicity, has served to reemphasize the peculiar susceptibility of the inner ear to injury by certain classes of drugs.

In this chapter we shall consider first the salicylates and quinine together, because of their historical association and their apparent similarity of action. They will be followed by chenopodium and the arsenicals, as belonging also to the preantibiotic period. Major emphasis will be placed on the ototoxicity of the aminoglycosides and the natriuretics as substances of current importance in both the clinic and the research laboratory. Other drugs with proven or suspected ototoxic action will be considered briefly.

II. The Salicylates and Quinine

The toxic manifestations associated with the salicylates and the cinchona alkaloids are sufficiently striking when fully developed to warrant the special designations *salicylism* and *cinchonism*. Both states are fully described in standard textbooks of pharmacology. Tinnitus and impaired hearing are characteristic effects of these drugs, appearing at a relatively early stage during the treatment of rheumatoid arthritis with salicylates (GRAHAM and PARKER, 1948) or of malaria with quinine (LAVERAN, 1898), and usually subsiding again when the medication is stopped. In most patients they belong, together with nausea and transient vomiting, to the group of symptoms characterized by SMITH and SMITH (1966) as "common but not clinically serious." Experiments on human subjects, such as those of ROOSA (1875), and POHLMAN and KRANZ (1922) with quinine, of MCCABE and DEY (1965) and MYERS and BERNSTEIN (1965) with acetyl salicylic acid, as well as those of FALBE-HANSEN (1941) with both drugs, have tended to confirm this impression of the customary reversibility of the auditory symptoms. For example, MYERS *et al.* (1965) recorded equal losses of 30–40 dB at all frequencies in patients given toxic doses of acetyl salicylic acid. Hearing returned to the pretreatment levels within 2 or 3 days after the drug was withdrawn. Nevertheless, there have been not a few exceptional cases of permanent loss of hearing recorded in the long history of their use in medicine.

MORTON (1696) mentioned temporary deafness as the only ill-effect he had observed during 25 years of treating fevers with cinchona bark. MÊLIER (1843) considered it the most common symptom produced by quinine sulfate and not a matter for concern, since it disappeared again quickly so long as doses were small or moderate. On the other hand, he had seen several patients given larger doses over a long period whose deafness had persisted. Menière, he wrote, had collected a number of similar cases which he planned to publish (apparently he never did so), and Itard had seen examples of the same sort, including one child who had become a deaf-mute as a result of quinine treatment.

Failure to recover from ototoxic hearing loss is also not unknown in patients receiving therapeutic doses of salicylates. SCHWABACH (1884) relates the history of such a case, as well as one in which persistent tinnitus caused by quinine was exacerbated by taking sodium salicylate. KIRCHNER (1883), who used quinine in what was apparently the earliest study of drug ototoxicity in experimental animals, also tells of a rheumatic patient who insisted that her salicylate therapy be stopped because she was convinced that it was ruining her hearing. Her deafness, tinnitus, and occasional dizziness gradually disappeared, but a moderate impairment of hearing remained for some time, alternately improving and worsening. If we can believe what must have been only the patient's subjective report, her case represents a rare instance of a fluctuation in hearing level associated with ototoxicity.

Severe salicylate intoxication from suicide attempts, accidental poisoning, or over-enthusiastic self-medication is all too frequent, but reports of permanent hearing loss in such patients are uncommon (WALTNER, 1955). GIGNOUX *et al.* (1966) describe a case involving a 16-year-old girl with normal hearing who became totally deaf after taking 40 aspirin tablets (12 gm). Recovery of hearing was asymmetrical, with a loss of 65–80 dB persisting in one ear as compared with 20 dB in the other, but no long-term follow-up is presented. JARVIS (1966) also reports an example of permanent unilateral deafness (90 dB at 2 kHz) in a patient who took two or three aspirin tablets every 2 hrs for 3 days after tooth extraction. On the other hand, KAPUR'S (1965) case of profound, sudden deafness in a boy who took only three tablets of aspirin during a minor indisposition seems more reasonably attributable to a viral infection than to the drug itself.

The similarities between the toxic actions of quinine and the salicylates have long been noted, especially the important fact that they both produce disturbances of vision (see GRANT, 1962) as well as of hearing. Their modes of action in the eye and ear have been much discussed, often with special attention to their effects on the blood vessels, but without any general agreement as to the primacy of vascular changes. KIRCHNER (1881) found hemorrhages in the semicircular cannals and the organ of Corti, from which he concluded that these compounds cause vasomotor disturbances affecting the entire labyrinth. ROOSA (1875) had seen vascular congestion in the vessels of the tympanic membrane after quinine and attributed the tinnitus and deafness to a similar "congestion of the terminal fibers of the auditory nerve in the cochlea." GRADENIGO (1892) and WITTMAACK (1903) postulated that the effect of quinine on the inner ear is caused by vasoconstriction similar to the retinal ischemia that is so clearly seen in the eye grounds of quinine-treated animals.

Later investigators have emphasized degenerative changes in the retinal ganglion cells as the primary cause of quinine amaurosis (GRANT, 1962), and loss of outer hair cells of Corti's organ as the cause of the deafness (LURIE, 1940; FALBE-HANSEN, 1941; RÜEDI *et al.*, 1952). COVELL (1936) attributed it to changes in the mitochondria of the stria vascularis and the hair cells, and later (1938) also to vascular stasis and distension in the stria. DE MOURA and HAYDEN (1968) found areas of strial atrophy, with no loss of hair cells beyond that to be expected as a result of aging, in the temporal bones of a 76-year-old woman who had shown a threshold shift during treatment with acetyl salicylic acid for rheumatoid arthritis. Her hearing level had improved by 25 dB after the treatment was stopped.

A. Animal Experiments

After acute injections of sodium salicylate in behaviorally-trained squirrel monkeys, MYERS and BERNSTEIN (1965) measured reversible hearing losses of 17–36 dB which showed reasonable correlation with the plasma salicylate levels, but they could demonstrate no cochlear changes by light or electron microscopy. In cats SILVERSTEIN *et al.* (1967) found a greater drop in the N_1 action potentials (AP) than in the microphonic potentials (CM). There were decreased malic dehydrogenase activity in the endolymph and perilymph and increased concentration of glucose, but no changes in sodium, potassium, or total protein.

HAWKINS (1950) and DAVIS *et al.* (1950), emphasized the acute selective effect of quinine on the cochlear AP response. MITCHELL *et al.* (1973) reported on the similar action of salicylates.

In guinea pigs acutely intoxicated by quinine, its dextrorotatory stereoisomer quinidine, and sodium salicyclate, vasoconstriction has been observed in capillaries of the suprastrial spiral ligament, the stria vascularis, and the tympanic lip and basilar membrane (inner and outer spiral vessels), when examined postmortem in surface preparations of these tissues (Figs. 1 and 2). The changes involve local narrowings of the capillary lumen by endothelial swelling with apparent participation of the pericytes, similar to those found in guinea pigs after noise exposure (HAWKINS, 1967, 1973). Figure 2 shows such an effect of quinidine on the spiral vessels. Similar changes after quinine injection have been demonstrated in vivo by LAWRENCE (1970) in his microcirculatory studies of the guinea pig cochlea. These findings support the inferences of GRADENIGO (1892) and of WITTMAACK (1903) concerning the role of ischemia in the action of quinine on the inner ear, as well as those of BLAU (1904) concerning the similar action of salicylates.

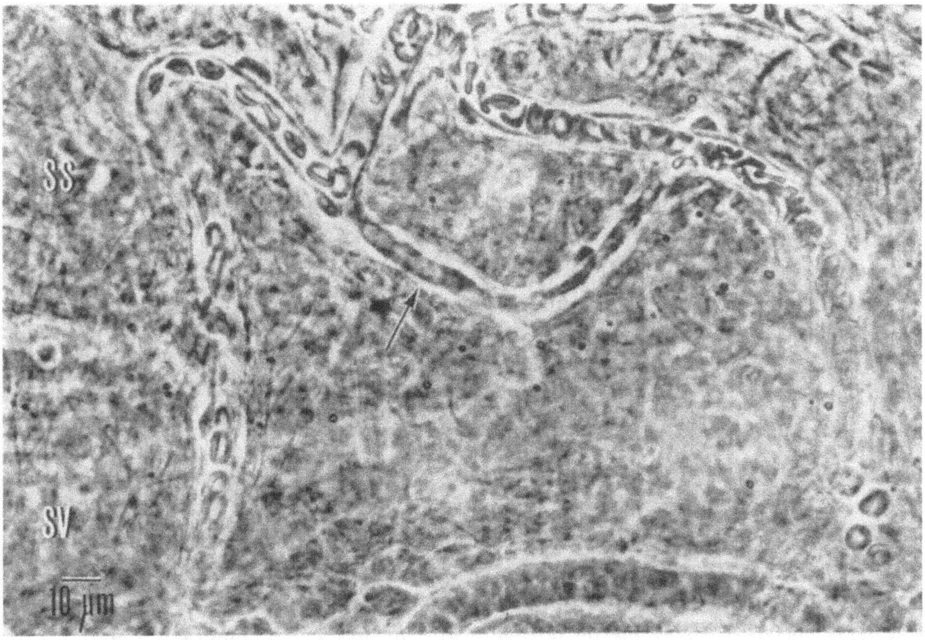

Fig. 1. Suprastrial capillary *(arrow)*, constricted and apparently degenerating, after single dose of quinidine 250 mg i.p. SS, suprastrial portion of spiral ligament. SV, stria vascularis. Guinea pig, 3rd turn. OsO_4

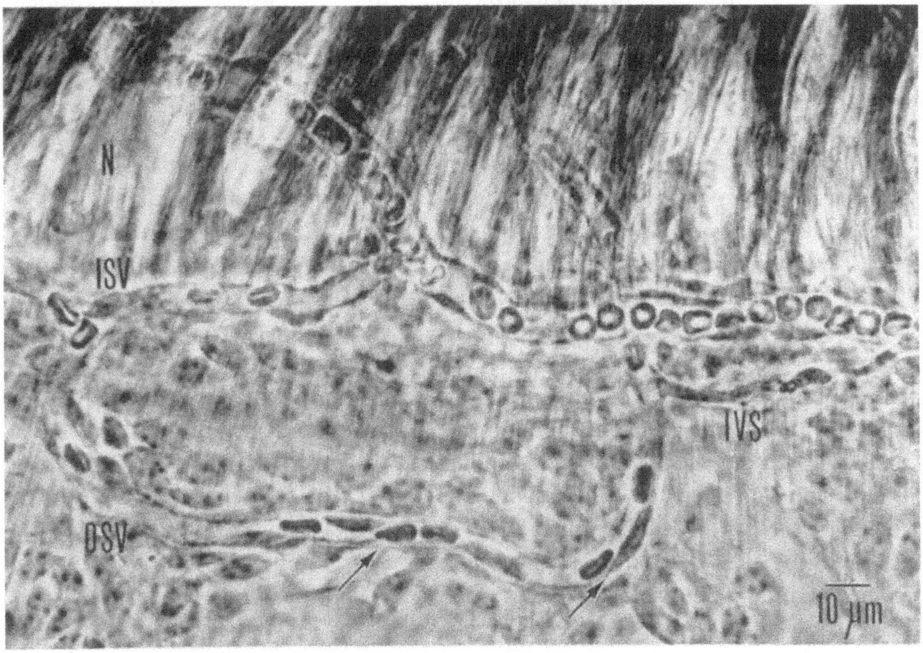

Fig. 2. Constriction of the capillary lumen by endothelial swellings *(arrows)* in the outer spiral vessel (OSV). The inner spiral vessel (ISV) appears less affected, but one arcade (IVS) is severely constricted and degenerating to form intervascular strand. N, nerve fibers in osseous spiral lamina. Guinea pig, quinidine 250 mg i.p. OsO_4

B. Possible Role of Prostaglandins

The biochemical basis for the action of salicyclates is still obscure. They are known to affect oxidative phosphorylation as well as transamination and dehydrogenation, but one may question whether the levels usually attained in the tissues are sufficient to inhibit the respective enzyme systems. Recent discoveries concerning the activities of the prostaglandins offer what may be an important lead. These extraordinary lipids are widely distributed in the body, apparently serving as local tissue hormones or modulators (WEEKS, 1973), and they may cause either vasoconstriction or vasodilatation. Those of the E series usually oppose vasoconstriction (McGIFF and NASJLETTI, 1973). It seems reasonable to assume that they are also present in the tissues of the cochlea, where they may be the local regulators of vascular tone and blood flow in the known absence of any vasomotor nerve supply to the vessels of the spiral ligament and stria. Since aspirin has been shown to inhibit prostaglandin synthetase (FERREIRA and VANE, 1974), it is tempting to speculate that the effect of salicylates on hearing is a reflection of their action on local prostaglandin synthesis and hence on the cochlear microvasculature. A similar mechanism might account for the reversible action of quinine. On the other hand, when ischemia is severe and prolonged, degenerative changes in the hair cells and spiral ganglion cells may occur, leading to permanent deafness.

III. Chenopodium

The oil of *Chenopodium anthelminticum* (American wormseed or Jerusalem oak) has a long history of use for ridding the intestine of nematodes such as hookworm and ascaris. Its active constituent is the pungent organic peroxide *ascaridole* (1,4-peroxido-p-menthene-2) which is present to the extent of 60–70%. Although once preferred as "the most certain, as well as the most innocent anthelmintic" (WILKINS, 1808) chenopodium has a narrow therapeutic range and can produce severe intoxication, with headache, CNS depression, coma, and sometimes death. The most striking symptoms associated with the inner ear are vertigo, ataxia, tinnitus, and deafness (BROWN, 1878; NORTH, 1880; SEXTON, 1880; ROTH, 1918; OPPIKOFER, 1919; ERB, 1949). Both transient and permanent effects on hearing have been described among the 15 cases of serious intoxication collected by OPPIKOFER, 10 of which had had a fatal outcome.

In animal experiments, Japanese investigators (OKA, 1929; OZAKI, 1935; OZENI, 1937) showed that chenopodium brought about degeneration of both the organ of Corti and the spiral ganglion, but they disagreed as to the order in which the degeneration occurred. The papers by OZAKI and OZENI, not available to the present writer, are cited by WERNER (1940) and by JUUL and VRAA-JENSEN (1947). In a study by the latter authors the cochlear microphonic response was reduced or abolished in guinea pigs, along with Preyer's reflex, by single or repeated doses of ascaridole 300 mg p. o. Complete loss of hair cells occurred in the animals most severely affected, but there was no clear-cut effect on the cells of the spiral ganglion. KREJCI and BEJDL (1954) were able to confirm these findings, showing that in chenopodium-intoxicated guinea pigs the uptake of ^{32}P by the damaged organ of Corti was reduced along with the microphonic response, whereas its incorporation into the spiral ganglion remained unaffected. The site of injury to the vestibular system may also be assumed to be peripheral, although it apparently has not been demonstrated experimentally. WERNER (1940), however, assumed that vestibular disturbance must be due to the central effects of chenopodium, which were prominent in the clinical cases cited above.

IV. The Arsenicals

Deafness or vestibular disturbance is rare in cases of industrial poisoning with inorganic arsenic. ROSENWASSER (1932) reported a single case of unilateral deafness in an otherwise healthy 34-year-old patient who had been given injections of iron arsenic as a tonic. Gradual, spontaneous recovery of hearing occurred after the injections were stopped. YAMAKAWA (1929) demonstrated loss of cochlear hair cells, outer sulcus cells, and spiral ganglion cells in the rabbit 3 days after subcutaneous injection of arsenous oxide (As_2O_3).

Interest in the ototoxic effects of the arsenicals derives from their formerly widespread use in the treatment of lues and trypanosomiasis. Since sensorineural deafness was known to occur in untreated lues, any harmful effect of arsphenamine (salvarsan) on the hearing was difficult to assess, and the question of its ototoxicity was vigorously debated. KOBRAK (1926) expressed the paradox, describing salvarsan as an inner ear poison which, when properly used, was capable of preventing injury to the inner ear by the disease. ROSS and LEDERER (1937) observed that in dogs both arsphenamine and neoarsphenamine are toxic for the vestibular system when injected into the middle ear. Intratympanic ototoxicity, however, does not necessarily imply ototoxicity by the usual parenteral routes of administration.

A vestibulotoxic action of atoxyl (sodium arsanilate) and arsacetin (sodium acetylarsanilate) was suggested when EHRLICH (1907) found that the latter compound caused a waltzing tendency in mice being treated for experimental trypanosomiasis. Although this phenomenon would seem to merit more intensive study than it has received, the chief interest in these compounds lies in their effects in the cochlea, which were studied in Japan during the 1930's by MIYAMOTO, NAKAMURA, and OZENI (all cited by WERNER, 1940). The remarkable finding was not so much the disappearance of Preyer's reflex and the degeneration of the organ of Corti and the spiral ganglion, but the effect on the stria vascularis. In the early stages of intoxication the stria appeared swollen, and Reissner's membrane bulged toward the scala vestibuli. Subsequently the strial cells were damaged, and the membrane sagged upon the organ of Corti, which at a later stage disappeared entirely. This sequence of events has been confirmed by CAUSSÉ *et al.* (1949, 1950), RÜEDI (1951), LEONARD *et al.* (1971), and ANNIKO and WERSÄLL (1975).

The last-named authors have shown by electron microscopy that both the marginal and intermediate cells become swollen and vacuolated within 12 hrs after the drug is administered, eventually being expelled into the lumen of the cochlear duct. Their degeneration leaves wide pericapillary spaces surrounding the strial vessels, which are normally closely invested by these cells. Whether hair cell loss and other degenerative changes in Corti's organ are caused by a direct action of the arsenical or indirectly as a result of its effect on the stria is not yet clear.

This strial ototoxicity of atoxyl appears to offer an important tool for studying the microhomeostatic role of the stria in the formation of the endolymph and the regulation of its ionic content, at least in the guinea pig. Whether it is applicable to other laboratory animals than rodents remains to be seen. Ototoxic effects of atoxyl seem to have been rare among the thousands of African patients treated for trypanosomiasis, but eye symptoms were fairly common (KOPKE, 1922). In discussing the toxicity of the arsenicals, FORDYCE (1911) lists not only optic neuritis and blindness from atoxyl, but also headache, vertigo, and nausea. SOLLMAN (1932) mentions deafness as well, but gives no reference. Further extensive but not exhaustive search has revealed a single report of hearing loss and tinnitus in a patient treated with atoxyl for lichen ruber planus. A week or two after the onset of the cochlear symptoms, vision also began to deteriorate to the point of complete blindness (BORNEMANN, 1905).

V. The Aminoglycosides

With the introduction of streptomycin in 1945 heralding the advent of the aminoglycosides, ototoxicity began to assume its rightful place as a phenomenon of widespread clinical concern rather than a pharmacologic curiosity or an obscure side-effect. The word *ototoxicity* itself first appears in the title of a brief paper on hydroxystreptomycin by HAWKINS (1951) but its adjectival form had been used once before in the report of a clinical trial of neomycin by WAISBREN and SPINK (1950). Even so, it does not occur as a separate entry in the index to *Excerpta Medica, Section 11: Otolaryngology* until 1963, when there were six items listed under that heading, related to three different antibiotics.

The association between prolonged or overzealous aminoglycoside treatment and disturbances of inner ear function was apparent from the first clinical trial of streptomycin and was repeatedly confirmed as other antibiotics of the group were introduced. Of the aminoglycosides that have had extensive clinical use, streptomycin (SM) has been predominantly vestibulotoxic. Its reduction product, dihydrostreptomycin (DHSM), which once enjoyed great popularity, sometimes gave rise to vestibular dysfunction in patients during prolonged administration, but it also showed an unfortunate tendency to cause hearing impairment. Because of this cochlear toxicity, approval for DHSM was withdrawn by the United States Food and Drug Administration and it has disappeared from the pharmacopeia. Kanamycin (KM) and neomycin (NM) are both toxic for the cochlea, the latter to the extent that it is approved only for oral or local use. Vestibular toxicity has rarely been reported with either of them. Gentamicin (GM) and tobramycin (TM), on the other hand, can show both types of ototoxicity, although the vestibular form is more usual in patients. The nonaminoglycoside antibiotic viomycin (VM) also shows a predilection for the vestibular system in man (DALY and COHEN, 1965).

A. Vestibular Toxicity

Vestibular ototoxicity has been reviewed in a recent chapter by HAWKINS and PRESTON (1975), to which the reader may refer for a more detailed discussion and a more extensive bibliography than can be included here. Vestibular disturbances had become extremely common by 1948 in tuberculous patients receiving SM treatment, and numerous descriptions are to be found in the literature of that period. Unfortunately, otoneurology and electronystagmography were not yet well developed, and few tuberculosis hospitals and sanatoria were prepared to take advantage of the unexpected wealth of material for research on human vestibular dysfunction that was suddenly placed at their disposal. Nevertheless, valuable descriptions of the vestibular disturbance were published, particularly those of FOWLER and SELIGMAN (1947), GLORIG and FOWLER (1947), BÉHAGUE *et al.* (1948), DIX (1948), GRAF (1949), BLOMKE (1950), JONGKEES and HULK (1950), KESER (1950), NORTHINGTON (1950), and BIGNALL *et al.* (1951), among others.

Most of these authors indicated that the characteristic feature of the disturbance was an unusual type of dizziness, which appeared sooner and was the more severe, the greater the daily dose of SM that the patient had received. Usually it made itself manifest after 3–4 weeks of intramuscular treatment, but if the drug was also given intrathecally, or if renal function was inadequate, the toxic effects were hastened and enhanced (JATHO, 1950).

Oddly enough, the patients' first complaints were usually related to vision rather than to equilibrium. Some described a blurring or mistiness of vision, especially when they tried to read, others a "jumping" or "jumbling" of objects in the field of view. These effects were noticed when the eyes were moved or their plane of focus shifted, or when the head was turned. The vertigo itself was often experienced only upon turning the head, which gave a sense of continued turning even after the motion had stopped.

The Romberg sign was often positive but not invariably so in patients with SM-intoxication. Their gait tended to be unsteady, on a wide base, with a tendency to fall to either side. Such patients found it especially difficult to walk in the dark, on uneven ground, or on a mattress. This last exercise was suggested as a simple test for the vestibular dysfunction by GLORIG and FOWLER (1947).

Tilt-table tests revealed responses that were delayed and inadequate to prevent falling (GLORIG and FOWLER, 1947; GRAF, 1948). Spontaneous nystagmus was rare, but a fine nystagmus could be observed on lateral gaze. Positional nystagmus was absent, and optokinetic nystagmus remained normal (DIX *et al.*, 1949; KESER, 1950).

When caloric and rotational tests were performed, the response was reduced in rate and duration, and in patients with severe intoxication it was sometimes entirely absent. The galvanic response tended to remain, supporting the hypothesis that site of action of SM is peripheral rather than central.

The symptoms of SM-intoxication sometimes gradually subsided, even when treatment was continued. Compensation for the loss of vestibular function was often good, especially in young children (MAJER, 1948). A few instances of partial recovery of the response to caloric stimulation were recorded, but this was an exceptional finding (KESER, 1950).

B. Site of action

A review of the uncertainty and controversy over the site of attack by SM on the vestibular system is given by HAWKINS and PRESTON (1975). The earliest animal experiments and neuropathologic examinations of materials from SM-treated patients suggested the presence of various brainstem or cerebellar lesions (MOLITOR *et al.*, 1946: HAWKINS, 1947; STEVENSON *et al.*, 1947; WINSTON *et al.*, 1940, 1949; and RÜEDI *et al.*, 1949). Experimental studies, however, showing unmistakable evidence of destruction of the neuroepithelia, both in the vestibular system and in the cochlea in SM-intoxicated animals, were reported by CAUSSÉ *et al.* (1948, 1949), BERG (1949), VANDERHAEGHE (1949), HAWKINS (1950), RÜEDI *et al.* (1951), and HAWKINS and LURIE (1952). Further histopathologic evidence of the peripheral site of SM-intoxication in man was furnished by GRAF (1951). In a combined behavioral and histopathologic study of SM-effects in cats, MCGEE and OLSZEWSKI (1962) found characteristic end-organ lesions in all of their treated animals, but no changes in the brainstem that could be attributed to the drug. Many other subsequent reports have described vestibular and cochlear injuries caused by the various aminoglycosides, but no convincing evidence has appeared of any primary lesions in the central nervous system.

C. Streptomycin vs. Dihydrostreptomycin

Vestibular disturbance was generally later in onset and less severe in patients treated with dihydrostreptomycin than in those treated with SM, bearing out initial laboratory findings (EDISON *et al.*, 1948). At first it seemed that DHSM, with antimicrobial activity equal to that of SM, promised even better therapeutic effects in tuberculosis, since treatment could be continued for a longer time without risk of vestibular involvement (HOBSON *et al.*, 1948; HINSHAW *et al.*, 1948). Unfortunately it soon became evident that DHSM possessed a cochlear toxicity which was unpredictable, sometimes delayed until after treatment had been stopped, and not infrequently progressive. The clinical literature on the ototoxic effects of DHSM and SM is too extensive for citation of more than a few major contributions. Those of GLORIG (1951), LIDÉN (1953), COHEN *et al.* (1953), and MAHADY *et al.* (1953), present direct comparisons of their cochlear and vestibular toxicities. The last two papers give the results of a carefully planned double-blind study carried out in eight hospitals with tuberculous patients receiving either SM or DHSM 1 gm daily for 120 days or longer. The results showed a greater incidence of vestibular disturbances with SM, and a greater incidence of high-frequency hearing loss with DHSM. The insidious nature of the cochlear toxicity of DHSM was emphasized in a publication by SHAMBAUGH *et al.* (1959), who had collected 37 cases of patients who had received a few injections of DHSM in combination with penicillin for minor infections and developed clinically significant sensorineural hearing loss some time later.

D. Dihydrostreptomycin in Experimental Animals

The greater cochlear toxicity of DHSM as observed in man has proved more difficult to reproduce in experimental animals than the vestibular toxicity.

HAWKINS and LURIE (1953) found that in cats treated with DHSM 200 mg/kg/day s.c. for as long as 120 days the cochlear microphonic potential (CM) recorded at the round window was unaffected or slightly enhanced, whereas the whole-nerve action potential (AP) was depressed. Degeneration of outer hair cells was seen in the upper basal turn, as well as in the middle and apical turns, but the inner hair cells appeared normal. There was a marked contrast between these effects of DHSM and the complete loss of cochlear potentials and degeneration of the organ of Corti seen in cats treated with neomycin 40 mg/kg/day for 60 days or 80 mg/kg for only 15 days.

MCGEE and OLSZEWSKI (1962) measured hearing thresholds in cats by avoidance conditioning and found greater losses in two of their animals 18–20 months after DHSM treatment (200–300 mg/kg/day for 21–60 days) than had been present at 1–2 months. With DHSM hair cells of the upper turns were destroyed, and thresholds for frequencies below 4 kHz were affected. With SM the effect was largely on the hair cells of the lower basal turn and thresholds were raised for frequencies of 4 kHz and higher.

Guinea pigs show little or no effect on CM or loss of hair cells when treated with DHSM 400 mg/kg/day s.c. for as long as 6 weeks (HAWKINS *et al.*, 1976). *Macaca nemestrina* monkeys tolerate DHSM 100 mg/kg/day s.m. for 8 months, without changes in hearing thresholds or hair cell loss. The patas monkey *(Erythrocebus patas)* is the only species examined thus far which shows a cochlear sensitivity to DHSM comparable to that observed in some patients. Monkeys of this species developed severe hearing losses for frequencies above 1 or 2 kHz, along with injury to Corti's organ throughout the basal turn, when treated with DHSM in doses as small as 20 mg/kg/day s.c. for 90 days (HAWKINS *et al.*, 1976).

E. Other Aminoglycosides

The four aminoglycosides NM, KM, GM, and TM constitute a group distinct from the streptomycins, in that they all contain the base deoxystreptamine linked to various aminohexoses, whereas the streptomycins contain streptidine. Other differences among them are indicated in Figs. 3 and 4. Unlike the rest, neomycin consists of three sugar rings rather than two, one of them being the pentose, *ribose* (ring III). For a succinct account of the chemical structures of these and other aminoglycosides in relation to their antimicrobial activity, see BENVENISTE and DAVIES (1973).

Variations in chemical configuration, including the number and placement of basic groups on the various sugars, affect the toxicity as well as activity of the aminoglycosides. A recent comparison of the cochlear toxicities of the four major deoxystreptamine-containing aminoglycosides in guinea pigs is shown in Fig. 5. Maximum CM-responses to a tone of 1 kHz recorded at the round window are shown as functions of the number of weeks of treatment with a dose of 100 mg/kg/day of each drug. On a weight-for-weight basis KM is the least ototoxic and GM the most ototoxic, at least for this species. In clinical use, the probability of ototoxic reactions from GM and TM is reduced in proportion to their greater antimicrobial activity, which makes possible the use of smaller doses and shorter courses of treatment. Other laboratory studies of the ototoxicity of GM have been published by AKIYOSHI and SATO (1967), BERNABEI *et al.* (1967), HAWKINS *et al.* (1969), IGARASHI *et al.* (1971), WATANUKI *et al.* (1972), FEDERSPIL (1972), and YLIKOSKI *et al.* (1973). The ototoxic effects of GM and TM have been compared in animals by BRUMMETT *et al.* (1972) and FEDERSPIL (1973). Gentamicin ototoxicity

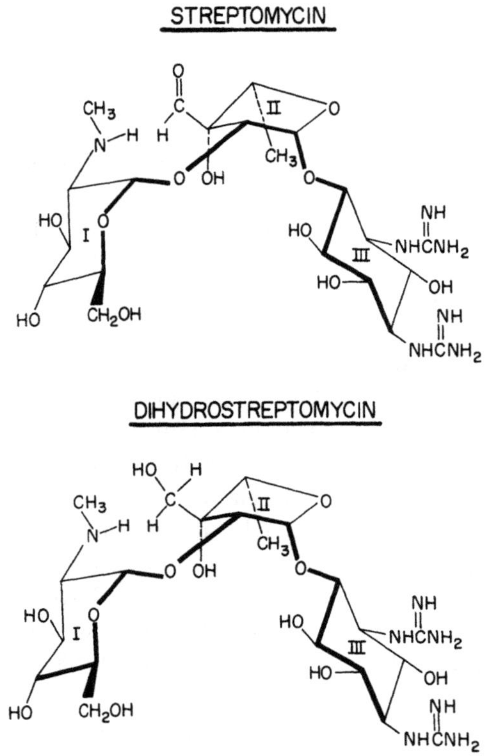

Fig. 3. Structural formulas of streptomycin and dihydrostreptomycin. Ring I is N-methyl-L-glucosamine, Ring III is guanidocyclitol streptidine. Ring II is pentose, streptose, which is reduced in the conversion of streptomycin to dihydrostreptomycin

in clinical use is reviewed by JACKSON and ARCIERI (1971). Both vestibular and cochlear effects of GM have been reported by DAYAL *et al.* (1974, 1975) in patients with thermal burns who were treated topically as well as parenterally.

F. Histopathological Findings

1. Neuroepithelia

Histopathologic evidence that the major targets of the ototoxic action of the aminoglycosides are the sensory endings of the cochlear and vestibular nerves was first obtained by CAUSSÉ (1949). His observation has been amply and repeatedly confirmed in light-microscopic studies by BERG (1949), RÜEDI *et al.* (1951), HAWKINS and LURIE (1952, 1953), WARD and FERNÁNDEZ (1961), DARROUZET and DELIMA SOBRINHO (1962), BECK and KRAHL (1962), TYBERGHEIN (1962), KOHONEN (1965), and many others. Early suggestions or suspicions of a primary action on the neurons of the VIIIth nerve or its nuclei in the brain stem (STEVENSON *et al.*,

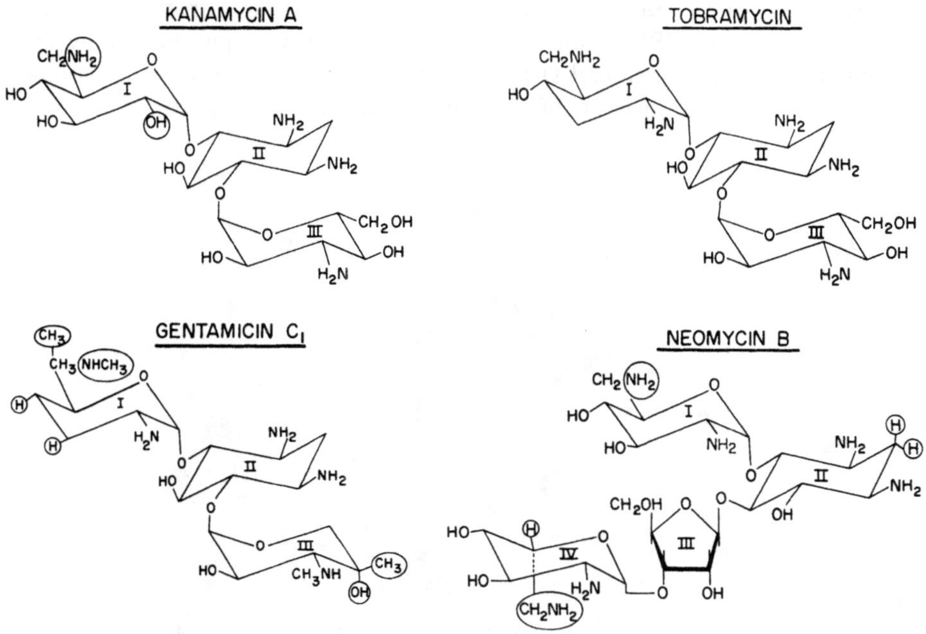

Fig. 4. Structural formulas of four aminoglycosides containing aminocyclitol 2-deoxystreptamine (Ring II). Groups circled are those which differ among various gentamicins, kanamycins, and similarly closely related families of antibiotics. (Based on Benveniste and Davies, 1973)

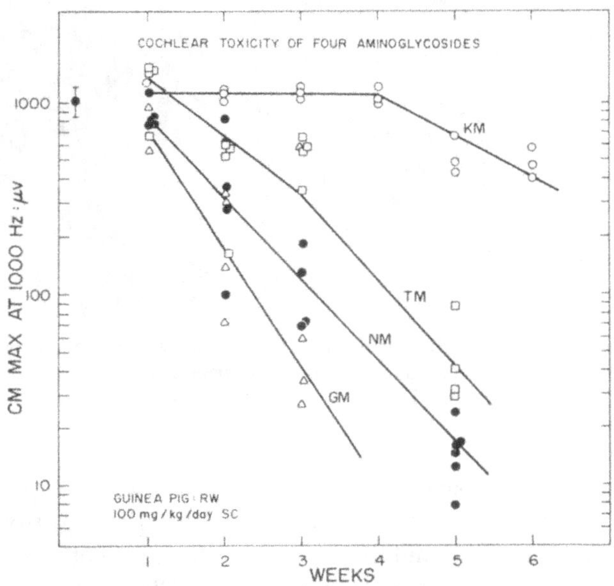

Fig. 5. Comparison of four aminoglycosides in terms of their effects on cochlear microphonic (round window) potential in guinea pigs. Ordinate, maximum rms voltage (CMmax) at 1 kHz. Single point at upper left shows mean CMmax for untreated controls ± S.D. Abscissa, duration of treatment. On this weight-for-weight basis, KM is least ototoxic. Dose used, however, is only 6—10 times that recommended for KM in clinical use, but 20—30 times that recommended for GM and TM

1947; HAWKINS and O'SHANNY, 1948; RÜEDI *et al.*, 1949; WINSTON *et al.*, 1948, 1949; FLOBERG *et al.*, 1949; CHRISTENSEN *et al.*, 1951) were put to rest by the negative findings of McGEE and OLSZEWSKI (1962) in their combined functional and neuropathologic comparison of SM and DHSM ototoxicity in cats.

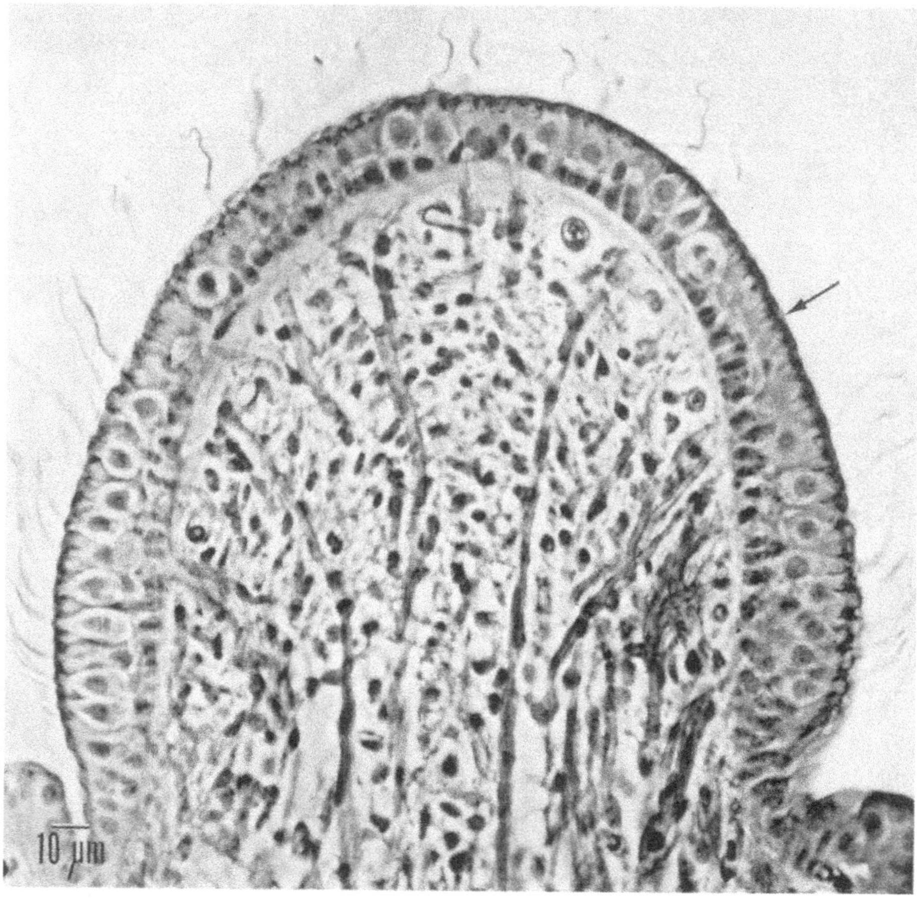

Fig. 6. Crista ampullaris of horizontal canal in a GM-treated squirrel monkey (40 mg/kg/day i.m. for 29 days). Many hair cells have disappeared *(arrow)*, others appear shrunken. Hair bundles are still present on type II cells of lower slopes. OsO_4, Araldite, phase-contrast

Studies of hair cell pathology at the electron-microscopic level produced by SM have been reported by WERSÄLL and HAWKINS (1962), FARKASHIDY *et al.* (1963), DUVALL and WERSÄLL (1964) and SPOENDLIN (1966) among others. The effects of GM have been described by WERSÄLL *et al.* (1969, 1973). In the vestibular neuroepithelia the hair cells of type I are usually damaged first and only later those of type II. The supporting cells tend to remain when the hair cells have been destroyed (Fig. 6). Fusion of stereocilia into "giant" hairs and degeneration of the mitochondrial cristae to typical myelin figures are early stages in the pathologic process.

Characteristic changes in hair cells of both types are seen in an ampullar crista from a TM-treated guinea pig in Fig. 7. Degeneration of the type I cell appears to be the more advanced. In Fig. 8 the dense population of hair bundles on the crista of the superior canal of a normal pigeon is contrasted with the almost bare surface

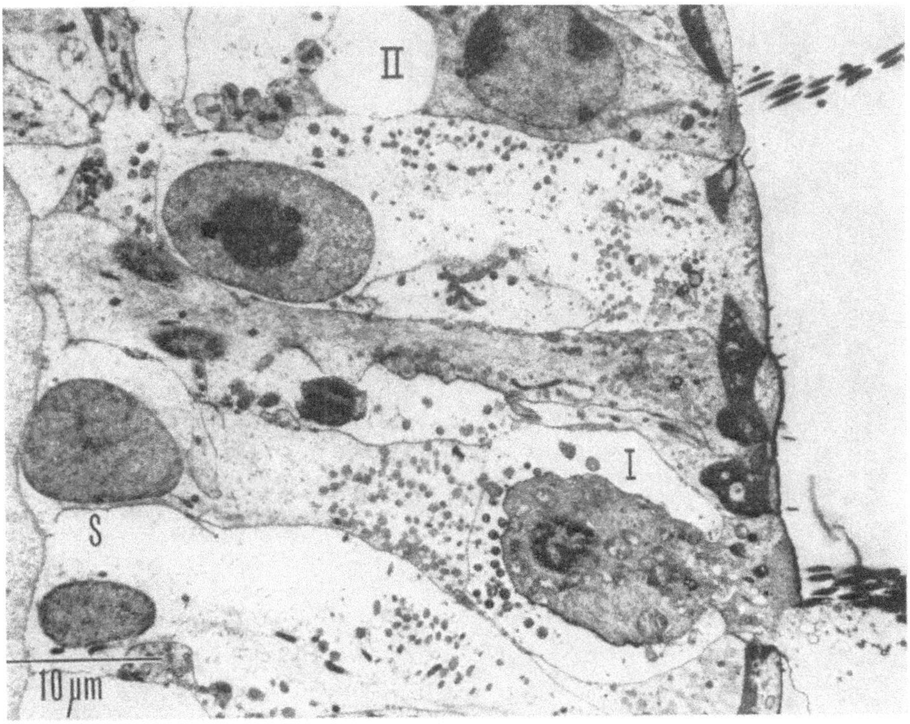

Fig. 7. Damage to hair cells on slope of crista in TM-treated guinea pig (100 mg/kg/day for 25 days). Contents of type I cell are being extruded; type II cell is less severely affected. S, supporting cell nuclei at basement membrane. EM

of the crista from a bird treated with SM. The hair bundles that remain appear fused and irregular. The acute labyrinthine intoxication produced by instilling an aminoglycoside solution into the middle ear brings with it the most spectacular changes in the hair cells (SPOENDLIN, 1966; WERSÄLL *et al.*, 1969) with rapid dissolution of the nuclei and extrusion of their cytoplasm and its organelles into the endolymph (*cf.* the type I cell of Fig. 7).

The chronic effects of repeated parenteral administration are less dramatic but equally lasting. In the cochlea they may be marked by a disturbance of the orderly pattern of the stereocilia (HAWKINS and ENGSTRÖM, 1964; KOHONEN, 1965), by nuclear swelling, and by vacuolization of the cytoplasm after disappearence of its subcuticular organelles (Fig. 9). The order in which these events occur is still not entirely clear. They may represent simply the stereotyped death-throes of the hair cell, regardless of the nature of the lethal insult (HAWKINS, 1973a).

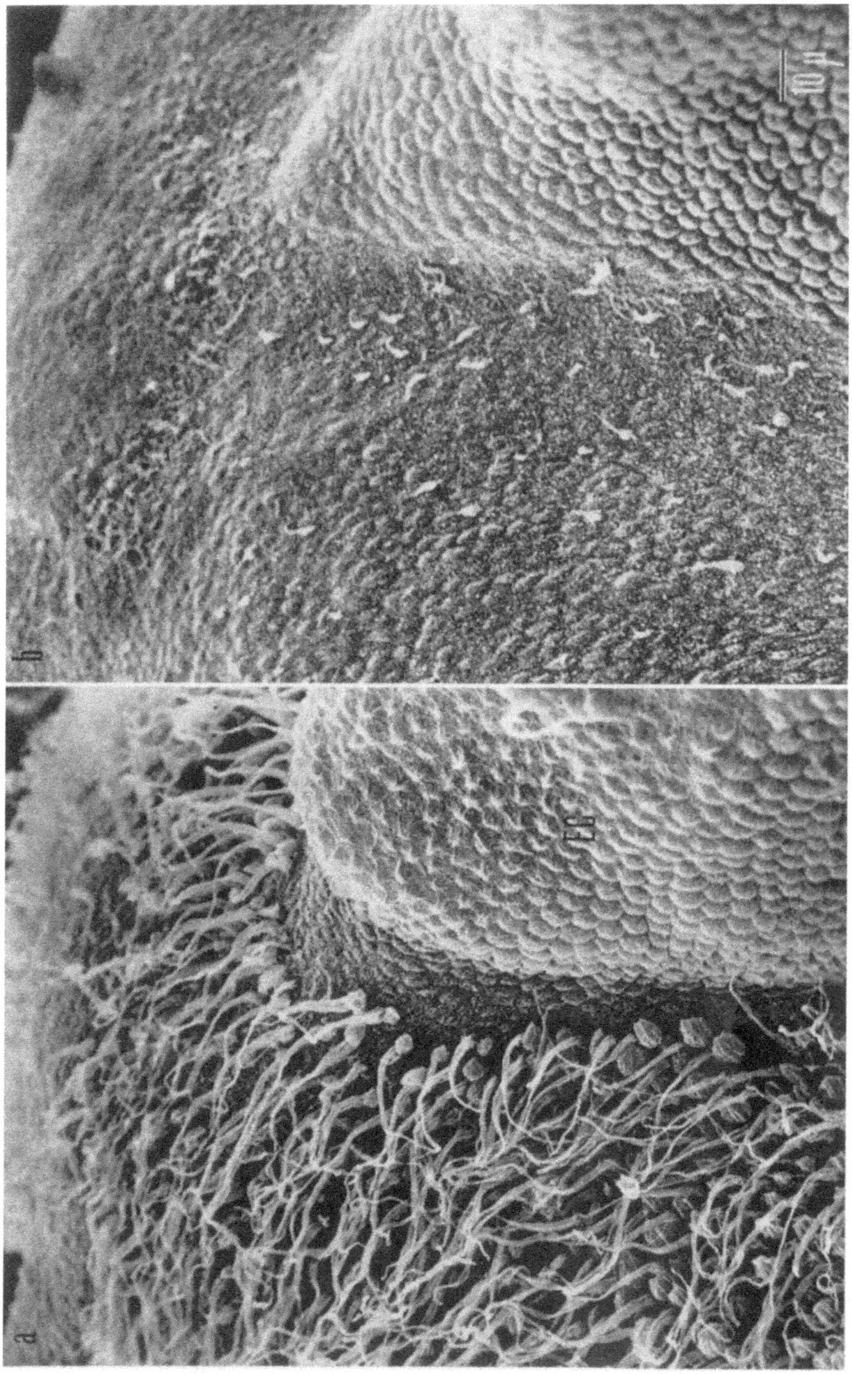

Fig. 8. Surface views of crista of superior semicircular canal in pigeons. a) normal, densely covered by hair bundles except on eminentia cruciata, EC. b) SM-treated, with loss of most hair bundles; those remaining appear fused. SM 200 mg/kg/day i.m. for 30 days. Unable to fly. SEM

DARROUZET and GUILHAUME (1974) have made a day-by-day EM study in guinea pigs of the changes in the hair cells resulting from treatment with KM 400 mg/kg/day for 7 days. They report first an increase in the Golgi apparatus in the subcuticular portion of the outer hair cells of the basal turn (3 days). Next,

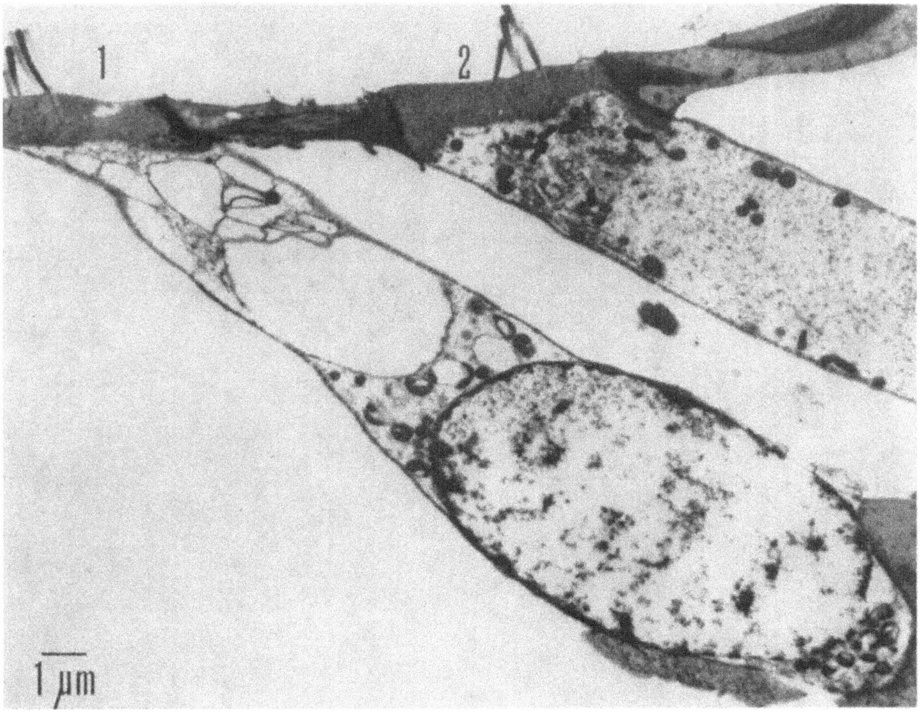

Fig. 9. Degenerating outer hair cell of row 1, from extreme basal end (hook) of spiral organ. At this early stage of GM-intoxication the hair cell of row 2 shows only an increase in Golgi apparatus and presence of subcuticular lysosomes. The parallel parietal membranes have disappeared. (Unpublished electron micrograph from guinea pig treated with GM 100 mg/kg/day s.c. for 7 days)

lysosomes appear in the same region (7 days). The lysosomes congregate beneath what one might term the *fonticulus* (fontanel), *i.e.* the circular area or "weak spot," where the cuticular plate is incomplete, with only a thin covering of plasma membrane on the hair cell surface (9th day). By this time the stereocilia have begun to fuse. A day later the cell bursts and its contents are extruded. What is left is presumably a phalangeal scar, as seen in the orderly array in Fig. 10.

With the degeneration of the hair cells, the reticular lamina "heals" itself by expansion of the phalangeal plates of the supporting cells. The result may be the characteristic, orderly pattern of phalangeal scars seen in surface preparations of the organ of Corti after KM intoxication (Fig. 10) or the disorderly scarring produced by GM or NM (Fig. 11). With prolonged treatment and severe injury, the organ of Corti may be replaced by an undifferentiated pavement epithelium covering the basilar membrane, at least in the lower basal turn.

A quantitative estimate of cochlear injury may be made by counting the missing hair cells and plotting the percentage of hair cells remaining on successive portions of the basilar membrane in the form of a cytocochleogram (ENGSTRÖM *et al.*, 1966). Such a plot is shown in Fig. 12, illustrating a loss of outer hair cells

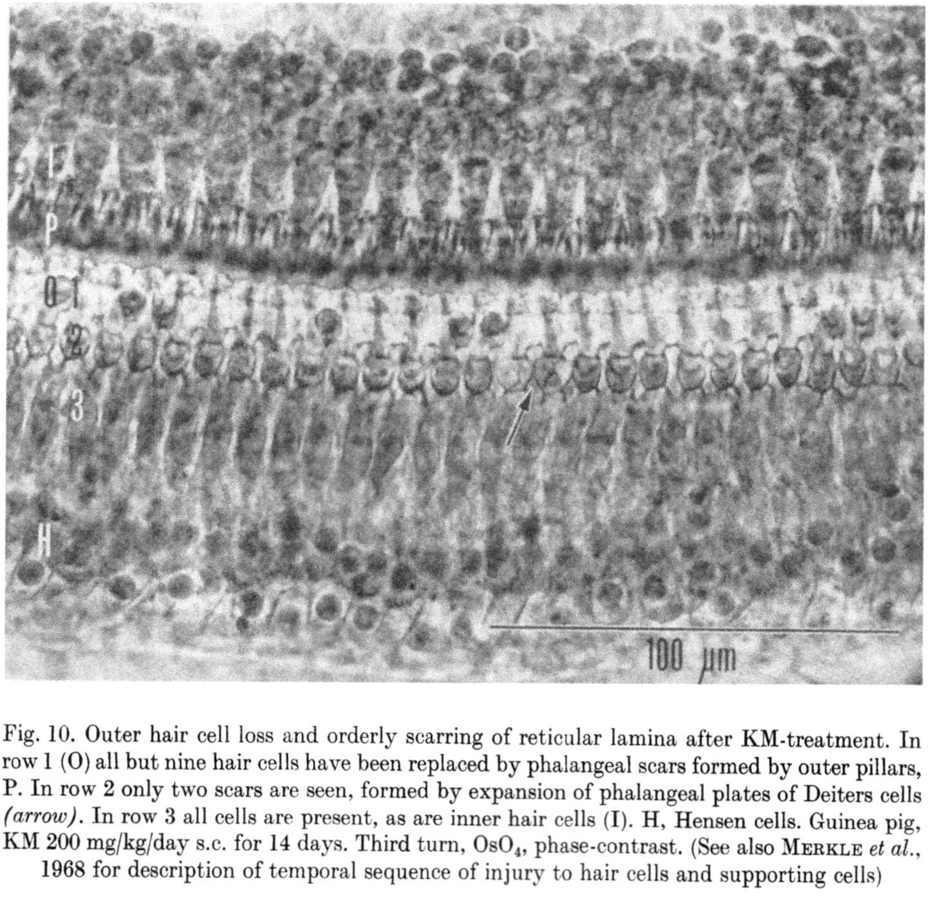

Fig. 10. Outer hair cell loss and orderly scarring of reticular lamina after KM-treatment. In row 1 (O) all but nine hair cells have been replaced by phalangeal scars formed by outer pillars, P. In row 2 only two scars are seen, formed by expansion of phalangeal plates of Deiters cells *(arrow)*. In row 3 all cells are present, as are inner hair cells (I). H, Hensen cells. Guinea pig, KM 200 mg/kg/day s.c. for 14 days. Third turn, OsO_4, phase-contrast. (See also MERKLE *et al.*, 1968 for description of temporal sequence of injury to hair cells and supporting cells)

from the most basal 4 mm of a guinea pig cochlea after 2 weeks of treatment with TM 100 mg/kg/day s.c. The cochlear microphonic potential recorded at the round window (RW) was severely depressed in the basal turn but it was more or less normal near the apex. The inner hair cells were still present in force, although their stereocilia may have become bent and swollen as seen by EM in an inner hair cell from a KM-treated guinea pig (Fig. 13).

Cochlear pathology can be related to hearing impairment in an aminoglycoside-treated animal by comparing the hair cell loss represented in the form of a cytocochleogram with the hearing loss plotted as an audiogram. This has been done for monkeys trained for behavioral audimetry and treated with KM, NM, or DHSM (STEBBINS *et al.*, 1969; HAWKINS *et al.*, 1976). Extensive loss of outer hair cells had

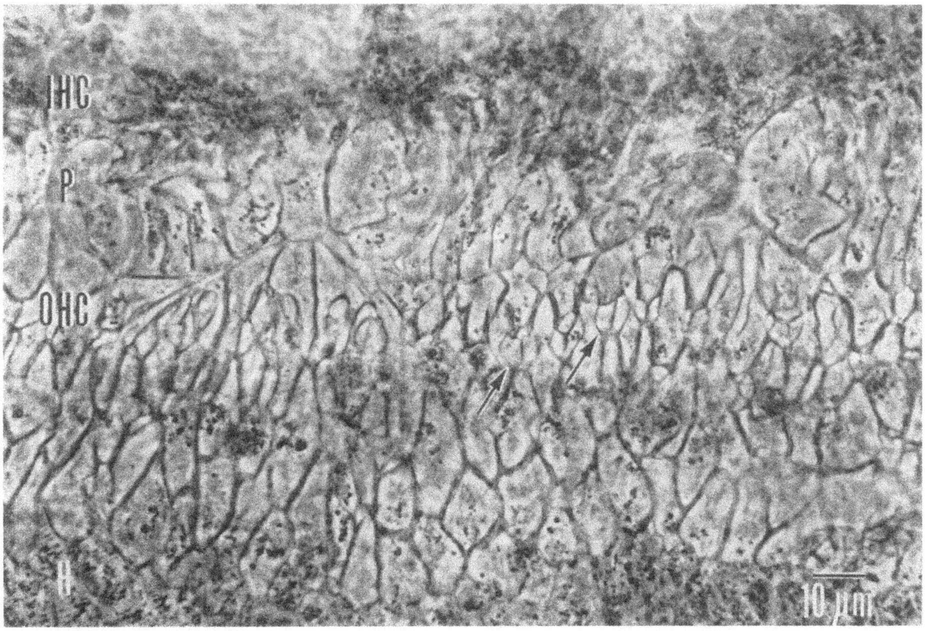

Fig. 11. Disorderly scarring of reticular lamina after NM-treatment. Rows of outer hair cells (OHC) are not easily distinguished, but a few, apparently recent scars can be seen *(arrows)* probably representing row 2. Head plates of pillars (P) are severely distorted, and no inner hair cells (IHC) remain. H, Hensen cells. Surface preparation from the upper second turn of a 12-year-old boy with oxalosis, who suffered a 60-dB hearing loss after receiving NM in course of renal transplant operation. OsO_4

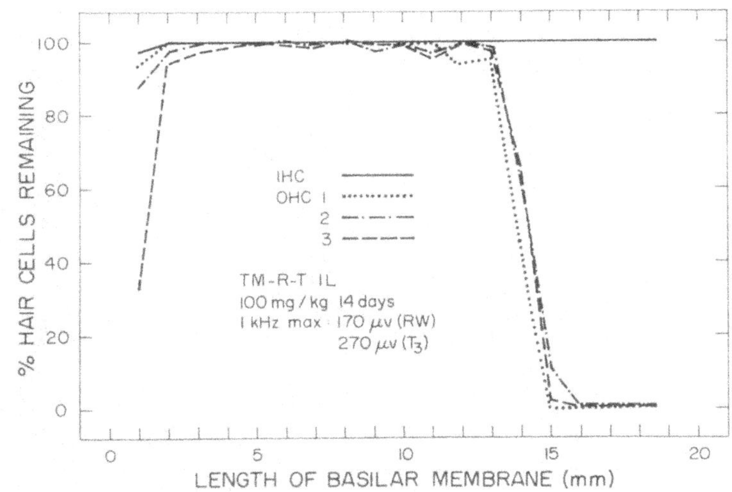

Fig. 12. Cytocochleogram of guinea pig showing loss of outer hair cells (OHC) of lower basal turn after TM-treatment. Inner hair cells (IHC) are still present in force. Apparent loss of 3rd-row OHC at 1 mm reflects normal, reduced, irregular pattern of hair cells near apex. CM max recorded at RW was reduced from ca. 1000 µV to 170 µV. CM voltage of 270 µV recorded from bony surface of third turn represents normal response

occurred in the ear depicted in Fig. 14. This patas monkey had incurred a 60–80 dB loss for all frequencies above 1 kHz as a result of DHSM-treatment. The inner hair cells were still present except in the lower basal turn.

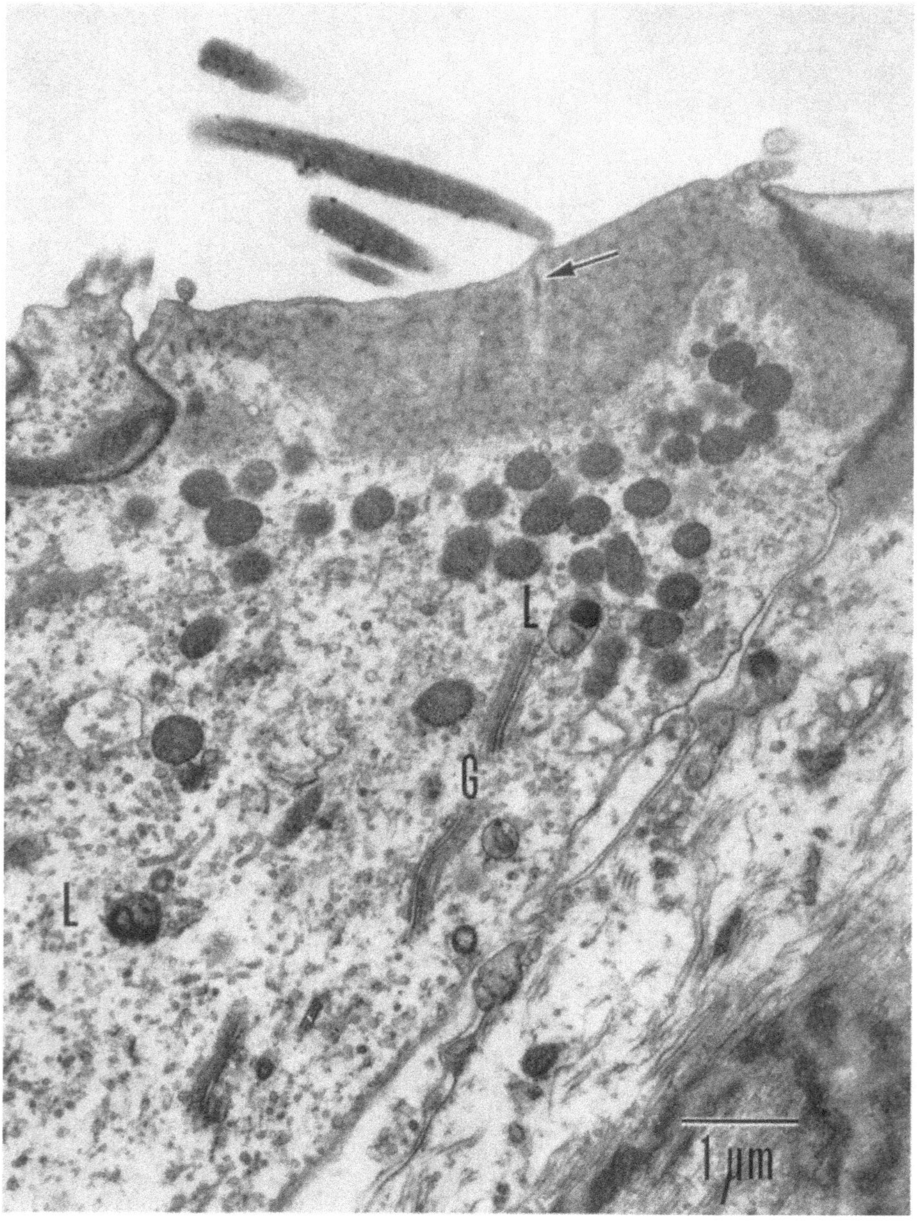

Fig. 13. Incipient degenerative changes in an inner hair cell of the basal turn remaining after loss of outer hair cells as a result of KM-treatment. Note bent sterocilium with crooked rootlet *(arrow)*, and small surface protuberance. L, lysosomes; G, Golgi apparatus. Guinea pig, upper basal turn, KM 400 mg/kg/day s.c. for 14 days. OsO_4, EM

2. Secretory Tissues

Injury to inner ear tissues by the aminoglycosides is not confined to the neuroepithelia. Changes in the stria vascularis after SM-treatment were described by RÜEDI *et al.* (1951) in guinea pigs and by GRAF (1951) in man. MÜSEBECK and

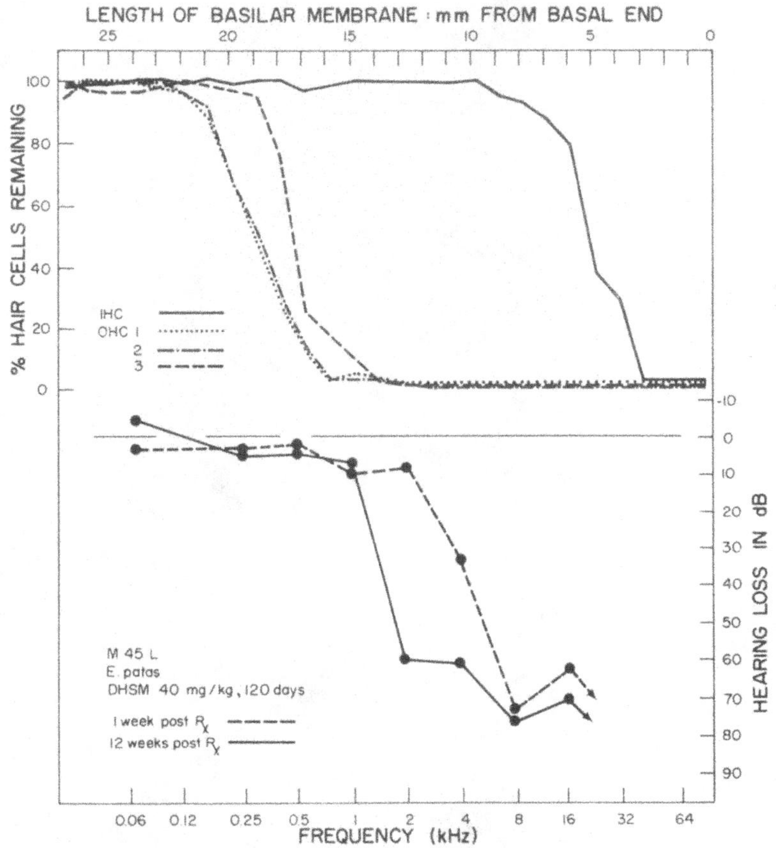

Fig. 14. Hair cell loss and progressive hearing loss in patas monkey after DHSM-treatment. Above, cytocochleogram showing loss of outer hair cells throughout basal and much of middle turn. Severe loss of inner hair cells is confined to the most basal 5 mm of cochlea. One week after end of treatment, hearing loss involved frequencies above 2 kHz. Twelve weeks later hearing for 2 kHz was also impaired. In terms of body weight the dose of DHSM 40 mg/kg/day for 120 days is equivalent to dose of 2 gm daily for 50-kg patient, dose lower than those used in initial clinical trial of DHSM (HOBSON *et al.*, 1948). (Unpublished data, HAWKINS *et al.*, 1976)

SCHÄTZLE (1962) in histochemical experiments had observed depletion of succinic acid dehydrogenase in the stria during DHSM-treatment before any change had occurred in the organ of Corti. They concluded that loss of hair cells must occur as a result of impairment of the respiratory metabolism of the stria.

JOHNSSON and HAWKINS (1972) described atrophic changes in the stria in animals treated with aminoglycosides. The marginal cells become shrunken with loss of mitochondria and reduction in the length of their basal processes. Since the

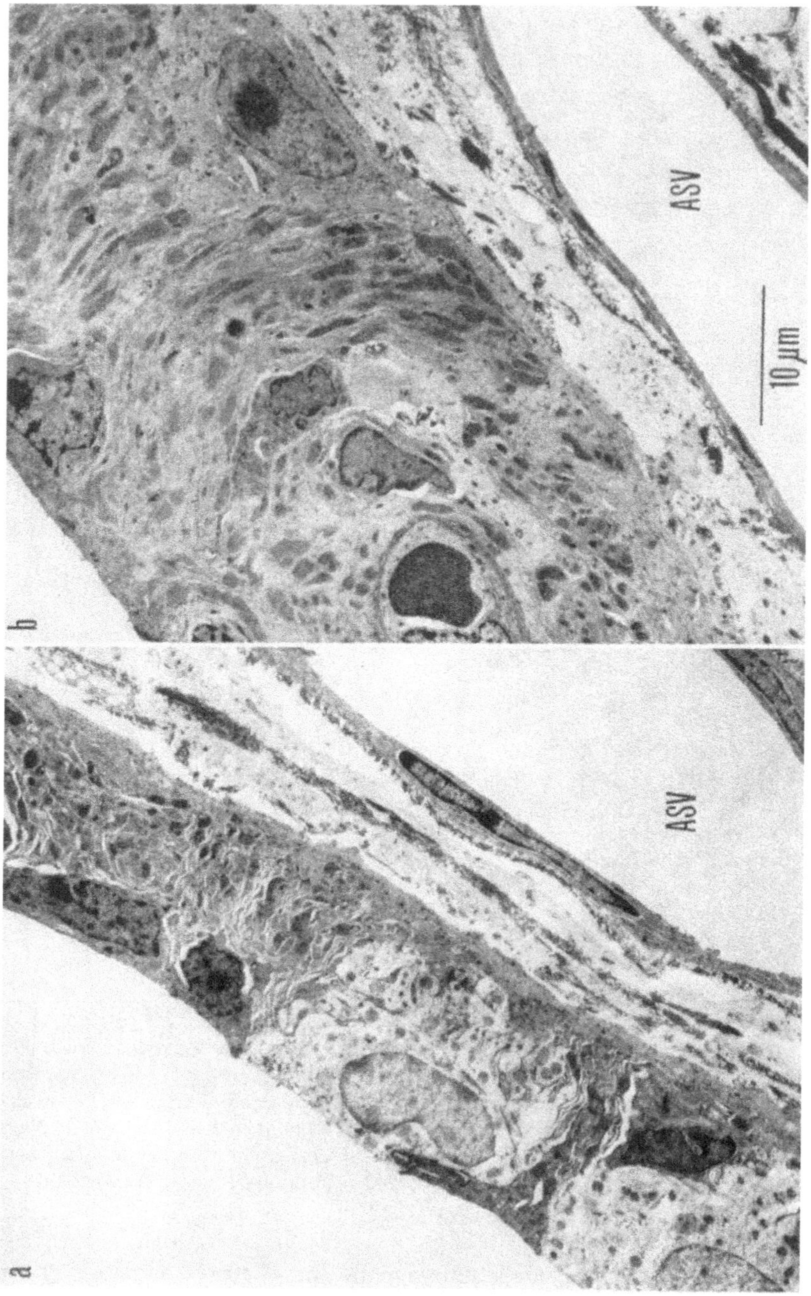

Fig. 15. Ototoxic changes in stria vascularis. a) After GM 100 mg/kg/day for 20 days. showing thin stria with atrophic changes, loss of basal processes of marginal cells. b) Normal stria, untreated control. ASV, adstrial vessel of spiral ligament. Both specimens from lower basal turn, guinea pig, same magnification. EM, OsO_4. (From HAWKINS, 1973b)

intermediate cells are also affected, the stria may be reduced to less than one-half its usual thickness. In Fig. 15 these changes are clearly seen in the stria of a GM-treated guinea pig, which looks pale and shrunken in comparison with that of a normal animal taken from the same cochlear turn. Such changes are more common with GM and NM, drugs having a strong nephrotoxic property, than with KM or SM.

The secretory tissues of the vestibular system corresponding to the stria are the dark-cell areas of the slopes of the ampullar cristae and the wall of the utricle, as well as the planum semilunatum. In the saccule they are entirely lacking. SPARWALD *et al.* (1971, 1972) have described degenerative changes in the dark cells of the crista in the guinea pig after SM-treatment. In the pigeon the dark cells are particularly well differentiated, and they show shrinkage and vacuolization after SM or GM (Fig. 16). Similar effects have been demonstrated in the squirrel monkey (HAWKINS and PRESTON, 1975). Other tissues which may be affected include the suprastrial portion of the spiral ligament, the pericapillary tissues of the spiral prominence, the outer sulcus, and Reissner's membrane (KANEKO, 1970; HAWKINS, 1971a, b; NOWAK, 1974).

G. Mode of Action

The peculiar toxicity of the aminoglycosides for only two organs of the body, namely, the inner ear and the kidney, has proved more difficult to explain than their mode of action in bacterial cells. Although initial biochemical studies with streptomycin had pointed to an interference with the citric acid cycle (UMBREIT, 1953) it has been shown that the antimicrobial effect depends upon the ability of aminoglycosides to inhibit protein synthesis. This is accomplished through an interaction with the 30 S ribosomal subunit (BENVENISTE and DAVIES, 1973). A similar inhibition was assumed to occur in eukaryotic cells, and biochemical studies for a while appeared to substantiate this inference (KRAUS and DOENNING, 1969). For a discussion of this question see BEARD *et al.* (1969).

1. Effects on Cell Membranes

Recent work by SCHACHT (1974, 1976) has revealed an interference with the lipids of the cell membrane rather than with the synthesis of protein. Specifically, NM has been found to inhibit phosphoinositide metabolism, which is believed to be essential in the control of membrane structure and permeability. Incorporation of [^{32}P]-orthophosphate into the phosphoinositides of the organ of Corti and stria vascularis is decreased by daily parenteral administration of NM. In homogenates of these tissues the presence of NM blocks the hydrolysis of phosphatidylinositol diphosphate and inhibits the binding of calcium. Apparently NM occupies the binding site for Ca^{++} with a part of its molecule, while other basic amino groups bind to anionic sites of the lipid. The membrane structure is disturbed, and the dephosphorylation/phosphorylation cycle is interrupted. As a result, the cell becomes unable to perform its normal duties and sooner or later dies.

The same mechanism has been demonstrated in renal tissue and in synaptosomes of the cerebral cortex. The brain itself is normally protected against the

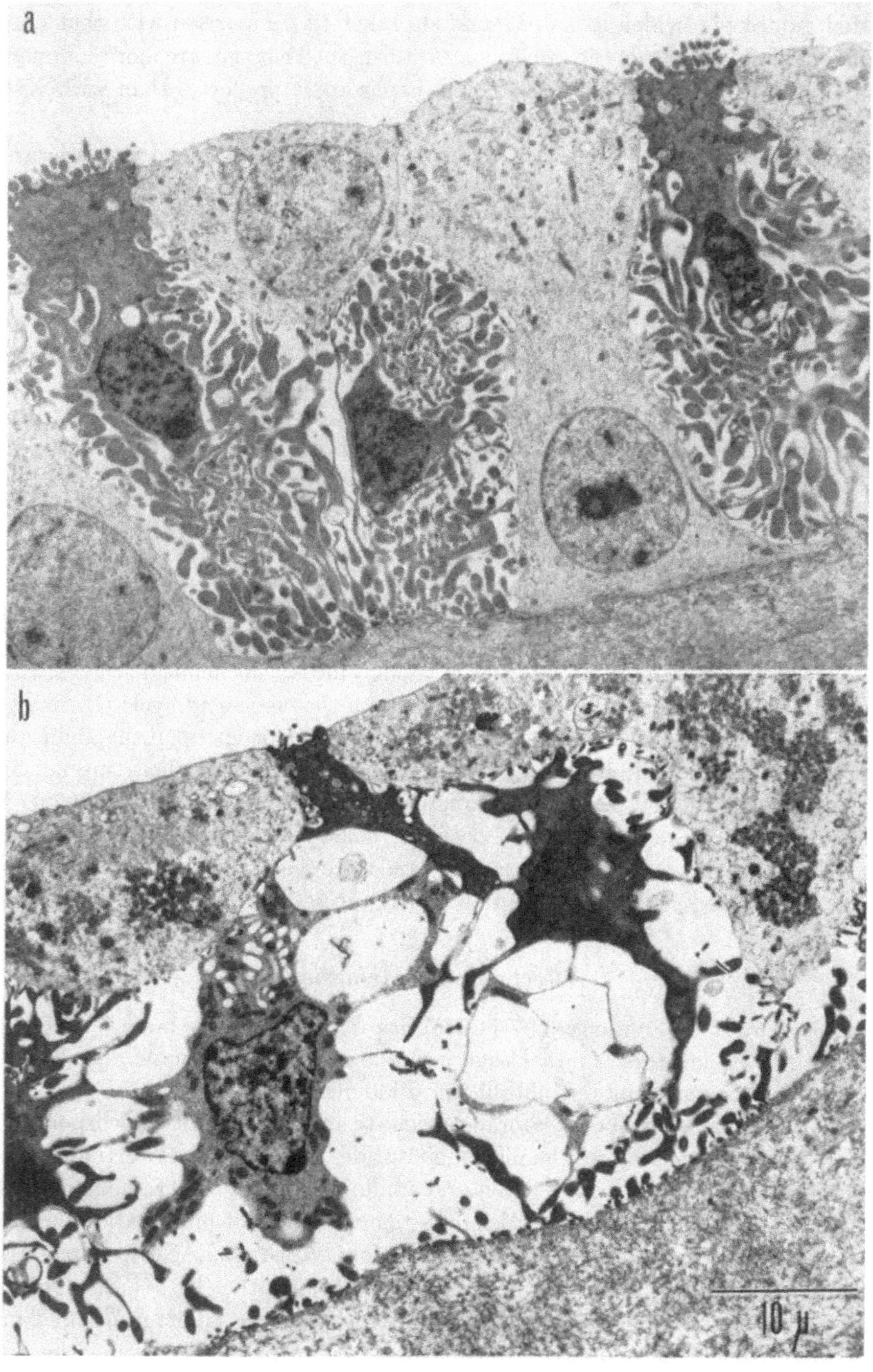

Fig. 16. Effect of SM on secretory cells of crista ampullaris in pigeon. a) Dark cell epithelia, untreated control. b) Edema and shrinkage of dark cells after SM 200 mg/kg/day i.m. for 30 days. Both specimens from posterior canal. EM, OsO_4

aminoglycosides, which do not easily pass the bloodbrain barrier, but intracisternal administration of SM in rabbits and cats can produce convulsions and respiratory paralysis (MOLITOR and KUNA, 1947).

The protection by ionized calcium against the acute toxic effects of streptomycin has been recognized almost since the antibiotic was first isolated. Other aspects of the pharmacology of the aminoglycosides which depend on their relation to calcium have been discussed by MÜCKTER (1961).

2. Route of Access to the Inner Ear

The aminoglycosides must reach the inner ear by way of the blood flowing through various capillary beds, since their concentration level in the cerebrospinal fluid remains low even when the plasma level is high (HAWKINS *et al.*, 1950). BALOGH *et al.* (1970) showed that tritium-labeled DHSM injected i.p. in guinea pigs appears in the vessels of the spiral ligament and stria within 15–30 min. It enters the perilymph via the spiral ligament, eventually reaching all cells of the cochlea as well as the endolymph. No preferential localization was demonstrated in their experiment, but v. ILBERG *et al.* (1971) found evidence of an accumulation of [^{3}H]-DHSM in the inner and outer hair cells after introducing it directly into the cochlea by perfusion. PORTMANN *et al.* (1974) injected the tracer into the carotid artery and found it mainly in the Deiters cells after 1 hr, in the outer hair cells after 4 hr.

Concentrations of aminoglycosides and other antibiotics in the inner ear fluids have been measured by VRABEC *et al.* (1965), VOLDRICH (1965), MURAVEISKAYA (1965), and STUPP *et al.* (1966), among others. STUPP (1970) found a gradual rise in aminoglycoside concentrations in the perilymph and endolymph after parenteral administration, and a slow clearance from them. Measurable amounts remained in the inner ear fluids after the drug had disappeared from the plasma. There was no direct correlation between plasma levels and perilymph levels. With KM the maximum perilymph concentration (ca. 20 µg/ml) was reached in 1–2 hrs, with SM and other aminoglycosides in 2–5 hrs, by which time the blood level had fallen sharply from its maximum. The half-life of KM in the perilymph was almost 15 hr, *i.e.*, about ten times that in the blood.

3. Relation to Nephrotoxicity

The kidney is the only other organ in which streptomycin has been found to persist in high concentration when its level in the plasma had fallen to zero (HAWKINS *et al.*, 1950; STAEMMLER and KARHOFF, 1956). It is tempting to account for the susceptibility of both organs to the aminoglycosides on the basis of the prolonged exposure to which they are subjected. In the kidney streptomycin has been shown to be bound to the tissue proteins. That a similar binding to the proteins of the spiral ligament and stria helps to prolong the stay of the aminoglycosides in the inner ear fluids is a reasonable inference.

It is axiomatic that a delay in excretion of an aminoglycoside as a result of nephrotoxic action or other renal failure must increase its level in the plasma and perilymph and thus enhance the probability of ototoxic injury (NAUNTON and WARD, 1959). In much the same way as the nephrotoxic action can disturb the macrohomeostasis of the body as a whole, so injury to the secretory and reabsorptive tissues of the labyrinth by prolonged exposure may disturb its microhomeostasis. This derangement may be a major factor in bringing about degeneration of the cochlear and vestibular hair cells (HAWKINS, 1973a). There are indications that degenerative changes in the suprastrial portion of the spiral ligament and other tissues of the outer wall, as produced by GM or NM, may precede the progressive loss of hair cells from the spiral organ as it advances from the base toward the apex. Nevertheless, much other evidence still points to a direct toxic action on the hair cells. Furthermore, the secretory tissues, especially the stria, have powers of recuperation from injury which are not shared by Corti's organ (QUICK and DUVALL, 1970; DUVALL *et al.*, 1974).

H. Electrophysiologic Studies

The first experimental indication of the cochlear toxicity of SM was the selective reduction in the voltage of the cochlear microphonic (CM) response in SM-treated cats (HAWKINS, 1950). The whole-nerve action potential (N1 or AP) in response to acoustic clicks was less affected. On the other hand, after DHSM, the amplitude of CM was enhanced and that of N1 reduced; NM eliminated both components (HAWKINS and LURIE, 1953). These effects can be understood in terms of the selective destruction of outer hair cells in the basal turn by SM, in the upper turns (of the cat) by DHSM (McGEE and OLSZEWSKI, 1962) and throughout the cochlea by NM. They should be worth reexamining by up-to-date methods of analysis for what additional information they might reveal about the components of the whole-nerve AP and their origins.

DAVIS *et al.* (1958) recorded the effects of SM in the various cochlear potentials of the guinea pig after intratympanic administration. They found that the endocochlear DC potential remained when CM was severely depressed, and that an AP response was still present when CM was very small. The summating potential (SP) appeared to be associated with the inner hair cells. Injury tended to enhance the negative SP and make it more regular. The more vulnerable positive SP was thought to have its source in the outer hair cells.

Dallos and his associates (DALLOS *et al.*, 1972; DALLOS and WANG, 1974) have used the selective destruction of the outer hair cells by KM in the guinea pig to make a close study of differences in the function of the outer and inner hair cells, and of their respective contributions to the summating and other cochlear potentials. DALLOS (1973) has presented their analysis and argument, which are too involved to be summarized here. They are based upon considerations of phase differences and distortion, and upon the assumption that the inner hair cells remain essentially intact after KM. Nevertheless, the changes in the stereocilia of the inner hair cells mentioned earlier (Fig. 13) suggest that they may not in fact retain their full functional integrity. The possibility must therefore be kept in mind that the negative SP may be largely of pathologic origin, the product of an injured organ of Corti.

Further investigations of cochlear nerve activity in aminoglycoside-injured ears have been concerned thus far with three general aspects of the neural responses to sound: a) adaptation of compound action potentials during stimulation at various rates; b) responses of single units, recorded with microelectrodes; and c) changes in compound action potentials during and after the development of ototoxic injury.

STANGE *et al.* (1964) measured adaptation rates of cochlear whole-nerve action potentials evoked by various rates of click stimulation in SM-treated cats. They found that the greater the dose of SM the animals received, the more rapid and complete was the adaptation of the AP responses. From their measurements they concluded that SM interferes with the formation and breakdown of a special excitatory substance in the hair cells, eliminating the more sensitive outer hair cells first. The condition of the hair cells was inferred from the adaptation data, but was not controlled histologically.

KIANG *et al.* (1970) used micropipette electrodes to record single unit responses from the cochlear nerves of anesthetized cats which had been treated with KM 200 mg/kg/day s.c. for 6–12 days. Examination of the cochlea postmortem revealed loss of both inner and outer hair cells from the first 5–10 mm of the basal turn in most of the animals. Units were first found by electrical stimulation, but many of those activated by shocks did not respond to sound, their hair cells presumably having been destroyed. Many units had abnormal tuning curves, some of such bizarre shape that no meaningful characteristic frequency (CF) could be assigned to them. Units unresponsive to sound were generally found at the periphery of the nerve, since that is the location of fibers from the lower basal turn. Fibers with low CF's located in the interior of the nerve trunk and representing the upper turns generally responded well. No evidence of hyperactivity was seen which might be correlated with tinnitus, any change in activity being in the direction of its reduction or elimination. A particular pattern of loss, with a sharp transition between absent and normal hair-cell activity was suggested as a possible explanation of tinnitus. Recruitment was more easily accounted for by noting the abnormal tuning curves of certain units tuned to high frequencies. These could no longer respond in their normal fashion to faint sound, but could still be activated when the intensity was increased.

The study of ARAN and DARROUZET (1975) is of interest not only for what it reveals of the long-term effect of cochlear injury by KM on the VIIIth nerve potentials, but also as an aid in the interpretation of electrocochleographic data in cases of sensorineural deafness in man. They recorded compound action potentials in response to clicks in guinea pigs with electrodes chronically implanted on the round window. Their technique was similar to that used by SIMMONS *et al.* (1960) and by OUCHI and OHTANI (1969) for following changes in CM in the course of aminoglycoside treatment.

During the brief but intensive administration of KM (400 mg/kg/day for 8 days) the responses were little altered, but they declined dramatically during the next 8–10 days. A phase of partial recovery lasting for about 2 months was followed by a long, slow decline until the end of the experiment at 7 months. During the initial period of rapid change thresholds increased by 20–40 dB, and latencies near threshold were markedly prolonged. At these levels N1 was absent, and the response was broad and slow. The overall amplitude was low, even at high intensities. These are characteristic features of the dissociated response seen in high-frequency hearing loss in man. Later with partial recovery the responses to filtered clicks at 4–8 kHz were of the recruiting type, with elevated thresholds but short latencies, and a rapid growth in amplitude as stimulus intensity was increased. With later deterioration of the response the thresholds became still higher, the latencies longer, and the amplitudes smaller. Cytocochleograms showed similar patterns of degeneration in all ears, with Corti's organ destroyed in the basal turn, inner hair cells present but many outer hair cells absent in the second turn, and scattered losses in higher turns. In general there was good agreement with histopathologic changes found by GONZALEZ *et al.* (1972) in KM-treated guinea pigs, some of which were killed immediately after treatment, others at 70 and 140 days. ARAN and DARROUZET distinguish between a period of acute intoxication by high concentrations of KM, and a period of metabolic impairment. During the partial recovery, KM is presumably cleared from the cochlea. The final slow decline, which the authors liken to an accelerated aging process (see also HAWKINS, 1973a) must represent the gradual degeneration of many of the cochlear nerve fibers following complete destruction of portions of the spiral organ.

I. Attempts to Minimize Ototoxicity

Over the years numerous attempts have been made, both in the laboratory and in the clinic, to reduce the ototoxicity of the aminoglycosides by administering them in combination with various other substances or in the form of special salts. Although many of the resulting preparations have achieved at least a passing vogue, it seems only prudent to admit that none of these praiseworthy efforts has been outstandingly successful.

The effect of calcium in reducing the acute toxicity of SM in the mouse has already been mentioned. The SM-calcium chloride complex, however, was no less vestibulotoxic than the hydrochloride or the sulfate (HAWKINS *et al.*, 1957). Hopes once placed in vitamins A (ESCHER and RUPP, 1953) and B (KLUYSKENS and VAN LINDT, 1953) as "detoxifying" agents proved ephemeral, and the same can be said for mercaptoethylamine (KLUYSKENS, 1953) and dimercaptopropanol (BAL) (HENNEBERT, 1953). More recent experiments by DARROUZET (1967) using surface preparations did not confirm his original impression (DARROUZET, 1963) of a protective action of "Otoneurine," a mixture of vitamin B-complex and aminoacids against KM in the guinea pig. Dexamethasone (Dectancyl) was found to be equally ineffective.

Special salts of SM and other antibiotics were introduced in the form of the glucuronate by ROSSI and OLIVIERI (1959) and the pantothenates by KELLER *ei al.* (1956). Although initial clinical reports about the reduced ototoxicity of the pantothenates were enthusiastic, the trials appear to have been inadequately controlled. A careful study by GLORIG (1958) revealed no significant difference in toxicity between DHSM-sulfate and a preparation of DHSM-pantothenate in tuberculous patients.

From an experimental investigation, HAWKINS *et al.* (1957) concluded that the vestibular toxicity of SM- and DHSM-pantothenates in the cat was not less than that of the sulfates. PLATTIG *et al.* (1967), using the three pantothenate salts of KM in an electrophysiologic study of adaptation of the AP response in cats, found the tri- and dipentothenates more ototoxic than KM-sulfate, but the monopantothenate less so in the conditions of the experiment. No data on hair cell loss were included in this report, but MERKLE *et al.* (1968) reached the same conclusions in their light-microscopic study using the Häutchenpräparat nethod of Neubert. According to STUPP (1970) these results are directly correlated with the levels reached by the various KM-pantothenates in the perilymph after parenteral administration. For KM-monopantothenate and KM-sulfate the maxima are lowest, but the monopantothenate shows the more rapid decline.

MORA *et al.* (1959) have shown that various polyanions are capable of reducing the acute toxicity of aminoglycosides by forming complexes with them. Such combinations may keep perilymph levels low but generally reduce antimicrobial activity as well (STUPP, 1973). This may be true of combinations with "Ozothine," an aqueous preparation of oxidation products of oil of turpentine, which has been found to reduce the ototoxicity of SM in animals (HOLZ *et al.*, 1967; STANGE *et al.*, 1967). Another is a depot preparation of SM, Streptomycin-Diactylpermoat (Hoechst) which gives prolonged low blood levels of SM with little or none appearing in the perilymph (RITTER *et al.*, 1971). LANGE (1972) has found SM with Ozothine useful in treating Menière's disease so as to affect the secretory tissues of the labyrinth with minimal loss of the hair cells.

With increasing knowledge not only of the pharmacokinetics but also of the mode of action of the aminoglycosides in the inner ear, one may hope for clearer understanding of structure-activity relationships with respect to their ototoxic action (BENVENISTE and DAVIES, 1973). With such information it may prove possible to select or devise with the aid of bacteria new or modified aminoglycosides with reduced ototoxicity while retaining satisfactory antimicrobial efficacy.

VI. Ethacrynic Acid and Furosemide

Ethacrynic acid (Edecrin, ETA) and furosemide (Lasix) are potent natriuretic agents introduced during the past decade which have furnished a forceful reminder of the close pathophysiologic kinship between the kidney and the inner ear (QUICK, 1973). Although the two drugs are quite different in chemical structure, the one being a derivative of phenoxyacetic acid, the other a relative of the sulfonamides, they have similar actions on the renal tubules, where they inhibit reabsorption of sodium and water in the proximal portion of the loop of Henle. The cellular mechanisms involved are not entirely clear, but three major possibilities have been put forward: a) inhibition of sodium-potassium dependent ATP-ase; b) reaction with protein-bound sulfhydryl groups; and c) a direct effect on energy metabolism in the mitochondria (SUKI *et al.*, 1973). The result has been described as an increase in tubular permeability rather than a decrease in ion transport, although BURG *et al.* (1973) found that the principal effect of furosemide in isolated perfused tubules is to inhibit active chloride transport in the ascending limb of Henle's loop.

A. Clinical Observations

Transient hearing loss in patients treated with ETA for oliguria was reported by Maher and Schreiner (1965) and by Schneider and Becker (1966). Pillay *et al.* (1969) showed that the loss was not always reversible, and that uremic patients might become permanently deaf as a result of ETA treatment. Similar reports soon began to appear about furosemide, at first emphasizing the transient character of the impairment (Vargish *et al.*, 1970; Schwartz *et al.*, 1970; Wigand and Heidland, 1970). More recently it has been recognized that permanent deafness can also occur after furosemide treatment (Quick and Hoppe, 1975). Furthermore, a patient who has had a severe transient deafness after furosemide can show a similar reaction to ETA (David and Hitzig, 1971) so that the two drugs resemble each other in their toxic actions on the inner ear as well as in their diuretic action on the kidney.

The conditions that determine whether diuretic-induced hearing loss in a given patient will be temporary or permanent are far from clear. Some authors have emphasized the severity of the uremia, others the oliguria itself as causative factors leading to retention and an irreversible ototoxic effect of the diuretic. Still others have made the important observation that permanent hearing loss can occur when patients being treated with an aminoglycoside are given either diuretic (Mathog and Klein, 1969; Meriwether *et al.*, 1971). Among the five cases reported by Johnson and Hamilton (1970) was one patient who developed a permanent hearing loss of 60–70 dB after receiving only 1 gm of KM followed by 50 mg of ETA. An even more remarkable case in their series was an oliguric patient who showed a similar hearing loss after only 1 gm of KM and 22.5 gm of mannitol given on the same day.

B. Animal Experiments

A number of laboratory studies of experimental animals have been made in an attempt to clarify the effects of ETA and furosemide on the inner ear. Although some authors have described a loss of cochlear hair cells after intravenous administration (Mathog *et al.*, 1970; Nakai, 1971; Crifò, 1973), others have found little or no change in the spiral organ (Kohonen *et al.*, 1970; Federspil and Hansen, 1973). It seems generally agreed that the initial action of ETA is on the stria vascularis (*cf.* Fig. 17), where extensive edematous swelling of the marginal and intermediate cells can be seen within minutes after an intravenous injection (Quick and Duvall, 1970; Nakai, 1971; Bosher *et al.*, 1973; Quick and Hoppe, 1975). The normally positive endocochlear potential rapidly becomes negative, as in anoxia. In some species there may be an increase in the concentration of Na^+ in the endolymph, with a fall in that of K^+ (Cohn *et al.*, 1971; Silverstein and Yules, 1971; Bosher *et al.*, 1973; Thalmann *et al.*, 1973). At present one cannot be sure whether the strial edema represents a temporary increase or a decrease in ion transport and water movements (Bosher *et al.*, 1973) but the net effect seems to be at least an interruption of normal strial function, and hence a disturbance of cochlear microhomeostasis. The strial changes are often reversible and do not necessarily give rise to a lasting injury to the hair cells (Federspil and Hansen,

1973). The stria itself has remarkable powers of recuperation (DUVALL *et al.*, 1974) and the edema produced by ETA slowly recedes. In cats SILVERSTEIN and BEGIN (1974) found its ototoxicity reversible, with only mild strial edema and cystic changes persisting $2^1/_2$ months after intracardiac injection of the diuretic.

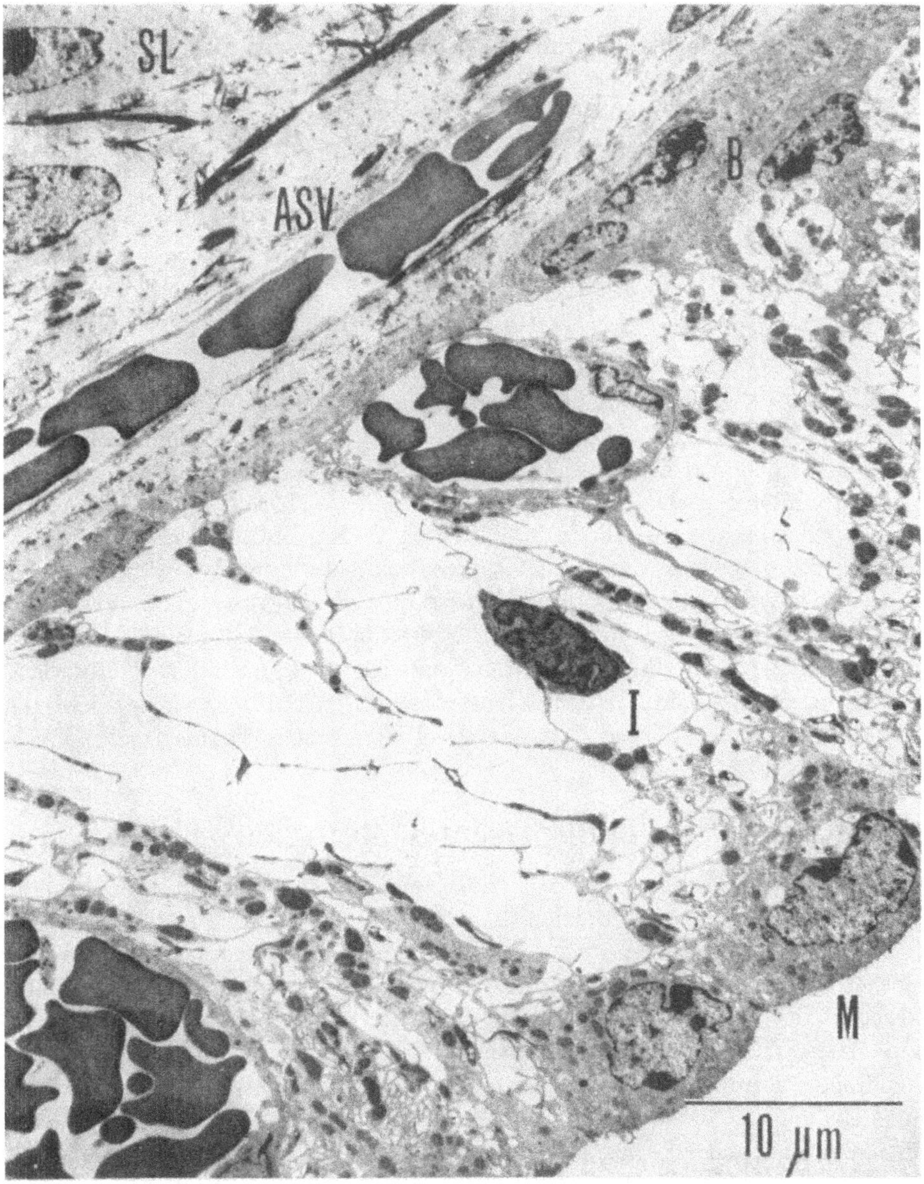

Fig. 17. Strial edema after combined treatment with ethacrynic acid and KM. Guinea pig killed 8 hrs after single dose of KM 200 mg/kg s.c., followed 2 hrs later by ETA 50 mg/kg i.v. M, marginal; I, intermediate; B, basal cells; ASV, adstrial vessel of spiral ligament, SL. EM, OsO_4

C. Interaction with Aminoglycosides

When given with a single dose of KM, an intravenous dose of ETA can cause extensive injury to the organ of Corti, although neither dose alone has any lasting effect on cochlear function (WEST *et al.*, 1973). There is a severe but apparently reversible strial edema (Fig. 17) followed 2 days later by injury to the suprastrial spiral ligament and destruction of hair cells. The potentiation is effective if the drugs are given within about 1 hr of each other. It presumably depends upon a breakdown of the hematolabyrinthine barrier for KM by ETA, or vice versa (HAWKINS *et al.*, 1975).

These experiments emphasize the need for the greatest caution in using diuretics of this class in patients who are receiving even a few doses of an aminoglycoside. Even furosemide alone given in large doses by "intravenous push" may cause a severe, irreversible hearing loss developing over a period of weeks (LLOYD-MOSTYN and LORD, 1971; QUICK and HOPPE, 1975).

D. Mode of Action

The biochemical mechanisms involved in the action of ETA and furosemide on the stria are presumably the same as those underlying the diuretic action. Although BROWN (1973) has suggested the possibility that strial carbonic anhydrase is affected, no similar acute ototoxic action has been seen with the carbonic anhydrase inhibitor acetazolamide (MENDELSOHN and MITTELMAN, 1971). Major emphasis has been placed on the inhibition of Na^+K^+-ATPase by ETA (PRAZMA *et al.*, 1972, among many others), but it is also a potent inhibitor of cochlear adenyl cyclase (KERR and SCHACHT, 1975). AHLSTRÖM *et al.* (1975) have found that the concentration of ETA required to reverse the sign of the endocochlear potential (10^{-5} molar) is much the same as that producing 50% inhibition of adenylate cyclase in mouse brain. A higher concentration (9.5×10^{-2} M) is required for inhibition of Na^+K^+-ATPase. Tissue levels of ETA in stria vascularis and kidney have not yet been determined.

VII. Transplacental Ototoxicity

Streptomycin has been shown to cross the placenta and to appear in the fetal blood, albeit in lower concentration than in the maternal (MOYA and THORNDIKE, 1963). KERN (1962) has reported a case of profound hearing loss in a child whose mother had received 20 gm of DHSM during the first 4 months of pregnancy. Other studies (ROBINSON and CAMBON, 1964; CONWAY and BIRT, 1965; VARPELA and HIETALAHTI, 1965) have discovered little evidence of ototoxic deafness acquired in utero by children whose mothers were treated with SM and DHSM.

A striking case of maternal and fetal ototoxicity attributed to combined treatment with KM and ETA has been reported by JONES (1973). The patient, in the 28th week of gestation, was given ETA when renal insufficiency developed while she was also receiving KM (1 gm/day, 4.5 gm total dose) for a Klebsiella infection. Two weeks later the mother suffered a complete sensorineural loss of hearing. The child, although normal in other respects, failed to develop speech. When tested at 3 years of age he appeared to be profoundly deaf.

VIII. Intratympanic Ototoxicity

Many substances can enter the perilymph via the round window membrane. All of the aminoglycosides tested and a number of other antibiotics (*e.g.*, chloramphenicol, tetracycline, erythromycin) have been shown to be ototoxic when placed in the middle ear (GULICK and PATTERSON, 1964; KOIDE *et al.*, 1966; D'ANGELO *et al.*, 1967; KOHONEN and TARKKANEN, 1969; STUPP *et al.*, 1973). Ethacrynic acid and furosemide, which have little permanent effect on the guinea pig cochlea when given parenterally, cause a dramatic edema of the stria and widespread destruction of Corti's organ when given intratympanically (HAWKINS and WRIGHT, unpubl.). The clinical use of ototopical antibiotics has been reviewed by KRAHL (1963) and MITTELMAN (1972). They find little evidence of inner ear injury by this route, presumably because of the low concentrations involved, but the risk is not to be regarded as merely hypothetical.

IX. Other Ototoxic Drugs

Space does not permit consideration of other representatives of the great variety of agents which have been reported to have ototoxic properties in man or in experimental animals. Useful reviews dealing with this broad range of substances have been published recently by BALLANTYNE (1973) and by AJODHIA and DIX (1975). One can hardly expect that the number of such drugs will grow measurably less in the near future. Increased awareness of their ototoxic potential should make it possible to contain the damage they may inflict on human ears.

Acknowledgments

Supported by USPHS Research Grant NS05065 and Program Project Grant NS05785 from the National Institute of Neurological and Communicative Disorders and Stroke. The electron micrographs were made by Mr. ROBERT E. PRESTON from sections prepared by Miss ANA LUISA RODRIGUEZ. Microdissection of human, monkey, and pigeon material was by L.-G. JOHNSSON, M. D. The technical assistance of Mrs. CAROLYN CLARK and Mrs. KAY CURRY is gratefully acknowledged, as are the secretarial and bibliographic labors of Mrs. JUNE LUDWIG, Miss JANET WILLIAMS, and Mrs. BARBARA DARNTON.

References

AHLSTRÖM, P., THALMANN, I., THALMANN, R., ISE, I.: Cyclic AMP and adenylate cyclase in the inner ear. Laryngoscope (St. Louis) **85**, 1241—1258 (1975).

AJODHIA, J.M., DIX, M.R.: Ototoxic effects of drugs. Minerva otorinolaring. (Torino) **25**, 117—131 (1975).

AKIYOSHI, M., SATO, K.: Histopathological and enzyme-histochemical studies on ototoxicity due to gentamicin and kanamycin in guinea pigs. Chemotherapy **15**, 501—512 (1967).

ANNIKO, M., WERSÄLL, J.: Damage to the stria vascularis in the guinea pig by acute atoxyl intoxication. Acta oto-laryng. (Stockh.) **80**, 167—179 (1975).

ARAN, J.-M., DARROUZET, J.: Observation of click-evoked compound VIII nerve responses before, during and over seven months after kanamycin treatment in the guinea pig. Acta oto-laryng. (Stockh.) **79**, 24—32 (1975).

BALLANTYNE, J.: Ototoxicity: A clinical review. Audiology **12**, 325—336 (1973).

BALOGH, K., HIRAIDE, F., ISHII, D.: Distribution of radioactive dihydrostreptomycin in the cochlea — an autoradiographic study. Ann. Otol. (St. Louis) **79**, 641—652 (1970).

BEARD, N.S., JR., ARMENTROUT, S.A., WEISBERGER, A.S.: Inhibition of mammalian protein synthesis by antibiotics. Pharmacol. Rev. **21**, 213—245 (1969).

BECK, C., KRAHL, P.: Experimentelle und feingewebliche Untersuchungen über die Ototoxicität von Kanamycin. Arch. Ohr-., Nas.-, u. Kehlk.-Heilk. **179**, 594—610 (1962).

BÉHAGUE, P., JULLIEN, W., GARDÈRES, M., DOUCET, P.: Action de la streptomycine sur l'equilibre chez les tuberculeux pulmonaires. Rev. neurol. **80**, 64—68 (1948).

BENVENISTE, R., DAVIES, J.: Structure-activity relationships among the aminoglycoside antibiotics: Role of hydroxyl and amino groups. Antimicrob. Agents Chemother. **4**, 402—409 (1973).

BERG, K.: The toxic effect of streptomycin on the eighth cranial nerve. Ann. Otol. (St. Louis) **58**, 448—456 (1949).

BERNABEI, L., DIBRINO, M., CONSALVO, P., PIERANGELI, C.E.: Contributo allo studio del danno labirintico sperimentale da gentamicina. Nota 1. Rilievi funzionali. Atti Accad. Fisiocr. Siena, Series 13, **16**, 445—467, 1221—1249 (1967).

BIGNALL, J.R., CROFTON, J.W., THOMAS, J.A.B.: Effect of streptomycin on vestibular function. Brit. med. J. **1**, 554—559 (1951).

BLAU, A.: Experimentelle Studien über die Veränderungen im Gehörorgan nach Vergiftung mit salizylsaurem Natrium. Arch. Ohrenheilk. **61**, 220—233 (1904).

BLOHMKE, A.: Über Schädigungen des 8. Hirnnerven bei Streptomycinbehandlung. Z. Laryng. Rhinol. **29**, 121—129 (1950).

BORNEMANN, W.: Ein Fall von Erblindung nach Atoxylinjektionen bei Lichen ruber planus. Münch. med. Wschr. **52**, 1043—1045 (1905).

BOSHER, S.K., SMITH, C., WARREN, R.L.: The effects of ethacrynic acid upon the cochlear endolymph and stria vascularis. A preliminary report. Acta oto-laryng. (Stockh.) **75**, 184—191 (1973).

BROWN, R.D.: Ototoxicity caused by ethacrynic acid and furosemide. Minerva otorinolaring. (Torino) **23**, 213—221 (1973).

BROWN, T.R.: Case of poisoning by oil of chenopodium. Maryland med. J. **4**, 20—28 (1878).

BRUMMETT, R.E., HIMES, D., SAINE, B., VERNON, J.: A comparative study of the ototoxicity of tobramycin and gentamicin. Arch. Otolaryng. (Chicago) **96**, 505—512 (1972).

BURG, M., STONER, L., CARDINAL, J., GREEN, N.: Furosemide effect on isolated perfused tubules. Amer. J. Physiol. **225**, 119—124 (1973).

CAUSSÉ, R.: Action toxique vestibulaire et cochléaire de la streptomycine au point de vue expérimental. Ann. Oto-laryng. (Paris) **66**, 518—538 (1949).

CAUSSÉ, R., GONDET, I., VALLANCIEN, B.: Action vestibulaire de la streptomycine chez la souris. C. R. Soc. Biol. (Paris) **142**, 747—749 (1948).

CAUSSÉ, R., BUU-HOI, N.P., GONDET, I., HOAN, N.: Modification des potentiels cochléaires du cobaye sous l'influence de l'acide acétylamino-phénylarsinique (arsacetine). C. R. Soc. Biol. (Paris) **143**, 68—70 (1949a).

CAUSSÉ, R., GONDET, I., VALLANCIEN, B.: Action de las streptomycine sur les cellules ciliées des organes vestibulaires de la souris. C. R. Soc. Biol. (Paris) **143**, 619—620 (1949b).

CAUSSÉ, R., GONDET, I., GRIBENSKI, A.: Lésions cochléaires accompagnant, chez le cobaye, la surdité caussée par l'arsacétine (acide acétyl-para-aminophényl-arsinique). C. R. Soc. Biol. (Paris) **144**, 63—66 (1950).

CHRISTENSEN, E., HERTZ, H., RISKAER, N., VRAA-JENSEN, G.: Histological investigation in chronic streptomycin poisoning in guinea pigs. Ann. Otol. (St. Louis) **60**, 343—349 (1951).

COHEN, S.S., JOHNSEN, L., LICHTENSTEIN, M.R., LYNCH, J.W.: A comparative study of streptomycin and dihydrostreptomycin in pulmonary tuberculosis. Amer. Rev. Tuberc. **68**, 229—237 (1953).

COHN, E.S., GORDES, E.H., BRUSILOW, S.W.: Ethacrynic acid effect on the composition of cochlear fluids. Science **171**, 910—911 (1971).

CONWAY, N., BIRT, B.D.: Streptomycin in pregnancy: Effect on the foetal ear. Brit. med. J. **2**, 260—263 (1965).

COVELL, W.P.: A cytologic study of the effects of drugs on the cochlea. Arch. Otolaryng. (Chicago) **23**, 663—641 (1936).

COVELL, W. P.: Effects of drugs on the stria vascularis. Arch. Otolaryng. (Chicago) **27**, 438—443 (1938).

CRIFÒ, S.: Ototoxicity of sodium ethacrynate in the guinea pig. Arch. Otorhinolaryngol. **206**, 27—38 (1973).

D'ANGELO, E. P., PATTERSON, W. C., MORROW, R. C.: Chloramphenicol. Topical application in the middle ear. Arch. Otolaryng. (Chicago) **85**, 682—684 (1967).

DALLOS, P.: Cochlear potentials and cochlear mechanics. In: Basic Mechanisms in Hearing. MØLLER, A. R. (ed.). New York and London: Academic Press, Inc. 1973.

DALLOS, P., WANG, C.-Y.: Bioelectric correlates of kanamycin intoxication. Audiology **13**, 277—289 (1974).

DALLOS, P., BILLONE, M. C., DURRANT, J. D., WANG, C.-Y., RAYNOR, S.: Cochlear inner and outer hair cells: Functional differences. Science **177**, 356—358 (1972).

DALY, J. F., COHEN, N. L.: Viomycin ototoxicity in man. A cupulometric study. Ann. Otol. (St. Louis) **74**, 521—534 (1965).

DARROUZET, J.: Essais de protection de l'organe de Corti contre l'ototoxicité des antibiotiques. Étude expérimentale. Rev. Laryng. (Bordeaux) **84**, 459—478 (1963).

DARROUZET, J.: Essais de protection de l'organe de Corti contre l'ototoxicité des antibiotiques. Acta oto-laryng. (Stockh.) **63** (appendix) 49—64 (1967).

DARROUZET, J., DE LIMA SOBRINHO, E.: Oreille interne, kanamycine et traumatisme acoustique: Étude expérimentale. Rev. Laryng. (Bordeaux) **83**, 781—806 (1962).

DARROUZET, J., GUILHAUME, A.: Ototoxicité de la kanamycine au jour le jour. Étude expérimentale en microscopie électronique. Rev. Laryng. (Bordeaux) **95**, 601—621 (1974).

DAVID, D. S., HITZIG, P.: Diuretics and ototoxicity. New Engl. J. Med. **284**, 1328—1329 (1971).

DAVIS, H., GERNANDT, B. E., RIESCO-MACCLURE, J. S.: Threshold of action potentials in ear of guinea pig. J. Neurophysiol. **13**, 73—87 (1950).

DAVIS, H., DEATHERAGE, B. H., RONSENBLUT, B., FERNÁNDEZ, C., KIMURA, R., SMITH, C. A.: Modification of cochlear potentials produced by streptomycin poisoning and by extensive venous obstruction. Laryngoscope (St. Louis) **68**, 596—627 (1958).

DAYAL, V. S., SMITH, E. L., MCCANIN, W. G.: Cochlear and vestibular gentamicin toxocity. Arch. Otolaryng. (Chicago) **100**, 338—340 (1974).

DAYAL, V. S., WHITEHEAD, G. L., SMITH, E. L.: Gentamycin—progressive cochlear toxicity. Canad. J. Otolaryng. **4**, 348—351 (1975).

DE MOURA, L. F. P., HAYDEN, R. C.: Salicylate ototoxicity. A human temporal bone report. Arch. Otolaryng. (Chicago) **87**, 368—372 (1968).

DIX, M. R.: The effects of streptomycin on the eighth nerve system. J. Laryng. **62**, 735—745 (1948).

DIX, M. R., HALLPIKE, C. S., HARRISON, M. S.: Some observations upon the otological effects of streptomycin intoxication. Brain **72**, 241—245 (1949).

DUVALL, A. J., WERSÄLL, J.: Site of action of streptomycin upon inner ear sensory cell. Acta oto-laryng. (Stockh.) **57**, 581—598 (1964).

DUVALL, A. J., WARD, W. D., LAUHALA, K. E.: Strial ultrastructure and vessel transport in acoustic trauma. Ann. Otol. (St. Louis) **83**, 498—514 (1974).

EDISON, A. O., FROST, B. M., GRAESSLE, O. E., HAWKINS, J. E., JR., KUNA, S., MUSHETT, C. W., SILBER, R. H., SOLOTOROVSKY, M.: An experimental evaluation of dihydrostreptomycin. Amer. Rev. Tuberc. **58**, 487—493 (1948).

EHRLICH, P.: Chemotherapeutische Trypanosomen-Studien. Berl. klin. Wschr. **44**, 280—283 (1907).

ENGSTRÖM, H., ADES, H. W., ANDERSSON, A.: Structural pattern of the organ of Corti. Stockholm: Almqvist and Wiksell 1966.

ERB, K.: Über Cochlear und Vestibularschädigungen nach Vergiftung mit Oleum Chenopodii. Z. Laryng. Rhinol. **28**, 449—454 (1949).

ESCHER, F., RUPP, F.: Die Schutzfunktion des Vitamin A bei der Streptomycin-intoxikation. Acta oto-laryng. (Stockh.) **43**, 311—321 (1953).

FALBE-HANSEN, J.: Clinical and experimental histological studies on effects of salicylate and quinine on the ear. Acta oto-laryng. (Stockh.) Suppl. **44** (1941).

FARKASHIDY, J., BLACK, R. G., BRIANT, T. D. R.: Effect of kanamycin on the internal ear: An electrophysiological and electron microscopic study. Laryngoscope (St. Louis) **73**, 713—727 (1963).

FEDERSPIL, P.: Über das Haarzellenschädigungsmuster nach parenteraler Gentamicin-Applikation beim Meerschweinchen. Z. Laryng. Rhinol. **51**, 845—866 (1972).

FEDERSPIL, P.: Morphologische Untersuchungen zur Ototoxizität von Gentamicin und Tobramycin. Arzneimittel-Forsch. **23**, 1739—1745 (1973).

FEDERSPIL, P., HANSEN, H.: Experimentelle Untersuchungen zur Ototoxicität des Furosemid. Res. exp. Med. **161**, 175—184 (1973).

FERREIRA, S. H., VANE, J. R.: Aspirin and prostaglandins. In: The Prostaglandins, Vol. 2. RAMWELL, P. W. (ed.). New York: Plenum Press 1974.

FLOBERG, L. E., HAMBERGER, C.-A., HYDÉN, H.: Inhibition of nucleic acid production in vestibular nerve cells by streptomycin. Acta oto-laryng. (Stockh.) Suppl. **75**, 36—52 (1949).

FORDYCE, J. A.: The modern treatment of syphilis, with reference to the recent synthetic preparations. J. Amer. med. Ass. **56**, 186—192 (1911).

FOWLER, E. P., JR., SELIGMAN, E.: Otic complications of streptomycin therapy. J. Amer. med. Ass. **133**, 87—91 (1947).

GIGNOUX, M., MARTIN, H., CAJGFINGER, H.: Troubles cochleo-vestibulaires apres tentative de suicide a l'aspirine. J. franç. Oto-rhinolaryng. **15**, 631—635 (1966).

GLORIG, A.: The effect of dihydrostreptomycin hydrochloride and sulfate on auditory mechanism. Ann. Otol. (St. Louis) **60**, 327—335 (1951).

GLORIG, A.: Report of a recent study on dihydroestreptomycin ototoxicity. Laryngoscope (St. Louis) **68**, 1013—1027 (1958).

GLORIG, A., FOWLER, E. P., JR.: Tests for the labyrinth function following streptomycin therapy. Ann. Otol. (St. Louis) **56**, 379—394 (1947).

GONZALEZ, G., MILLER, N., WASILEWSKI, V.: Progressive neuro-ototoxicity of kanamycin. Ann. Otol. (St. Louis) **81**, 127—131 (1972).

GRADENIGO, G.: Krankheiten des Labyrinths und des Nervus acusticus. In: Handbuch der Ohrenheilkunde. II. F. C. W. VOGEL, Leipzig, hrsg. H. Schwartze, pp. 352—353, 474—479, 1892.

GRAF, K.: Die Schädigungen des Vestibularis und Kochlearis durch Streptomycin. Pract. oto-rhino-laryng. (Basel) **10**, 527—533 (1948).

GRAF, K.: Streptomycindosierung und neurotoxische Nebenwirkungen. Schweiz. med. Wschr. **35**, 793—814 (1949).

GRAF, K.: Histologische Veränderungen des Innenohres nach Behandlung der Meningitis Tuberculosa mit Streptomycin. Acta oto-laryng. (Stockh.) **39**, 121—131 (1951).

GRAHAM, J. D. P., PARKER, W. A.: The toxic manifestations of sodium salicylate therapy. Quart. J. Med. **41**, 153—163 (1948).

GRANT, W. M.: Toxicology of the eye. Springfield: C. C. Thomas, pp. 452—455, 1962.

GULICK, W. L., PATTERSON, W. C.: The effects of chloramphenicol upon the electrical activity of the ear. II. Long. term data. Ann. Otol. (St. Louis) **73**, 204—209 (1964).

HAWKINS, J. E., JR.: Disturbances of vestibular function produced in animals by streptomycin. Fed. Proc. **6**, 125 (1947).

HAWKINS, J. E., JR.: Cochlear signs of streptomycin intoxication. J. Pharmacol. exp. Ther. **100**, 38—44 (1950).

HAWKINS, J. E., JR.: The ototoxicity of hydroxystreptomycin. In: Transactions of the tenth conference on the chemotherapy of tuberculosis. Veterans Administration, Washington pp. 224—226, 1951.

HAWKINS, J. E., JR.: Vascular patterns of the membranous labyrinth. In: Third symposium on the role of vestibular organs in space exploration. GRAYBIEL, A. (ed.). Washington, D. C.: National Aeronautics and Space Administration 1967.

HAWKINS, J. E., JR.: Comparative otopathology: aging, noise and ototoxic drugs. Advanc. Oto-rhino-laryng. **20**, 125—141 (1973a).

HAWKINS, J. E., JR.: Ototoxic mechanisms: a working hypothesis. Audiology **12**, 383—393 (1973b).

HAWKINS, J. E., JR., ENGSTRÖM, H.: Effect of kanamycin on cochlear cytoarchitecture. Acta oto-laryng. (Stockh.) suppl. **188**, 100—106 (1964).

HAWKINS, J. E., JR., LURIE, M. H.: The ototoxicity of streptomycin. Ann. Otol. (St. Louis) **61**, 789—806 (1952).

HAWKINS, J.E., JR., LURIE, M.H.: The ototoxicity of dihydrostreptomycin and neomycin in the cat. Ann. Otol. (St. Louis) **62**, 1128—1148 (1953).

HAWKINS, J.E., JR., O'SHANNY, W.: Functional analysis of the chronic neurotoxic action of streptomycin. Fed. Proc. **7**, 225 (1948).

HAWKINS, J.E., JR., PRESTON, R.E.: Vestibular ototoxicity. In: The vestibular system. NAUNTON, R.F. (ed.). New York: Academic Press 1975.

HAWKINS, J.E., JR., WRIGHT, C.G.: Irreversible ototoxicity of ethacrynic acid and furosemide after intratympanic injection, (unpublished).

HAWKINS, J.E., JR., BOXER, G.E., JELINEK, V.C.: Concentration of streptomycin in brain and other tissues of cats after acute and chronic intoxication. Proc. Soc. exp. Biol. (N. Y.) **75**, 759—761 (1950).

HAWKINS, J.E., JR., JOHNSSON, L.-G., ARAN, J.-M.: Comparative tests of gentamicin ototoxicity. J. infect. Dis. **119**, 417—426 (1969).

HAWKINS, J.E., JR., JOHNSSON, L.-G., STEBBINS, W.C., MOODY, D.B., MURASKI, A.: The patas monkey as a model for dihydrostreptomycin ototoxicity. (In preparation, 1976).

HAWKINS, J.E., JR., MARQUES, D.M., CLARK, C.S., PRESTON, R.: Ototoxic potentiation between ethacrynic acid and aminoglycoside antibiotics in guinea pigs. J. acoust. Soc. Amer. **57**, Suppl. 1, S60 (1975).

HAWKINS, J.E., JR., WOLCOTT, H., O'SHANNY, W.J.: Ototoxic effects of streptomycin and dihydrostreptomycin pantothenates in the cat. In: Antibiotics annual 1956—1957. New York: Medical Encyclopedia, Inc., pp. 554—563, 1957.

HENNEBERT, M.P.E.: Traitment par le B.A.L. des intoxications streptomyciniques de l'oreille interne. Ann. Oto-laryng. (Paris) **70**, 473—477 (1953).

HINSHAW, H.C., FELDMAN, W.H.: Streptomycin in the treatment of clinical tuberculosis: a preliminary report. Proc. Mayo Clin. **20**, 313—318 (1945).

HINSHAW, H.C., FELDMAN, W.H., CARR, D.T., BROWN, H.: The clinical administration of dihydrostreptomycin in tuberculosis: a preliminary report. Amer. Rev. Tuberc. **58**, 525—530 (1948).

HOBSON, L.B., TOMPSETT, R., MUSCHENHEIM, C., MCDERMOTT, W.: A laboratory and clinical investigation of dihydrostreptomycin. Amer. Rev. Tuberc. **58**, 501—524 (1948).

HOLZ, E., HOFFMAN, M., BECK, C.: Morphologische und bakteriologische Befunde zur Minderung der Ototoxicität basischer Streptomycesantibiotika. Arch. klin. exp. Ohr.-, Nas.- u. Kehlk.-Heilk. **188**, 236—242 (1967).

v. ILBERG, C., SPOENDLIN, H., ARNOLD, W.: Autoradiographical distribution of locally applied dihydrostreptomycin in the inner ear. Acta oto-laryng. (Stockh.) **71**, 159—165 (1971).

IGARASHI, M., LUNDQUIST, PER-G., ALFORD, B.R., MYATA, H.: Experimental ototoxicity of gentamicin in squirrel monkeys. J. infect. Dis. Suppl. **124**, S 114—S 124 (1971).

JACKSON, G.G., ARCIERI, G.: Ototoxicity of gentamicin in man: a survey and controlled analysis of clinical experience in the United States. J. infect. Dis. **124**, Suppl. S 130—S 137 (1971).

JARVIS, J.F.: A case of unilateral permanent deafness following acetyl salicylic acid. J. Laryng. **80**, 318—320 (1966).

JATHO, K.: Über Vestibularis- und Cochlearisschädigungen bei Streptomycinbehandlung und deren Bedeutung für die Otologie. Arch. Ohr.-, Nas.- u. Kehlk.-Heilk. **157**, 276—300 (1950).

JOHNSON, A.H., HAMILTON, C.H.: Kanamycin ototoxicity—possible potentiation by other drugs. Sth. med. J. (Bgham, Ala.) **63**, 511—513 (1970).

JOHNSSON, L.-G., HAWKINS, J.E., JR.: Strial atrophy in clinical and experimental deafness. Laryngoscope (St. Louis) **82**, 1105—1125 (1972).

JONES, H.C.: Intrauterine ototoxicity: A case report and review of literatur. J. nat. med. Ass. **65**, 201—203 (1973).

JONGKEES, L.B.W., HULK, J.: The action of streptomycin on vestibular function. Acta oto-laryng. (Stockh.) **38**, 225—232 (1950).

JUUL, A., VRAA-JENSEN, G.: On the effect of ascaridole on the inner ear. Electrobiological and histological studies on the localization of the cochlear microphone effect. Acta pharmacol. (Kbh.) **3**, 51—72 (1947).

KANEKO, Y., NAKOGAWA, T., TANAKA, K.: Reissner's membrane after kanamycin administration. Arch. Otolaryng. (Chicago) **92**, 457—462 (1970).

KAPUR, Y. P.: Ototoxicity of acetylsalicylic acid. Arch. Otolaryng. (Chicago) **81**, 134—138 (1965).

KELLER, H., KRÜPE, W., SOUS, H., MÜCKTER, H.: Versuche zur Toxizitätsminderung basischer Streptomyces-Antibiotika. 1. Mitteilung: Streptomycin und Dihydrostreptomycin. Arzneimittel-Forsch. **5**, 170—176 (1955).

KERN, G.: Zur Frage der intrauterinen Streptomycinschädigung. Schweiz. med. Wschr. **92**, 77—79 (1962).

KERR, T. P., SCHACHT, J.: Adenyl cyclase in the guinea pig cochlea. J. acoust. Soc. Amer. **57**, S61 (1975).

KESER, H.: Nystagmographie der Streptomycinschädigungen des Vestibularis. Arch. Ohr.-, Nas.- u. Kehlk.-Heilk. **156**, 475—478 (1950).

KIRCHNER, W.: Über die Einwirkung von Chinin und Salicylsäure auf das Gehörorgan. Berl. klin. Wschr. **18**, 725—726 (1881).

KIRCHNER, W.: Extravasat im Labyrinth durch Chinin- und Salicylwirkung. Mschr. Ohrenheilk. **17**, 85—88 (1883).

KIANG, N. Y. S., MOXON, E. C., LEVINE, R. A.: Auditory-nerve activity in cats with normal and abnormal cochleas. In: Sensorineural hearing loss. WOLSTENHOLME, G. E. W., KNIGHT, J. (eds.). London: J. & A. Churchill, pp. 241—237, 1970.

KLUYSKENS, P.: La mercaptoethylamine et l'intoxication a la dihydrostreptomycine. C. R. Soc. Biol. (Paris) **147**, 733—735 (1953).

KLUYSKENS, P., LINDT, P. v.: Peut-on diminuer les effets toxiques de la dihydrostreptomycine? Acta oto-rhino-laryng. belg. **7**, 371—376 (1953).

KOBRAK, F.: Die Salvarsanschäden des inneren Ohres. Klin. Wschr. **5**, 1572—1573 (1926).

KOIDE, Y., HATA, A., HANDO, R.: Vulnerability of the organ of Corti in poisoning. Acta oto-laryng. (Stockh.) **61**, 332—344 (1966).

KOHONEN, A.: Effect of some ototoxic drugs upon the pattern and innervation of cochlear sensory cells in the guinea pig. Acta oto-laryng. (Stockh.) Suppl. **208**, 1—70 (1965).

KOHONEN, A., TARKKANEN, J.: Cochlear damage from ototoxic antibiotics by intratympanic application. Acta oto-laryng. (Stockh.) **68**, 90—97 (1969).

KOHONEN, A., JAUHIAINEN, T., TARKKANEN, J.: Experimental deafness caused by ethacrynic acid. Acta oto-laryng. (Stockh.) **70**, 187—189 (1970).

KOPKE, A.: Les troubles oculaires dans la maladie du sommeil. Bull. Soc. Path. exot. **15**, 139—146 (1922).

KRAHL, P.: Ototoxische Antibiotica in Ohrentropfen, ihre Vorzüge und Gefahren. Arch. klin. exp. Ohr.-, Nas.- u. Kehlk.-Heilk. **182**, 591—593 (1963).

KRAUS, H., DOENNING, A.: Cytophotometrische RNA — und Eiweißbestimmungen am häutigen Innenohr des Meerschweinchens als Grundlagen zur Beurteilung des Eiweißstoffwechsels und der Streptomycin-Ototoxicität. Arch. klin. exp. Ohr.-, Nas.- u. Kehlk.-Heilk. **194**, 551—557 (1969).

KREJCI, F., BEJDL, W.: Analytische Untersuchungen mit radioaktivem Phosphor (P^{32}) über die Hörschädigung bei Oleum-Chenopodii-Vergiftung. Arch. Ohr.-, Nas.- u. Kehlk.-Heilk. **164**, 539—542 (1954).

LANGE, G.: Ergebnisse der Streptomycin-Ozothin-Behandlung beim Morbus Menière. Arch. klin. exp. Ohr.-, Nas.- u. Kehlk.-Heilk. **203**, 16—22 (1972).

LAVERAN, A.: Traité du paludisme. Paris, Masson et Cie. p. 368, 1898.

LAWRENCE, M.: Circulation in the capillaries of the basilar membrane. Laryngoscope (St. Louis) **80**, 1364—1375 (1970).

LEONARD, J. E., NAKASHIMA, D., SNOW, J. B., JR.: The effects of damage to the organ of Corti and the stria vascularis on endolymphatic cationic changes. Arch. Otolaryng. (Chicago) **94**, 541—547 (1971).

LIDÉN, G.: Loss of hearing following treatment with dihydrostreptomycin or streptomycin. Acta oto-laryng. (Stockh.) **43**, 551—572 (1953).

LLOYD-MOSTYN, R. H., LORD, I. J.: Ototoxicity of intravenous frusemide. Lancet **2**, 1156—1157 (1971).

LURIE, M. H.: Studies of acquired and inherited deafness in animals. J. acoust. Soc. Amer. **11**, 420—426 (1940).

MAHADY, S.C.F., ARMSTRONG, F.L., BECK, F., HORTON, R., LINCOLN, N.S.: A comparative study of streptomycin and dihydrostreptomycin in pulmonary tuberculosis. Amer. Rev. Tuberc. **68**, 238—248 (1953).

MAHER, J.F., SCHREINER, G.E.: Studies on ethacrynic acid in patients with refractory edema. Ann. intern. Med. **62**, 15—29 (1965).

MAJER, E.H.: Ergebnisse der Cochlear- und Vestibularprüfung nach Streptomycinbehandlung. Wien. klin. Wschr. **60**, 844—845 (1948).

MATHOG, R.H., KLEIN, W.J., JR.: Ototoxicity of ethacrynic acid and aminoglycoside antibiotics in uremia. New Engl. J. Med. **280**, 1223—1224 (1969).

MATHOG, R.H., THOMAS, W.G., HUDSON, W.R.: Ototoxicity of new and potent diuretics. A preliminary study. Arch. Otolaryng. (Chicago) **92**, 7—13 (1970).

MCCABE, P., DEY, F.: The effect of aspirin upon auditory sensitivity. Ann. Otol. (St. Louis) **74**, 312—324 (1965).

MCGEE, T.M., OLSZEWSKI, J.: Streptomycin sulfate and dihydrostreptomycin toxicity. Behavioral and histopathologic studies. Arch. Otolaryng. (Chicago) **75**, 295—311 (1962).

MCGIFF, J.C., NASJLETTI, A.: Renal prostaglandins and the regulation of blood pressure. In: Prostaglandins and cyclic AMP. Biological actions and clinical applications. KAHN, R.H. and LANDS, W.E.M. (eds.). New York: Academic Press, Inc. pp. 119—151, 1973.

MÊLIER, F.: Expériences et observations sur les propriétés toxiques du sulfate de quinine. Mém. Acad. Méd. (Paris) **10**, 722—745 (1843).

MENDELSOHN, M., MITTELMAN, J.: Diuretics and the cation content of guinea pig endolymph. Ann. Otol. (St. Louis) **80**, 186—191 (1971).

MERIWETHER, W.D., MANGI, R.J., SERPICK, A.A.: Deafness following standard intravenous dose of ethacrynic acid. J. Amer. med. Ass. **216**, 795—798 (1971).

MERKLE, U., PLATTIG, K.H., KEIDEL, U.O.: Histologische Untersuchungen zur ototoxischen Wirkung des Kanamycins am Cortischen Organ der Katze. Z. mikr.-anat. Forsch. **78**, 441—460 (1968).

MITCHELL, C., BRUMMETT, R., HIMES, D., VERNON, J.: Electrophysiological study of the effect of sodium salicylate upon the cochlea. Arch. Otolaryng. (Chicago) **98**, 297—301 (1973).

MITTELMAN, H.: Ototoxicity of ototopical antibiotics. Past, present and future. Trans. Amer. Acad. Ophthal. Otolaryng. **76**, 1432—1443 (1972).

MOLITOR, H., KUNA, S.: The significance of neurotropic properties of commercial streptomycin. Arch. int. Pharmacodyn. **74**, 334—342 (1947).

MOLITOR, H., GRAESSLE, O.E., KUNA, S., MUSHETT, C.W., SILBER, R.H.: Some toxicological properties of streptomycin. J. Pharmacol. exp. Ther. **86**, 151—173 (1946).

MORA, P.T., YOUNG, B.G., SHEAR, M.J.: Reduction of toxicity of cationic macromolecules by complexing with anionic derivatives of synthetic polyglucoses. Nature (Lond.) **184**, 431—432 (1959).

MORTON, R.: Exercitationes de morbis universalibus acutis. Ed. ult. Venice: Typis Hieronymi Albuzzi, 1696.

MOYA, F., THORNDIKE, V.: Passage of drugs across the placenta. Amer. J. Obstet. Gynec. **84**, 1778—1798 (1963).

MÜCKTER, H.: Zur Pharmakologie der basischen Streptomyces-Antibiotika. Antibiot. et Chemother. (Basel) **9**, 83—144 (1961).

MURAVEISKAYA, V.S.: Opredelenie konsentratsii streptomitsina, digidrostreptomitsina, kolimitsina, i monomitsina v labirintnoi zhidkosti morskikh svinok. Antibiotiki **10**, 249—250 (1965).

MÜSEBECK, K., SCHÄTZLE, W.: Experimentelle Studien zur Ototoxicität des Dihydrostreptomycins. Arch. Ohr.-, Nas.- u. Kehlk.-Heilk. **181**, 41—48 (1962).

MYERS, E.N., BERSTEIN, J.M.: Salicylate ototoxicity: A clinical experimental study. Arch. Otolaryng. (Chicago) **82**, 483—493 (1965).

MYERS, E.N., BERNSTEIN, J.M., FOSTIROPOLOUS, G.: Salicylate ototoxicity. A clinical study. New Engl. J. Med. **273**, 587—590 (1965).

NAKAI, Y.: Electron microscopic study of the inner ear after ethacrynic acid intoxication. Pract. oto-rhino-laryng. (Basel) **33**, 366—376 (1971).

NAUNTON, R.F., WARD, P.H.: The ototoxicity of kanamycin in the presence of compromised renal function. Arch. Otolaryng. (Chicago) **69**, 398—399 (1959).

NORTH, A.: Two cases of poisoning by the oil of chenopodium. Amer. J. Otol. **2**, 197—200 (1880).

NORTHINGTON, P.: Syndrome of bilateral vestibular paralysis and its occurrence from streptomycin therapy. Arch. Otolaryng. (Chicago) **52**, 380—396 (1950).

NOWAK, R.: Submikroskopische Veränderungen der Reissnerschen Membran nach Streptomycinapplikation. Acta oto-laryng. (Stockh.) **77**, 37—43 (1974).

OKA, N.: Über die Ascaridolvergiftung. Pharmacologie **4**, 201—232 (1929).

OPPIKOFER, E.: Chenopodiumölvergiftung und Gehörorgan. Korresp.-Bl. schweiz. Ärz. **49**, 161—172 (1919).

OUCHI, J., OHTANI, I.: Studies on the ototoxicity of kanamycin. The correlation between electrophysiological findings and histopathological changes. Pract. oto-rhino-laryng. (Basel) **31**, 218—233 (1969).

OZAKI: Z. Otol. (Tokio) **41**, 1935 (cit. WERNER 1940a).

OZENI: Z. Otol. (Tokio) **43**, 1937 (cit. WERNER 1940b).

PILLAY, V. K. G., SCHAWARTZ, F. D., AIMI, K., KARK, R. M.: Transient and permanent deafness following treatment with ethacrynic acid in renal failure. Lancet **1**, 77 (1969).

PLATTIG, K. H., KEIDEL, U. O., DAVID, E.: Minderung der Ototoxizität des Kanamycins durch Pantothensäure. Elektrophysiologische Untersuchungen an der Katze. Dtsch. Med. Wschr. **92**, 1391—1397 (1967).

POHLMAN, A. G., KRANZ, F. W.: On the effect of certain drugs, notably quinine on the acuity of hearing. Proc. Soc. exp. Biol. (N. Y.) **20**, 140—151 (1922).

PORTMANN, M., DARROUZET, J., COSTE, C.: Distribution within the cochlea of dihydrostreptomycin injected into the circulation. Arch. Otolaryng. (Chicago) **100**, 473—475 (1974).

PRAZMA, J., THOMAS, W. G., FISHER, D., PRESLAR, M. J.: Ototoxicity of the ethacrynic acid. Arch. Otolaryng. (Chicago) **95**, 448—456 (1972).

QUICK, C. A.: The relationship between cochlea and kidney. Laryngoscope (St. Louis) **83**, 1469—1482 (1973).

QUICK, C. A., DUVALL, A. J., III: Early changes in the cochlear duct from ethacrynic acid: An electronmicroscopic evaluation. Laryngoscope (St. Louis) **80**, 954—965 (1970).

QUICK, C. A., HOPPE, W.: Permanent deafness associated with furosemide administration. Ann. Otol. (St. Louis) **84**, 94—100 (1975).

RITTER, R., CHOU, J., ILBERG, C. v., WAGNER, W. H.: Eine neue Möglichkeit zur Verhinderung der Ototoxicität des Streptomycins. Arch. klin. exp. Ohr.-, Nas.- u. Kehlk.-Heilk. **199**, 573—577 (1971).

ROBINSON, G. C., CAMBON, K. G.: Hearing loss in infants of tuberculous mothers treated with streptomycin during pregnancy. New Engl. J. Med. **271**, 949—951 (1964).

ROOSA, D. B., JOHN, ST.: Experiments concerning the effects of quinine upon the ear. Trans. Amer. otol. Soc. **2**, 93—97 (1875).

ROSENWASSER, H.: Neuritis of the auditory nerve occurring during intravenous arsenic medication. Arch. Otolaryng. (Chicago) **15**, 284—288 (1932).

ROSS, E. L., LEDERER, L. G.: Influence of some toxic substances on the inner ear. Laryngoscope (St. Louis) **47**, 555—571 (1937).

ROSSI, G., OLIVIERI, A.: The salts derived from the combination of streptomycin and neomycin with glucuronic acid. A.M.A. Arch. Otolaryng. **69**, 188—196 (1959).

ROTH, D. A.: Some dangers of the chenopodium treatment. Sth med. J. (Bgham, Ala.) **11**, 733—734 (1918).

RÜEDI, L.: Some animal experimental findings on the functions of the inner ear. Ann. Otol. (St. Louis) **60**, 993—1023 (1951).

RÜEDI, L., FURRER, W., ESCHER, F., LÜTHY, F.: Toxische Wirkungen des Streptomycins. Acta oto-laryng. (Stockh.) Suppl. **78**, 66—77 (1949).

RÜEDI, L., FURRER, W., GRAF, K., NAGER, G., TSCHIRREN, B., LUTHY, F.: Nouvelles constatations sur la toxicité de la streptomycine et de la quinine à l'égard de l'oreille du cobaye. Rev. Laryng. (Bordeaux) **72**, 238—264 (1951).

RÜEDI, L., FURRER, W., LUTHY, F., NAGER, G., TSCHIRRER, B.: Further observations concerning the toxic effects of streptomycin and quinine on the auditory organ of guinea pigs. Laryngoscope (St. Louis) **62**, 333—357 (1952).

SCHACHT, J.: Interaction of neomycin with phosphoinositide metabolism in guinea pig inner ear and brain tissues. Ann. Otol. (St. Louis) **83**, 613—618 (1974).

SCHACHT, J.: Biochemistry of neomycin ototoxicity. J. acoust. Soc. Amer. **59**, 940—944 (1976).

SCHNEIDER, W. J., BECKER, E. L.: Acute transient hearing loss after ethacrynic acid therapy. Arch. intern. Med. **117**, 715—717 (1966).

SCHWABACH, D.: Über bleibende Störungen im Gehörorgan nach Chinin und Salicylgebrauch. Dtsch. med. Wschr. **10**, 163—166 (1884).

SCHWARTZ, G. H., DAVID, D. S., RIGGIO, R. R., STENZEL, K. H., RUBIN, A. L.: Ototoxicity induced by furosemide. New Engl. J. Med. **282**, 1413—1414 (1970).

SEXTON, S.: A note on the aural phenomena produced by chenopodium poisoning. Amer. J. Otol. **2**, 292—294 (1880).

SHAMBAUGH, G. E., JR., DERLACKI, E. L., HARRISON, W. H., HOUSE, H., HOUSE, W., HILDYARD, V., SCHUKNECHT, H., SHEA, J. J.: Dihydrostreptomycin deafness. J. Amer. med. Ass. **170**, 1657—1660 (1959).

SILVERSTEIN, H., BEGIN, R.: Ethacrynic acid — its reversible ototoxicity. Laryngoscope (St. Louis) **84**, 976—989 (1974).

SILVERSTEIN, H., YULES, R. B.: The effect of diuretics on cochlear potentials and inner ear fluids. Laryngoscope (St. Louis) **81**, 873—888 (1971).

SILVERSTEIN, H., BERNSTEIN, J. M., DAVIES, D. G.: Salicylate ototoxicity. A biochemical and electrophysiological study. Ann. Otol. (St. Louis) **76**, 118—128 (1967).

SIMMONS, F. B., GALAMBOS, R., ALBRIET, J. P.: Serial studies of the onset and progression of drug-induced cochlear damage in cats. Arch. Otolaryng. (Chicago) **72**, 233—239 (1960).

SMITH, M. J. H., SMITH, P. K.: The salicylates. A critical bibliographic review. New York: Interscience, 1966.

SOLLMAN, T.: A manual of pharmacology. 4th ed. Philadelphia: Saunders 1932.

SPARWALD, E., LANGE, G., LEUPE, M.: Veränderungen an den dunklen Zellen der Crista ampullaris nach Streptomycin-Medikation beim Meerschweinchen. Arch. klin. exp. Ohr.-, Nas.- u. Kehlk.-Heilk. **199**, 587—590 (1971).

SPARWALD, W., MERCK, W., LEUPE, M.: Über den zeitlichen Zusammenhang zwischen Schädigung der Sinneszellen und der dunklen Zellen der Crista ampullaris des Meerschweinchenlabyrinthes bei Streptomycinintoxikation. Arch. klin. exp. Ohr.-, Nas.- u. Kehlk.-Heilk. **202**, 687—689 (1972).

STAEMMLER, M., KARHOFF, B.: Die akuten Nephrosen. II. Nierenschäden durch Antibiotica. Virchows Arch. path. Anat. **378**, 481—502 (1959).

STANGE, G., SPRENG, M., KEIDEL, U. O.: Die Wirkung von Streptomycinsulfat auf Erregung und Adaptation der Haarzellen des Cortischen Organs. Pflügers Archiv. ges. Physiol. **279**, 99—120 (1964).

STANGE, G., SODA, T., BECK, C.: Elecktrophysiologische Ergebnisse bei Ototoxicitätsminderung basischer Streptomyces-Antibiotica. Arch. klin. exp. Ohr.-, Nas.- u. Kehlk.-Heilk. **188**, 242—249 (1967).

STEBBINS, W. C., MILLER, J. M., JOHNSSON, L.-G., HAWKINS, J. E., JR.: Ototoxic hearing loss and cochlear pathology in the monkey. Ann. Otol. (St. Louis) **78**, 598—602 (1969).

STEVENSON, L. D., ALVORD, E. C., JR., CORRELL, J. W.: Degeneration and necrosis of neurons in eighth cranial nuclei caused by streptomycin. Amer. J. Path. **23**, 875—876 (1947).

STUPP, H.-F.: Untersuchung der Antibiotikaspiegel in den Innenohrflüssigkeiten und ihre Bedeutung für die spezifische Ototoxizität der Aminolykosidantibiotika. Acta oto-laryng. (Stockh.) Suppl. **262**, —85 (1970).

STUPP, H., RAUCH, S., SOUS, H., LAGLER, F.: Untersuchungen über die Ursache der spezifisch ototoxischen Wirkung der basischen Streptomyces-Antibiotika unter besonderer Berücksichtigung des Kanamycins. Acta oto-laryng. (Stockh.) **61**, 435—444 (1966).

STUPP, H., KÜPPER, K., LAGLER, F., SOUS, H., QUANTE, M.: Inner ear concentration and ototoxicity of different antibiotics in local and systemic application. Audiology **12**, 350—363 (1973).

SUKI, W. N., EKNOYAN, G., MARTINEZ-MALDONADO, M.: Tubular sites and mechanisms of diuretic action. Ann. Rev. Pharmacol. **13**, 91—106 (1973).

THALMANN, R., MIYOSHI, T., KUSAKARI, J., THALMANN, I.: Quantitative approaches to the ototoxicity problem. Audiology **12**, 364—382 (1973).

TYBERGHEIN, J.: Influence of some streptomyces antibiotics on the cochlear microphonics in the guinea pig. Acta oto-laryng. (Stockh.) Suppl. **171**, 1—56 (1962).

UMBREIT, W. W.: The action of streptomycin. V. A new metabolic intermediate. J. Bact. **66**, 74—81 (1953).

VANDERHAEGHE, H.: Sur les troubles de l'équilibre provoqués par la streptomycine. Arch. int. Pharmacodyn. **79**, 269—272 (1949).

VARGISH, T., BENJAMIN, R., SHENKMAN, L.: Deafness from furosemide. Ann. intern. Med. **72**, 761 (1970).

VARPELA, E., HIETALAHTI, J.: Streptomycin medication during pregnancy and the child's hearing. Ann. Paediat. Feen. **11**, 38—45 (1965).

VOLDŘICH, L.: The kinetics of streptomycin, kanamycin and neomycin in the inner ear. Acta oto-laryng. (Stockh.) **60**, 243—248 (1965).

VRABEC, D. P., CODY, D. T. R., ULRICH, J. A.: A study of the relative concentrations of antibiotics in the blood, spinal fluid, and perilymph in animals. Ann. Otol. (St. Louis) **74**, 688—705 (1965).

WAISBREN, B. A., SPINK, W. W.: A clinical appraisal of neomycin. Ann. intern. Med. **33**, 1099—1119 (1950).

WALTNER, J. G.: Effect of salicylates on iner ear. Ann. Otol. (St. Louis) **64**, 617—622 (1955).

WARD, P. H., FERNÁNDEZ, C.: The ototoxicity of kanamycin in guinea pigs. Ann. Otol. (St. Louis) **70**, 132—142 (1961).

WATANUKI, K., STUPP, H. F., MEYER ZUM GOTTESBERGE, A.: Toxic effects of gentamicin upon the peripheral sensory vestibular organs. Laryngoscope (St. Louis) **82**, 363—371 (1972).

WEEKS, J. R.: The prostaglandins: their nature, formation and general pharmacology. In: Prostaglandins and cyclic AMP. KAHN, R.H., LANDS, W.E.M. (eds.). New York: Academic Press, Inc., pp. 1—14, 1973.

WERNER, C. F.: Das Labyrinth. Bau, Funktion und Krankheiten des Innenohres vom Standpunkte eines experimentellen und vergleichenden Pathologie. Leipzig: Georg Thieme Verlag 1940.

WERSÄLL, J., HAWKINS, J.E., JR.: The vestibular sensory epithelia in the cat labyrinth and their reactions in chronic streptomycin intoxication. Acta oto-laryng. (Stockh.) **54**, 1—22 (1962).

WERSÄLL, J., LUNDQUIST, P.-G., BJÖRKROTH, B.: Ototoxicity of gentamicin. J. infect. Dis. **119**, 410—416 (1969).

WERSÄLL, J., BJÖRKROTH, B., FLOCK, Å., LUNDQUIST, P.-G.: Experiments on ototoxic effects of antibiotics. Advanc. Oto-Rhino-Laryng. **20**, 14—41 (1973).

WEST, B. A., BRUMMETT, R. E., HIMES, D. L.: Interaction of kanamycin and ethacrynic acid. Arch. Otolaryng. (Chicago) **98**, 32—37 (1973).

WIGAND, M. E., HEIDLAND, A.: Akute reversible Hörverluste durch rasche, hochdosierte Furosemidinfusionen bei terminaler Niereninsuffizienz. Arch. klin. exp. Ohr.-, Nas.- u. Kehlk.-Heilk. **196**, 314—319 (1970).

WILKINS, H.: Account of the oil of the chenopodium anthelminticum. Philadelphia Medical Museum. **V**, 252—256 (1808).

WINSTON, J., LEWEY, F. H., PARENTEAU, A., MARDEN, P. A., CRAMER, F. B.: An experimental study of the toxic effects of streptomycin on the vestibular apparatus of the cat. Ann. Otol. (St. Louis) **57**, 738—753 (1948).

WINSTON, J., LEWEY, F. H., PARENTEAU, A., MARDEN, P. A., CRAMER, F. B.: Further experimental studies of the toxic effects of streptomycin on the central vestibular apparatus of the cat. Ann. Otol. (St. Louis) **58**, 988—1105 (1949).

WITTMAACK, K.: Beiträge zur Kenntnis der Wirkung des Chinins auf das Gehörorgan. Pflügers Arch. ges. Physiol. **95**, 209—233 (1903).

YAMAKAWA, K.: Die Wirkung der arsenigen Säure auf das Ohr. Arch. Ohrenheilk. **123**, 238—296 (1929).

YLIKOSKI, J., WERSÄLL, J., BJÖRKROTH, B.: Hearing loss and cochlear pathology in gentamicin intoxicated guinea pigs. Acta path. microbiol. scand. Section B. Suppl. **241**, 30—47 (1973).

Author Index

Page numbers in *italics* refer to the bibliography

Subject Index